Exploring the Dimensions of Human Sexuality

Sixth Edition

Jerrold S. Greenberg,
EdD, FASHA, FAAHE

Professor Emeritus
University of Maryland

Clint E. Bruess, EdD,
CHES, FASHA, FAAHE

Dean Emeritus
University of Alabama at Birmingham
Professor Emeritus
Birmingham-Southern College

Sara B. Oswalt, MPH,
PhD, CSE

Associate Professor
University of Texas at San Antonio

JONES & BARTLETT
LEARNING

World Headquarters
Jones & Bartlett Learning
5 Wall Street
Burlington, MA 01803
978-443-5000
info@jblearning.com
www.jblearning.com

Jones & Bartlett Learning books and products are available through most bookstores and online booksellers. To contact Jones & Bartlett Learning directly, call 800-832-0034, fax 978-443-8000, or visit our website, www.jblearning.com.

Substantial discounts on bulk quantities of Jones & Bartlett Learning publications are available to corporations, professional associations, and other qualified organizations. For details and specific discount information, contact the special sales department at Jones & Bartlett Learning via the above contact information or send an email to specialsales@jblearning.com.

08263-0

Production Credits

VP, Executive Publisher: David D. Cella
Publisher: Cathy L. Esperti
Editorial Assistant: Sara J. Peterson
Senior Production Editor: Nancy Hitchcock
Director of Marketing: Andrea DeFronzo
VP, Manufacturing and Inventory Control: Therese Connell
Composition: Cenveo® Publisher Services

Cover Design: Kristin E. Parker
Associate Director of Rights & Media: Joanna Lundeen
Rights & Media Specialist: Jamey O'Quinn
Media Development Editor: Shannon Sheehan
Cover Image: © Gayvoronskaya Yana/Shutterstock
Printing and Binding: RR Donnelley
Cover Printing: RR Donnelley

Library of Congress Cataloging-in-Publication Data

Names: Greenberg, Jerrold S., author. | Bruess, Clint E., author. | Oswalt, Sara B., author.
Title: Exploring the dimensions of human sexuality / Jerrold S. Greenberg, EdD, FASHA, FAAHE, Professor Emeritus, University of Maryland, Clint E. Bruess, EdD, CHES, FASHA, FAAHE, Dean Emeritus, University of Alabama at Birmingham, Professor Emeritus, Birmingham-Southern College, Sara 　Oswalt, MPH, PhD, CSE, Associate Professor, University of Texas at San Antonio.
Description: Sixth edition. | Burlingt　　A : Jones & Bartlett Learning, [2017]
Identifiers: LCCN 2015042707 | ISBN 9　　4081541 (pbk. : alk. paper)
Subjects: LCSH: Sex (Psychology) | Hygiene, Sexual. | Interpersonal relations. | Sexual ethics.
Classification: LCC HQ21 .G67118 2017 | DDC 155.3—dc23 LC record available at http://lccn.loc.gov/2015042707

6048

Printed in the United States of America
20 19 18 17 16   10 9 8 7 6 5 4 3 2 1

Dedication

This book is dedicated to three of the cutest grandchildren possible: Jonah, Zoe, and Garrett. The joy they bring is unsurpassed.

—*Jerrold S. Greenberg*

To Susan J. Laing, with appreciation for her part in a wonderful relationship.

—*Clint E. Bruess*

To M . . . for everything.

—*Sara B. Oswalt*

Brief Contents

Contents

Communication Dimensions

Multicultural Dimensions

Global Dimensions

Gender Dimensions

Ethical Dimensions

A Message from the Authors

Human sexuality is an important component of a healthy lifestyle. It is not a topic to be hidden or avoided, as this can lead to serious consequences for one's health and overall life satisfaction. When human sexuality is understood, the result is a healthier lifestyle and an increased ability to achieve consistency between one's actions and moral principles. The authors of this text have seen the effects of both approaches to human sexuality in their own families.

The benefit of perceiving sexuality as a topic of discussion and understanding can be seen in one example of a telephone call from one of the author's daughters. She said that her 14-year-old daughter asked about noises she sometimes heard coming from her parents' bedroom. Her mother explained that the noises were her mom and dad enjoying physical contact as part of showing love for each other. Fortunately, she had previously talked with her daughter about sexuality and reproduction, so she was able to refer back to that conversation. She asked her father for advice regarding how she handled the situation and what she should do further. He responded that she should be pleased that her daughter felt comfortable enough to talk with her about the noises, and that it was good that she had explained sexuality and reproduction to her daughter so she had accurate information that was appropriate for her age. Beyond that, the author simply said that his daughter was on the right track related to the sexuality education of her daughter, and the best thing to do moving forward was to continue to keep the lines of communication open.

In contrast, an example of how human sexuality is inappropriately conceptualized occurred when the son of a different author was entering fifth grade. School personnel organized a committee of parents to review instructional materials for the sexuality education course. As luck would have it, the author was selected to serve on this committee. At the first committee meeting, he was surprised to learn that the program focused exclusively on reproductive anatomy and physiology. He asked, "How will you help students process their feelings pertaining to sexuality?" The answer was that the reproductive system would be taught just as any other body system would, with no plans to include a discussion of feelings associated with sexuality. At that point the author volunteered to resign from the parent review committee and asked to join the "Digestive System Parent Review Committee." Of course, there was none. That allowed the author to point out that there really is a distinction between education regarding sexuality and education pertaining to other health issues, and that this distinction needed to be addressed with students. We do that in this text by exploring the varied dimensions of human sexuality.

In fact, we have known students who would have liked to enroll in our human sexuality courses but did not due to their discomfort regarding sexuality. Some were embarrassed to have their friends or relatives find out that they did not know *everything* about sexuality. Others felt uncomfortable discussing sexuality in a class with their peers. And still others believed they knew more than they actually did, although in reality they did not know enough to live a sexually healthy life. Consequently, in *Exploring the Dimensions of Human Sexuality, Sixth Edition* we make a special effort to engage students in a nonjudgmental manner and make the content interesting, resulting in enhanced learning.

The Dimensions of Human Sexuality

In many regards, human sexuality today does not differ from that of our ancestors' times. Biologically, human reproduction occurs in the same way. As in the past, religion and culture have a significant impact on our sexuality, as does public policy. As long-time sexuality educators, we know that no single aspect of sexuality can be separated from the others, and no single aspect is more important than the others. Therefore, we have chosen to write a text that presents all aspects of sexuality as interconnected and significant. Throughout this text you will find an emphasis on health and well-being based on the assumption that we are all sexual beings from birth until death and that sexuality should be viewed in its totality—with biological, psychological, and sociocultural dimensions.

The Organization of the Book

The dimensions discussed in the text can be broken down into biological, psychological, and sociocultural categories. Some examples are described here.

Biological Dimensions

Physiology

The basis of understanding sexuality is knowledge about the physiology of our bodies. Factual information lays the foundation for critical thinking—without the facts, you cannot begin to think critically about your sexuality. The greater your knowledge, the more likely you are to take responsibility for your sexual health.

Gender

The physiological differences between the sexes create the foundation for the development of psychological and social wellness and strongly influence our perceptions of sexual wellness. Gender dimensions receive a chapter of their own as well as a boxed treatment in every chapter.

Psychological Dimensions

Psychology

Developing a positive image of self and sexuality is critical to developing sexual wellness. A positive body image lends itself to overall wellness; a negative self-image can lead to drug abuse (steroids or diet pills) or psychological disorders (anorexia, bulimia, binge eating disorder, or muscle dysmorphia). Body image is so important that we devote a chapter to the topic—the most comprehensive coverage in the market!

Spirituality

Religious and spiritual beliefs influence feelings about sexual behavior, premarital sexual activity, adultery, divorce, contraception, abortion, and masturbation. Spiritual issues are discussed in Multicultural Dimensions boxes and in the opening chapter.

Sociocultural Dimensions

Multicultural

Cultures within the United States and around the world differ in their views of sexuality. From semi-nude beaches in the south of France to Middle Eastern Muslim communities where women are covered from head to toe, ours is a world of diversity. Sometimes these diverse behaviors are a part of the culture, and other times they are given legal sanction. A good example of this is the many ways in which abortion is viewed. Views on abortion range from strict prohibition, including strong laws, to simply as a method of birth control, such that it is common for women to have as many as four or five abortions in her lifetime. Your ability to respect your sexual partner's cultural beliefs and feelings will result in a higher level of satisfaction for both of you. To help students better understand sexual diversity, each chapter contains boxed examples of sexual beliefs or practices pertaining to a culture within the United States or a culture elsewhere in the world.

Ethics

Ethical considerations are the basis of legal and moral decision making concerning sexuality. The law and courts regulate such sexual issues as access to abortion clinics, workplace sexual harassment, and ownership of frozen embryos. Moral implications of ethical decisions include sexual coercion and underscore the importance of taking responsibility for your sexual wellness. Ethical Dimensions boxes appear in every chapter, and the *Sexual Ethics, Morality, and the Law* chapter covers these issues in depth.

Public Policy

Public policy also affects our sexual behavior. For example, national health objectives promote sexual health awareness pertaining to acquired immune deficiency syndrome (AIDS) and sexually transmitted infections (STIs), unwanted teenage pregnancies, and prenatal care. Furthermore, public policy on free speech continues to allow the uncontrolled distribution of sexually explicit material on the Internet. Unfortunately, as a result of public policy, access to proper health care, birth control, and sexually related choices is often unavailable to some people.

Integration of Dimensions

Given the many factors influencing our sexual behavior, we have created a striking full-page feature that recognizes their interwoven nature: *Exploring the Dimensions of Human Sexuality.* It serves as an integrated approach that ties all these strands together. This feature, found at the end of each chapter, assists students in understanding how many different aspects of sexuality affect their sexual health and influence their sexual behavior. Our intent is to help students envision the convergence of the many aspects of sexuality and help them make sexual decisions that lead to a lifetime of positive sexual health and wellness.

■ Pedagogy

Because we realize that learning best occurs when students are actively involved, we have created a text that goes beyond merely presenting factual knowledge about the varied dimensions of human sexuality.

We provide numerous ways for students to explore the dimensions of human sexuality and determine how each affects their *personal* sexuality. This exploration is facilitated through the pedagogical features described next.

Body Image Chapter

We offer a comprehensive look at the concept of body image. It is rare to find so much detail on this subject together in one place. The *Body Image* chapter discusses how body image affects self-esteem and sexuality, how the quest for a perfect body creates problems ranging from eating disorders to cosmetic surgery and steroid abuse, and how body image affects both sexes.

Dimensions of Human Sexuality Boxed Features

A carefully designed program reinforces the dimensions theme of the text with five distinct types of boxes: Multicultural Dimensions, Global Dimensions, Gender Dimensions, Communication Dimensions, and Ethical Dimensions. *Please refer to page xxi of the Visual Walkthrough for detailed descriptions of these features.*

Critical Thinking

Exploring the Dimensions of Human Sexuality, Sixth Edition requires students to think critically about how the multifaceted dimensions of human sexuality relate to them. To that end, we have embedded critical thinking questions within the text to help students reflect on the subject matter and understand its implications for their sexual health. Critical thinking questions are found in boxes, in photo captions, and in the end-of-chapter section—including application questions related to the chapter-opening story, critical thinking questions about material, and a critical thinking mini-case. Critical thinking questions help students recall information and synthesize new material with existing knowledge and stimulate students to make informed judgments about the information provided.

"Myth vs Fact" and "Did You Know..." Boxes

Students' sexual health and wellness are also influenced by sexual myths and folklore. Many of our brief sidebars are designed to set students straight on such myths. "Did You Know. . ." boxes add whimsical and high-interest information to engage the student further.

Chapter-Opening Story

Each chapter opens with an engaging story that explores the concepts to be discussed in the chapter. Students are drawn into the chapter material with a high-interest case and introduced to the topics that will be discussed. At the end of the chapter, students are asked to relate the chapter's information to application questions about the opening story.

Reviewing the Dimensions of Human Sexuality

Each chapter ends with an interactive feature designed to help students take responsibility for their sexual health and wellness. This section includes an interactive self-assessment designed to help students understand and clarify their own feelings about sexuality issues presented in that chapter. It also includes discussion questions, application questions pertaining to the opening story, critical thinking questions, a critical thinking mini-case, and a self-assessment.

■ New to this Edition!

Throughout this new edition, extensive updates have been made to focus on information and statistics about recent developments. Information from hundreds of new references has been added—almost all of these references were published in the last few years. Suggested readings at the end of each chapter have been updated, as have the Web Resources sections at the end of each chapter. Some sections within chapters have been moved to improve organization, others have been deleted, and new sections have been added to reflect changes related to human sexuality. New and more appropriate photos and illustrations have replaced older ones as needed.

In addition, the sixth edition includes 22 chapters, as compared to the 18 chapters found in previous editions. The new chapters were created through the expansion of earlier editions' "In Focus" features on unexpected pregnancy outcomes, body image, alternative sexual behavior, and HIV and AIDS.

Chapter-Specific Changes and Updates

- **Chapter 1** offers a summary of selected research from the UCLA Higher Education Research Institute related to college freshmen and their opinions about issues related to sexuality. In addition, updated research findings from the Youth Risk Behavior Surveillance are included.

- **Chapter 2** includes the latest research related to sexuality. There are 26 new references in the chapter.

- **Chapter 3** examines newer electronic modes of communication related to sexuality. It also includes a new Multicultural Dimensions box about female and male subcultures, a revised Ethical Dimensions box about ethics, communication, and date rape, and a new list of possible barriers to good sexual communication.

- **Chapter 4** contains a new Global Dimensions box on female mutilation in various parts of the world, a new figure on temperature and mucus changes during the menstrual cycle, the latest recommendations regarding cervical cancer screening, and the latest research on both female ejaculation and the safety of silicone breast implants.

- **Chapter 5** provides the latest American Academy of Pediatricians' policy statement on circumcision, additional discussion of prostate cancer incidence and screening for African American males, and the latest recommendations for preventing pressure on the perineum when bicycling.

- **Chapter 6** includes an updated table detailing the percentage of people having unprotected sexual intercourse without knowing their partners' history. In addition, there are added recommendations related to tantric sex techniques.

- **Chapter 7** includes updated information on the availability of emergency contraception and other contraceptive methods, such as Skyla and Liletta, two new IUDs. The public health emphasis on *long-acting reversible contraception (LARC)* is also discussed.

- **Chapter 8** includes a revised story introducing the chapter and an expanded section that covers the work of midwives and doulas. The chapter coverage also includes expanded discussion of home births, a revised section on nutrition during pregnancy, and an updated section on drugs' effects on the fetus during pregnancy, including a new section on methamphetamine.

- **Chapter 9** provides updated rates and procedures for abortions. It also includes a revised summary of state laws regarding abortion availability and restrictions, along with a revised section on domestic and international adoption practices and challenges. A new Ethical Dimensions box on crisis pregnancy centers is also included.

- In **Chapter 10**, a new Gender Dimensions box on terminology covers 11 important terms. There is also a new "Did You Know..." box on gender relations and the prospects for more fairness and equity. Recent gender issues and potential controversies are included as well. Information about transgender has been updated and greatly expanded.

- **Chapter 11**, on body image, includes updated information about the relationship between sexuality and body image, including discussion of self-image, partner preference, and beliefs and behaviors. A new "Did You Know..." box on the pros and cons of Barbie dolls has been added, as well a new Gender Dimensions box on self-esteem and body image. In addition, the role of the Internet in influencing concepts of body image is discussed. An update on developments and issues related to cosmetic surgery and body image is included.

- **Chapter 12** is now titled *Sexual Orientation, Identity, and Expression* to better reflect the content and issues covered. Terms in the chapter are defined even though some of their meanings are very fluid—that is, they have changed over time and continue to change. The chapter content includes a new Multicultural Dimensions box focusing on race and ethnicity identities among LGBT adults, a section on disparities that bisexual people often experience, a new "Did You Know . . ." box on Native Americans' concepts of gender and sexual orientation, and current statistics about LGBT people. In addition, the chapter provides new information on the topic of intersex, a new "Did You Know . . ." box on animals and homosexuality, a new Global Dimensions box on attitudes toward LGBT rights in various countries, and abundant information from experts on LGBT information and issues.

- **Chapter 13** includes updated information about the effectiveness of comprehensive sexuality education programs. A new Ethical Dimensions box focuses on vaccination of children against HPV, and the content includes updated statistics about sexual behaviors of teens, recent information about teen pregnancies and births, and a summary of new information about child sexual abuse and sexual harassment.

- **Chapter 14** explores information and opinions about the "hookup culture." The influence of technology on the behavior of college students is described, and recent research on the sexual behavior of young adults is discussed. Information about cohabitation is also provided. A new Communication Dimensions box entitled "How to Make Someone Fall in Love with You" is included, along with information about how to promote healthy relationships and marriages. A "Did You Know . . ." box related to chances of divorce has been added as well.

- **Chapter 15** contains the latest research related to the existence of the G spot and the controversy surrounding its existence. Research on sexual fantasies and the differences in sexual fantasies between males and females is included as well. A table was added that delineates the time spent (in minutes) during sexual intercourse, on a state-by-state basis. Updated data are also included on the prevalence and frequency of various sexual behaviors, the sexual behavior of LGBT people, and sexual activity of the elderly.

- **Chapter 16** has a new "Did You Know . . ." box focusing on theories about paraphilias. Updated information is also included about many alternative sexual behaviors, such as exhibitionism, voyeurism, sexual masochism, and sexual sadism, among others. New information about treatments for sexual offenders is included.

- **Chapter 17** includes a number of new photos. This chapter now offers increased emphasis on preventing and dealing with sexual violence on campus, including important elements of a campus sexual violence policy. A new "Did You Know . . ." box deals with the controversy over "gray rape," and a new Global Dimensions box gives examples of attitudes toward child sexual abuse outside the United States. The various types of relationship abuse are also explained, and updated information on domestic violence is included.

- **Chapter 18** covers self-testing for STIs in more depth. Social determinants of health are covered more extensively than in previous editions, including how they relate to STI rates. More discussion of HPV and oral sexual activity is included as well.

- **Chapter 19** includes a refreshed introductory story. Multicultural, Gender, and Ethical Dimensions boxes were added on three topics: HIV and American Indians/Alaskan Natives, transgender people and HIV, and the roles of recovering drug addicts in peer education for HIV prevention. The discussion of treatment for HIV and AIDS, including the importance of linkage when caring for HIV-infected individuals, has been expanded as was the discussion on pre-exposure prophylaxis related to HIV. Information is now included on post-exposure prophylaxis as well, and the discussion on prevention of HIV infection has been extensively revised.

- **Chapter 20** is updated to be consistent with *DSM-5* terminology and criteria for sexual disorders (including deletion of sexual aversion disorder). While not listed in the *DSM-5*, persistent genital arousal disorder (PGAD) is now covered in this chapter as well. The Multicultural Dimensions box on Latino culture and sexual dysfunction has been updated, as has the Ethical Dimensions box on sexual surrogacy. A new box has been included detailing the world's first FDA approved drug designed to treat Hypoactive Sexual Desire Disorder (HSDD) for women.

- **Chapter 21** contains a great deal of updated information about sexuality and advertising. A new table on the top 25 dating and relationship reality TV shows was added.

Discussions related to the media and sexuality were extensively updated, along with information on technology and sexuality. A new Gender Dimensions box on male and female use of pornography has been added, as was extensive new information related to pornography in general. Information about sex work and sex workers has been significantly updated as well.

- **Chapter 22** updated the information about differences in the sexual language used in different cultures and countries. A new discussion focuses on sexting, its implications, and relevant precautions. Data on the prevalence of extramarital affairs were also added.

- In the Epilogue, the scenario has been updated to reflect changes since the last edition.

When appropriate, boxed material has been changed and updated throughout the sixth edition. Statistics have also been updated throughout the text—for example, the most current statistics regarding STIs, adoptions, abortions, birth rates, marriage and divorce rates, and prevalence of sexual behaviors are presented. There is also a significant increase in the number of references cited to reflect the latest research and recommendations by experts. All boxed material has been updated as appropriate, and photos have been added or deleted to make them more appropriate to current issues.

Writing this text has been a service-learning activity for us. We did abundant and thorough research to identify state-of-the-art knowledge and attitudes pertaining to sexuality, and learned a great deal in doing so. That was the "learning" part of the service-learning equation. The "service" part relates to our interest in helping to enhance the sexual health and wellness of our readers. As such, we hope you find the information we included, the issues we raised and discussed, and the myths we debunked useful as you live, express your sexuality, and make decisions related to your sexuality. If you do, the time, effort, and energy we have devoted to writing this text will have been well worth that investment.

About the Authors

Jerrold S. Greenberg, EdD, FASHA, FAAHE

Dr. Greenberg is Professor Emeritus in the School of Public Health at the University of Maryland. He earned his baccalaureate and master's degrees from the City College of New York and then continued his education at Syracuse University, where he earned his doctorate. Dr. Greenberg taught at Syracuse University, Boston University, and the State University of New York at Buffalo before accepting a professorship at the University of Maryland in 1979.

Dr. Greenberg has written more than 50 books on such topics as elder care, health, stress management, physical fitness, sexuality, and methods of health education. In addition, he has published more than 80 articles in professional journals and lay magazines.

Among Dr. Greenberg's honors are the University of Maryland Service-Learning Advocate of the Year award for 2003–2004; the American School Health Association's Distinguished Service Award; selection as Alliance Scholar by the American Alliance for Health, Physical Education, Recreation, and Dance; the Presidential Citation, the Certificate of Appreciation, and the Scholar Award of the American Association for Health Education; selection for inclusion in *Who's Who in America*, *Outstanding Young Men of America*, and *Who's Who in World Jewry*. Dr. Greenberg has also served on the editorial boards of the professional journals *Health Education* and *The Journal of School Health*, and as a reviewer for other professional journals. In addition, Dr. Greenberg has conducted stress management workshops for professional, business, and lay organizations throughout the United States.

Clint E. Bruess, EdD, CHES, FASHA, FAAHE

Dr. Bruess is Dean Emeritus of the School of Education and Professor Emeritus of Health Education at the University of Alabama at Birmingham. He is also Professor Emeritus at Birmingham–Southern College. He earned his baccalaureate degree at Macalester College, his master's at the University of Maryland, and his doctorate at Temple University.

Dr. Bruess was a professor at West Chester University, Towson University (also department chair), and the University of Alabama at Birmingham (also department chair and later Dean of the School of Education), before becoming Division Chair and Professor at Birmingham–Southern College. He also directed the School Health Education Project for the National Center for Health Education for 3 years.

Dr. Bruess has coauthored more than 15 textbooks in the areas of human sexuality, sexuality education, personal health, and school health programs. In addition, he has published numerous articles in professional journals and served in elected and appointed positions for the American School Health Association (also a Fellow), American Association for Health Education (also a Fellow), and Society of Public Health Educators. Dr. Bruess continues to review professional articles for *Health Education*, *The Journal of School Health*, *The International Journal of Health Education*, *The American Journal of Health Behavior*, and *The American Journal of Sexuality Education*. He currently teaches a Human Sexuality Course at Samford University and a graduate-level Sexuality Education course at the University of Alabama.

Sara B. Oswalt, MPH, PhD, CSE

Dr. Oswalt is an associate professor in the Department of Kinesiology, Health and Nutrition at the University of Texas at San Antonio. She attended Pennsylvania State University for her undergraduate degree, Indiana University for her master's degree, and the University of Georgia for her doctorate degree. She worked as a college health educator for 8 years, spending 6 of those years as the sexual health coordinator for the University of Georgia.

Dr. Oswalt has authored more than 35 journal articles. Her research interests are directed at college students, assessing their health status and the evaluation of college and university efforts to address those health issues. She has a special interest in sexual health issues for the college population. She regularly teaches sexuality courses for undergraduate students and is also an American Association of Sexuality Educators, Counselors, and Therapists (AASECT) Certified Sexuality Educator (CSE).

Acknowledgments

We would like to thank Sue Tendy, EdD, of the U.S. Military Academy at West Point for her contributions to the material on sexual harassment in the military. Our sincere thanks and appreciation go to the Jones & Bartlett Learning Health Science team: Cathy Esperti, Publisher; Sara Peterson, Editorial Assistant; Julie Bolduc, Production Manager; Nancy Hitchcock, Senior Production Editor; and Andrea DeFronzo, Director of Marketing. We would like to acknowledge the dedication and hard work of these individuals, for without them this project would never have been realized. Finally, we would like to thank the many reviewers who guided us throughout the various stages of this project. Their voices, criticism, and support have truly made this a better text.

Dr. Cindy Allen
Lock Haven University

Robert E. Braun, MPH, CHES
The University of Toledo

Eric R. Buhi, MPH, PhD
University of South Florida

Dr. Charles Chase
West Texas A&M University

Laura Gowen, PhD
Portland State University

Erin Hutzelman, MEd
University of Toledo

Deneen Long-White, MS, CHES
Howard University

Dr. Kirsten Lupinski
Albany State University

Maureen E. McGarry, PhD, RN, NCC
Community College of Rhode Island

Molly A. McKinney
Eastern Kentucky University

Rizwana Rahim, PhD
East-West University

Ina Ramos, MPH, PhD
Bowie State University

Marco Torres, MPH
Moreno Valley College

A Visual Walkthrough

Exploring the Dimensions of Human Sexuality, Sixth Edition is designed around the central theme that our feelings, attitudes, and beliefs regarding sexuality are continually influenced by our internal and external environments. All aspects of sexuality—biological, spiritual, psychological, and sociocultural—are interconnected and significant. The boxed feature program, additional pedagogy, and ancillaries of this new text have been designed around these core concepts.

■ Boxed Features

Communication Dimensions
These boxes discuss communication issues that arise around sexuality between the genders, partners from different ethnic groups, and others.

Multicultural Dimensions
To better appreciate how various people view sexuality, we offer a multicultural boxed feature. These boxes deal exclusively with diversity issues within the United States.

Global Dimensions
Sexuality is viewed very differently outside of the United States. Issues such as divorce in China and international differences in discussing sexuality are discussed in the Global Dimensions boxes.

Gender Dimensions
Issues arising from gender are integrated throughout the text, discussed in detail in the *Gender Dimensions* chapter, and featured in the Gender Dimensions boxes found in each chapter. Topics covered in these boxes include communication breakdown between genders, responsibility for contraception, and many others.

Ethical Dimensions
The importance of ethics in sexuality is underscored in the Ethical Dimensions boxes. This is where topics such as abstinence-only education and the ethics surrounding technological advances are discussed.

■ Pedagogical Design

Chapter-Opening Pedagogy

Each chapter-opening page gives the reader a glimpse of the content with chapter objectives and a list of the Dimensions of Human Sexuality boxed features that will follow. In addition, a high-interest and engaging real-life story draws students into the chapter material and introduces them to the topics that will be discussed. This opening story is revisited at the end of the chapter in the application questions.

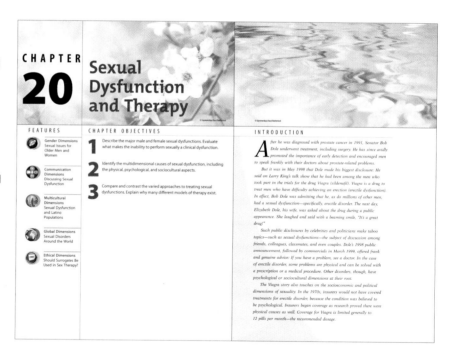

Exploring the Dimensions of Human Sexuality

This feature organizes the multifaceted issues in each chapter into biological, psychological, and sociocultural factors.

Reviewing the Dimensions of Human Sexuality

This end-of-chapter activity gives students the opportunity to review and apply key chapter concepts. Items in this section include discussion questions, critical thinking questions, and application questions that relate to the chapter-opening story. The Exploring Personal Dimensions section directs students to focus on personal choices and take responsibility for their sexual health and well-being.

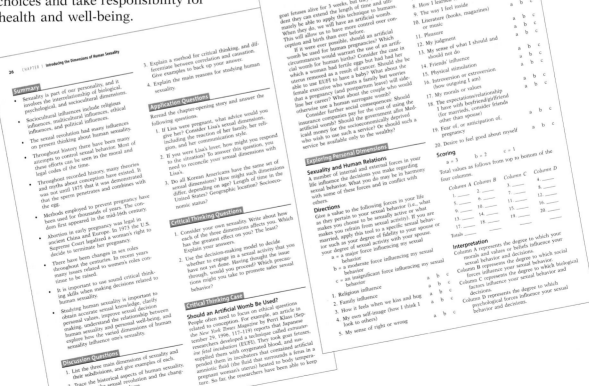

▨ Special Features

Myth vs Fact

Students' sexual health and wellness are influenced by sexual myths and folklore. "Myth vs Fact" boxes identify myths associated with the material presented in each chapter along with the fact to dispel each myth.

Did You Know . . .

Brief "Did You Know . . ." sidebars add whimsical and high-interest information to further engage the student.

Myth vs Fact

Myth: Sexual dysfunctions occur because someone either has been sexually abused or raped or has masturbated too often.

Fact: It is true that sexual abuse, such as rape and child abuse, can contribute to the development of a sexual dysfunction. Yet, there are many people who experience those traumatic events and never develop a sexual dysfunction. Regarding masturbation, there is no evidence that the frequency of masturbation is in any way related to the subsequent development of a sexual dysfunction.

Myth: Guys who "can't get it up" are not real men.

Fact: Many cases of erectile dysfunction are caused by physiological problems. To classify these men as less than real men is analogous to characterizing any man who has any physical illness as not a real man. The inability to achieve and maintain an erection is in no way related to manliness.

Myth: Women are not naturally interested in sex, so a woman who cannot be sexually aroused is quite normal.

Fact: Males and females have a natural interest in and capacity for sex, although the level of desire and arousal differs between people. When males or females are experiencing less desire or arousal than they would like and this experience distresses them, they should seek professional help.

? Did You Know . . .

Where to Find Help
The following numbers can be helpful if you want to find out more about reporting abuse or if you want more information about abuse:
Child abuse: (800) 4-A-CHILD (422-4453)
Elder abuse: (800) 677-1116
Sexual assault: (800) 656-4673
Domestic violence: (800) 799-7233

Teaching and Learning Aids

Instructor resources such as PowerPoint lecture presentations, a TestBank, and an instructor's manual assist in classroom preparation.

An Interactive Online Workbook allows students to review chapter topics and assess their own sexuality behaviors in relation to these topics. Exercises and activities include Chapter Summary, Fill in the Blanks, Review the Dimensions, Focus on the Facts, Quick Questions, and Test Your Knowledge.

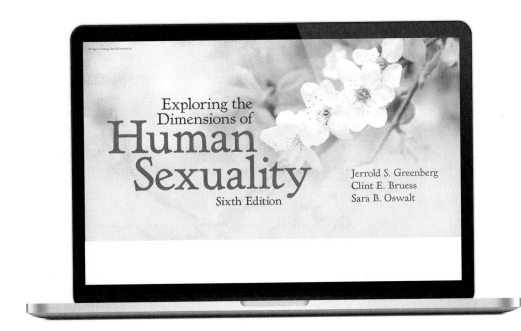

CHAPTER 1

Introducing the Dimensions of Human Sexuality

© Gayvoronskaya Yana/Shutterstock

CHAPTER OBJECTIVES

1 Identify and discuss the dimensions of human sexuality, including biological, psychological, and sociocultural factors.

2 Discuss the historical aspects of human sexuality, including the sexual revolution, the role of gender, and the role of culture.

3 Apply critical thinking methods to human sexuality.

4 Outline the reasons to study human sexuality, including the steps of the decision-making process.

INTRODUCTION

*L*et us begin our exploration of the many dimensions of human sexuality by examining how they affect the life of one person: Lisa, an 18-year-old college freshman, involved in her first serious—and sexual—relationship. After several months of dating, Lisa experiences the scare of her life: Her period is late. After a few days she purchases a home-pregnancy kit. As she waits until the morning to take the test, she begins to think about the role of sexuality in her life.

Like most people who grow up in the United States today, Lisa received basic sexuality education in public school. But that brief overview—which Lisa and her friends giggled through—touched only on the physical aspects of reproduction. Nothing prepared her for the emotions she felt during her current relationship, or how her social and cultural upbringing would affect her sexual behavior.

Lisa is a Korean American, a member of a family who respect heritage and tradition. Her parents, a university professor and a homemaker, were born in Korea and had an arranged marriage. The traditional Korean view of sexuality is conservative, and virginity is highly prized for marriage. Although Lisa holds on to many traditional views, she also struggles with the permissive attitude toward sexuality that prevails in the U.S. culture today—an attitude that her boyfriend shares (Brennan, 1999).

An unexpected pregnancy for Lisa would be a major tragedy in her family. Pregnancy outside marriage would shame not only the individual (and make her an "unperson") but also the entire family. Her family could choose to exile her.

Korean Americans tend not to tolerate secrecy by children and exert strict parental control. The Korean culture discourages open discussion of feelings and seeking out of psychological counseling. Thus Lisa is in a *crisis because she feels she cannot tell her parents, but she also cannot tell anyone else (who may in turn tell her parents). In fact, Lisa has yet to tell her boyfriend what is upsetting her.*

Religion plays a major role in many people's sexuality. For Lisa's parents, whose cultural traditions in Korea can be traced to Confucianism, abortion may be a possibility (as a means of saving face for the family). But many Korean American immigrants are members of fundamentalist Christian groups, who often prohibit abortion. Lisa wonders what she will do if, in fact, she is really pregnant.

Lisa is lucky: She is not pregnant. But Lisa has realized that she has to start taking greater responsibility for her sexual behavior. How can she incorporate the many dimensions affecting her sexuality into her personal sexuality?

This chapter begins our exploration of the many dimensions of sexuality and how they affect our lives.

■ The Dimensions of Human Sexuality

When you think about human sexuality, what do you think of? Some form of physical contact? Human reproduction? Feelings when you see an attractive person? Human sexuality is all that and more. **Human sexuality** is a part of your total personality. It involves the interrelationship of biological, psychological, and sociocultural dimensions.

The Sexuality Information and Education Council of the United States (SIECUS) defines human sexuality as encompassing the sexual knowledge, beliefs, attitudes, values, and behaviors of individuals. Its various dimensions include the anatomy, physiology, and biochemistry of the sexual response system; identity, orientation, roles, and personality; and thoughts, feelings, and relationships. The expression of sexuality is influenced by ethical, spiritual, cultural, and moral concerns (SIECUS, 2014).

The Alberta Society for the Promotion of Sexual Health (ASPSH) indicates that sexuality means many things: feelings about ourselves, roles we play in society, and reproduction. It is not limited to how we behave sexually. It is the total of our physical, emotional, and spiritual responses, thoughts, and feelings. Sexuality is more about who we are than about what we do (ASPSH, 2015).

Sexuality is a natural part of life. The concepts of human sexuality are learned. From our viewpoint, human sexuality involves at least three dimensions—biological, psychological, and sociocultural. Each dimension has many subdimensions. The interactive relationship of these dimensions describes an individual's total sexuality.

The Interactive Nature of Sexual Dimensions

A complex set of biological, psychological, and sociocultural variables plays a role in all our sexual interactions. The decision to be sexually active is a result of many factors. Sexual arousal is a physiological function. Psychologically, our body image and feelings of self-worth may inhibit getting involved ("I'm not good enough for her"; "I'm not attractive enough for him"). A lack of self-worth may also inhibit arousal. Our culture helps us develop a sense of what is attractive—height, weight, hair style, skin tone. In addition, religious beliefs affect our sexual undertakings, as do legal and ethical considerations. Role models set by family and friends influence us as well.

All these dimensions constantly interact and influence our sexuality. Although we discuss them

---

human sexuality   A part of your total personality. It involves the interrelationship of biological, psychological, and sociocultural dimensions.

Gender
DIMENSIONS

The Multifaceted Dimension of Gender

The first words our parents heard after we emerged from the womb declared our biological gender: "It's a boy!" or "It's a girl!" Our parents bought crib sheets and clothes that were pink or blue to match our gender.

We soon learned the sociocultural meanings of gender: Boys and girls are socialized to play in different styles and usually learn to prefer different sets of toys. Our moms and/or dads tended to do gender-specific chores. Teenage boys are somehow allowed to be sexually active, whereas girls are discouraged from such activities (a concept known as the "double standard").

Psychologically, girls are encouraged to show their emotions, whereas boys learn to suppress emotions. This leads to differing communication styles as well: Females are generally more expressive verbally than males. (Of course, there are many expressive men and inexpressive females. Remember that Lisa in our opening story has been culturally socialized to suppress open discussion of feelings.)

One couple announced the birth of their baby, Storm, but decided not to share the baby's sex. They felt that their decision gave Storm the freedom to choose who he or she wanted to be. They said that kids receive messages from society that encourage them to fit into existing boxes, including those with regard to gender. To other people they simply said, "Please, can you just let Storm discover for him/herself what s(he) wants to be?" (Roth, 2011).

Socially, there are many gender issues that will be covered in detail throughout this text. In the workplace, a woman often earns less than a man earns (a concept known as the "wage gap") and often faces a tougher time getting promoted into upper management (a concept known as the "glass ceiling"). After a woman goes home from work, she usually does more household chores (known as the "second shift") than her spouse.

Why are such topics covered in a human sexuality course? Because our gender—who we are as men and women and how we experience ourselves as male and female—is an essential component of our sexuality.

---

separately for clarity, remember that almost all sexuality-related decisions we make are influenced by more than one dimension.

Biological Dimension

The basis of understanding sexuality is physiological knowledge about how our bodies work. Factual information lays the foundation of decision making—without the facts, you cannot begin to think critically about your sexuality. The greater your knowledge, the more likely you are to take responsibility for your sexual health.

Until relatively recently, most of the research into human sexuality focused on physiology. For example, a model of the human sexual response cycle, published by the well-known researchers Masters and Johnson in 1966, focused mainly on physiology.

Fisher (1992) emphasizes the genetic aspects of behavior. In her view, humans have a common nature, a set of unconscious tendencies that are encoded in our genes. She believes that although we are not aware of these predispositions, they still motivate our actions. Although she recognizes that culture plays a role in one's sexuality, she also seems to support **essentialism**, the belief that the essence of sexuality is biological.

The biological dimension of our sexuality involves our physical appearance, especially the development of physical sexual characteristics; our responses to sexual stimulation; our ability to reproduce or to control fertility; and our growth and development in general. Although human reproductive function does not begin until puberty, human sexual–erotic functioning begins immediately after birth and lasts a lifetime. It is important to realize that biological functioning, as it relates to sexuality, is a part of the natural functioning of human beings. These biological aspects also relate to the other dimensions of sexuality, and all the dimensions work together to produce an individual's total sexuality—which, in turn, is part of the total personality (Bruess & Schroeder, 2014).

The physiological differences between the sexes help to lay the groundwork for the development of psychological and social wellness, and our gender strongly influences our perceptions of sexual wellness. For example, the sexual double standard, in which men are expected to be promiscuous and women are not, is a belief held by many people in the United States. In our human sexuality classes we always ask students to complete the sentences

essentialism Belief that once the cultural and historical aspects are taken away, the essence of sexuality is biological.

Myth vs Fact

Myth: Human sexuality relates mainly to biological functioning.
Fact: Human sexuality includes a biological dimension but also includes psychological and socio-cultural dimensions.

Myth: Most people are well informed about human sexuality.
Fact: Unfortunately, most people still have relatively poor

knowledge of sexuality. Therefore, many myths about human sexuality still exist.

Myth: Sexual "normality" is similar among various cultures.
Fact: Sexual attitudes and behaviors differ greatly among cultural groups. There is no set standard for "normality."

"A man who carries a condom in his wallet is _____" and "A woman who carries a condom in her purse is _____." The man is routinely described as "responsible," the woman as "a slut."

Psychological Dimensions

Although sexual activity is definitely physical, it also involves psychology—our sense of being. The noted sexual therapist Dr. Ruth Westheimer has a favorite saying, that sexual behavior "is all between the ears."

A major psychological factor that affects our sexual wellness is body image. A positive body image lends itself to a feeling of overall wellness; a negative self-image can lead to drug abuse (use of steroids or diet pills) or psychological disorders (anorexia, bulimia, binge eating disorder, or muscle dysmorphia).

The psychological dimension of sexuality is probably the clearest example of learned aspects of sexuality. Our attitudes and feelings toward ourselves and other people begin to develop very early in life. From the time we are born, we get signals from all around us telling us how to think and act. We learn that some words are "wrong" or "dirty" and that certain parts of our body are "unmentionable." We even learn to be careful about what conversational topics we enter into with certain people. If we feel one way about ourselves but think others would find these feelings unacceptable, we learn to hide our true feelings and to pretend. After all, thinking or talking about sexuality is not a good idea anyway (or so we have learned). Some of us are lucky enough to grow up with a more positive set of experiences. Regardless of whether our experiences are positive or negative, however, our learned responses to them become integral to our sexuality.

social constructionism The belief that sexual identities are acquired from and influenced and modified by an ever-changing social environment.

Sociocultural Dimensions

The biological and psychological components of sexuality are affected by society and culture. The sociocultural dimension of sexuality is the sum of the cultural and social influences that affect our thoughts and actions.

In contrast to a perception of sexuality's being controlled mainly by biological or genetic characteristics, Tiefer (1995) promotes the idea of **social constructionism**, which proposes that sexual identities and experiences are acquired from and influenced and modified by an ever-changing social environment. According to social constructionists, people acquire and assemble meanings, skills, and values from the people around them. This dimension of sexuality is the sum of the cultural influences that affect our thoughts and actions, both historical and contemporary. For example, historical influences become evident when one considers roles of males and females as well as certain customs.

Indeed, we are surrounded by social influences on our sexuality. Among the sources of influence are religion, multiculturalism, socioeconomic status, ethics, the media, and politics. We will look at each influence here briefly and will revisit them throughout the text.

© Evan Agostini/Invision/AP Photos

Romance reality shows have been successful with television viewers. With so many people looking for love, networks have no shortage of candidates, but it remains to be seen whether real romance can blossom in front of the camera. Do you watch romance reality shows? Why do you think society has embraced them? Do you think it's healthy to make a game out of love?

TABLE 1.1

Summary of Selected Research from the UCLA Higher Education Research Institute

TOPIC A: Is it OK for two people who like each other to have sexual intercourse?

FINDINGS: In 1999, 40% of freshmen agreed this was OK even if they had known each other for only a short time. By 2005 this increased to 46.2% (59.8% of males and 35.1% of females). This was lower support for casual sexual intercourse than the all-time high of 52% in 1987.

TOPIC B: Should abortion be legal?

FINDINGS: Support for laws protecting abortion peaked in 1990 at 65% About half of the 1999 freshman class said abortion should be legal. By 2012, support for legal abortion rose to 60.7%—about equal for males and females. It was 61% in 2013.

TOPIC C: Should gay couples have the right to marry?

FINDINGS: The percentage supporting the legal rights of gay couples to marry was 57.9% in 2002 and 71.3% in 2012 (58.8% of males and 72.4% of females). It was 75% in 2013—up 24 points from 1997. In 2007, 24.3% of the freshmen supported laws prohibiting gay relationships.

TOPIC D: Should gays and lesbians have the legal right to adopt a child?

FINDINGS: In 2011, the percentage supporting this right was 48% agreeing strongly and 28.5% agreeing somewhat. Women supported the rights of gays and lesbians to adopt more than men. In 2013, 83.3% of freshmen were supportive of these rights (86.8% of women and 69.8% of men).

TOPIC E: Should married women confine their activities to the home and family?

FINDINGS: The proportion who supported this reached a 15-year low of 21.5% in 2002 and was 21% in 2005.

Sources: Characteristics of freshmen, 2001; The nation: Attitudes and characteristics of freshmen at 4-year colleges, 2002; Rooney, 2003; This year's freshmen at 4-year colleges: A statistical profile, 2005; The American freshmen: National norms for fall 2007, 2008; This year's freshmen at 4-year colleges: A statistical profile, 2009; The American freshmen, 2011; Survey tracks changes in political views of freshmen, 2012; The American freshman: National norms, fall 2013.

Religious Influences

Religious and spiritual beliefs influence feelings about morality, sexual behavior, premarital sexual behavior, adultery, divorce, contraception, abortion, and masturbation.

It is hard to know for sure what influences the attitudes of college students toward many controversial issues, but religion is certainly one of the important influences. It is interesting to note the findings of the UCLA Higher Education Research Institute. Since 1966, this group has done a comprehensive survey of college freshmen. Unfortunately, they do not include all of the same questions related to sexuality each year, but the available findings related to sexuality are found in **Table 1.1**.

Religion plays a major role in many people's sexuality, including Lisa from the opening story. For Lisa's parents, whose cultural traditions in Korea can be traced to Confucianism, abortion might have been a possibility (as a means of saving face for the family).

Religion can also play a role in use or nonuse of medical services related to sexuality. It can even influence the availability of such services when policies allow service providers to refuse to provide services that are against their personal beliefs. For example, a pharmacist might refuse to sell contraceptives because he does not believe in their use, or a doctor

© CBS Broadcasting Inc. All Rights Reserved/CBS Photo Archive/Landov

In its infancy, television was reluctant to show a biracial couple. When Lucille Ball and Desi Arnaz proposed the *I Love Lucy* show in the early 1950s, television executives wanted a white actor to play opposite Lucy, fearing problems of showing a white-and-Latino couple. Lucy and Desi were forced to put up $5,000 of their own money to create a pilot, which was, of course, a success.

© Eric Risberg/AP Photos

The cast of the movie *Rent*. Considered revolutionary in the mid-1990s, the story dealt frankly with HIV/AIDS and gay relationships. Such sensitivity has become commonplace in almost all media today.

might refuse to perform an abortion because she does not believe abortions are morally appropriate.

Through the years, religiosity (an intense religious belief) has been found to influence the number of sexual partners, the frequency of various forms of sexual behavior, the age at first sexual intercourse, types of sexual behaviors, standards related to sexual activity before marriage, and even marital satisfaction. Religiosity also seems to influence the sexual behaviors of college students. A study conducted at a southeastern university showed that both males and females who reported less frequent worship attendance and weaker religious feelings were more likely to participate in sexual behaviors than those with more frequent worship attendance and stronger religious feelings (Penhollow, Young, & Denny, 2005).

Multicultural Influences

Cultures within the United States differ in their views of sexuality. Your ability to respect your sexual partner's cultural beliefs and feelings will result in a higher level of satisfaction for both of you.

First we must distinguish between ethnic background and ethnicity. A person's ethnic background is usually determined by birth and is related to country of origin, native language, race, and religion. **Ethnicity** refers to the degree of identification an individual feels with a particular ethnic group.

Our opening story underscores this concept. Had Lisa been pregnant, she would have found herself torn between her parents' strong ethnicity and the individual cultural beliefs and practices that she learned in school and college. Such difficult cultural conflicts might place some people in a position like Lisa's at high risk for potential serious problems.

Cultural influences from citizens of other countries also play a dramatic role in U.S. culture. This is especially important for college students in the United States, because 1 in 10 students is from another country. These students' local cultural understandings of the body, health, and morality shape their use of contraceptive methods and abortion. For example, in the United States, abortion is not viewed as a method of contraception. In some other countries, however, abortion is viewed as a primary method of birth control. Some women from these countries might have as many as four or five abortions. In some countries, it has been reported that men who are not members of evangelical religions are more likely to have had an extramarital partner and unprotected extramarital intercourse than those who are more deeply religious. There might even be differences in various regions of a given country. Also, in some countries, women whose beliefs and experiences reflect traditional norms can be at increased risk of intimate-partner violence.

Another multicultural example deals with the topic of genolercide. In some cultures, women are aborted, killed, and neglected to death. In China and northern India, 120 males are born for every 100 females. The destruction of baby girls is a product of three forces: the ancient preference for sons, a modern desire for smaller families, and ultrasound scanning and other technologies that identify the gender of a fetus. Unborn daughters are often sacrificed in pursuit of a son (Gendercide, March 6, 2010).

Socioeconomic Influences

Socioeconomic status and education also influence sexual attitudes and behaviors, at least within the same ethnic group. Examples of this influence include low-income individuals often thinking and acting differently than middle-class individuals, being more likely to engage in sexual intercourse at an earlier age, and having children outside of marriage.

Educational levels also seem to influence sexual behavior. Examples include people with more education masturbating more and people with at least some college education having more sexual partners than those who did not attend college.

---

ethnicity The degree of identification an individual feels with a particular ethnic group.

Socioeconomic status influences more than just sexual activities. The poor have less access to proper health care, birth control, care during pregnancy, day care for children, and positive sexual role models.

Lisa, from our opening story, is affected by her family's high socioeconomic status. The prevailing indicator of success among second-generation Korean Americans is high academic achievement at prestigious universities, followed by pursuit of professional careers. Lisa's academic performance to this point has reflected this cultural value. An unexpected and unwanted pregnancy would create a major obstacle to achieving the expected success and thus create an added intergenerational cultural conflict.

All people are sexual beings, and our experiences influence our thinking about sexuality.

Ethical Influences

The ethics of sexuality involves questioning the way we treat ourselves and other people. Examples of sexually oriented ethical dilemmas include the following:

- Should I or should I not participate in a certain sexual behavior?

- Is it ethical to use a prostitute?

- Is it ethical not to disclose my full sexual history to a new partner?

- Is it ethical to engage in sexual behaviors with a person who is underage?

- Is it ethical to use a position of power to obtain sexual partners?

Ethical issues are not necessarily the same as legal concerns. For example, prostitution is illegal in the United States except in a few counties in Nevada. However, the ethical question of prostitution would look at the morality of hiring a prostitute—who may be selling her body as a last resort to survive. Also, the age of maturity in your state (the age at which you are deemed legally of age to engage in sexual activity) is probably 16 or 17 years old. Thus, it would be illegal to have a sexual partner younger than that age. However, in Tokyo, Japan, the legal age for girls is 12 years. Is it ethical for you to have a sexual partner who is of age in the country you are visiting, even if she is very young?

How we consider such questions and ultimately decide what is right and wrong profoundly shapes our sexuality. Ethical decision making underscores the importance of taking responsibility for your sexual wellness.

Media Influences

It has long been recognized that the media help shape public attitudes on many topics—especially sexuality, sex roles, and sexual behaviors. The depictions of sexuality we encounter in the media are there mainly to entertain and sell products. Consequently, the media do not provide us with realistic depictions.

Television shows are filled with portrayals of sexual activity and "double-meaning" comments. The music industry has countless sexual images. Listen to the words of many currently popular songs and you will hear the sexual content. Magazines, tabloids, many online sources, and books contribute to the many sexual themes that bombard us. Next time you are in the checkout line at the supermarket, take a look at the number of magazine covers that relate to sexuality. Numerous advertisements also use sexual themes to sell products. We are told that if we buy the right soap, toothpaste, clothes, or cars we will look sexier and be more attractive.

Some people have argued that, if they would so choose, the media could promote sexual health by communicating accurate information and portraying realistic situations. For example, they might show effective communication about sexuality and

Ethical DIMENSIONS

Should Human Embryos Be Used for Stem Cell Research?

In 2005 the National Academies released guidelines for embryonic stem cell research. They were amended in 2007, 2008, and 2010. Stem cells are harvested 3 to 5 days after a sperm and egg unite—before implantation in the uterus. Such stem cells have the capacity to develop into almost any type of tissue in the body. Although it is also possible to extract "adult" stem cells from bone marrow, skin, blood, and other types of tissue, adult stem cells have more limited applications than stem cells from embryos. The National Academies developed guidelines because such research is controversial.

Supporters of stem cell research point out that stem cells can be used to treat many human conditions—such as diabetes, Parkinson's disease, and multiple sclerosis. Someday stem cells might even be used to grow spare body parts. Supporters believe researchers should press on to find "cures" for such conditions because the results could be helpful to so many people. Opponents are strongly against research in which embryos are destroyed. Pro-life groups and others believe government funding should not be provided for such research and that it should not be done at all.

For many years stem cell research has been an important political and ethical issue. Many issues, such as whether a woman should become pregnant to produce stem cells to be used for research, have been heavily debated. Others argue about whether stem cell research results in the taking of a human life.

The guidelines of the National Academies prohibit not only the cloning of human beings, but also payments to egg donors and use of eggs without the donor's informed consent. Debates about stem cell research are likely to continue for years to come.

Source: Data from Stem cells at the National Academies. Washington, DC: National Academies, 2011. Available: http://dels-old.nas.edu/bls /stemcells.

On the surface, *Sex and The City* presented four successful, single women living, loving, and having it all in New York City. Beneath the shoes, clothes, and beautiful faces in beautiful places, some saw the show as an insightful commentary on loss, loneliness, and the failure of sexual liberation.

relationships, interactions as verbally and physically respectful, more examples of responsible sexual activity, more instances where healthy sexual encounters are anticipated and not last-minute responses to the heat of passion, and the importance of having good information and using contraceptives and condoms to prevent unwanted pregnancies and diseases.

Political Influences

Even public policy affects our sexual behavior. For example, the U.S. government's *Healthy People 2020* projects attempt to use health promotion to establish AIDS and sexually transmitted infection (STI) awareness, decrease unwanted teenage pregnancies, and increase the number of women who receive prenatal care. Also, the U.S. constitutional right to free speech allows the uncontrolled distribution of some pornographic material on the Internet.

Even political elections—including choosing elected officials and voting on ballot initiatives—can have a profound effect on policies and on thinking about human sexuality. Consider the political ramifications of election results.

As a result of the 2002 elections, for the first time in decades the same political party (in this case, the Republicans) that occupied the White House also controlled the U.S. House and the Senate. This provided an opportunity for that political party to strongly influence various policy issues, including those related to sexuality. The Republican Party has openly supported limiting the right of women to get abortions. It also has clearly desired to emphasize abstinence from sexual activity as the major way to control pregnancies and STIs among young people. It has gone so far as to provide federal funding for certain types of educational programs only if they

Global DIMENSIONS

The Islamic Influence

Islam is the world's fast-growing religion, and its followers are called Muslims. Islam is very common in the Middle East, but it also exists in many other parts of the world. One-fifth of the world's population is Muslim, and 2 to 8 million Muslims live in the United States.

As with other religions, Muslims have differing beliefs on many aspects of sexuality. However, generally Muslims oppose intercourse before marriage, but value it highly within marriage. Both sexes are considered to have high interest in sexual behavior and get great satisfaction from it. Both males and females are encouraged to show modesty in public by wearing loose-fitting, body-covering clothing.

Controversy sometimes occurs among Muslims over traditions, such as, women wearing headscarves. Trying to support secularism, the Muslim country of Turkey for decades banned women from wearing head-scarves in universities. In early 2008, Turkey's parliament lifted the ban, allowing university women to wear head-scarves.

However, the issue remains controversial. Those opposed to women wearing headscarves protested at some campuses, while some university leaders continued to enforce the ban that parliament had removed.

In 2013, the Turkish government relaxed its decades-long restriction on wearing the headscarf in all government offices and universities. Women who want to wear the hijab—a traditional headscarf covering the head and hair, but not the face—will be able to do so. While the controversy continues, this policy was put into place because of concerns that restrictions on the hijab were discouraging women from conservative backgrounds from seeking employment in the government or higher education.

Source: Data from Hodge, D., R. & Nadir, A. Moving toward culturally competent practice with Muslims: Modifying cognitive therapy with Islamic tenets. *Social Work, 53*(1) (2008), 31–41; Martin, C. A head scarf is not just a scarf. *Christian Science Monitor* (February 25, 2008) 9–11. Smith, R. Why Turkey lifted its ban on the Islamic headscarf. *National Geographic.com*, 2013. Available: http://news.nationalgeographic.com/news/2013/10/131011-hijab-ban-turkey-islamic-headscarf-ataturk/.

Even Miss America can be involved in politics related to sexuality.

emphasize abstinence. It also has not been very supportive of rights for LGBTQ people.

Many issues in the 2008 elections related to sexuality. There was the first female major party candidate for president. It was announced that the teenage daughter of the female candidate for Vice President of the United States was pregnant and not married. During the presidential campaign, platforms and debates included discussions about the legality of abortion, rights for gay people (including marriage and adoption), stem cell research, and abstinence-only versus comprehensive sexuality education. After Barack Obama was inaugurated as president in 2009, these issues, along with many others, continued to influence politics. Political issues, in turn, continued to influence human sexuality in many ways. These relationships continued to be seen in the 2014 election, when both the House of Representatives and the Senate ended up being controlled by Republicans.

It remains common for political candidates to be questioned about their views on a number of issues related to sexuality. Abortion, LGBTQ rights, and some medical advances (e.g., genetic engineering, stem cell research, and variations of artificial insemination) are often the most common sexuality topics discussed in political circles. However, the context

? Did You Know . . .

During the first seven to eight decades of the 1900s, there was a steady increase in the rates of premarital sexual intercourse for 15- to 19-year-old students. In 1991, 54.1% had ever engaged in sexual intercourse. The rates then gradually declined, reaching 45.6% in 2001. Then they again increased to 47.8% in 2007 (49.8% of males and 45.9% of females).

In 2007, the number of teens who have had sexual intercourse increased dramatically with grade level: from 32.8% of ninth graders, to 43.8% of tenth graders, to 55.5% of eleventh graders, to 64.6% of twelfth graders. Nationwide, 7.1% of students had sexual intercourse for the first time before 13 years of age. Overall, the proportion of students who had ever had sexual intercourse was higher among black (66.5%) and Hispanic (52.0%) students than among white (43.7%) students.

However, as reported in 2010, the numbers of each group who participated in sexual intercourse again went down. Overall, the number having ever had sexual intercourse was 31.6% for ninth graders, 40.9% for tenth graders, 53% for eleventh graders, and 62.3% for twelfth graders. Nationwide, 5.9% of students had had sexual intercourse for the first time before

age 13 years. Overall, the population of students who ever had sexual intercourse was higher among black (65.2%) and Hispanic (49.1%) students than among white (42%) students.

Note that in each case the numbers were *smaller* in 2010 than in 2007. This is mentioned because many people think that these numbers keep going up, and that is not necessarily the case.

The numbers reported in 2013 were similar to those reported in 2010. The number having ever had sexual intercourse was 30% for 9th graders, 41.4% for 10th graders, 54.1% for 11th graders, and 64.1% for 12th graders. Nationwide, 5.6% had had sexual intercourse for the first time before age 13 years. Overall, the population of students who had ever had sexual intercourse remained higher among black (60.6%) and Hispanic (49.2%) students than among white (43.7%) students.

Source: Data from Youth risk behavior surveillance—United States, 2007. *Morbidity and Mortality Weekly Report, 57, no. SS-4* (June 6, 2008), 21–23; Youth risk behavior surveillance—United States, 2009. *Morbidity and Mortality Weekly Report, 59, no. SS-5* (June 4, 2010), A–142. Youth risk behavior surveillance—United States 2013. *Morbidity and Mortality Weekly Report, 63, no. 63* (June 13, 2014), 1–168.

Myth vs Fact

Myth: Rates of premarital intercourse increased rapidly in the first 60–70 years of the 20th century.
Fact: There was a rather steady rate of premarital sexual intercourse during the first six to seven decades of the 20th century.

Myth: We have long known that early childhood experiences are important to sexual development.
Fact: It was not until at least the middle of the 20th century that it was recognized that early childhood experiences are important to a child's healthy development.

and focus of such discussions change periodically. For example, a discussion about health insurance might focus on whether abortion services and/or contraceptives should be covered. A discussion about LGBTQ rights might focus on tax issues or the future of gays and lesbians in the military. We can be confident that politics will continue to influence thinking about human sexuality, and vice versa.

▓ Historical–Cultural Influences on Sexuality

Just as many sociocultural influences have affected human sexuality, so have some interesting

historical–cultural influences. Because we cannot consider all of them, and because most of these topics are covered in greater depth elsewhere in this text, we briefly focus on some from a historical standpoint—namely, the sexual revolution, control of sexual behavior, conception, contraception, and sex roles. As you read about these historical–cultural influences, think about how you and people you know may have been affected by them.

The Sexual Revolution

No doubt you have heard references to the sexual revolution. The meaning of this term varies according to the speaker; however, it is clear that many changes related to sexuality have occurred in the past 80 to 100 years. Whether there has been an actual revolution—or perhaps an evolution—is for you to decide after considering some facts and observations.

Many people talk about a sexual revolution in reference to rates of sexual intercourse before marriage. Many of our history books would lead us to believe that in the past, Americans were sexually chaste before marriage. If we read between the lines, however, we find that this is not necessarily true. Reiss (1973) informs us that in the late 1700s in Massachusetts, one of three women in a particular church confessed fornication to her minister (the actual number was probably higher yet). The U.S. western frontier society relied heavily on prostitution. The women's liberation movement of the 1870s revealed numerous sexual affairs. And the first vulcanized rubber condom was displayed at the Philadelphia World's Fair in 1876. These are not isolated events, and they should make us question what we think about the sexual purity and innocence of our forebears (Bruess & Schroeder, 2014).

Studies done between 1920 and 1945 do seem to indicate that the greatest increases in rates of premarital sexual intercourse occurred in the early 1900s (Bell, 1966). This means that the so-called sexual revolution began early in the 20th century and not in more recent years. Many older people who seem so concerned about changes in sexual behavior were in the middle of the sexual revolution themselves. Our best research tells us that approximately 35% to 45% of females and 55% to 65% of males participated in sexual intercourse before marriage during most of the first six to seven decades of the 20th century (Bruess & Schroeder, 2014).

Many changes that influence our thinking about sexuality occurred in the first six to seven decades of the 20th century. For example, as traditional moral viewpoints were questioned, people began to wonder about whether any one standard of morality could apply universally. Social scientists talked about people defining their own morality, while religious leaders often saw morality as determined by an order higher than mere humans.

Several events also occurred during this period that contributed to a trend toward more receptivity to the topic of sexuality. For example, wars exposed many people to other cultures, and the uncertainty of survival contributed to a philosophy of "Live tonight, for tomorrow we may die." The result was a change in the concept of sexual morality. In addition, there was a rise in the status of women as they became better educated, a more significant part of the workforce, more aggressive, and more active partners in sexual activity.

Myth vs Fact

Myth: Contraceptive methods were not available until the 20th century.

Fact: Methods used to prevent pregnancy are as old as recorded history.

Rapid improvements in communication and transportation also had a tremendous effect on sexuality. First the telephone became a convenient way to promote interpersonal relationships, and today the Internet provides a means for people to meet, send quick love messages, and stay in touch. Magazines, TV, and films continued to have many sexual themes, and the car became a "bedroom on wheels," providing a way to have private sexual activity.

It became accepted that early childhood experiences are important to the development of young children—including their sexual development. This understanding has had ramifications for sexuality education programs for children of all ages.

Important events that influenced sexuality include the research of Alfred Kinsey in the 1940s and 1950s related to sexual behavior, the first nationwide appearance of Elvis Presley in 1956 (considered obscene by many), and the introduction of the bikini swimsuit in 1959. The lyrics of popular songs became more sexually suggestive, and record smashing by opponents of these songs occurred in an attempt to censor the music.

The 1960s work of William Masters and Virginia Johnson on human sexual response also greatly contributed to our knowledge of how we function sexually and how and why we sometimes do not function. In addition to basic information about sexual functioning, their research provided the foundation for sexual counseling and methods for dealing with human sexual inadequacy.

Increasingly reliable contraceptives, especially the pill (introduced in the United States in 1960), were developed and accepted by large numbers of

Some people thought this performance by Elvis Presley was obscene.

people. Today many reliable and relatively safe contraceptive methods are available, and the vast majority of married couples use contraception.

In the late 20th century and early 21st century, books, classes, and radio and television programs about sexuality, as well as numerous websites related to sexuality, became common. The press reports the findings of virtually every new study, and discussions about sexuality in American society are out of the closet and into public forums.

Control of Sexual Behavior

Throughout the history of Western culture, there have been many attempts to control sexual behavior. Most of these are found in moral and legal codes of the time. For example, early Christian moralists taught that because sexual activity outside marriage had a purpose other than **procreation**, it was a sin. Even within marriage, sexual union was lawful only if it was performed for the purpose of begetting children. Almost all medieval theologians emphasized that it was a mortal sin to embrace one's spouse solely for pleasure (Aries & Bejin, 1985, 115).

There were many other religious influences and restrictions. For example, intercourse was objectionable on all fast or feast days, during the days a female was menstruating, for 40 days after childbirth, during pregnancy, and during breastfeeding. Also, intercourse between husband and wife was supposed to take place in the "natural" position, with the wife on

her back and the husband on top. All other positions were considered "unnatural."

Many religious people thought that only the lowest type of people engaged in oral–genital sexual activity or anal intercourse. Homosexuality was considered an abomination and punishable by death.

A belief in witchcraft was another means of controlling sexual behavior. Strong feelings, especially lust and passion, were believed to arise from evil spirits, and because women (and not men) inspired lust, some religious leaders saw women as witches or agents of the devil. Witches were tortured, ostensibly to drive the devil out of them, or killed. Bewitchment was said to account for the mysterious and overwhelming emotional effects that women had on men, sometimes driving them to irrational acts. Witch trials were held throughout the Middle Ages, particularly during the 15th century (Sadock, Kaplan, & Freedman, 1973).

In 17th-century England, the Puritan influence was responsible for legislation to prevent amusements such as dancing, singing, and the theater. Women were treated as prostitutes if they wore long hair or makeup. On Sundays any activities not related to worship were banned.

By the end of the 18th century, sexual behavior was subdued and spontaneity inhibited. People conducted their lives very discreetly. Harsh negative attitudes toward same-sex sexual behavior were common during this time, and many people who practiced that behavior were reportedly put to death. So strong were fears and feelings during the period that people who asked for leniency for those convicted of sodomy (which includes almost any sexual behavior one wishes to prohibit) were themselves in danger of persecution. Eighteenth-century studies of sexuality emphasized physiology and generally concluded that excessive sexual activity—specifically, expelling of semen to excess—had debilitating physical consequences.

In the 19th century, during Victorian times, sexual drives were generally repressed. Though it was believed that men had natural and spontaneous sexual desires, women supposedly had dormant sex drives unless subjected to undue excitation. Children, it was believed, had no sexual feelings.

Much was done to protect the people of Victorian times from sexual arousal. Sexual references in literature and general conversation were suppressed, as were most sexual feelings. Masturbation, a particularly repudiated activity, was called the "secret sin," "self-pollution," and the "solitary vice." Devices were even developed to place around the male's penis at night to prevent **spermatorrhea** (more commonly called **nocturnal emissions** or **wet dreams**) (Figure 1.1).

In the early 20th century, as conservative morality about sexuality diminished and people argued that sexual expression was natural and normal, some secular

procreation Sexual intercourse for the purpose of reproduction.

spermatorrhea (wet dreams, or nocturnal emissions) Emission of semen during sleep.

FIGURE **1.1** Devices designed to prevent wet dreams. One device caused a bell to ring when erection occurred (a). For some devices, no bell was needed (b and c).

attempts were made to legislate sexual morality. This resulted in censorship, prohibition, and the revival of old statutes against certain sexual behaviors, such as same-sex behavior, oral–genital relations, and sodomy.

© The Kobal Collection at Art Resource, NY

Woody Allen's farcical treatment of sperm cells in *Everything You Always Wanted to Know about Sex …* reflects what was once thought true. When sperm cells were discovered by a magnifying glass in 1677, scientists believed that they saw tiny men (called *animalcules*) inside sperm cells. Other scientists even claimed to see microscopic horses in horse sperm!

Theoretically, in the United States there is a separation of church and state, but legal debates about such subjects as abortion, access to sexual information and services, LGBTQ issues, and sexual behaviors have prompted some people to wonder about that separation.

Conception

Much of our information about prehistoric people is obtained by analyzing the remains of their art. In addition, we can make inferences about primitive cultures from the art that exists today. Prehistoric cave paintings indicate that more than 30,000 years ago sexuality was an important part of culture. Some of these stone engravings suggest human intercourse, and some show women and men with exaggerated body parts.

Despite the attention to sexuality in their art and perhaps their religion, prehistoric people apparently did not understand its role in reproduction. Consequently, theorists believe that a number of explanations for childbirth existed. One notion may have been that children were sent by ancestral deities; sexual intercourse was reserved solely for pleasure. Or a woman became pregnant by sitting over a fire on which she had roasted a fish received from the prospective father. An Australian tribe believed that a woman conceived by eating human flesh. Some cultures thought it was possible for a man to become pregnant (Tannahill, 1980). Some of these theories might seem humorous, but they are really no more peculiar, or at least no more wrong, than such modern superstitions as "You can't get pregnant if you do it only once." By the time of the first written records, however, it appears that humans were aware that they played some part in reproduction, even if they did not know how.

Throughout recorded history, many theories and myths about conception existed. For example, Aristotle theorized that the human fetus resulted from the mixture of menstrual blood and seminal fluid.

One hundred years before Aristotle, the Greek poet Aeschylus believed that a child was conceived by a male alone (Where do babies come from?, 1987).

The microscope allowed scientists to see sperm for the first time. In 1677, the Dutch naturalist Anton van Leeuwenhoek described the human sperm discovered by one of his students. Many scientists, however, refused to accept that sperm could be responsible for creating human life. Other scientists claimed they had seen tiny humans inside sperm. This thinking led to the belief that a tiny, fully formed person would not grow until he or she reached the female "nest." At the same time other scientists, known as **ovists**, claimed that the preformed baby was contained in the female and the sperm served only to activate its development. It was not until 1875 that it was demonstrated that the sperm penetrates and combines with the egg (Where do babies come from?, 1987).

It is impossible to know the overall effect of the accurate understanding of conception; however, it would seem that such knowledge was useful to both males and females. The understanding that sexual intercourse could result in conception must have influenced sexual behavior and made it possible to have at least some control over whether or not to procreate. The control of reproduction is possible today; throughout most of history it was not.

Contraception

Although the process of reproduction was not understood until relatively recently, **contraception**—methods employed to prevent pregnancy—is as old as recorded history. More than 4,000 years ago Egyptian women used medicated tampons as contraceptives. Lint, moistened in a mixture of acacia tips ground with honey, was placed into the vagina. Many other practices, some of them dangerous, were used in the centuries that followed (*The ecology of birth control*, 1971). Among these were inserting spongy or absorbent fabrics into the vagina or mixing crocodile dung with a paste and inserting the mixture into the vagina. It is said that Persian women placed lemon-soaked sponges in the vagina to prevent pregnancy. It is interesting to note that these methods have some merit. Most of them attempted to form a barrier or alter the acid–base relationship within the vagina. In fact, many of today's contraceptive methods are based on these same principles.

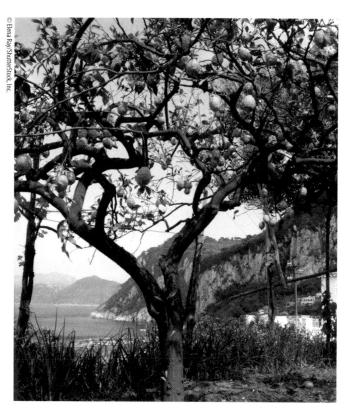

Humans have sought and used contraceptives from the present day to ancient times, when ingredients ranged from lemons to crocodile dung.

The first modern contraceptive device, which was eventually called the condom, appeared in the mid-16th century. It was designed to protect the wearer against the plague of syphilis then spreading throughout Europe. The condom was first made of fine linen, then of animal intestine, and finally of rubber. Even though its original use was for protection from disease, its potential as a contraceptive was quickly noticed (*The ecology of birth control*, 1971).

In the middle of the 19th century, the German physician Mensinga perfected the rubber diaphragm. He believed that women should have equal rights with men and that their lives would be improved by controlling the number of children they conceived. In the United States, the diaphragm was generally unknown until after World War I. Although condoms were not as effective as diaphragms, and although they depended on the male's willingness to use them, they were manufactured in great quantities at the end of the 19th century and thus became cheaper and more available (Bullough, 1976a, 651). Today, 5.5 billion condoms are manufactured in the United States each year.

The idea of the intrauterine device (IUD) was borrowed from an ancient practice of camel drivers, who put a round stone (or an apricot pit, according to some accounts) into the uterus of a female camel to prevent pregnancy on long trips. During the 1920s,

ovist Adherent to the 17th-century belief that the preformed baby was contained within the female body and that the male's sperm simply activated its development.

contraception Means of preventing pregnancy in spite of sexual intercourse.

Communication
DIMENSIONS

The CERTS Model Wendy Maltz developed the CERTS model for healthy sexuality. The letters stand for Consent, Equality, Respect, Trust, and Safety. Consent means you can freely and comfortably choose whether or not to engage in sexual activity. Equality means your sense of personal power is on an equal level with your partner. Respect means you have positive regard for yourself and for your partner. Trust means you trust your partner on physical and emotional levels. Safety means you feel secure and safe within the sexual setting.

Maltz suggests that spending time together and engaging in lots of honest, open communication are good ways to make sure that the CERTS conditions are operating in your relationship. Meeting the CERTS conditions does not guarantee that everything will be perfect, but it can help you feel secure knowing that you've minimized the possibility of something bad resulting from your sexual experiences.

Source: Data from *The CERTS model for healthy sex.* 2011. Available: http://www.healthysex.com/page/certs-model.

a German gynecologist modernized the idea by substituting a ring of surgical silk or silver (The ecology of birth control, 1971). It was not until experiments with IUDs were performed in Israel and Japan in 1959, however, that their use became widespread.

A number of effective spermicides appeared on the market at the end of the 19th century. The early ones, marketed in a suppository form, probably worked by blocking the cervix with an oily film. Numerous other chemicals soon appeared on the market (Bullough, 1976a, 651). Foams and jellies were introduced in the early 20th century. Research on an oral contraceptive was widespread in the 1950s, but it was not until 1960 that the first oral contraceptive was approved for public use. It can probably be said that this event marked the beginning of the modern era of contraception.

It was 30 years later, in 1990, that the U.S. Food and Drug Administration approved levonorgestrel (Norplant). This hormonal contraceptive implant system was six capsules 34 mm long, inserted beneath the skin of a woman's upper arm. Its release marked the first time long-term (in this case, up to 5 years) hormonal control of conception was available in the United States (FDA OKs hormonal implant, 1990).

Not necessarily considered a form of contraception, abortion is a means of controlling births. Abortion early in pregnancy was legal in ancient China and Europe. In the 13th century the Roman Catholic church indicated that the soul developed 40 days after conception in males and 90 days after conception in females, and abortion was allowed within those intervals. In the late 1860s the Catholic church declared that life begins at conception; that doctrine led to its abortion ban (O'Keefe, 1995).

Early American law allowed abortion until the woman felt fetal movement, but during the 1860s abortion became illegal in the United States except to save the woman's life. In addition to the religious

Myth vs Fact

Myth: Open discussion about sexuality will have negative results—people will be more likely to be sexually permissive.
Fact: Healthy communication about sexuality will help people develop into sexually healthy adults—open discussions do not have negative results.

Myth: The relatively open attitudes in thinking about sexuality in Sweden have resulted in higher rates of teen pregnancy and sexually transmitted infections.
Fact: Swedish attitudes and practices related to sexuality have resulted in lower rates of teen pregnancy and sexually transmitted infections.

Myth: Abortion has been illegal throughout most of the history of the United States.
Fact: Early American law allowed abortion until a woman felt fetal movement. In the 1860s abortion became illegal in the United States, but in 1973 the Supreme Court legalized a woman's right to terminate her pregnancy.

Myth: What is sexually arousing to people is very much the same regardless of the culture.
Fact: In different cultures the idea of what is sexually arousing varies a great deal.

beliefs of some people, reasons for this included health problems related to crude abortion procedures, the belief that population growth was needed for economic reasons, and maybe a male-dominated political system's response to more women seeking independence and equality (Sheeran, 1987). It was not until 1973 that the U.S. Supreme Court in its famous *Roe* v. *Wade* decision legalized a woman's right to decide to terminate her pregnancy before the fetus could survive independently of the woman's body. Debates about this issue continue.

Sex Roles

"The paramount destiny and mission of women are to fulfill the noble and benign offices of wife and mother. This is the law of the Creator." Words of a time long past? Not quite. This is actually an excerpt from a Supreme Court opinion rendered in the first case tried under the Fourteenth Amendment in 1873. The court's decision upheld the denial of the right of women to practice law (Bardes, Shelley, & Schmidt, 1998).

Historically, the role of the woman as a sexual partner has been to satisfy male needs. In India, for example, women were viewed as nothing without men. In the West, women who enjoyed sexual activity dared not speak of it publicly because of the severe penalties for doing so. Throughout the ages women were viewed as property of men (Spielvogel, 1997). In most societies, if a woman committed adultery, was raped, or lost her virginity, she was considered damaged property. A woman's father or husband could expect to gain compensation for this damage, or, in the case of adultery, he might even kill her and her partner if they were caught (Bullough, 1976b, 677–679).

In many societies men enjoyed a status vastly superior to that of women. This status can probably be accounted for by (1) men's greater physical strength, (2) women's repeated pregnancies in the absence of reliable contraceptive methods, and (3) the ideology that disparity in male and female roles was divinely ordained. Men used their greater physical strength to trap animals and handle livestock, to defend themselves, and to intimidate women. Because women were often pregnant and spent much of their time caring for children, little time was left to alter their inferior status. Those who felt male and female roles had a divine origin saw any attempts to change these roles as antireligious (Murstein, 1974, 566).

The ancient Greeks believed that men were primarily mental and spiritual in their makeup and that women were primarily physical and earthy. Because the Greeks believed the mind and body were separate entities, this meant men had a higher nature and deserved greater privileges. Several centuries later, however, Jesus insisted on the basic equality of the sexes. He opposed Jewish divorce law, which allowed women to be disposed of as property (Nelson, 1978).

Throughout medieval times, women were thought to be inferior to men. Their motives were suspect, they were thought to be sinful, and their female functions were belittled. Some still believed Aristotle's earlier claim that the female was little more than an incomplete male. Both religious and scientific thinking seemed to support these ideas (Bullough, 1976b).

In the early 1800s there were more male children than female children in the western states and territories of the United States. Some researchers have thought this was because nutrition and health of young females were neglected because their labor was not as economically valued. Others have indicated that this imbalance simply occurred because more boys were born in, survived childhood in, or moved to western regions (Courtwright, 1990). This presents another example in which it is difficult to determine the real reasons for the situation.

However, the mid- to late 1800s and the early 1900s witnessed many advances in the status of women in the United States. After the first major organized meeting on the rights of women in 1848, there was a sort of legal emancipation, an opening of work opportunities, and an ideological acceptance of the equality of the sexes. Actual changes in behavior, however, did not keep pace with this verbal acceptance. The average woman was probably more interested in receiving greater respect and consideration, and in receiving the right to vote, than in having equal professional rights. Most articles advocating the causes important to women today were written by highly educated men and women, and probably the majority of Americans were not even aware of these new ideas (Murstein, 1974, 379). Nonetheless, the seeds of the women's rights movement were planted.

The women's suffrage movement began in the late 19th century with the goal of obtaining the right to vote for women. The passage in 1920 of the Nineteenth Amendment to the U.S. Constitution guaranteed women the right to vote. World War II created an environment for increased gender equality. As men were required to leave home for military duty, thousands of women left their traditional roles in the home and took paying jobs for the first time. It was not until the 1960s, however, after many postwar marriages, the baby boom, and continued disappointment about women's roles, that a new movement for gender equality became evident.

Some people had thought that the ratification of the Nineteenth Amendment would end the struggle

Women did not get the right to vote in the United States until 1920.

Multicultural DIMENSIONS

Pregnancy and Health

When speaking of culture, sociologists generally refer to the "learned values, beliefs, norms, behaviors, and even material objects that are passed from one generation to the next." Within the culture of the United States, however, are many subcultures—groups of people with shared values within the overall culture. Each subculture has a distinctive way of looking at life that sets it off from the prevalent culture. In the United States, these groups may be defined by ethnicity, age, religion, sexuality, geographical location, and national origin. The Multicultural Dimensions boxes look at varied subcultures within the United States.

The first multicultural issue we explore relates to teen pregnancy in developing countries. Approximately 16 million girls younger than age 18 give birth each year, according to the United Nations Population Fund. Another 3.2 million have unsafe abortions. For many of these girls, pregnancy has little to do with informed choice. The youngest mothers face an increased risk of maternal complications, death, and disability. Their children face higher risks as well. After one intervention program, teen pregnancy rates were 26% lower. Condom usage increased by 28%.

It is obvious that better medical intervention is a key to improving the health of mothers and their children. But more than just medical intervention is required: There also needs to be a change in how women are viewed and how things get done to really make a difference. For example, it is essential to have a stable environment that empowers women and respects their rights. Educating girls and women is one of the most fundamental ways to improve maternal and newborn health and benefits both families and societies. Essential interventions will be guaranteed only within the context of improved education and the abolition of discrimination.

Source: World Population Day focuses on teen pregnancy. United Nations, July 2013. Available: http://www.un.org/en/development /desa/news/population/world-population-day.html. 2014 International Day of the Girl Child. UNICEF, 2014. Available: http://www.unicef.org/gender/gender_70474.html.

for women's rights, but this had not happened. In 1963 the Equal Pay Act, which stated that women must receive pay equal to that of men if they perform the same work, was enacted. In 1964 women were included in the protections of the Civil Rights Act. This made it clear that equality of opportunity for women was endorsed by the federal government (Degler, 1980, 442). Still, women today earn an average of less than 90 cents for every dollar men earn.

In 1963 Betty Friedan published *The Feminine Mystique,* which helped create a widespread movement for women's rights. She urged women to make a life for themselves in addition to their homes and families. The case for women's equality was also championed in a number of other books. In 1966 Friedan organized the National Organization for Women (NOW), which has consistently advocated women's rights. By 1970 a number of other organizations that pushed for women's equality were formed, including the Women's Equity Action League and the Women's Political Caucus. So successful was the women's movement that it has been considered "possibly the most lasting legacy of the … period of protests" (Degler, 1980, 446).

In recent years many issues related to women's roles have been raised. Women now work in a variety of jobs previously thought to be only for males, and there are more women in positions of authority. Discrimination against pregnant women in the workplace has lessened, many women delay having children to pursue other interests, and there is an increased acceptance of child care while women work. Varied opinions about women's roles continue. Studies about gender and leadership style, gender differences in work, family conflict, gender and the influence of achievement evaluations, gender in the college classroom, among others, continue to provide reams of information about women and their roles and status. But whether we have achieved equality between the sexes is still a matter of debate.

▨ Thinking Critically About Human Sexuality

You have probably observed that, when it comes to many topics related to health and sexuality, there are "experts" everywhere. The concept of critical thinking is important to being able to judge the accuracy of what these people say as well as lots of other information you hear related to sexuality. In this case, the word *critical* does not mean being negative or criticizing people or things. It means being careful and somewhat analytical.

In essence, then, **critical thinking** is thinking that prevents blindly accepting conclusions or arguments (or headlines) and instead closely examines all assumptions. This includes carefully evaluating existing evidence and cautiously assessing all conclusions (Baron, 1998).

Critical thinking is like the scientific methods you may have used in other classes. In practice, it involves guidelines such as these (Baron, 1998):

1. Never jump to conclusions; gather as much information as you can before making up your mind about any issue.

2. Keep an open mind; do not let your existing views blind you to information or new conclusions.

3. Always ask "How?" as in "How was this evidence gathered?"

4. Be skeptical; always wonder about *why* someone is making an argument, offering a conclusion, or trying to persuade you.

5. Never be stampeded into accepting some view or position by your own emotions—or by arguments and appeals designed to play on your emotions.

Not every guideline will apply in every situation, but the important goal is to develop a style of thinking using as many of the guidelines as seems appropriate in a given situation.

Correlation Versus Causation

A research study found that for people 60 years and older, the 62% who drank coffee still enjoyed active sex lives, compared with only 37% of those who were not coffee drinkers. Does coffee lead to a better sex life for seniors? Or are the two events just coincidental? The study shows a **correlation**, a relationship between two events. But it does not show a **causation**, a relationship in which one event causes the other.

It is easy to show that a correlation exists, but correlations do not show cause and effect. There is a high correlation between the winning conference of the Super Bowl and the stock market: When the NFC wins, the stock market goes up in most years; when

the AFC wins, the market goes down in most years. However, no scientific study is needed to understand that the Super Bowl does not cause the stock market to go up or down.

Returning to the coffee example, perhaps people older than 60 years old who are in good health enjoy both coffee and sexual activity. However, there does not appear to be a causal link between caffeine use and sexual activity. In contrast, a study showing a correlation between the drug Viagra and an active sex life would appear to have a causal link. So, correlations can sometimes help predict behavior and point to possible causes of behavior. Further studies can help validate the causation.

Being a Good Consumer of Sexual Information

We are bombarded with information—and misinformation—about sexuality issues. In fact, most best-selling newsstand periodicals lure readers with information about "new" sexual techniques or sex surveys. It is important to keep the principles of the scientific method in mind when reading popular literature.

Consider a study that garnered a great deal of media attention: The medical anthropologists Soma Grismaijer and Sidney Ross Singer (2002) surveyed 4,700 women and concluded that their odds of having breast cancer increased the longer women wore bras. Their hypothesis was that the cinching effect of a bra suppresses the lymphatic system below a woman's armpit, blocking an internal network of vessels that are intended to flush toxic wastes from the body. Over time, these toxins accumulate in the breast tissue and create an environment in which cells can turn cancerous.

The results of the survey appear to confirm their hypothesis: Of women who wore bras 24 hours a day, in three of four breast cancer developed; of women who wore bras less than 12 hours a day, in one in seven breast cancer developed; of women who rarely wore bras, in only 1 in 168 did breast cancer develop.

The study appears to have found a *correlation* between length of bra-wearing time and breast cancer. However, few medical scientists would agree that a *causation* exists; many would even question the correlation. First, consider the design of the survey on which the conclusion was based: Participants were not randomly selected, following accepted statistical guidelines. For example, women who have had breast cancer might be more willing to participate in a breast-cancer study. Nor were participants questioned about preexisting breast-cancer risks. In addition, participants answered only 12 questions regarding their bra-wearing habits.

---

critical thinking   Thinking that avoids blind acceptance of conclusions or arguments and closely examines all assumptions.

correlation   A relationship between two events.

causation   A relationship in which one event causes another event to occur.

A scientific approach to the correlation of bra use and breast cancer would be to find a large, randomly selected sample of women who wear bras for specific lengths of time each day. The women would need to be prescreened for breast-cancer risk and would need to undergo medical exams before participating. Family history of cancer, age, race, body mass, weight, diet, exercise, alcohol or drug consumption, and other factors would have to be controlled in some manner. A matching control group (not selected by bra-wearing time) would add further validity. The study could follow the women across a long period, perhaps 15 to 25 years.

Thus a critical review of the study quickly calls into doubt the causal factor between bra use and breast cancer. Even the correlation appears to be contrived. However, it does open the door for further studies.

A final point about the scientific method should be made here: When this study first appeared in popular print media, the information provided varied by the source. News media presented the story as provocative and quirky but with powerful opposition voiced by medical doctors and cancer specialists. But one popular "health" magazine reported the study in a way that suggested a causal link—and placed an ad on the opposite page for a "health drug" claiming to lower risk of breast cancer. Always remember to think about why someone is publishing the study. In this case, it was clearly done to help sell a product.

▪ Why Study Sexuality?

There are many reasons for studying human sexuality, including obtaining accurate sexual knowledge, clarifying personal values, improving sexual decision making, learning the relationship between human sexuality and personal well-being, and exploring how the varied dimensions of human sexuality influence one's sexuality.

Sexual Knowledge

A major reason for studying human sexuality is to acquire a sound foundation of sexual knowledge. Only knowledge can dispel sexual myths, superstitions, and misinformation that block understanding, inhibit communication, and create confusion. Correct information lays the groundwork for sexual decision making. The greater your knowledge, the more likely you are to take responsibility for your sexual health. College students want specific factual information (probably pertaining to a sexual encounter), as well as the answer to the age-old question, "Am I normal?"

The issue of sexual and physical normality underscores the psychological dimensions of human sexuality. It is normal to wonder whether your appearance and/or sexual desires are normal. Many men worry about the size and shape of their penis, and women often worry about the size and shape of their breasts. Learning about the wide variety in appearances may help you feel better about yourself. Learning more about sexuality can often increase your sense of personal worth, or **self-esteem**.

Factual knowledge can also help you interpret sociocultural traditions or myths. History is filled with examples of myths about the biological nature of sexuality. Aristotle, for example, thought that menstrual fluid was the substance from which the embryo was formed, a belief held for centuries. Leonardo da Vinci's anatomical drawings show a tube running from the uterus to the breasts of a woman, depicting the common belief that the menstrual fluid that did not flow during pregnancy was diverted to the breasts to make milk—this in spite of the fact that he had dissected female cadavers and certainly never saw such a tube! The U.S. culture is by no means free of sexual myths, as you will discover throughout this text.

A major issue relating to sexual knowledge involves how to engage in "safer sex." Which activities can lead to the transmission of STIs and HIV? Is your partner, for example, in a high-risk group? What can be done to lower the risk of transmitting STIs and HIV? Does your partner share your knowledge—and concern—about such issues? If not, should you be willing to engage in sexual activity with that person?

Personal Values

A second reason for studying sexuality is to clarify personal sexual **values**, those beliefs to which we attach the most worth. By exploring your own dimensions of human sexuality, you may come to understand the origins and nature of your sexual values, as well as the values of others.

Remember Lisa from our opening story. She began to understand how sexuality fit into her personal values, especially those involving her family. The values that her family and culture held were very important to Lisa, and she fretted over the prospect of becoming an "unmember" of her family, were she to become pregnant outside marriage.

self-esteem Sense of personal worth.

values Those beliefs to which we attach the most worth.

Many values influence sexual decision making.

Sound knowledge influences sexual decision making.

Responsible Sexual Decision Making

A third reason for studying sexuality is to improve your sexual decision-making skills. Most people have had some sexual experience. A large majority of college students have had sexual intercourse, and almost all have participated in some form of sexual activity. But experience alone does not necessarily provide wisdom or skill in sexual decision making. The study of sexuality provides a sound foundation of sexual information, promotes an understanding of sexual attitudes, and examines a broad range of sexual issues.

For example, assume you were dating Lisa in the opening story. Without an understanding of the many social and cultural factors that influence her sexuality, you would find it hard to understand her feelings. Her communication style is restricted by her cultural background, which discourages openly discussing feelings and seeking psychological counseling. Lack of understanding of why Lisa holds in her feelings could lead to a deterioration of your relationship.

Dr. Drew, the dry-witted host of *Loveline*, a radio and TV talk show that answers viewers' sexuality questions, often suggests that listeners think about their actions before they get involved in sexual situations.

A frequently occurring situation on the show is that of having sexual activity with a roommate's lover, which callers often claim "just happened." Dr. Drew responds that, in most cases, it does not just happen—the two parties consciously flirt, possibly dress enticingly, and in the end must find a time and place to be alone. Dr. Drew suggests that had the parties stopped to think about the actions they were taking, they could have made the sexually responsible decision not to engage in sexual activity. In addition to the radio and TV shows, the Loveline podcast is available at http://podcastone.com/Loveline.

A Decision-Making Model

A simple but formal model of the decision-making process consists of the following steps (Bruess & Richardson, 1995).

1. *Recognition.* Only with the recognition of an issue can a decision be made. For example, a couple who consider engaging in sexual intercourse need to recognize the risk of pregnancy, transmission of STIs or HIV, and overstepping of a partner's personal dimensions.

    The best decision making requires defining the issue as precisely as possible: For example, which forms of contraception are acceptable? Which forms are unacceptable? What can be done to promote safer sexual activity? How does my partner feel about this? Which physiological or cultural dimensions might influence my partner's decisions?

2. *Evaluation.* Having recognized a need to make decisions, it is time to gather relevant information, analyze the possible choices, and decide on the best alternative. For example, the latex condom might be a

Communication
DIMENSIONS

Talking About Your Human Sexuality Class

Expect to find a great deal of interest when you tell people you are taking a class in human sexuality. Inevitably, many of your friends, colleagues, neighbors, and family members will ask, "What are you learning?" How you answer that question says a great deal about your tactfulness, how people perceive your knowledge, and how interestingly and humorously you can present delicate information. We have dealt with this question for years, and here are some suggestions:

- Be careful talking about sexual information at work. One *Seinfeld* episode revolved around Jerry being unable to remember a new girlfriend's name—except that it rhymed with a female body part. Eventually, he remembers her name is Dolores—which rhymes (sort of) with clitoris. One man embarrassed a sexually inhibited female colleague by describing the episode at work. The woman, who did not know the term *clitoris,* was further embarrassed when the man showed her the definition in a dictionary (in front of several colleagues). She complained to human resources, and he was fired. He sued the company and won a settlement, which is currently in the appeals process. Do not give people sexual information they do not want to hear! As illustrated in the *Seinfeld* case, it is best to change subjects—or even apologize—if someone is uncomfortable with what you are saying. Watch for nonverbal cues as well. Pressing a point may cost you friends.

- Do not go into detail. Use the KISS method (Keep It Simple and Sincere). If you find the human sexual response cycle interesting, discuss it in general terms: "I was surprised to learn that males and females have the same physiological response to sexual activity." If asked further questions, simply arrange for the person to borrow your book.

- Do not gross people out. In general, people do not want to hear sordid stories relating to sexuality. Information on atypical sexual behaviors, female genital mutilation, or sexual slavery is not usually dinnertime conversation. Recognize diversity. In fact, many people will be highly offended by hearing such information.

- Do not be afraid to say something in a straightforward manner. Show comfort with the subject matter by using sexual terminology in a polite, accurate manner. No one will be offended by the use of the word *penis* or *vagina* if used in context—especially if you are answering someone's question.

- Do not lecture. No matter how hard you try (or how sincere you are), you simply will not change friends' sexual behavior by telling them what they are doing wrong.

---

choice for contraception and lowering of the possibility of STI transmission. But the condom also has a lower rate of contraception effectiveness than some other methods. Another choice might be using a contraceptive method with a higher effectiveness rate—such as the pill—combined with a latex condom for STI protection. Further consideration might be necessary if one person is unwilling to use contraceptives because of religious beliefs. Or perhaps one partner has an allergy to latex condoms (in which case polyurethane condoms could be substituted). The decision to remain abstinent could also be discussed.

3. *Implementation.* When a decision has been reached, the plan needs to be put into action. A decision to combine the pill with latex condoms is not effective unless you can delay intercourse until the woman has received a prescription for the pill and taken it for about a month and the man has purchased latex condoms (and learned how to use them).

4. *Review.* After putting the decision into practice, there should be a periodic review. Are the desired results being achieved, or should another alternative be tried? Perhaps after making the decision, something new is learned about the issues that raises questions about the choice. For example, Lisa's pregnancy scare would likely make her seek out a more effective contraceptive method. If so, the decision-making process can be started again. In fact, you will find yourself renewing the decision-making process throughout your life, according to how your circumstances change.

Sexual Health and Wellness

Finally, sexual education can contribute to safer sexual behavior. Given that some sexual behaviors can result in pregnancies and/or the spread of STIs (including HIV), it is important for people of all ages to understand which practices can result in safer sexual behavior and to incorporate such practices into personal relationships.

Note that although we use the term *safer sex*, no sexual activity can be deemed *perfectly* safe. Although knowing a partner's sexual history, using latex condoms consistently, and avoiding certain sexual behaviors can *reduce* your risk of STIs and HIV, they do not *eliminate* the risk. Condoms can break or be improperly used. Your partner may not wish to disclose a complete sexual history (especially embarrassing or abusive situations). Alcohol can also get in the way of judgment.

Following safer sexual practices does not end with youth. The number of older Americans with HIV/AIDS is rising steadily. In a recent year, almost 38% of those diagnosed with HIV were 45 years and older (Centers for Disease Control and Prevention, 2014).

Practicing safer sexual behavior can promote sexual health and wellness, as well as improve self-esteem. The failure to practice safer sexual behavior can result in physiological, psychological, and social trauma. Although many STIs are "curable," some (such as genital herpes) can only be controlled. Knowing that you have herpes or genital warts may lead to lower self-esteem and a reluctance to seek out partners. Contracting HIV would mean a lifetime of treatment to prevent contracting AIDS. An unwanted pregnancy can have devastating results for both the parents and the child. For Lisa, pregnancy outside marriage could have resulted in losing her family.

So how do we know if someone is sexually healthy? The Alberta (Canada) Society for the Promotion of Sexual Health lists 17 criteria for sexually healthy individuals. Among the criteria are: appreciate their own bodies, avoid exploitative relationships, interact with both sexes in appropriate and respectful ways, demonstrate tolerance for people with different values, decide what is personally "right" and act upon these values, talk with a partner about sexual activity before it occurs, and seek further information about sexuality as needed.

Service–Learning Projects in Your Community

While we focus on how you can develop a healthy and sexually responsible lifestyle, we recognize that all of us also have a responsibility to contribute to the health of our communities. We live in a college community, and in a city, town, or village. We live in a state and in this country. And, of course, we are part of a global community as well. With the knowledge you learn in your sexuality course and by reading this book, you have a unique opportunity to contribute to the sexual health of the communities with which you are associated. One of the best ways to do that is through service–learning. **Service–learning** is an educational method that involves students applying what they learn in their coursework in the community so as to contribute to the welfare of that community. For example, after studying the effects of gangster rap music on the sexual attitudes of young people, you might choose to write to local government representatives advocating that warnings be provided with music of this nature. Or you might volunteer at a rape crisis center. As a result of our commitment to you, and to help you organize to meet your commitment to your communities, we provide suggestions for sexuality-related service–learning activities on the website for this text.

---

service–learning Educational method that involves students applying what they learn in their coursework in the community to contribute to that community's welfare.

Exploring the Dimensions of Human Sexuality

Case Study

Many factors influence our sexuality. For example, consider your physical appearance. At first glance, it appears to be a biological factor, set by genetics. But your body image, or self-concept of your appearance, is psychological. Sociocultural factors also come into play—your perception is influenced by the culture in which you live and conveyed by the media that surround you.

Biological Factors

- Sex
- Genetics
- Reproduction
- Fertility control
- Sexual arousal and response
- Physiological cycles and changes
- Physical appearance
- Growth and development

Sociocultural Factors

- Socioeconomic status
- Laws
- Religion
- Culture
- Ethnic heritage
- Media and ad information
- Family, neighbors, and friends
- Ethics

Psychological Factors

- Emotions
- Experience
- Self-concept
- Motivation
- Expressiveness
- Learned attitudes and behaviors
- Body image

Summary

- Sexuality is part of our personality, and it involves the interrelationship of biological, psychological, and sociocultural dimensions.

- Sociocultural influences include religious influences, multicultural influences, ethical influences, and political influences.

- The sexual revolution had many influences on present thinking about human sexuality.

- Throughout history there have been many attempts to control sexual behavior. Most of these efforts can be seen in the moral and legal codes of the time.

- Throughout recorded history, many theories and myths about conception have existed. It was not until 1875 that it was demonstrated that the sperm penetrates and combines with the egg.

- Methods employed to prevent pregnancy have been used for thousands of years. The condom first appeared in the mid-16th century.

- Abortion in early pregnancy was legal in ancient China and Europe. In 1973 the U.S. Supreme Court legalized a woman's right to decide to terminate her pregnancy.

- There have been changes in sex roles throughout the centuries. In recent years many issues related to women's roles continue to be raised.

- It is important to use sound critical thinking skills when making decisions related to human sexuality.

- Studying human sexuality is important to obtain accurate sexual knowledge, clarify personal values, improve sexual decision making, understand the relationship between human sexuality and personal well-being, and explore how the varied dimensions of human sexuality influence one's sexuality.

Discussion Questions

1. List the three main dimensions of sexuality and their subdivisions, and give examples of each.

2. Trace the historical aspects of human sexuality, including the sexual revolution and the changing roles of sex and culture.

3. Explain a method for critical thinking, and differentiate between correlation and causation. Give examples to back up your answer.

4. Explain the main reasons for studying human sexuality.

Application Questions

Reread the chapter-opening story and answer the following questions.

1. If Lisa were pregnant, what advice would you give her? Consider Lisa's sexual dimensions, including the reaction of her family, her religion, and her communication style.

2. If you were Lisa's lover, how might you respond to the situation? To answer this question, you need to reconcile your sexual dimensions with Lisa's.

3. Do all Korean Americans have the same set of sexual dimensions? How might such dimensions differ, depending on age? Length of time in the United States? Geographic location? Socioeconomic status?

Critical Thinking Questions

1. Consider your own sexuality. Write about how each of the three dimensions affects you. Which has the greatest effect on you? The least? Explain your answers.

2. Use the decision-making model to decide whether to engage in a sexual activity that you have not yet done. Having thought the issue through, would you proceed? Which precautions might you take to promote safer sexual behavior?

Critical Thinking Case

Should an Artificial Womb Be Used?

People often need to focus on ethical questions related to conception. For example, an article in the *New York Times Magazine* by Perri Klass (September 29, 1996, 117–119) reports that Japanese researchers developed a technique called *extrauterine fetal incubation* (EUFI). They took goat fetuses, supplied them with oxygenated blood, and suspended them in incubators that contained artificial amniotic fluid (the fluid that surrounds a fetus in a pregnant woman's uterus) heated to body temperature. So far, the researchers have been able to keep goat fetuses alive for 3 weeks, but they are confident they can extend the length of time and ultimately be able to apply this technique to humans. When they do, we will have an artificial womb. This will allow us to have more control over conception and birth than ever before.

If it were ever possible, should an artificial womb be used for human pregnancies? Which circumstances would warrant the use of an artificial womb for human births? Consider the case in which a woman had fertile eggs but had had her uterus removed as a result of cancer. Should she be able to use EUFI to have a baby? What about the female executive who wants a family but worries that a pregnancy (and postpartum leave) will sideline her career? What about the couple who would otherwise use a human surrogate womb?

Consider further social consequences: Should insurance companies pay for the cost of using the artificial womb? Should the government allot Medicaid money for the socioeconomically deprived who wish to use such a service? Or should such a service be available only to the wealthy?

Exploring Personal Dimensions

Sexuality and Human Relations
A number of internal and external forces in your life influence the decisions you make regarding sexual behavior. What you do may be in harmony with some of these forces and in conflict with others.

Directions
Give a value to the following forces in your life as they pertain to your sexual behavior (i.e., what makes you choose to be sexually active or what makes you refrain from sexual activity). If you are married, apply this tool to a specific sexual behavior such as your degree of fidelity to your spouse or your degree of sexual activity with your spouse.

   a = a major force influencing my sexual behavior
   b = a moderate force influencing my sexual behavior
   c = an insignificant force influencing my sexual behavior

1. Religious influence   a   b   c
2. Family influence   a   b   c
3. How it feels when we kiss and hug   a   b   c
4. My own self-image (how I think I look to others)   a   b   c
5. My sense of right or wrong   a   b   c
6. Radio, television, Internet, or movies   a   b   c
7. How it feels to touch someone   a   b   c
8. How I learned to act   a   b   c
9. The way I feel inside   a   b   c
10. Literature (books, magazines) or music   a   b   c
11. Pleasure   a   b   c
12. My judgment   a   b   c
13. My sense of what I should and should not do   a   b   c
14. Friends' influence   a   b   c
15. Physical stimulation   a   b   c
16. Introversion or extroversion (how outgoing I am)   a   b   c
17. My morals or values   a   b   c
18. The expectations/relationship I have with boyfriend/girlfriend (for marrieds, consider friends other than spouse)   a   b   c
19. Fear of, or anticipation of, pregnancy   a   b   c
20. Desire to feel good about myself   a   b   c

Scoring
   a = 3   b = 2   c = 1

Total values as follows from top to bottom of the four columns.

Column A	Column B	Column C	Column D
1._____	2._____	3._____	4._____
5._____	6._____	7._____	8._____
9._____	10._____	11._____	12._____
13._____	14._____	15._____	16._____
17._____	18._____	19._____	20._____
Totals _____	_____	_____	_____

Interpretation
Column A represents the degree to which your morals and values or beliefs influence your sexual behavior and decisions.
Column B represents the degree to which social forces influence your sexual behavior.
Column C represents the degree to which biological factors influence your sexual behavior and decisions.
Column D represents the degree to which psychological forces influence your sexual behavior and decisions.

The relative influences can be compared directly with each other to see which area is the strongest or whether they are equal. You may interpret the results as follows:

11–15   major influence

6–10   moderate influence

1–5   insignificant influence

Suggested Readings

Alberta Society for the Promotion of Sexual Health. *Definitions of sexual health*, 2015. Available: http://www.aspsh.ca/definitions_of_sexual _health.

Bruess, C. E. Sexuality education, in *Battleground schools*, Mathison, S., & Ross, W. eds, Westport, CT: Greenwood/Praeger, 2008.

Bruess, C. E., & Schroeder, E. *Sexuality education: Theory and practice*, 6th edition. Boston, MA: Jones and Bartlett, 2014.

Defining sexual health. World Health Organization, 2015. Available: http://www.who.int /reproductivehealth/topics/sexual_health /sh_definitions/en/#.

Edwards, W. M., & Coleman, E. Defining sexual health: A descriptive overview. *Archives of Sexual Behavior, 33, no. 3* (June 2004), 189–195.

Report of the Task Force on the Sexualization of Girls. Washington, DC: American Psychological Association, 2007.

Rice, S. What does it mean to be healthy? *American Journal of Sexuality Education, 1, no. 2* (2006), 75–82.

Taverner, W. J. Sexual health in prime time. *American Journal of Sexuality Education, 1, no. 4* (2006), 71–82.

Web Resources

For links to the websites below, visit *go.jblearning .com/dimensions5e* and click on Resource Links.

Sexuality Information and Education Council of the United States
www.siecus.org

Source for the Consensus Statement on Adolescent Sexual Health and other information related to healthy sexuality.

Alberta Society for the Promotion of Sexual Health
www.aspsh.ca

Source for an excellent definition of sexuality.

Sex & Sexuality
www.plannedparenthood.org/health-topics /sexuality-4323.htm

Information from Planned Parenthood about how understanding our sexuality can help us enjoy our lives more.

Sexual Health Network
www.sexualhealth.com/aboutus.php

A network dedicated to providing easy access to sexuality information, education, support, and other resources.

Teens Health
http://kidshealth.org/teen/sexual_health

Designed to help both males and females learn the facts about sexual health.

References

The American freshman. *Research Brief*, Higher Education Research Institute, UCLA, January 2011.

The American freshman: National norms for fall 2007. *Chronicle of Higher Education, 54, 24* (February 1, 2008), A34.

The American freshman: National norms, fall 2013. Los Angeles: Higher Education Institute, UCLA, 2013.

Aries, P., & Bejin, A. *Western sexuality*. New York: Basil Blackwell, 1985.

ASPSH. *Definitions of sexual health*, 2015. Available: http://aspsh .ca/definitions_of_sexual_health.

Bardes, B. A., Shelley II, M. C., & Schmidt, S. W. *American government and politics today: The essentials.* Belmont, CA: West/Wadsworth, 1998.

Baron, R. A. *Psychology*, 4th ed. Needham Heights, MA: Allyn & Bacon, 1998.

Bell, R. R. *Premarital sex in a changing society.* Englewood Cliffs, NJ: Prentice-Hall, 1966.

Brennan, J. Reconciling immigrant values, in *Case studies in cultural diversity*, Ferguson, V. D., ed. Sudbury, MA: Jones and Bartlett, 1999, 185–189.

Bruess, C. E., & Richardson, G. *Decisions for health.* Dubuque, IA: Brown & Benchmark, 1995, 1.14–1.16.

Bruess, C. E., & Schroeder, E. *Sexuality education: Theory and practice*, 6th ed. Boston: Jones & Bartlett, 2014.

Bullough, V. L. *Sex, society & history.* New York: Science History Publications, 1976a.

Bullough, V. L. *Sexual variance in society and history*, New York: John Wiley & Sons, 1976b.

Centers for Disease Control and Prevention. *HIV among older Americans*. Atlanta, GA: Centers for Disease Control and Prevention, 2014. Available: http://www.cdc.gov/hiv/risk/age /olderamericans/index.html.

Characteristics of freshmen, 2001. *Chronicle of Higher Education, 68, no. 1* (August 31, 2001), 22–23.

Courtwright, D. T. The neglect of female children and childhood: Sex ratios in nineteenth century America: A review of the evidence. *Journal of Family History, 15* (1990), 313–323.

Degler, C. N. *At odds: Women and the family in America from the revolution to the present*. New York: Oxford University Press, 1980.

The ecology of birth control. Chicago: G. D. Searle, 1971.

FDA OKs hormonal implant. *Family Planning Perspectives, 20, no. 6* (November/December 1990), 1–4.

Fisher, H. E. *Anatomy of love*. New York: W. W. Norton, 1992.

Gendercide. *The Economist* (March 6, 2010), 13.

Grismaijer, S., & Singer, S.R. *Dressed to kill*. Pahoa, HI: ISCD Press, 2002.

Murstein, B. L. *Love, sex, and marriage*. New York: Springer, 1974.

The nation: Attitudes and characteristics of freshmen. *Chronicle of Higher Education, 49, no. 1* (August 30, 2002), 26.

Nelson, J. B. *Embodiment: An approach to sexuality and Christian theology*. Minneapolis: Augsburg, 1978.

O'Keefe, M. The times are trying politicians' souls. *The Oregonian* (April 20, 1995), A1.

Penhollow, T. M., Young, M., & Denny, G. Predictors of quality of life, sexual intercourse, and sexual satisfaction among active older adults. *American Journal of Health Education, 40, 1* (January/February 2009), 14–22.

Reiss, I. L. Changing trends, attitudes and values on premarital sexual behavior in the U.S., in *Human sexuality and the mentally retarded*, de la Cruz, F. F., & La Vock, G. D., eds. New York: Brunner/Mazel, 1973, 286–289.

Rooney, M. Freshmen show rising political awareness and changing social views. *The Chronicle of Higher Education, 49, no. 21* (January 31, 2003), A35–A38.

Roth, Z. Parents keep child's gender under wraps. Yahoo! News, May 26, 2011. Available: http://news.yahoo.com/blogs /lookout/parents-keep-child-gender-under-wraps-170824245 .html.

Sadock, B. J., Kaplan, H. I., & Freedman, A. M. *The sexual experience*. Baltimore: Williams & Wilkins, 1973.

Sheeran, P. *Women, society, the state and abortion: A structuralist analysis*. New York: Prager, 1987.

SIECUS position statements on human sexuality, 2014. Available: http://siecus.org/index.cfm.

Spielvogel, J. J. *Western civilization*, 3rd ed. St. Paul, MN: West, 1997.

Survey Tracks Changes in Political Views of Freshmen. *Chronicle of Higher Education, 58, no. 22* (February 3, 2012), A11.

Tannahill, R. *Sex in history*. New York: Stein & Day, 1980.

This year's freshmen at 4-year colleges: A statistical profile. *Chronicle of Higher Education, 51, no. 22* (February 4, 2005), A34.

This year's freshmen at 4-year colleges: A statistical profile. *Chronicle of Higher Education, 55, 21* (January 30, 2009), A19.

Tiefer, L. *Sex is not a natural act*. Boulder, CO: Westview Press, 1995.

Where do babies come from? *Family Life Educator* (Winter 1987), 5–7.

CHAPTER 2

Sexuality Research

FEATURES

Ethical Dimensions
Permission to
Do Research on
Sexual Behavior

Multicultural Dimensions
Differences in Sexual
Attitudes and
Behavior Among
Different Races

Global Dimensions
The Liu Report:
Sexual Behavior in
Modern China

Gender Dimensions
Differences in
Research Results

Communication Dimensions
Talking About
Sexuality Research
Results

CHAPTER OBJECTIVES

1 Describe the various methods used in sexuality research, including the steps in the scientific process.

2 Identify the ethical issues involved in sexuality research.

3 Describe the work of early sexuality researchers, including how they set the stage for modern research.

4 Summarize the contributions of major modern sexuality researchers.

INTRODUCTION

Y ou have probably heard the joke, "My mind is made up; don't confuse me with the facts." Unfortunately, when it comes to sexuality research, this attitude too often prevails. For example, a few years ago one of our students mentioned that one of his parents had asked him how his courses were going that term. When he mentioned he was learning about research on human sexuality, there were a few seconds of silence.

He explained that he had been raised in a home where sexuality was not discussed. He asked his parent about the silence, and the answer came back that it was a little difficult to think about research on such a topic. What did the researchers do? How did they do it? Why would they even want to do research on sexuality?

Our student explained that for a few minutes he felt he was the parent while he tried to answer these questions. Fortunately, he had already read information on this topic, so he thought he did a pretty good job.

This is not an isolated instance of lack of understanding, or even of repression, when it comes to sexuality research. For instance, in many places in this chapter you will find references to the National Health and Social Life Survey (NHSLS). In 1988, a team of researchers at the University of Chicago won a federal government grant competition to conduct an extensive research study on sexual behavior. In 1989, however, conservative members of Congress attacked its research for a number of reasons (Laumann, Michael, & Gagnon, 1994). They said it was a plot by homosexuals to legitimate the normality of gay and lesbian lifestyles; it was an unwarranted intrusion by the government in private matters; it was not needed; it should not be supported with taxpayers' money; and the project staff had an antifamily agenda.

During a federal governmental review, facts about the research were widely misrepresented. It was also claimed that the researchers had published statements that they had not, and statements were taken out of context in an attempt to show that the researchers should not be doing the research. As a result, the previously approved government grant was cancelled. The research was then completed with private funding. Since the study of human sexuality still prompts anxiety and even fear in some people, as well as a hesitancy to talk about the subject with other people, sexuality research can be difficult.

In this chapter we present some of the major 20th- and 21st-century research on sexuality to show you how knowledge about human sexuality is obtained and to discuss some of the findings that researchers believe can aid individuals in accepting and understanding the sexual parts of their personalities. We turn to the findings after identifying some of the methodology used in sexuality research.

Research Methods

Research is undertaken to expand our knowledge about specific factors in our environment. Our current knowledge of human sexuality is based on relatively few studies. Perhaps by reading about issues and techniques related to research in general, you will better understand and evaluate the studies we discuss, as well as ask yourself how valid the findings are.

The first task of any researcher, regardless of the subject, is to ask an explicit question. The next is to design a way of gathering the relevant information. In sexuality research the most common methods used are surveys, case studies, and experimental research. Less common is the method of direct observation, a method used more in sexual research clinics but also used extensively in the research of Masters and Johnson (discussed shortly). Each method of research has its advantages and disadvantages, some of which are discussed here.

A good researcher chooses a method according to the particular problem and population being studied. For example, a survey would be used when a large number of responses are desired, as in a study of adolescent behavior. Observation might be desirable when a small number of subjects are involved, as in measuring responses of people who are engaging in a sexual behavior while being electrically monitored.

The Scientific Method

Sexology is the study of sexuality. To study sexuality appropriately, it is necessary to use the **scientific method**—that is, research conducted in an atmosphere free from bias—because it is the most objective way to establish new knowledge in any field. Scientists must always approach research studies without preconceived ideas of what their studies will show. In addition, they cannot have preconceived agendas to show what sexual behavior *should* be. Researchers do not set out to "prove" something but instead conduct research scientifically to discover what *is*—not necessarily just what they want it to be. Researchers follow proper procedures and discover information through research that can then be generalized to the real world outside the study.

As we will explain, the scientific method involves the following steps:

1. *Identifying a research question* (which could be based on personal interest or experience, on social concerns, or on the interests of those funding the research, such as government agencies or private industry)

---

sexology The study of sexuality.

scientific method Research conducted in an atmosphere free from bias.

2. *Reviewing the literature*

3. *Formulating a hypothesis (or two or more hypotheses)*

4. *Operationalizing variables*

5. *Collecting data*

6. *Analyzing the data to test the hypotheses*

The scientific method first involves identifying a research question. Not all questions about sexuality lend themselves to scientific research, because many involve subjective values, morals, and philosophical questions. (However, scientific research can provide information that can help us address even these types of questions.)

Second, to inform themselves adequately, researchers must review literature related to the research question. Thus the researchers learn what is already known about the topic, think of ways to conduct the desired research, and possibly even come up with new research questions.

Third, a hypothesis is formulated. A **hypothesis** is a tentative proposal or an educated guess about the results of a research study. It often deals with the relationship between two variables. A **variable** is a measurable event that varies or is subject to change (such as frequency of sexual behavior, use of contraceptives, or amount of alcohol ingested).

Fourth, operationalizing the variables means specifying how they are going to be measured. For example, some variables, such as gender or income level, are easy to measure. Others, such as sexual desire or satisfaction in a relationship, are not. There are many ways to measure these variables, and the research has to state clearly how this will be done.

Fifth, collecting the data involves using methods such as survey research, case studies, experimental research, and direct observation. Each of these is explained in greater detail shortly.

Sixth, the data are analyzed to test the hypotheses. Data can be analyzed to describe situations, to show a relationship between variables, or to show that one situation causes another. Each of these methods of analysis demands the use of appropriate statistical methods.

Various forms of bias can be problematic. For example, in addition to possible bias of researchers, there could be bias of research subjects. If all subjects are college educated, they will probably be biased. Or, if some subjects are really not willing to participate or to be honest even if they agree to participate, they will also be biased. This type of bias is referred to as **volunteer bias**—characteristics of volunteers that are likely to influence research results.

One of the goals of the scientific method is to find information that can be generalized to the real

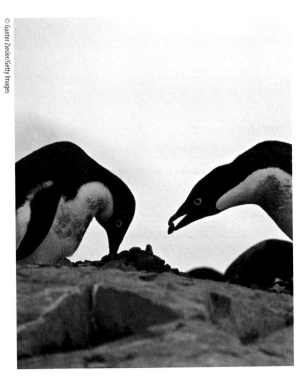

© Gunter Ziesler/Getty Images

Researchers on Antarctica's Ross Island have noted that female penguins, desperate for stones for their real nest, were willing to engage in "courtship" with an unpaired male penguin in exchange for stones. The penguin expert Eric Bennett decided to try an experiment at the Baltimore Zoo: He dressed up as a penguin and surrounded himself with lots of rocks. Within minutes, female penguins began presenting themselves for courtship. Does Bennett's experiment reflect the scientific method?

world outside the study. Obviously, when researchers are trying to learn more about human sexuality, they cannot get information from *all* human beings. Therefore, they must study a relatively small group of people from which the results may be generalized to a larger population. **Generalization**, the ability to conclude that the same results would be obtained outside the study, can occur only if all aspects of the scientific method are properly planned, carried out, and controlled as much as possible.

The **population** is the group being studied in a research project. Usually only a **sample** (a segment of the larger population) participates, because the total

---

hypothesis   A tentative proposal or an educated guess about the results of a research study.

variable   A measurable event that varies or is subject to change.

volunteer bias   Characteristics of volunteers that are likely to influence research results.

generalization   The ability to conclude that the same results would be obtained outside the study.

population   The group being studied in a research project.

sample   A segment of the larger population.

population would be too large and unwieldy. A **random sample** represents the larger population and is chosen in a way that eliminates bias. If the sample is selected properly, the researcher can generalize findings to the larger population.

Survey Research

Much information about human sexuality has been obtained by **surveys** asking people about sexual attitudes and experiences. This kind of data can be obtained orally (face-to-face interviews) or in written form (pencil-and-paper questionnaires). Researchers use surveys when information from a large number of people is desired. For example, they might use a survey to find out how people feel about condom advertisements on television.

The **interview** allows the interviewer to explain the purpose and value of the survey, to clarify and explain the questions, and to report answers clearly. However, some individuals may not report their sexual experiences and views honestly because they may be embarrassed to admit particular behaviors and thoughts to a stranger. Also, the subjects being interviewed may be equally embarrassed to admit they do not participate in certain sexual activities.

Questionnaires are less expensive than interviews, which require many people to conduct the interviews. A questionnaire that the subject can fill out at his or her convenience makes many people feel more relaxed and reinforces anonymity; the privacy may also ensure more honest answering. In addition, the questionnaire eliminates the subject's being influenced by the interviewer's facial or bodily gestures.

The major concern with any **self-report data** is that subjects may include inaccuracies. Accuracy is obviously necessary for reliable research. For instance, people often have difficulty recalling past events, and events can become highly embellished or minimized the longer the time between experience and reporting. Recall involves estimating **frequency** and/or **duration** of behaviors, and many people have problems remembering numbers.

Case Studies

Case studies are in-depth studies of individuals or small, select groups of individuals. Those under study are generally followed over a period of months or years. Case studies provide a chance to look at specific behaviors or characteristics in great depth. Also, because case studies generally cover a relatively long period, the researcher is able to explore cause-and-effect relationships in detail. For example, much information about sex offenders and people with sexual-response difficulties has been obtained through case studies.

With case studies, however, there is no way to use proper sampling techniques, making it difficult to generalize case-study results to the rest of the population. For instance, how do we know that sex offenders or those receiving treatment for sexual-response problems are like the rest of the population?

Experimental Research

In an **experiment**, behavior can be studied under controlled conditions. A common experimental design is one in which two groups are matched and compared. The groups are identical but for one important difference—the **experimental group** is subjected to a particular event or condition, whereas the **control group** is not. Both groups are observed, and the results are compared to determine whether the experimental condition had an effect. For example, a researcher could compare the responses of different groups of people (perhaps grouped by gender or age) to erotic materials.

Experimental research allows control over variables thought to influence responses or behavior. At the same time, the somewhat artificial setting may influence behavior or response. Merely knowing you are in a study or being in a laboratory might alter your reaction.

Direct Observation

Observation is a method in which subjects are watched in a laboratory, a class, a natural setting, or the workplace. It can be an accurate way to collect

---

random sample A sample that represents the larger population and that is chosen without bias, so that every member of the larger population has an equal chance to be selected.

survey Research in which people complete questionnaires or are personally interviewed.

interview Oral research method designed to gather information.

questionnaire Written instrument designed to gather information.

self-report data The respondents' descriptions of something.

frequency How often something occurs or has occurred.

duration How long something occurs or has occurred.

case study In-depth study of individual(s) or small groups.

experiment Observation of behavior (or effects) under controlled conditions.

experimental group In an experiment, the group subjected to a particular event or condition.

control group In an experiment, the group not subjected to a particular event or condition.

observation Watching subjects in a particular setting.

Ethical DIMENSIONS

Permission to Do Research on Sexual Behavior

A faculty member at a small university was told by the president of the university that he could not conduct research in the form of a survey of sexual behavior of undergraduate students at the university. The president said the project was not appropriate at their institution.

The president was concerned that the survey's explicit questions might offend students and their parents. Even though a 13-member campus review board unanimously approved the survey, top university administrators said that the survey was also subject to their approval. This procedural step had never before been invoked. One of the vice presidents said that such a survey could have negative impacts on admissions and parents' attitudes about the school.

Taking the opposite position, the researchers said that better safe-sex programs were needed for their undergraduates, and that a well-done survey would be a good place to start. The faculty and students working together on the project hoped to publish the results in a scholarly journal. They said that preventing them from conducting the survey denied them academic freedom. They were upset that the result was an apparently arbitrary decision of senior administrators.

What do you think? Was it ethical for the researchers to conduct the survey? Was it ethical for the president to tell them they could not conduct the survey? Should the senior administrators have allowed the survey to be conducted even if they did not like the idea of the survey being done on their campus?

sexual information—particularly if the researcher controls the setting. A prime example of observational research has been the human sexual-response research of Masters and Johnson.

The major drawback of direct observation is the required expenditure of time and money. In addition, people are likely to be reluctant to perform sexual activity in a laboratory where they are being observed. Some people also question the ethics of participating in observational research either as the researcher or as the subject. When people do feel relatively comfortable and volunteer for observational research related to sexuality, one must always ask whether their sexual responses in such a setting replicate those obtained in the privacy of their normal environment. Another important question is whether people who are comfortable doing this are similar to the majority of people who aren't: Put another way, can the findings be generalized?

Focus Groups

A **focus group** is a form of research where a group of approximately 6 to 10 people are asked about their feelings or attitudes toward a topic and then discuss related issues. For example, the participants might be asked what they think about equal rights for people with various sexual orientations. The leader usually has a focus-group script that guides the discussion (it includes questions, follow-up questions,

and other instructions). A typical focus-group session might last for 1–2 hours. It is important to have extensive interchange among the participants to get as many thoughts and ideas as possible from the group. Focus-group members sometimes talk among themselves in reaction to a topic or question from the focus-group leader—with the leader listening and taking notes for analysis later.

There are arguments both for and against focus groups. Some experts believe they are valuable ways to get important information from a group of people in a relatively inexpensive way. Other experts think they can be very time-consuming, the group cannot possibly be large enough to be a representative sample of the population, and the group can be unduly influenced by the researcher. Traditionally, most focus groups meet in person, but today there are also teleconference focus groups and online focus groups.

Interpreting Statistics

In many kinds of sexuality research, statistics related to the results will be presented. When we hear about statistical results, we have to differentiate between

focus group A form of research where a group of 6 to 10 people are asked about a topic and then discuss related issues.

correlation and causation. **Correlation** is a statistical measure that shows how variables are naturally related in the real world. For example, studies might show that youth who watch more television also participate in more sexual behavior. That is interesting information, but it tells us nothing about *why* that relationship exists; it only tells us that the relationship *does* exist.

How do we know if the results of a study are accurate? Perhaps the findings just happened to occur in this study, but wouldn't occur in other similar studies. We can use statistics to help us determine how likely it is that the results will also occur in other studies. A number of statistical methods can be used to determine statistical significance. **Statistical significance** refers to the likelihood that a study's results are due to chance. If the results are significant at the .05 level, for example, there is only a 5% chance those results are due to chance. If it has been reported that people who don't use condoms develop HIV to a greater extent than those who do use condoms, and that finding is significant at the .05 level, we can be confident that the difference is attributable to not using condoms rather than to chance. In other words, not using condoms "caused" more people to develop HIV as compared to the rate found among people who did use condoms.

How can you use this information to contribute to your sexual health? When you are deciding whether to engage in a sexual behavior, you can read studies to see if there are statistically significant differences between those who engage in that behavior and those who do not. This will give you confidence that these differences are a result of that behavior, and that you can expect similar results if you decide to engage in that sexual behavior.

Issues in Sexuality Research

Despite the care and planning that go into implementing a research project, the success of a project depends on the cooperation of the subjects. The most difficult task in studying humans is finding a large group who will stay with the project to completion. When mail questionnaires are used, for example, the response rate is generally less than 40% of the total number distributed—and often close to 20%.

Interviews are expensive, but the response rate can be high, depending on the interviewer's expertise and awareness. The interviewer must establish rapport with the subjects so that they are not embarrassed, intimidated, or totally unresponsive.

When asked to be surveyed about sexual behavior, many people will refuse, but others will participate. Therefore, those who do participate may be more or less sexually experienced and liberated than those who choose not to take part. This volunteer bias may allow us to draw conclusions from the study results about how some people view sexual matters, but it does not allow us to conclude that people in general behave or believe that way. When people answer surveys or consent to be interviewed, there are always problems of reporting accuracy, ability to recall past experiences as they really occurred, and willingness to be truthful, particularly about sexual matters, when facing an interviewer. Consider, for example, that reporting and evaluating how we feel now are easier than reporting how we felt sometime in the past. In recalling how and where we learned about sexuality or what sexual activities we were involved in as children, we are easily influenced by events that took place in intervening years, by changes in behavior socially defined as normal (or at least permissible), and by our own maturity. Even if subjects want and intend to give honest responses, they may feel reluctant to share the intimate details of their activities with a stranger, worry about the researcher's attitude toward their sexual behavior—particularly in an interview—or be afraid that their responses are not genuinely confidential.

Research on sexuality faces some additional problems. Many conditions affect our sexuality, including broad cultural and social definitions of sexuality roles and proper sexual behavior, as well as characteristics such as ethnic origin, religion, personal experience, and education. Such conditions and their effects may be too complex to measure or control. Also, cooperative subjects may be hard to find, because in our culture people feel anxiety, self-consciousness, and a reluctance to share private thoughts, experiences, and memories about sexuality. For example, many people would not want to talk about their experiences with forcible sexual behavior. Even talking about whether one masturbates and, if so, how frequently, is not something most people are eager to do.

There can also be some limitations in sexuality research. For example, nonresponse (refusal to participate) can make it difficult to get responses from the desired subjects. Also, self-selection volunteer bias may be a problem. Volunteers for sexuality research may be more sexually experienced and hold more positive attitudes toward sexuality than nonvolunteers. Finally, there may be a demographic bias. As seen in Kinsey's work and even today, it is often easier to get

correlation A statistical measure that shows how variables are naturally related to each other.

statistical significance The likelihood that a study's results are due to the relationship uncovered between the study's variables as opposed to chance.

Multicultural DIMENSIONS

Differences in Sexual Attitudes and Behavior Among Different Races

You will sometimes see research findings indicating differences in sexual behaviors and attitudes among people of different races. Care is needed when interpreting such findings, because it is often hard to differentiate between what may be a result of racial culture, what may be a result of socioeconomic differences, and what may be random or coincidental. A good example of this is provided by statistics about births to unmarried women.

According to *National Vital Statistics Reports* (Martin et al., 2013), the birth rate for unmarried women in the United States was 45.3 births per 1,000 unmarried women (down from a historical peak of 51.8 per 1,000 in 2008).

Approximately 40.7% of all births occurred to unmarried women.

The proportions of nonmarital births varied widely by race and Hispanic origin. The percent of nonmarital births for non-Hispanic black (72%) and American Indian or Alaska native (67%) mothers was more than three times that of Asian or Pacific Islander (17%) mothers, and more than twice that of non-Hispanic white mothers (29%). A little more than half (54%) of births to Hispanic mothers were to unmarried women. These proportions were essentially unchanged since 2011.

Source: Martin, J. A., Hamilton, B. E., Osterman, M. J. K., Curtin, M. A., & Mathews, T. J. Births: Final data for 2012. *National Vital Statistics Reports 62, 9* (December 30, 2013), 1–87.

---

subjects for sexuality research who are white, middle-class, white-collar workers and college students.

Adding to the difficulty of gathering accurate information is the influence of the researcher's own values and biases. The researcher may have very strong opinions about issues in the study and may—perhaps unintentionally—phrase questions in favor of his or her views, emphasize certain words in a face-to-face interview, and/or have certain racial, ethnic, or cultural views that affect rapport with the subjects in the study. Interviewers and writers of questionnaires may have perceptions about the group they are surveying, which can also influence how questions are asked or phrased. When the information is collected and interpreted, the researcher must consciously prevent personal feelings and attitudes from affecting analysis and reporting. For example, a researcher who might be either strongly for or strongly against abortion would need to be very careful when asking questions about abortion and recording the answers of a research subject. It would be wise to have several researchers with different views work together to check questionnaires and procedures to be sure there is as much **objectivity** as possible—that is, be sure the results are the same no matter who asks the questions or records the answers.

Ethical Issues in Sexuality Research

Recently there has been increased attention to the need to protect the people participating in any form of human research. Because of the intimate nature of sexual research, the ethical issues involved in this field are particularly important.

An ethical issue of particular concern is obtaining the **informed consent** of participants; subjects of research studies must agree in writing to participate *after* the purposes, risks, and benefits of the study have been explained to them. Consent is obtained to ensure that subjects both understand what the project entails and agree to undergo the experience as described. This requirement protects subjects against physical and psychological abuse by irresponsible researchers and protects researchers against claims that subjects were taken advantage of. Investigators are now required by law to obtain an individual's consent to be subjected to the project as described; those testing minors must also obtain parental or guardian permission.

Researchers do not have the right to coerce people to participate in a study, and they must be honest when presenting information about the research. They also have a responsibility to protect the confidentiality of their participants. They must be sure that personal facts can never be connected to a given

objectivity Being sure the results are the same no matter who asks the questions or records the answers.

informed consent Document required to participate in a research study after the purposes, risks, and benefits of the study have been explained.

Courtesy of Behavioral Technology, Inc., Salt Lake City, Utah

The vaginal plethysmograph is used to measure sexual response by detecting changes in the amount of blood in the vaginal walls. The device is used in sexuality research.

Courtesy of Behavioral Technology, Inc., Salt Lake City, Utah

The penile strain gauge is used to measure erectile response by detecting changes in the circumference of the penis. The device is used in sexuality research.

individual. It is obvious that participants must also be protected from physical and psychological harm. Many methods must be used to guarantee the anonymity of participants and to be sure confidential information is never released.

Human-research review committees commonly exist in government agencies and in universities. These committees must review and approve any research designs and procedures that will use human subjects. Such committees consider the value of the research and compare it to any potential risks to the participants. It can be difficult for committees to decide whether to allow a researcher to carry out a particular study—especially if children are involved. This is one reason why we do not have better information about the sexual thoughts and experiences of young people.

Additional ethical questions arise in studies of the sexual behaviors and attitudes of various racial groups. Some people argue that such research is important to better understanding of diverse feelings and practices. In contrast, others believe that describing sexual behaviors and attitudes according to racial groups contributes to stereotypical thinking.

Another interesting ethical issue arises from the ways that have been developed to measure physiological changes in the vagina or the penis due to sexual stimulation. **Vaginal plethysmography** involves inserting a probe into a woman's vagina to measure increased blood volume, an indication of sexual arousal. Changes in blood volume over time can be charted with this device. Similarly, a **penile strain gauge** can be used. This is a wire or cuff placed around the penis that is attached to a **plethysmograph**, a laboratory measuring device that charts physiological changes over time and records changes in the girth of the penis as it responds to sexual arousal or loss of arousal.

Plethysmography has been used to see whether a person has certain sorts of sexual interests, such as a sexual interest in children. For example, if it were suspected that a person were sexually attracted to children, the device might provide additional information that could lead to a referral for possible treatment. Following treatment, the device could be used again to see whether the degree of sexual interest in children has decreased. However, because people can sometimes learn to control their physiological responses, this is not a foolproof test. Also, it would be a mistake to base too many assumptions about a person's future sexual behaviors on one measure of physiological response. Use of penile and vaginal plethysmography is likely to be debated for years to come.

Finally, it is crucial to be sure a test has **validity**—that is, that it tests what it is supposed to test. For example, a sexual-knowledge test must be a good representation of overall sexual knowledge. This might be shown by a comparison to a known good test or by expert ratings.

Most research on sexual feelings, attitudes, responses, and behavior depends on participants' reporting about themselves. Some people believe that sexuality research is useless and meaningless because subjects can lie about their sexual behavior, exaggerate their experiences, or feel too embarrassed to discuss personal sexual matters openly and honestly. Others believe that we need information about sexual matters and must encourage research, even while acknowledging its limitations. Although it is difficult to validate information that people include on a questionnaire or divulge in an interview, validation is frequently done by asking for the same information in another part of the survey or in conversation and cross-checking whether the information given is the same in both instances.

Given the variety of attitudes toward sexuality in our society, the many different opinions concerning

vaginal plethysmography   Insertion of a probe into the vagina to measure changes in blood volume.

penile strain gauge   A wire or cuff placed around the penis to measure physiological changes over time.

plethysmograph   A laboratory measuring device that charts physiological changes over time.

validity, validation   Demonstration that tests measure what they are designed to measure.

moral and ethical issues related to sexuality, and even the disagreement as to whether sexuality should be researched at all, researchers have a difficult job. They must design a scientifically sound study, create confidence in that study, and guarantee their subjects' privacy.

Evaluating Sexuality Information on the Internet

Anyone who uses a search engine to look for information about "sex" or "sexuality" finds so many hits that it is not humanly possible to review all of the sites mentioned. In addition, although accurate and reliable information about sexuality can be found on the Internet, so can a preponderance of information about sexuality that is incorrect or misleading. How can you determine whether information about sexuality found on the Internet is accurate? Here are some suggestions (National Center for Complementary and Alternative Medicine, 2011);

1. *Who runs the site?* Any good website related to sexuality should make it easy for you to learn who is responsible for the site and its information.

2. *Who pays for the site?* The source of a site's funding should be readily apparent. The funding source can affect what content is presented, how the content is presented, and what the site owners want to accomplish on the site.

3. *What is the purpose of the site?* An "About This Site" link appears on many sites; if it's there, use it. The purpose of the site should be clearly stated and help you evaluate the trustworthiness of the information.

4. *Where does the information come from?* If the person or organization in charge of the site did not create the information, the original source should be clearly labeled. This identification allows others to easily find original sources of information.

5. *What is the basis of the information?* The site should describe the evidence on which the material is based. Facts and figures from valid research should have references. Also, opinions or advice should be clearly set apart from information that is based on research results.

6. *How is the information selected?* Is there an editorial board? Do people with excellent professional and scientific qualifications review the material before it is posted?

7. *How current is the information?* Websites should be reviewed and updated on a regular basis, and the most recent update or review date should be clearly posted. Even if the information is still accurate, you want to know whether the site owners have reviewed it recently to ensure that it is still valid.

8. *How does the site choose links to other sites?* What is the policy of the website owner about how links to other sites are established? What are the criteria for the sites that are linked to the website?

9. *What information about you does the site collect, and why?* Any credible website should tell you exactly what it will and will not do with personal data gathered about you. Many commercial sites sell data about their users to other companies. Don't sign up for anything you don't fully understand.

10. *How does the site manage interactions with visitors?* There should be a way for you to contact the site owners with problems, feedback, and questions. Information about the terms for using any site services should be readily available as well.

■ Early Sexuality Researchers

We have some information about sexual practices throughout human history. Although not all of the information was gathered in a systematic way, in Western civilization attempts to study human sexual behavior systematically date back at least to the ancient Greeks. Physicians, such as Hippocrates, and philosophers, such as Plato and Aristotle, are the forefathers of sexuality research. They made extensive observations and offered the first elaborate theories regarding sexual responses and dysfunctions, reproduction and contraception, abortion, legislation related to sexuality, and sexual ethics (The Kinsey Institute, 1998).

In Rome, Greek physicians such as Soranus and Galen further advanced sexual knowledge. Their work prompted later Islamic scholars to spend much time on sexual questions. These studies, together with the Greek and Roman manuscripts, became standard texts at medical schools and stimulated a rebirth of anatomical research in the 16th, 17th, and 18th centuries. In the 19th century, new concerns about overpopulation and sexual psychology intensified efforts to study the topic of sexuality. Finally, at the turn of the 20th century, the investigation of sexuality became a legitimate endeavor in its own right (The Kinsey Institute, 1998).

Richard von Krafft-Ebing

Richard von Krafft-Ebing (1840–1902) wrote during a period when Victorian standards strongly suppressed thinking about human sexuality. Because he was a product of this period, and because he was a physician who worked primarily with sexually disturbed people, von Krafft-Ebing's writings (1902) indicated that sexual activity is something to fear.

He supported what we now know as the double standard, whereby men have sexual freedoms that women do not. He may have supported this perspective because of his apparent discomfort with the sexuality of women.

Von Krafft-Ebing's writings had a tremendous influence on many physicians as well as the public. Even though he seemed to be biased and made some false assumptions, his writings convinced some physicians and researchers that the study of sexuality was legitimate. This helped prepare the way for Ellis and Freud.

Henry Havelock Ellis

Henry Havelock Ellis (1859–1939), an English psychologist and physician who studied human sexuality, grew up in fear of what he had been told about the danger of nocturnal emissions. He was also concerned about his general ignorance of human sexuality. Between 1896 and 1910 Ellis published a six-volume series entitled *Studies in the Psychology of Sex*, which included the following beliefs:

1. Masturbation is common for both sexes.

2. Orgasm in males and females is very much the same.

3. Homosexuality and heterosexuality are a matter of degree.

4. Women do have sexual desire, contrary to Victorian thought.

5. There is no one norm for human sexuality. Thoughts and acts vary among individuals and cultures.

6. There should be sexuality education for both sexes starting at early ages.

7. There should not be laws against contraception or private sexual behavior.

It is clear that Ellis's ideas were controversial and ahead of their time, particularly his support of sexuality

education. In fact, some people today still have difficulty accepting his beliefs. Ellis's work influenced the later pursuits of many sexuality researchers and writers.

Sigmund Freud

Sigmund Freud (1856–1939), a psychological researcher, developed theories about human development, personality, and psychopathology that have influenced our thinking today. To develop into a well-adjusted person, according to Freud, one had to progress successfully through a number of psychosexual stages.

Freud viewed sexuality and sexual pleasure as a central part of human life and felt that people naturally sought to have as much pleasure and as little pain as possible. He indicated that sexual activity was natural and that procreation was secondary to pleasure, and he cautioned against severe restrictions on sexual instincts. People, he maintained, could become neurotic if denied natural expression of their sexual instincts.

One of Freud's important contributions was his suggestion that early childhood experiences had strong consequences for adult functioning. Largely because of Freud's work, sexual thoughts and behaviors are still considered to be major influences on contemporary life in general.

© Everett Collection/age fotostock

Freud's theories have influenced thinking about sexuality for more than 100 years.

Magnus Hirschfeld

Magnus Hirschfeld (1868–1935) was a German physician who started his career in medicine and was soon drawn to the study of human sexuality. He was a transvestite (he coined the word "transvestism") in addition to being a homosexual. He believed that sexual orientation was a naturally occurring trait worthy of scientific study rather than social hostility. He urged homosexuals from all walks of life to come out and get involved in a growing campaign for emancipation. He promoted the idea that sexual honesty was necessary for healthy living.

Hirschfeld produced many books and papers concerning sexuality and succeeded in bringing the discussion of homosexuality into the halls of government as well as the homes of everyday people. As German fascists gained power in the 1920s, however, he was physically attacked at least twice and there were political attempts to suppress his work. By 1930 he was forced into exile and made his home in France.

Katherine Davis

Katherine Davis (1860–1935) was born in Buffalo, New York, and educated in the United States. She taught high school science for 10 years, then went on to earn a Ph.D. degree in economics in 1900. In 1901 she began working in the field of corrections, and in 1914 became the commissioner of corrections for New York City.

She quickly moved to improve conditions in the penal institutions, then became interested in topics related to the well-being of women. From 1918 to 1928 she was general secretary of the New York Bureau of Social Hygiene board of directors, where she directed research on many topics related to public health. In 1929 she published *Factors in the Sex Life of Twenty-Two Hundred Women*. In addition, she was the author of many articles in professional and popular journals (Women in American history, 2005).

Her survey of married Caucasian women of above-average intelligence, education, and social position revealed some interesting results (History of sex surveys: Factors in the sex life of 2200 women, 2005). For example, contraception (then called "voluntary parenthood") was approved in principle by almost 90% of the respondents and practiced by 73%. Of those who claimed to have "happy" marriages, only one out of four worked outside the home. Based on this fact, the researchers concluded that working was not conducive to marital happiness.

Ninety percent of the married women considered their husband's sex drives to be as strong as or stronger than their own. A little over 3% believed their sex drives were stronger. Masturbation was admitted to by 65% of the unmarried women and 40% of the married women, but 2 out of 3 of these women considered the habit "morally degrading." Slightly more than 50% of the single women said they had experienced "intense emotional reactions" with other women, and over 25% admitted that the relationship involved overt homosexual expression.

Dr. Davis's research included some opinion questions. She found that 39% of the women thought sexual intercourse was necessary for complete physical and mental health, 19% thought a young woman was justified in having intercourse before marriage, 21% thought a young man was justified in having intercourse before marriage, 85% thought married people were justified in having intercourse for reasons other than having children, 63% thought information regarding birth control methods should be available for unmarried people, and 72% felt that it was acceptable for an abortion to be performed.

Clelia Mosher

Clelia Mosher (1863–1940) was born in Albany, New York. She was educated at Stanford University, where in her master's thesis she debunked a widespread myth of that time: the belief that women breathed differently than men, and were therefore unfit for exercise. Mosher found that this difference was caused by women being laced into tight-fitting corsets, and that there was no reason that they could not otherwise participate in strenuous exercise.

Mosher completed medical school at Johns Hopkins in 1899. In 1923 she wrote a book entitled *Women's Physical Freedom*. She explained her views on women's health, menstruation, and breast care. She promoted a positive view of women's potential and argued against many Victorian attitudes.

Over a period of 30 years, she surveyed Victorian women, most of whom were born about the time of the Civil War, about their sexual lives. This was probably the first known survey of sexual attitudes and behaviors. She gave her nine-page survey to a total of 47 women. Therefore, the sample size was small and the women were not representative of Victorian women in general. Most were faculty wives at universities and also well educated for that era. Even though it was a biased sample, it is noteworthy because it is the only known survey of Victorian women. This was a period when women were not supposed to be sexual. Interestingly, her findings were not published until 1980. Here are some of them:

- Although Victorian women were not supposed to feel sexual desire, 35 of the 47 women indicated that they liked sexual intercourse.

- Thirty-four of the women had experienced orgasms.

- Many of the women indicated that it could be a problem because it took them longer to reach orgasm than their male partner. They said there was a need for men to know about this.

- More than two-thirds of the women used some kind of birth control. Douching was the most common, followed by withdrawal and "timing." Obviously, we do not consider these methods very reliable today. Some husbands used a "male sheath" (a condom), and two women used a "rubber cap over the uterus" (either a diaphragm or a cervical cap). One woman said she used "cocoa butter," but she did not explain why or how.

- Three of the women said that their ideal would be to never have sexual intercourse at all. But most of the women expressed their sexual desires and experienced orgasms. Most seemed to enjoy sexual relations with their husbands.

It is impressive that Mosher was able to accomplish her research at the height of the Victorian era. It seems that she was a talented woman who tried hard to improve the status of women at the same time she was doing groundbreaking research.

20th-Century Sexuality Researchers

The 19th-century model of sexuality and sexual behavior was a medical one. Individuals who differed from the accepted norms were considered ill or, in scientific terms, deviant or pathological; however, little was known about sexual attitudes, behaviors, and activities. There was a dearth of knowledge about human sexuality from the psychological, psychosocial, and physiological perspectives. Research into sexual attitudes and behaviors lacked respectability, and many institutions would not fund or support it. In the 1930s changes in public attitudes in the United States, desire for contraception (both for child spacing and for population control), and a more open interest in the scope of sexual behavior led to greater acceptance of human sexuality as a legitimate field for research.

What follows is an overview of the more prominent research in human sexual behavior during the 20th century. Although some of this work was done in the late 1930s, you will find that many of the issues are not very different from those you are concerned with and possibly are experiencing now.

Alfred Kinsey and his colleagues were at the forefront of using scientific methodology to study human sexuality. His research, begun in 1938, was revolutionary in that it covered a wide range of sexual activities and applied statistical methods to sexuality research.

Our overview covers two categories—scientific literature and popular literature. In most instances it is obvious which category applies, but admittedly in a few cases the point is arguable. We hope that a review of these studies will not only add to your sum of information but also help you to expand and develop your sexuality and interpersonal relationships.

Scientific Literature

Alfred C. Kinsey: Establishing Scientific Sex Research

Alfred Kinsey, a biologist and zoologist, joined the faculty of Indiana University in 1920. He gained academic recognition early in his career through his writings in biology. In 1937 Kinsey became the teacher of a newly introduced course in marriage and sexuality education. As his interest in the subject grew, he began to amass information concerning sexual activities and beliefs about sexuality. Kinsey eventually gathered the largest amount of information on human sexuality ever collected.

The interviews conducted by Kinsey and his colleagues covered six ways in which males and females achieve orgasm in our culture: masturbation, nocturnal sex dreams and emissions, heterosexual petting, heterosexual premarital intercourse, homosexual intercourse, and sexual contact with animals. Using highly specific interviews, Kinsey and his associates collected data from only white males and females. The sample contained a disproportionately high number of better-educated people living in cities. All subjects were volunteers. Kinsey's studies may be the best-known example of survey research related to sexuality, but his sample cannot be viewed as representative of the U.S. population. *Sexual Behavior in the Human Male* (1948) is based on interviews with 5,300 males; *Sexual Behavior in the Human Female* (1953) on interviews with 5,900 females.

Americans had little knowledge about sexual behavior in this culture until Kinsey presented his findings. His conclusions generated a great deal of public reaction. In males, the lower the educational level, the higher the premarital activity. For women, the findings were the opposite—the higher the educational level, the more likely the premarital activity. Most of the married females reported orgasm response through coital and noncoital sexual behavior. Only about 2% of women reported a complete lack of sexual arousal. A great many of Kinsey's subjects reported childhood sexual experiences, which reinforced Freud's belief that sexual expression is experienced in childhood. Kinsey concluded from all the data that people are sexual from early childhood through adulthood. Despite its limitations, Kinsey's work was hailed as the first large-scale study of sexual behavior. Some of Kinsey's major findings are described in the following paragraphs.

Masturbation   Close to 92% of males in Kinsey's sample stated that they had masturbated at some point in their lives, with the highest incidence reported between 16 and 20 years of age; about 62% of all females reported that they had masturbated. The higher the educational level, the greater the incidence of masturbation in both men and women. In both males and females, the stronger the religious adherence, the lower the incidence of masturbation.

Nocturnal Dreams About Sex   Dreams about sex were experienced by both sexes. From the data Kinsey concluded that 70% of females had dreams about sex. The highest incidence of nocturnal emissions was reported by 71% of single males aged 21 to 25 years.

Premarital Intercourse   With regard to heterosexual premarital intercourse, Kinsey found that 22% of all adolescent males had experienced intercourse. Among college males 67% had experienced premarital intercourse. Males of lower social class reported greater frequency of premarital intercourse than those of higher social class. Nearly 50% of the females reported premarital intercourse. At all social levels, males and females who were devoutly religious reported much less premarital intercourse than nondevout subjects.

Homosexual Activity   Kinsey found homosexual incidence highest in high school males. About 37% of all males had some homosexual experience between adolescence and old age. Twenty-five percent of females aged 30 years and over had been erotically aroused by other females, and 17% had experienced sexual contact with other females.

The Kinsey Institute is still operating. It is called the Kinsey Institute for Research in Sex, Gender, and Reproduction and is located at Indiana University. In 2004 Kinsey's life was the subject of a popular movie.

William Masters and Virginia Johnson: The Physiology of Sexual Response

The research efforts and studies of Masters and Johnson are probably the most widely known and cited of all sex-related data. These researchers were the first to observe people's sexual behaviors in a laboratory setting and to identify physiological changes during sexual arousal. William Masters was a gynecologist and Virginia Johnson a psychologist. Together they were the directors of what was the Reproductive Biology Research Foundation in St. Louis and is now the Masters and Johnson Institute. In 1966 they published their data in *Human Sexual Response,* and in 1970 they published *Human Sexual Inadequacy.*

Once the two started their research, they informed university contacts and professionals that they were in search of volunteer study subjects. Of the 1,273 volunteers who initially applied, Masters and Johnson selected 694—276 married couples, 106 unmarried women, and 36 unmarried men. Ninety-eight of the single people had been married previously.

The investigators obtained social and sexual histories for all their subjects, gave them information to explain the studies, and introduced them to the laboratory setting. For experiments involving sexual intercourse, married couples were used as subjects; in studies other than intercourse (such as masturbation and controlled vaginal tests with an artificial phallus), unmarried subjects participated.

Through direct observation, filming, and monitoring with instruments, Masters and Johnson recorded a variety of changes in the physiology of the body in general and in the genitals and reproductive organs in particular. Their major finding was the existence of a cycle of physiological events in response to sexual

Global
DIMENSIONS

The Liu Report: Sexual Behavior in Modern China

Dalin Liu and associates (1997) interviewed 23,000 Chinese people over a period of 18 months. The nationwide survey about sexual attitudes and behavior, a Chinese "Kinsey Report," was the first conducted in China. Liu reported the following:

1. For high school students, the mean age of first ejaculation was 14.4 years.
2. College students were highest in their masturbation rates (59% for males and 17% for females) as compared to high school students (13% for males and 5% for females), city married subjects (33% for males and 12% for females), and village married subjects (9% for males and 11% for females).
3. Thirteen percent of the college student males and 6% of the college student females had experienced premarital sexual activity. This compared with 22% of the city married men and 16% of the city married women, and 35% of the village married men and 15% of the village married women.
4. Among all groups, college students had the highest proportion of those who had homosexual behavior (8%) as compared to less than 1% of city married

subjects and just over 2% of village married subjects.

5. Sexual satisfaction was reported by 55% of married males and 67% of married females.
6. Ninety-five percent of the college students and 67% of the married subjects felt positively about the female's initiating sexual activity. Four percent of the college students and 11% of the married subjects felt negatively about this idea.
7. Fifty-six percent of college students, as compared to 10% of married subjects, approved of extramarital sexual activity. Thirty-nine percent of the college students and 79% of the married subjects felt very negative about extramarital sexual activity.
8. Most Chinese couples engage in little or no foreplay before initiating intercourse. Many wives report some discomfort during intercourse as a result of insufficient vaginal lubrication.
9. Women are more likely than men to initiate divorce proceedings (three of five divorces are requested by women).

Source: Data from Liu, D., Man Lun Ng, Li Ping Zhou, & Haeberle, E. J. *Sexual behavior in modern China.* New York: Continuum, 1997.

---

stimulation. The whole cycle, known as the *human sexual response,* occurs in both sexes in four phases, always in order: excitement, plateau, orgasm, and resolution. This research showed that males and females have many similar responses, as well as responses specific to the physiology of each sex. The research of Masters and Johnson now serves as the basis for modern therapy, education, and counseling; cross-disciplinary research; and general information about sexual functioning.

As well developed as it is, Masters and Johnson's research is not without criticism. Some professionals believe that their model of human sexual response ignores psychological and cognitive aspects of arousal. However, it could also be argued that their original model was intended to only demonstrate what happens biologically and that other factors could be considered later. It is interesting, however, that their second study was expanded to consider a broader range of factors related to human sexual response.

The second major Masters and Johnson study, *Human Sexual Inadequacy,* was published in 1970. This study of sexual dysfunction put the relationship

of the physiology and the psychology of sexual response in sharper focus. Causes of sexual dysfunction, the relationship of the partners who experienced dysfunction, and sexual interaction in general were the concerns of this book. Masters and Johnson defined *sexual dysfunction* as an inability to respond emotionally and physically to sexual arousal. The physiological, psychological, and emotional (or situational) causes were suggested and defined, with treatment developed to deal with the causes and symptoms presented.

In 1979 Masters and Johnson published *Homosexuality in Perspective.* This study of the sexual response of gays and lesbians added much information to the human sexuality literature. The data were gathered by studying the sexual response cycles of 38 lesbian couples and 42 gay couples between 1957 and 1970. The researchers reported that there was little difference between gays and lesbians and heterosexuals in sexual functioning and response to sexual stimulation. However, gays and lesbians appeared to communicate with partners more effectively during sexual activity than did heterosexuals.

William Masters and Virginia Johnson were the first sexuality researchers to observe people's sexual behaviors in a laboratory setting. Among their many contributions to sexuality research is the human sexual response cycle.

Masters and Johnson and You The work of Masters and Johnson affects your sexual life in many ways. Both you and your partner can now better understand your bodies' responses to sexual stimulation. Knowing that you proceed through several identifiable phases during your sexual response cycle will make you and/ or any sexual partner more willing to proceed at a sexual pace in synchrony with your physiology. The results will be greater sexual satisfaction and less sexual dysfunction. Because of the work of Masters and Johnson and that of others motivated by Masters and Johnson's studies, a person experiencing problems with sexual functioning has access to a whole warehouse of effective sexual therapy modalities. As with the work of Kinsey, the studies of Masters and Johnson not only broke ground for sexual research as a profession, but also produced some very useful information for the general public.

The National Health and Social Life Survey

A University of Chicago research team conducted the first comprehensive survey of adult sexual behavior since Kinsey's research (Laumann et al., 1994). The National Health and Social Life Survey (NHSLS) was designed to assess the incidence and prevalence of a broad range of sexual practices and attitudes within the U.S. population. It was originally funded by the U.S. Department of Health and Human Services.

The broadest conclusion reported in this publication was that homosexuality is not a disease and that gays and lesbians, like heterosexuals, are individuals who have sexual concerns.

Myth vs Fact

Myth: Most women prefer a sexual partner who has a large penis.
Fact: Surveys indicate this is not true. Plus, we know that a female's vagina can adjust to different size penises and that there is far less difference in the sizes of erect penises than of soft penises.

Myth: Sexual activity usually ends soon after age 60.
Fact: Most people older than 60 years in relatively good health continue to participate in many forms of sexual activity.

Myth: Masturbation is physically harmful.
Fact: Masturbation does not harm the body in any way.

Myth: Anal intercourse between uninfected people can transmit human immunodeficiency virus (HIV).
Fact: If there is no infection, there will be no HIV transmission. To contract acquired immunodeficiency syndrome (AIDS), a person must first be infected with HIV.

Myth vs Fact

Myth: Most husbands have extramarital affairs.
Fact: The rates may vary in different studies, but the National Health and Social Life Survey reported that 25% of men and 15% of women had extramarital affairs.

Myth: Few women masturbate.
Fact: Most men and women, married and unmarried, occasionally masturbate. About 50% to 68% of females masturbate at least once a month.

Myth: Most normal women have orgasms from penile thrusting alone.
Fact: Different women prefer different kinds of stimulation. Many do not reach orgasm from penile thrusting alone.

Myth: A man cannot have an orgasm without an erection.
Fact: He can have an orgasm even if he does not have an erection.

Myth: Erectile dysfunction (sometimes referred to as "impotence" by the layperson) usually cannot be treated successfully.
Fact: With counseling, medical treatments, surgical treatments, and better sexual knowledge alone or in combination, most instances of erectile dysfunction can be treated.

Gender
DIMENSIONS

Differences in Research Results

When reviewing research results, researchers have often found relatively large differences between genders in the amount of heterosexual sexual behavior. Even when comparing the amounts for males and females of the same age, it is common to see much higher rates for males than females. The reasons for this are not known, but this situation makes for interesting discussion because one must wonder who the males are having heterosexual behavior with if the numbers are much smaller for females.

Some experts feel that at least some of these differences may be because women don't always answer such surveys honestly, but give answers that they believe are expected of them. Women's sensitivity to social expectations for their sexual behavior might cause them to be less than honest when asked about their sexual behavior. It might also be that men claim more sexual behavior than they actually had because they feel that is expected of them. In some studies, men and women were asked about their sexual behavior when they believed they were connected to a lie detector machine. Although there were still some gender differences, women's answers were much closer to men's under these circumstances.

Watch for these kinds of comparisons as you consider research on sexual behavior and think about reasons why gender differences might exist.

After 2 years of planning, federal funds for the project were withdrawn. In 1991, because conservative members of Congress were offended by the idea of using government funds for research on sexual behavior, legislation was passed to eliminate federal funding for such studies.

The research team then obtained funding from several private foundations. They were able to proceed, but with a much smaller sample. The research team trained 220 professional interviewers, and all 3,432 subjects were interviewed face-to-face. Their smaller sample size resulted in a population that was representative of white Americans, black Americans, and Hispanic Americans; however, there were too few representatives of other groups to provide useful information about them.

Here are a few examples of their findings: (1) Of married persons, 93.7% had had only one sexual partner in the last year as compared with 38% of those never married and not cohabitating; (2) married people were much more likely than singles to report being extremely or very happy; (3) 9.1% of men and 4.3% of women reported engaging in any same-sex activity since puberty (for nearly half of these men the behavior occurred only before the age of 18 years). About 1.4% of the women and 2.8% of the men reported a gay/lesbian identity.

The NHSLS found that married people are much more likely than singles to report being very happy.

Popular Literature

Shere Hite: Women's Sexuality, Men's Sexuality, and Women and Love

Between 1972 and 1976, when her findings were published in *The Hite Report*, Shere Hite mailed more than 100,000 60-item essay-type questionnaires to such women's groups as the National Organization for Women, university women's organizations, and women's newsletters. She also placed notices in *The Village Voice*, *Mademoiselle*, *Brides*, *Ms.*, and *Oui* magazines asking women to send for questionnaires. Hite received completed questionnaires from 3,109 women, who expressed their personal feelings about masturbation, orgasm, intercourse, clitoral stimulation, lesbianism, sexual slavery (satisfying males' needs

Shere Hite completed several important research projects about sexual behavior.

during sexual activity and ignoring their own needs), and the sexual revolution. Many women reported that they experienced orgasm more frequently from clitoral stimulation than from coitus and that they achieved deep orgasm from masturbation. Furthermore, they described a history of orgasm in general. Of the sample, 8% preferred sexual activity with other women, 53% said that they preferred sexual activity with themselves, and 17% preferred no sexual activity at all. Although the question was not directly asked, many women offered the information that they were curious about and might be interested in a sexual encounter with another woman. The majority of older women said that sexual pleasure increased with age, but many respondents older than 45 years reported difficulty in finding new sexual partners.

The findings published in *The Hite Report* were of great interest, for despite the fact that only a relatively small portion of the total female population was reached, no study had previously afforded such large numbers of women the opportunity to

express their preferences and desires in matters of sexuality. However, remember that Hite recruited her subjects by inserting a notice in magazines such as *Oui, The Village Voice, Ms.,* and *Mademoiselle.* Rather than being representative of all women, this small, select group of women is considered to be what is called a biased sample. Hite did not statistically analyze her data; rather, she used what are described as anecdotal reports—essays written by individuals describing their sexual activities and the feelings they experienced.

In 1981 Hite published *The Hite Report on Male Sexuality* using the same anecdotal analysis, this time presenting the views of 7,200 men. Men preferred intercourse to masturbation or oral–genital sexual activity. They were generally unaware that women could achieve orgasm by means other than intercourse. They expressed ignorance of when a female orgasm occurs and expressed anxious feelings about not knowing. Some of the males expressed anger over always being the initiators of sexual activity yet volunteered that sexually aggressive women were difficult for them to deal with. Many men stated that they grew up not being allowed to express themselves emotionally, for the culture demanded that men be strong and showing emotion was not defined as indicating strength. Again, because the Hite study of males was anecdotal, it is not considered to be of statistical note.

In 1987 Hite published *Women and Love: A Cultural Revolution in Progress.* After spending 7 years analyzing surveys from 4,500 women, she concluded that women are fed up with men. Despite women's liberation and the sexual revolution, Hite reported that women remain oppressed, and even abused, by men. Four of five women in her study said they still had to fight for their rights within relationships, 87% said that men became more emotionally dependent than women, 92% complained that men communicate with women in language that indicates "condescending, judgmental attitudes," 95% reported forms of "emotional and psychological harassment," 79% said they seriously question whether they should put so much energy into love relationships, 98% wished for more verbal closeness with male partners, 70% of the women married 5 years or more said they had extramarital affairs more often for emotional closeness than for sexual activity, and 87% of the married women said they have their deepest emotional relationship with a woman friend.

Many respectable researchers, both male and female, questioned Hite's findings. Criticisms pointed to a highly self-selected sample—only a 4.5% return from more than 100,000 questionnaires distributed to a variety of women's groups in 43 states—and a likely disproportion of unhappy people, because unhappy people were probably more willing to

? Did You Know . . .

Remember that the main purpose of sexual themes in newspapers, in magazines, on the Internet, and on radio and TV may be to sell newspapers and magazines and raise ratings of the programs. Also, there is a motivation to entertain people. It may be possible to get some sound information about sexuality through these sources; however, caution is needed if you are going to be a wise consumer. It is probably healthy to be skeptical until you have a chance to verify the information in accepted professional journals.

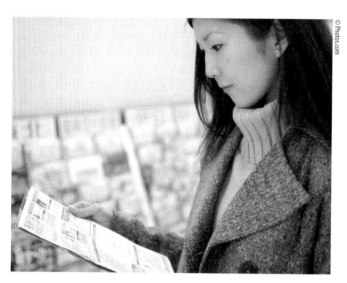

Readers must carefully evaluate information about human sexuality found in popular literature.

answer the questions than were happy people. Hite indicated a desire for men to see what women feel works in relationships, but others feared that Hite's book encouraged women to take the easy way out and blame everything on men.

Lorna Sarrel and Philip Sarrel: The Redbook Report on Sexual Relationships

In 1980 *Redbook* magazine published a sexuality questionnaire to which approximately 20,000 women and 6,000 men responded. The questionnaire was primarily concerned with the quality of relationships and the interpersonal communication of couples. More than half of the men (60%) and less than half of the women said that sharing feelings was very important to their relationships. Seventy-five percent of those who answered the questionnaire rated their current sexual relationships as being good or excellent. Fifteen percent reported sexual dysfunction, and these people said that they spoke very little about sexuality with their partner. Of particular interest is the fact that 40% of men and women who were parents said that lack of privacy interfered in some way with their enjoyment of sexual activity. Many individuals accepted sexual activity to satisfy a partner even if they did not want to make love at the time, and half of those who did said they "end up enjoying it."

This study is not indicative of sexual relationships of the population in general, because the readership of *Redbook* in 1980 tended to be youthful, married, better educated, and financially more secure than the general population. However, these people do represent a very large group of our population and they certainly do show an interest in sexual matters, are comfortable with the subject, and possess a willingness to discuss sexuality and interpersonal relationships. It is fair to believe that they did represent many couples in the society (Sarrel & Sarrel, 1980).

June Reinisch and Ruth Beasley: The Kinsey Institute New Report on Sex

The inclusion of a 1991 book within our popular literature section may be debatable, but it is indeed written for the general public. In fact, one of its authors said, "It's a great book to have in the bathroom, when you have time to read bits and pieces. It is designed to be a 'friendly encyclopedia,' telling readers in question-and-answer format almost everything they wanted to know about sexuality" (Dolan, 1990).

Research from the Kinsey Institute and the results of a Roper poll of 2,000 adults show that knowledge about sexuality is still at a very low level. For example, half of the adults tested did not know that a lubricant such as Vaseline or baby oil can cause microscopic holes in a condom or a diaphragm in as little as 60 seconds. This lack of understanding hardly contributes to safer sex practices.

Of women aged 30 to 44 years, only 55% received a passing grade on the test, and 52% of men in the same age group did. Men answered correctly more often on matters of sexual practices, and women knew more about their own sexual health. People living in the Midwest had the highest scores, and those in the South and the Northeast had the lowest.

Communication
D I M E N S I O N S

Talking About Sexuality Research Results

It is not easy to analyze findings of sexual research, and it is common to hear others talking about some "new findings" they just heard about. What if someone tells you about some sexual "research" and some interesting findings? What can you suggest to help the person (and you) analyze whether the research seems sound? Here are some possibilities for questions and conversational points.

- Was the scientific method used? This method does not rely just on testimonials or someone's opinion. It requires proper sampling techniques, accurate measurement and observation, and appropriate statistical analysis of the findings to reach valid conclusions.
- Is the study replicable? One study, taken alone, seldom proves anything. To be valid, one researcher's findings must be repeatable by others.
- Have the research findings been properly used? For example, conclusions based on data from one population may not apply to another population, and the

results from animal studies cannot be applied with certainty to humans.

- Were the proper statistics used and were they used correctly? Many people tend to accept statistical data without question, although statistical errors do occur.
- What is the competency of the author or researcher? Does the person have a record of excellent previous research? What kinds of expertise does the author or researcher have?
- Has the research been reviewed by peers? Peer review is the process in which the work of a scientist is reviewed by others who have equal or superior knowledge. It may be done while the study is being developed or afterward, as when results of the study are being considered for publication in a scientific journal.

Even these questions will not guarantee appropriate judgments about the accuracy of sexual research, but it can be very helpful to see whether there are good answers to them. They may also inspire some very interesting conversation.

Seventeen Magazine and The Kaiser Family Foundation: SexSmarts Survey on Teen Sexual Behavior

One of the latest in a series of surveys of teens aged 15–17 years found that only 1 in 10 teens who have had sexual intercourse discussed his or her sexual plans with parents ahead of time, and more than a third did not tell their parents about their sexual history at all. Forty-eight percent of all survey respondents and 56% of sexually active respondents never talked with a parent about "how to know when you are ready to have sex." Eighty percent of respondents said teens do not discuss sexual issues with their parents because they worry that their parents will disapprove or will assume that they are already participating in sexual behavior if they discuss the subject with them (Kaiser Family Foundation and *Seventeen* magazine release latest SexSmarts Survey on teen sexual behavior, 2002).

Eighty-four percent of all respondents said they had never talked with a healthcare provider about how to know when one is prepared for sexual behavior. More than two-thirds had not discussed contraception, HIV and AIDS, condoms, or STIs with a healthcare provider. Nearly two-thirds had spoken

with a sexual partner about "what they are comfortable doing sexually." Fifty-eight percent had never discussed STIs with a partner, 56% had never discussed HIV and AIDS with a partner, and 53% of all respondents and 28% of sexually active teens had never discussed contraception with a partner. Most cited lack of knowledge about sexual issues, fear of what a partner might think, and embarrassment as reasons they do not discuss sexual issues with partners.

NBC News and People Magazine: National Survey of Young Teens Sexual Attitudes and Behavior

NBC News and *People Magazine* had the Princeton Survey Research Associates International conduct a survey of 1,000 young teenagers (ages 13–16) and their parents. The results were reported in 2004 and updated in 2005 (Nearly 3 in 10 young teens sexually active, 2005). Teens were asked about their sexual health, behavior, and attitudes, and parents were asked for their views on the sexual lives of today's teens.

The survey showed that parents and teens have somewhat different opinions on the pressure teens

By the time they finish high school, the percentage of females who have had sexual intercourse is about 62%, with about 38% who have not.

face and their attitudes. For example, 85% of parents strongly or somewhat agreed that "there is a lot of pressure on teenagers to have sex by a certain age," compared with 66% of the teens. Forty-seven percent of parents strongly or somewhat agreed with the statement, "for teens oral sex is not as big a deal as sexual intercourse," compared with 75% of teens.

The survey confirmed that teens engage in a wide range of sexual behavior, from kissing to sexual intercourse. For example, 58% of all teens (ages 13–16) reported having "kissed someone romantically," 27% reported having "been with someone in an intimate or romantic way," 21% reported having "touched someone's genitals or private parts," 13% reported having engaged in sexual intercourse, and 12% reported having engaged in oral sex. Among the 12% of all teens who reported having had oral sex, 1% first had oral sex at age 11, 8% at age 12, 19% at age 13, 22% at age 14, 29% at age 15, and 16% at age 16.

As might be expected, older teens (ages 15–16) reported higher rates of sexual behavior. Seventy-two percent had "kissed someone romantically," 41% had "been with someone in an intimate or romantic way," 37% had "touched someone's genitals or private parts," 21% had engaged in sexual intercourse, and 19% had engaged in oral sex.

Parents seemed to underestimate whether their teens had engaged in sexual behavior. When asked about their own child, 83% believed he or she had not engaged in sexual activity beyond kissing.

According to the study, many teens were not protecting themselves from pregnancy or STIs. Thirty percent who had oral sex reported "always" using "protection such as a condom" during oral sex, 14% reported using protection "most of the time," 13%

"some of the time," and 42% reported "never" using protection during oral sex.

Thirty-six percent of teens who had sexual intercourse used birth control every time, 6% used it "almost every time," 8% used it "most of the time," 7% used it "only sometimes," 1% "hardly ever," and 40% never used birth control.

The survey showed that many factors, from parent's reactions to curiosity to sexual desire, play a role in teens' decisions about sexual behavior. Eighty-two percent of teens who had engaged in sexual intercourse cited having met the right person as a major or minor reason for their decision, 71% cited curiosity, 68% cited sexual desire, 56% cited a hope that it would make their relationship even closer, 34% cited pressure from their partner, and 18% cited a desire "to be more popular and accepted" as a major or minor reason for their decision.

For those who had never engaged in sexual intercourse, 89% cited feeling they were too young as a major or minor reason for their decision, 88% cited "a conscious decision to wait," 86% cited worries about STIs, 85% cited worries about pregnancy, 84% cited worries about what their parents would think, 75% cited not having met the right person yet, 63% cited religious or moral beliefs, 54% cited worries about what their friends would think, and 49% cited not having had the opportunity as a major or minor reason for their decision.

Among those who had engaged in oral sex, 76% cited "the other person wanted to" as a major or minor reason for their decision, 71% cited having met the right person, 69% cited the belief that "you are still a virgin if you have oral sex," 68% cited not having to worry about pregnancy, 64% cited curiosity, 40% cited wanting to avoid sexual intercourse, 35% cited the belief you can't get STIs from oral sex, 24% cited wanting to avoid being touched or undress, and 21% cited "wanting to be more popular and accepted" as a major or minor reason for their decision.

■ Examples of Research in the 21st Century

It is almost impossible to count the many research studies related to human sexuality done in recent years. And until these studies stand the test of time, it is difficult to tell which, if any, might become classics. The following is a chronological summary of selected, more recent, research studies.

Sexual standards are influenced by culture and gender.

Rates of sexual activity vary with differences in ethnicity.

Studies on Premarital Sexual Attitudes and Behavior
Dailard (2001) reported on the findings of the National Longitudinal Study of Adolescent Health (more commonly called the "Add Health Survey"). She indicated that teens' reports of ever having had sexual intercourse increase dramatically with grade level, from 16% among 7th and 8th graders to 60% among 11th graders. Teenagers who are African American or in low-income or single-parent families are more likely to have had sexual intercourse than their peers. In addition, the Add Health Survey strongly indicates that whether a teenager has ever had sexual intercourse is largely explained by that individual's own sexual history and his or her perceptions about the costs and benefits of having sexual intercourse. In sharp contrast, the data indicate that other major risk behaviors—such as cigarette smoking, drug and alcohol use, weapons-related violence,

and suicidal thoughts and attempts—are shaped more by factors such as problems with school or work or the number of friends who regularly smoke or drink.

Dennison and Russell (2005) pointed out that more than 1,000 published reports employed data from the Add Health Study. Findings from these reports indicate that adolescents at the upper and lower ends of the intelligence distribution were less likely to have engaged in intercourse, religiosity reduced the risk of coital debut in both males and females, youth from intact families were less likely to have engaged in intercourse, greater parental involvement was related to a lower likelihood of sex initiation, and most teens had their first sexual experience within the context of a romantic relationship. The average waiting time before engaging in sexual intercourse within these romantic relationships was 5 months. In addition, students who felt connected at school reported later ages at sexual initiation, girls participating in sports tended to delay sexual activity, and students who took abstinence pledges were less likely than nonpledgers to practice safe sex once they became sexually active.

In 2002 the Kaiser Family Foundation reported the results of a national survey of 1,200 adolescents and young adults 13–24 years old (Substance use and risky sexual behavior, 2002). It concluded that for many teens and young adults, alcohol use and drug use are closely linked to sexual decision making and risk taking. Nearly 90% said their peers used alcohol or drugs before having sexual intercourse at least some of the time, and many young people reported that condoms are often not used when people are drinking or using drugs. More than a third of sexually active young people reported that alcohol or drugs had influenced their decisions about sex. Almost as many had "done more" sexually than they had planned while under their influence. As a result, they reported they worried about STIs and pregnancy.

It is interesting that most sexually active teenagers had sexual intercourse for the first time in their parents' homes, late at night (Most sexually active teens first had sex at home, 2002). On the basis of a national survey that had tracked 8,000 children aged 12–16 years since 1997, the study found that 56% of those who had been sexually active said they first had sexual intercourse at their family's home or at the family home of a partner, 12% said at a friend's house, 4% said in a vehicle, 3% said at an outdoor location, 3% said at a hotel or motel, and 10% said at another location. In addition, 42% said they first had sexual intercourse between 10 P.M. and 7 A.M. and 28% said between 6 P.M. and 10 P.M. Only 15% of respondents said they had intercourse for the first time between 3 P.M. and 6 P.M. This study dispels the myth that teens most often have sexual intercourse after school, when parents are at work.

Changes in sexual risk behavior among U.S. high school students (grades 9–12) over a 10-year period were reported in 2002 (Trends in sexual risk behaviors among high school students, 2002). The percentage who reported ever having had sexual intercourse decreased by 16%. In 1991, 56% had participated, but in 2001 only 46% had done so. Also, the overall proportion who had had four or more partners dropped by 24%—from 19% in 1991 to 14% in 2001.

The overall prevalence of "current sexual activity"—defined as having intercourse at any point during the 3 months preceding the survey—did not change between 1991 and 2001. It was reported by about one-third of the respondents. Condom use rose between 1991 and 1999 but had "leveled off" since then. In 2001 about 58% of sexually active teens used condoms, compared to about 46% in 1991. The percentage of sexually active students who had used drugs or alcohol before their most recent intercourse increased 18% between 1991 and 2002.

For a number of years the U.S. Centers for Disease Control has periodically conducted a Youth Risk Behavior Surveillance (YRBS). A portion of the questions within the survey of health behaviors of students in grades 9–12 relate to sexual behavior. Some of the YRBS results reported in 2004, 2010, and 2013 are shown in Table 2.1.

In 2005 Halpern-Felsher et al. reported that ethnically diverse 9th-grade adolescents evaluated oral sexual activity as significantly less risky than vaginal intercourse on health, social, and emotional consequences. They also believed that oral activity is more acceptable than vaginal intercourse for adolescents their own age in both dating and nondating situations, oral sexual activity is less of a threat to their values and beliefs, and more of their peers will have oral sexual activity than vaginal intercourse in the near future. More study participants reported having had oral sexual activity (20%) than vaginal intercourse (14%), and more intended to have oral sexual activity in the next 6 months (32%) than vaginal intercourse (26%).

In 2005, South et al. studied the effect of residential mobility on the timing of first premarital sexual intercourse. They found that adolescents who had recently moved were about one-third more likely than nonmobile adolescents to experience first premarital intercourse. They further found that much of the difference between adolescents who moved and those who didn't in the onset of sexual activity was attributable to the greater propensity for delinquency and weaker academic performance among members of movers' school-based friendship networks.

In 2008, Lescano et al. studied factors associated with anal intercourse among adolescents and young adults. Recent heterosexual anal intercourse was reported by 16% of the 1,348 respondents. Females who engaged in anal intercourse were more likely to be living with a sexual partner, to have had two or more partners, and to have experienced coerced intercourse. For males, only a sexual orientation other than heterosexual was a significant predictor of engaging in heterosexual anal intercourse.

In 2010, Sanders et al. asked a random sample of 486 adults ages 18–96 which sexual behaviors fit the definition of "having had sex." In general, there was not a significant difference between men and women, yet there was no real consensus on which behaviors fit the definition. Although nearly all respondents concurred that penile–vaginal intercourse (PVI) fit the criteria, two out of 10 people did not concur that penile–anal intercourse did. Three out of 10 said

TABLE 2.1

Youth Risk Behavior Surveillance (YRBS) Results, 2004, 2010, and 2013

Sexual Behavior	2004	2010	2013
Percent of high school students (grades 9–12) who had sexual intercourse	47%	46%	47%
Percent of sexually active students who used a condom at last sexual intercourse	63%	61%	59%
Incidence of intercourse for African American males	74%	72%	68%
Incidence of intercourse for Hispanic males	57%	53%	52%
Incidence of intercourse for white males	41%	40%	44%
Incidence of intercourse for African American females	61%	54%	53%
Incidence of intercourse for Hispanic females	46%	45%	47%
Incidence of intercourse for white females	42%	45%	45%
Incidence of intercourse for 9th grade students	33%	34%	30%
Incidence of intercourse for 10th grade students	44%	41%	41%
Incidence of intercourse for 11th grade students	53%	53%	54%
Incidence of intercourse for 12th grade students	62%	62%	64%
Had first intercourse before age 13 years	7%	6%	6%
Had sexual intercourse during their lifetime with four or more partners	14%	14%	15%

Source: Data from Grunbaum, J., Kann, L., Kinchen, S., Ross, J., Hawkins, J., Lowry, R., Harris, W. A., McManus, T., Chyen, D., & Collins, J. Youth risk behavior surveillance—United States, 2003. In: *Surveillance Summaries, Morbidity and Mortality Weekly Report, 53, no. SS-2* (2004), 1–20; Eaton, D. K., Kann, L., Kinchen, S., Shanklin, S. Ross, J., Hawkins, J., Harris, W. A., Lowry, R., McManus, T., Chyen, D., Lim, C., Whittle, L., Brener, N. D., & Wechsler, H. Youth risk behavior surveillance—United States, 2009. In: *Surveillance Summaries, Morbidity and Mortality Weekly Report, 59, no. SS-5* (2010), 1–143. Kahn, L., Kinchen, S., Shanklin, S. L., Flint, K. H., Hawkins, J., Harris, W. A., Lowry, R., Olsen, E. O., McManus, T., Chyen, D., Whittle, L., Taylor, E., Demissie, Z., Brener, N., Thornton, J., Moore, J., & Zaza, S. Youth risk behavior surveillance—United States, 2013. *Mortality and Morbidity Weekly Report, 63, 4* (2014), 1–168.

"no" to oral–genital activity, as did half of the respondents about manual–genital contact. Many disagreed that having PVI without the man ejaculating could be called "having sex." Findings demonstrated that we cannot assume that our own definitions of having "had sex" are shared with others.

In 2011, Chandra et al. reported on data collected through in-person interviews with a national sample of more than 13,000 males and females. Among adults 25–44, approximately 98% of females and 97% of males had ever had vaginal intercourse, 89% of females and 90% of males had ever oral sex with an opposite-sex partner, and 36% of females and 44% of males had ever had anal sex with an opposite-sex partner. Twice as many women reported any same-sex contact in their lifetimes compared with men (13% of women and 5.2% of men). Among teenagers aged 15–19, 7% of females and 9% of males had had oral sex with an opposite sex partner, but no vaginal intercourse.

In 2011, Lehmiller et al. reported on gender differences in approaching friends with benefits (FWB) relationships. They defined FWB relationships as consisting of friends who are sexually, but not romantically,

involved. They engage in sexual activity on occasion, but otherwise have a basic friendship. Their results indicated many similarities in terms of how males and females approached FWB relationships, but several important differences emerged. Sexual activity was a more common motivation for men to begin such relationships, whereas emotional connection was a more common motivation for women. Also, men were more likely to hope that the relationship stayed the same over time, whereas women expressed more desire for it to change into either a full-fledged romance or a basic friendship. Both men and women were more committed to the friendship than to the sexual aspect of the relationship. The researchers felt their findings were largely consistent with the notion that traditional gender role expectations and the sexual double standard may influence how men and women approach FWB relationships.

In 2014, Houck et al. analyzed self-reported data on sexting and sexual behavior from more than 400 teens who attended five urban public schools in Rhode Island. All were in the seventh grade and between the ages of 12 and 14. Students were identified by school personnel as having "symptoms of behavioral

or emotional difficulties" and were therefore considered to be at risk for sexual health concerns, including HIV/STI or unintended pregnancy. Among middle
school students in this study, 5% reported texting
or emailing a sexual picture of themselves to someone else in the preceding 6 months. An additional
17% reported texting or emailing sexual messages
(with no photo). Middle schoolers who had texted
or emailed sexual messages or photos were 4 to 7
times more likely to have engaged in sexual activity
with another person compared to their non-sexting
peers. The authors concluded that pediatricians and
other clinicians should initiate conversations about
sexting with parents and their early-adolescent
patients.

In 2014, Simpson et al. compared hip width and
sexual behavior. The study was conducted among 148
women between 18 and 26 years old who had at least
one sexual partner previously. Overall, women in the
study with hips wider than 14.2 inches had more
sexual partners and more one-night stands than
women with hips less than 12.2 inches wide. More
specifically, the women for whom one-night stands
accounted for three out of every four of their sexual
relationships had hips at least 0.8 inches wider than
those of their counterparts in whose lives such fleeting relationships were not as prevalent. The researchers surmised that women with wider hips are more
likely to engage in sexual intercourse because the
birth process is generally easier and less traumatic
for them than for smaller-hipped women. They concluded that women's sexual activity is at least in part
influenced by hip width.

Studies on Ethnic Differences in Sexual Attitudes and Behavior

Only relatively recently have researchers looked at
the influence of ethnic differences in sexual attitudes
and behavior. Examples of such studies are given in
the following discussion.

Ford and coworkers (2001) reported that the sexual partners of white and black adolescents are likely
to be similar to them. In contrast, the sexual partners
of Latino adolescents and of adolescents of "other"
race or ethnicity are more likely to be of a different
racial or ethnic group. As adolescents get older, their
partners become more heterogeneous.

Cavanagh (2004) studied the sexual debut of girls
in early adolescence. She found that among white
girls, those who matured early were more likely to
have sexual intercourse in early adolescence, and this
was partially due to the friendship groups of which
they were a part. Early puberty seemed to draw white
girls into larger friendship groups characterized by
riskier behavior and lower academic achievement.
Hispanic girls were similar to white girls in key ways,

but different in others. For them, as for whites, both
early puberty and friendship group characteristics
were closely related to sexual debut, but unlike whites,
friendship group characteristics did not mediate the
association between early pubertal timing and sexual
debut. Early pubertal timing mattered for Hispanics
in other ways not captured in the model used in the
study. There was also another factor uniquely characterizing Hispanics—the presence of older boys. Interestingly, among African American girls, there were no
meaningful associations among early pubertal timing,
the friendship group, and sexual debut.

Other studies have shown a variety of ethnic differences related to sexuality. For example, Connell et
al. (2004) found that African American groups are
more aware of STIs and HIV than either white or
Hispanic groups. However, African Americans tend
to have a higher percentage of people testing positive
for HIV/AIDS (Johnson & Jackson, 2004). The prevalence rate of HIV has been found to be 16% for African Americans, 7% for Hispanics, and 3% for whites
(Harawa et al., 2004). Also, Hispanic youth seem to
be at a greater risk for experiencing early intercourse
than white youth (Adam et al., 2005).

Regarding birth control, use of injectable contraceptives is high among African American women,
but not as high among Asian Indian or white women
(Burgard, 2004). Knowledge disparities can also be
seen when comparing ethnic groups. For example,
41% of Hispanic women and 75% of African American women have heard of emergency contraception
as compared to 99% of white women (Chuang &
Freund, 2005).

As indicated in the Multicultural Dimensions box
earlier in this chapter (Martin et al., 2013), the proportions of nonmarital births vary widely by race and
Hispanic origin. They range from a low of 17% for
Asian or Pacific Islander mothers to a high of 72%
for non-Hispanic black mothers.

Also, as shown in Table 2.1, the incidence of sexual intercourse among high school students was 68%
for African males, 52% for Hispanic males, and 44%
for white males. For females, it was 53% for African
Americans, 47% for Hispanics, and 45% for whites
(Kahn et al., 2014).

Studies on the Use of Contraception

Ford and colleagues (2001) reported that the less
similar adolescents and their sexual partners are to
one another—whether because of a difference in age,
grade, or school—the less likely they are to use condoms and other contraceptive methods. The likelihood
of having sexual relations with adolescents with different characteristics increases as adolescents get older.

Oncalem and King (2001) reported that many
college students either have tried to talk their sexual

partners out of using a condom or have had a partner try to dissuade them from condom use. Nearly 14% of women and nearly 17% of men who had engaged in sexual intercourse admitted to having actively tried to dissuade a partner from the couple's using condoms. Thirty percent of men and 41% of women said that a sexual partner had tried to dissuade them. The most frequent reasons cited were (1) that sexual intercourse feels better without a condom, (2) that the woman will not get pregnant, and (3) that the person will not get a sexually transmitted infection.

While it may seem obvious, Bruckner et al. (2004) reported that the factor most strongly associated with the risk of pregnancy among young women is contraceptive use, with nonusers being significantly more likely than inconsistent and consistent users to become pregnant. However, these researchers also indicated that adolescents who become pregnant do not sufficiently appreciate the negative consequences, and that prevention programs should target participants' attitudes toward pregnancy. If more positive attitudes toward contraception can be developed, this will help shape effective contraceptive use.

While there are many reasons for close involvement between parents and adolescents, Frisco (2005) pointed out an interesting relationship to contraceptive use. Her research showed that parental involvement in education shapes teenagers' attitudes about school and work by encouraging achievement and by providing a home environment that values education. Such parental involvement also increases the odds that young women will use contraception, especially increasing the likelihood of using specific reliable birth control methods.

Manlove et al. (2008) examined a sample of sexually experienced 15- to 19-year-old males to identify factors associated with condom use. They found that Hispanic males and those who did not receive formal sexuality education had lower odds of condom use and/or consistency. African American males and those with more positive attitudes about condoms had greater odds of both using condoms and using them consistently. Males who were older at most recent sexual intercourse, who had an older sexual partner or a casual sexual partner, who were in longer relationships, or who engaged in more frequent sexual intercourse had reduced odds of contraceptive use.

In 2010, the Guttmacher Institute (Facts on contraceptive use in the United States, 2010) reported that of the 43 million fertile, sexually active women who do not want to become pregnant, 89% use a method of contraception. Sixty-three percent of reproductive-age women who practice contraception

© John Birdsall/age fotostock

Adolescents give many reasons why they did not use contraception.

use nonpermanent methods, including hormonal methods (such as the pill, patch, implant, injectable, and vaginal ring), the IUD, and condoms. The remaining women rely on female or male sterilization. For women younger than age 30, the most common method is the pill. Among women aged 30 and older, more rely on sterilization. Overall, pills are used by 28% of users, tubal sterilization by 27%, male condoms by 16%, a vasectomy by 10%, an IUD by 6%, withdrawal by 5%, an injectable by 3%, a vaginal ring by 2%, an implant by 1%, and periodic abstinence (calendar method) by a little less than 1%.

Related to control of births, in 2011 it was reported (Facts on induced abortion in the United States, 2011) that the overall U.S. abortion rate declined after 1981. The abortion rate among U.S. women of childbearing age declined from about 29.3 per 1,000 women in 1981 to about 19 in 2011. Sixty-one percent of abortions are obtained by women who have one or more children; 18% are obtained by teenagers. Women in their twenties account for more than half of all abortions, and women who have never married and are not cohabiting account for 45% of all abortions.

Among the 34.2% of currently sexually active high school students (grades 9–12) in the United States, 61% reported that either they or their partner used a condom during the last sexual intercourse, 20% used birth control pills, 3% used Depo-Provera, 23% used either birth control pills or Depo-Provera, and 9% used both a condom and birth control pills or Depo-Provera (Eaton et al., 2010).

In 2014, Kahn et al. reported on the Youth Risk Behavior Surveillance results related to contraceptive use among high school (grades 9–12) students. Among the 34% of currently sexually active students nationwide, 59.1% reported that either they or their partner had used a condom during the last sexual intercourse, 19% reported that either they or their partner had used birth control pills, 1.6% reported that either they or their partner had used an intrauterine device or contraceptive implant, and 4.7% reported that either they or their partner had used a contraceptive shot, patch, or ring to prevent pregnancy before last sexual intercourse. However, 13.7% reported that neither they nor their partner had used any method to prevent pregnancy during last sexual intercourse.

By preventing unintended pregnancies, contraception provides significant health, social, and economic benefits for women. Correct and consistent contraceptive use, however, is critical (New infographic: Contraception is highly effective, 2013). The two-thirds of U.S. women at risk of unintended pregnancy who use contraception consistently and correctly in any given year account for only 5% of all unintended pregnancies. By comparison, the 19% of women at risk who use contraception inconsistently account for 43% of unintended pregnancies, while the 16% of women at risk who use no contraceptive method at all for a month or more during the year account for 52% of such pregnancies. These simple statistics demonstrate how effective contraceptive use can be.

Lindberg and Kost (2013) reported that 40% of births are intended by men. Unintended births were more common among younger men and men with lower levels of education than among older and more educated men, respectively. Unintended births are especially prevalent among black men (51%), with smaller rates found among Hispanic men (38%) and white men (34%). Not surprisingly, men who planned the birth were more likely to be happy about the birth than were those who had not planned the birth. The authors pointed out the need to include men in discussions about unintended pregnancy and use strategies to help men work as individuals and with their partners to control when and if they have children.

Milhausen et al. (2014) assessed the prevalence and individual predictors of condom use at last PVI in a national sample of 654 Canadian university students. Fewer than half of these students (47.2%) reported condom use at last PVI. The main reason cited for having used a condom was birth control. The strongest predictor of condom use at last PVI was a preference for condoms as a contraceptive method. Female students who reported that their most recent sexual encounter occurred with a more committed partner had slightly lower odds of reporting condom use at last PVI. The results indicated that rates of condom use are low among Canadian university students, and that many students are likely at high risk

Young people say they get a lot of their sexual information from their peers.

for STIs. The authors indicated that interventions to raise awareness of STIs are needed on Canadian university campuses.

Frost et al. (2014) reported that publicly supported family planning visits helped clients avoid myriad negative health outcomes. Also, the financial investment resulted in a net government savings of $13.6 billion, or $7.09 for every public dollar spent. These savings were a result of three factors: (1) contraceptive care that prevented unintended pregnancies, unplanned births, abortions, and preterm or low-birth-weight births; (2) STI testing that prevented many STIs, ectopic pregnancies, and infertility cases; and (3) Pap testing and HPV vaccinations that prevented many cervical cancer cases and cervical cancer deaths.

Other Representative Studies

The Guttmacher Institute (Facts on American teens' sexual and reproductive health, 2011) reported that each year almost 750,000 U.S. women ages 15–19 become pregnant. Two-thirds of all teen pregnancies are among 18- and 19-year-olds. The peak rate of teen pregnancies was 117 per 1,000 women ages 15–19, which occurred in 1990. Since then, there has been a steady decline to about 70 per 1,000. However, the U.S. teen pregnancy rate continues to be one of the highest in the developed world—more than twice as high as rates in Canada (28 per 1,000) or Sweden (31 per 1,000). About 59% of U.S. teen pregnancies end in birth, 27% in abortion, and 14% in miscarriage.

In 2011, Pazol et al. reported that approximately 410,000 teens ages 15–19 gave birth in 2009. The national teen birth rate was 39.1 per 1,000 females, a 37% decrease since 1991, and the lowest rate ever recorded. State-specific teen birth rates varied from 16.4 to 64.2 births per 1,000 females and were highest among southern states. Birth rates for black and Hispanic teens were 59.0 and 70.1 births per 1,000 females, respectively, compared with 25.6 for white teens.

In 2011, Torian et al. reported that sharp increases were reported from 1981 to 1995 in the number of new AIDS cases and deaths in the United States, reaching highs of over 75,400 in 1992 and 50,600 in 1995, respectively. However, with the introduction of highly active antiretroviral therapy, AIDS diagnoses and deaths declined substantially from 1995 to 1998 and remained stable from 1998 to 2008, at an average of just over 38,200 AIDS diagnoses and 17,400 deaths per year, respectively. Despite the decline in AIDS cases and deaths, at the end of 2008 an estimated 1,178,350 persons were living with HIV, including 236,000 (20.1%) whose infection was undiagnosed. Most (75%) persons living with HIV were male, and 65.7% of the males were men who have sexual activity with men. HIV prevalence rates for blacks or African Americans (1,819 per 100,000 population) and Hispanics or Latinos (593) were approximately eight times and two and a half times the rate among whites (238), respectively.

Daniel and Balog (2009) reported that the age of female puberty seems to have decreased in the United States and western countries as child health and nutrition have improved and obesity has become more common. Environmental contaminants, particularly endocrine disruptors, may also play a role in lowering the age of puberty. Puberty at an early age increases the risk of stress, poor school performance, teen pregnancy, eating disorders, substance abuse, and a variety of health issues that may appear later in life, including breast cancer and heart disease. The age of first breast development is dropping faster than that of first menstrual period (menarche). While the age of menarche dropped from a mean of 17.5 years in the middle of the 19th century to 12.5 years by the middle of the 20th century, girls begin menstruating only a few months earlier today than girls 40 years ago.

Biro et al. (2010) indicated that 15% of U.S. girls have breast development, an early sign of puberty, by age 7. Black girls are more likely to have early breast development, with 23% starting by age 7 compared to almost 15% of Hispanic girls. They found that 10% of white girls began developing breasts by age 7, which is twice the rate of a 1997 study.

Examinations of associations between religiosity and sexual behaviors and attitudes have shown interesting results. In 2004 Lefkowitz et al. found relationships between religiosity (group affiliation, attendance at religious services, attitudes, perceptions of negative sanctions, and adherence to sanctions) and sexuality. They reported that religious

behavior was the strongest predictor of sexual behavior. In 2005 research by Penhollow et al. indicated that religiosity variables, especially frequency of religious attendance and religious feelings, were significant predictors of sexual behavior.

Interestingly, in 2011 McFarland et al. reported that among older married adults religion is largely unrelated with frequency of sexual behavior and satisfaction, although religious integration in daily life shares a weak, but positive, association with pleasure from sexual activity.

In 2004 Vlassoff et al. assessed the costs and benefits of sexual and reproductive health interventions. Their study showed that poor sexual and reproductive health account for a substantial share of the global burden of disease. Their research indicated that the benefits of sexual and reproductive health interventions are far-reaching. For example, in addition to medical benefits, maternal health care lowers death and disability due to pregnancy-related causes, helps families remain intact, enables higher household savings and investment, and encourages higher productivity. Prevention and treatment for STIs and treatments for medical conditions also help reduce social stigma and help parents remain healthy so they are better able to care for and invest in their children. Contraceptives, together with maternal health services, minimize the adverse health effects of unintended pregnancy and high-risk births, including unsafe abortion, hemorrhage, infection, anemia, low birth weight, and malnutrition. These researchers concluded that sexual and reproductive health interventions are a good investment.

Koch (2006) reported on women's bodies being a "puzzle" for college men. She found that college men believed women and their bodies are complex "puzzles" that are difficult to understand. The college men also felt ignorance about women's bodies, particularly their genital/reproductive anatomy and menstruation. Confusion over how to deal with women's body image was another major theme. The men believed that women are too concerned about their body image. Most felt that having better knowledge of women's bodies and the experiences they go through would improve their relationships with women.

As electronic devices have played much larger roles in the lives of college students, some issues related to electronic devices and sexuality have arisen. For example, the National Campaign to Prevent Teen and Unplanned Pregnancy and CosmoGirl.com commissioned a survey of teens and young adults to explore electronic activity (Sex and Tech, 2008). The key findings showed that a significant number of teens have electronically sent, or posted online, nude or semi-nude pictures or videos of themselves. Sexually suggestive messages were even more prevalent than sexually suggestive images. Most respondents knew that it was potentially dangerous to post sexually suggestive content, but did it anyway. Many of the teens and young adults said they were pressured by friends to send or post sexual content. Most said it was a "fun and flirtatious" activity.

The National Survey of Sexual Health and Behavior (NSSHB) (2010) included data from the largest nationally representative study of sexual-health behaviors ever fielded. It included information about sexual experiences and condom-use behaviors of 5,865 adolescents and adults ages 14–94. This survey generated so much information that the initial findings were presented in nine separate research articles in a special issue of *The Journal of Sexual Medicine* published on October 1, 2010. According to the study's findings, 1 in 4 acts of vaginal intercourse in the United States are condom protected (1 in 3 among singles). Information was obtained on the percentage of Americans (by age group) performing certain sexual behaviors in the past year. Behaviors included masturbated alone, masturbated with partner, received oral from woman, received oral from man, gave oral to woman, gave oral to man, vaginal intercourse, received penis in anus, and inserted penis in anus. As one example, percentages for vaginal intercourse by age group were as follows: 14–15 (9% for males and 11% for females); 16–17 (30% for males and 30% for females); 18–19 (53% for males and 62% for females); 20–24 (63% for males and 80% for females); 25–29 (86% for males and 87% for females); 30–39 (85% for males and 74% for females); 40–49 (74% for males and 70% for females); 50–59 (58% for males and 51% for females); 60–69 (54% for males and 42% for females); and 70+ (43% for males and 22% for females).

Here is a sampling of other findings from the NSSHB:

- Condoms are used twice as often with casual sexual partners as with relationship partners.

- The sexual repertoires of U.S. adults are extremely variable, with more than 40 combinations of sexual activity described at adults' most recent sexual event.

- Many older adults continue to have pleasurable sex lives, reporting a range of different behaviors and partner types.

- About 85% of men report that their partner had an orgasm at the most recent sexual event; this compares to 64% of women who report having had an orgasm at their most recent sexual event. (A difference that is too large to be accounted for by some of the

men having had male partners at their most recent event.)

- Men are more likely to have an orgasm when sexual activity includes vaginal intercourse; women are more likely to have an orgasm when they engage in a variety of sexual acts and when oral sexual activity or vaginal intercourse is included.

- Whereas about 7% of adult women and 8% of men identify as gay, lesbian, or bisexual, the proportion of individuals in the United States who have had same-gender sexual interactions at some point in their lives is higher.

- At any given time, most U.S. adolescents are not engaging in partnered sexual behavior. While 40% of 17-year-old males reported vaginal intercourse in the past year, only 27% reported the same in the past 90 days.

- Adults using a condom for intercourse were just as likely to rate the sexual event positively in terms of arousal, pleasure, and orgasm than when having intercourse without one.

In 2011, Mark, Jansen, and Milhausen assessed the relative importance of demographic, interpersonal, and personality factors in predicting sexual infidelity in heterosexual couples. Almost one-fourth of men (23.2%) and one-fifth of women (19.2%) indicated they had "cheated" during their current relationship (i.e., engaged in sexual interactions with someone other than their partner). Men had an increased tendency to engage in regretful sexual behavior during negative affective states. For women, low relationship status and low compatibility in terms of sexual attitudes and values were predictive of infidelity. Overall, these researchers concluded that, for both men and women, sexual personality characteristics and, for women, relationship factors are more relevant to the prediction of sexual infidelity than are demographic variables such as marital status and religiosity.

In 2014, Gray et al. studied dating and sexual behavior among single parents of young children in the United States. They pointed out that theory and research on partnered parents suggests trade-offs between parenting and sexuality, with those trade-offs most pronounced among mothers of young children. Without the help of a partner, singles often have to divert more energy to parenting, so one might think that single parents would not be dating as much. But that is not what the researchers found. In this study, the sample consisted of 5,481 single Americans 21 years of age and older, of whom 4.3% were parents of a child age 5 or younger. The researchers reported greater frequency of sexual activity and first dates among single parents with a child aged 5 years or younger, but no differences in other outcomes compared with single parents of older children.

Research on Sexuality Education

Research has been done to evaluate the effect of sexuality education programs. For example Kirby (2001) reported that some sexuality and HIV education programs can delay the onset of intercourse, reduce the number of partners, reduce the frequency of sexual intercourse, increase condom or contraceptive use, and thereby decrease sexual risk taking. Also, some programs that have addressed nonsexual risk or protective factors (such as attachment to family, parental monitoring, and attachment to school) have reduced sexual risk taking. Characteristics of effective programs include the following: (1) They focus on reducing one or more behaviors that lead to unintended pregnancy or STIs; (2) they provide basic, accurate information about the risks of teen sexual activity and about ways to avoid intercourse or use methods of protection against pregnancy and STIs; (3) they provide examples of practice with communication, negotiation, and refusal skills; (4) they continue for a sufficient length of time; and (5) they employ teaching methods designed to involve the participants and induce them to personalize the information.

In 2004 Albert reported on a poll that showed a divide among parents and teenagers on whether comprehensive sexuality education encourages young people to engage in sexual activity. Forty-four percent of the parents said that messages beyond abstinence-only education might encourage sexual activity, but 68% of the teens said that "more information does not automatically translate into more sex." The survey also showed that teenagers most often seek information about sexuality from their parents, but most parents don't believe their kids listen to them. Ninety percent of the parents said they do not know how to discuss sexuality with their children.

Unfortunately, evaluations of comprehensive sexuality education have tended to focus mainly on whether the programs have helped young people delay sexual activity and prevent unwanted pregnancy and disease (Haffner & Goldfarb, 1998). Other goals, such as helping young people develop an appreciation of their bodies or communicate effectively with peers and partners, are often overlooked. Evaluations of sexuality education need to be improved so they reflect broad program goals. In the meantime, many evaluations have found that high-quality sexuality education programs increase knowledge, clarify values, increase parent–child communication, help young people delay the initiation of sexual intercourse, increase the use of contraception and condoms, do not encourage young people to begin intercourse, and do not increase the frequency of sexual intercourse.

Kohler et al. (2008) found that young people who received comprehensive sexuality education were significantly less likely to report a teen pregnancy compared to those who received no sexuality education. Abstinence-only programs were not significantly associated with a risk reduction for teen pregnancy when compared with no sexuality education. In comparing abstinence-only programs with comprehensive sexuality education, comprehensive programs were associated with a 50% lower risk of teen pregnancy. Also, teaching about contraception was not associated with an increased risk of adolescent sexual activity or an STI.

Kirby (2008) found that most abstinence programs did not delay initiation of sexual activity and that only 3 of 9 had any significant positive effects on any sexual behavior. In contrast, two-thirds of comprehensive programs showed strong evidence that they positively affected young people's sexual behavior, including both delaying initiation of sexual activity and increasing condom and contraceptive use for those who decided to become sexually active. He concluded that abstinence programs have little evidence to warrant their widespread replication; conversely, strong evidence suggests that some comprehensive programs should be disseminated widely.

In their publication *Comprehensive Sex Education: Research and Results* (2009), Advocates for Youth summarized what the research indicates. They stated that evaluations of comprehensive sexuality education programs show that such programs can help youth delay onset of sexual activity, reduce the frequency of sexual activity, reduce the number of sexual partners, and increase condom and contraceptive use. Also, those who receive comprehensive sexuality education are "NOT more likely to become sexually active, increase sexual activity, or experience negative sexual health outcomes." Conversely, they also indicated that there is little, if any, evidence to show that abstinence-only programs are effective—even at achieving abstinence among teens.

Related to sexuality education, some professionals have promoted virginity pledges. Rosenbaum (2009) found that 5 years after giving pledges, 82% of pledgers denied having ever pledged. Pledgers and nonpledgers did not differ in premarital sexuality activity, sexually transmitted diseases, and anal and oral sex variables. Pledgers were less likely to protect themselves from pregnancy and disease before marriage.

Grose, Grabe, and Kohfeldt (2014) pointed out that youth are seldom granted access to sexuality education programs that address social factors that are linked to negative sexual health outcomes, such as traditional social norms surrounding gender and sexuality. Using a sample consisting of 95 eighth graders, their study assessed the links between several components of sexual empowerment, including gender ideology, sexual knowledge, and contraceptive beliefs. Findings correlated participation in the program with more progressive attitudes toward girls and women, less agreement with the idea that males should be dominant, and increases in sexual health and resource knowledge. Participation in the sexual education program also led to safer beliefs related to contraception.

Gowen and Winges-Yanez (2014) explored the issue of whether current sexuality education materials are tailored to fit the needs of lesbian, gay, bisexual, transgender, and queer/questioning (LGBTQ) youth. They investigated the sexuality education experiences of 30 LGBTQ youth and solicited suggestions for improving the inclusiveness of sexuality education curricula. Results indicated that LGBTQ youth perceived current sexuality education as primarily "exclusive," although examples of "inclusive" sexuality education were provided. In addition, suggestions for creating a more inclusive experience included directly discussing LGBTQ issues, emphasizing STI prevention over pregnancy prevention, and addressing healthy relationships. The researchers felt that these suggestions would make sexuality education more inclusive for all young people.

Grossman et al. (2014) looked at protective effects of comprehensive sexuality education. They also included a family component in their intervention. These researchers followed a cohort of 2,453 sixth graders through the eighth grade. In schools where the comprehensive program was taught, 16% fewer boys and 15% fewer girls had had sexual intercourse by the end of eighth grade. Completing family activities during the first year of the program also predicted delayed sexual debut for boys. The researchers pointed out that greater family involvement may encourage parents to talk with their children earlier and more frequently about sexuality.

The Future of Sexuality Research

More sexuality research is definitely needed. Not only do we need to have more information on sexual behavior itself, but we also need to explore how we make decisions to engage in sexual activity, how the quality of relationships can be improved, and which factors will be important in helping people achieve sexual satisfaction throughout the life cycle. A variety of cultural and societal factors (age, religion, education) have always affected sexual decision making, but recently a change in societal attitudes toward marriage, divorce, childbearing, and sexual relationships has become evident. The stresses these new attitudes bring to bear on personal relationships need to be explored in the near future.

There are real challenges related to sexuality research. Tiefer (1994), in her presidential address to the International Academy of Sex Research, emphasized three crises facing sexology. First, the media are inundating the public with sexual topics. Second, many people in academic circles still hesitate to accept sexuality research as being as legitimate as other forms of research. Finally, there is a tendency for sexuality research to focus only on medical topics and not on the comprehensive nature of people and society. We have learned a great deal through sexuality research; however, even better research methods are needed to fit together the psychological, the biological, and the sociological aspects of sexuality research.

In closing, Tables 2.2 and 2.3 summarize the sexuality research of selected researchers.

TABLE 2.2

Selected Sexuality Researchers and Their Studies (Grouped by Type of Method)

Author(s)	Date	Title
Interview survey		
Scientific literature		
Kinsey, Pomeroy, & Martin	1948	*Sexual behavior in the human male*
	1953	*Sexual behavior in the human female*
Laumann, Gagnon, Michael, & Michaels	1994	*The social organization of sexuality*
Carolina Population Center	2001	National longitudinal study of adolescent health (The "Add Health Survey")
Karofsky	2001	Parent–teen communication and the initiations of sexual intercourse

(Continues)

TABLE 2.2

Selected Sexuality Researchers and Their Studies (Grouped by Type of Method) (Continued)

Author(s)	Date	Title
Interview survey		
Scientific literature		
Bancroft et al.	2004	Sexual activity and risk taking in young heterosexual men: The relevance of sexual arousability, mood, and sensation seeking
Burgard	2004	Factors associated with contraceptive use in late and post apartheid South Africa
Bruckner & Bearman	2004	Ambivalence and pregnancy: Adolescents' attitudes, contraceptive use and pregnancy
Cavanagh	2004	The sexual debut of girls in early adolescence: The intersection of race, pubertal timing, and friendship group characteristics
Connell & Freund	2004	Investigating ethnic differences in sexual health: Focus groups with young people
Harawa et al.	2004	Associations of race/ethnicity with HIV prevalence and HIV related behaviors
Johnson & Jackson	2004	What is the significance of black–white differences in risky sexual behavior?
U.S. Centers for Disease Control and Prevention (Grunbaum et al.)	2004	Youth risk behavior surveillance system
Adam et al.	2005	Acculturation as a predictor of the onset of sexual intercourse among hispanic and white teens
Chuang & Freund	2005	Emergency contraception knowledge among women in a Boston community
Frisco	2005	Parental involvement and young women's contraceptive use
Halpern Fisher et al.	2005	Oral versus vaginal sex among adolescents: Perceptions, attitudes, and behavior
South et al.	2005	Residential mobility and the onset of adolescent sexual activity
Sanders et al.	2010	Which sexual behaviors fit the definition of "having sex"?
Chandra et al.	2011	Sexual behavior, attraction, and identity in the United States
Houck et al.	2014	Adolescent sexting and sexual behavior
Simpson et al.	2014	Influence of hip width on women's sexual behavior
Popular literature		
Hite	1976	*The Hite report*
	1981	*The Hite report on male sexuality*
	1987	*Women and love: A cultural revolution in progress*
Sarrel & Sarrel	1980	The *Redbook* report on sexual relationships
Reinisch & Beasley	1991	*The Kinsey Institute new report on sex*
Kaiser Family Foundation and *Seventeen* magazine	2002	SexSmarts survey on teen sexual behavior
NBC News and *People Magazine*	2004	National Survey of Young Teens Sexual Attitudes and Behavior
Direct observation		
Scientific literature		
Masters & Johnson	1966	*Human sexual response*
	1970	*Human sexual inadequacy*
	1979	*Homosexuality in perspective*

TABLE 2.3

Examples of Additional Research

Author(s)	Date	Title
Oncalem & King	2001	Comparison of men's and women's attempts to dissuade sexual partners from the couple using condoms
Kirby	2001	Emerging answers: Research findings on programs to reduce sexual risk taking and teen pregnancy
Ford et al.	2001	Characteristics of adolescents' sexual partners and their association with use of condoms and other contraceptive methods
Kaiser Family Foundation	2002	Substance use and risky sexual behavior: Attitudes and practices among adolescents and young adults
Child Trends	2002	National longitudinal survey of youth (Most sexually active teens first had sex at home, late at night, survey shows)
Greenbaum et al.	2004	Youth Risk Behavior Surveillance—United States, 2003
Lefkowitz et al.	2004	Religiosity, sexual behaviors, and sexual attitudes during emerging adulthood
Vlassoff et al.	2004	Assessing costs and benefits of sexual and reproductive health interventions
Penhollow et al.	2005	The impact of religiosity on the sexual behaviors of college students
Koch	2006	Women's bodies as a "puzzle" for college men: Grounded theory research
Kirby	2008	Impact of sexuality education programs on adolescent sexual behavior
Kohler et al.	2008	Sexuality education and the initiation of sexual activity
Lescano et al.	2008	Correlates of heterosexual anal intercourse among at-risk adolescents and young adults
Manlove et al.	2008	Condom use and consistency among male adolescents in the United States
Sex and Tech	2008	Results from a survey of teens and young adults
Daniel & Balog	2009	Early female puberty
Rosenbaum	2009	Patient teenagers? A comparison of the sexual behavior of virginity pledgers and matched nonpledgers
Biro et al.	2010	Pubertal assessment and characteristics
Eaton et al.	2010	Youth Risk Behavior Surveillance—United States, 2009
Guttmacher Institute	2010	Facts on contraceptive use in the United States
National Survey of Sexual Health and Behavior (NSSHB)	2010	Research about sexual-health behaviors
Guttmacher Institute	2011	Facts on induced abortion in the United States
Guttmacher Institute	2011	Facts on American teens' sexual health
Lehmiller et al.	2011	Friends with benefits relationships
McFarland et al.	2011	Role of religion on sexual behavior and satisfaction
Pazol et al.	2011	U.S. teen pregnancy statistics
Torian et al.	2011	U.S. HIV statistics
Mark et al.	2011	Factors predicting infidelity in heterosexual couples
Guttmacher Institute	2013	Infographic on contractive effectiveness
Lindberg et al.	2013	Exploration of men's birth intentions
Martin et al.	2013	Incidence of sexual intercourse for high school students
Milhausen et al.	2013	Prevalence and predictors of condom use
Frost et al.	2014	Financial savings from family planning programs
Gowen et al.	2014	Sexuality education materials and LGBTQ youth
Gray et al.	2014	Dating and sexual behavior of single parents
Grose et al.	2014	Sexuality education and sexual empowerment
Grossman et al.	2014	Protective effects of sexuality education
Kahn et al.	2014	Youth Risk Behavior Surveillance—United States, 2013

Exploring the Dimensions of Human Sexuality

© Gayvoronskaya Yana/Shutterstock

It's amazing how many factors are involved in even basic research on sexuality. Political forces have banned the use of government money for research dealing with sexuality, so monies must be provided by private foundations or companies, which may have a political or financial agenda of their own.

Learned behaviors prompt many people to answer questions as they think they should be answered, instead of with the truth, and that tendency can create survey bias. The limited number of people willing to respond to a sexuality survey, especially in lower socioeconomic classes, also hinders researchers.

Finally, cultural, ethnic, and religious biases may hinder researchers from getting the data needed. For example, a survey of sexual behavior based on religious affiliation would do poorly, because many Muslim (the number-two religion in the United States) women would not allow interviews or would do so only with their husband present.

Biological Factors

- The medical model was the focus of sexuality research in the 19th century.
- The sexual response cycle was discovered by the researchers Masters and Johnson.
- Physiological changes in the vagina or penis can be monitored by the vaginal plethysmograph and penile strain gauge, respectively.

Sociocultural Factors

- The gender "double standard" research goes back to the 19th century, when discomfort with women's sexuality prompted such beliefs.
- Education leads to both a later age of first intercourse and a higher likelihood of using contraception at first intercourse.
- Religious adolescents are less likely to participate in sexual intercourse; when they do, they are less likely to use reliable contraceptives.
- Ethical considerations abound in sexuality research.

Psychological Factors

- The NHSLS data found that married people were much more likely than single people to report being extremely or very happy.
- Behaviors and practices, as well as frequency of sexual activity, need to be accounted for in sexuality research.
- Motivation to respond to a sexual research survey may create a bias in the sample.
- Learned attitudes and behaviors may influence answers given on sexuality surveys.

Summary

- The scientific method involves identifying a research question, reviewing literature, formulating a hypothesis, operationalizing the variables, collecting data, and analyzing the data to test the hypothesis.

- Research in sexuality can involve surveys, case studies, experimental research, and direct observation.

- Ethical issues in sexuality research include informed consent, confidentiality, anonymity, and protection of subjects.

- Evaluating information about sexuality found on the Internet is often difficult. We need to ask ourselves important questions, such as the purpose of the site or the source of the information, to better evaluate Internet sexuality content.

- Early sexuality researchers included Richard von Krafft-Ebing, Henry Havelock Ellis, Sigmund Freud, Magnus Hirschfeld, Katherine Davis, and Clelia Mosher.

- In the mid-20th century, Alfred Kinsey did extensive research on sexual attitudes and behavior of males and females.

- The research of Masters and Johnson gave us a great deal of information about human sexual response.

- Many studies have been done to help us know more about premarital sexual attitudes and behavior, teen pregnancy, ethnic differences in sexual attitudes and behaviors, use of contraception, changes in selected statistical relationships, and the effects of sexuality education.

- More sexuality research is definitely needed. Needs include knowing more about how we make decisions about sexual behavior, how to improve the quality of relationships, and which factors will help achieve sexual satisfaction throughout the life cycle.

Discussion Questions

1. Compare and contrast the varied methods of sexuality research.

2. Describe the ethical issues involved in sexuality research, citing examples of each.

3. Who were the early sexuality researchers, and what did they figure out? Is their research still considered valid?

4. List the major modern sexuality researchers and describe their contributions. How has their research changed sexuality?

Application Questions

Reread the story that opens the chapter and answer the following questions.

1. Imagine your parents asked you to explain what sexuality researchers do—and why. Prepare a brief response to their query.

2. Explain which dimensions of human sexuality would influence congressional funding for a study on sexuality. Would representatives from some states be more willing to support sexuality research? Explain your answer.

3. For over a year, allegations of sexual relations between former President Clinton and White House intern Monica Lewinsky rocked the news. Evaluate why, in light of a sexual scandal, the president's approval ratings continued to climb.

Critical Thinking Questions

1. What motivates a person to take the time and effort to respond to a human sexuality research questionnaire? Could that motivation lead to a sample bias?

2. Masters and Johnson were not the only team to discover a human sexual response cycle. How is it possible that different research groups obtained different results regarding a physiological response?

3. In 1991, the U.S. federal government pulled support from the NHSLS research project and passed legislation prohibiting the spending of federal funds on sexuality research. Although this was clearly a political move, it raises the question, Why should the government support such research? Put another way, how does sexuality research help the American people?

4. Imagine that you and/or your lover read a popular magazine sex survey that showed that a large percentage of people were doing a sexual activity that you had never tried. Would that motivate you to try something new? Would you encourage your lover to try it? How would you feel if your lover asked you to try it?

Critical Thinking Case

Years ago it was widely reported that Russian track and field athletes were encouraged to have sexual relations the night before a major meet. In fact, reports claimed that those who did so performed better (closer to their potential). Imagine that the coach of your college's track team has just learned this information. He has asked you to design a sexuality research project, using scientific methodology, to prove or disprove the hypothesis that sexual activity leads to improved athletic performance.

Which method(s) of research would give you the best results? Explain why. Is it possible to prove the validity of such a hypothesis? Which other factors might be involved? Which ethical issues might you encounter? How could those issues be overcome?

Exploring Personal Dimensions

Sexuality Research
Mark each of the following statements "true" or "false."

_____ 1. All research completed as part of the National Health and Social Life Survey was financially supported by the U.S. federal government.

_____ 2. The first step in the scientific method is identifying a research question.

_____ 3. A hypothesis is a statement based on research results.

_____ 4. Kinsey's research is an example of survey research.

_____ 5. The research of Masters and Johnson is an example of experimental research.

_____ 6. A plethysmograph is used in the laboratory to measure and chart physiological changes over time.

_____ 7. Most normal women have orgasms from penile thrusting alone.

_____ 8. The Sex and Tech study in 2008 showed that a significant number of teens have electronically sent, or posted online, nude or semi-nude pictures or videos of themselves.

_____ 9. The Liu Report can be correctly referred to as a Chinese National Health and Social Life Survey.

_____10. More than half the U.S. students in grades 9–12 have participated in sexual intercourse.

_____11. Both the proportion of adolescent females in the United States who have experienced sexual intercourse and their likelihood of pregnancy have increased in recent years.

_____12. Good sexuality education programs do not hasten the onset of sexual intercourse and may increase the use of contraception—particularly condoms.

Interpretation
All of the even-numbered statements are true and all of the odd-numbered statements are false. If you were correct on at least 10 statements, you did well. If you were not correct on at least 10 statements, find the correct answers in the chapter. All of the correct answers are in this chapter on sexuality research.

Suggested Readings

Brecher, E. *The sex researchers*. New York: Signet Books, 1969.

Chandrda, A., Mosher, W.D., Copen, C, & Sionean, C. Sexual behavior, sexual attraction, and sexual identity in the United States: Data from the 2006–2008 National Survey of Family Growth. National *Health Statistics Report, 36* (March, 2011),1–36. Available: *http://www.cdc.gov/nchs/data/nhsr/nhsr036.pdf.*

Cox, S., Pazol, K., Warner, L., Romero, L., Spitz, A., Gavin, L., & Barfield, W. Vital signs: Births to teens aged 15–17 years—United States, 1991–2012. *Morbidity and Mortality Weekly Report, 64* (April 8, 2014). Available: http://www.cdc.gov/mmwr/pdf.

Dodge, B., Reece, M., Herbenick, D., Schick, V., Sanders, S., & Fortenberry, J.D. Sexual health among U.S. black and Hispanic men and women. A national representative study. *The Journal of Sexual Medicine, 7, Issue Supplement a5* (October 2010), 330–345.

Kahn, L., Kinchen, S., Shankin, S. L., Fint, K. H., Hawkins, J., Harris, W. A., Lowry, R., O'Malley, E., McManus, T., Chyen, D., Whittle, L., Taylor, E., Demissie, Z., Brener, N., Thornton, J., Moore, J., & Zaza, S. Youth risk behavior surveillance—United States, 2013. *Morbidity and Mortality Weekly Report, 63, 4,* (June 13, 2014). Available: http://www.cdc.gov/mmwr/pdf.

Pomeroy, W. *Dr. Kinsey and the Institute for Sex Research*. New York: Harper & Row, 1972.

U.S. Department of Commerce and the Executive Office of the President. *Women in America: Indicators of social and economic well-being*. March 2011. Available: http://www.whitehouse.gov/sites/default/files/rss_viewer/Women_in_America.pdf.

Web Resources

Information on Marie Stopes, an early sexuality researcher
www.encyclopedia.com/topic/Marie_Carmichael_Stopes.aspx

Contains additional information about an early sexuality researcher.

Society for the Scientific Study of Sexuality: Annual Review of Sex Research
www.sexscience.org

Provides updated information on various sexuality research topics.

The Kinsey Institute Research Program
www.kinseyinstitute.org/research/surveylinks.html

Information about many present and past sexuality research studies.

The Alan Guttmacher Institute: New Research and Analysis
www.agi-usa.org

With emphasis on research related to pregnancy and to abortion, the Guttmacher Institute has information on many sexuality research topics.

Sexuality Information and Education Council of the United States
www.siecus.org

Information and publications on numerous sexuality topics are available from the Sexuality Information and Education Council of the United States (SIECUS).

References

Advocates for Youth. *Comprehensive sex education: Research and results,* 2009. Available: http://www.advocatesforyouth.org/publications-a-z/1487-publications.

Albert, Bill. *With one voice 2004: America's adults and teens sound off about teen pregnancy.* Washington, D.C.: National Campaign to Prevent Teen Pregnancy, December 2004.

Biro, F. M., Galvez, M. P., Greenspan, L. C., Succop, P. A., Vangeepuram, N., Pinney, S. M., Teitelbaum, S., Windham, G. C., Kushi, L. H., & Wolff, M. S. Pubertal assessment method and baseline characteristics in a mixed longitudinal study of girls. *Pediatrics, 126, no. 3* (September 1, 2010), e583–e590.

Bruckner, H., Martin, A., & Bearman, P. S. Ambivalence and pregnancy: Adolescents' attitudes, contraceptive use and pregnancy. *Perspect Sex Reprod Health, 36, no. 6* (November/December 2004), 248–257.

Burgard, S. Factors associated with contraceptive use in late- and post-apartheid South Africa. *Studies in Family Planning, 35, no. 2* (June 2004), 91–104.

Cavanagh, S. E. The sexual debut of girls in early adolescence: The intersection of race, pubertal timing, and friendship group characteristics. *Journal of Research on Adolescence, 14, no. 3* (September 2004), 285–312.

Chandra, A., Mosher, W. D., Copen, C., & Sionean, C. (2011). Sexual behavior, sexual attraction, and sexual identity in the United States: Data from the 2006–2008 National Survey of Family Growth. *National Health Statistics Reports 36* (March 2011), 1–49.

Chuang, C. H., & Freund, K. M. Emergency contraception knowledge among women in a Boston community. *Contraception, 71, no. 2* (Feb. 2005), 157–160.

Connell, P., McKevitt, C., & Low, N. Investigating ethnic differences in sexual health: Focus groups with young people. *Sexually Transmitted Infections, 80, no. 4* (August 2004), 300–305.

Dailard, C. Recent findings from the "Add Health" survey: Teens and sexual activity. *The Guttmacher Report, 4, no. 4* (August 2001), 1–3, 2–4.

Daniel, E., & Balog, L. F. Early female puberty: A review of research on etiology and implications. *The Health Educator, 41, no. 2* (Fall 2009), 47–53.

Dennison, R. P., & Russell, S. T. Positive perspectives on adolescent sexuality: Contributions of the National Longitudinal Study of Adolescent Health. *Sexuality Research & Social Policy, 2, 4* (December 2005), 54–59.

Dolan, B. No sex please, we're ignorant. *Time* (September 17, 1990), 71.

Eaton, D. K., Kann, L., Kinchen, S., Shanklin, S., Ross, J., Hawkins, J. Harris, W. A., Lowry, R., McManus, T. Cheyen, D., Lim, C., Whittle, L., Brener, N. D., & Wechsler, H. Youth risk behavior surveillance—United States, 2009. In: *Surveillance Summaries*, June 4, 2010, *Morbidity and Mortality Weekly Report, 59, no. SS-5* (2010), 1–143.

Facts on American teens' sexual and reproductive health. Guttmacher Institute, January 2011. Available: http://www.guttmacher.org/pubs/FB-ATSRH.html.

Facts on contraceptive use in the United States. Guttmacher Institute, May 2011. Available: http://www.guttmacher.org/pubs/fb_contr_use.html.

Facts on induced abortion in the United States. Guttmacher Institute, June 2010. Available: http://www.guttmacher.org/pubs/fb_induced_abortion.html.

Ford, K., Woosung, S., & Lepowski, J. Characteristics of adolescents' sexual partners and their association with use of condoms and other contraceptive methods. *Family Planning Perspectives, 33, no. 3* (May/June 2001), 100–105, 132.

Frisco, M. Parental involvement and young women's contraceptive use. *Journal of Marriage and Family, 67, no. 1* (February 2005), 110–121.

Frost, J. J., Sonfield, A., Zolna, M. R., & Finer, L. B. Return on investment: A fuller assessment of the benefits and cost savings of the U.S. publicly funded family planning program. *Milbank Quarterly*. 2014. Available: http://onlinelibrary.wiley.com/enhanced/doi/10.1111/1468-0009.12080/gt.

Gowen, L. K., & Winges-Yanez, N. Lesbian, gay, bisexual, transgender, queer, and questioning youths' perspectives of inclusive school-based sexuality education. *Journal of Sex Research, 51, 7* (2014), 788–800.

Gray, P. B., Garcia, J. R., Crosier, B. S., & Fisher, H. E. Dating and sexual behavior among single parents of young children in the United States. *Journal of Sex Research* (2014). DOI: 10.1080/00224499.2014.941454.

Grose, R. G., Grabe, S., & Kohfeldt, D. Sexual education, gender ideology, and youth sexual empowerment. *Journal of Sex Research, 51, 7* (2014), 742–753.

Grossman, J. M. Tracy, A. J., Charmaraman, L., Ceder, I., & Erkut, S. Protective effects of middle school comprehensive sex education with family involvement. *Journal of School Health, 84* (2014), 939–747.

Haffner, D. W., & Goldfarb, E. S. *But, does it work? Improving evaluations of sexuality education.* Sexuality Information and Education Council of the United States, 1988.

Halpern-Felsher, B. L., Cornell, J. L., Kropp, R. Y., & Tschann, J. M. Oral versus vaginal sex among adolescents: Perceptions, attitudes, and behavior. *Pediatrics, 115, no. 4* (April 2005), 845–851.

Harawa, N. T., et al., Associations of race/ethnicity with HIV prevalence and HIV-related behaviors. *Journal of Acquired Immune Deficiency Syndrome, 35, no. 5* (March 2004), 526–536.

History of sex surveys: Factors in the sex life of 2200 women. Trivia-Library.com (2005). Available: www.trivia-library.com.

Hite, S. *The Hite report.* New York: Macmillan, 1976.

Hite, S. *The Hite report on male sexuality.* New York: Alfred Knopf, 1981.

Hite, S. *Women and love: A cultural revolution in progress.* New York: Alfred Knopf, 1987.

Houck, D., Barker D., Rizzo, C., Hancock, E., Norton, A., & Brown, L. K. Sexting and sexual behavior in at-risk adolescents. *Pediatrics, 132, 2* (2014), e276–e282. DOI: 10.1542/peds.2013-1157.

Johnson, E. H., & Jackson, L. A. What is the significance of black–white differences in risky sexual behavior? *Journal of the National Medical Association, 86, no. 10* (October 2004), 745–759.

Kahn, L., Kinchen, S., Shanklin, S. L., Flint, K. H., Hawkins, J., Harris, W. A., Lowry, R., Olsen, E. O., McManus, T., Chyen, D., Whittle, L., Taylor, E., Demissie, Z., Brener, N., Thornton, J., Moore, J., & Zaza, S. Youth risk behavior surveillance—United States, 2013. *Mortality and Morbidity Weekly Report, 63, 4* (2014), 1–168.

Kaiser Family Foundation and *Seventeen* magazine release latest SexSmarts survey on teen sexual behavior. Kaiser Family Foundation (July 9, 2002). Available: http://kff.org/womens -health-policy/poll-finding/sexsmarts-survey-teens-and -sexual-health-communication/.

Kinsey, A. C., Pomeroy, W. B., & Martin, C. E. *Sexual behavior in the human female*. Philadelphia: Saunders, 1953.

Kinsey, A. C., Pomeroy, W. B., & Martin, C. E. *Sexual behavior in the human male*. Philadelphia: Saunders, 1948.

The Kinsey Institute. *The history and concept of sexology*, 1998.

Kirby, D. *Emerging answers: Research findings on programs to reduce sexual risk-taking and teen pregnancy*. Washington, DC: National Campaign to Prevent Teen Pregnancy, 2001.

Kirby, D. H. The impact of abstinence and comprehensive sex and STD/HIV education programs on adolescent sexual behavior. *Sexuality Research Social Policy, 5, no. 3* (September 2008), 18–27.

Koch, P. B. Women's bodies as a "puzzle" for college men: Grounded theory research. *American Journal of Sexuality Education, 1, 3* (2006), 51–72.

Kohler, P. K., Manhart, L. E., & Lafferty, W. E. Abstinence-only and comprehensive sex education and the initiation of sexual activity and teen pregnancy. *Journal of Adolescent Health, 42, no. 4* (April 2009), 344–351.

Laumann, E. O., Michael, R. T., & Gagnon, J. H. A political history of the National Sex Survey of Adults. *Family Planning Perspectives, 26, no. 1* (1994).

Lefkowitz, E. S., Gillen, M. M., Shearer, C. L., & Boone, T. L. Religiosity, sexual behaviors, and sexual attitudes during emerging childhood. *Journal of Sex Research, 41, no. 2* (May 2004), 150–159.

Lehmiller, J. J., VanderDrift, L. E., & Kelly, J. R. Sex differences in approaching friends with benefits relationships. *Journal of Sex Research, 48, no. 2–3* (March 2011), 275–284.

Lescano, C. M., Houck, C. D., Brown, L. K., Doherty, G., DiClemente, R. J., Fernandez, M. I., Pugatch, D., Schlenger, W. E., & Silver, B. J. Correlates of heterosexual anal intercourse among at-risk adolescents and young adults. *American Journal of Public Health, 99* (2009), 1131–1136.

Lindberg, L. D., & Kost, K. Exploring U.S. men's birth intentions. *Maternal and Child Health Journal, 18, 3* (June 22, 2013), 625–633.

Manlove, J., Ikramullah, E., & Terry-Humen, E. Condom use and consistency among male adolescents in the United States. *Journal of Adolescent Health, 43, 4* (October 2008), 325–333.

Mark, K. P., Janssen, E., & Milhausen, R. R. Infidelity in heterosexual couples: Demographic, interpersonal, and personality-related predictors of extradyadic sex. *Archives of Sexual Behavior, 40, 5* (2011), 971–982.

Martin, J. A., Hamilton, B. E., Osterman, M. J. K., Curtin, M. A., & Mathews, T. J. Births: Final data for 2012. *National Vital Statistics Reports, 62, 9* (December 30, 2013), 1–87.

Masters, W. H., & Johnson, V. E. *Homosexuality in perspective*. Boston: Little, Brown, 1979.

Masters, W. H., & Johnson, V. E. *Human sexual inadequacy*. Boston: Little, Brown, 1970.

Masters, W. H., & Johnson, V. E. *Human sexual response*. Boston: Little, Brown, 1966.

McFarland, M. J., Uecher, J. E., & Regerus, M. D. The role of religion in shaping sexual frequency and satisfaction: Evidence from married and unmarried older adults. *Journal of Sex Research, 48, no. 2 & 3* (March 2011), 297–308.

Milhausen, R. R., McKay, A., Graham, C. A., Crosby, R. A., Yarber, W. L., & Sanders, S. A. Prevalence and predictors of condom use in a national sample of Canadian university students. *Canadian Journal of Human Sexuality, 22, 3* (December 2013), 142–151.

National Center for Complementary and Alternative Medicine. *10 things to know about evaluating medical resources on the Web*, 2011. Available: http://nccam.nih.gov/health /webresources/.

National Survey of Sexual Health and Behavior. Center for Sexual Health Promotion, Indiana University, 2010. Available: http://www.nationalsexstudy.indiana.edu.

Nearly 3 in 10 young teens sexually active: NBC News, *People* magazine commission landmark national poll. *NBC News* (January 19, 2004, updated January 31, 2005). Available: http://www.msnbc.msn.com/id/6839072.

New infographic: Contraception is highly effective. Guttmacher Institute Media Center. June 5, 2013. Available: www .guttmacher.org/media/interviews/2013/06/05/.

Oncalem, R. & King, B. Comparison of men's and women's attempts to dissuade sexual partners from the couple using condoms. *Archives of Sexual Behavior, 30, no. 4* (August 2001), 379–391.

Pazol, K., Warner, L., Gavin, L., Callaghan, W. M., Spitz, A. M., Anderson, J. E., Barfield, W. D., & Kann, L. Vital signs: Teen pregnancy—United States, 1991–2009. *Morbidity and Mortality Weekly Report, 60, no. 13* (April 8, 2011), 414–420.

Penhollow, T., Young, M., & Denny, G. The impact of religiosity on the sexual behaviors of college students. *American Journal of Health Education, 36, no. 2* (March/April 2005), 75–83.

Rosenbaum, J. E. Patient teenagers? A comparison of the sexual behavior of virginity pledgers and matched nonpledgers. *Pediatrics, 123, 1* (January 2009), e110–e120.

Sanders, S. A., Hill, B. J., Yarber, W. L., Graham, C. A., Crosby, R. A., & Milhausen, R. R. Misclassification bias: Diversity in conceptualisations about having "had sex." *Sexual Health, 7, 1* (2010), 31–34. DOI: 10.1071/SH09068.

Sarrel, P., & Sarrel, L. The *Redbook* report on sexual relationships, part I. *Redbook* (October 1980), 73–80.

Sex and Tech. Washington, DC: *National Campaign to Prevent Teen and Unplanned Pregnancy,* 2008. Available: http://www .thenationalcampaign.org/sextech/PDF/SexTech_Summary.pdf.

Simpson, V. J., Brewer, G., & Hendrie, C. A. Evidence to suggest that women's sexual behavior is influenced by hip width rather than waist-to-hip ratio. *Archives of Sexual Behavior, 43* (2014), 1367–1371. DOI: 10.1007/s10508-014-0289-z.

South, S. J., Haynie, D. L., & Bose, S. Residential mobility and the onset of adolescent sexual activity. *Journal of Marriage and Family, 67, no. 2* (May 2005), 499–514.

Substance use and risky sexual behavior: Attitudes and practices among adolescents and young adults. *American Journal of Health Education, 33, no. 5* (September/October 2002), 278–281.

Tiefer, L. Three crises facing sexology. *Archives of Sexual Behavior, 23, no. 4* (1994), 361–373.

Torian, L., Chen, M., Rhodes, P., & Hall, H. I. HIV surveillance—United States, 1991–2008. *Morbidity and Mortality Weekly Report, 60, no. 21* (June 3, 2011), 689–693.

Trends in sexual risk behaviors among high school students—United States, 1991–2001. *Morbidity and Mortality Weekly Report, 51, no. 38* (September 27, 2002), 856–859.

Vlassoff, M., Singh, S., Darroch, J. E., Carbone, E., & Bernstein, S. *Assessing costs and benefits of sexual and reproductive health interventions.* New York: Guttmacher Institute, 2004.

von Krafft-Ebing, R. *Psychopathia sexualis.* Stuttgart, Germany, 1902.

Women in American history. *Britannica Online.* Available: http:// www.britannica.com.

CHAPTER 3

Sexual Communication

© Gayvoronskaya Yana/Shutterstock

FEATURES

Multicultural Dimensions
Female and Male Subcultures?

Communication Dimensions
Adult Sexting

Ethical Dimensions
Ethics, Communication, and Date Rape

Gender Dimensions
Sexual Behavior in Marriage

Communication Dimensions
Clarity in Sexual Communication

Global Dimensions
International Differences in Discussing Sexuality

Communication Dimensions
Guidelines for Healthy Sexual Communication

CHAPTER OBJECTIVES

1 Describe the process of sexual communication, including nonverbal communication.

2 Identify barriers to sexual communication, including gender differences, attitudes about sexuality, and sexual language.

3 Discuss techniques for improving sexual communication.

INTRODUCTION

*I*magine watching a movie that follows the life of a young couple together—through courtship and marriage, infidelity, and parenthood. The film presents a lovely portrayal of a young couple growing in—and eventually out of—love. It not only shows the life cycle of a 12-year relationship, but also brilliantly portrays how communication changes during that life cycle.

As the couple meets and falls in love at a dizzying pace, conversation flows. It seems there is nothing that they cannot talk about. They openly share their worlds together, delighting in the pleasure of each other. They communicate with touch, holding hands, kissing, and intimate sexual activity.

In one blissful scene, the young lovers are shown to their table in a nice restaurant. They hold hands, giggle, smile, make eye contact while walking across the restaurant. But they notice an older married couple who are eating their dinner. The couple is simply eating—no conversation, no touching, no eye contact. One of the young lovers turns and suggests to the other, "I guess married people don't talk."

But as their relationship and life change, so does their communication style. In time, they have experienced life together, and they do not talk about it as much as they used to talk about their lives before they met. The mistakes they made as youths disappear into their sophisticated adulthood. There are no silly mistakes to giggle about anymore.

In time, they begin to know each other so well that each can antici- pate what the other is going to say or wants to do. Verbal expression becomes infrequent, because it no longer seems very important.

And their lives change, too: They become parents, and do well in their chosen professions. Children and work decrease the amount of time they have for each other. Again, life changes alter communication styles.

Eventually, the couple is back in the same restaurant, but this time as a married couple—no talk, no touch, no eye contact. A young couple, holding hands and giggling, looks at them; one whispers something in the other's ear. The older couple have come full circle—they are the married couple who do not talk!

Of course, one of the pleasures of being in a long-term relationship is that there is such a high level of comfort that sometimes you do not have to talk. Yet the very essence of a relationship is communication. Over time, if you rely on your assumptions about what the other per- son wants, needs, or thinks, the relationship begins to break down—and knowing what your partner wants all the time can become old hat. As people do in real life, our couple fails to bridge the gap between not need- ing to talk constantly and not communicating.

Their relationship deteriorates. They meet new people, have affairs—all in an effort to relive those days of carefree expression, of newness and excite- ment. Eventually the marriage ends; the full cycle of the relationship has been portrayed in less time than it may take you to read this chapter!

Many of you who have had long-term relationships can probably relate to this story. When partners fail to communicate freely about sexu- ality or other topics, their relationship is bound to be limited—in scope and time. You have a great opportunity to enrich your relationships and sexual experiences when you can communicate with your partner about arousing mind and body experiences, your feelings about each other, and the other's preferences in life and in sexuality.

■ The Process of Communicating Sexually

Effective communication begins with an understand- ing of how communication works. The basic com- munication model (Figure 3.1) illustrates the five steps of the communication process. Let us consider how the basic communication model might work in a relationship in which partners are participating in some sexual activity.

First, the sender has an idea. Partner A (the sender) does not want to have sexual intercourse. The nature of the idea is influenced by many factors, such as the context of the situation and the sender's mood, background, culture, and frame of reference. For example, Partner A may be too tired or upset, perhaps it is already too late at night, or perhaps Partner A does not know enough about Partner B. Whatever the reasons, Partner A does not want to participate.

Second, the sender encodes the idea in a message. **Encoding** means converting the idea into words or gestures to convey meaning. Partner A says, "I do not want to have sexual intercourse." A potential problem is that words have different meanings for different people. If misunderstandings result from missed meanings, that process is called **bypassing**. For example, Partner B may think all forms of sexual behavior except sexual intercourse are acceptable to Partner A. It may also be possible that Partner B thinks Partner A is just "saying" this and does not really mean it.

Third, the message travels over a channel. Channels include speech, phones, computers, and written correspondence. In this case, the channel contains speech and gestures. Partner A's voice tones, inflections, and gestures are part of the channel.

Fourth, the receiver (Partner B) decodes the message. **Decoding** means translating the message from its symbol form into meaning. Communication can be successful only when decoding is accurate. Various forms of "noise," however, can distort the message. In its simplest sense, the noise of a crowded room makes hearing difficult. Noise can also be represented by misinterpretation of words, voice tones, or gestures; emotional reactions; or the use of alcohol or other drugs. In our example, after having several drinks, Partner B hears, "Come and convince me."

Fifth, the receiver responds verbally or nonverbally—this is called **feedback**. Feedback helps the sender know whether the message was received and understood. In view of what Partner B

Basic Communication Model

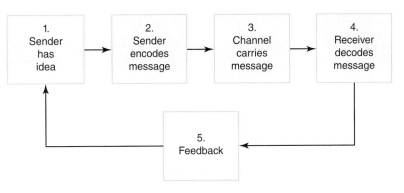

FIGURE **3.1** The basic communication model.

heard, feedback is sent in the form of further sexual advances, because "noise" disturbed the transmission of Partner A's message.

Note that in Figure 3.1 the model provides for continual sending, receiving, and feedback. In our example, it is likely that the feedback provided by Partner B will result in additional communication from Partner A, and so the process continues.

Nonverbal Communication

Nonverbal communication includes all unwritten and unspoken messages. These may be sent intentionally or unintentionally. These silent signals exert a strong influence on the receiver in our basic communication model, but interpreting them can be difficult. For example, does the fact that Person A is looking down indicate modesty or just fatigue? Do crossed arms indicate that a person is unwilling to communicate or that a person feels cold?

The vast majority of message meaning (some experts say more than 90%) is sent nonverbally. Messages can be difficult to decipher when verbal and nonverbal messages seem to contradict each other. For example, if Person A says it is acceptable to participate in sexual intercourse but then is not very responsive, Person B may have a problem knowing what Person A is really communicating.

When verbal and nonverbal messages conflict, receivers often have more faith in the nonverbal cues than what is said. It is important to recognize the

Communication can change in the course of a relationship. From your personal experience, has communication changed over the long term of a relationship?

encoding Converting an idea into words or gestures to convey meaning.

bypassing When misunderstandings result from missed meanings.

decoding Translating the message from its symbol form into meaning.

feedback When the receiver responds verbally or nonverbally.

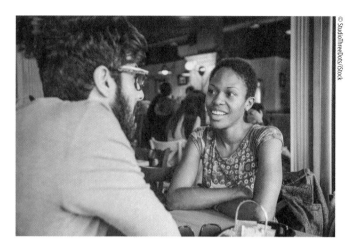

You can show interest in your partner with nonverbal communication. Gazing into each other's eyes, leaning in toward each other, smiling, and touching are all ways of conveying interest in one another.

significance of nonverbal communication, but it is unwise to attach a specific meaning to each gesture in every situation.

Note the body posture of your classmates. During an interesting class activity, most of them will probably be leaning or looking toward the lecturer or the center of the group, indicating that they are involved in what is happening. During a boring class, they will probably be leaning away from the lecturer or group. We call this physical behavior *body language*. Communicating by body posture often conveys as much as, or more than, the spoken word. When people feel uncomfortable about expressing their thoughts or feelings verbally, body language may be the only form of communication in which they participate.

We all recognize the importance of communicating nonverbally: We smile when we say hello, scratch our heads when perplexed, and hug a friend to show affection. (We also have an array of body terms to describe our nonverbal behavior: "Keep a stiff upper lip," "I can't stomach him," "She has no backbone," "I'm tongue-tied," "He caught her eye," "I have two left feet," "That was spine-tingling.") We show appreciation and affection, revulsion and indifference with expressions and gestures. We tell people we are interested in them by merely making eye contact and, as the male peacock displays his feathers, we display our sexuality by the ways we dress and walk and even by the way we stand.

Unfortunately, the nonverbal expression of feelings and thoughts is easy to misinterpret. College students often indicate that they think there are differences in male and female nonverbal communication. Many males and females say that women are

more expressive and better at sending and receiving nonverbal messages. This might include smiling, having an expressive face, using hands to communicate, and having an expressive voice. In contrast, men might be louder, more likely to interrupt, and be more uneasy about the use of nonverbal behaviors.

Consequently, to depend on nonverbal communication alone to express yourself sexually is to risk being misunderstood. Furthermore, if your partner is depending on nonverbal communication to express feelings to you, it is up to you to find out—verbally—whether you are getting the right message. Without such a reality check, your partner, although totally failing to connect, might assume that he or she is communicating effectively. For example, imagine that a man and woman on their first date begin hugging, kissing, and caressing each other after a movie. The woman's breathing speeds up, and the man, taking this as a sign of sexual arousal and interest, presses onward. When the woman suddenly pushes free and complains that the man is too impatient, he is confused. The problem here is one of interpretation rather than incompatibility: The rapid breathing that the man took as a sign of arousal was really a sign of nervousness. If these people had been more effective verbal communicators, they would have been able to clarify the situation in the beginning. Instead they reached a silent impasse, with him confused and her resentful. It can work the other way around, too; both people may want to touch each other but feel too awkward to show it and thus are disappointed.

There are many forms of nonverbal communication. Lists of the types often include eye contact, facial expression, tone of voice, posture, touch, intensity, timing and pace, and sounds that convey understanding (such as "ahhh," "ummm," and "ohhh") as the most important nonverbal clues. Probably three

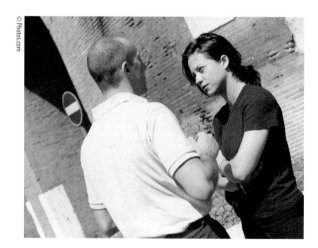

Misinterpretation of your partner's body language can often lead to conflict in a relationship.

Multicultural
DIMENSIONS

Female and Male Subcultures? Male–female communication is related to gender issues. In the business world sometimes males and females seem to be members of different subcultures: Even though business meetings are increasingly coed gatherings, there are often real differences in the behavior of females and males.

Men seated around conference tables often put on a show of bravado while trading "witty" put-downs to protect themselves from the pain of criticism. As a prerequisite to success, their culture has taught them to be both self-effacing and self-promoting.

Women, by contrast, have learned from their culture to be perfectionists, eager to show they have done all their homework by explaining every point; yet they are quick to admit mistakes. A woman executive reported seeing this at a meeting where a female colleague began her presentation with many apologies, telling the group that needed information was not available, that her slides probably contained typos, and so on. But she went on to give a flawless presentation with perfect slides. The man who followed her launched right into his presentation with no apologies and his slides were much less well put together.

On average, men talk more at meetings than women, and so their ideas typically are adopted more often. Men also are more comfortable making up things, so if someone asks about a particular financial figure, for example, they may offer one. A woman is more likely to say, "I'm not sure about that." Women sometimes give the impression that they do not know what they are talking about, whereas many men seem confident whether they know a little or a lot.

However, it is probably possible to change behaviors and expectations in different cultures. For example, at some companies, female executives report a "comfort level" about speaking freely at meetings that they did not feel working at other places.

Of course, we cannot assume that all males or females will behave exactly as those described do. We also have to remember that possible communication differences are not always a result of being a male or a female. For example, the differences might be related to status rather than sex. The point is that we need to be aware of possible subcultural differences in our personal relationships as well as in our business relationships. Understanding these possible differences can be helpful in improving communication in all relationships.

On a very different note related to possible female and male subcultures, it is known that many women pretend, or "fake," orgasm, but is this also true for men? Among 180 male and 101 female college students, it was found that both men and women pretended orgasm (28% and 67%, respectively). Most pretended during penile–vaginal intercourse, but some pretended during oral sexual activity, manual stimulation, and phone sex. Frequently reported reasons for faking were that orgasm was unlikely, they wanted the sexual activity to end, and they wanted to avoid negative consequences (for example, hurting their partner's feelings) and to obtain positive consequences (for example, pleasing their partner). Results also suggest a sexual script in which women should orgasm before men and that men are responsible for women's orgasms.

Note the implications in this study related to communication between sexual partners before and during sexual activity.

Source: Muehlenhard, C. L., & Shippee, S. K. Men's and women's reports of pretending orgasm. *Journal of Sex Research, 47, no. 6* (Nov.–Dec. 2010), 552–567.

---

of the most important forms of nonverbal communication are proximity, eye contact, and touching.

Another name for proximity is *nearness*. Even in our example of students' leaning in the direction of the speaker if they are interested, they are showing nearness. Most often, however, proximity refers to the face-to-face distances between people. Although there are differences, in most cultures moving closer indicates increased interest or intimacy, and moving farther away indicates the opposite.

Making eye contact with another person shows interest. This can be true when one is simply listening to another person; however, making eye contact with another person for a little longer than usual can also be a signal of interest in a relationship.

Touching can be very important in a relationship, and it can show interest, intimacy, and emotional closeness. It can range from a slight touch to show concern or connection to the intimate touching associated with sexual relationships. Touch must be

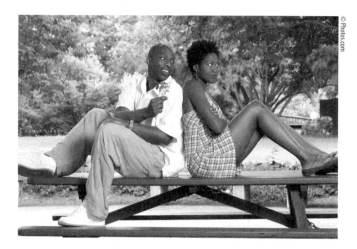

Body position can be a barrier to effective communication.

used with caution. For example, if someone you do not know very well touches you, that action could be offensive to you. Also, in social and work situations it is important to be careful in using touch to prevent appearing overly intimate and to avoid giving any suggestion of sexual harassment.

Van Wagner (2009) provides some nonverbal communication tips. Here are a few of them:

1. Pay attention to nonverbal signals. This will help improve communication for both the sender and the receiver.

2. Look for incongruent behaviors. When words don't match up with nonverbal signals, people tend to ignore what is said and focus instead on nonverbal expressions of moods, thoughts, and emotions.

3. Use good eye contact. Do not stare fixedly into someone's eyes—but note that failing to look others in the eye makes it seem like there is something to hide.

4. Ask questions about nonverbal signals. If there is confusion about a person's nonverbal signals, it can help to ask questions.

5. Be aware that signals can be misread. A person's overall demeanor tells a lot more than a single gesture.

Barriers to Effective Sexual Communication

For many people, it is sometimes hard to talk about sexuality. Keeping silent about it, however, helps promote ignorance and can lead to bad sexual health

outcomes. Keeping silent also helps people promote myths about sexuality that might sound accurate in the absence of honest and open sexual communication. To help improve sexual communication, it can be helpful to consider common obstacles to good sexual communication (Barriers to good sexual communication, 2014):

- *Sex myths.* Lies we have been told about sexuality present a barrier to good sexual communication. One of the keys to good sexual activity is an ability to talk about it.

- *Sexual fear.* Our various fears (such as sexual rejection, making a fool of oneself, disclosing sexual desires) can be obstacles to good communication. They can make it hard to talk about sexuality honestly with the people around us.

- *Negative beliefs about sexuality.* Most people are raised with some negative beliefs. These can be personal (e.g., your body is ugly or dirty) or more universal (e.g., sexuality is bad; sexual activity should be used only for procreation, it leads to immorality). These beliefs act as a strong deterrent to talking about sexuality.

- *Lack of sexuality information.* To talk about sexuality, it helps to have some basic information. Many people do not have accurate information, which poses another barrier to communication.

- *Sexual vocabulary.* Children are rarely taught the correct names for genitalia or sexual behaviors. Some people find it hard to talk about sexuality because they do not know the words to express what they want to say. Having a basic sexual vocabulary can make it easier to talk about sexuality.

- *Privacy.* We are told that sexuality is private, and you need privacy to talk about it. But it can often be hard to get privacy. Carving out privacy in terms of both space and time will make sexual communication go more smoothly.

- *Boundaries.* One of the reasons talking about sexuality may feel threatening is that you are putting yourself "out there" in some way. Good sexual communication usually means having a clear sense of personal boundaries. Without this, you may disclose more than you are comfortable with or even take more responsibility for the person you are talking to than you really should.

Male/Female Communication Issues

There can be disagreements about possible differences between male and female communication patterns. However, we would all probably agree that if we want to promote high-quality relationships, we need to do all we can to reduce the potential for miscommunication. Through the years, there have been many studies done and articles written about male and female communication patterns. A few examples are summarized here in chronological order.

Do males and females naturally communicate differently, or are their communication behaviors learned just as other behaviors are? Some people believe that males are socialized to be more assertive and direct, in both verbal and nonverbal communication. Eye contact, body placement, and rough physical contact by males can communicate intention, superiority, and territoriality. Historically, women have generally been socialized to have a less pronounced presence. They tend, for example, to listen empathetically, communicate and elicit emotions, and process conflict. As a result, a familiar complaint of women in heterosexual relationships is that male partners "never want to talk about things," "aren't sensitive to their needs," and "just don't understand." Conversely, males often wonder how a seemingly innocuous comment could cause their female partner's sudden silence or desire to talk about where the relationship is going. People internalize the values attached to communication to the point that men become used to living within conflict and women prefer the roles of peacemaker and relationship builder. Some people argue that looking at sex exclusively as the source of different communication styles is a mistake and that such elements as upbringing, socioeconomic status, culture, and ethnicity must be considered within this context (Do women and men communicate differently?, 2003).

Reeder (2005) pointed out that research findings regarding communication differences related to sex are simply contradictory. For example, some studies show men to be more assertive, while others find women to be as assertive or even more assertive than men. When it comes to most communication behaviors, such as leadership style, sociability, or displays of power in intimate relationships, Reeder indicated that academic research reveals little to no difference between sexes. Mehl et al. (2007) reported further evidence that there may not be the sex differences previously thought. They had 396 participants wear voice recorders for several days. It was found that women and men both spoke about 16,000 words per day. Overall, communication research suggests that male–female differences are actually quite small.

Being male or female seems to account for only 1% of the variation in communication behaviors. Other factors play a more significant role, such as the type of relationship and the context within which the communication takes place.

According to Harris (2011), because males and females are often brought up differently related to communication, it is important to understand the basic differences in how we talk to each other. She described the various communication styles. A lot of men, according to Harris, tend to use *competitive communication*. The way they talk sends a message that they are oriented toward power and dominance. They are very direct when it comes time to make decisions, and they like to make decisions without the help of anyone else. Women, in contrast, tend to use *affiliate communication*. They bring many others into the communication process and want to bounce ideas off of others.

Also, a lot of men use *direct communication*. When they want something, they quickly voice their opinion. This leaves little possibility of misunderstanding. Women may not want to be so bold as to come right out and say what they want, so they may use *indirect communication*. Such statements are often more vague and leave room for various interpretations. In a conversation, it can be very frustrating and confusing if one person is being more direct and the other is being more indirect.

Barr (2013) summarized some interesting points about male and female communication styles. She pointed out that women tend to connect through conversation, whereas men more likely connect through action. Women like to share emotions and thoughts, whereas men share ideas, suggestions, and facts but often avoid talking about feelings. Also, women use a lot of nonverbal communication, such as making eye contact, gesturing, and using animated facial expressions. A woman often prefers talking while sitting or standing in a group of people where everyone is face-to-face. A man, in contrast, commonly prefers talking shoulder-to-shoulder in an angled pattern where he and his friends can take in the room. A man often prefers a relaxed, sprawled pose and keeps the body language and facial expressions more contained. A woman may punctuate the conversation with affirmative noises such as "OK" and "Uh huh" to let you know she is listening, but a man often prefers to sit quietly and focus on what is being said.

Lieberman (2014) gave some examples of typical differences in male and female styles of communication. Here are a few of them:

1. Women are more likely to talk to other women when they have a problem or need

Communication
DIMENSIONS

Adult Sexting   In recent years there have been a number of examples of adult sexting—even some that involved prominent politicians, sports stars, and other celebrities. Is adult sexting just a new form of pornography? When is it a harmless way to communicate, and when is it damaging or even dangerous? Is it different for people in their 20s as opposed to older adults? Six experts gave their opinions on some of these questions.

Pepper Schwartz, professor of sociology at the University of Washington, said that adult sexting is a form of flirtation. It is a dangerous flirtation if pictures are being sent that you might not want 200 million people to see, but it can be sexy and playful among mutually consenting adults. If sexting is not performed in the context of a mutually collaborative and intimate relationship, it can feel like an act of sexual aggression. People should have the right to block unwanted pictures and gross messages.

Michelle Drouin, assistant professor of psychology at Indiana University-Purdue University Fort Wayne, indicated that her research with 745 U.S. college students showed that sexting is a popular means of sexual communication within both committed romantic relationships and casual sexual relationships. For those with insecure attachments, sexting may help fulfill relationship needs and demands. This may be especially true for emotionally distant men, who were less likely to call, text, or engage in face-to-face sexual conversations with a partner.

S. Craig Watkins, professor at the University of Texas at Austin, said that he is not convinced that the raunchy behavior online is equivalent to porn. However, sexting certainly reveals how our sexual norms and the expression of our sexual selves are evolving in ways that make all of us vulnerable.

Susan Lipkins, a psychologist in Port Washington, New York, said that for most people sexting is a form of flirting. For some, it is a form of gossip; for others a form of harassment. For those born around 1987 or later, sexting is simply a form of communication. However, for those a little older sexting may have different implications. Adults who sext may be doing so to assert their power within a group or toward a particular person, to increase their popularity, to use their status and enhance it, or to display their aggression. In general, sexters view sexting as harmless and fun, whereas nonsexters see it as dangerous.

Finally, K. Jason Krafsky and Kelli Krafsky, coauthors of *Facebook and Your Marriage*, indicated that there is a double standard that applies to the virtual world and real world, with two different sets of rules, acceptable behavior, and consequences. Making unwanted sexual advances virtually is called "cyberflirting", but in the real world it is sexual harassment. Being sexually active with multiple partners on the Internet is called "virtual sex," but in the real world it is engaging in high-risk and irresponsible behavior. Sending lewd pictures of your private parts online is called "sexting," but in the real world it is a crime called indecent exposure. They point out that we should not buy the lie that we can have dual citizenship in both worlds, breaking the rules in one without consequence in the other.

What do you agree with or disagree with that these six experts have said? What does all of this have to do with communication about sexuality?

The preceding information from the six experts is important for understanding why adult sexting occurs. It may become even more important as the number of people who sext continues to increase. Across all age groups, the proportion of cell phone owners who say they send and receive sexts continues to increase. The largest increases in these rates have been reported among those aged 18–24. This group is the most likely to both send and receive sexts (44%). By comparison, in 2012, only 26% of this group said they received sexts (Pew Research Center, 2014).

Source: Data from Room for debate: A running commentary on the news. What's wrong with adult sexting? *The New York Times* (June 9, 2011). Available: http://www.nytimes.com/roomfordebate/2011/06/09/whats-wrong-with-adult-sexting?nl=todaysheadlines&emc=thab1. Pew Research Center. *Couples, the Internet, and social media*, 2014. Available: http://www.pewinternet.org/2014/02/11/couples-the-internet-and-social-media/.

Ethical DIMENSIONS

Ethics, Communication, and Date Rape

One example of potential communication difficulties is sexual behavior on a date. Let us consider some ethical issues related to communication and date rape.

Some men and women believe there are women who like to be talked into having sexual intercourse. A misunderstanding can easily occur if a mixed message is sent or received. There is an ethical responsibility for a male or female to be sure messages are accurately interpreted.

Some cultural images of romantic interaction in sexual situations may lead to many ethical questions about date rape. For example, is it part of a dating ritual for a woman to resist a man's initial sexual advances? What is her ethical responsibility to be sure she is sending accurate—and not misleading—messages?

If a woman is drunk or has used other chemical substances that can influence judgment, what is the ethical responsibility of her partner in regard to their actions? Should the female have considered the ethics of putting herself (and the partner) in that situation in the first place? If she is under the influence of chemical substances, she may send a message in a way she does not intend.

If a partner is drunk or has used other chemical substances that can influence judgment, this can interfere with the ability to understand the message being sent accurately. What is his/her ethical responsibility for accurate communication in this situation?

The feedback being sent is very important. If a woman goes to a partner's apartment or invites the partner to her apartment for a drink and then participates in heavy petting, do her actions suggest consent? Is it ethical for her to do these things if she has no intent of participating in sexual intercourse? How should she provide accurate feedback so there is accurate communication?

How about if a woman is dressed in revealing clothing? Is it ethical for her to do this if she is not interested in sexual activity? Is it ethical for a partner to interpret the wearing of revealing clothing as an invitation for sexual activity?

Date rape may be a result of miscommunication. There are many ethical issues related to communication and date rape to consider. Clear communication is needed to help prevent date rape.

Relatedly, what is the prevalence of implied versus verbal consent at first intercourse among U.S. college students? Higgins et al. (2010) found that among those with consensual first intercourse experiences, 49% provided nonverbal consent. Respondents who used condoms at first intercourse were more likely to provide verbal consent, suggesting that condoms may prompt sexual discussion (or vice versa). In contrast, those who provided nonverbal consent were less likely to have used contraception. It seems, then, that college students who do not discuss whether to engage in vaginal intercourse for the first time are less likely to use contraception.

Source: Higgins, J. A., Trussell, J., Moore, N. B., & Davidson, J. K. Sr. The language of love?—Verbal versus implied consent at first heterosexual intercourse: Implications for contraceptive use. *American Journal of Health Education, 44, no. 4* (July/August 2010), 218–230.

to make a decision. Men tend to keep their problems to themselves and do not see the point in sharing personal issues.

2. Women get things done at work by building relationships. Men build relationships while they are working on tasks with each other.

3. Women focus on building rapport, by sharing experiences and asking questions. Men like to give information rather than ask questions.

4. At meetings women tend to nod their head to show they are listening. Men tend to nod their heads only when they agree.

Attitudes About Sexuality

Some people are prevented from communicating openly by attitudes learned at home. Some parents "protect" young children from references to sexuality. When as teenagers these children are exposed to talk about sexuality—on the street or at school—they often feel guilty for participating in or eavesdropping on such forbidden conversations. When parents fail to acknowledge our sexuality as children, we should not be surprised if suppressed feelings permeate our adult sexual lives.

Some writers suggest that men often do not communicate well with women because they have a "fear

Gender
DIMENSIONS

Sexual Behavior in Marriage

Listen to this couple in their mid to late 20s, married 9 years:

Wife: I don't understand him. He's ready to go any time. It's always been a big problem with us right from the beginning. If we've hardly seen each other for two or three days and hardly talked to each other, I can't just jump into bed. If we have a fight, I can't just turn it off. He has a hard time understanding that. I feel like that's all he wants sometimes. I have to know I'm needed and wanted for more than just jumping into bed.

Husband: She complains that all I want from her is sex, and I try to make her understand that it's an expression of love. I'll want to make up with her by making love, but she's as cold as the inside of the fridge. I get mad when that happens. Why shouldn't I? Here I'm trying to make up and make love, and she's holding out for something—I don't know what.

Wife: He keeps saying he wants to make love, but it just doesn't feel like love to me. Sometimes I feel bad that I feel that way, but I just can't help it.

Husband: I don't understand. She says it doesn't feel like love. What does that mean, anyway? What does she think love is?

Wife: I want him to talk to me, to tell me what he's thinking. If we have a fight, I want to talk about it so we could maybe understand it. I don't want to jump in bed and just pretend it didn't happen.

Husband: Talk! Talk! What's there to talk about? I want to make love to her and she says she wants to talk. How's talking going to convince her I'm loving her?

In sexual behavior, as in other matters, the barriers to effective communication are high and the language people use only further confuses and mystifies them. He says he wants to make love, but she says, "It doesn't feel like love." Neither quite knows what the other is talking about; both feel vaguely guilty and uncomfortable, aware only that somehow they're not connecting. He believes that he has already given her a profound declaration of love: He married her and they share a home.

Yet she says, "Just once, I'd like him to love me without it ending up in sex. But when I tell him that, he thinks I'm crazy."

For him, perhaps, it does seem crazy. Sexual activity may be the one way in which he can allow himself the expression of deep feeling. His wife, however, finds it difficult to be comfortable with her feelings in the same area. She keeps asking for something that she can understand and is comfortable with—a demonstration of his feelings in nonsexual ways. He keeps giving her the one thing he can understand and is comfortable with—his feelings wrapped up in a blanket of sex. Thus some husbands and wives find themselves in an impossibly difficult bind, one that stems from the cultural context in which girls and boys grow to adulthood.

We are suggesting that the man's ever-present sexual readiness is not simply an expression of urgent sexual need but is also a complex response to a socialization process that restricts the development of the emotional side of his personality. Conversely, the woman's insistent plea for a nonsexual emotional statement is a response to a process that encourages the development of the emotional side of her personality.

of intimacy" that is really a fear of rejection. One way to deal with this is for men to learn to talk about their lives more openly, as women have learned to do. Developing their own friendships with other men can help men acquire personal skills that will also improve their relationships with women.

Parent–Teen Communication

When it comes to communicating with their children about sexuality, many parents consider the task a daunting one, for which they feel ill equipped. Parents often do not have meaningful conversations with sons and daughters because they do not know what to say or how to begin, fearing that talking to children about sexuality might either scare them or encourage them in sexual behaviors at a young age. Most parent–child discussions about sexuality seem to be limited, indirect, and uncomfortable. Unfortunately, parents' failure to effectively communicate with their children about sexuality may place teens at risk for negative outcomes.

Many teens would welcome communication with their parents about sexuality.

Kitchen and Huberman (2011) summarized reasons that it is important for parents to be knowledgeable and become comfortable as sexuality educators. Good parent–teen communication helps young people establish individual values and make healthy decisions. Young people who feel a lack of parental warmth are more likely to report emotional distress, school problems, drug use, and sexual risk behaviors. In contrast, loving parent–child communication about sexuality leads to improved contraceptive and condom use, improved communication about sexuality, delays in the initiation of sexual intercourse, and lower sexual risk behaviors. Teens who discuss sexuality with their parents are also more likely to talk with their partner about HIV/AIDS.

Many programs have been developed to help parents improve their comfort and ability in speaking with children and teens about sexuality. These programs commonly deal with topics such as building the relationship with the child, new ways of communicating, listening skills for talking about sensitive topics, getting past roadblocks when talking about sexuality, coping with conflict, and helping the child make sound decisions.

El-Shaieb and Wurtele (2009) surveyed 214 parents of young children about their plans for sexual discussions with their children. Parents reported being educated mostly by their mothers and rated both of their parents as ineffective educators. Compared to a similar survey of parents conducted over 25 years earlier, these parents intended to discuss sexual abuse at an earlier age, but to delay discussing genital differences, birth, and reproduction. Compared

to fathers, mothers intended to discuss sexuality at earlier ages and anticipated this to be more effective. Parents' intentions to discuss varied between sons and daughters for certain topics, and there were two topics (masturbation and nocturnal emissions) many parents did not intend to discuss with their children.

As the years have gone by, it seems that communication about sexuality between parents and their children has gotten somewhat better. For example, Sifferlan (2014) reported new data that showed while parents and their children are perfectly willing to chat about sexuality, they may not be doing it as often as they should. A nationally representative sample of 1,663 pairs of parents and their children, ages 9–21, was surveyed to get a sense of how American families of all backgrounds are communicating about sexuality and healthy relationships. Approximately half of the parents said they started talking about sexuality with their children by age 10, and 80% started by age 13. While 80% talked to their children about sexuality beyond the basics, such as how to handle peer pressure and how to stay safe online, responses indicated that they were not doing so frequently. As Sifferlan noted, there is a lot of incomplete or incorrect information about sexuality out there, and if parents and young people really are willing to have these conversations, it is time to break the ice.

Because many college students eventually decide to become parents, here are some tips about talking with kids about sexuality (Silverberg, 2008). Perhaps the most important one is to make talking with your children about sexuality a lifelong conversation. Instead of just having a "big sex talk," recognize that many small moments of learning and teaching about sexuality happen throughout a child's development. El-Shaieb and Wurtele (2009) indicated that parents need guidance about when and how best to discuss sexual issues with their children. To help them get ready, parents need to: (a) learn about healthy sexual development, (b) consider the influence of their own experiences learning about sexuality, (c) understand the impact of ineffective sexuality education in one generation leading to poor sexuality education in the next, (d) understand the role of demographic influences on their communication styles, and (e) discuss with other parents various dilemmas confronting them in their sexuality education efforts. Also, it is important to be comfortable when it comes to talking about sexuality. Many things, such as reading this book and taking a sexuality class, can greatly help to increase your comfort level with this topic. It is also good to make it OK for your kids to ask about sexuality. All children have such questions, and it helps to create an environment where they feel comfortable asking them. Finally, it is important to use age-appropriate information. A number of excellent resources, such as many of those mentioned throughout this text, are available that can help people understand more about age-appropriate sexuality information.

Sexual Language

One of us was invited to speak with a group of elderly people about sexuality. Proceeding with undaunted courage, he began the session with exercises designed to neutralize the emotional impact of sexual words. He showed slides containing one or two words and instructed the participants to shout in unison the word appearing on the slide. The first slide was shown and the audience shouted *love* with much enthusiasm. Buoyed up by the group's cooperation and interest, he projected the next slide—*hug*. The audience again shook the room with their shouts. From that point on, however, it was all downhill. With each successive word, the decibel level of the voices lowered—no small wonder, considering the remaining words: *kiss, caress, pet, sexual intercourse, oral sex, penis,* and *vagina*. The point was made. Many people are uncomfortable with sexual language. How can sexual communication be effective if we cannot even speak the language?

When discussing sexual topics, people often find that the words themselves prevent rational, thoughtful, comfortable interaction. Some words evoke such strong emotions—embarrassment, guilt, shame, or anger—that they interfere with thoughtful discourse. Generally, the greater the emotion, the greater the interference.

For example, it may be that the term used influences what a partner hears: "penis," "dick," and "cock" may all have different connotations for different people. Calling a vagina a "vagina" may sound very clinical to one person, whereas calling it a "pussy" or a "cunt" may sound sexy, dirty, or just fine to someone else. The sexual language used can promote communication and relationships, or it can inhibit them.

In addition to being comfortable with language related to sexuality, it is also important to be sure we are talking about the same thing when we use sexual terms. For example, what does "having sex" mean? It can be interesting to discuss this question with college students. Does "having sex" include only penile–vaginal intercourse? Does anal sexual activity count? How about oral sexual activity? Mutual masturbation? Does intense petting and body contact constitute having sex? It is common to hear college students as well as other people refer to "having sex." But to be sure we are communicating clearly we have to be sure we have the same definitions for the terms we are using.

Techniques for Improving Sexual Communication

As we have discussed, there are many reasons for good sexual communication. One of these includes a need to communicate about desires related to sexual activity. Miller and Byers (2004) interviewed 153 heterosexual couples about their actual and ideal duration of foreplay and intercourse, as well as their partners' desired duration of foreplay and intercourse. Both men's and women's perceptions of their partners' ideal duration of foreplay and intercourse were found to be more strongly related to their own sexual stereotypes than to their partners' self-reported sexual desires. This suggested that people rely on sexual stereotypes when estimating their partners' ideal sexual scripts. Improving communication about sexuality could help eliminate such misperceptions. There are no magical methods for attaining free, open, and comfortable communication about sexual topics, but we do have some suggestions.

First, Owen (2008) provides some suggestions to improve the overall atmosphere for communication. She indicates that it is important to realize that one does not know everything. This leads to asking good questions. Also, it helps to ask the right questions. For example, "Is this what you like?" can be a great question that also shows concern about the other person. Being open-minded and nonjudgmental is helpful as well. Maintaining care and trust also leads to better communication. One person is much more likely to open up to another if there is confidence that the information will not be shared with others. Other suggestions for improving communication are found in the following pages.

Planning

One common barrier to good sexual communication is the complete avoidance of the subject by both partners. We suggest that partners set aside time to discuss sexuality as they would any other topic of mutual interest and of significance to their relationship. In setting up a time for such a discussion, it is wise to make the following plans.

1. Make sure you have plenty of time for your discussion. Do not be cut short when one of you has to run off somewhere.

2. Do not allow others to interrupt your discussion by calling you or by barging in on you.

3. Accept all feelings and the right to express these feelings verbally. For example, it is just as appropriate to say, "I feel angry when …" as it is to say, "I feel terrific when …"

Communication
DIMENSIONS

Clarity in Sexual Communication

In the communication process, the idea sent and the message actually received are ideally the same. But as you likely know from experience, matters do not always work that way. Often, the words chosen, the tone of voice, the body language, or the context in which the message is delivered blurs the true intent of the sender. When you add the ambiguity of sexual language, communicating clearly becomes even more difficult. Consider how such language ambiguity might affect a newer relationship.

Let us say that you suggest beginning a more "serious relationship" with someone. Your partner responds that the relationship is not ready for "sexual relations." At this point, it is not clear what either party has said. A "serious relationship" could imply having sexual activity, but it could also imply seeing each other more often or not seeing other people. The "sexual relations" comment in the context of an intimate conversation could be construed to refer to any sexual activity.

Thus it is important to be clear in communicating about sexuality with a partner. If you or your partner cannot talk about sexuality, that may be a sign that you are not ready to be involved in a sexual relationship.

A good way to start a conversation is to talk about sexual histories. By starting the conversation and opening it up for participation, you will make it more comfortable for your partner. Talk about sexual activities that you have enjoyed and would like to share with your partner.

Before entering into a sexual relationship, you should talk about any STIs that you or a partner may have had, and any STI and/or HIV testing you have had (and why you had it done). In addition, you should discuss using latex condoms to prevent STI transmission as well as using a contraceptive method to prevent pregnancy.

---

4. Take a risk—really describe your thoughts and needs. Do not expect your partner to guess what they are.

5. Approach the discussion with both people understanding that the goal is to improve your relationship rather than to see who can shock whom.

6. Expect changes but not miracles. Sexual communication requires continued dialogue. You might want to seek the help of other family members, friends, peer counselors, members of the clergy, psychologists, sexuality counselors, or others who can contribute to your ability to communicate sexually.

Working to improve your sexual communication will help you and your partner develop a deeper trust, a greater sense of intimacy, and a feeling of adventure about your relationship.

Flooding

A technique for learning to use and become comfortable with sexual language is called **flooding**. In one use of this technique, people stand in front of a mirror, look themselves in the eye, and repeat over and over again the words they feel uncomfortable using.

We are not necessarily referring to profanity. We are talking about sexual language. Learning to feel comfortable with these words and being able to use them should be your goals.

© Galina Barskaya/ShutterStock, Inc.

It can take work to have good sexual communication.

flooding Experiencing something so frequently that you no longer are aroused by it. This is a technique used to become more comfortable with sexual terminology.

Learning Assertiveness

Some people just have a tough time communicating—period. Inevitably they have trouble communicating sexually. When this is the case, working to improve only the sexual side of communication is a mistake. Therefore, we turn now to a topic that concerns one's ability to express oneself with confidence in all areas—the quality of assertiveness and the means to develop it.

The first step toward grasping what it means to be assertive is to distinguish assertive, aggressive, and nonassertive behaviors. **Assertiveness** means standing up for your basic rights *without violating* anyone else's. **Aggressiveness** means standing up for your basic rights (or more) *at the expense* of someone else's rights. **Nonassertiveness** means *giving up* your basic rights so that other people can achieve theirs.

For example, an assertive style of verbal sexual communication would be one in which you stand up for your own sexual rights and needs by expressing your wishes, while allowing your partner the same freedom.

Body language, too, can be aggressive, non-assertive, or assertive. Aggressive body language includes a pointing finger, leaning toward the other person, glaring, and using a loud, angry tone of voice. Nonassertive body language is characterized by slumped posture, a lack of eye contact, hand-wringing, hesitant speech, nervous whining or laughing, and not saying or doing what you want to. Assertive behavior, by contrast, entails sitting or standing tall, looking directly at the person you are talking to, speaking in explicit statements with a steady voice, and using the gestures or physical contact that is right for you.

There are certainly benefits in using assertive communication. It can keep people from walking all over you, for example. At the same time, it can help you from steamrolling others. In addition, assertive communication can help you gain self-confidence and self-esteem, understand and recognize your feelings, improve communication, create win–win situations, and engage in honest relationships. Tips to help people to become more assertive include the following (Being assertive: Reduce stress, communicate better, 2015):

- *Assess your style.* Do you voice your opinions or remain silent? Do people seem to fear talking to you? Are you quick to judge or blame?

- *Use "I" statements.* This lets others know what you are thinking without sounding accusatory. For example, say "I disagree," rather than "You're wrong."

- *Rehearse what you want to say.* This can include saying things aloud to yourself to practice, writing things out in advance, or even role-playing with a friend and asking for blunt feedback.

- *Use body language.* As stated earlier, communication involves more than just verbal conversation. Act confident even if you aren't feeling it, keep an upright posture and lean forward a little, and make regular eye contact.

- *Keep emotions in check.* Conflict can be hard, and you may feel like crying or being upset in some other way. Breathe slowly and keep your voice even and firm.

Expressing Yourself Nonverbally

Words are important, but they do not say it all. Do not be afraid to smile, wink, hug, touch, kiss, or in other ways communicate your affection for another. As we said earlier, in the way you walk, sit, gesture, and so on, you are "talking" to your partner, whether you intend to or not. But you can also consciously use those gestures to help get your message across.

Seeking Information (Listening)

Verify your interpretation of the other person's verbal, and especially nonverbal, communication. Listen actively, and ask whether your understanding of your partner's feelings and intentions is accurate. Listening is often hard and takes real skill. If you want to hear what others say effectively, make sure you are not a

- *Mind reader:* You hear little or nothing as you think, "What is this person really thinking or feeling?"

- *Rehearser:* Your mental tryouts for "Here's what I'll say next" tune out the speaker.

- *Filterer:* Some call this selective listening—hearing only what you want to hear.

- *Dreamer:* Drifting off during a face-to-face conversation can lead to an embarrassing "What did you say?" or "Could you repeat that?"

---

assertiveness Standing up for one's basic rights without violating anyone else's rights.

aggressiveness Standing up for one's basic rights, but at the expense of someone else's basic rights.

nonassertiveness Giving up one's basic rights so others may achieve theirs.

Sitting close together, touching, and smiling are all ways to show you care. Nonverbal communication is important; expressing feelings in words is also vital.

Good listeners show they are mentally engaged.

- *Identifier:* If you refer everything you hear to your experience, you probably did not hear what was said.

- *Comparer:* When you get side-tracked assessing the messenger, you are sure to miss the message.

- *Derailer:* Changing the subject too quickly tells others you are not interested in anything they have to say.

- *Sparrer:* You hear what is said but quickly belittle it or discount it. That puts you in the same class as the derailer.

- *Placater:* Agreeing with everything you hear just to be nice or to prevent conflict does not make you a good listener (Why don't we hear others?, 2005).

Listening makes others feel worthy, appreciated, interesting, and respected. When we listen, we foster the same skill in others by acting as a model for positive and effective communication. Active listening is really an extension of the Golden Rule. To know how to listen to someone else, think about how you would want to be listened to. Here is what good listeners know (Cortright, 2015):

- *Face the speaker.* Sit up straight and lean forward slightly to show your attentiveness through body language.

- *Maintain eye contact* to the degree that you can all feel comfortable.

- *Minimize external distractions.* Turn off the TV, put down reading materials, and ask the speaker and other listeners to do the same.

- *Respond appropriately* to show you understand. Raise your eyebrows, nod, and give prompts such as "Really" or "Interesting."

- *Focus solely on what the speaker is saying.* Try not to think about what you will say next.

- *Minimize internal distractions.* Refocus on the speaker if your thoughts keep interrupting.

- *Keep an open mind.* Wait until the speaker is finished before deciding if you agree.

- *Engage yourself.* Ask questions for clarification, but wait until the speaker is finished.

Hostile settings and other communication hindrances can defeat even the best listeners. Here are a few steps to avoid those pitfalls:

1. Choose the physical environment. Find a quiet, nonthreatening place to talk if you want to ensure true understanding.

2. Cut the interruptions. It can be difficult to communicate if the phone rings or if a person pops in at the door.

3. Recognize differences. People communicate best in different ways. Some of us are primarily auditory, whereas others are visual or "hands-on."

4. Persist. Refuse to believe that you cannot understand another person's message.

Steps Toward Change

Counselors often work with couples to help them improve their communication skills. In summary, the

International Differences in Discussing Sexuality

International differences exist related to the topic of human sexuality. One way to gain an understanding of these differences is to consider how sexuality education is viewed in some countries. Chances are, those who are more open about sexuality education will also be more ready to discuss the topic of sexuality. Obviously, the situation in various countries can change with time, but here are a few traditional examples:

1. In Chile, sexuality is generally not a topic that is talked about by family members or in schools.
2. In Denmark, sexuality and social-life education has been a compulsory subject in schools since 1970, and it was a tradition long before then.
3. In India, sexuality education has generally not been offered in schools because society believed it would "spoil the minds" of children.
4. In Japan, sexuality education in schools (typically focused on reproductive issues) has been mandated, beginning at age 10 or 11 years.

5. In Romania, sexuality education was removed from the schools in the early 1980s. The major sources of sexuality information are friends, mass media, and healthcare providers.
6. In Sweden, sexuality education has been a compulsory subject in schools since 1955. It is well integrated into the school curriculum. In addition, Swedish children receive their first sexuality education at home, from their parents.
7. In the United Kingdom, sexuality education has been required in secondary schools since 1993. There are varied practices in schools within England, Ireland, and Scotland.

Although it can be difficult to draw definite conclusions from this information, it appears that there can be real differences in the ability of people from various countries to engage in effective communication about human sexuality. Of course, we cannot generalize about all people from any country, because many differences are possible within countries. But these differences can strongly influence communication about sexuality.

Source: Data from Carson, S. L. *Cross-cultural perspectives on human sexuality.* Boston: Allyn & Bacon, 1998.

---

counselor (1) encourages **active listening**; (2) elicits feedback from each partner by asking each to summarize what he or she just heard; (3) facilitates the expression of feelings and thoughts directly and succinctly; (4) requests the use of **"I" statements** (beginning each sentence with "I" to express personal feelings better and avoid blaming the other partner) instead of questions; and (5) prohibits interruptions and blaming. These techniques will help all of us communicate much more effectively.

Resolving Conflicts

In relationships—even the best of relationships—conflicts arise. Too often poor communication skills (such as improper listening), a combative or offensive stance geared toward winning rather than communicating, an inability to acknowledge another's point, or a refusal to consider alternative solutions

interferes with the healthy resolution of these conflicts. As a result, conflicts threaten the continuation of the relationship and, at the least, tear little pieces from it, potentially leaving the relationship bankrupt. To gain a sense of how these poor communication skills impair effective conflict resolution, consider the following dialogue.

Paul: *Well, Barbara, as you know, I really care for you, and I hope we can continue to develop our relationship. We can't go any further tonight, though, because I'd like you to be tested for HIV.*
Barbara: *Now you ask—right in the middle of this romantic time! Why didn't you say something about this before?*
Paul: *You've got some nerve. You should have realized this is something we need to consider.*
Barbara: *I should have realized? How was I supposed to know you were concerned about HIV status? You never said anything about it.*
Paul: *Why should I take the chance of getting HIV? You're pretty selfish, aren't you?*

---

active listening Paraphrasing what someone has said to demonstrate interest and understanding.

"I" statement Statement that begins with an "I" to express personal feelings.

Barbara: *I've had it! Either we're going to trust each other and move ahead in our relationship or you can say good-bye right now.*
Paul: *In that case, GOOD-BYE!*

In this example, both Paul and Barbara are trying to win: Paul wants Barbara to have an HIV test, and Barbara wants Paul to have faith and move ahead with their relationship. Neither Paul nor Barbara can possibly win this battle, although they are probably unaware of this. If they proceed with their relationship (including sexual intercourse and other intimate behaviors), Paul will be uneasy because of his concern about HIV. He will probably feel his concerns are not very important to Barbara, will resent her lack of concern, and will have a difficult time participating freely in the relationship.

However, if Barbara agrees to the HIV test, she will feel that Paul did not trust her and "forced" her to take the test. She may also feel he waited to spring the idea on her and wonder why it did not arise earlier.

It becomes evident, then, that regardless of which way they go, one or the other will be resentful. This resentment will probably result in a weakening, or possibly a dissolution, of their relationship. So, no matter who wins, both really lose.

This situation is not totally hopeless, though. Consider the effect on resolving their conflict if Paul and Barbara had communicated as follows:

Paul: *Well, Barbara, as you know, I really care for you, and I hope we can continue to develop our relationship. We can't go any further tonight, though, because I'd like you to be tested for HIV.*
Barbara: *Now you ask—right in the middle of this romantic time! Why didn't you say something about this before?*
Paul: *You feel we should have discussed this earlier?*
Barbara: *Yes, and HIV status is something we both need to be concerned about.*
Paul: *You have a concern about my HIV status, too?*
Barbara: *You bet! And I think it is only fair that we treat ourselves and each other equally in this situation.*
Paul: *You think that it would be a problem if you got the HIV test and I didn't?*
Barbara: *Yes.*
Paul: *Would you be embarrassed if other people knew you had taken the test?*
Barbara: *Yes, I guess I would.*
Paul: *It sounds like my request might have hurt you at least a little?*
Barbara: *Yes, I guess it did.*
Paul: *I'm glad that you also care about our relationship. But HIV is really a serious health problem today, and I am worried about it. And I'm bothered that you didn't understand my concern.*

Barbara: *I guess you do have a reason to be concerned. I'm sorry.*
Paul: *Well, let's see what alternatives we have.*
Barbara: *Maybe I should just go ahead and be tested.*
Paul: *Or perhaps we should both be tested.*
Barbara: *How about agreeing that we will honestly share the results with each other but also that the results are private and not anyone else's business?*
Paul: *That's fine with me. In fact, we don't even need to tell anyone else we took the tests. That is our private matter.*
Barbara: *Would it make sense to agree to take the tests as soon as possible so we both know the results as soon as we can?*
Paul: *That seems sensible, and since your schedule in the next couple of weeks is so busy, I'll be happy to work around your schedule.*
Barbara: *Okay. Remember, though, the next time either of us has concerns or suggestions we need to bring them up as early as possible.*

In this example, Paul took the initiative in resolving his interpersonal conflict with Barbara. He began by employing a technique known as *active listening*, or *reflective listening*. The key to this technique is that the listener paraphrases the words of the speaker to indicate that he or she comprehends the meaning of the speaker's message. The listener tries to pick up on hidden messages and feelings not actually verbalized and paraphrases those as well. For example, Paul understood that Barbara would be embarrassed if other people knew she had taken the test, even though she never explicitly stated that. When Paul was able to understand and listen so well to Barbara—well enough to identify feelings she had not verbalized—Barbara was convinced that Paul cared enough to understand her needs. *Then* Barbara was ready to hear about Paul's needs and became more receptive to his viewpoint. Paul next expressed his opinion and the reasons for his feelings. The point of reflective listening is to enable each participant to acknowledge the other's view and to be less insistent in arguing for his or her own.

The next step in this technique is to propose as many alternative solutions as possible through brainstorming. The result is a win–win, rather than a no–win, situation, reached through a mutual agreement that it is possible to agree. Paul agrees that they both will be tested and that they will treat the testing and the results confidentially. He also shows respect for Barbara's busy schedule and says he is willing to work around it.

In addition, Paul and Barbara have improved their relationship *because* of this conflict. The conflict instigates a discussion about their needs and, therefore, provides the opportunity for them to

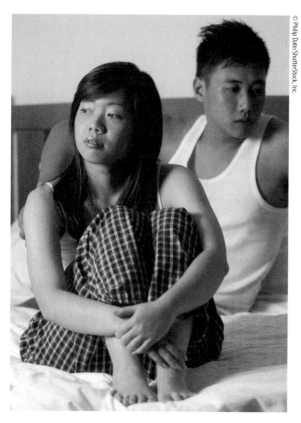

Communication about HIV status can be difficult, but it is very important.

Myth vs Fact

Myth: For most people, good communication comes naturally.
Fact: Although some people may seem to be naturally better than others at communication, good communication is a lot of work for almost everyone.

Myth: Because sexuality is such an open topic today, most people can discuss it rather easily.
Fact: Even though sexuality seems more open, many people still experience much difficulty in talking about sexual topics and personal relationships.

Myth: Communication skills are basically the same in all cultures.
Fact: Although most skills may be quite similar, communicating with people from another culture can be challenging. Even though the language may be the same, communication methods and meanings may greatly differ.

Myth: Because men and women now have the same rights and are equal, they communicate in the same ways.

Fact: Conditions can be slow to change. Even though men and women have equal rights, we still need to be sensitive to differences in learning and motivation related to communication.

Myth: The most important part of communication is the meaning of the words we use.
Fact: It has often been said that "actions speak louder than words." It is also true that nonverbal communication is often more important, and revealing, than words used.

Myth: It is a bad idea to take a risk when trying to communicate with another person. The technique may backfire.
Fact: There are risks in most things we do, and developing and using good communication skills can involve disclosing personal feelings and desires. In a trusting relationship, this should not be too risky.

---

demonstrate their feelings for each other by organizing to satisfy those needs. Instead of threatening the relationship, the conflict has actually improved it.

To reiterate, the steps in this conflict resolution process are as follows:

1. *Active listening:* Reflecting to the other person his or her own words and feelings.

2. *Identifying your position:* Stating your own thoughts and feelings about the situation, and explaining why you feel this way.

3. *Proposing and exploring alternative solutions:* First brainstorming and then evaluating the possibilities.

Although you may feel awkward using this technique initially, and your conversations may seem stilted, with practice it will become a part of your style and will be very effective. The payoffs are huge; do not give up on it.

Giving and Receiving Criticism

Imagine a "sex critic" planned to evaluate your sexual functioning as a movie critic critiques movies! All of us would probably feel threatened, and because of that, our abilities to function normally would most likely be compromised. Well, in a very real sense, our sexual partners are our sex critics. They evaluate what we do in terms of how pleasing it is for both them and us. It would be nice if we could receive our "sex critique" without feeling threatened by it, without feeling that it denigrated our self-esteem. It would also be nice if we were open enough both to give and to receive feedback about our sexual functioning in a way that enhanced our sexual lives and those of our partners. Well, we can learn both to receive and to give criticism in a way that is truly constructive. Here are a few hints:

1. Find a private, relaxing place to discuss thoughts and feelings about your sexual relationship. You do not want to feel uncomfortable in your environment while discussing such a sensitive topic. Feeling uncomfortable will not be conducive to either receiving or giving feedback on such a sensitive issue.

2. Devote sufficient time to such a discussion. It would be unfortunate if you were beginning to communicate well on significant matters just as one of you had to leave.

3. Limit distractions so that your attention is focused on the conversation. Rather than wondering who might overhear you or who might inadvertently hit you in the head with a Frisbee, find a quiet, private place for your discussion.

4. It is probably not wise to do these things just before or just after a sexual encounter. Plan a relaxed time for this discussion.

In addition to these general suggestions, when *giving criticism* try to remember to

1. Begin your comments on a positive note. "You know, when you kiss me I really feel great." Then move to the behavior you would like to change. "I enjoy your touches so much that it would be terrific if you could ...."

2. Be specific regarding the change you are recommending. Rather than announcing, "You don't hold me enough," suggest, "When we watch television, I'd really like it if you would put your arm around me."

3. Be aware of the limitations of your partner. Do not expect more than your partner is able to give. To critique something that cannot or will not be changed may harm the relationship. If your partner is slow to arouse, asking him or her to speed up is unrealistic and, we might add, unfair. It is criticism given for no useful purpose.

Myth vs Fact

Myth: Being assertive means standing up for your basic rights at the expense of someone else's rights.
Fact: Being aggressive is standing up for your basic rights at the expense of someone else's. Being assertive means standing up for your basic rights without violating anyone else's.

Myth: Conflicts will always get in the way of good relationships.
Fact: It is true that conflicts are a part of life, but if we learn how to deal with them effectively they can help us grow and have better relationships.

When *receiving criticism* try to remember to

1. Separate your partner's suggestions and recommendations from your self-worth. You are no less of a person because you might need to adjust some of your sexual behavior. In fact, if you were not open to suggestion, then you might suspect you have a problem.

2. Assume a nondefensive attitude. Rather than attempting to justify your present actions, ask questions to understand the criticism better. Then, if you disagree, you will know why you disagree.

3. If the criticism is too general, ask for specific suggestions to help you make the recommended change. In addition, inquire as to how your partner can help make this change more likely to occur. Ask your partner to participate in remedying the situation or action being criticized.

Communication DIMENSIONS

Guidelines for Healthy Sexual Communication

A great source of information about sexual communication is Healthy Sex.com. Wendy and Larry Maltz provide insights related to many aspects of sexuality. They provide 15 communication guidelines for healthy sexual communication. In addition to the points already mentioned in this chapter, they include the following points directly related to sexuality:

- Both partners need to make a commitment to engage in a discussion about intimate concerns.
- When discussing sexual intimacy concerns, keep in mind that partners are apt to feel scared, embarrassed, or hurt. Emphasize what you like and what works well before making a new request or discussing something that bothers you.
- See intimate problems as a normal and natural part of a relationship. Turn them into opportunities to learn and grow as a couple.
- Seek professional help when needed. Don't allow unresolved sexual issues to fester and erode your positive feelings for each other.

Source: Data from Maltz, W., & Maltz, M. Communication guidelines for healthy sex. Healthy Sex.com. Available: http://bigbrother_2000.tripod.com/guideline.html.

4. Whether or not you agree with the criticism, thank your partner for being honest enough to express the concern to you. Acknowledge that it is not easy to discuss such matters and you appreciate the opportunity to consider something you have been doing or not been doing that is causing a problem. Encourage future suggestions that have the potential to improve your relationship.

With these recommendations for giving and receiving criticism, your relationship should improve. That is because not only will the specific suggestions lead to actual changes, but the practice of opening up your relationship to discussions of problems will, in itself, help foster a style of communicating that will serve you well in all aspects of your relationship. It will then be easier to discuss matters that bother you, and it will be easier to express emotions such as love, caring, and wonderment. The relationship will improve with this style of communication.

When trying to communicate effectively, it can be helpful to have some ground rules. Silverberg (2009) suggests that talking with a partner about these rules can help in developing your own set of rules. Here are some examples:

1. Check in and check out. At the beginning of the conversation, spend a minute talking about your day and how you are feeling so you know what each person is bringing into the conversation. It can also help to take a minute at the end of the conversation to say how it went.

2. Define safety for yourselves and to each other. Discuss what is needed to feel safe so partners can talk honestly and openly.

3. Listen without interrupting. This can be a hard rule to follow, but it is a very important one.

4. Respect differences in interests and desires. If one person exposes personal information, the other person should consider that a compliment, even if the desire is not something he or she is interested in doing.

5. Bring a sense of goodwill to the conversation. Neither partner should be trying to intentionally hurt the other or be mean to the other.

6. Anyone can call time-out at any time. To have a safe conversation, partners need to feel they can stop the conversation at any time. This doesn't mean that one partner should storm out in the middle of a sentence,

but rather that either partner can ask for a time-out to end the conversation at that time with the agreement to pick it up at a later point.

Final Thoughts on Sexual Communication

In this chapter we have discussed the importance of word meanings, nonverbal communication, cultural and personal backgrounds, and attitudes toward communication about sexuality. We have also seen that there are many ways to improve our ability to communicate significantly but that doing so usually takes a great deal of effort.

At the same time, however, to be effective, communication must be truthful. In practice, this is often not the case.

Communication difficulties may even increase the level of risk—especially for females. Some women believe they never have the right to stop foreplay, including at the point of intercourse; refuse to have sexual intercourse, even if they have had intercourse with that partner before; make their own decisions about contraception, regardless of their partner's wishes; ask their partner whether they have been examined for STIs; or tell their partner that they want to make love differently or that the partner is being too rough. Moreover, some young women believe that they never have or only sometimes have the right to tell a relative they are not comfortable with being hugged or kissed in certain ways. These findings show that some young women may be unable to communicate their sexual beliefs and desires clearly and are therefore at risk for undesired outcomes.

Finally, it is interesting to note what a number of leading sexologists have said about communication. They were asked to relate the most important information they had learned about sexuality over the years. Here are some of their thoughts:

1. It is hard to be honest about past sexual experiences with a new partner.

2. Some sexual secrets—unless they pose a health threat—are better left unshared.

3. Nonverbal communication often works better than words in bed.

4. Talking during sexual activity—sharing fantasies, using forbidden words—can be very sexy.

5. Couples who have nothing to say to each other in restaurants are usually married—and they may be in trouble.

Appropriately giving and receiving criticism will enhance communication in a relationship.

6. Open, honest communication is the most important foundation for a relationship.

7. You cannot underestimate the value of humor.

8. After humor, consideration is the second most important ingredient in a sexual relationship. Most people appreciate a sensitive and thoughtful partner.

9. Most people are not comfortable talking about sexual issues.

10. Consent requires communication.

11. It is better to talk about sexual feelings, desires, and boundaries in relationships.

12. Talking about scenes in movies or books can sometimes be a good way to communicate what you like in sexual behavior and relationships.

Exploring the Dimensions of Human Sexuality

© Gayvoronskaya Yana/Shutterstock

Your ability to communicate sexually plays an important role in your sexual wellness and self-image. Your capacity to discuss sexual histories, contraceptives, and safer sexual activities can help prevent unwanted pregnancy and transmission of STIs and HIV.

From a psychological standpoint, a positive self-image as a communicator gives you confidence. A negative self-image may hinder your ability to ask for dates, to ask for sexual activities that you like, or to ask for safer sexual activities.

Sexual communication is influenced by virtually all social and cultural phenomena, including religion, ethnic heritage, language, family traditions, peers, geographical region, and even mass media.

Being male or female plays a pervasive role: Men and women communicate in different styles and express emotions differently.

Consider the confusion of sexual language: If your partner suggested that you were not close enough to engage in "sexual relations," you might back off any type of physical contact. It is important to talk with your partner to make sure each of you understands what the other wants.

Biological Factors

- Physiological reactions—such as blushing or erections—are nonverbal means of communicating sexual attraction.
- Alcohol or drugs can distort the communication process.
- Physical touching can indicate interest, intimacy, and emotional closeness.
- Hearing loss over time can inhibit communication and frustrate a partner.

Sociocultural Factors

- Media strongly influence sexual communication.
- Being male or female affects style of communication.
- Sexuality education may increase confidence.
- Cultures influence communication style.
- Religion may influence the sexual activities in which one participates.
- Family and peers set an example of sexuality.

Psychological Factors

- Emotions can overwhelm the ability to communicate.
- The role of the double standard in thinking may alter the communication process.
- Ego may get in the way of listening to a partner.
- Self-image and body image may distort communication.

Summary

- The process of communication consists of having an idea, the sender encoding a message, sending the message over a channel, the receiver decoding a message, and the receiver providing feedback.

- Nonverbal communication includes all unwritten and unspoken messages. It is a very important part of effective communication, but it can also be easy to misinterpret.

- Barriers to communication include bypassing, the frame of reference, lack of language skills, lack of listening skills, and use of mind-altering drugs.

- There are many things that parents can do to improve communication about sexuality with their children, including making conversations about sexuality ongoing, knowing individual comfort levels, and making it acceptable for children to ask about sexuality.

- Communication can be improved by planning, using flooding, learning assertiveness, using effective nonverbal communication, and using good listening skills.

- Counselors often help people improve their communication skills by encouraging active listening, eliciting feedback from each partner, facilitating the expression of thoughts directly, using "I" statements, and not allowing interruptions and blaming.

- It can be helpful to establish ground rules to help promote good sexual communication. Examples include listening without interruption and respecting differences in desires and interests.

Discussion Questions

1. Describe the steps of the communication process. Explain how they would work in discussing specific relationship or sexuality issues.

2. What are the barriers to effective sexual communication? How can they be overcome?

3. How can you improve your communication abilities? Which techniques would work best for you? Which would not work for you? Explain why.

Application Questions

Reread the chapter-opening story and answer the following questions.

1. If you were teaching this course, and the young couple in the story were students, what information would you want them to leave with from your course?

2. The changes in communication style across the life cycle of the relationship can enhance or harm it. For example, anticipating what your partner wants can lead to a strengthened relationship, but it can also lead to deterioration of communication. What could the young couple have done to maintain interest in their relationship? (You may want to think about what successful couples you know do to stay happy.)

Critical Thinking Questions

1. Should sexual partners communicate all they think and feel so that they can better respond to each other's needs? Or should sexual partners be selective in relating their innermost thoughts and feelings? Explain why or why not. Would your opinion change from situation to situation?

2. You are excited about an upcoming first date when you overhear a conversation describing your date as someone who has had many sexual partners in the past. You have no idea whether the information is correct. Later, on your date, your partner implies a willingness to engage in sexual activity. Although you like the person and are sexually attracted, you are unable to forget what you overheard. How can you open the discussion of sexual histories without offending your date?

3. On the last episode of MTV's *Road Rules Latin America*, all five of the campers (three males and two females) climb naked into a Jacuzzi as a final "gathering of friends." In real life, if you climbed naked into a Jacuzzi with some "close friends," what kind of sexual message might that be sending? What if you climbed into the Jacuzzi with just one other person whom you wanted to get to know better?

Critical Thinking Case

The following is a true date-rape case that occurred at Georgetown University years ago. Kim and Mark (names changed) decided to go to the senior black-tie dance together. Both had agreed beforehand that it would not be a "real date." But during the long evening of drinking and dancing, their plans changed.

They met at 8:30 and went to two parties, the dance, and a bar before returning to Mark's apartment at about 4:00 A.M. Kim had lost her key and had agreed to go back to his apartment. "I decided I wouldn't mind kissing him." They kissed, undressed, and climbed into his bed. Kim said later that she had frequently shared a bed with her previous boyfriend without having sexual intercourse and assumed she could do the same with Mark. When Mark asked whether he should get a condom, Kim said they did not know each other well enough to have sex. At that point, the stories diverge.

Kim said she told Mark, "I've never had sex before, and I don't want to have it on a whim." Then, "all of a sudden, he was on top of me, forcing himself into [me].... I kept trying to push him off with my hands and squirming around, and I kept saying I didn't want to have sex."

Mark said in an affidavit that she was "kissing me and thrusting her pelvis against me.... At no time during our sexual activity did I use any kind of physical force against Kim. Nor did I threaten Kim verbally."

How could communication have gone so awry? Consider the dimensions of human sexuality as you explain what went wrong. Then describe what could have been done to prevent the incident.

Exploring Personal Dimensions

Measure Your Assertiveness

Indicate how characteristic or descriptive each of the following statements is of you by using the code given.

+3 very characteristic of me, extremely descriptive

+2 rather characteristic of me, quite descriptive

+1 somewhat characteristic of me, slightly descriptive

–1 somewhat uncharacteristic of me, slightly nondescriptive

–2 rather uncharacteristic of me, quite nondescriptive

–3 very uncharacteristic of me, extremely nondescriptive

_____ 1. Most people seem to be more aggressive and assertive than I am.

_____ 2. I have hesitated to make or accept dates because of "shyness."

_____ 3. When the food served at a restaurant is not done to my satisfaction, I complain about it to the waiter or waitress.

_____ 4. I am careful to avoid hurting other people's feelings, even when I feel that I have been injured.

_____ 5. If a salesperson has gone to considerable trouble to show me merchandise that is not quite suitable, I have a difficult time saying no.

_____ 6. When I am asked to do something, I insist upon knowing why.

_____ 7. There are times when I look for a good, vigorous argument.

_____ 8. I strive to get ahead as well as most people do.

_____ 9. To be honest, people often take advantage of me.

_____10. I enjoy starting conversations with new acquaintances and strangers.

_____11. I often don't know what to say to attractive persons of the other sex.

_____12. I will hesitate to make phone calls to business establishments and institutions.

_____13. I would rather apply for a job or for admission to a college by writing letters than by going through personal interviews.

_____14. I find it embarrassing to return merchandise.

_____15. If a close and respected relative were annoying me, I would smother my feelings rather than express my annoyance.

_____16. I have avoided asking questions for fear of sounding stupid.

_____17. During an argument I am sometimes afraid that I will get so upset that I will shake all over.

_____18. If a famed and respected lecturer makes a statement that I think is incorrect, I will have the audience hear my point of view as well.

_____19. I avoid arguing over prices with clerks and salespeople.

_____20. When I have done something important or worthwhile, I manage to let others know about it.

_____21. I am open and frank about my feelings.

_____22. If someone has been spreading false and bad stories about me, I see him or her as soon as possible to "have a talk" about it.

_____23. I often have a hard time saying "no."

_____24. I tend to bottle up my emotions rather than make a scene.

_____25. I complain about poor service in a restaurant and elsewhere.

_____26. When I am given a compliment, I sometimes just don't know what to say.

_____27. If a couple near me in a theater or at a lecture were conversing rather loudly, I would ask them to be quiet or to take their conversation elsewhere.

_____28. Anyone attempting to push ahead of me in a line is in for a good battle.

_____29. I am quick to express an opinion.

_____30. There are times when I just can't say anything.

Scoring

To score this scale, first change the signs (+ or –) to the opposite for items 1, 2, 4, 5, 9, 11, 12, 13, 14, 15, 16, 17, 19, 23, 24, 26, and 30. Next, total the plus (+) items, then total the minus (–) items, and, last, subtract the minus total from the plus total to obtain your score. This score can range from –90 through 0 to +90. The higher the score (closer to 190), the more assertively you usually behave. The lower the score (closer to +90), the more nonassertive is your typical behavior. This particular scale does not measure aggressiveness.

Source: Rathus, S. A. A 30-item schedule for assessing assertive behavior, _Behavior Therapy, 4_ (1973), 398, 406. Copyright © 1973 Academic Press, Orlando, FL.

Suggested Readings

Barr, K. R. Male and female communication styles. _Livestrong.com,_ November 2013. Available: http://www.livestrong.com/article/188130 -male-and-female-communication/.

Cherry, K. Top 10 nonverbal communication tips. About.com Psychology, 2014. Available: http://psychology.about.com/od/nonverbal communication/tp/nonverbaltips.htm.

Hinchliff, S., Gott, M., & Galena, E. "I daresay I might find it embarrassing": General practitioners' perspectives on discussing sexual health issues with lesbian and gay patients. _Health & Social Care in the Community, 13, no. 4_ (July 2005), 345–353.

Merchant, K. How men and women differ: Gender differences in communication styles, influence tactics, and leadership styles. _CMC Senior Theses,_ 2012. Available: http://scholarship .claremont.edu/cgi/viewcontent.cgi?article =1521&context=cmc_theses.

Savitsky, D., Keysar, B., Epley, N. Carter, T., & Swanson, A. The closeness-communication bias: Increased egocentrism among friends versus strangers. *Journal of Experimental Social Psychology, 47* (2011), 269–273.

Segal, J. Nonverbal communication. *Helpguide Newsletter* (November, 2014). Available: http://helpguide.org/articles/relationships/nonverbal-communication.htm.

Silverberg, C. How to talk with your kids about sex. *About.com Sexuality*, 2014. Available: http://sexuality.about.com/od/sexeducationforparent1/a/talk_sex_kids.htm.

Silverberg, C. Sexual communication ground rules. About.com Sexuality, 2014. Available: http://sexuality.about.com/od/improvingsexcommunication/a/ground_rules.htm.

Tannen, D. *You just don't understand*. New York: Morrow, 1990 (also available in paperback from Ballantine, 1991).

Web Resources

For links to the websites below, visit go.jblearning.com/dimensions5e and click on Resource Links.

Planned Parenthood: Tools for Parents
www.plannedparenthood.org/parents

Gives ideas that can help communication between parents and their children.

Double Your Dating: Sexual Communication Workbook
www.freewebs.com/maestro_mr/SCW.pdf

Gives hints about many aspects of sexual communication within relationships.

MindTools: Communication Skills
www.mindtools.com/page8.html

Contains numerous articles related to communication skills in many different situations.

Queendom: The Land of Tests
www.queendom.com/tests/access_page/index.htm?idRegTest=2288

You can find out how your interpersonal skills rate by taking a Communication Skills Test.

Sexual Communication & Relationships: About.com Sexuality
http://sexuality.about.com/od/communication/

Gives suggestions related to talking about sexuality with kids and teens, talking with partners, talking with medical personnel, communication in alternative relationships, and communication quick tips.

Sexual Communication: Health 24
http://www.health24.com/Sex/Great-sex/Sexual-communication-20120721

Provides an overview of ways to help improve communication about sexuality with a partner.

References

Barr, K. R. Male and female communication styles. *Livestrong .com*, November 5, 2013. Available: www.livestrong.com /article/188130-male-and-female-communication/.

Barriers to good sexual communication. *Healthism*, 2014. Available: http://healthism.blogspot.com/2011/11/barriers-to -good-sexual-communication.html.

Being assertive: Reduce stress, communicate better. Mayo Clinic, 2015. Available: http://www.mayoclinic.org/healthy-living /stress-management/in-depth/assertive/art-20044644.

Bower, S. A., & Brower, G. *Asserting yourself: A practical guide for positive change*. Reading, MA: Perseus Books, 1976.

Cortright, S. M. 10 tips to effective & active listening skills. *Power to Change*, 2015. Available: http://powertochange .com/students/people/listen/.

DePaulo, B. M., Kirkendol, S. E., Kashy, S. E., Wyer, M. M., & Epstein, J. A. Lying in everyday life. *Journal of Personality and Social Psychology, 70, no. 5* (1996), 979–997.

Do women and men communicate differently? In *Taking sides: Issues in family and personal relationships*, Schroeder, E., ed. Guilford, CT: McGraw-Hill/Dushkin, 2003.

El-Shaieb, M., & Wurtele, S. K. Parents' plans to discuss sexuality with their children. *American Journal of Sexuality Education, no. 4* (April–June 2009), 103–115.

Haffner, D. W., & Schwartz, P. *What I've learned about sex*. New York: Perigee Books, 1998.

Harris, E. K. *Differences in male and female communication: Ways we communicate*, September 9, 2011. Available: http://ezinearticles.com/?Differences-in-Male-and-Female -Communication—Ways-We-Communicate&id=6550397.

Kitchen, E., & Huberman, B. Parent–child communication programs. Advocates for Youth, 2011. Available: http:// www.advocatesforyouth.org/parent-child-communication -programs.

Lieberman, S. *Differences in male and female communication styles*, October 2014. Available: http://www .simmalieberman.com/articles/maleandfemale.html.

Listening to understand. *The Pryor Report Success Workshop*, a supplement to *The Pryor Report Management Newsletter* (August 1998).

Miller, S. A., & Byers, E. S. Actual and desired duration of foreplay and intercourse: Discordance and misperceptions within heterosexual couples. *Journal of Sex Research, 41, no. 3* (August 2004), 301–309.

Owen, C. The importance of sexual communication. *suite101. com*, July 2008. Available: http://improving-relationships .suite101.com.

Reeder, H. M. Exploring male–female communication: Three lessons on gender. *Journal of School Health, 75, no. 3* (March 2005), 115–117.

Rickert, V. I., Sanghvi, R., & Wiemann, C. M. Is lack of sexual assertiveness among adolescent and young adult women a cause for concern? *Perspectives on Sexual and Reproductive Health, 34, no. 4* (July/August 2002), 16–28.

Saxe, L. Lying: Thoughts of an applied social psychologist. *American Psychologist, 46, no. 4* (1991), 409–415.

Segal, J. Nonverbal communication. *Helpguide Newsletter*, October 2008. Available: http://www.helpguide.org/mental /eq6_nonverbal_communication.htm.

Sifferlan, A. *Parents and teens aren't embarrassed by the sex talk anymore*, October 2014. Available: http://time.com/3503458 /parents-teens-sex-talk-smart-phones-internet/.

Silverberg, C. How to talk with your kids about sex. *About.com Sexuality*, March 2008. Available: http://sexuality.about .com/od/sexeducationforparent1/a/talk_sex_kids.htm?p=1.

Silverberg, C. Sexual communication ground rules. *About.com Sexuality*, January 2009. Available: http://sexuality.about .com/od/improvingsexcommunication/a/ground_rules.htm.

Van Wagner, K. Top 10 nonverbal communication tips. *About. com Psychology*, 2009. Available: http://psychology.about .com/od/nonverbalcommunication/tp/nonverbaltips.htm.

Why don't we hear others? *Communication Briefings, 22, no. 1* (July 2005), 1.

CHAPTER 4

Female Sexual Anatomy and Physiology

FEATURES

Global Dimensions
Female Genital Mutilation in Various Parts of the World

Ethical Dimensions
Should PMS Be Used as an Excuse for Unacceptable Behaviors?

Gender Dimensions
Breast Self-Examination

Multicultural Dimensions
Breast Cancer More Deadly in African Americans

CHAPTER OBJECTIVES

1 Name and describe the parts of the female reproductive system, to include external and internal genitalia.

2 Discuss the role of breasts in sexual arousal and response, as well as in the reproductive function of lactation.

3 Explain the role of hormones as they pertain to sexuality.

4 Describe what occurs during menstruation, to include menarche, the menstrual cycle, and problems associated with each.

5 Cite various diseases that can affect the female reproductive system and the self-care procedures, as well as medical treatments, associated with these diseases.

INTRODUCTION

*O*ne of the authors of this text was sitting at his desk preparing for an upcoming class. On the desk were diagrams of the female and male reproductive systems, colored pictures with various parts differentiated from others by different pastel colors and shading. Before long, a colleague walked into the office. The visitor was a professor of educational administration and the proud recipient of a baccalaureate degree in mathematics, a master's degree in counseling, and a doctorate in educational administration. In short, this was an educated man, one on whom students and family relied and whose opinions were accorded the respect someone of his stature deserves. As he entered the office, he glanced at the desk and was fascinated with the reproductive system diagrams. When he inquired as to their purpose, he was told that they were to be used in a sexuality education class to help students learn about their sexual organs. It was then that he sheepishly admitted his own ignorance about the structure and function of the reproductive system. For the next 20 minutes, he and his colleague proceeded to discuss the reproductive systems of females and males, referring to the diagrams on the desk.

The only surprising aspect of this incident was the openness with which this educated man admitted his ignorance. In general, people know less about themselves, both physically and psychologically, than they know about cars or ecology or sports or politics or contemporary musicians or any of the hundreds of topics people care about or find fascinating. The less we know about our bodies, the less well equipped we are to keep them healthy. The more we know, the more choices we have and the better decisions we can make. Appropriate health maintenance should be valued similarly by males and females, and both genders need to adopt certain behaviors, such as periodic medical screenings, to *maintain their health. However, men's and women's reproductive health issues are not the same.*

The purpose of this chapter is to describe the anatomy and physiology of the female reproductive system as a step toward creating a comprehensive picture of human sexuality.

External/Vulva

FIGURE 4.1 Female external reproductive organs.

The Female Reproductive System

Both females and males have external and internal genitals, or reproductive organs. We begin with the external female genitals and progress inward.

The External Genitals

The external female genitals are the mons pubis, labia majora, labia minora, clitoris, vestibule, and urethral opening (Figure 4.1). All of these organs together are called the **vulva**.

---

vulva The female external genitalia.

mons pubis (mons veneris, mount of Venus) The rounded, soft area above the vaginal opening that becomes covered with hair at puberty.

labia majora Two large folds of skin whose main function is to protect the external genitalia and the opening of the vestibule (defined later).

labia minora Two folds of skin lying inside the labia majora, which contain numerous blood vessels and nerve receptors.

The Mons Veneris

The **mons pubis** (also called the **mons veneris**, or **mount of Venus**) is the rounded, soft area above the pubic bone that becomes covered with hair at puberty. Since the mons contains numerous nerve endings, it can be sexually stimulated.

The Labia Majora

The **labia majora** (major lips) are two large folds of skin whose main function is to protect the external genitalia. Unless the labia majora are spread apart, the other external genitalia are not visible. The outer surfaces of the labia majora also grow hair after puberty, and the inner surfaces remain smooth. Within the tissue of the labia majora are smooth muscle fibers, nerves, and vessels for blood and lymph.

The Labia Minora

The **labia minora** (minor lips) are two folds of skin lying inside the labia majora. Loaded with blood vessels and nerve receptors, the labia minora and their upper part, the clitoris, are very sensitive to stimulation. During sexual arousal, blood fills the labia minora, causing them to spread, making the vagina

Female Genital Mutilation in Various Parts of the World

Female genital mutilation has been used throughout the world for various reasons. Primary among them is the quest to diminish sexual stimulation. The result, the argument goes, is that fewer women participate in sexual intercourse outside of marriage and fewer masturbate. Other reasons cited for female genital mutilation include (1) the belief that female genitalia are unsightly and dirty, and that unmutilated girls are unclean; (2) the belief that mutilation is necessary for a girl to be considered a woman—in some cultures, the clitoris and labia are considered the "male parts" of a woman's body; (3) initiation into adulthood; and (4) religious beliefs and practices (Amnesty International, 2009).

Female mutilation can take several different forms. The most simple form is *circumcision*, whereby the clitoral hood is removed. In a *clitoridectomy*, the clitoris itself is surgically removed. Genital *infibulation* is the most complex procedure: The clitoris and the labia minora are removed, and both sides of the vulva are scraped raw and then stitched together. When the tissue grows together, only a small opening remains through which urine and the menstrual flow pass. During these procedures, it is unusual for sterile instruments to be used. Most of the time razor blades or broken glass is used to do the cutting, without the benefit of pain-reducing medications or disinfectants. Therefore, as you might imagine, aside from causing psychological trauma, female mutilation can result in serious medical complications. The combination of infections, bleeding, and pain can cause shock, gangrene, and even death.

According to the World Health Organization (2014), 125 million girls and women alive today have been genitally mutilated in the 29 countries of Africa and Middle East where the practice is concentrated.

Mutilated women are also increasingly found in Europe, Australia, Canada, and the United States, primarily among immigrants from Africa and southwestern Asia (UNICEF, 2011a).

In response, several international organizations have attempted to end this practice. In 1997, the World Health Organization (WHO), the United Nations Population Fund (UNFPA), and the United Nations Children's Fund (UNICEF) issued a statement opposed to female genital mutilation. In 2008, WHO, with nine other United Nations partners, issued a new statement on the elimination of female genital manipulation and provided evidence of its frequency and scope, while also offering recommendations for its elimination. More recently, in 2012, the United Nations General Assembly adopted a resolution on the elimination of female genital mutilation; WHO, in collaboration with key United Nations agencies, also published global strategies to stop healthcare providers from performing female genital mutilation.

Numerous other organizations and governments have publicly opposed female genital mutilation, even though the tendency is to avoid interference in cultural practices of sovereign countries. Grass-roots organizations, such as the Kenyan women's organization Maendeleo ya Wanawake, and Tostan in Senegal, have also sprung up around the world with the goal of eliminating female genital mutilation. These groups conduct educational campaigns encouraging women to break the generational cycle of female genital mutilation by preventing their daughters from experiencing it. The prevalence of female genital mutilation is declining. It is measurably less common among younger women than older ones, and among daughters compared with their mothers. But progress is slow, and millions of girls remain threatened by the practice (UNICEF, 2011b).

---

more accessible. Within the labia minora lie **Bartholin's glands**. The glands slightly lubricate the labia during coitus (intercourse).

The Clitoris

The **clitoris** is the most sensitive structure in the female body. This small organ contains two spongy bodies, the **corpora cavernosa**, that have the capacity to fill with blood during arousal. (The penis, a similar organ, contains spongy bodies that react to arousal in a similar way.) During sexual stimulation,

the corpora cavernosa fill with blood, causing the clitoris to become erect. Popular knowledge about the

---

Bartholin's glands Small glands located within the labia minora that secrete a few drops of fluid during sexual arousal.

clitoris The structure located at the upper part of the labia minora that is homologous to the penis and is very sensitive to stimulation.

corpora cavernosa A cavernous structure located within the clitoris or the penis that fills with blood during sexual excitement, causing erection.

Many variations exist in the female external genitals.

sensitivity of the clitoris has led some to seek out and stimulate it to arouse their female sexual partners. Here is a case in which knowledge can have either a positive or a negative effect on sexual relationships. Those who carefully and delicately stimulate the clitoris may sexually arouse their partner, but those who rub incessantly will only irritate the clitoris and thereby irritate their partner.

The clitoris is covered by the **clitoral hood**. As can be seen in Figure 4.1, the hood is attached to the labia minora. One function of the clitoral hood is to protect the glans of the clitoris. When we discuss the male reproductive organs, we will observe that the foreskin of the penis protects the glans penis in a similar way.

Knowing about the anatomy of the reproductive system offers guidance for sexual functioning, and the relationship of the clitoris, the clitoral hood, and the labia minora provides a case in point. During sexual excitement, the clitoris retracts under the clitoral hood. Therefore, stimulating the clitoris requires pulling back the clitoral hood, pulling the labia majora upward, or putting pressure on the hood or clitoris itself. For example, during sexual intercourse, the clitoris can be stimulated if the penis is positioned correctly. One position that will stimulate the clitoris is called "riding high." With the female lying on her back, the male places his penis into the vagina so that its upper shaft rubs on the clitoris. Another option is for the penis to be pressed, thrusting downward, on the lower part of the labia minora so as to create downward movement of the hood and its contact with the clitoris. Many women, however, require additional manual stimulation of the clitoris to cause orgasm during intercourse.

The Vestibule
When the clitoris is erect and the labia minora spread, the urethral and vaginal openings (called the **vestibule**) become visible.

The Urethral Opening
The urethral opening, where urine is excreted, is not generally considered a part of the reproductive system in females, although there is some evidence that women who do experience something akin to ejaculation do so through the urethra.

The Hymen
The **hymen**, a thin connective tissue containing a relatively large number of blood vessels, covers the opening of the vagina in women who have an intact hymen. The function of this tissue is unknown. Hymens vary in shape and size: A hymen may surround the vaginal opening (an **annular** hymen), bridge it (a **septate** hymen), or form a sievelike covering (a **cribriform** hymen) (Figure 4.2).

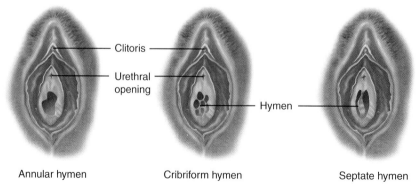

Annular hymen   Cribriform hymen   Septate hymen

FIGURE **4.2** The various types of hymens.

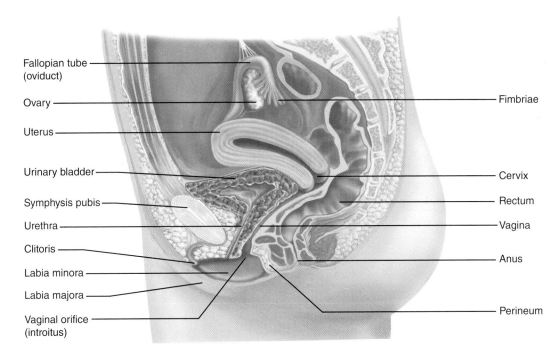

Fallopian tube (oviduct)
Ovary
Uterus
Urinary bladder
Symphysis pubis
Urethra
Clitoris
Labia minora
Labia majora
Vaginal orifice (introitus)

Fimbriae
Cervix
Rectum
Vagina
Anus
Perineum

FIGURE 4.3 Organs of the female reproductive system.

Normally all forms of hymens have openings that are large enough to permit menstrual flow or the insertion of a tampon or a finger, but that are usually too small to permit an erect penis to enter without the hymen tearing. Historically the presence of an intact hymen was considered proof that a woman had never had intercourse. But the hymen can be ruptured by accident or by normal exercise, as well as by intercourse, so a tear in the tissue is not a reliable indication that a woman is no longer a virgin. The rupturing of the hymen during first intercourse generally does not result in a great deal of pain and bleeding, although some people expect it to. Pain is usually related to muscular tension due to anxiety or to entry of the penis into the vagina before the vagina is sufficiently lubricated; care and attention can ordinarily prevent it. A few drops of blood may be noticeable.

The Internal Genitals

The female internal genitals consist of such structures as the vagina, uterus, fallopian tubes, and ovaries. These structures of the female internal genitalia, as well as relevant surrounding structures, are depicted in Figures 4.3 and 4.4.

The Vagina

The **vagina** is a hollow, tunnel-like structure, about 4.5 inches (11.4 centimeters) long, that opens outward to the vestibule and at the opposite end into the uterus. The vagina has several reproductive functions: It surrounds the penis and receives its ejaculate during intercourse, serves as the route of exit for the newborn, and provides an exit for menstrual flow. When the vagina is empty, its lips and walls are in contact, but during childbirth the vagina can expand wide enough for the baby to pass through, and during intercourse it can both expand and close tightly enough on a penis to provide sexual satisfaction. Soft transverse folds in the vaginal wall enable the vagina to expand, and muscle fibers within the walls enable it to contract, as they do in orgasm. No muscles surround the vaginal entrance (the **introitus**); however, the **pubococcygeal**

clitoral hood The skin covering the clitoris.

vestibule The area containing the vaginal and urethral openings.

hymen A thin connective tissue covering the opening of the vagina.

annular Type of hymen that surrounds the vaginal opening.

septate Type of hymen that bridges the vaginal opening.

cribriform Type of hymen that creates a sievelike covering for the vaginal opening.

vagina A hollow, tunnel-like structure of the female internal genitalia whose reproductive functions are to receive the penis and its ejaculate, serve as a route of exit for the newborn, and provide an exit for menstrual flow.

introitus The vaginal entrance.

pubococcygeal muscle A muscle that encircles the vagina and supports it.

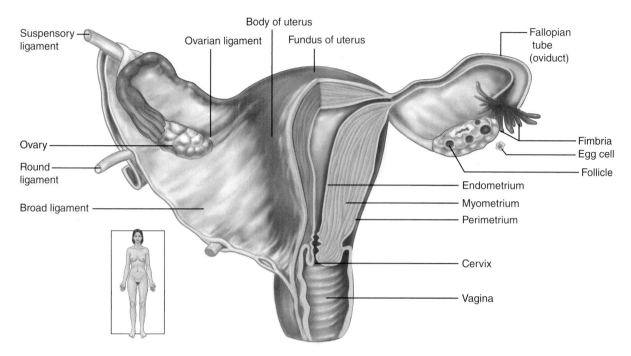

FIGURE 4.4   An anterior view of the female reproductive organs showing the relationships of the ovaries, fallopian tubes, uterus, cervix, and vagina.

and **bulbocavernosus muscles** that support the vagina can be voluntarily contracted so as to intensify sexual responsiveness by forcing the vaginal walls to close on the penis. Exercises to help women develop greater control of these muscles (called **Kegel exercises** after their proponent) are frequently recommended by sexual counselors (Kegel, 1952). To learn to control the pubococcygeal muscles, try the following:

1. Insert a finger into the vagina and contract muscles in that area until you feel the vagina squeeze the finger.

2. Practice squeezing and then relaxing these muscles—first slowly, then rapidly.

3. Practice the preceding exercise about three times daily until you feel you have voluntary control of the pubococcygeal muscles.

The Grafenberg Spot
One would think that after centuries of studying the human body and its sexual nature there would be

little room for disagreement regarding its function. Not so. The existence and the effect of the **Grafenberg spot (G spot)** provide a case in point.

The stimulation of an area along the anterior (front) wall of the vagina, several inches into the vaginal canal and just below the bladder, appears to be sexually exciting for many females. This area is known as the Grafenberg spot, named after Ernest Grafenberg, the gynecologist who first noted its erotic potential (Figure 4.5) (Grafenberg, 1950). The presence of glands in this area has been known for some time (Skene, 1980), and it is these glands—called **Skene's glands**—through which a type of ejaculate is expelled in some women when they experience orgasm by stimulation of the G spot (Grafenberg, 1950; Sevely & Bennett, 1978; Addiego et al., 1981; Belzer, 1981; Perry & Whipple, 1981; Zaviacic et al., 1988).

Others maintain that there is no one particular spot in the vagina that is more sensitive than others to stimulation (Kilchevsky et al., 2012; Puppo & Gruenwald, 2012). For example, the noted sexual therapist Helen Singer Kaplan believed there are many spots within the vagina that are sexually arousing, and the G spot is merely one of those (Kaplan, 1983). Masters and Johnson agreed with Kaplan; they reported that only 10% of the women they studied "had an area of heightened sensitivity in the front wall of the vagina or a tissue mass that fit the various descriptions of this area" (Masters, Johnson, & Kolodny, 1985). Although some women reported sensitivity in the front wall of the vagina, a study by Alzate and Londono (1984) could not locate a specific spot such as that described by

bulbocavernosus muscle A muscle that encircles and supports the vagina.

Kegel exercises Exercises to help women develop greater control of muscles supporting the genitalia.

Grafenberg spot (G spot) An area located along the anterior wall of the vagina, several inches into the vaginal canal, that when stimulated in some women may result in sexual excitement and/or orgasm.

Skene's glands Glands located along the walls of the vagina that are thought to be analogous to the male prostate gland, and the site from which some women eject a fluid during orgasm.

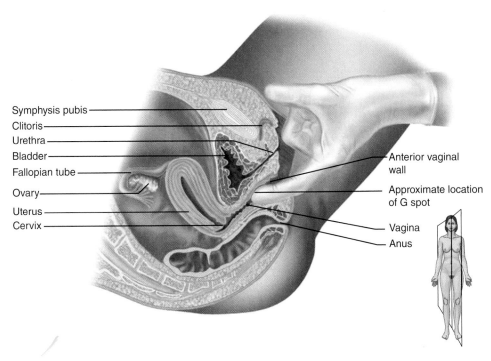

Symphysis pubis
Clitoris
Urethra
Bladder
Fallopian tube
Ovary
Uterus
Cervix

Anterior vaginal wall
Approximate location of G spot
Vagina
Anus

FIGURE 4.5 The location of the Grafenberg spot.

Grafenberg. Heath (1984) found an area of erotic sensitivity and concluded that it is larger than previously described: about the width of the middle two fingers and at least two-thirds the length.

In a more recent study of female twins, 56% of the women studied reported having a G spot, even though there was determined to be no genetic basis for its existence (Burri, Cherkas, & Spector, 2010). However, there still remain skeptics. For example, some researchers explain the sensation on the anterior wall of the vagina as pressure and movement of the clitoris during vaginal penetration and not a distinct G spot area (Foldes & Buisson, 2009). At the 2009 meeting of the International Society for the Study of Women's Sexual Health Congress, the *Journal of Sexual Medicine* held a debate among experts regarding the existence of the G spot. The conclusion was that more research is needed to determine whether the G spot actually exists (Jannini et al., 2010).

The Female Prostate

The existence of a female prostate and ejaculate, although controversial, was first described centuries ago. In the 4th century, several Chinese Taoist texts mentioned female ejaculation. In the 7th century, the Indian *Kamasutra* mentioned it, as did Aristotle (in 300 B.C.) and Galen (in the 2nd century) (Korda, Goldstein, & Sommer, 2010).

That glandular tissue exists in the area of the G spot is not debatable. The pathologist Robert Mallon (1984) conducted autopsies on women and found evidence of

this glandular tissue, as did Heath (1984). Both of these researchers found prostatelike glandular tissue in the front wall of the vagina. When the substances within these glands were analyzed, they were found to contain fluids similar to those found in the male prostate. Hence, some sexuality experts have concluded that there are a female prostate (the Skene's glands) and a female ejaculate. Further evidence for a female ejaculate is offered by Addiego and colleagues (1981), who analyzed the fluid expelled by females at the time of orgasm and found it to contain an enzyme (prostatic acid phosphatase, or PAP) characteristic of semen. However, when Goldberg and associates (1983) studied this ejaculate, they concluded that it was similar to urine. Alzate and Hoch (1986) also found ejaculate secreted through the urethra. To complicate matters further, a study conducted by Belzer and associates (1984) concluded that the ejaculate obtained from women contained significantly more prostatic acid phosphatase than did their urine. More recently, researchers using ultrasound and biochemical analysis concluded that there is glandular tissue surrounding the length of the female urethra containing a duct that secretes fluid during orgasm. Upon analysis, that fluid was more similar to prostate secretions than urine (Wimpissinger et al., 2007). Obviously, further study is needed to confirm the existence of a female ejaculate beyond any doubt.

That some women expel a fluid from the vagina during orgasm has been demonstrated. The prevalence of this phenomenon is between 10% and 54% (Castleman, 2014; Pastor, 2012). In a series of studies,

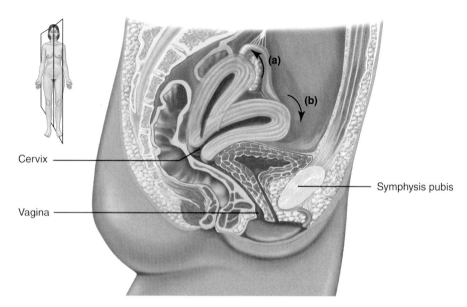

Cervix

Vagina

Symphysis pubis

FIGURE 4.6 Various positions of the uterus: (a) retroflexed and (b) anteflexed.

Zaviacic and colleagues professed to clarify the confusion surrounding female ejaculation and the female prostate (Zaviacic et al., 2000; Zaviacic & Ablin, 2000). In summarizing Zaviacic's research, Castleman (2014) cites several conclusions that support the existence of a female prostate and female ejaculation from this prostate. First, microscopic studies of the Skene's glands have identified cells that secrete fluid. Second, women produce prostate-specific antigen (PSA), a compound unique to the prostate gland. When men develop prostate cancer, PSA levels rise. When women develop cancer of the Skene's glands, their PSA levels also rise. Therefore women must have tissue analogous to the male prostate. Zaviacic and colleagues concluded that the Skene's glands are, in fact, the female prostate and that female ejaculate is similar to male semen.

Whether this fluid is similar to that of the male prostate remains a matter of much research and debate. What is not discussed or researched, however, is the concern first expressed by the Boston Women's Health Collective (1998) regarding the possibility that the G spot orgasm will become a new "ideal" for the sexually liberated woman. It would indeed be unfortunate if this new ideal created pressure on women who do not experience erotic feelings when the Grafenberg spot is stimulated and, therefore, perceive themselves to be inadequate sexually. When the media popularize sexual information, as they did with the Grafenberg spot, often education is needed to remind the public about the many paths to sexual fulfillment. This is particularly true today.

The Uterus

At the top of the vagina lies the **uterus**, a pear-shaped hollow organ with muscular walls. Its function is to nurture the developing embryo and fetus. Except during pregnancy, the uterus is about 3 inches (8 centimeters) long, 3 inches wide at the top, and 1 inch (2.5 centimeters) thick. The uterus extends into the vagina at its **cervix**; the actual opening to the uterus in the cervix is called the **os**. The upper two-thirds of this cavity is called the **corpus**, and the top end is called the **fundus**. Most uteruses tilt forward (that is, they are *anteflexed*) over the bladder; approximately 20% tilt backward (*retroflexed*) (Figure 4.6). Women with retroflexed uteruses are more likely to experience discomfort during menstruation and may have more difficulty in inserting a diaphragm as a result of the angle of the cervix. Contrary to widespread belief, however, the ability to conceive is in no way affected by the position of the uterus.

The uterus consists of three layers. The outermost layer, the **perimetrium**, is very elastic, enabling the uterus to accommodate a growing embryo during pregnancy. The middle layer, the **myometrium**, consists of

uterus A pear-shaped hollow structure of the female genitalia in which the embryo and fetus develop before birth.

cervix The mouth of the uterus, through which the vagina extends.

os The opening to the uterus.

corpus The upper two-thirds of the uterus.

fundus The upper end of the uterus closest to the opening of the fallopian tubes.

perimetrium The outermost layer of the uterus, sometimes termed the *serosa*, a very elastic layer that allows the uterus to accommodate a growing embryo and fetus.

myometrium The middle layer of the uterus, consisting of smooth muscle that aids in the pushing of the newborn through the cervix.

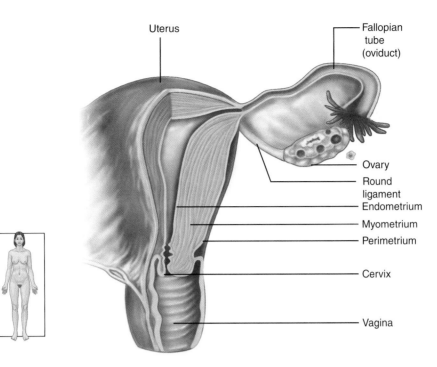

FIGURE **4.7** Layers of the uterine wall.

smooth muscles, whose ability to contract helps push the newborn through the cervix and into the vagina (which during childbirth acts as the birth canal). The innermost layer of the uterus is the **endometrium**. This layer is loaded with blood vessels and can therefore provide the nourishment necessary to sustain a developing fetus. It builds up and partly sloughs off as the menstrual flow in every menstrual cycle, unless fertilization takes place. Figure 4.7 depicts the anatomical relationships of the three layers of the uterus.

The Fallopian Tubes and the Ovaries
At the fundus, the uterus opens into the two **fallopian tubes** (we will use this more common name, although **oviduct** might be more appropriate). At the other end of each tube is an **ovary**, the organ that produces and stores the *ova*, or eggs. When a female is born, each of her ovaries contains approximately 40,000 to 400,000 eggs. Every egg has the potential to be fertilized by a sperm to become an embryo. After the girl reaches puberty, one of these eggs is usually discharged through the wall of one of her ovaries during each menstrual cycle. The egg develops inside a capsule called a **Graafian follicle** and is discharged when it has matured. The discharged egg, now matured and freed from its capsule and the ovary, is ready to be fertilized by a male's sperm. When the follicle ruptures to discharge its egg, the empty follicle, now a yellowish structure called the **corpus luteum**, secretes a hormone (**progesterone**) that signals the endometrium to prepare for a fertilized egg. Progesterone and **estrogen**, another

hormone produced by the ovaries, play significant roles in menstruation, birth, growth, and aging.

When the ovum is discharged from the ovary, it is directed into the fallopian tubes. As shown in Figure 4.4, these tubes serve as routes for ova to reach the uterus. The newly released ovum is caught by the fingerlike end of the fallopian tube, called a **fimbria**, and is guided into the cone-shaped open end of the tube. If fertilization takes place, it usually takes place there.

endometrium The innermost layer of the uterus, to which the fertilized egg attaches and by which it is nourished as it develops before birth, which is partly discharged (if pregnancy does not occur) with the menstrual flow.

fallopian tubes (oviduct) The routes through which eggs leave the ovaries on their way to the uterus, in which fertilization normally occurs.

ovary A structure of the female genitalia that houses ova before their maturation and discharge and that produces estrogen and progesterone.

Graafian follicle A part of the ovary from which a mature egg ruptures, allowing the corpus luteum to develop in the location where the egg was released.

corpus luteum A yellowish structure that develops in the Graafian follicle at the discharge of an ovum and that produces progesterone and estrogen.

progesterone A hormone secreted by the corpus luteum signaling the endometrium to develop in preparation for a zygote.

estrogen A hormone produced by the ovaries whose level in the blood helps control the menstrual cycle.

fimbria The fingerlike ends of the fallopian tubes that catch the ova when they are discharged from the ovaries.

FIGURE 4.8 The female breast.

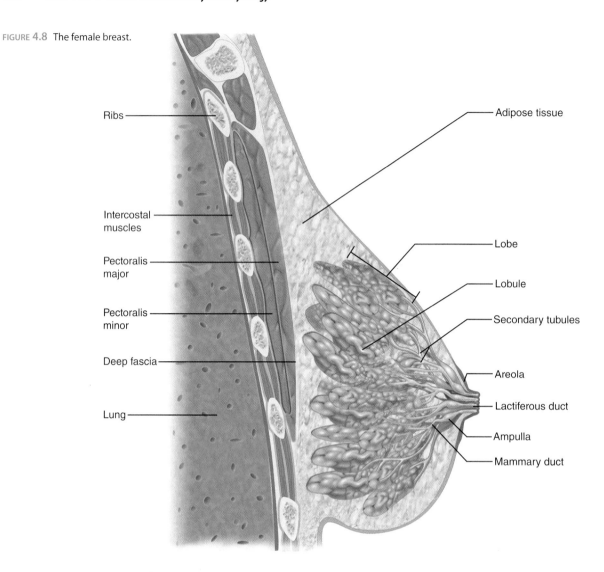

Ribs

Intercostal muscles

Pectoralis major

Pectoralis minor

Deep fascia

Lung

Adipose tissue

Lobe

Lobule

Secondary tubules

Areola

Lactiferous duct

Ampulla

Mammary duct

Whether fertilized or not, the ovum continues on its journey through the tube, moved along in a sweeping motion by tiny hairlike structures called **cilia**. The destination of the fertilized ovum is the endometrium in the uterus, where it becomes attached and continues its development. An unfertilized ovum also travels to the endometrium, then disintegrates, and eventually is expelled through the vagina, along with some of the endometrium, in the process called *menstruation*. (Once an ovum is expelled, the menstrual cycle is completed. Soon an ovary will discharge another mature egg and the process will begin again.)

It should be noted that occasionally a woman may produce more than one egg per cycle, thereby becoming prone to multiple births. Fertility drugs, which may result in multiple births, are suspected of causing the maturation of several eggs per cycle. Sometimes the fertilized egg may attach in the abdominal cavity or the fallopian tube rather than in the uterus. This is termed an **ectopic pregnancy**.

▌ The Breasts

Although the female breasts are not reproductive organs, they do have significance in sexual arousal and response, and they serve an important reproductive function in providing milk for the newborn infant. Each breast contains about 15 to 20 clusters of milk-secreting structures called **mammary glands** (Figure 4.8). Each of these mammary gland clusters has an opening to the nipple, where the milk ducts open. The stimulation of the newborn's sucking on the nipple causes the pituitary gland to secrete a

cilia Hairlike structures that guide objects, such as ova, moving past them.

ectopic pregnancy The attachment and development of the zygote in a location other than in the uterus.

mammary glands Milk-secreting glands located in the female breast.

The size and shape of breasts vary among women.

hormone called **prolactin**, which in turn stimulates the production of breast milk.

Most of the breast is fat and connective tissue. Except for small muscles in the area of the nipple and **areola** (the darkened skin around the nipple), there are no muscles in the breast. Because the breast is muscle-free, exercises to increase breast size are ineffective. Over the years the breasts may hang lower than normal if the ligaments are stretched by lack of support or by jostling (for example, not wearing a bra while jogging).

The nipples—of men as well as women—are richly supplied with nerve endings that respond with pleasurable sexual feelings when stimulated. During sexual arousal the nipples become erect. The size of the breasts or their shape is not related to sensitivity. Women with either small or large breasts may be equally sexually stimulated by the fondling of the breasts. Though some have characterized our society as making a fetish of large breasts, preferences in breast size and shape vary from individual to individual. It should be noted, however, that although breast size varies, extent of glandular tissue is comparable in all women's breasts. Because the amount of glandular tissue is the same, women with small breasts produce the same amount of breast milk after childbirth as women with larger breasts and are therefore as successful breastfeeding their babies as are women with larger breasts.

Our society has so emphasized breast size that many women have their breasts reconstructed. In the past, liquid silicone was injected to enlarge the breast, but approximately 60% of women experienced problems such as infection, deformity, or exceptional hardness of the breast. More recently, silicone pouches containing saline solution have been implanted to reshape the breast. However, in 1992, in response to reported breakage of the pouches, the Dow Chemical Company, the largest manufacturer of silicone pouches, stopped manufacturing them and agreed to pay for their removal for women who so desired. The most recent research, however, indicates that silicone implants are not the health issue previously thought. In a study of the research related to silicone breast implants, the Institute of Medicine (a subgroup of the National Academy of Sciences) found no convincing evidence that chronic disease was more likely to develop in women with silicone breast implants

than women without implants (Reuters, 1999). Furthermore, during a lawsuit against breast implant manufacturers, a federal judge appointed a panel of scientists to study the issue and report their findings to the court. The court-appointed panel found no convincing evidence that silicone breast implants cause disease of the immune system as alleged in the lawsuit. The Food and Drug Administration (FDA) also approved silicone-gel implants for breast enhancement in 2003.

In 2011, the FDA announced that subsequent study had verified the safety of silicone breast implants, but stated that women should fully understand the risks before considering getting them. Among the risks cited by the FDA (2011) are the following:

- Breast implants are not lifetime devices. The longer a woman has them, the more likely she is to have complications and need to have the implants removed or replaced. Women with breast implants will need to monitor their breasts for the rest of their lives.

- The most frequently observed complications and adverse outcomes are tightening of the area around the implant, additional surgeries, and implant removal. Other complications include a tear or hole in the outer shell (implant rupture), wrinkling, uneven appearance (asymmetry), scarring, pain, and infection.

- Studies to date do not indicate that silicone gel-filled breast implants cause breast cancer, reproductive problems, or connective tissue disease, such as rheumatoid arthritis. However, no study has been large enough or long enough to completely rule out these and other rare complications.

---

prolactin A pituitary hormone that stimulates the production of milk from the mammary glands.

areola The darkened part of the breast immediately surrounding the nipple.

TABLE 4.1

Functions of the Female Reproductive Organs

Organ	Function
Ovary	Production of egg cells and female sex hormones
Fallopian tube	Conveying of egg cell toward uterus; site of fertilization; transport developing zygote to uterus
Uterus	Protection and sustaining of life of embryo and fetus during pregnancy
Vagina	Conveying of uterine secretions to the outside of body; receiving of erect penis during sexual intercourse; transport of fetus during birth process
Labia majora	Enclosing and protection of other external reproductive organs
Labia minora	Formation of margins of vestibule; protection of openings of vagina and urethra
Clitoris	Organ richly supplied with sensory nerve endings associated with feeling of pleasure during sexual stimulation
Vestibule	Space between labia minora that includes vaginal and urethral openings
Vestibular glands	Secretion of fluid that moistens and lubricates vestibule

We also need to be concerned about other health issues regarding the breast, such as cancer of the breast. (We discuss this in greater detail later in the chapter.) Suffice it to say here that women need to obtain periodic medical checkups by a health professional to make sure that any abnormalities are identified early, thereby increasing the likelihood that treatment will be successful and as noninvasive as possible.

Table 4.1 reviews the functions of the female reproductive organs.

▇ The Hormones

What happens at the sight of an attractive person in a skimpy bathing suit? If the stimulus is sufficiently interesting, it can result in the first stages of sexual response—for example, increased heart rate, vaginal lubrication, and erection of the penis or clitoris. How does the visual image result in these physical changes? The chain of events is rather complex. It starts with the **hypothalamus**, a structure in the brain that, either through direct nerve pathways or through chemicals called **releasing factors**, can instruct various body parts to function. The hypothalamus might be said to serve as a bridge between external stimuli and physiological responses. But let us go back to the bathing suit. Two things happen: (1) When the individual perceives the external stimulus as sexually exciting, the hypothalamus "tells" the pituitary gland to secrete its hormones, and (2) these chemicals stimulate the adrenal gland to secrete its hormones and the testes and ovaries to secrete their hormones. These secretions change the blood flow (producing vasocongestion), the heart rate, breathing, vaginal moistness, and so on.

These powerfully acting **hormones** are chemical substances that influence organs and tissues. They are produced by **endocrine glands**, glands that secrete their products into the bloodstream. The thyroid, for example, secretes a hormone that travels to the heart and increases the heart rate. The adrenal gland secretes the hormone adrenalin, which travels to the bronchial tubes of the lungs and dilates them. As we have just seen, the secretions of several glands are involved in sexual response.

The **pituitary**, a pea-shaped gland located at the base of the brain, serves as a sort of master gland to the others in the system. It stimulates the other glands to release their hormones. The front part of the pituitary secretes three sexual hormones, called **gonadotropins**, which act on or stimulate the **gonads** (the testes and ovaries). The

hypothalamus A structure in the brain that controls the pituitary gland and is directly connected by nerve pathways to various organs of the body.

releasing factors Chemicals released from the hypothalamus that affect the function of various body parts.

hormone A chemical substance secreted by a ductless gland, which is carried to an organ or tissue where it has a specific effect.

endocrine glands Glands that secrete their products into the bloodstream.

pituitary The "master gland," an endocrine gland located at the base of the brain that stimulates the other endocrine glands to produce their hormones.

gonadotropins Sexual hormones secreted by the pituitary that stimulate the gonads to produce their hormones.

gonads The male testes and the female ovaries, which produce gonadotropin hormones responsible for the development of secondary sexual characteristics.

gonads are also endocrine glands, and they produce their own hormones. The three gonadotropins are **follicle-stimulating hormone (FSH)**; **luteinizing hormone (LH)**, often called the **interstitial-cell-stimulating hormone (ICSH)** in males; and prolactin (produced only during pregnancy and breastfeeding). Once stimulated by these gonadotropic hormones, the gonads produce their own hormones: estrogens, progesterones, and androgens. The adrenal gland also secretes androgen directly.

In women, estrogens and progesterones regulate the menstrual cycle, with estrogens important in producing vaginal lubrication. Although estrogens and progesterones have no known function in men, the presence of too much estrogen in the male body can lower interest in sexual activity and may result in enlargement of the breasts. **Androgens** affect the sex drive of both men and women: The presence of too much causes excessive sexual appetite, the presence of too little androgen decreases sexual interest. FSH stimulates cells in the seminiferous tubules (called **spermatocytes**) to produce sperm.

Despite the fact that hormones account for and influence sexual differences, males and females produce the same hormones. Estrogens and progesterones are considered female hormones and androgens male hormones, but both males and females produce all three. They do differ in the amounts they produce, however. For example, males have levels of the strongest androgen (**testosterone**) 10 times those of females, and females have significantly more estrogens than males. Obviously, too, males and females differ in the organs activated by the hormones. Long before we begin to think about hormones and our sexuality, hormones have already had significant effects.

▩ Menstruation

At some time during puberty, a girl reaches **menarche**; that is, she has her first menstrual cycle. Then, and cyclically thereafter unless she is pregnant, blood (actually the blood-enriched endometrium) is discharged (or flows) from her uterus through her vagina for several days. The Latin origin of the word **menstruation** is *mensis*, meaning "month," because the menses, or periods, supposedly occur monthly. Actually they are not so predictable. Between menarche and menopause, when menstruation ceases, a woman's menstrual cycle may stabilize in a 28- to 30-day pattern (20- to 40-day cycles are also quite normal), or it may never stabilize. Cycles may vary in length from period to period, or they may be stable for a long time, fluctuate, and become stable again. Menstruation has been called the "curse," the "monthly sickness," and

worse, but it is a normal physiological response to hormonal activity.

Menarche

The reason menstruation begins when it does is not exactly known. One hypothesis relates to the increase in body fat at puberty as a result of hormonal secretions. Evidence for this hypothesis can be found in long-distance runners. Many women who jog long distances lose considerable weight and body fat. It is not uncommon for such women to experience secondary **amenorrhea**; that is, they no longer menstruate regularly. In fact, some experts estimate that as many as 50% of women runners experience a cessation of menstruation (Barrack et al., 2010). Athletes involved in "lean sports" (those that emphasize weight categories or aesthetics, such as ballet, gymnastics, or endurance running) are at highest risk (Javed et al., 2013). In addition, women suffering from anorexia nervosa—a condition in which the woman is so preoccupied with being thin that she eats very little and loses a great deal of body weight and fat—often lose their periods. In truth, though, no one really knows why women joggers or anorexics cease to menstruate, and, at least for the joggers, there appears to be more going on than just a loss of body fat. Other studies have found that many thin female joggers continue to menstruate, and many heavier ones do not.

Menstrual Physiology

The menstrual cycle begins when the pituitary gland secretes two hormones: FSH, which stimulates the

---

follicle-stimulating hormone (FSH) A hormone, secreted by the anterior portion of the pituitary gland, that "instructs" the ovaries to prepare an egg to be released from a follicle.

luteinizing hormone (LH) A hormone, secreted by the anterior portion of the pituitary gland, that stimulates ovulation.

interstitial-cell-stimulating hormone (ICSH) A hormone, secreted by the anterior portion of the pituitary gland in males, that stimulates the production of sperm.

androgens Male sex hormones.

spermatocytes Cells that develop through several stages to form sperm.

testosterone The male sex hormone produced in the testes that is responsible for the development of male secondary sexual characteristics.

menarche The time when a female begins her first menstrual cycle, usually at 8 to 16 years of age.

menstruation The cyclical emission of the blood-enriched endometrium when pregnancy does not occur.

amenorrhea The absence of menstruation in a woman who should be menstruating.

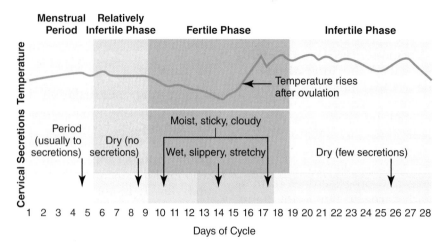

FIGURE **4.9** Temperature and Mucus Changes During the Menstrual Cycle

growth, or "ripening," of follicles in the ovary; and LH, which stimulates the ovary to release one egg, that is, to *ovulate*. Once the egg is released, the area from which it was released (the Graafian follicle) becomes a yellow body (corpus luteum). The Graafian follicle secretes the hormone estrogen, and the yellow body secretes progesterone and estrogen. Progesterone causes the lining of the uterus to thicken and store nutrients in preparation to receive, implant, and nourish a fertilized egg, called a **zygote**. If the egg is not fertilized, the yellow body degenerates and thus becomes unable to secrete progesterone any longer. The lack of progesterone is a signal to expel the unneeded endometrium. This tissue, which is gradually shed over the course of a few days, is the menstrual flow. The cycle is then ready to begin anew.

Phases of the menstrual cycle can be recognized by changes in body temperature and in the type of secretions from the cervix (Figure 4.9).

zygote A fertilized egg.

proliferative phase The first part of the menstrual cycle, during which FSH production is increased and the follicles are maturing.

secretory phase The second part of the menstrual cycle, during which ovulation occurs and the production of LH stimulates the development of the corpus luteum.

menstrual phase The part of the menstrual cycle during which the endometrial lining is sloughed off as the menstrual flow.

follicular phase The part of the menstrual cycle during which menstruation occurs and the pituitary increases the production of FSH so the follicles mature; a combination of the menstrual and proliferative phases.

ovulation The part of the menstrual cycle when the ovum is discharged from the ovary.

luteal phase The same phase of the menstrual cycle as the secretory phase, which includes ovulation and the production of LH from the corpus luteum.

Phases of the Menstrual Cycle

Figures 4.10 and 4.11 depict the roles of hormones in the menstrual cycle and its phases. The first phase is termed the **proliferative phase**. It is during this phase that FSH production is increased by the pituitary gland, which in turn stimulates the follicles in the ovaries to mature. The follicles then can produce estrogen, which causes the endometrial lining of the uterus to thicken and prepare for the implantation of the zygote. The pituitary then increases production of LH in response to the elevated levels of estrogen in the bloodstream, causing one follicle to prepare to expel an ovum (the Graafian follicle), and the proliferative phase proceeds until ovulation.

The **secretory phase** of the menstrual cycle begins once ovulation occurs and entails continued secretions of LH, which stimulate the development of the corpus luteum. The corpus luteum secretes progesterone, causing further thickening and engorgement of blood of the endometrium. If implantation does not occur, the pituitary shuts down production of FSH and LH, causing degeneration of the corpus luteum. The result is a decrease in the secretions of estrogen and progesterone.

The next phase of the menstrual cycle is the **menstrual phase**, in which the endometrial lining of the uterus is sloughed off as the menstrual flow.

Some sexuality experts divide the menstrual cycle into three different phases: the **follicular phase**, **ovulation**, and the **luteal phase**. The follicular phase coincides with the menstrual and proliferative phases, ovulation is marked by the discharge of the ovum from the Graafian follicle, and the luteal phase is the same as the secretory phase. This categorization pertains to changes in the ovaries, whereas the previous categorization refers to changes in the uterus.

FIGURE **4.10** Hormones from the hypothalamus control the release of hormones from the pituitary gland, which in turn regulates production of ova and sex hormones from the ovaries. Note how the rise and fall of the hormone level is related to the building up and sloughing off of the uterine lining.

FIGURE **4.11** Changes in relative concentrations of hormones during ovulation and menstruation.

As noted in Figure 4.11, in a 28-day cycle ovulation occurs on day 14, with the menstrual flow lasting for 4 days. The great variation in the menstrual cycle—among women and even in any one woman—should be emphasized. The 28-day cycle, although often spoken of as *the* cycle, is not very common. Furthermore, in spite of menstrual cycles' differing in length, there is little difference in the luteal phase of these cycles. That is, regardless of the length of the menstrual cycle, once ovulation occurs, it basically takes 14 days until menstruation begins. For example, if a woman's cycle is 42 days long, she will ovulate on day 28, and 14 days later she will menstruate; if her cycle is 30 days long, she will ovulate on day 16 and will still menstruate 14 days later.

Effects of Menstruation on the Body and Mind

Menstruation can have several physical and emotional effects, which vary greatly from woman to woman and from one cycle to another. Eighty-five percent of women of reproductive age experience physical or emotional changes associated with their menstrual cycle, and between 40% and 50% of women are bothered by menstrual cycle–related conditions such

© Adam Gregor/ShutterStock, Inc.

Menstruation can affect a woman's body and mind. Cramps and backaches can occur, as well as feelings of nervousness or depression. Different women are affected differently by menstruation—some women have minor symptoms whereas others have symptoms that are more severe.

function of what she expects to experience. Evidence for this hypothesis does exist. For example, when researchers conducting studies of menstruating women inform the women of what the study is about, women report more of these symptoms than when they do not know what is being studied (Brooks, Ruble, & Clark, 1977; Ruble & Brooks-Gunn, 1979). Because many of these symptoms cannot be objectively measured, what a woman expects to feel may create a self-fulfilling prophecy. That is not to say women do not experience real discomfort; rather, the mind may affect the amount of discomfort experienced.

Stress researchers have determined that the mind–body connection is a real one. That is, with certain actual illnesses and diseases, either the mind affects the body so as to prepare it to become ill or the mind changes the body in a way that makes the illness worse than it might otherwise be (Greenberg, 2013). Other factors that might influence menstrual symptoms include diets too high in saturated fats, a lack of regular exercise, work in extremely cold environments, eating disorders, and stress (Barnard et al., 2000; Medicine.Net.com, 2014; National Institute of Child Health and Human Development, 2014).

The preceding discussion is not meant to negate the real physical and emotional effects of menstruation. For example, depending on one's age, and whether one has given birth to a child or not, cramping associated with menstruation can vary. Teenagers and perimenopausal women—those in the period between the beginning of menopause and the complete cessation of a woman's period—report worse cramping than is usual, whereas women who have given birth to a child report less cramping.

Menstrual Problems

Several conditions associated with menstruation require special attention. Among these conditions are dysmenorrhea, amenorrhea, and premenstrual syndrome.

Dysmenorrhea

Painful menstruation is termed **dysmenorrhea**. Many women experience some discomfort and pain during some menstrual cycles, and other women experience discomfort and pain regularly. It has been estimated that 70% to 90% of menstruating women have some degree of menstrual problems on a regular basis (Sommerfield, n.d.). Women may experience severe abdominal cramping, a bloated feeling, headaches, backaches, and nausea. An estimated 10% to 15% of women experience menstrual pain each month severe enough to prevent normal daily function at school, work, or home (Smith, 2012).

The cause of **primary dysmenorrhea**—that is, pain during menstruation—is not specifically known.

as premenstrual syndrome or premenstrual dysphoric disorder (Ballagh & Heyl, 2008; MedicineNet.com, 2014). It is estimated that 2.5 million women are affected by menstrual disorders each year (Clayton, 2008). There is evidence that some 10% of women take time off from work, school, or other activities because of menstrual discomfort (Patterson, 1990). Some women report cramps, backaches, and pimples; others report none of these symptoms. Some women report feeling depressed, bloated, nervous, or weak, and others do not.

Whether a woman experiences any of these effects—be they physical or emotional—may be a

dysmenorrhea Painful menstruation.

primary dysmenorrhea Painful menstruation, the cause of which is unknown.

Many health practitioners identify the cause as **prostaglandins**, substances produced by body tissues that act as hormones. Prostaglandins, which are found in unusually high amounts in women with dysmenorrhea, cause the muscles in the uterus to contract. This contraction causes pain and cuts off some of the blood supply (with its oxygen) to the uterus, thereby causing more discomfort.

To treat primary dysmenorrhea, physicians sometimes prescribe antiprostaglandin medications such as naproxen (Aleve), Anaprox, or Ponstel. These medicines inhibit the production of prostaglandins and relieve pain, dizziness, headache, nausea, vomiting, and irritability in many women. Many women who do not use prescription drugs find aspirin or ibuprofen helpful in relieving pain (these also somewhat inhibit prostaglandin production). Other remedies proposed for dysmenorrhea include eating more fish and vegetables and less animal fats and taking calcium, vitamin B, and magnesium supplements. Drinking plenty of fluids has also been recommended, because it seems that when the body is dehydrated, the hormone vasopressin is secreted. Vasopressin conserves body fluids, an effect that is not what a woman feeling bloated needs. Oral contraceptives can also help relieve menstrual pain by eliminating ovulation and thereby decreasing the amount of prostaglandin produced (American College of Obstetricians and Gynocologists, 2012). In addition, placing a heating pad on the abdomen, lightly massaging the abdomen with the fingertips (effleurage), drinking warm beverages, taking a warm shower, doing waist-bending exercises, having an orgasm, and walking may alleviate some menstrual pain.

Secondary dysmenorrhea is painful menstruation caused by some other identifiable condition. For example, **endometriosis** (a condition in which endometrial cells attach and develop on some body tissue other than the uterus) can cause secondary dysmenorrhea, as can pelvic inflammatory disease, uterine tumors, and blockages of the opening to the uterus (the os). In these cases, treatment consists of finding and removing the cause of the menstrual pain, which may require surgery or medication.

Amenorrhea

Amenorrhea is the absence of menstrual flow. If a woman has never menstruated and is 18 years or older, her condition is called **primary amenorrhea**. If menstruation ceases after menarche, the condition is called **secondary amenorrhea**. Amenorrhea may be caused by pregnancy, malfunctioning of the ovaries, cysts or tumors, disease, hormonal imbalance, poor nutrition, or emotional distress. It may also be caused by strenuous exercise of the sort done by runners and young dancers (Koutedakis & Jamurtas, 2004; Mayo Clinic Staff, 2014; Torstveit &

Sundgot-Borgen, 2005). The causes of amenorrhea in physically active women are not known. Some experts hypothesize that exercising women experience a decrease in body fat that may contribute to the cessation of their periods, as it does in anorexic women (Medline Plus, 2012). Lower body fat may interfere with production of the amount of estrogen needed to menstruate. Among female athletes, amenorrhea is quite common (Mayo Clinic, 2007a), and it is suspected the cause is a combination of low body fat, the stress upon the body as a result of strenuous physical exercise, and the psychological stress associated with competition. Although the actual cause of amenorrhea in female athletes is difficult to determine, it does not follow that some physical condition does not exist in any one woman—athlete or not—that can be identified as the cause of her menstrual problem. It is advised that women whose menses cease consult their physicians to discuss any conditions or illnesses that are treatable.

The fear of pregnancy also has been known to create enough anguish and anxiety in sexually active women to cause a cessation of menses. Fearing pregnancy, many couples wait with bated breath for the evidence that the woman is not pregnant—menstruation. A slight delay in her period (not unusual) makes the woman anxious about the possibility of an unwanted pregnancy. Her anxiety can then further delay menstruation or create amenorrhea. Thus a vicious cycle develops that only a pregnancy test or the menstrual flow can break. Any woman who has been sexually active and has missed more than one period should have a pregnancy test.

Premenstrual Syndrome

Some women experience mood changes and other physical and emotional discomforts just before their menstrual periods. This condition is referred to as **premenstrual syndrome (PMS)**. In fact, more than 150 disorders have been associated with premenstrual syndrome; some of the more common ones are depression, tension, anxiety, mood swings, irritability

---

prostaglandins Hormonelike substances produced by body tissue that may cause dysmenorrhea.

secondary dysmenorrhea Painful menstruation caused by some identifiable condition such as endometriosis.

endometriosis The growth of the endometrium uterine lining at a location other than in the uterus.

primary amenorrhea A condition in which a woman of age 18 years or older has never menstruated.

secondary amenorrhea A condition in which a woman has ceased menstruating after menarche.

premenstrual syndrome (PMS) Marked mood fluctuation during the week before menstruation, accompanied by physical symptoms.

TABLE 4.2

Premenstrual Symptoms

The Office of Women's Health of the U.S. Department of Health and Human Services lists the following symptoms of PMS:

- Acne
- Feeling tired
- Upset stomach
- Constipation
- Diarrhea
- Appetite changes or food cravings
- Trouble with concentration or memory
- Depression

- Swollen or tender breasts
- Trouble sleeping
- Bloating
- Anxiety
- Headache or backache
- Joint or muscle pain
- Tension, irritability, mood swings, crying spells

Source: Office of Women's Health. *Premenstrual syndrome (PMS) fact sheet,* 2012. Available: http://www.womenshealth.gov/publications/our-publications /fact-sheet/premenstrual-syndrome.html.

or anger, difficulty in concentrating, lethargy, weight gain, fluid retention, bloating, breast soreness, joint or muscle pain, nausea, vomiting, and headaches (Mayo Clinic, 1998). It has been estimated that at some time during their reproductive years 75% of women experience PMS (Mayo Clinic, 2007b).

Premenstrual syndrome was described by Katharina Dalton, a leading researcher in the treatment of PMS, in *Once a Month* (1979): "Once a month with monotonous regularity, chaos is inflicted on American homes as premenstrual tension and other menstrual problems recur time and again with demoralizing repetition." Reading this, many women found solace in the fact that other women had similar experiences each menstrual cycle. It is undeniable that many women do experience something akin to PMS fairly regularly (see Table 4.2).

There is no laboratory test or other sure way to diagnose premenstrual syndrome. Doctors rely on the woman's menstrual history, often requesting that patients keep a diary of the onset, duration, and the nature and severity of symptoms for at least two menstrual cycles. If symptoms such as those cited are present in the week before a woman's period, subside as her period starts, and are absent the week after her period, she is diagnosed as having PMS. This diagnosis is important not only to determine the treatment to recommend but also to help screen out other conditions commonly confused with PMS, such as contraceptive side effects, dysmenorrhea, eating disorders, substance abuse, depression, and other psychiatric disorders.

There have been numerous theories about the causes of PMS. These are described in the following list, along with the recommended treatment based on the theory of causation.

1. *Prostaglandins.* As a woman's uterine lining begins to shed during the menstrual cycle, prostaglandins (hormones) are released into her bloodstream. As the prostaglandins build up, they cause the uterine walls to become tense and to contract, resulting in cramping. As with dysmenorrhea, antiprostaglandin medications are recommended, such as aspirin, acetaminophen (for example, Tylenol or Datril), naproxen (Aleve), or ibuprofen (Motrin, Advil, or Nuprin).

 Did You Know . . .

When the American Psychiatric Association included PMS in its *Diagnostic and Statistical Manual of Mental Disorders IV* as an illness, terming it **late luteal phase dysphoric disorder (LLPDD)**, some people objected to the potential negative economic and social impact for all women. They believed it promoted a view of women as unreliable and unstable. However, others were grateful that women could then collect health insurance for treating PMS and that research would be focused on the condition.

In 2013, *Diagnostic and Statistical Manual of Mental Disorders, Fifth Edition (DSM-5)* was published. It reaffirmed LLPDD as an illness, and defined it as physical and/or behavioral symptoms that occur repetitively in the second half of the menstrual cycle and often the first few days of the menses.

2. *Progesterone.* Progesterone builds up during the menstrual cycle, causing PMS symptoms. Antiprogesterone medications are recommended to alter the menstrual cycle (speeding or delaying the onset of bleeding).

3. *Natural opiates.* Women experience a drop in the level of the neurotransmitter beta-endorphin, which is manufactured in the brain the week before the menstrual flow. This neurotransmitter has been described as the body's natural opiate in that it alleviates pain and generally makes you feel good. Treatment involves administering the drug naloxone, which maintains high levels of beta-endorphins.

4. *State of mind.* The symptoms of PMS are the result of brain activity—that is, the mind. Moods, perceptions, thoughts, ideas, self-confidence, and self-image are "choreographed" by the brain premenstrually. Treatment, therefore, entails counseling and other means to help women change their states of mind.

Other treatments include the following:

1. Birth control pills to stop ovulation.

2. Medications such as injectable medroxyprogesterone acetate (Depo-Provera) to stop ovulation and menstruation temporarily in severe cases.

3. Antidepressants in lower dosages than usually prescribed for depression, such as fluoxetine hydrochloride (Prozac), sertaline hydrochloride (Zoloft), paroxetine hydrochloride (Paxil), and venlafaxine hydrochloride (Effexor), if symptoms are mainly emotional.

4. A vegetarian diet.

5. Naturopathic medicine that includes lifestyle and dietary changes and may consist of nutritional supplements, botanical medicines, homeopathy, Chinese medicine, acupuncture, hydrotherapy, manipulation, physical therapy, or minor surgery (Phalen, 2000).

In addition, the following is recommended (Mayo Clinic, 2012):

1. Maintain a healthy body weight.

2. Lower the intake of salt and salty foods, especially before the period, to reduce fluid retention and bloating.

3. Avoid alcohol before the period to minimize depression and mood swings.

4. Avoid caffeine, such as in coffee, cola, and tea, to reduce moodiness, tension, and breast tenderness.

5. Increase the intake of carbohydrates such as breads, potatoes, cereals, vegetables, and rice.

6. Exercise regularly to enhance the sense of well-being.

7. Reduce stress by getting plenty of sleep, practicing a relaxation technique regularly, and trying yoga or massage.

Premenstrual Dysphoric Disorder

As many as 10% of women experience premenstrual symptoms so severe they cannot maintain their daily routines (Mayo Clinic, 2008). Some experts believe this is a result of a condition they term *premenstrual dysphoric disorder* (PMDD). PMDD has been

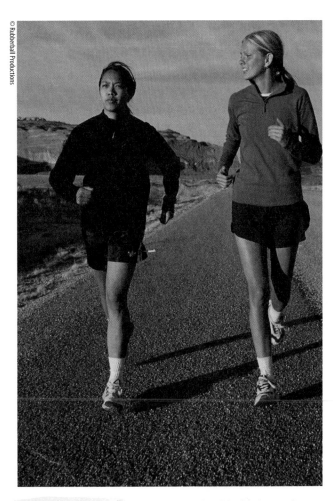

© Rubberball Productions

Exercising regularly and maintaining a healthy body weight are two strategies that are recommended to help women limit the severity of their menstrual and premenstrual symptoms.

late luteal phase dysphoric disorder (LLPDD) A type of premenstrual syndrome in which mental and emotional symptoms occur the week before menstruation. This is the name given to that condition by the American Psychiatric Association.

Ethical
DIMENSIONS

Should PMS Be Used as an Excuse for Unacceptable Behaviors?

Ever since British courts in the 1980s lessened the charges against two women who admitted to murder, sentencing them based on charges of manslaughter instead, because they were judged to suffer from PMS, various legal defenses have been mounted based on similar arguments. The legal basis for these defenses is "diminished responsibility," which attorneys have argued is grounds to either lessen a client's sentence or excuse the client from punishment altogether. Those supportive of this view argue that the symptoms of PMS—for example, trouble concentrating, irritability, mood swings, anxiety and depression, anger, headache or backache, insomnia, and many others—are consistent with an *insanity* defense, which claims that a crime is committed unconsciously, even if the individual is only temporarily insane. Another defense relies on claims of *diminished capacity*. That is, offenders are said to be unable to comprehend the criminal act they are committing. PMS, it is argued, as a result of its symptoms, results in an inability to fully understand the criminality of the woman's actions.

Those opposed to the use of PMS as a defense resent PMS sufferers being branded as insane or of diminished capacity. This perception, they argue, merely reinforces the stereotype that claims all women act irrationally during menses. Further, the great majority of women who experience PMS do not behave antisocially, insanely, or with diminished capacity. In addition, opponents question whether any ill person might then be excused for his or her criminal behavior if women who experience PMS are excused. Extending this logic, sick people could sign contracts and not be held responsible for them, could steal items and not be prosecuted for that theft, and could even sexually abuse children without fear of reprisal. If this was allowed to occur, anarchy would ensue.

If you were a judge, would you rule that "diminished responsibility" was a justifiable defense for these actions? In addition to PMS, which other physical or emotional conditions would you allow to be similarly used to explain or excuse people's actions?

described as a supercharged PMS, and is cited in the *Diagnostic and Statistical Manual of Mental Disorders, Fourth Edition.* PMDD's symptoms include

- A marked depressive mood

- A decreased interest in usual activities

- Lethargy, fatigability, or lack of energy

- Hypersomnia (falling asleep when not wanting to) or insomnia (difficulty falling asleep)

There is disagreement among women's health specialists about whether PMDD should be categorized as a "mental disorder." Some believe that classifying menstrual problems as a mental disorder stigmatizes women. As one psychologist argued: "It's a label that can be used by a sexist society that wants to believe that women go crazy once a month" (Daw, 2002). Others believe a PMDD classification acknowledges women's feelings and focuses researchers' attention on developing medications to help premenstrual women. The medications now used to treat PMDD include ibuprofen (Advil, Motrin, Midol Cramp), ketoprofen (Orudis KT), naproxen (Aleve), or aspirin (Office of Women's Health, 2012).

Endometriosis

Sometimes tissue resembling the inner lining of the uterus (the endometrium) is found outside the uterus. This condition is known as *endometriosis*. Endometriosis is found most often on the lining of the pelvic cavity, the ovaries, the rectum, and the colon, and in the uterus and on the bladder. Sometimes it is also found on the small intestine, liver, spleen, and lymph nodes. Endometriosis is, unfortunately, not an uncommon occurrence. In fact, it affects 63 million women and girls in the United States, 1 million in Canada, and millions more worldwide (Endometriosis Association, 2010). Although it can affect all women, endometriosis is most common among 25- to 30-year-olds, and it has also occurred in girls as young as 11 years of age.

The causes of endometriosis are not known, although there are several theories. One theory holds that pieces of the endometrium somehow find themselves in the fallopian tubes and are transported into the pelvic cavity. This is called *retrograde menstruation*. The endometrium pieces then adhere to one another to form adhesions, which cause pain. Another theory is based on the realization that in the early stages of fetal development there are but a few cells present and that these cells eventually differentiate into different tissue. This theory posits that perhaps cells outside the uterus, for some unknown reason, take on the function of cells in the endometrium. Still another theory argues that endometrial cells are transported through the bloodstream or through the lymph system to sites elsewhere in the body. Finally, some researchers believe that endometriosis is caused by a breakdown in the function of the immune system, resulting in an inability to destroy endometrium cells that manage to leave the uterus.

Women who acquire endometriosis usually experience a great deal of pelvic pain. This pain most often occurs just before or during menstrual bleeding, and usually abates after bleeding ceases. Pain may also be experienced in the lower back or lower abdomen and may be associated with urination. Fatigue and/or bloated feelings may occur, there may be blood in the urine and/or heavy menstrual bleeding, and diarrhea or constipation may result. In addition to causing these uncomfortable symptoms, endometriosis can lead to serious health consequences. For example, scar tissue can form and result in infertility. Or, adhesions can connect organs such as the uterus, fallopian tubes, ovaries, and intestines.

Endometriosis is treated in several ways, depending on the severity of the symptoms and the location of the tissue. Laparoscopic surgery—in which two small incisions are made in the abdomen through which is inserted a viewing instrument to perform the surgical cut—can be helpful in identifying the existence of endometrial tissue outside the uterus and determining its location. Then the tissue can be surgically removed before the procedure is completed. Sometimes the tissue has spread so extensively that the surgeon needs to open the abdomen to remove it rather than merely inserting a laparoscope. This procedure is called a *laparotomy.*

In addition to surgery, there are medications that result in lower levels of estrogen than normal and, therefore, alleviate much of the pain associated with endometriosis. Some of these drugs are synthetic hormones that stop the ovaries from producing estrogen, causing cessation of menstruation. These are known as *gonadotropin-releasing hormone analogues (GnRH analogues).* Another drug sometimes used is a synthetic hormone derived from testosterone (Danazol). More frequently, oral contraceptives are prescribed to prevent ovulation and reduce (when estrogen and progestin are used in combination) or eliminate menstrual bleeding. Finally, relief from pain may be obtained temporarily with ibuprofen or other analgesics (pain relievers).

Myth vs Fact

Myth: The menstrual cycle is 28 days long and does not fluctuate in length for any one woman.
Fact: The most prevalent menstrual cycle happens to be 30 days long. Even so, the cycle varies greatly from woman to woman and even for any one woman.

Myth: Women are usually emotionally "low" premenstrually and emotionally "high" at ovulation.
Fact: This has not been conclusively determined. There are conflicting research findings and criticism of the methodology researchers have employed to answer this question.

Myth: Women's work activity needs to be adjusted during their periods.
Fact: Though this myth has been used to support job discrimination practices against women, there is no evidence that women cannot function normally in their jobs when menstruating.

Myth: Women should not swim or exercise as usual during their periods.
Fact: With the usual hygienic practices used by women, there are no known physical reasons for not exercising as usual. For some women, iron supplementation may be necessitated by the iron lost in the menstrual blood, but that precaution is a simple one.

Myth: Women's sexual desire is at a peak just before and just after menstruation.
Fact: For some women and for some cycles this may be true. However, sexual desire involves more than one's physical condition—the nature of the relationship, the setting, one's comfort with sexuality, one's health, and so on—so that expecting sexual desire to be determined solely by the menstrual cycle is unrealistic.

The Menstrual Cycle and Sex

Many researchers have searched for a relationship between sexual interest and the time of the menstrual cycle. Findings of these studies have, for the most part, been contradictory (Bullivant et al., 2004). Some researchers report that women are more interested in sex just *before* menstruation (AskMen, 2011), and others find them most interested *during* menstruation (Friedman et al., 1980). Still others report the *middle* of the menstrual cycle to be the most sexually active (Adams, Gold, & Burt, 1978) or the time just *after* the menses to be when most sexual fantasizing occurs (Matteo & Rissman, 1984). Several other studies have not found the midcycle related in any way to heightened sexual arousal (Slob et al., 1991; van Goozen et al., 1997).

When are women most sexually aroused? The answer to this question probably varies from one woman to another and, in addition to menstrual physiology, depends on such factors as one's lover, the setting, and numerous psychosocial factors such as the woman's comfort with her body, her level of self-esteem, and her religious and cultural beliefs regarding menstruation. The bottom line is that

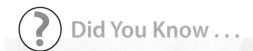

? Did You Know . . .

If a couple decides to engage in sexual intercourse when the woman is menstruating, they should realize that transmission of HIV is probably more likely at this time of the menstrual cycle than at any other. That is because of the blood present and the probability that some of that blood will have contact with an opening (albeit microscopic) into the body. If HIV is in that blood, it can infect the sexual partner. The "safer sex" practice of refraining from sexual intercourse while a woman is menstruating is usually overlooked. From the woman's perspective, participating in coitus while menstruating can facilitate HIV entry into her body.

women can be sexually aroused at any time during their menstrual cycle (menstruation.com.au, 2008).

Although there are no medical reasons to refrain from coitus during menstruation (if one or both partners are HIV-negative, see the Did You Know box on this page), many couples do so. At least one study found over half the men and women surveyed believed couples should not engage in sexual intercourse when the woman is menstruating (Research Forecasts, 1981). According to a 1996 study, 16 percent of women 20 to 37 years of age reported that they had had sexual intercourse during their last menstrual period (Tanfer & Aral, 1996). Some people refrain from coitus during menstruation because of religious taboos (Menstrual Taboo, 2014). For example, in Orthodox Judaism menstruating women are considered unclean and are supposed to sleep in a separate bed. When they are through menstruating, Jewish women are supposed to cleanse themselves in a ritual bath called a *mikvah*. Others refrain from sexual intercourse during menstruation because of the potential messiness. Still others refrain because of the physical discomfort they feel—bloating, cramping, or fatigue. And, finally, there are women who are ashamed of their menstrual flow and prefer to keep it a private matter not shared with anyone. A couple who refrains from sexual intercourse during menstruation should be comfortable with their decision, whatever the reason; likewise, a couple who decides to engage in coitus during this time should be comfortable with their decision.

A couple who decide to engage in sexual intercourse during the menstrual period can take several actions to make that experience as enjoyable as possible. First, they should discuss any concerns they may have—for example, the potential messiness or any religious inhibitions. Second, the woman can wear a diaphragm or cervical cap to hold back the menstrual flow. A menstrual cup, such as the Softcup, which blocks menstrual flow, can also be used during sexual intercourse without being felt by either partner (Sex on your period, 2013). Because the menstrual fluid can sometimes irritate the penis, the man should wear a condom (a good idea anytime coitus occurs). With these simple actions, coitus during menstruation can be a positive and rewarding experience.

▉ Menopause

Usually between the ages of 40 and 55 years, women produce progressively less estrogen and progesterone, as an effect of aging on the ovaries. Whereas the pituitary continues to produce FSH and LH, the ovaries can no longer respond to these pituitary hormones as they once could. This decrease in estrogen and progesterone occurs over approximately a 5- to 10-year period and results in a cessation of menstruation. The period when these changes take place is called the **perimenopause**, or the **climacteric**; when menstruation has not occurred for a year, we call that **menopause**.

▉ Sexually Related Diseases: Self-Care and Prevention

Some diseases are not transmitted by sexual activity but do affect sexual organs. These are termed sexually related diseases (SRDs). Advances in chemical and surgical treatment of diseases of the sex organs have improved 5- and 10-year survival rates and made restoration of function more attainable than ever before. Maintaining reproductive health means following safer sexual practices, paying attention to your body, monitoring it for certain signs, using the

perimenopause (climacteric) The period just before menopause when the production of estrogen and progesterone is decreasing, usually a 5- to 10-year period.

menopause The time when a woman's menstrual cycle ceases, usually between 40 and 55 years of age.

specialized health services available, and seeking information—from organizations and publications—on issues related to reproductive health. Successful treatment of SRDs generally depends on early diagnosis of potential problems.

The Female Reproductive System

Self-care and disease prevention activities for the female involve many of the sexual organs, including the breasts, cervix, uterus, ovaries, and vagina.

The Breasts

The most common breast disorders are cancer, cystic mastitis (mammary dysplasia), fibroadenoma, nipple discharge, and breast abscess. Most of these disorders occur only in women, but men are susceptible to breast cancer, too.

Breast Cancer The breast is the leading site of cancer in American women and the second major cause of cancer death (the first is lung cancer). At the time of this writing, it is estimated that 232,670 new cases of **breast cancer** will have been diagnosed in women in 2014, and 2,360 cases will have been diagnosed in men (American Cancer Society, 2014a). After increasing about 4% per year in the 1980s, breast cancer incidence rates have dropped slightly. Still, 40,000 women and 430 men will probably have died of breast cancer in 2014. And yet, death rates from breast cancer continue to decline, especially among younger women. The 5-year survival rate for localized breast cancer increased from 72% in the 1940s to 99% in 2014. If the cancer has spread regionally, however, the 5-year survival rate drops to 84%, and, if the cancer has spread to distant locations (metastasized), the survival rate drops to 24%. However, there are large differences in breast cancer survival by race. Whereas the 5-year survival rate is 90% for white women, it is 79% for African American women.

No specific cause of breast cancer is known, but epidemiological studies have identified certain risk factors that predispose women to breast cancer. One of these risk factors is age. As women get older, the risk increases. The risk is also higher in women who have a family history of breast cancer, who experienced an early menarche or a late menopause, who recently used oral contraceptives or postmenopausal estrogens, and who never had children or had the first live birth at a late age. Other suspected risk factors are being overweight or obese; exposure to pesticides and other selected chemicals; alcohol consumption; weight gain; heavy smoking; and physical inactivity. In addition, two genes that appear to make women susceptible to breast cancer have been discovered, BRCA1 and BRCA2. However, only 5% to

It is recommended by several organizations that women older than age 40 get a mammogram annually. Younger women should have annual clinical breast exams every 3 years.

10% of breast cancers are thought to be inherited, and only 5% of breast cancer patients were found to have the gene BRCA1 or BRCA2. One study found that 75% of women in whom breast cancer develops have no identifiable risk factor other than gender and age (Hortobagyi, McLelland, & Reed, 1990). This makes it especially important for all women to have regular breast examinations by a physician.

Breast self-examination (BSE) is a self-care procedure women can adopt. Although medical specialists actively check for breast cancer in routine examinations, some experts believe that checking one's own breasts every menstrual cycle increases the chances of early detection. The technique is simple. If cancer is present, the earlier it is diagnosed, the better the chance for survival.

In April 1987 a committee of the United States Public Health Service (which had been established to recommend those medical procedures with demonstrated effectiveness and those without) caused concern among cancer prevention specialists by citing BSE as a procedure whose value had not been clearly

breast cancer The most common type of cancer in women.

breast self-examination (BSE) A periodic self-care procedure that involves feeling the breast for any abnormalities. The test is performed once every menstrual cycle or every month after menopause.

Gender
DIMENSIONS

Breast Self-Examination

By regularly examining her own breasts, a woman may notice any changes that occur. The best time for breast self-examination (BSE) is about a week after your period ends, when your breasts are not tender or swollen. If you are not having regular periods, do BSE on the same day every month.

1. Lie down with a pillow under your right shoulder and place your right arm behind your head.
2. Use the finger pads of the three middle fingers on your left hand to feel for lumps in the right breast.
3. Press firmly enough to know how your breast feels. A firm ridge in the lower curve of each breast is normal. If you are not sure how hard to press, talk with your doctor or nurse.
4. Move around the breast in a circular, up-and-down line, or wedge pattern (a, b, c). Be sure to do it the

same way every time, check the entire breast area, and remember how your breast feels from month to month.

5. Repeat the exam on your left breast, using the finger pads of the right hand. (Move the pillow to below your left shoulder.)

6. If you find any changes, see your doctor right away.
7. Repeat the examination of both breasts while standing, with one arm behind your head. The upright position makes it easier to check the upper and outer part of the breasts (toward your armpit). This is where about half of breast cancers are found. You may want to do the standing part of the BSE while you are in the shower. Some breast changes can be felt more easily when your skin is wet and soapy.

For added safety, you can check your breasts for any dimpling of the skin, changes in the nipple, redness, or swelling while standing in front of a mirror right after your BSE each month.

(a)   (b)   (c)

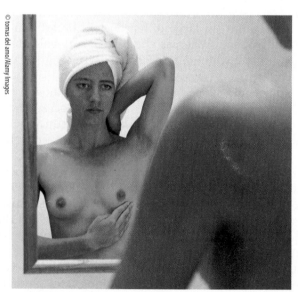

shown. The committee was charged with reviewing the scientific evidence for many medical screenings and examination procedures and eliminating those that contributed to the increasing cost of health care. As such they decided that BSE was not employed by enough women and cancers not found in enough quantity to warrant public health campaigns to encourage women to perform the examination. Other cancer experts, who argued that BSE does not cost a woman any money and that it can uncover early treatable cancers, recommended that women ignore the committee's finding and continue doing monthly BSEs. Canadians have also weighed in on this issue. The Canadian Task Force on Preventive Health Care (Baxter, 2001) studied the benefits and harms associated with breast self-examinations and found no evidence of effectiveness and evidence of harm. The harm included an increase in the number of physician visits for the evaluation of benign breast lesions and significantly higher rates of benign breast biopsy findings. As a result, the Canadian Task Force recommended that women not perform breast self-examinations. The American Cancer Society (2014a) takes a neutral stance, stating in their guidelines that breast self-exam is an option for women starting in their 20s. In addition, after conducting an extensive review of the research literature, the U.S. Preventive Services Task Force (2009) concluded there were more risks than benefits associated with breast self-exams and, therefore, recommended against teaching women how to perform breast self-examination.

If choosing to perform BSE, for best results, perform the exam when the skin is wet or moist—after showering or after applying body lotion. Menstruating women should perform this test 1 week after their period; postmenopausal women should check their breasts at least once a month. All women should check their breasts visually in the mirror and by means of this exam. Consult a gynecologist if you find a lump, a thickening, or any other unusual feature. These symptoms may include pain in the breast, discharge from the nipple, a change in the character of the nipple itself, or changes in the character of the breast.

In addition, the American Cancer Society, the American Medical Association, and the National Comprehensive Cancer Network recommend that women have regular breast examinations by a physician. These examinations include both **clinical breast exams** and **mammography** screening, depending on a woman's age and medical history. A clinical breast exam is similar to BSE, except that it is conducted by a physician trained to detect any abnormalities. It is suggested that women aged 20 years and older have a clinical breast examination regularly, preferably every 3 years between ages 20 and 40 years and annually

thereafter. However, the U.S. Preventive Services Task Force also questioned the value of clinical breast exams (2009).

Mammography is also recommended. A mammogram is an X ray of the breast that often allows physicians to detect breast lumps before they would be palpable by a physician (see Figure 4.12). Some organizations argue that women older than age 40 years should have a mammogram annually. However, whether women in their 40s or women over 74 years old receive benefit from mammograms has been called into question by the U.S. Preventive Services Task Force (2009). (See Table 4.3.) The Centers for Disease Control and Prevention (2010) reported that in 2008, 67% of women aged 40 years and older had had a mammogram within the previous 2 years. Obviously, we have a long way to go in educating women about the need to get mammograms and the benefits they can expect.

There is increasing interest in using breast magnetic resonance imaging (MRI) as a screening test for breast cancer. The use of MRI to detect breast cancer is being studied at the time of this writing. Some studies have shown that MRI is associated with higher false-positive rates. Thus women who are screened with MRI may have more unnecessary surgical biopsies. At the present time, it is still undetermined whether the increase in cancer

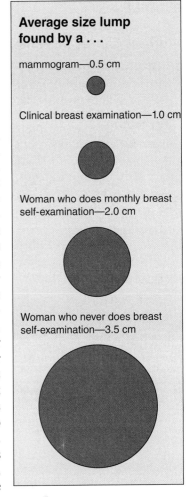

Average size lump found by a . . .

mammogram—0.5 cm

Clinical breast examination—1.0 cm

Woman who does monthly breast self-examination—2.0 cm

Woman who never does breast self-examination—3.5 cm

FIGURE **4.12** The sizes of breast masses detectable by mammography, physical examination, and self-examination illustrate the importance of screening mammography in the early detection of breast cancer.

clinical breast exam A breast examination conducted by a physician to detect any abnormalities.

mammography An X ray of the breasts to detect any abnormality before it is visible or palpable.

TABLE 4.3

Breast Cancer Screening Controversy*

In November of 2009, the U.S. Preventive Services Task Force issued new guidelines regarding breast cancer screening. These guidelines generated a good deal of discussion with some experts and organizations agreeing and others disagreeing with the task force. The recommendations of the task force and several other organizations are summarized below.

Procedure	Organization(s)	Recommendation
Breast self-exams	USPSTF	Not recommended
	American Cancer Society	Optional
	American Medical Association	Recommended
	National Comprehensive Cancer Network	Recommended
	Canadian Task Force on Preventive Services	Not recommended
	American College of Obstetrics and Gynecology	Optional
	World Health Organization	Not recommended
Clinical breast exams	USPSTF	Not recommended
	American Cancer Society	Recommended
	American Medical Association	Recommended
	National Comprehensive Cancer Network	Recommended
	Canadian Task Force on Preventive Services	Not recommended
	American College of Obstetrics and Gynecology	Optional
	World Health Organization	Not recommended
Mammograms	USPSTF	Only for ages 50–74
	American Cancer Society	For age 45+
	American Medical Association	For age 40+
	National Comprehensive Cancer Network	For age 40+
	American College of Physicians	Optional for age 40+
	Canadian Task Force on Preventive Services	For age 40+
	American College of Obstetrics and Gynecology	For age 40+
	World Health Organization	Only ages 50–69

Given the variance in these recommendations, it is suggested that women discuss the best screening procedures for their individual circumstances with their physicians considering such factors as their family history, health status, and age.

* These recommendations are currently under review, and updates are expected to be published at the conclusion of that review.

Source: Data from U.S. Preventive Services Task Force. Screening for breast cancer: U.S. Preventive Services Task Force recommendation statement. *Annals of Internal Medicine, 151* (2009), 716–726.

detection achieved with MRI, in conjunction with the as-yet-undemonstrated decrease in death rates as a result, conveys enough of a benefit to warrant recommendations for wider use of this technology,

biopsy (open biopsy) Usually referred to as an open biopsy, a minor surgical procedure during which tissue of a tumor is removed and examined for presence of cancer.

needle biopsy Insertion of a needle into a lump in a breast to see whether fluid (which indicates a cyst rather than a tumor) can be removed.

carcinoma A type of cancer emanating from epithelial cells.

given the large increase in false-positive rates and the possibility of overdiagnosis (American Cancer Society, 2013a).

When breast cancer is suspected, a **biopsy** is performed. In a **needle biopsy** a fine needle is inserted into the tumor and fluid or cells are withdrawn. If the lump dissipates as soon as fluid is obtained, the lump is confirmed as a cyst and generally no further procedure is needed. An **open biopsy** is a minor surgical procedure during which tissue of the tumor is removed and examined for possible cancer (**carcinoma**).

Patients who have breast cancer are classified in terms of stages. These stages are determined by the

Multicultural DIMENSIONS

Breast Cancer More Deadly in African Americans

Although breast cancer develops more often in white women, African American women are more likely to die of it (American Cancer Society, 2014a). Researchers and epidemiologists have been perplexed as to why. It was originally assumed that this difference was due to the disproportionately high number of African American women who live in poverty, resulting in lack of access to health care. That, in turn, would lead to later diagnosis and, consequently, less effective treatment. However, having studied this dilemma for several years, scientists have concluded that, although poverty status plays a role (it is estimated that poverty accounts for approximately 50% of the cause), biology is significantly involved. Tumors in African American women are just more virulent.

Evidence for this conclusion can be found in a study that compared African American and white women who belonged to health maintenance organizations (HMOs) in which health care was readily available (access to mammograms and other medical care). Still, the African American women HMO members had larger and more advanced tumors when diagnosed. The suspicion was that these tumors grew faster, and that is why at the time of diagnosis they were larger and more advanced.

Research also indicates that African American women do not wait any longer to seek medical diagnosis when identifying a breast abnormality than do white women. Consequently, that is not a significant variable in the difference in tumor size or death rates between African American and white women.

A review of research of breast cancer in African American women published in the *New York Times* (Kolata, 1994) summarized what is known about this situation. Cited are several studies in which tumors in African American women were found to be more actively dividing than those in white women, and more lacked hormone receptors and had tissue features indicative of unfavorable diagnosis.

Although it is wise for all women to obtain regular medical examinations, given what we know about tumors in African American women, it is particularly prudent for them to do so.

characteristics of the tumor and the lymph nodes and whether **metastasis**—spread of the cancer to other body sites—has occurred. Treatment naturally depends on the stage of the cancer. The treatment of breast cancer may involve **lumpectomy**, in which only the breast lump and lymph nodes under the arm are removed, usually followed by radiation therapy; **mastectomy**, in which the breast and lymph nodes under the arm are removed; **chemotherapy**, treatment with drugs; **radiation therapy**; and **hormone therapy**. There are three kinds of mastectomy: *simple mastectomy*, in which the whole breast is removed, sometimes along with lymph nodes under the arm; *modified radical mastectomy*, the most common form of mastectomy, in which the breast, many of the lymph nodes under the arm, the lining over the chest muscles, and sometimes part of the chest wall are removed; and *radical mastectomy* (also called the *Halstead radical mastectomy*), in which the breast, chest muscles, and all lymph nodes under the arm are removed. Radical mastectomy used to be the most frequently performed operation for breast cancer but now is used only when the tumor has spread to the chest muscles.

For patients with no lymph node involvement, hormone therapy may be prescribed as a preventive measure against recurrence of cancer. The most commonly used hormones are tamoxifen and special "designer estrogens," which may be administered for 5 years. There presently remains a question regarding the increased risk of development of cancer of the uterus for women on hormonal therapy. For early-stage breast cancer, long-term survival rates after lumpectomy plus radiation therapy are similar to survival rates after modified radical mastectomy, and,

metastasis Spread of cancer from a primary site to other parts of the body.

lumpectomy Removal of a lesion, benign or malignant.

mastectomy Removal of the breast and/or other tissue. *Simple:* Removal of only the breast (sometimes with removal of lymph nodes under the arm). *Modified radical:* Removal of the breast, lymph nodes, lining of the chest muscle, and sometimes part of the chest wall. *Radical:* Removal of the breast, lymph nodes, and chest muscle.

chemotherapy Use of chemicals (medication) to treat disease; may be oral, intravenous, intramuscular, or topical.

radiation therapy A form of treatment for cancer that uses carefully directed radiation to destroy cancer cells.

hormone therapy Form of treatment for cancer that uses hormones to combat cancer cell growth.

After mastectomy.

After reconstructive surgery after mastectomy.

therefore, this less invasive procedure is being used more often—except for those women who choose not to experience the side effects of radiation and thus choose mastectomy.

We live in a society in which breast size and shape are mistakenly seen as contributing greatly to a woman's sexuality. Thus a woman who loses a breast through amputation can be devastated. Many women who have had mastectomies, whether or not they are sexually active, suffer feelings of loss, fear of rejection, and, of course, fear of the cancer's recurrence. Community support systems such as the Reach to Recovery Project of the American Cancer Society (ACS) and the Breast Referral Service, founded by Rose Kushner, who herself recovered from a mastectomy, give invaluable support to women in adjusting to the treatment of their cancers. The involvement of lovers or husbands and children is of great importance, because all of them, not just the woman, must adjust to her changed appearance and emotional sensitivity. Breast reconstruction after a mastectomy is also available. It offers a woman a more normal appearance and often eases her acceptance of the change in her body. This option should be discussed with the surgeon before breast surgery, if possible.

Reconstructive breast surgery can create a breast-like structure by using saline (salt) water encased in a silicone pouch that is implanted under a woman's skin and chest muscle.

Cystic Mastitis　Also called *chronic cystic mastitis, fibrocystic condition*, and *mammary dysplasia* (cell change), **cystic mastitis** is the most common breast condition.

---

cystic mastitis　Known also as fibrocystic disease, a condition characterized by fluid-filled lesions (cysts) that are tender and believed to be related to estrogen activity.

fibroadenoma　A benign (noncancerous) tumor that is firm, round, and somewhat movable.

It is usually found in women 40 to 60 years of age (California Pacific Medical Center, 2008). Because cystic mastitis is uncommon in postmenopausal women, it is believed to be related to estrogen activity. In cystic mastitis small and large cysts form in the breast tissues. The cysts are generally filled with fluid and may have to be drained frequently. Sometimes the cysts must be removed. Studies have concluded that "fibrocystic breasts" occur frequently in women and are not associated with significant increases in risk for breast cancer (Mayo Clinic Staff, 2010). One research report indicated a possible link between cystic mastitis and coffee, tea, cola, and chocolate consumption. On the basis of this study, some practitioners recommend that women decrease or eliminate the consumption of these products. But because this treatment approach has not been tested by using randomized double-blind studies, medical researchers and practitioners have questioned its validity.

Fibroadenoma　**Fibroadenoma** is a benign (noncancerous) tumor that may develop in white women in their early 30s and in black women somewhat earlier (there are no data on other groups). The tumor is usually firm, round, and somewhat movable. Generally the treatment is surgical removal.

Nipple Discharge　A discharge from the nipples of women who are not nursing can be due to cystic mastitis, to a small benign tumor (called a *papilloma*) in a duct leading to the nipple, or to an uncommon condition *(ectasia)* in which the ducts of the breast enlarge and distend, allowing fluid to accumulate and escape. Occasionally the use of hormones—such as oral contraceptives and postmenopausal estrogen supplements—can cause nipple discharge, which should cease when the drugs are discontinued. Any discharge from the nipples should be checked by a physician.

Breast Abscess Generally **breast abscesses** (infections) are seen in nursing women, but they occur in nonnursing women as well, and in either case should be treated by a physician. Redness, swelling, or a tender, painful mass is symptomatic of breast infection. If the infection is not stopped, an abscess can develop. These are usually treated by incision and drainage, antibiotics, or both.

The Cervix

Rates of **invasive cervical cancer**, which involves deep-tissue layers of the cervix and sometimes spreads to other organs, have decreased steadily over the past several decades. This decline is attributed to the increase in Pap smear screening, which leads to early detection and subsequent early treatment. Still, an estimated 12,360 cases of invasive cervical cancer were diagnosed in 2014 with 4,020 deaths (American Cancer Society, 2014a), in spite of a steady decline in death rate from cervical cancer since 1982. Cervical cancer death rates declined for African Americans more rapidly than for whites. However, in 2010 the mortality rate for African American women (4.6 per 100,000) was twice as high as it was for white women (2.2 per 100,000). The 5-year relative survival rate for the earliest stage of invasive cervical cancer is 91%. The overall (all stages combined) 5-year survival rate for cervical cancer is about 68% (American Cancer Society, 2014a).

Although the exact cause of cervical cancer is unknown, several factors can put you at risk. Among these are having your first intercourse at an early age, having multiple sex partners, having many pregnancies, having a mother who took diethylstilbestrol (DES) while pregnant with you, and having a sexually transmitted infection caused by the human papillomavirus (HPV).

The American Cancer Society (2013b) recommends that all women begin cervical cancer screening at age 21. Women aged 21 to 29 should then have a Pap test every 3 years. Beginning at age 30, women should have a Pap test combined with a human papillomavirus (HPV) test every 5 years. This so-called *co-testing* should continue until age 65, although the American Cancer Society allows for another option—that is, women aged 30 to 65 may get tested every 3 years with just the Pap test. Women older than 65 years of age who have had regular screening in the previous 10 years should stop cervical cancer screening as long as they have not had any serious precancers found in the last 20 years.

Pap smear screening is a simple procedure that involves swabbing a small sample of cells from the cervix, transferring these cells to a slide, and examining them under a microscope. Regular gynecological screening is advised for all women, particularly because early cell changes in the cervical tissue do not present symptoms a woman can recognize herself—although invasive cervical cancer sometimes does cause a bloody discharge between periods and/or bloody spotting after intercourse. Unfortunately, data indicate that not enough women are getting regular Pap tests. In 2008, only 73% of women had a Pap smear within the past 3 years (Centers for Disease Prevention and Control, 2014).

Other procedures have been developed to screen for cervical cancer. One of these is called *PapSure* (Redfran, 2002). This procedure involves a visual inspection of the cervix using a scope and a blue chemical light, and is performed in conjunction with a traditional Pap smear. Another cervical cancer detection test is the experimental *LUMA Cervical Imaging System* (McMillan, 2004). In this procedure, the cancerous tissue absorbs light differently than healthy tissue, showing possible problematic areas. Certainly, even more advanced screening techniques will be developed in the coming years.

Treatment for invasive cervical cancer generally consists of surgery; radiation, and/or chemotherapy. Eighty-seven percent of patients survive 1 year after diagnosis, and 68% survive 5 years. When detected at an early stage, invasive cervical cancer is one of the most successfully treated cancers, with a 5-year survival rate of 91% for cancers that have not spread. Unfortunately, only 49% of invasive cervical cancer in white women and only 39% in African American women are diagnosed at this stage. Again, this points to the value of getting a Pap test regularly (American Cancer Society, 2014).

At the time of this writing, it was estimated that 52,630 cases of cancer of the uterus, most often of the endometrium, would be diagnosed in 2014. Incidence rates of uterine cancer have varied since the mid-1980s. In 2010, the incidence rate for white women was 27.4 per 100,000, and 24.4 per 100,000 for African American women (National Center for Health Statistics, 2014). Although incidence rates are higher among white women than African American women, the relationship is reversed for mortality rates: The overall 5-year relative survival for whites (84%) is 23 percentage points higher than that for African Americans (61%).

Estrogen is the major risk factor for uterine cancer. Women who choose estrogen replacement therapy to combat the effects of menopause, who are

---

breast abscess Infection of the breast characterized by redness, swelling, and a painful or tender mass.

invasive cervical cancer Cancer that has invaded a wide area of cervical tissue.

Pap smear A test of the tissue of the cervix for cervical cancer (named after its founder, Dr. Papanicolaou).

administered tamoxifen to prevent breast cancer or its recurrence, who experience an early menarche, who have a late menopause, who never have children, or who do not ovulate have been shown to be at increased risk. Conversely, pregnancy and the use of oral contraceptives appear to provide protection against uterine cancer.

The Pap test is rarely effective in detecting uterine cancer early. It is with this realization that the American Cancer Society recommends that women older than 40 years have an annual pelvic exam and that women at high risk have an endometrial biopsy at menopause and periodically thereafter. Early warning signs include uterine bleeding or spotting; pain is a later symptom. Treatment, which depends on the stage of the cancer, consists of surgical removal of the uterus and/or ovaries, radiation therapy, hormonal therapy, and chemotherapy. The 5-year survival rate is 95% if the cancer is discovered at an early stage, when it is contained regionally. Survival rates for whites exceed that for African Americans.

The Ovaries

Ovarian cysts and tumors can occur when a female is any age. A cyst is an abnormal cavity that is filled with fluid. The most common ones are called **functional cysts**; these occur on the follicle or corpus luteum and are usually caused by the failure of the follicle to rupture and discharge the egg. Generally they are small and not particularly significant. They usually disappear spontaneously within a month or two.

Dermoid cysts are common in young women. They contain hard, fatty material, and sometimes remnants of teeth. These are believed to be embryonic in nature and are considered benign. Most ovarian cysts and tumors are usually benign, but if they cause symptoms such as pain, tenderness, and internal bleeding, they can require surgery. Because there is always the possibility of future problems, such as malignancy, a woman should remain under medical supervision once cysts or tumors have been diagnosed.

In the **Stein–Leventhal syndrome** the ovaries become enlarged and have cysts on them. Infertility and secondary amenorrhea also result. This condition affects one in ten women of childbearing age

and is the most common cause of female infertility. Although its causes are not specifically known, genes are thought to be one factor because women experiencing this condition tend to have a mother or sister with it as well. Researchers also think insulin could be a cause given that Stein–Leventhal syndrome affects the ovaries and ovulation (The National Women's Health Information Center, 2010). Symptoms include infrequent menstrual periods, no menstrual periods, and/or irregular bleeding; infertility; increased hair growth on the face, chest, stomach, back, thumbs, or toes; and pelvic pain. Treatment may include birth control pills; medications such as Clomid and Serophene to stimulate ovulation; surgery ("ovarian drilling") that involves puncturing the ovary and administers an electrical current to destroy a small portion of the ovary; and lifestyle changes (eating a healthy diet, exercise, and weight loss) to improve the body's use of insulin. Most patients respond to therapy, and frequently fertility is restored to normal.

Ovarian cancer killed an estimated 14,270 American women in 2014. In fact, ovarian cancer causes more deaths than any other cancer of the female reproductive system. An estimated 21,980 new cases of ovarian cancer were diagnosed in 2014. One of the reasons ovarian cancer is so deadly is that its symptoms are "silent": They may go unnoticed until late in development. Rarely does abdominal swelling occur and even more rarely abnormal vaginal bleeding. Stomach gas, discomfort, and distention that cannot be explained by other causes may indicate a need to have a thorough medical examination with ovarian cancer in mind.

Risk factors include never having children, being older (ovarian cancer occurs more frequently in women in their 80s), and having had certain other cancers such as colon and endometrial cancers. As with all cancers, early detection is important. Pelvic exams are most valuable, because Pap tests rarely are effective in uncovering ovarian cancer. In 2000 a new technique using sonography was developed that has the potential of diagnosing ovarian cancer earlier than is presently possible. This new method, *transvaginal ultrasonography*, was able to diagnose stage 1 ovarian cancer in 59% of women, whereas other methods could detect only 30% of these stage 1 cancers (Sato et al., 2000). Treatment can include surgical removal of one or both of the ovaries and/or the fallopian tubes (called a *salpingo-oophorectomy*) and the uterus (*hysterectomy*). If disease is detected early and the tumor is small, only the involved ovary is removed. This consideration is especially important to young women who want to have children. Radiation therapy and chemotherapy are also used in the treatment of ovarian cancer. The 5-year survival rate varies by the stage when

---

functional cyst An ovarian cyst that occurs on the follicle or corpus luteum, usually caused by the failure of the follicle to rupture and release an egg.

dermoid cyst A type of benign ovarian cyst commonly found in young women.

Stein–Leventhal syndrome Reproductive malfunction in women; a syndrome of endocrine origin that involves ovarian cysts, amenorrhea, and infertility.

ovarian cancer Cancer of the ovaries; it causes more cancer deaths than any other cancer of the female reproductive system.

© Custom Medical Stock Photo

Sexual health begins with routine self-exams.

diagnosed. If cancer is diagnosed and treated early, the survival rate goes up to 92%. Unfortunately, only 15% of cases are detected in their localized stage. Five-year survival rates vary from 27% to 92%, depending on the stage of the cancer.

The Vagina

Normal vaginal secretions are odorless, and the acidity of the vagina helps it to cleanse itself. Nevertheless, some women choose to cleanse the vagina by **douching**—that is, by rinsing with water or a vinegar and water solution. A vaginal douche, the value of which has been questioned, is not recommended and can be harmful if not done correctly. Damage can occur in two main ways: (1) Improper insertion of the douching material may actually damage the tissue, resulting in an increased chance of infection; (2) the chemical balance of the vagina can be altered, affecting contraceptive function. For instance, if a woman is using a spermicidal cream or other form of spermicide as a means of contraception, douching may destroy its effectiveness.

Smegma, a cheeselike substance secreted by the glans penis of males, may have effects on women's health. A female engaging in coitus with a male who has not washed away smegma could be subjecting herself to vaginal infections. There is also some concern that smegma may contribute to cancer of the cervix. It seems prudent, therefore, for sexually active women to make sure that their male sexual partners engage in the routine hygiene care necessary to remove smegma. Although it may be embarrassing, this may be a small price to pay for the prevention of vaginal infection and cervical cancer. Signs of sexually transmitted infections should also be given attention. Make sure to check your vulva routinely. See a healthcare provider if you have unusual discharges, abdominal pain, or open sores on your genitalia.

Toxic Shock Syndrome (TSS)

In the late 1970s several young women died of a previously little-known disease called **toxic shock syndrome (TSS)**. The toxins that cause this syndrome are produced by the *Staphylococcus aureus* bacteria, which may grow in the vagina and are absorbed by the body. These toxins enter the bloodstream and cause high fever (above 102°F), nausea, vomiting, diarrhea, a rapid drop in blood pressure, and sometimes aching muscles and peeling skin on the palms and feet. The exact mechanism of transmission is unknown. The syndrome appears to be linked to the use of tampons—particularly those made of superabsorbent material. It is thought that the presence of the tampon in the vagina for a prolonged period (6 hours or more) may provide an environment conducive to proliferation of the toxin-producing bacteria. When some tampons are inserted into the vagina, small irritations of the vaginal mucosa may occur and promote entry of the bacteria.

It is recommended that superabsorbent tampons not be used because they pack the vagina tightly, prevent air circulation, and allow bacteria to proliferate. It has also been suggested that women using other types of tampons leave them in place for no longer than 2 hours and not use them at all during the night while sleeping.

Toxic shock syndrome has been seen in both genders among postsurgical patients, burn victims, and

douche Cleansing of the vagina by inserting a nozzle that secretes a recommended cleansing substance, a controversial procedure.

toxic shock syndrome (TSS) A syndrome caused by *Staphylococcus aureus* bacteria in which symptoms include high fever, nausea, vomiting, diarrhea, and a drop in blood pressure; a potentially fatal syndrome that has been linked with the use of superabsorbent tampons.

FIGURE **4.13** Medical examination with speculum and spatula in place.

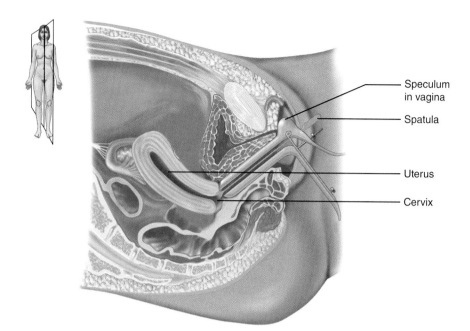

- Speculum in vagina
- Spatula
- Uterus
- Cervix

patients with boils and abscesses. Nonmenstrual cases constitute about half of all reported cases (Nemours Foundation, 2007).

Care from Medical Specialists

All health-related specialists agree that you should report any unusual signs or symptoms related to the reproductive system to a specialist in women's reproductive health—a **gynecologist** or a gynecological nurse practitioner. Furthermore, the American College of Obstetrics and Gynecology recommends that women have a routine gynecological exam every year, even when no signs or symptoms appear. Routine checkups, usually conducted on a special table with the woman's knees up and her feet in stirrups, consist of the following procedures:

1. An inspection of the external genitals for any irritations, discolorations, unusual discharges, or other abnormalities.

2. An internal check for cystoceles (bulges of the bladder into the vagina) and rectoceles (bulges of the rectum into the vagina). The examiner also looks for pus in the Skene's glands and for the strength of the pelvic and abdominal muscles. He or she also tests urine control by asking the patient to cough while checking to see whether urine flows involuntarily.

3. An inspection of the vagina and cervix by means of a **speculum**, a plastic or metal instrument that is inserted into the vagina to hold the walls apart during the examination (Figure 4.13). (At this point and throughout the remainder of the examination, if you are interested in seeing your genitals and watching the exam, ask the examiner to set up a mirror for you and to point out the various organs. If the examiner is not sympathetic to this request, you might consider looking for another practitioner.) The examiner will look for anything unusual, such as lesions (sores) or inflammation affecting the vagina or cervix. Next the practitioner will scrape a tiny amount of tissue from the cervix by using a small wooden instrument called a *spatula*. This tissue will be used for the Pap smear. *If requested by the patient*, the smear can also be tested for signs of gonorrhea.

4. A bimanual examination (Figure 4.14). By sliding the index and middle fingers of one hand into the vagina and pressing down on the abdominal wall from the outside, the examiner feels for the uterus, fallopian tubes, and ovaries to determine their position, their size, and the presence of pain or inflammation. The examiner may also examine the internal genitals by inserting one finger into the rectum and another into the vagina.

5. An examination of the breasts for lumps or thickenings.

Two additional points should be noted about the routine gynecological exam. First, although the

---

gynecologist   A physician specializing in women's reproductive health.

speculum   A metal (or plastic) instrument that is inserted into the vagina to hold the walls apart, allowing for medical examination.

FIGURE **4.14** Bimanual examination.

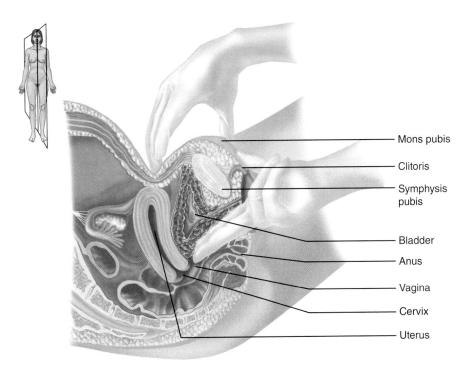

Mons pubis
Clitoris
Symphysis pubis
Bladder
Anus
Vagina
Cervix
Uterus

Speculum and spatula.

checkup may be uncomfortable, it should not be painful. Second, before beginning the physical examination, the practitioner should take a gynecological history. Noted on the history should be information regarding the regularity, flow, and any changes in the menstrual cycle; any pregnancies, miscarriages, or abortions; all birth-control methods used; the incidence of breast cancer in close female relatives; and whether the woman's mother took the drug DES during her pregnancy with the patient—that is, whether the patient is a "DES daughter." DES is a drug that was given in the 1940s and 1950s to women with a history of miscarriage. It is no longer used for miscarriages, because it has been found that vaginal

cancer is more prevalent in DES daughters than in other women (Centers for Disease Control and Prevention, 2011a), and that women who took DES have breast cancer in greater numbers than non-DES women. If the patient's mother did take DES, a periodic **colposcopy**, a check for changes in the vagina and cervix, should be conducted. The examiner uses an instrument called a *colposcope* to view the vagina for abnormal tissue growth. The examiner might also perform a biopsy.

The most consistent research finding for DES sons is that they have an increased risk for noncancerous epididymal cysts, which are growths on the testicles (Centers for Disease Control and Prevention, 2011b).

Care from Organizations and Available Publications
For women, the ACS, the National Organization for Women, the March of Dimes, the National Women's Health Network, women's health centers and clinics, as well as local organizations of women who have had breasts removed due to cancer are but a few of the groups devoted to improving women's reproductive health. These groups function in various ways: Some publish written material, others lobby for legislation and funds, and still others provide social support for women with reproductive health problems. In addition, clinics conduct medical examinations, test and care for STIs, and offer premarital blood tests and other services for women.

colposcopy An examination of the vagina and cervix using an instrument—a colposcope—to detect abnormal tissue growth.

Exploring the Dimensions of Human Sexuality

The physiological development of a female starts when a sperm with an X chromosome fertilizes an egg. But socioeconomic status of the mother influences whether prenatal care is received, good nutrition will be available, and medical help will be sought. If the mother smokes, drinks, or abuses drugs during pregnancy, the fetus will be affected.

A woman's physiology is further altered during puberty and menopause. The increased fat content at puberty negatively affects many women's body image, which in turn negatively affects self-concept.

Unable to control the changes taking place within her body, the pubertal girl sometimes resorts to controlling the one thing she can control: food intake. Dieting is common, but excessive food control, or self-induced vomiting after meals, can result in a serious eating disorder.

Biological Factors

When a sperm with an X chromosome meets an egg (all of which have X chromosomes), a female will develop. Biological factors continue to influence development throughout life.

- Genetic coding affects physical appearance, including height; coloration of skin, hair, and eyes; breast size; and many aspects of health.
- Female physical appearance changes at puberty, when the lean-body-mass-to-fat ratio changes from about 5:1 to about 3:1, signaling the body to commence menarche.
- Hormonal changes affect mood.
- At menopause, lower estrogen levels increase a female's risk for heart attack.

Sociocultural Factors

Sociocultural factors interact with biological factors to influence health.

- Socioeconomic status influences prenatal care and nutrition.
- Ethnic heritage influences health. African American women tend to get a more virulent form of breast cancer, resulting in a higher death rate. Jewish women are genetically at risk for scoliosis (curvature of the spine).
- Culture influences women's health. Fear of Western medicine prevents some immigrants from seeking treatment at early stages of a problem.
- Media and ads that present ultrathin women as ideals can influence the eating patterns and health of women.

Psychological Factors

Psychological factors interact with other factors and can influence health.

- Women tend to have nearly twice the rate of depression of men.
- Teen women with low self-concept have a higher probability of having an unwanted pregnancy and birth.
- Expressiveness of emotions helps women stay mentally and physically healthy.
- Learned attitudes and behaviors about gender roles can prevent a woman from fulfilling her potential.
- Body-image problems in women can lead to long-term disorders, such as bulimia and anorexia nervosa.

Summary

- The external female genitals (the vulva) consist of the mons pubis, labia majora, labia minora, clitoris, vestibule, and urethral opening.

- The clitoris is protected by the clitoral hood and is very sensitive because it contains many nerve endings.

- The internal female genitals consist of the vagina, uterus, fallopian tubes, and ovaries.

- In the vagina, the outer one-third contains the most nerve endings. As a result, the length of the penis is generally irrelevant to sexual satisfaction. Furthermore, the vagina contracts around an object inserted in it, making the width of the penis also generally irrelevant to sexual satisfaction.

- The uterus consists of three layers: the perimetrium, which is elastic, thereby enabling the uterus to stretch during pregnancy; the myometrium, which is made up of smooth muscle, thereby helping to push the baby through the cervix; and the endometrium, which is loaded with blood vessels, thereby providing the nourishment needed to sustain a developing fetus.

- Hormones control menstruation. Follicle-stimulating hormone (FSH) stimulates the ovary to ripen an ovum, luteinizing hormone (LH) signals the Graafian follicle to release the ripened ovum, estrogens signal the pituitary gland to release LH, and progesterone released by the corpus luteum prepares the uterus for implantation of the fertilized ovum.

- Menstrual problems include dysmenorrhea (painful menstruation), which can be either primary or secondary; amenorrhea (a lack of menstruation); and premenstrual syndrome (menstruation associated with bloating cramping, fatigue, depression, headache, and other symptoms).

- The breast is the leading site of cancer in women, and breast cancer is the second leading cause of cancer deaths among women. Breast care consists of breast self-exams (although some groups recommend not doing breast self-exams), annual clinical breast exams, and mammograms as recommended. In addition, women should have gynecological exams and Pap smears as recommended.

Discussion Questions

1. List and describe the parts of the female reproductive system, including external and internal genitalia.

2. Compare the roles of breasts as child nurturer and sexual organ.

3. Describe how hormones react to sexual stimuli and make a person aroused.

4. Which physiological changes occur in a woman's body during the menstrual cycle? What are the resulting psychological effects?

5. For which diseases of the reproductive system is a woman at risk? How can she prevent these diseases?

6. Describe the self-care and preventive medicine that a woman should practice to ensure her sexual health.

Application Questions

Reread the anecdote that opens the chapter and answer the following questions.

1. How could you use your understanding of the parts of the human body to improve your sexuality? Is such knowledge as important as the ability to communicate or to understand the diverse needs of a partner? Put another way, would an expert on sexuality be a better lover?

2. Describe how you feel when you look at anatomical drawings of genitalia. Do you feel sexually excited? Embarrassed? Bored? Explain why you feel that way.

Critical Thinking Questions

1. Some women argue that only another woman can really understand the feelings and sensations that a woman feels, that male gynecologists are likely to discount some female concerns, and that it is easier to talk with another woman than a man about their sexual health. Others argue that medical competency and compassion are not limited by gender. Should a gynecologist be a woman? Explain your answer.

2. If you look at the women on TV, in movies, and in magazines, the pervasive image is clear: lean and busty. Yet the psychologist G. Terence Wilson, an eating disorder specialist, points out that a woman cannot be lean and have large breasts—it is not biologically possible. As a woman loses fat, her breasts reduce in size.

Should a woman who finds herself lean and flat get breast implants or regain weight so her breasts will be larger? Explain your answer.

Critical Thinking Case

As discussed in the chapter, some researchers believe that onset of menarche occurs on the basis of body composition—namely, when a woman reaches a certain percentage of body fat. It also appears that amenorrhea (cessation of menstruation) occurs in women athletes with low body fat and in women with anorexia nervosa.

Consider the negative connotations associated with body fat in our society, especially as portrayed in the mass media. What reaction might prepubescent girls have to learning that they will gain body fat and then reach menarche? How could middle and high school students be taught in a positive manner about the body composition changes associated with the onset of menarche? Would such knowledge lead young girls to diet to prevent menarche?

One final question: A very athletic person in your dormitory tells you that she has heard about the relationship between body fat and amenorrhea. She tells you that she does strenuous aerobic exercise as a means of what she calls "natural birth control." What would you tell her?

Exploring Personal Dimensions

For Women Only

Taking charge of self-care and prevention greatly increases your chance of achieving sexual health and wellness. If you are a female, for the following statements, circle YES or NO. Then fill in the dates to help you keep track of your self-care activities.

I do vaginal self-examinations on a   YES   NO
regular basis.
 My last vaginal exam was on _____.
 My next vaginal exam is due on _____.

I have regular gynecological   YES   NO
examinations.
 My last gynecological exam was on _____.
 My next gynecological exam is due on _____.

I have regular Pap smears.   YES   NO
 My last Pap smear was on _____.
 My next Pap smear is due on _____.

I have regular mammograms   YES   NO
(if applicable).
 My last mammogram was on _____.
 My next mammogram is due on _____.

I keep track of my menstrual cycle.   YES   NO
 My last period began on _____.
 My next period is due on _____.

I practice safer sexual activities.   YES   NO

I understand that vaginal intercourse   YES   NO
during menstruation increases the
risk of transmitting HIV.

I have a family medical tree listing   YES   NO
diseases.

I discussed my family's medical   YES   NO
history with my doctor.

Suggested Readings

Alexander, L. L., LaRosa, J. H., Bader, H., & Garfield, S. *New dimensions in women's health*. Burlington, MA: Jones & Bartlett Learning, 2013.

Heffner, L. J., & Schust, D. J. *The reproductive system at a glance*, 3rd ed. Hoboken, NJ: Wiley-Blackwell, 2010.

Kolander, C., Ballard, D., & Chandler, C. *Contemporary women's health: Issues for today and the future*. New York: McGraw-Hill, 2010.

Norsigian, J. *Our bodies, ourselves*. New York: Touchstone, 2011.

Pruthi, S. *Women's health encyclopedia: The essential companion every woman needs for a healthy life*. Rochester, MN: Mayo Clinic, 2010.

Schuiling, K. D., & Likis, F. E. *Women's gynecologic health*. Sudbury, MA: Jones and Bartlett, 2011.

Youngkin, E. Q., Davis, M. S., Schadewald, D. M., & Juve, C. *Women's health: A primary care clinical guide*. 4th ed. Englewood Cliffs, NJ: Prentice Hall, 2012.

Web Resources

Inner Body: Your Guide to Human Anatomy Online: Female Reproductive System
www.innerbody.com/image/repfov.html

An overview of the female reproductive system with diagrams and detailed information about each structure, including the mammary glands, cervix, fallopian tubes, labia minor, ovary ligaments, ovaries, uterus, vagina, and vulva.

SexualHealth.com
www.sexualhealth.com/channel/view/women-sexual-health/

Presents information on women's sexual health topics such as desire, pleasure, orgasm, medications and supplements, gynecological concerns, pain during intercourse, menopause, menstruation and breast health, infertility, pregnancy and childbirth, masturbation, body image, and contraception.

National Woman's Health Network
http://nwhn.org/

The National Women's Health Network seeks to improve the health of women by developing and promoting a critical analysis of health issues in order to affect policy and support consumer decision making. The Network aspires to a healthcare system that is guided by social justice and reflects the needs of diverse women. On the website, women's health information and resources, as well as health alerts, are provided.

National Women's Health Information Center
www.migrantclinician.org/toolsource/resource /4womengov-national-womens-health-information -center.html

A website maintained by the U.S. government that provides resources and information about women's health issues. Includes health topics, health organizations, statistics, publications, and other links.

International Society of Men's Health (ISMH)
www.ismh.org/en/

ISMH is an international organization dedicated to the field of men's health. The comprehensive scope of men's health brings together multiple disciplines such as urology, cardiology, endocrinology, oncology, gerontology, psychiatry, psychology, sexual and reproductive medicine, public health, and others. IMSH also publishes *Journal of Men's Health*, which presents the latest findings to keep men healthy.

References

Adams, D. B., Gold, A. R., & Burt, A. D. Rise in female-initiated sexual activity at ovulation and suppression by oral contraceptives. *New England Journal of Medicine, 299* (1978), 1145–1150.

Addiego, F., Belzer, E., Perry, J., & Whipple, B. Female ejaculation: A case study. *Journal of Sex Research, 17* (1981), 13–21.

Alzate, H., & Hoch, Z. The G spot and female ejaculation: A current appraisal. *Journal of Sex and Marital Therapy, 12* (1986), 211–220.

Alzate, H., & Londono, M. Vaginal erotic sensitivity. *Journal of Sex and Marital Therapy, 10* (1984), 49–56.

American Cancer Society. *American Cancer Society recommendations for early breast cancer detection in women without breast symptoms*, 2013a. Available: http://www.cancer.org/cancer/breastcancer/moreinformation /breastcancerearlydetection/breast-cancer-early-detection -acs-recs.

American Cancer Society. *Breast cancer screening: The American Cancer Society and Living Well, October module*, 2007a.

American Cancer Society. *Can cervical cancer be prevented?* 2013b. Available: http://www.cancer.org/cancer /cervicalcancer/detailedguide/cervical-cancer-prevention.

American Cancer Society. *Cancer facts & figures 2014*. Atlanta, GA: Author, 2010a.

American College of Obstetricians and Gynecologists. *Dysmenorrhea*. Washington, DC: American College of Obstetricians and Gynecologists, 2012. Available: http://www.acog.org/Patients/FAQs/Dysmenorrhea#help

Amnesty International. *Why is it practiced?* 2009. Available: http://endfgm.eu/en/female-genital-mutilation/what-is-fgm /why-is-it-practiced/.

American Psychiatric Association. *Diagnostic and statistical manual of mental disorders, fourth edition, text revision*. Washington, DC: American Psychiatric Association, 2000.

AskMen. *Have great sex while she's menstruating*, 2011. Available: http://www.askmen.com/dating/love_tip_60/61_love_tip .html.

Ballagh, S. A., & Heyl, A. Communicating with women about menstrual cycle symptoms. *Journal of Reproductive Medicine, 53* (2008), 837–846.

Barnard, N. D., Scialli, A. R., Hurlock, D., & Bertron, P. Diet and sex-hormone binding globulin, dysmenorrhea, and premenstrual symptoms. *Obstetrics and Gynecology, 95* (2000), 245–250.

Barrack, M. T., Van Loan, M. D., Rauh, M. J., & Nichols, J. F. Physiologic and behavioral indicators of energy deficiency in female adolescent runners with elevated bone turnover. *American Journal of Clinical Nutrition, 92* (2010), 652–659.

Baxter, N. Preventive health care, 2001 update: Should women be routinely taught breast self-examination to screen for breast cancer? *Canadian Medical Association Journal, 164, no.13* (2001), 1837–1846.

Belzer, E. G. Orgasmic expulsions of women: A review and heuristic inquiry. *Journal of Sex Research, 17* (1981), 1–12.

Belzer, E. G., Whipple, B., & Moger, W. On female ejaculation. *Journal of Sex Research, 20* (1984), 403–406.

Boston Women's Health Collective. *Our bodies, ourselves: For the new century*. New York: Simon & Schuster, 1998.

Brooks, J., Ruble, D., & Clark, A. College women's attitudes and expectations concerning menstrual-related changes. *Psychosomatic Medicine, 39* (1977), 289–298.

Bullivant, S. B., Sellergren, S. A., Stern, K., Spencer, N. A., Jacob, S., Mennella, J. A., & McClintock, M. K. Women's sexual experience during the menstrual cycle: Identification of the sexual phase by noninvasive measurement of luteinizing hormone. *Journal of Sex Research, 41* (2004), 82–93.

Burri, A. V., Cherkas, L., & Spector, T. D. Genetic and environmental influences on self-reported G-spots in women: A twin study. *Journal of Sexual Medicine, 7* (2010), 1842–1852.

California Pacific Medical Center. *Breast cysts*. San Francisco, CA: Author, 2008. Available: http://www.cpmc.org/services /women/breast/breast_cyst.html.

Castleman, M. Female ejaculation: What's known and unknown. *All About Sex*. January 2, 2014. Available: http://www .psychologytoday.com/blog/all-about-sex/201401/female -ejaculation-what-s-known-and-unknown.

Centers for Disease Control and Prevention. *About DES: Known health effects for DES daughters*, 2011a. Available: http://www.cdc.gov/DES/consumers/about/effects _daughters.html.

Centers for Disease Control and Prevention. *About DES: Known health effects for DES sons*, 2011b. Available: http://www .cdc.gov/DES/consumers/about/effects_sons.html.

Centers for Disease Control and Prevention. *Mammography/breast cancer*, 2014a. Available: http://www.cdc.gov/nchs/fastats /mammography.htm.

Centers for Disease Control and Prevention. *Pap test and cervical cancer*, 2014b. Available: http://www.cdc.gov/nchs/fastats /pap-tests.htm.

Clayton, A. H. Symptoms related to the menstrual cycle: Diagnosis, prevalence, and treatment. *Journal of Psychiatric Practice, 14* (2008), 13–21.

Dalton, K. *Once a month*. Ramona, CA: Hunter House, 1979.

Daw, J. Is PMDD real? *Monitor on Psychology, 33* (2002). Available: http://www.apa.org/monitor/oct02/pmdd.html.

Endometriosis Association. What is endometriosis? *Endo-Online* (2005). Available: http://www.endo-online.org/endo.html.

Foldes, P., & Buisson, O. The clitoral complex: A dynamic sonographic study. *Journal of Sexual Medicine, 6* (2009), 1223–1231.

Friedman, R., Hurt, S., Arnoff, M., & Clarkin, J. Behavior and the menstrual cycle. *Signs, 5* (1980), 719–738.

Goldberg, D. C., Whipple, B., Fishkin, R., Waxman, H., Fink, P., & Weisberg, M. The Grafenberg spot and female ejaculation: A review of initial hypotheses. *Journal of Sex and Marital Therapy, 9* (1983), 27–37.

Grafenberg, E. The role of urethra in female orgasm. *International Journal of Sexology, 3* (1950), 145–148.

Greenberg, J. S. *Comprehensive stress management*, 13th ed. New York: McGraw-Hill Higher Education, 2013.

Heath, D. An investigation into the origins of a copious vaginal discharge during intercourse—enough to wet the bed— that is not urine. *Journal of Sex Research, 20* (1984), 194–215.

Hortobagyi, G. N., McLelland, R., & Reed, F. M. Your key role in breast cancer screening. *Patient Care, 24* (1990), 82–113.

Jannini, E. A., Whipple, B., Kingsberg, S. A., Buisson, O., Foldès, P., & Vardi, Y. Who's afraid of the G-spot? *Journal of Sexual Medicine, 7* (2010), 25–34.

Javed, A., Tebben, P. J., Fischer, P. R., & Lteif, A. N. Female athlete triad and its components: Toward improved screening and management. *Mayo Clinic Proceedings, 88* (2013), 996–1009.

Kaplan, H. S. *The evaluation of sexual disorders*. New York: Brunner/Mazel, 1983.

Kegel, A. Sexual functions of the pubococcyngeus muscle. *Western Journal of Surgery, Obstetrics, and Gynecology, 60* (1952), 521–524.

Kilchevsky, A., Vardi, Y., Lowenstein, L., & Gruenwald, I. Is the female G-spot truly a distinct anatomic entity? *Journal of Sexual Medicine, 9* (2012), 719–726.

Kolata, G. Deadliness of breast cancer in blacks defies easy answer. *The New York Times* (August 3, 1994), C10.

Korda, J. B., Goldstein, S. W., & Sommer, F. The history of female ejaculation. *Journal of Sexual Medicine, 7 (2010):*1965–1975.

Koutedakis, Y., & Jamurtas A. The dancer as a performing athlete: Physiological considerations. *Sports Medicine, 34* (2004), 651–661.

Mallon, R. *Demonstration of vestigial prostate tissue in the human female.* (October 1984). Paper presented at the Annual Regional Conference of the American Association of Sex Educators, Counselors, and Therapists, Las Vegas, NV.

Masters, W. H., Johnson, V. E., & Kolodny, R. C. *Human sexuality*, 2nd ed. Boston: Little, Brown, 1985.

Matteo, S., & Rissman, E. Increased sexual activity during the midcycle portion of the human menstrual cycle. *Hormones and Behavior, 18* (1984), 249–255.

Mayo Clinic. *Amenorrhea*, 2014. Available: http://www.mayoclinic .org/diseases-conditions/amenorrhea/basics/causes/con -20031561.

Mayo Clinic. *Ask a women's health specialist: Premenstrual dysphoric disorder (PMDD): A severe form of PMS.* Rochester, MN: Author, 2008. Available: http://www .mayoclinic.com/health/pmdd/AN01372.

Mayo Clinic. *Fibrocystic breasts*, 2010. Available: http://www .mayoclinic.com/health/fibrocysticbreasts/DS01070 /DSECTION=complications.

Mayo Clinic. *Premenstrual syndrome (PMS)*, 2012. Available: http://www.mayoclinic.org/diseases-conditions /premenstrual-syndrome/basics/symptoms/con-20020003.

Mayo Clinic. *Women's health: Amenorrhea*. Rochester, MN: Author, 2007a. Available: http://www.mayoclinic.com /health/amenorrhea/DS00581/DSECTION=causes.

Mayo Health Clinic. *Dietary suggestions for premenstrual syndrome*, 1998.

McMillan, M. Cervical scanner. *Washington Post* (September 14, 2004), HE2.

MedicineNet.com. *Menstrual cramps*, 2014. Available: http://www .medicinenet.com/menstrual_cramps/page3.htm.

MedlinePlus. *Secondary amenorrhea*, 2012. Available: http://www .nlm.nih.gov/medlineplus/ency/article/001219.htm.

Menstrual taboo. *Wikipedia*, 2014. Available: http://en.wikipedia .org/wiki/Menstrual_taboo.

menstruation.com.au. *Libido and your cycle*, 2008. Available: http://www.menstruation.com.au/periodpages/libido.html.

National Cancer Institute. *Breast cancer screening modalities: Mammography.* Washington, DC: Author, 2008a. Available: http://www.cancer.gov/cancertopics/pdq/screening/breast /HealthProfessional/page5.

National Center for Health Statistics. *Health, United States, 2013.* Hyattsville, MD: Author, 2014.

National Institute of Child Health and Human Development. *What causes menstrual irregularities?* 2014. Available: http://www.nichd.nih.gov/health/topics/menstruation /conditioninfo/Pages/causes.aspx.

Nemours Foundation. *Toxic shock syndrome*. Jacksonville, FL: Author, 2007. Available: http://kidshealth.org/teen/sexual _health/girls/tss.html.

Office of Women's Health. *Premenstrual syndrome (PMS) fact sheet*, 2012. Available: http://www.womenshealth.gov /publications/our-publications/fact-sheet/premenstrual -syndrome.html.

Pastor, Z. Female ejaculation orgasm vs. coital incontinence: a systematic review. *Journal of Sexual Medicine, 10* (2013), 1682–1691.

Patterson, J. Killer cramps. *Shape* (August 1990), 20–22.

Perry, J. D., & Whipple, B. Pelvic muscle strength of female ejaculators: Evidence in support of a new theory of orgasm, *Journal of Sex Research, 17* (1981), 22–39.

Phalen, K. F. PMS: Pretty miserable symptoms. *Washington Post Health* (August 1, 2000), 19.

Puppo, V., & Gruenwald, I. Does the G-spot exist? A review of the current literature. *International Urogynecological Journal, 23* (2012), 1665–1669.

Redfran, S. Pap plus: Some ob-gyns are adding a visual screen to aid cancer detection. *Washington Post* (April 4, 2002), F1.

Research Forecasts, Inc. *The Tampax report: A summary of survey results on a study of attitudes toward menstruation*. New York: Tampax, 1981.

Reuters. Study again clears silicone, *Washington Post* (June 22, 1999), A2.

Ruble, D., & Brooks-Gunn, J. Menstrual myths. *Medical Aspects of Human Sexuality, 13* (June 1979), 110–127.

Sato, S., et al. Transvaginal ultrasonography screening detects early-stage ovarian cancer. *Cancer 2000, 89* (2000), 582–587.

Sevely, J., & Bennett, J. Concerning female ejaculation and the female prostate. *Journal of Sex Research, 14* (1978), 1–20.

Sex on your period. *SexInfo Online*. 2013. Available at: http:// www.soc.ucsb.edu/sexinfo/article/sex-your-period.

Skene, A. Two important glands of the urethra. *American Journal of Obstetrics, 265* (1980), 265–270.

Slob, A. K., Ernste, M., & Van der Werff ten Bosch, J. J. Menstrual cycle phase and sexual arousability in women. *Archives of Sexual Behavior, 20* (1991), 567–577.

Smith, H. S. *How common are menstrual cramps?* 2012. Available at http://www.sharecare.com/question/common -menstrual-cramps.

Sommerfield, J. Lifting the curse: Should monthly periods be optional? *MSNBC Online*.

Tanfer, K., & Aral, S. Sexual intercourse during menstruation and self-reported sexually transmitted disease history among women. *Sexually Transmitted Diseases, 23* (1996), 395–401.

Torstveit, M. K., & Sundgot-Borgen, J. Low bone mineral density is two to three times more prevalent in non-athletic premenopausal women than in elite athletes: A comprehensive controlled study. *British Journal of Sports Medicine, 39* (2005), 282–287.

U.S. Food and Drug Administration. *Silicone gel-filled breast implants: Updated safety information, 2011*. Available: http://www.fda.gov/forconsumers/consumerupdates /ucm259825.htm.

U.S. Preventive Services Task Force. Screening for breast cancer: U.S. Preventive Services Task Force recommendation statement. *Annals of Internal Medicine, 151* (2009), 716–726.

UNICEF. *Female genital mutilation/cutting*, 2011a. Available: http:// www.unicef.org/protection/index_genitalmutilation.html.

UNICEF. *The state of the world's children, 2011*. New York: United Nations, 2011b.

Van Goozen, S. H. M., Wiegart, V. M., & Helmond, F. A. Psychoendocrinological assessment of the menstrual cycle: The relationship between hormones, sexuality, and mood. *Archives of Sexual Behavior, 26* (1997), 359–382.

Wimpissinger, F., Stifter, K., Grin, W., & Stackl, W. The female prostate revisited: Perineal ultrasound and biochemical studies of female ejaculate. *Journal of Sexual Medicine, 4* (2007), 1388–1393.

World Health Organization. *Fact sheet: Female genital mutilation*. Geneva, Switzerland: Author, 2008. Available: http://www .who.int/mediacentre/factsheets/fs241/en/print.html.

World Health Organization. *Female genital mutilation*, 2014. Available: www.who.int/mediacentre/factsheets/fs241/en/

Zaviacic, M., & Ablin, R. J.. The female prostate and prostate-specific antigen: Reasons for using the term "prostate" in the human female. *Histology and Histopathology, 15* (2000), 131.

Zaviacic, M., Jakubovská, V., Belosovic, M., & Breza, J. Ultrastructure of the normal adult female human prostate gland (Skene's gland). *Anatomy and Embryology, 201* (2000), 51.

Zaviacic, M., Zaviacicova, A., Holoman, I. K., & Molcan, J. Female urethral expulsions evoked by local digital stimulation of the G-spot: Differences in the response patterns. *Journal of Sex Research,24* (1988), 311.

CHAPTER 5

Male Sexual Anatomy and Physiology

© Gayvoronskaya Yana/Shutterstock

CHAPTER OBJECTIVES

1 Name and describe the parts of the male reproductive system to include the external and internal genitalia, including the pathway of the sperm.

2 Discuss the role of hormones in males as they enter puberty.

3 Cite various diseases that can affect the male reproductive system and the self-care procedures, as well as medical treatments, associated with these diseases.

INTRODUCTION

*A*n economics professor recently told me that a father had come in to talk about his son's mediocre academic performance. The father asked for a second chance for his son, explaining that "too often he thinks with his other head." Of course, this is not the first time I had heard this suggestion that men "think with their penises."

The notion goes back to the fifth century. In the Greek comedy Lysistrata, *the women of the city decide to withhold sex from their men until all wars are ended. The men quickly put their civic pride aside in favor of their women—thinking with their "other heads," no doubt!*

However, today's man may think more about *his penis than* with *it. And the great obsession seems to be size. In the mid-1900s a national sex survey found that men thought the average length of a penis was 14 inches; women thought it was 12 inches. However, the average length is really about 6 inches!*

Magazines like Penthouse Forum *did not help. Chock-full of large appendages—10 inches here, 8 inches there, a "foot long" here, as "thick as his arm" there—the stories were meant to present fantasy, not reality.*

The writer Susan Minot provides an interesting perspective in her short story "Lust."

> Tim's was shaped like a banana, with a graceful curve to it. They're all different. Willie's like a bunch of walnuts when nothing was happening, another's as thin as a thin hot dog. But it's like faces; you're never really surprised.

As you will read in this chapter, for all the worry that men may feel, it is quite natural for men's penises to vary considerably, just as their faces do.

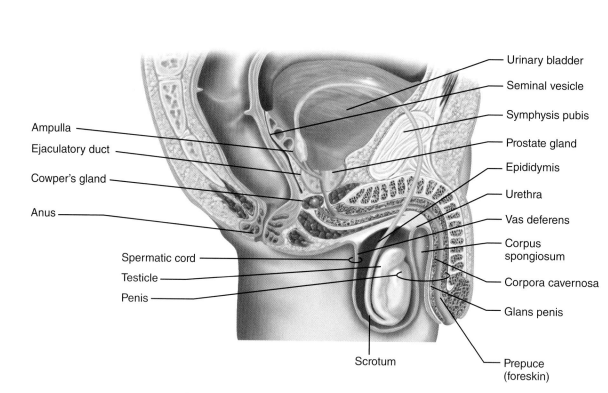

FIGURE 5.1 Side view of the male reproductive organs.

The Male Reproductive System

As females do, males have both external and internal genital organs. Figure 5.1 depicts a side view of the male external and internal genitalia, and Figure 5.2 shows a view from the rear. We begin our study of the male reproductive system with the external genitals.

The External Genitals

The male external genitals are the penis and the scrotum.

The Penis

The **penis** is a male sexual organ consisting of the root, the shaft, and the glans. As we have mentioned, penis

penis Structure of the male external genitalia consisting of the root, shaft, and glans; also contains the urethra, through which urine is excreted.

glans penis The head of the penis.

meatus The opening of the urethra in the head of the penis, where both seminal fluid and urine are passed.

coronal ridge (corona) The raised ridge where the glans penis ends and the penile shaft begins.

Kamasutra Ancient sex manual from India.

flaccid The relaxed, unerect state of the penis.

size concerns many students, who often ask about the "average-size penis." As a *general* guideline, the average penis is about 2–5 inches long when relaxed (flaccid) and about 4–7 inches long when erect. When sexually aroused, the penis becomes stiff and enlarged (erect) because its tissues fill with blood. The penis shaft is attached to the body by its root. The head of the penis is called the **glans penis**. The glans contains the urethral opening, or **meatus**, where both seminal fluid (which contains sperm) and urine are passed. Marking the end of the glans is a raised ridge called the **coronal ridge**, or **corona**. The coronal ridge helps to form a seal with the walls of the vagina during sexual intercourse. Below the corona the body, or shaft, of the penis begins. Although the entire penis is sensitive and sexually excitable, the glans and corona are particularly sensitive; in fact, they are the most sensitive parts of the male anatomy.

Historically penis size has been a matter of fascination. The **Kamasutra**, an ancient Indian book on erotica, classified men according to penis size in three categories: hare-men (erect penises of approximately 4.5 inches [11 centimeters]), bull-men (erect penises of approximately 6.75 inches [17 centimeters]), and horse-men (erect penises of approximately 9 inches [23-centimeters]). Other sources correlated penis size with personality traits or with the size of some other part of the body. Penises that are short when **flaccid**

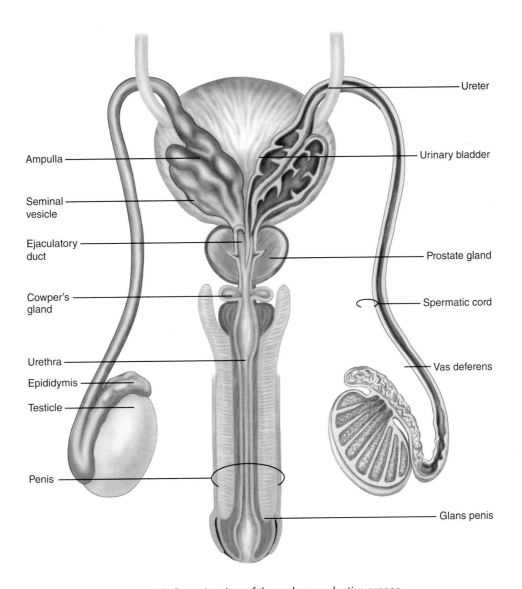

Ureter

Urinary bladder

Prostate gland

Spermatic cord

Vas deferens

Glans penis

Ampulla

Seminal vesicle

Ejaculatory duct

Cowper's gland

Urethra

Epididymis

Testicle

Penis

FIGURE 5.2 Posterior view of the male reproductive organs.

gain more size during **erection** than those that are longer when flaccid. Thus, although flaccid penises may differ significantly in length, erect penises are of similar lengths (Delvin & Webber, 2008). One way this has been described is that some men are "showers" and others are "growers" (Haffner & Schwartz, 1998).

Two contradictory views regarding penile size flourish in our time: "The larger the penis, the more satisfied the sexual partner" and "Sexual partners don't care about the size of a man's penis." It is not clear which is nearer the truth. Because the vagina adapts to the penis regardless of its size, some people have argued that size is unrelated to the sexual satisfaction of the female. However, part of our response to another's body is visual, and it seems reasonable to assume that if people have preferences for breasts of certain sizes and shapes, so might they react differently to penises of different shapes and sizes. None

of these preferences has anything to do with function unless it causes anxiety. The vagina contracts around the penis, regardless of its width or circumference. Furthermore, the inner two-thirds of the vagina has very little sensitivity. Both of these facts lead most authorities to conclude that penile width or length is unrelated to sexual satisfaction. Some people do, however, report preference for penises of a certain width or length. Whether these preferences are physiological or psychological is unknown at this time.

Just as women can strengthen the pelvic musculature with Kegel exercises, so can men strengthen the muscles surrounding the penis. Because these muscles are usually contracted only during ejaculation,

erection The extension of the penis and its engorgement with blood when the male is sexually stimulated.

Many variations exist in the size and shape of the male genitals.

they tend to be weak. By strengthening the muscles surrounding the penis, men may experience more satisfying orgasms and maintain better control of ejaculation. To do male Kegel exercises (National Kidney and Urologic Diseases Information Clearinghouse, 2012):

1. Identify the right muscles by imagining that you are trying to stop yourself from passing gas or urinating. Squeeze the muscles you would use. If you sense a "pulling" feeling, those are the right muscles for pelvic exercises.

2. Do not squeeze other muscles at the same time or hold your breath. Also, be careful not to tighten your stomach, leg, or buttock muscles. Squeezing the wrong muscles can put pressure on your bladder control muscles. Squeeze just the pelvic muscles.

3. Pull in the pelvic muscles and hold for a count of 3. Then relax for a count of 3. Repeat, but do not overdo it. Work up to 3 sets of 10 repeats.

4. Start doing your pelvic muscle exercises lying down. This position is the easiest for doing Kegel exercises because the muscles then do not need to work against gravity. When your muscles get stronger, do the exercises sitting or standing. Working against gravity is like adding more weight.

5. Be patient. Do not give up. It takes just 5 minutes, 3 times a day. Your ejaculatory control may not improve immediately, but most people notice an improvement in approximately 1 month.

Circumcision

The glans penis is covered by a **foreskin** (sometimes called the **prepuce**). For hygienic, cultural, or religious reasons, the foreskin is sometimes surgically removed. Removal of the foreskin—called **circumcision**—is more usual in the United States than in European countries. Circumcision takes place in the hospital approximately 2 days after birth or, if performed according to Jewish custom, 8 days after birth. In addition to Judaism, the Muslim faith requires circumcision. Figure 5.3 shows how circumcision is performed.

Hygiene also provides a rationale for circumcision. Several preputial glands—glands that secrete hormones only after puberty—are located in the foreskin and under the corona (Tyson's glands). These glands secrete an oily substance that, if not removed from under the foreskin, can combine with dead skin cells to form a cheesy substance called **smegma**. If this smegma is not regularly removed from under the foreskin, it becomes granular and irritates the glans penis, causing discomfort and possibly infection. Removing the smegma requires washing the glans penis. This becomes more difficult if the foreskin is not removed, because it has to be retracted manually to expose the glans.

Since 1971, the American Academy of Pediatrics (AAP) has released several statements noting that there is no medical reason for circumcision. As a result, circumcision rates in the United States dropped from a high of 95% of newborn males in the mid-1960s to an estimated 58% in 1987 (Rovner, 1990). However, in 1990, the Academy (Brower, 1989)

foreskin (prepuce) The covering of the glans penis, which is removed during circumcision.

circumcision Surgical removal of the foreskin covering the glans penis.

smegma A cheeselike substance secreted by the glans penis that must be removed from below the foreskin of uncircumcised males to prevent irritation and/or infection.

FIGURE **5.3** Methods of performing circumcision. (a) In this method, a piece of plastic is placed over the glans, and the foreskin is stretched over the plastic and trimmed off. (b) In this method, the foreskin is carefully cut "freehand" and then stitched.

(a)

(b)

reversed its position, citing advantages based on the work of Dr. Thomas Wiswell and colleagues (1985). Wiswell found that uncircumcised infants were 10 times more likely to have urinary tract infections than circumcised babies. Wiswell also reported that of 50,000 cases of cancer of the penis over a 50-year period, only 10 occurred in circumcised men.

However, not everyone agrees with the AAP's 1990 position. For example, Smith and colleagues (1987) found no difference in rates of urinary infections, and other researchers have reached similar conclusions over the years (Samuels & Samuels, 1983; Wallerstein, 1980). However, in 1999, AAP advised that the benefits of circumcision are not significant enough to recommend it as a routine procedure (American Academy of Pediatrics, 1999). The current AAP policy is somewhat less prescriptive, as evidenced in the accompanying box.

But another argument attempts to justify circumcision: The foreskin interferes with sexual stimulation because it serves as a barrier to the glans penis. There are no data to support this argument and, in fact, logic would indicate otherwise. The foreskin retracts when the penis becomes erect, and the glans penis is, therefore, able to be stimulated just as it is for the circumcised male. Furthermore, some people have argued the opposite: That is, if the glans is not usually protected by a foreskin, it may become insensitive because of its repeated contact with clothing. Therefore, the circumcised penis may, in fact, be *less* sensitive than the uncircumcised penis. Neither viewpoint is conclusive.

Still other reasons have been offered to justify circumcision. For example, uncircumcised males may be at greater risk of penile cancer, and their female sexual partners may be at greater risk of vaginal infections, cervical cancer, genital warts, and other sexually transmitted infections. However, for every study that supports these concerns, there appear to be studies that refute them.

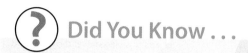

? Did You Know . . .

American Academy of Pediatricians' Policy Statement on Circumcision

Systematic evaluation of English-language peer-reviewed literature from 1995 through 2010 indicates that preventive health benefits of elective circumcision of male newborns outweigh the risks of the procedure. Benefits include significant reductions in the risk of urinary tract infection in the first year of life, and subsequently in the risk of heterosexual acquisition of HIV and the transmission of other sexually transmitted infections. The procedure is well tolerated when performed by trained professionals under sterile conditions with appropriate pain management.

Complications are infrequent; most are minor, and severe complications are rare. Male circumcision performed during the newborn period has considerably lower complication rates than when performed later in life. Although health benefits are not great enough to recommend routine circumcision for all male newborns, the benefits of circumcision are sufficient to justify access to this procedure for families choosing it and to warrant third-party payment for circumcision of male newborns. It is important that clinicians routinely inform parents of the health benefits and risks of male newborn circumcision in an unbiased and accurate manner.

Parents ultimately should decide whether circumcision is in the best interests of their male child. They will need to weigh medical information in the context of their own religious, ethical, and cultural beliefs and practices. The medical benefits alone may not outweigh these other considerations for individual families.

Source: Task Force on Circumcision. Policy statement: Circumcision policy statement. *Pediatrics, 130* (2012), 585.

There are more reasons for not being circumcised. First is concern about the trauma the infant experiences. Because infants cannot be administered general anesthesia or pain-relieving narcotic agents, circumcision is often performed without the benefit of anesthesia. To respond to this concern, some physicians inject a local anesthetic directly into the penis in an attempt to diminish or eliminate the pain associated with circumcision. Another issue is the risk of infection, hemorrhage, emotional trauma, and other effects associated with any surgical procedure.

Yet, there is agreement among medical experts that when the foreskin is so tight that an erection hurts or pain is experienced during sexual intercourse, removal of the foreskin is recommended. This condition is known as **phimosis**.

To summarize, here are reasons parents might consider circumcising their son:

- They are Jewish or Muslim. Infant circumcision is part of these religious traditions.
- If the father is circumcised, parents might want their son's penis to be like his father's penis.
- Parents do not want to have to teach their sons to clean their foreskins.
- Circumcised men may have a lower incidence of urinary tract infections.

Global DIMENSIONS

Male Genital Mutilation and Circumcision Practices

Around the world and throughout history there have been many societies that have practiced male genital mutilation. For example, castration, the removal of the testes, was common in ancient Rome; eunuchs, castrated men, dressed as women and became priests. Islamic societies are forbidden by the Koran to castrate men. Yet they used men castrated by the Christians as keepers of the harem, because they posed no threat of engaging in sexual activities. In addition, boys were castrated in the Middle Ages in Europe to maintain their soprano singing voices after puberty.

In some societies in the Pacific, men are circumcised, but the foreskin is not totally removed; instead, it is slit lengthwise and folded back. This is called *supercision*. Sometimes the foreskin is stretched tightly over a piece of bamboo, and then the incision is made. Circumcision is often associated with entry into manhood in these cultures and is usually celebrated with a ceremony of some sort.

- Some uncircumcised men have problems as they grow up, for example, pain during intercourse, requiring circumcision during adulthood. This is much more painful and dangerous than newborn circumcision.

- The rate of cancer of the penis, though extremely rare, is higher in uncircumcised men.

- Uncircumcised men may be more susceptible to sexually transmitted infections.

Here are reasons parents might not want to circumcise their son:

- Circumcision is not part of their cultural tradition.

- Circumcision is painful for infants.

- If the father is not circumcised, parents might want their son's penis to be like his father's penis.

- As with any surgery, circumcision poses some risks. In rare cases (less than two times in 1,000) infection or even damage to the penis occurs.

- They think circumcision is not natural. Boys are born with penises with foreskins; their intact penises should be left alone.

- Circumcision is done without the infant's permission. This should be an adult choice.

- The child is ill at birth. Circumcision should never be done on a sick or medically unstable infant.

The Scrotum

The other external structure of the male reproductive system is the **scrotum**, which is located below the penis. The scrotum is a sac of skin containing the **testes** and the **spermatic cords**. It comprises two layers: the outer layer, which is covered with hair and sweat glands, and the inner layer (called the *tunica dartos*), which contains muscle and connective tissue. This organ regulates the temperature in the testes by drawing them up toward the body when the body is cold and letting them hang lower, away from the body, when it is hot. As a consequence the temperature of the testes is always approximately 5.6°F (3.1°C) cooler than the internal body temperature. This temperature-control function is necessary for the production of viable sperm. The scrotum also contracts when the inner thigh is stimulated or when it is chilled. This effect, is due to the contraction of the cremasteric muscles located in the spermatic cord, which is known as the *cremasteric reflex*.

Myth (vs) Fact

Myth: Whereas females can strengthen their pelvic muscles, thereby exercising better control of their sexual response, there is not much males can do.
Fact: Males can strengthen their pelvic muscles also. They can perform Kegel exercises to strengthen the muscles surrounding the penis, thereby achieving more satisfying orgasms and maintaining better control of ejaculation.

Myth: There is no medical reason for males to be circumcised.
Fact: Recommendations regarding circumcision have changed over the years. More recently, it has been suggested that uncircumcised males may be at greater risk of penile cancer and that their female partners may be at greater risk of reproductive health problems. However, circumcision poses the risk of infection, hemorrhage, emotional trauma, and other conditions. Whether to be circumcised is a decision that needs a great deal of consideration.

Myth: Breast cancer affects women; men do not have to worry about contracting it.
Fact: Men can also contract breast cancer. In 2014 approximately 2,360 new cases of breast cancer were diagnosed, and 430 men died of it.

Myth: The ejaculate is made up predominantly of sperm.
Fact: The ejaculate, semen, consists mostly of seminal vesicle and prostate gland secretions. The volume of sperm is approximately the size of a pinhead.

Myth: A male with a small flaccid penis has much to worry about.
Fact: First, small flaccid penises tend to expand more during erection than do large flaccid penises. Second, the nerve endings in the vagina are in the outer third, making the length of the penis somewhat superfluous, at least as far as sexual satisfaction is concerned.

The Internal Genitals

The male internal genitals contain numerous organs housed within the penis, the scrotum, and the pelvis (refer again to Figure 5.1).

The Urethra

The **urethra** is a tube through the penis that begins at the bladder and ends at the meatus. Its function is to provide a route for both semen and urine to exit

phimosis Condition resulting when penile erection causes pain because the foreskin is too tight.

scrotum (scrotal sac) A sac of skin that contains the testes and spermatic cords.

testes Male gonads contained within the scrotal sacs that produce sperm cells and the male sex hormone testosterone. Singular form: testicle.

spermatic cord The cord from which the testicle is suspended that contains the vas deferens (defined later), blood vessels, nerves, and muscle fibers.

urethra The tube through which the bladder empties urine outside the body and through which the male ejaculate exits.

Organs

Testicle vertical cross section

Seminiferous tubules horizontal cross section

FIGURE 5.4 Testicle cross section.

the body. **Urine** is a waste product of the body that is stored in the bladder until it is expelled through the urethra. **Semen**, which is discussed later in this section, contains **spermatozoa**, or **sperm**, as well as other substances.

The Corpora Cavernosa and the Corpus Spongiosum

In addition to the urethra, the penis contains three spongy bodies: two **corpora cavernosa** and the **corpus spongiosum**, which are structures filled with networks of blood vessels and nerves. It is these columns of tissue, which fill with blood during sexual arousal, that make the penis grow hard and erect. During ejaculation the muscle surrounding the corpus spongiosum (the bulbocavernosus muscle) contracts and forces semen outward through the urethra.

The Testes

As mentioned, the testes (Figure 5.4) are suspended in the scrotal sac by spermatic cords, the **vas deferens** (through which sperm leave the testes), blood vessels, nerves, and muscle fibers. The testes produce sperm (about 50,000 every minute) and **testosterone**, a male sex hormone generally responsible for male secondary sexual characteristics (for example, deep voice, facial hair, and body hair). Within each testicle are approximately 1,000 **seminiferous tubules**, which are responsible for producing sperm, in a process called **spermatogenesis**. The cells between the seminiferous tubules, called **interstitial cells**, produce testosterone.

Once sperm are produced in the seminiferous tubules, they travel through the **vasa efferentia** to the **epididymis**, where they are stored and nourished for up to 6 weeks.

The Pathway of the Sperm

A mature sperm is about 0.0024 inch (0.0060 centimeter) long, with a head, neck, midpiece, and tail. The normal sperm contains 23 chromosomes. Each sperm contains a sex chromosome that determines the sex of the offspring. Sperm can be stored for up to 6 weeks in the epididymis before proceeding up the vas deferens to the **ampulla** (an enlarged portion of the vas deferens). Here in the ampulla the sperm receive more nutrients from the **seminal vesicles**, two sacs, each about 2 inches (5 centimeters) long, that secrete

urine The body-waste product stored in the bladder and eliminated through the urethra.

semen The male ejaculate, which contains sperm and other secretions.

spermatozoa (sperm) The mature male sperm cell.

corpora cavernosa A spongy body in the penis that contains a network of blood vessels and nerves.

corpus spongiosum A spongy body in the penis that contains a network of blood vessels and nerves.

vas deferens The duct, through which sperm stored in the epididymis (discussed later) is passed, that is cut or blocked during vasectomy.

testosterone The male sex hormone produced in the testes that is responsible for the development of male secondary sex characteristics.

seminiferous tubules The structures located within the testes that actually produce the sperm.

spermatogenesis The manufacturing of sperm in the seminiferous tubules.

interstitial cells The cells (sometimes called Leydig's cells) between the seminiferous tubules, where testosterone is produced.

vasa efferentia The duct through which sperm produced in the seminiferous tubules travel to the epididymis.

epididymis The location where sperm are stored in the testes and where nutrients are provided to help the sperm develop.

ampulla The enlarged portion of the vas deferens where sperm are provided nutrients from the seminal vesicles; also, the part of the fallopian tube of women containing the cilia.

Did You Know . . .

1. Testosterone causes bones to thicken and for this reason is sometimes administered to elderly people who have osteoporosis.

2. Excessive concentrations of sex hormones are metabolized primarily in the liver, with the products excreted in the bile and urine. Consequently, people with liver disorders experience the effects of excessive sex hormones (for example, the development of excessive body hair, development of breasts, or aggressiveness).

3. Sex hormones stimulate growth, thereby explaining the rapid growth that occurs during puberty. However, they also stimulate ossification (hardening) of the epiphyseal disks (a band of cartilage at the end of the bone), which causes bones to stop growing. Because estrogens produce greater effects on the disks than androgens, females stop growing earlier than males.

a substance believed to activate the sperm's **motility** (ability to move spontaneously).

With sufficient sexual stimulation, the ejaculatory process begins. Fluid from the **prostate gland** mixes with the sperm and with the secretions of the seminal vesicles, further aiding sperm motility and prolonging sperm life. The prostate fluid is an alkaline medium that offsets the acidity in the vagina that would otherwise kill the sperm. The **Cowper's glands**, two pea-sized glands adjacent to the urethra, empty into the urethra another alkaline fluid, which serves to neutralize the acidity caused by the urethra's transport of urine. The Cowper's glands secretions are the tiny droplets that sometimes appear on the tip of the penis before ejaculation. This secretion may contain some sperm left over from a previous ejaculation; therefore, it can cause pregnancy to occur even if the penis is withdrawn before ejaculation.

Ejaculation itself is the expulsion through the penis of semen, the mixture in which the sperm are carried. Ejaculation results from muscular contractions of the glands and ducts of the reproductive system. The expelling of semen is usually accompanied by **orgasm**, the climax of a growing complex of pleasurable sensations. Both the ampulla and seminal vesicles contract, as does the bulbocavernosus muscle surrounding the corpus spongiosum in the penis. The ejaculated semen contains sperm (the volume is about the size of a pinhead) and about a teaspoonful of secretions from the seminal vesicles, the prostate gland, and the Cowper's glands. Approximately 300 million sperm are expelled in a single ejaculation. According to some authorities, semen contain at least 20 to 35 million sperm per cubic centimeter in a male who is fertile—that is, able to fertilize an ovum.

During ejaculation a valve at the bladder's entrance closes to prevent urine from entering the urethra.

Table 5.1 reviews the functions of the male reproductive system.

Hormones

At some time during puberty, boys become capable of reproduction. This capability is accompanied by the ability to ejaculate, although initially the male's ejaculate does not contain mature sperm. The cause of male reproductive capacity is the increased secretion of androgens, followed by the development of secondary sex characteristics. Accompanying male reproductive capacity, and also a result of increased androgen production, is a heightened interest in sex. This can be considered double jeopardy, because an increase in sexual appetite in a person newly capable of fertilizing an ovum can create problems—such as unplanned pregnancy or frustrated **libido**. The majority of both males and females seem to adjust to this new condition and pass through this phase of life unscarred. Unfortunately some do not, as evidenced by the high rate of pregnancy in unmarried teenage girls.

During puberty, increased testosterone level leads to growth of the penis, prostate, seminal vesicles, and epididymis. The reason males cannot ejaculate before puberty is that the prostate and seminal vesicles are not

seminal vesicles Two sacs of the male internal genitalia that secrete nutrients to nourish sperm.

motility The ability to move spontaneously, which is required for fertilization.

prostate gland A structure of the male internal genitalia that secretes a fluid into the semen before ejaculation to aid sperm motility and prolong sperm life.

Cowper's glands Two pea-sized glands adjacent to the urethra that secrete a lubricating fluid before ejaculation.

ejaculation The ejection of semen from the penis during orgasm.

orgasm The peak release of sexual tension, accompanied by sensory pleasure and involuntary rhythmic muscular contractions; ejaculation in the male.

libido Sexual desire or drive.

TABLE 5.1

Functions of the Organs of the Male Reproductive System

Organ	Function
Testes	
Seminiferous tubules	Produce spermatozoa
Interstitial cells	Produce and secrete male sex hormones
Epididymis	Stores and allows maturation of spermatozoa; conveys spermatozoa to vas deferens
Vas deferens	Conveys spermatozoa to ejaculatory ducts
Ejaculatory ducts	Receive spermatozoa and additives to produce seminal fluid
Seminal vesicles	Secrete alkaline fluid containing nutrients and prostaglandins
Prostate gland	Secretes alkaline fluid that helps neutralize acidic seminal fluid and enhances motility of spermatozoa
Cowper's gland	Secretes fluid that lubricates urethra and end of penis
Scrotum	Encloses and protects testes
Penis	Conveys urine and seminal fluid outside the body; acts as the organ of copulation

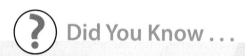

Did You Know . . .

Androstenedione is the supplement that Mark McGwire made famous during his 70-home-run season. Touted as an artificial steroid, it was said to raise testosterone levels. But researchers at the University of Iowa found that it did not raise testosterone levels or increase strength. A side effect was lower levels of "good" cholesterol (high-density lipoproteins), raising the risk of heart disease. Preliminary results of a further study by the Harvard researcher Hoel Finkelstein for Major League Baseball showed that androstenedione raised estrogen levels in men—and could result in breast enlargement!

Source: Data from Body-building aid questioned, CBSNews (June 3, 1999). Available: www. cbsnews.com/2100-204_162-493000.html.

Ethical DIMENSIONS

What Are a Dead Man's Rights?

The Center for Bioethics at the University of Pennsylvania documented 25 cases in which sperm were taken from dead men and preserved by deep-freezing. Furthermore, a survey of 273 fertility centers in the United States identified 82 requests for taking sperm from dead men, of which 25 had been honored. It is possible to remove sperm up to 24 hours after death, and the person most often making the request is the widow. However, there also are records of social workers and even an intensive care nurse who made such a request.

Who has a right, if anyone at all does, to have such a request honored? Only the spouse, or a parent as well?

Should men have the right to decide whether they will have children and with whom, even after they are dead?

Should sperm taken from dead men be used by women unrelated to them, whose husbands do not produce viable sperm? Who else should have access to this sperm?

Should the sperm be sold and the proceeds go to the man's family? What should be done with the frozen sperm if the dead man's family decides not to use them?

These are tough decisions that should be guided by ethical principles.

functional until they are "turned on" by the increased level of testosterone. Late-developing boys (15 to 16 years old) have been found to experience less sexual activity during adolescence than do early developers (Kinsey, Pomeroy, & Martin, 1948; Masters, Johnson, & Kolodny, 1982, 169; Zimmer-Gembeck & Helfand, 2008). This difference has been attributed to the effect of testosterone on increasing the sexual appetite in males. No long-lasting effect on sexual behavior has been reported, however.

Hormone Therapy

Hormone therapy is sometimes administered to men. For instance, testosterone supplements are sometimes administered to treat erectile dysfunction in older men (although testosterone levels are not low in all men who have trouble maintaining erection). Sometimes this treatment for erectile dysfunction is effective; other times it is not. The reason for this inconsistency is unclear; however, it is safe to say that the complex nature of sexuality makes it only partially responsive to hormone treatment. Testosterone supplements may not have much effect when personality, past experiences, the sexual partner, effectiveness in communication, setting, and so on, continue to have negative effects.

Self-Care and Prevention

Male reproductive care is as specialized as female reproductive care. Men should learn proper hygiene and methods of monitoring their reproductive health. When problems arise, males should consult their own medical specialists (internists or urologists). As with females, there are many organizations and publications that focus exclusively on issues of male reproductive health.

Breast Cancer in Men

Cancer of the breast occurs in men as well as women, although it is considered rare. An estimated 2,360 new cases of male breast cancer were diagnosed in 2014, and 430 men died of it that same year (American Cancer Society, 2014). Breast cancer is seen in men as early as their 30s. Although this cancer is rare, men are wise to examine their breasts for lumps. The procedure is the same for men and women.

It appears that several factors are related to the development of breast cancer in men. Among these are obesity, a lack of regular physical activity, and tobacco use (Brinton et al., 2008; Susan G. Komen, 2014). Also, African American males have a higher incidence of breast cancer than do white males (Fred

Should Physicians Have to Provide Care Regardless of Their Personal Values or Moral Convictions?

One month before George W. Bush's presidency was to end, he finalized a regulation allowing health professionals to refuse to provide any medical service they objected to on moral grounds (Meckler, 2008). This "right of conscience" regulation was interpreted to mean that abortion, family planning, providing prescriptions for emergency contraception (the "morning after pill"), giving certain information or advice, or any other service the medical provider deemed immoral—even referrals for such services—could be withheld from the patient.

Those favoring such a regulation argue that no one—not even a health professional—should be required to behave in a manner that the person considers immoral. Furthermore, if the patient is denied a medical service, there will always be other medical staff willing to provide the desired service. Lastly, medical providers should not face the threat of being fired or losing a promotion because they refuse to do something they believe to be against their religious or moral beliefs.

Those opposed to the "right of conscience" regulation believe that because medical providers are licensed by the state, they are obligated to serve the medical needs of *all* citizens of that state. They also argue that the rule sacrifices the patient's health to the religious belief of the providers (Savage, 2008). Furthermore, not providing a medical service requested by a patient, and not referring the patient to another healthcare provider from whom those services could be obtained, is doing harm to the patient and, therefore, is itself immoral and unethical.

Would you support a "right of conscience" regulation or do you agree with President Obama who rescinded it in 2011? What reasoning would you use when making this decision?

Source: Stein, R. Obama administration replaces controversial "conscience" regulation for health-care workers. *Washington Post,* February 11, 2011.

During a rectal digital exam, the physician feels for the size and texture of the prostate gland in an attempt to discover any abnormalities that need follow-up evaluation.

Hutchinson Cancer Research Center, 2014; Nahleh et al., 2007). In addition, as with women, breast cancer is more prevalent in men who carry the BRCA1 and BRCA2 genetic mutations (Breastcancer.org, 2013; National Cancer Institute, 2014). Another cause of concern is that male breast cancer is associated with a higher incidence of prostate cancer, suggesting careful screening for prostate cancer should be performed in men with breast cancer (Lee & Jones, 2008). In one large-scale study (Nahleh et al., 2007), male breast cancer patients survived an average of 7 years as compared to 9.8 years for female breast cancer patients. However, males in this study were diagnosed with breast cancer at a more advanced stage and with more lymph node involvement compared to the female patients. Furthermore, the male

patients were diagnosed at a mean age of 67 years, whereas the female patients were diagnosed at a mean age of 57 years.

Treatment for male breast cancer is similar to that of female breast cancer with one major difference: The psychological and emotional consequences of breast removal are not as significant for males as for females. Consequently, men seldom need counseling or a cosmetic means of disguising breast-tissue removal.

The Prostate

An important self-care procedure involves the prostate gland. The symptoms of **prostatitis** (inflammation of the prostate) are pain in the lower back, pain in defecation, pain during a rectal exam, and pus in the urine. Prostatitis usually affects younger men and

prostatitis Infection of the prostate gland.

Multicultural
DIMENSIONS

PSA Cancer Screening

As stated elsewhere in this chapter, the incidence rate for prostate cancer is higher in African American men than in white men. From 2005 to 2009, the overall age-adjusted incidence rate was 236 cases per 100,000 African American men and 146.9 cases per 100,000 white men (Howlader et al., 2012). African American males also have a higher death rate from prostate cancer, even after adjusting for access-to-care factors. As such, some caring physicians might recommend PSA screening for their African American patients, despite most medical organizations' recommendations that clinicians discuss the potential benefits and known harms of PSA screening with their patients and consider their patients' preferences rather than routinely ordering PSA screening.

One ethical principle guiding this kind of decision making is *paternalism*. Medical care providers who are advocates of paternalism argue that they are experts in health and, therefore, know more than their patients. It follows, then, that they can make a more informed and appropriate medical decision than can their patients. As a result, they are reluctant to discuss the pros and cons of screening *with* their patients and more comfortable making these decisions *for* their patients. This feeling of paternalism becomes even more pronounced when patients are minorities, or poorly educated. Given that some studies have found African American males are less knowledgeable about prostate cancer screening than white males (Chan et al., 2003; Barber et al., 1998), in spite of their higher incidence and mortality rates, the paternalism argument takes on added validity for some healthcare providers.

It seems to your authors that all men deserve to be informed about medical procedures available to them. After all, it is the patient—not the healthcare provider—who has to live with the outcomes of these procedures. If there is potential harm associated with PSA screening, we believe the patient should know that before consenting to the procedure.

can be cured with antibiotic drugs. If you experience these symptoms, consult a physician.

An estimated 233,000 new cases of prostate cancer were diagnosed in the United States in 2014, and an estimated 29,480 men died of it that same year. Prostate cancer is the second leading cause of cancer deaths in men in the United States (lung cancer is the first). Between 1989 and 1992, prostate cancer rates increased dramatically, probably because of the use of a blood test developed to identify an antigen produced when prostate cancer is present. The blood test measures the presence of prostate-specific antigen (PSA). Since 1993, prostate cancer incidence rates have declined. It should be pointed out that prostate cancer incidence rates are one and one half times as high for African American men as they are for white men, and the death rate is almost two and a half times as high (Prostate Cancer Foundation, 2012). The reason for this difference is not known, but some experts have conjectured that diets high in fat and/or the presence of a gene that may make the prostate more susceptible to the effects of testosterone may be the cause.

There are several factors that place a man at risk of development of prostate cancer. One of these is age. As a man gets older he becomes more susceptible to prostate cancer, although the cancer may have been present at a younger age but not fully developed. More than 70% of prostate cancers are diagnosed in men who are older than 65 years of age. Heredity is suspected of playing a role in perhaps 5% to 10% of cases.

Signs and symptoms include weak or interrupted urine flow; the need to urinate frequently, especially at night; blood in the urine; pain or burning when urinating; and persistent pain in the lower back, pelvis, or upper thighs. However, some of these symptoms may be caused by an enlargement of the prostate, which is common as men age, without the presence of a tumor. This condition is called *benign prostatic hyperplasia (BPH)* and can be treated with medications. The only way to distinguish BPH from prostate cancer is by a medical examination that includes a **digital rectal examination (DRE)**, PSA blood test, and biopsy of the prostate. On June 12, 1997, the American Cancer Society published updated guidelines for prostate cancer screening (American Cancer Society, 1997). The guidelines state, "Both prostate specific antigen (PSA) and digital rectal examination (DRE) should be offered annually, beginning at age 50 years, to men who have a life expectancy of at

digital rectal examination (DRE) A rectal examination whereby a physician inserts a finger into the rectum of a male patient to check for any abnormalities of the prostate.

least 10 years. Men at high risk (African American men and men with a family history of one or more first-degree relatives diagnosed with prostate cancer at an early age) should begin treatment at age 45." The reason a 10-year life expectancy is cited is that prostate cancer is usually a slow-growing cancer; thus it is thought prudent for men to refrain from having treatment if they are not expected to live long enough to benefit from that treatment. These men would likely die of some other condition before the prostate cancer killed them. An abnormal PSA test result is one with a value above 4 ng/mL (some suggest above 2 ng/mL), which would then lead to follow-up evaluation and subsequent procedures. These may include a biopsy of tissue extracted from the prostate gland.

In 2008, the U.S. Preventive Services Task Force, which evaluates medical screenings and makes recommendations regarding those screenings, published new guidelines for the use of the PSA test. It stated that men age 75 years of age and older should not be screened for PSA because the length of time one would die of prostate cancer is greater than 10 years, and a 75-year-old man's average life expectancy is only 10 years. Therefore, older men should not be subjected to the test, as it could lead to other medical procedures. For men younger than 75 years, the Task Force stated, "Current evidence is insufficient to assess the balance of benefits and harms of screening." In 2011, the Task Force went further and stated that all men, regardless of age, should not be routinely tested for PSA because the exam does not save lives and subjects men to unnecessary harm. The harms referred to relate to unnecessary medical procedures, such as biopsies and surgery; anxiety; and medical complications. The reasoning behind these recommendations pertains to the lack of evidence of the validity of PSA screening when a cutoff score of 4.0 ng/mL is used, as was standard practice. To respond to the lack of sensitivity of the screening at a score of 4.0 ng/mL, lowering the score to 2.5 ng/mL has been increasingly used. However, lowering the score leads to more false positives and, therefore, subjects men to more unnecessary biopsies and other medical procedures. Furthermore, two large-scale, long-term studies have concluded that PSA screening does not affect the prostate cancer death rate (Andriole et al., 2009; Schroder et al., 2009). The researchers found that the rate of death from prostate cancer was very low and did not differ significantly between the group of men who were screened and the group of men who were not.

Recognizing the controversy and lack of clear guidance, most major medical organizations recommend that clinicians discuss the potential benefits and known harms of PSA screening with their patients, and consider their patients' preferences rather than routinely ordering PSA screening. Among these organizations are the American Academy of Family Physicians, American College of Physicians, American College of Preventive Medicine, and American Medical Association.

If cancer is suspected, treatment consists of surgery, radiation, and/or hormonal therapy and chemotherapy if the cancer is in a late stage. However, because there is significant potential for serious side effects of these treatments (such as erectile dysfunction and/or incontinence), if the cancer is classified as low-grade and/or at an early stage, careful observation over a period without immediate treatment (called "watchful waiting") may be advised.

Ninety-three percent of all prostate cancers are diagnosed while still localized, and these patients have a 100% 5-year survival rate. During the past 25 years, the 5-year survival rate for all prostate cancers increased from 68% to 100%. Ninety-nine percent of men with prostate cancer survive 10 years, and 94% survive 15 years.

The Testes

Testicular cancer is the most common form of cancer in men during late adolescence and early adulthood. Most cases occur in men aged 15 to 40 years. It is estimated that about 8,820 new cases of testicular cancer were diagnosed in 2014 and that 380 men died of testicular cancer that year (American Cancer Society, 2014). The testicular cancer risk is four times greater for white men than it is for African American men (American Cancer Society, 2013c). The rate has doubled among white Americans in the past 40 years and has remained the same for African Americans.

Among the risk factors for testicular cancer are undescended testes (cryptorchidism). Other risk factors include a family history of testicular cancer, certain occupations (miners, oil and gas workers, leather workers, food and beverage processing workers, janitors, and utility workers), cancer of the other testicle, and infection with HIV. Testicular cancer is not related to injury or to vasectomy.

Treatment consists of surgery, radiation therapy, and/or chemotherapy. Surgery involves removal of the testicle. A cut is made in the groin, and the spermatic cord and the testicle are withdrawn from the scrotum through the opening. This procedure is called a *radical inguinal orchiectomy*. Depending on the stage of the cancer, some lymph nodes may also be removed. With only one testicle removed, the patient remains

testicular cancer Cancer of the testicles; the most common form of cancer in men aged 29 to 35 years.

Gender DIMENSIONS

Testicular Self-Examination

In the recent past, males were advised to perform testicular self-examinations in the hope of identifying testicular cancer at its earliest stage. However, after examining the pros and cons of such self-exams, the United States Preventive Services Task Force (2011) recommended that such tests not be performed. As with breast self-exams, the Task Force concluded that the potential harms outweighed the potential benefits of testicular self-exams. Still, any abnormalities found in the testicles should be immediately reported to a physician.

fertile. However, if two testicles need to be removed, the patient will no longer be able to produce sperm. Another side effect of the surgery is the possibility of damage to the nerves that control ejaculation. Damage to these nerves may also cause infertility. Men who still wish to have biological children can store sperm in a sperm bank for use after the surgery.

Treatment is highly effective if the cancer is diagnosed early. Ninety-nine percent of stage 1 cancers can be cured, 96% of stage 2 cancers can be cured, and 74% of stage 3 cancers can be cured. The lower the stage number, the earlier the cancer was diagnosed.

Any lumps, masses, or thickened areas may be symptoms of abnormality, not always cancerous; however, medical diagnosis and consultation are imperative. As with other forms of cancer, early diagnosis increases your chance of survival.

The Penis

Penile discharges of pus, painful urination, itching, or sores or warts on the genitals may indicate the presence of a sexually transmitted infection. Also, as suggested earlier in this chapter, men should make sure that smegma is washed away daily to prevent irritation or infection in themselves and their partners. For circumcised males, keeping the penis smegma-free is easy, involving rolling only a little of the remaining foreskin out of the way during normal showering. Uncircumcised men have to be more careful, pulling back the foreskin and washing the glans and the inside of the foreskin.

Care from Organizations and Available Publications

Several organizations aid men in caring for their reproductive health: The American Cancer Society publishes brochures and pamphlets; local health departments operate clinics providing medical examinations, testing, and care for STIs, premarital blood tests, and counseling about birth control and sexual problems. Other organizations, such as the National Cancer Institute, keep track of the incidence and frequency of diseases related to reproductive health. And still other organizations, such as the Health Research Group, a nonprofit group devoted to studies to improve health care, conduct research to prevent and treat various conditions affecting the male reproductive system.

? Did You Know . . .

The area between the penis and the anus is called the perineum; it is where the perineal nerve is located. Researchers have found that the perineal nerve is compressed during bicycle riding of three hours per week or longer and that blood flow to the area can be impaired as a result (Huang, Munarriz, & Goldstein, 2005). That can lead to numbness in the penis and perineum and is associated with the onset of erectile dysfunction (Marceau et al., 2001). Erectile dysfunction is the inability to achieve penile erection.

The possibility that this problem might occur does not mean, however, that men should not ride bicycles for protracted periods of time. A minor adjustment in the bicycle saddle can prevent this condition. The bicycle saddle should be changed from the traditional one with a protruding nose to no-nose saddle (Lowe, Schrader, & Breitenstein, 2004). In a study of bicycle police officers, who spend a considerable amount of time riding their bicycles, a no-nose saddle was found to reduce perineum pressure and decrease symptoms (Schrader, Breitenstein, & Lowe, 2008).

Other ways to prevent this problem include (MedicineNet.com, 2014):

1. Stand up frequently on the pedals to take pressure off the perineum.
2. Change your position on the saddle while biking. Shifting forward and backward when riding can eliminate pressure on just one part of the perineum.
3. Wear bike shorts. They have chamois padding in the perineal area that will help relieve pressure.
4. Adjust the height of the handlebars slightly until they are in a comfortable position.
5. Make sure that the seat post is adjusted to the proper height. The knees should be just slightly bent at the bottom of the pedal cycle.

© Shadd, Dirk/ZUMA Press/Corbis

Exploring the Dimensions of Human Sexuality

Biological Factors

When a sperm with a Y chromosome meets an egg, a male offspring will develop. Biological factors continue to influence development throughout life.

- Genetic coding affects physical appearance, including height; coloration of skin, hair, and eyes; muscularity; and many aspects of health.
- Physiological changes result at puberty from the hormone testosterone, which in turn affects muscle development and body size. Testosterone also increases aggression and leads to increased rates of heart attacks.
- Toward middle age, testosterone levels begin to drop, resulting in decreased muscle mass, increased fat, and a reduced sex drive.

Sociocultural Factors

Sociocultural factors interact with biological factors to influence health.

- Religion may affect the decision as to whether to circumcise the penis.
- The cultural bias allowing men to be sexually permissive can compromise a man's sexual health and wellness.
- Ethnic heritage influences health; for example, African American males tend to have higher levels of cancer and heart disease than white males.
- Media and ads portray the ideal man with extreme muscularity, achievable only with tremendous work and, in many cases, illegal steroids.
- Family, neighbors, and friends often reinforce gender stereotypes.
- Behavior proscribed by society as illegal can influence health; for instance, a man can compromise his health by using anabolic steroids.

Psychological Factors

Biological and sociocultural factors combine to influence psychological factors.

- Body image and self-concept are enhanced for many ... rcise and competitive sports.
- ... ress their emotions, increased levels ... lt.
- ... s and behaviors about gender roles ... ealthy lifestyles for men.

Case Study

The physiological development of a male starts when a sperm with a Y chromosome fertilizes an egg. More male than female pregnancies occur, but because male fetuses are weaker, a greater number of miscarriages result. Also, more male infants die than do femal

Socioeconomic stat mines whether prenatal ate prenatal and postn and medical help is sou drinks, or abuses dru fetus can be adversely

A man's physiolog The increased testost muscularity and a slir also causes increase

Male gender ro men to uphold a behaviors. Repressi increased stress.

Summary

- The male external genitals consist of the penis and the scrotum. The penis contains the urethra, through which urine and the ejaculate is omitted; the scrotum houses the testes.

- Surgical removal of the foreskin (prepuce) is called circumcision. Over the years there have been differing views on the necessity for circumcision. In some cultures and religions, circumcision is recommended and, therefore, frequently performed.

- The male internal genitals contain numerous structures. The urethra is the tube through which the ejaculate is ejected. The corpora cavernosa and corpus spongiosum fill with blood during sexual arousal, resulting in erection of the penis. Sperm are produced in the seminiferous tubules in the testes, stored in the epididymus, and travel out of the testes through the vasa efferentia.

- The ejaculate consists of secretions from the prostate gland, the seminal vesicles, and sperm. It travels through the vas deferens to the urethra, where it is eventually ejected through the meatus of the penis.

- During puberty, boys become capable of reproduction. This is a result of increased secretion of androgens, followed by the development of secondary sex characteristics. Males are not capable of reproduction before puberty because the prostate and seminal vesicles are not functional until they are activated by the increased production of testosterone that occurs during puberty.

- Males are susceptible to a variety of reproductive system illnesses and conditions. Among these are breast cancer, inflammation of the prostate (prostatitis), enlargement of the prostate (benign prostatic hyperplasia), and prostate cancer.

- Males should regularly care for their reproductive systems. These measures include screenings as appropriate, medical examinations by healthcare providers, and behaviors to prevent illnesses and diseases (for example, eating a nutritional diet, maintaining the recommended weight, exercising regularly, and adjusting the bicycle seat if one is a bicycle rider).

Discussion Questions

1. Name and describe the parts of the male reproductive system, including external and internal genitalia.

2. Explain how the increase and decrease of testosterone level affect the male reproductive system, including physiological and psychological effects.

3. Describe the self-care and preventive practices that a man should use to ensure his sexual health.

Application Questions

Reread the story that opens the chapter and answer the following questions.

1. The phrase "Most men think with their penis" clearly derives from the belief that hormones (physiology) control the man, and not vice versa. Do you believe this is correct? Or do sociocultural and psychological factors help balance a man's thinking?

2. The notion of penis size has generally been shown in research to be of little importance to women. Why does size continue to be a matter of jokes and of apprehension among men?

3. Can the male concern with penis size be compared to a woman's concern about her breast size? (After all, more than 100,000 women have breast enhancements each year.) If men could get relatively safe penis-enlargement surgery, do you believe that many would?

Critical Thinking Questions

1. In many schools throughout the country, sexuality education classes mention the concept of menstruation in a mixed-gender group. But the real discussion of menstruation occurs only in the follow-up "girls only" groupings. Consider whether boys should be taught about menstruation. Without factual knowledge, how can boys comprehend the physical and emotional issues surrounding menstruation? How can they be prepared for safer sexual practices during menstruation if they have not learned about it? Finally, how would you explain menstruation to a group of fifth-grade boys?

Critical Thinking Case

Dad has not been feeling like himself lately. He is unusually tense and easy to upset. It may be due to his lack of sleep. He goes to bed at the same time he always has, but he wakes up often in the middle of the night to urinate. When you ask him about it, he says that he really does not excrete a great deal of urine, just enough to relieve the feeling of having to urinate. As you try to help Dad, answer the following questions.

1. What are some possible causes of Dad's waking up often in the middle of the night to urinate?

2. What would you suggest Dad do about his dilemma? How could you help facilitate his taking this action?

3. What other reproductive system health issues would you expect Dad to encounter as he gets older? What can he do to prevent or postpone the occurrence of these conditions? What can he do to respond to them as they arise?

Exploring Personal Dimensions

For Men Only
Taking charge of self-care and prevention greatly increases your chances of achieving sexual health and wellness. For the following statements, circle YES or NO. Then fill in the dates to help you keep track of your self-care activities.

I have regular physician's examinations. YES NO
    My last physician's exam was on _____.
    My next physician's exam is due on _____.
    My physician perfoms a digital   YES NO
    rectal exam.

I practice safer sexual activities.   YES NO

I have a family medical tree listing   YES NO
diseases.

I discussed my family's medical history   YES NO
with my doctor.

Suggested Readings

Danoff, D. S. *Penis power: The ultimate guide to male sexual health*. Beverly Hills, CA: Del Monaco Press, 2011.

Danoff, D. S. *Penis power: The ultimate guide to male sexual health*. Bloomington, IN: Author House, 2011.

Leone, J. E. *Concepts in male health: Perspectives across the lifespan*. Hoboken, NJ: Wiley, 2012.

Padmanaban, K. *Men's sexual health*. Amazon Digital Services, 2012.

Vergel, N. *Testosterone: A man's guide*. Newburg, PA: Milestones Publishing, 2010.

Watson, L. *Unspeakable mutilations: Circumcised men speak out*. Amazon Digital Services, 2014.

Weis, M. *Total male: Save your life by taking charge of your sexual health*. CreateSpace Publishing, 2014.

Zilbergeld, B. *The new male sexuality: The truth about men, sex, and pleasure*. New York: Bantam Books, 2014.

Web Resources

Male Reproductive System
www.training.seer.cancer.gov/anatomy/reproductive/male

Diagram of the male reproductive system with links providing more information. Links include testes, duct system, accessory glands, penis, and male sexual response and hormonal control.

National Cancer Institute

www.cancer.gov

A federal government website providing information about cancer, including prostate and testicular cancers. Includes links to cancer topics, clinical trials, cancer statistics, research and funding, and current news pertaining to cancer.

American Cancer Society

www.cancer.org

A resource for all matters pertaining to cancer, including prostate and testicular cancers. Includes links to types of cancers, making informed treatment decisions, statistics, resources, and recent news.

The Male Health Center

www.malehealthcenter.com

An Internet education site providing information about male health. Included is information about sexual dysfunction, male sexual health problems, sexually transmitted infections, sexual hormones, and sexual aging issues.

Men's Health Network

www.menshealthnetwork.org

Men's Health Network (MHN) is a nonprofit educational organization comprised of physicians, researchers, public health workers, individuals, and other health professionals. MHN is committed to improving the health and wellness of men through education campaigns, partnerships with retailers and other private entities, workplace health programs, data collection, and work with healthcare providers to provide better programs and funding for men's health needs.

References

American Academy of Pediatrics. Circumcision policy statement. *Pediatrics, 103* (1999), 686–693.

American Cancer Society. *American Cancer Society updates prostate cancer screening guidelines*, June 12, 1997.

American Cancer Society. *Cancer facts & figures 2014*, 2014.

American Cancer Society. *Testicular cancer*, 2013c. Available: http://www.cancer.org/cancer/testicularcancer/detailedguide /testicular-cancer-risk-factors.

Andriole, G. L., et al. Mortality results from a randomized prostate-cancer screening trial. *New England Journal of Medicine, 360* (2009), 1310–1319.

Barber, K. R., et al. Differences between African American and Caucasian men participating in a community-based prostate cancer screening program. *Journal of Community Health, 23* (1998), 441–451.

Breastcancer.org. *The risk factors for male breast cancer*, 2013. Available: http://www.breastcancer.org/symptoms/types /male_bc/risk.

Brinton, L. A., Richesson, D. A., Gierach, G. L., Lacey, J. V., Park, Y., Hollenbeck, A. R., & Schatzkin, A. Prospective evaluation of risk factors for male breast cancer. *Journal of the National Cancer Institute, 100* (2008), 1477–1481.

Brower, V. Circumcision's back. *American Health* (September 1989), 126.

Chan, E. C. Y., Vernon, S. W., O'Donnell, F. T., Ahn, C., Greisinger, A., & Aga, D. W. Informed consent for cancer screening with prostate-specific antigen: How well are men getting the message? *American Journal of Public Health, 93* (2003), 779–785.

Delvin, D., & Webber, C. Facts about penis size. *Net Doctor*, 2008. Available: http://www.netdoctor.co.uk/sex _relationships/facts/penissize.htm.

Fred Hutchinson Cancer Research Center. *African Americans and cancer*, 2014. Available: http://www.fhcrc.org/en/events /cancer-in-our-communities/african-americans-and-cancer .html.

Haffner, D. W., & Schwartz, P. *What I've learned about sex*. New York: Perigee Books, 1998.

Howlader N., Noone, A. M., Krapcho, M., et al., eds. *SEER cancer statistics review, 1975–2009 (Vintage 2009 populations)*. Bethesda, MD: National Cancer Institute, 2012.

Huang, V., Munarriz, R., & Goldstein, I. Bicycle riding and erectile dysfunction: An increase in interest (and concern). *Journal of Sexual Medicine, 2* (2005), 594–595.

Kinsey, A. C., Pomeroy, W. B., & Martin, C. E. *Sexual behavior in the human male*. Philadelphia: Saunders, 1948.

Lee, U. J., & Jones, J. S. Incidence of prostate cancer in male breast cancer patients: A risk factor for prostate cancer screening. *Prostate Cancer and Prostatic Diseases* (May 27, 2008).

Lowe, B. D., Schrader, S. M., & Breitenstein, M. J. Effect of bicycle saddle designs on the pressure to the perineum of the bicyclist. *Medicine and Science in Sports and Exercise, 36* (2004), 1055–1062.

Marceau, L., Kleinman, K., Goldstein, I., & McKinlay, J. Does bicycling contribute to the risk of erectile dysfunction? Results from the Massachusetts Male Aging Study (MMAS). *International Journal of Impotence Research, 13* (2001), 298–302.

Masters, W. H., Johnson, V. E., & Kolodny, R. C. *Human sexuality*. Boston: Little, Brown, 1982.

Meckler, L. Bush-era abortion rules face possible reversal. *The Wall Street Journal* (December 17, 2008), A5.

MedicineNet.com. *Groin numbness and bike riding*, 2014. Available: http://www.medicinenet.com/script/main/art.asp?articlekey=84072&page=2.

Nahleh, Z. A., Srikantiah, R., Safa, M., Jazieh, A. R., Muhleman, A., & Komrokji, R. Male breast cancer in the Veterans Affairs population: A comparative analysis. *Cancer, 109* (2007), 1471–1477.

National Cancer Institute. *General information about male breast cancer*, 2014. Available: http://www.cancer.gov/cancertopics/pdq/treatment/malebreast/Patient/page1.

National Kidney and Urological Diseases Information Clearinghouse. *Urinary incontinence in men*. Bethesda, MD: 2012. Available: http://kidney.niddk.nih.gov/kudiseases/pubs/index.aspx.

Prostate Cancer Foundation. *African Americans: At higher risk for prostate cancer*, 2012. Available: http://www.pcf.org/site/c.lejriroreph/b.8368629/k.d6c1/african_americans_at_higher_risk_for_prostate_cancer.htm.

Rovner, S. A reversal on circumcision. *Washington Post Health* (May 15, 1990).

Samuels, M., & Samuels, N. All about circumcision. *Medical Self-Care* (Spring 1983), 20–23.

Savage, D. "Conscience" rule for doctors may spark abortion controversy. *Los Angeles Times* (December 2, 2008).

Schrader, S. M., Breitenstein, M. J., & Lowe, B. D. Cutting off the nose to save the penis. *Journal of Sexual Medicine, 5* (2008), 1932–1940.

Schroder, F. H., et al. Screening and prostate-cancer mortality in a randomized European study. *New England Journal of Medicine, 360* (2009), 1320–1328.

Smith, G. L., Greenup, R., & Takafuji, E. T. Circumcision as a risk factor for urethritis in racial groups. *American Journal of Public Health*, 77 (1987), 452–454.

Susan G. Komen. *Breast facts for men*, 2014. Available at: http://ww5.komen.org/BreastCancer/FactsForMen.html.

U.S. Preventive Services Task Force. Screening for prostate cancer: U.S. Preventive Services Task Force recommendation statement. *Annals of Internal Medicine, 149* (2008), 185–191.

U.S. Preventive Services Task Force. *Testicular cancer: Screening*, 2011. Available: http://www.uspreventiveservicestaskforce.org/Page/Topic/recommendation-summary/testicular-cancer-screening.

Wallerstein, E. *Circumcision*. New York: Springer, 1980.

Wiswell, T. E., Smith, F. R., & Bass, J. W. Decreased incidence of urinary tract infections in circumcised male infants. *Pediatrics*, 75 (1985), 901–903.

Zimmer-Gembeck, M. J., & Helfand, M. Ten years of longitudinal research on U.S. adolescent sexual behavior: Developmental correlates of sexual intercourse, and the importance of age, gender and ethnic background. *Developmental Review, 28* (2008), 153–224.

CHAPTER 6

Sexual Response and Arousal

FEATURES

Gender Dimensions
Male–Female
Differences in
Sexual Response

Global Dimensions
Aphrodisiacs and
Tigers: A Strange Mix

**Communication
Dimensions**
Discussing Sexual
Desires

Ethical Dimensions
Should Sexual
Enhancements
Be Used to Increase
Sexual Arousal?

Global Dimensions
Age of First
Intercourse

CHAPTER OBJECTIVES

1 Describe the role of the brain in sexual response, including the hormones involved and the role they play.

2 Describe the four phases of the Masters and Johnson sexual response cycle, as well as other theoretical models of sexual response.

3 Describe the physiology of orgasm in both males and females, differentiating between the different types of orgasm.

INTRODUCTION

*B*rian was sitting in his social studies class paying more attention to the attractive Tanya than to the teacher's lecture. Since he had entered high school he found himself more and more interested in girls, whose presence distracted him from his school work at times that were inappropriate. It was during one of these times that his social studies teacher asked Brian to identify a particular geographical region on the map in the front of the room. This was a problem for two reasons, both related to Tanya. First, Brian had no idea where that geographical region was, and, second, Brian's infatuation with Tanya and the accompanying fantasies resulted in Brian's having an erection. Now, erections are not something that high school students, or anyone else for that matter, choose to display before peers, so understandably Brian was embarrassed. What was he to do?

This has happened to many high school males, who somehow manage to use textbooks to shield their erections or find some excuse to delay walking to the front of the room until "it is safer." Some high school girls and older females also experience sexual excitement that results in an erection, in this case, of the clitoris. Yet, they are not as vulnerable as males to being exposed because clitoral erection is not evident through women's clothes. Women also experience vaginal lubrication when sexually excited, but this too is not readily identifiable when one is dressed.

If this reaction has happened to you, perhaps you wondered whether you are "normal"—you are. Perhaps you discussed this concern with your close friends. Most of us probably did not discuss it with our parents. That would have been too embarrassing. Maybe you read about these reactions in a magazine or saw them depicted in a movie. Unfortunately, too many young people rely on these sources for information about *sex—and magazines and movies often relay misconceptions and misinformation. But how were you to know that? Where else could you go? Whom else could you speak with?*

This chapter provides the information you may have wondered about since that time when your body first responded sexually. Included is a description of the typical human sexual response and the means of eliciting that response. Our goal is to help you establish and maintain a satisfying and effective sexual relationship when you decide you are ready for one. We begin with the study of the usual human sexual response.

Sexual Arousal and Response

When unaroused, the penis is flaccid; the skin of the scrotal sac is wrinkled, thin, and loose; and the testes hang down from the body. In females, the labia are thin and enclose the vestibule, the clitoris extends from under the clitoral hood, the inner part of the vagina remains elongated, and the nipples of the breast are not erect.

After sexual excitement diminishes, these structures return to their prearoused state. This takes some time, which varies from person to person.

Sexual pleasure and satisfaction are both psychologically and physiologically based. Without the subjective feeling of pleasure, physiological arousal will not occur. For example, if you dislike the body odor of your partner, it will be difficult for you to develop an erection if you are a male or lubrication of the vagina if you are a female. As we shall soon see, pleasurable sexual stimulation will lead to an identifiable sexual response cycle. Knowing what this response cycle is can help you view your sexuality as a normal part of your functioning, for it suggests that sexual responses can be understood, predicted, and studied in the same way that other physiological processes can. Furthermore, learning to discern and distinguish your own bodily responses can enable you to pay attention, tell your partner about your responses, and thus increase your enjoyment.

How the Mind and Body Control Sexual Response

When a person becomes sexually aroused, several different parts of the body work together to create the psychological feeling of arousal and the accompanying physiological reactions. When Brian fantasized about Tanya, his brain, glands, nervous system, circulatory system, and reproductive system were only some of the bodily parts involved. Before we discuss the particular response to sexual stimulation, let us look more closely at what happens between the body and mind on such occasions.

The Brain: The Master of the Body

As with most vital functions, the brain is a key player during sexual arousal (Greenberg, 2013). It is the brain that interprets the stimulation—be it visual, olfactory, or other—and begins the process of "activating" other body parts.

The brain includes two major components: the **cerebral cortex** (the upper part) and the subcortex (the lower part). Figure 6.1 shows the structures of the brain and their locations. The subcortex includes the cerebellum (coordinates body movements), the medulla oblongata (regulates heartbeat, respiration, and other such basic physiological processes), the pons (regulates the sleep cycle), and the diencephalon. The diencephalon has many purposes, including the regulation of the emotions. It is made up of the thalamus and hypothalamus. The thalamus relays sensory impulses from other parts of the nervous system to the cerebral cortex. The hypothalamus, a key structure in sexual arousal, is the primary activator of the autonomic nervous system, which controls basic body processes such as hormone balance, temperature, and the constriction and dilation of blood vessels.

The **limbic system**, called the "seat of emotions," consists of the thalamus and hypothalamus (the diencephalon) and other structures important in sexual arousal. The limbic system is connected to the diencephalon and is primarily concerned with emotions and their behavioral expression. The limbic system is thought to produce such emotions as fear, anxiety, and joy in response to physical and psychological signals.

cerebral cortex The part of the brain called the *gray matter* that controls higher-order functioning such as language and judgment.

limbic system The part of the brain referred to as the "seat of emotions," which produces emotions in response to physical and psychological signals.

FIGURE **6.1** Many areas of the brain are involved in interpreting and determining each person's reaction to sexual stimulation.

The cerebral cortex (called the *gray matter*) controls higher-order abstract functioning, such as language and judgment. The cerebral cortex can also control more primitive areas of the brain. When the diencephalon recognizes fear, for instance, the cerebral cortex can use judgment to recognize the stimulus as nonthreatening and override the fear.

Last is the **reticular activating system (RAS)**. In the past, cortical and subcortical functions were considered dichotomized; that is, human behavior was thought to be a function of one area of the brain or the other. Now, brain researchers believe that neurological connections between the cortex and subcortex feed information back and forth. This network of nerves, the RAS, can be considered the connection between mind and body. The reticular system is a kind of two-way street, carrying messages perceived by the higher-awareness centers to the organs and muscles and also relaying stimuli received at the muscular and organic levels up to the cerebral cortex. In this manner, a sexually stimulating touch can generate physiological responses.

The Brain and Sexual Response

When you encounter a sexual stimulus of whatever kind, this message is passed to the brain via nerves. Once it reaches the brain, the message passes through the reticular activating system either from or to the limbic system and the thalamus. The limbic system is where emotion evolves, and the thalamus serves as the switchboard, determining what to do with the incoming messages. Next, the hypothalamus is activated and, in turn, activates the autonomic nervous system and the endocrine system through messages sent via nerves or substances released into the bloodstream.

All of this is generalized, of course. No two people are exactly the same, so no two people should be expected to react in exactly the same manner to sexual stimulation. First, what one person finds sexually arousing, another might not. As a result, one person might experience erection or vaginal lubrication when seeing pictures of people engaged in sexual activities, whereas another person might be "turned off" by this material. Second, because of illness or injury, some typical responses may be precluded for some people. For example, a male with a spinal cord injury might not be able to achieve an erection in spite of what might usually be sexually arousing for others. Furthermore, some people have little control over apparently involuntary responses; however, other people are able to exercise some control. For example, although ejaculation is considered an involuntary response to sexual stimulation, we know that people can learn to control (that is, delay) ejaculation should they choose to. So, in general, there is a great deal of variation in sexual response, even though there are certain typical means of reacting to sexual stimulation.

The Autonomic Nervous System

The autonomic nervous system consists of the sympathetic nervous system and the parasympathetic

reticular activating system (RAS) A network of nerves that connect the cortex and the subcortex—the connection between mind and body.

nervous system. These "subnervous systems" connect to various parts of the body through nerves. Consequently, as sexually arousing stimuli are experienced, messages are sent via the nerves to body parts, instructing them to react. The heart rate increases, muscles tense, perspiration occurs, and the mind starts racing. In addition, certain arteries are instructed to open (dilate) and allow more blood to flow through. That is why, for instance, the penis and the clitoris become erect. Arteries in these structures dilate, allowing blood to flow to the area; the nerves instruct veins to constrict, thereby holding the blood in that one place. The result is erection. The increase of blood to the genital area, called *engorgement*, also creates pressure on the walls of the vagina, resulting in vaginal lubrication. Furthermore, muscles contract as a result of messages sent through the nerves that make up the autonomic nervous system. For men, for example, contractions of the Cowper's gland, the seminal vesicles, and the prostate gland result in fluids being secreted into semen; contractions of the abdominal muscles and the muscles surrounding the reproductive organs are experienced by women.

The Role of Hormones in Sexual Arousal

The endocrine system is responsible for the secretion of hormones that travel to various body parts, instructing them how to behave. For example, when you are "stressed out," hormones are deposited into the bloodstream by the pituitary, adrenal, thyroid, and other glands and transported around the body, resulting in an increase in heart rate, muscle tension, blood pressure, and perspiration.

Sexual arousal works similarly. When you encounter a sexually arousing stimulus, your endocrine system is activated; hormones are secreted and changes occur in your body. That is what happens when someone fantasizes about a sexual experience. The fantasy translates into a sexual response that depends on the release of hormones that target certain body parts and bodily functions.

Sexual hormones are produced in the testes and ovaries. Testosterone, an androgen produced predominantly in the interstitial cells of the testes in men and in the ovaries in women (although a small amount is also produced in the adrenal glands), affects sexual interest, or *libido*. The more testosterone, the greater the interest in sex. Conversely, the less testosterone, the less interest in sex. Islamic societies once used castrated men to watch the women in the harem because their lowered interest in sex made them no threat to the women.

Recognizing the influence of testosterone on sexual interest, and in an attempt to enhance sexual satisfaction, some people turn to chemical aids. One of these "aids" is the substance used by the baseball player Mark McGwire during his record-breaking home run season. Popularly referred to as "andro," androstenedione was marketed as a dietary supplement; thus it was not regulated by the U.S. Food and Drug Administration (FDA). Athletes employed androstenedione to help them recover from weight-training workouts. Chemically, androstenedione is a steroid hormone and a near cousin of testosterone. The association with testosterone was enough to convince some people to use it to enhance sexual satisfaction. The problem with doing so is twofold: (1) The amount of testosterone may not be sufficient for the desirable effects, and (2) its use may result in harmful side effects, especially over the long term. Among other potential side effects, steroid use can lead to liver cancer, mood swings, hair growth, masculinization in women, and atrophied testes in men. In spite of these problems, androstenedione's possible effects on sexual arousal seem to override good judgment for some people hell-bent on making their sex lives ever richer.

The Role of Culture in Sexual Arousal

Whereas sexual arousal involves a physiological reaction to sexual stimulation, that reaction depends on the interpretation of the stimulant. For example, penis and clitoral erections are physiological responses to something interpreted as sexually stimulating. And yet, what someone finds sexually stimulating in one culture may have just the opposite reaction in another culture. For example, one culture might

© SusIO/Shutterstock

In a study of body shape preferences, African Americans chose a more full-figured body to be ideal whereas Caucasians chose a thinner body type to be ideal. Which body shape do you prefer?

value a "full-bodied" woman, whereas another might value thinness. Furthermore, perceptions of what is sexually stimulating may differ within the same culture over time. In the United States, for instance, the actress Marilyn Monroe was a sexual icon in the 1950s. Today, she would probably be viewed differently because we now place a higher value on thinness than we did back then.

Subcultures also may have different perceptions of what is sexually stimulating. One of your authors' graduate students conducted a study of what African Americans and Caucasians considered to be the ideal body type. Research subjects were given silhouettes to evaluate. Whites reported that a thinner silhouette was more attractive, whereas African Americans stated a more full-figured body type was more desirable.

In some Muslim societies, women are required to be covered from head to toe. In contrast, in many Western societies, scantily clad women evoke a sexual response. In some subcultures, pornographic material is sexually stimulating while in others it is considered disgusting.

Thus, although sexual stimulation is a physiological process, it has a cultural and societal component to it that starts the physiological reaction in the first place.

The Masters and Johnson Sexual Response Cycle

The research of Masters and Johnson (1966) revealed a great deal about human sexuality. One of their major contributions was their description of the four phases of the human sexual response.

Excitement Phase

During the first phase of the Masters and Johnson **sexual response cycle**, the *excitement phase*, sexual stimuli result in a number of specific changes in the bodies of men and women. Heart rate, blood pressure, and muscle tension all increase. Blood engorges the abdominal area, resulting in an increase in penile and clitoral erection, as well as an increase in size of the labia minora, vagina, and nipples. The testes move closer to the body, and the scrotal skin thickens and tightens during the excitement phase. In women, vaginal lubrication occurs, and the labia majora spread and separate so as to make the vestibule more accessible. Some of these structures also deepen in color as a result of the increased blood to the area. The engorgement of blood is also responsible for the darkening of the skin on the chest and breasts called the *sex flush*. Although the sex flush occurs in both genders, it is more common in women and occurs in

all ethnic groups, although it may be more evident in whites than in people of color.

Transudation is the process resulting in vaginal lubrication. When a female is sexually aroused, blood flows into the area surrounding the walls of the vagina in a process called *vasocongestion*. The pressure of the increased blood causes a seepage of moisture from the spaces between the cells. This moisture crosses the vaginal lining, first appearing as droplets. Eventually the fluid builds up in sufficient quantity to moisten the entire inner walls of the vagina. The amount of moisture may even be enough, depending on the woman's position, to leak out of the vagina and lubricate the labia and introitus.

The excitement phase may be short or last for several hours. The longer it lasts, the more variability occurs. For example, changes in the penis and the vagina vacillate over time during an extended excitement phase, so that the penis may occasionally become less erect, and vaginal lubrication may diminish periodically as well. The exciting aspect of excitement (pun intended) is the great variability among people. Some respond quickly; others need more time. Some favor moving to the next phase quickly; others desire more time. Some focus on their own reactions and feelings and satisfaction; others are more concerned with the partner's satisfaction. Furthermore, any one person may experience the excitement phase differently from one sexual encounter to another.

Plateau Phase

The second phase of Masters and Johnson's sexual response cycle is called the *plateau phase*. During the plateau phase, excitement becomes enhanced. Heart rate quickens, blood pressure rises, muscle tension increases, and breathing is faster. In men, Cowper's gland secretions may result from muscular contractions. The penis becomes fully erect, and the testes move closer to the body cavity. In women, the clitoris retracts under the clitoral hood; the inner two-thirds of the vagina fully extends, forming a "tenting" effect and creating a receptacle for semen; and the outer third of the vagina engorges with blood, forming the orgasmic platform. Although the plateau phase usually lasts but a few minutes, there are reports of more intense orgasms by people who have purposefully extended the plateau phase. And yet, orgasm is not the necessary follow-up to plateau. Although for men

---

sexual response cycle The sequence of physiological and psychological reactions as a result of sexual arousal.

transudation The process of vaginal lubrication resulting from engorgement of blood that creates pressure that forces moisture to seep from the spaces between the cells.

the loss of erection is unlikely once plateau is reached, in women as we shall soon see, reaching the plateau phase may be sufficient for sexual satisfaction.

Orgasm Phase

The *orgasm phase* for males consists of two stages: the *emission stage* and the *expulsion stage*. During the emission stage, muscular contractions of the vas deferens, the seminal vesicles, and the prostate gland create a buildup of semen in the urethral bulb located at the base of the penis. At the same time, the external urethral sphincter contracts, holding in the semen. Concurrently, the internal urethral sphincter contracts, thereby preventing semen from entering the bladder (a condition known as *retrograde ejaculation*) and urine from entering the urethral bulb where the semen has accumulated. The accumulation of semen in the urethral bulb creates a sensation of imminent and inevitable ejaculation, which usually lasts only a few seconds. Soon the second stage, expulsion, occurs.

During the expulsion stage, the **internal urethral sphincter** remains contracted, so urine and semen do not mix. However, the **external urethral sphincter** relaxes, and muscles surrounding the urethral bulb and the urethra contract, with the result that the accumulated semen is expelled from the urethral opening. Although there is some variation from one person to another, males generally experience intense sensations during the first couple of contractions and less sensation during later contractions. The degree of sensation appears also to be related to the amount of semen expelled.

In women, the orgasm phase also consists of muscular contractions and intense sensations. The pelvic muscles that surround the vagina, in particular those that make up the **orgasmic platform**, contract 3 to 15 times, each contraction lasting less than 1 second. Other weaker and slower contractions follow. In addition, uterine contractions occur, beginning from the top of the uterus and proceeding downward.

In both males and females, other changes occur during orgasm. For example, heart rate increases dramatically, blood pressure rises, and breathing becomes rapid and shallow. Muscles throughout the body contract, and perspiration is evident. And an intense, pleasant psychological feeling associated with the release of sexual tension afforded by orgasm occurs.

Resolution Phase

During the *resolution phase*, there is a return to the unaroused state. In males, there is a decrease in the size of the penis as the erection is lost. This occurs in two stages: The first lasts about 1 minute as the blood exits the corpora cavernosa; the second takes several minutes as the blood leaves the corpus spongiosum. This is a result of the opening of the veins in the penis, which allows blood to be removed from the area. The testes become smaller and move down from the body cavity, and the scrotal skin becomes thinner and looser.

In women, muscles relax, and the uterus, vagina, and labia return to their unaroused positions and color. As a result of the uterus's returning to its unaroused position, the cervix lowers into the seminal pool. If sperm is present in the seminal pool, the cervix is likely to have contact with them, and fertilization is possible. If one is trying to become pregnant, then the woman should lie on her back after intercourse to encourage this contact. Of course, the best way to prevent

---

internal urethral sphincter The valve that prevents urine from entering the urethra and sperm from entering the bladder during ejaculation.

external urethral sphincter The valve that closes during the emission stage, resulting in a buildup of semen, and that opens during the ejaculation stage, allowing semen to be expelled.

orgasmic platform The narrowing of the outer third of the vagina during orgasm caused by contractions of the muscles in that area.

sex flush A darkening of the skin of the neck, face, forehead, or chest during sexual stimulation.

myotonia Muscle tension occurring during sexual arousal.

hyperventilation Deep and rapid breathing that occurs during sexual excitation.

tachycardia An increase in heart rate that occurs during sexual activity.

vasocongestion Increased blood flow to an area of the body; occurs in the pelvic area during sexual arousal.

Females and males have many sexual responses in common, as well as many that differ. One of the differences is that males need a refractory period in which to recover before being capable of another orgasm, whereas females do not.

Male–Female Differences in Sexual Response

There are many similarities and many differences in how males and females respond to sexual arousal. Masters and Johnson found the following similarities in the response cycle of men and women:

1. *Nipples.* Both males' and females' nipples become erect and wider in diameter when sexually stimulated.
2. *Sex Flush.* Males and females both experience a darkening of the skin of the neck, face, forehead, or chest during sexual stimulation, known as the **sex flush**. This darkening of the skin is a result of the accumulation of blood in these areas.
3. *Muscle Tension.* Commencing during the plateau phase and involving the legs, arms, abdomen, neck, and face, muscle tension (**myotonia**) appears in both sexes. During orgasm, muscles of the abdomen, chest, and face are also tensed. After orgasm, during the resolution phase, there is a release of all muscular tension in both sexes.
4. *Breathing.* During sexual excitation, both sexes experience deep and rapid breathing, called **hyperventilation.**
5. *Heart Rate.* Heart rate increases from a normal resting rate of about 72 up to 180 or more beats per minute during orgasm are not unusual in either sex. Such an increase is termed **tachycardia.**
6. *Blood Pressure.* Blood pressure rises in both males and females during sexual excitation.
7. *Perspiration.* Approximately one-third of both males and females perspire after orgasm.
8. *Blood Flow.* Increased blood flow to the pelvic area results in clitoral and penile erection and vaginal lubrication. This increased blood flow is termed **vasocongestion.**
9. *Orgasm.* During orgasm there is a rapid contraction of muscles in both sexes, with a relaxing of the muscles after orgasm.

The following listing describes the differences in the sexual responses of males and females:

1. *Nipples.* Whereas females are most likely to experience nipple erection during the excitement phase, males usually experience it during the plateau phase. Further, female nipple erection appears to disappear soon after orgasm (although this is an illusion caused by the swelling of the areolae), whereas male nipple erection is often obvious long after.
2. *Sex Flush.* Whereas males experience sex flush only in the plateau phase, in females sex flush can occur either late in the excitement phase or in the plateau phase. And though it may occur on the neck, forehead, and chest of both males and females, the sex flush occurs over the lower abdomen, thighs, lower back, and buttocks of females only.
3. *Muscle Tension.* In females, muscular tension causes an increase in the length and width of the vagina and expansion of the diameter of the cervix. In males, it causes elevation of the testes; that is, they are moved closer to the body by the contraction of muscles supporting them.
4. *Breathing.* Hyperventilation has different effects on males and females. After orgasm, males must wait for hyperventilation to diminish before being able to have another orgasm or even to achieve another erection; this period while breathing slows is referred to as a *refractory period.* Females, however, may have another orgasm before hyperventilation subsides—that is, without a refractory period and without entering a resolution phase. Consequently some females are capable of many orgasms in a short period.
5. *Blood Pressure.* Blood pressure increases somewhat more in males than in females. In males systolic blood pressure has been found to increase 40 to 100 mm Hg and diastolic blood pressure 20 to 50 mm Hg during sexual stimulation. In females the increase ranges from 30 to 80 mm Hg systolic and 20 to 40 mm Hg diastolic.
6. *Perspiration.* In men, sweating is usually limited to the soles of the feet and palms of the hands. Women are more likely to perspire over the back, thighs, chest, and sometimes the trunk, head, and neck.
7. *Orgasm.* Women are more likely than men to be multiorgasmic. Further, orgasm for the woman usually lasts longer than for men. There is disagreement about female ejaculation; it is sufficient to say here that, at the very least, female ejaculation does not occur as often during orgasm as does male ejaculation.

pregnancy if engaging in sexual intercourse is to use some method of contraception.

In addition to the preceding changes, during the resolution phase the clitoris returns from under the clitoral hood and the sex flush dissipates. In both males and females, heart rate, blood pressure, and breathing rate return to normal, and muscle tension decreases. Males then experience a **refractory (recovery) period** during which they are incapable of another orgasm. This period may be only several minutes for young males but is usually longer in older males. Females, however, are capable of having **multiple orgasms** before needing to recover.

Each of us, male and female, progresses sequentially through the preceding four phases if we experience orgasm. Clearly, many body processes are involved during sexual activity, and each phase of the response affects the body somewhat differently. Even if we do not reach the orgasmic phase, we may pass through the earlier phases. For example, you may be engaged in sexual stimulation and quickly reach the excitement phase. The plateau stage may occur next, but—just your luck—the telephone rings and your excitement dissapates when you find out a loved one needs your help.

In studying the sexual response cycle in males and females, Masters and Johnson found both startling differences and amazing similarities. Knowing how females and males compare and contrast sexually is important to reinforcing the notion that we all have much in common while still preserving our differences.

If any of these responses is new to you, do not be surprised. You probably do not know everything about your digestive functions or nervous system, for instance, so why would you know everything about your sexual responses without studying them? The next time you are sexually aroused (either physically or by thoughts or fantasies), stop for a moment and attempt to identify the responses just discussed—or reflect now on some past sexual experience. Remember, no two of us are exactly alike. Consequently you may not experience all the sexual responses as we have described them. This is to be expected. Generally, though, you will find that your sexual responses are similar to the ones described.

Figure 6.2 depicts the typical male sexual response according to Masters and Johnson. Males start with the excitement phase, move to the plateau phase, proceed to have an orgasm, and then either move through the resolution phase, in which they return to the pre-aroused state, or to a refractory period (a part of the resolution phase), during which they recover from the orgasm and prepare themselves for another orgasm. Masters and Johnson found this pattern to be standard, although men report variations on this model.

Females were described by Masters and Johnson as being more varied in their sexual responses. Figure 6.2 also shows this variability. Pattern (a) is similar to the male pattern with a progression from excitement to plateau to orgasm and then resolution, except that it depicts a female's ability to have multiple orgasms without a refractory period. Pattern

(a) Phase of Sexual Response Cycle for Males

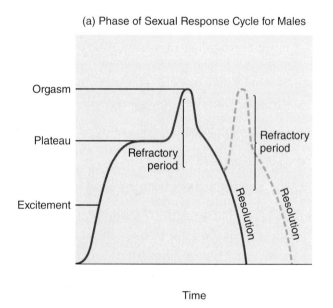

(b) Phase of Sexual Response Cycle for Females

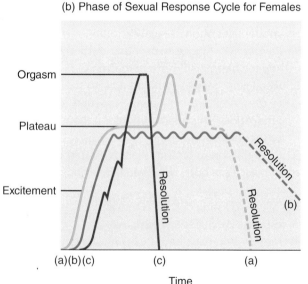

FIGURE 6.2 According to Masters and Johnson, the male sexual response cycle (a) is much more predictable than is the female response cycle (b), and females can have a similar response to males—that is, moving through the four phases and experiencing orgasm—or can maintain the plateau phase without orgasm. Females can also be multiorgasmic without experiencing a refractory period.
Source: Data from Masters, W. H., & Johnson, V. E. *Human sexual response.* Boston: Little Brown, 1966.

(b) shows the woman's progressing from excitement to an enhancement of this excitement during the plateau phase and then moving directly to resolution (bypassing orgasm). This pattern implies that women may be sexually satisfied without experiencing an orgasm. Pattern (c) depicts another possible female sexual response cycle in which there is no definitive plateau phase but a rapid escalation to orgasm and a very quick resolution.

Figures 6.3 and 6.4 summarize changes that occur in males and females during the four phases of the Masters and Johnson sexual response cycle.

Other Theoretical Models of Sexual Response

Other models descriptive of the human sexual response have been proposed. These models are the product of years of experience in sexual counseling and therapy.

Kaplan's Triphasic Model

Originally, the noted sex therapist Helen Singer Kaplan (1974) proposed a biphasic model of the human sexual response. That model conceptualized sexual response as having two identifiable phases. The first phase involved vasocongestion of the genitals, and the second phase consisted of the reflexive muscular contractions of orgasm. Kaplan argued that the two phases were each controlled by a different part of the nervous system: vasocongestion, by the parasympathetic nervous system, and orgasm, by the sympathetic nervous system (both are components of the autonomic nervous system). Furthermore, she explained, different structures are involved in each of these phases: the blood vessels for vasocongestion and the muscles for orgasm. Kaplan gave other justifications for the biphasic model, but space limits our discussion to the justification that derived from Kaplan's observations in her professional practice. Kaplan noted that the interference with vasocongestion resulted in erection problems in the male, whereas different sexual dysfunctions (premature ejaculation and retarded ejaculation) were the result of orgasm impairment. In some females, normal vasocongestion and sexual excitement were experienced in spite of the presence of orgasm problems. Because problems with vasocongestion were quite different from and mutually exclusive with problems with orgasm, Kaplan believed the biphasic model to be valid.

Over the years Kaplan's biphasic model evolved into a triphasic one. Kaplan (1979) now conceptualizes human sexual response as consisting of a **desire phase**, an **excitement phase**, and a **resolution phase**. During her practice as a sex therapist Kaplan had found that sexual dysfunctions fall into one of these three categories and that these categories are separate and distinct (that is, it is possible to function well in one or two phases while having problems in another). The unique component of Kaplan's triphasic model is the desire phase—a psychological prephysical sexual response stage. Masters and Johnson's model ignores this part of the sexual response.

Sexual desire is not always present during sexual activity, however. Sometimes a person may engage in sexual activity to satisfy his or her partner rather than because he or she feels desire. A speaker in one of our sexuality classes described how when his wife complains of some ache or pain (or the proverbial headache) when he is interested in sex, he asks where she feels bothered. When he finds the spot, he gently massages that area, soon turning the massage into a sensual experience. Shortly, he relates, the desire phase is reached.

Zilbergeld and Ellison's Model

Another model of human sexual response consists of five components. The therapists Bernie Zilbergeld and Carol Ellison (1980) were concerned that Masters and Johnson's model ignored the cognitive and subjective aspects of the sexual response, while focusing exclusively on the physiological aspects. They argued that the subjective elements of sexual desire and sexual arousal were omitted from the Masters and Johnson model. *Sexual desire* is defined in this five-component model as the frequency with which a person wants to engage in sexual activity; *sexual arousal* is defined as how excited one becomes during sexual activity. The five components of this model are as follows.

1. Interest, or desire

2. Arousal

3. Physiological readiness (for example, erection or vaginal lubrication)

4. Orgasm

5. Satisfaction (one's evaluation of how one feels)

refractory (recovery) period   The time needed by males for recovery between orgasms.

multiple orgasms   Orgasms that occur without the need for a refractory, or recovery, period.

desire phase   The first stage of the sexual response cycle, as described in Helen Singer Kaplan's model, which consists of psychologically becoming interested in sex before any physical changes occur.

excitement phase   The second stage of Kaplan's model of sexual response, which consists of physiological arousal and changes and, possibly, orgasm.

resolution phase   A stage of the sexual response cycle consisting of a return to the prearoused state.

(a) Unaroused State

Vas deferens
Internal urethral sphincter
Urethral bulb
Urethra
Penis
Testicle
Urethral opening
Scrotum

Bladder
Seminal vesicle
Prostate gland
External urethral sphincter
Anus
Cowper's gland

(b) Excitement Phase

Urethral opening dilates slightly

Partially aroused penis becomes erect

Scrotal skin thickens and tightens

Testicles begin to engorge and move closer to the body

(c) Plateau Phase

Possible Cowper's gland secretions

Glans engorgement

Testicles become engorged and elevated farther

Scrotal skin still is thick and tight

(d) Orgasm Phase: Emission Stage

Contractions of ampulla of vas deferens

Internal urethral sphincter contracts

Urethral bulb expands

External urethral sphincter contracts

Contractions of prostate gland

Contractions of seminal vesicle

(e) Orgasm Phase: Expulsion Stage

Semen expelled

Internal urethral sphincter stays contracted

Contractions of urethra

External urethral sphincter relaxes and opens

Contractions of muscles around base of penis

Contractions of rectal sphincter

(f) Resolution

Rapid partial decrease in size of penis; then slow return to unaroused state and size

Testicles become smaller and move down from the body

Scrotal skin thins and becomes more loose

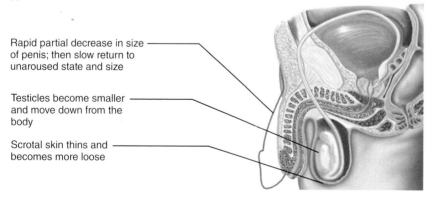

FIGURE **6.3** Male sexual response cycle, in detail.

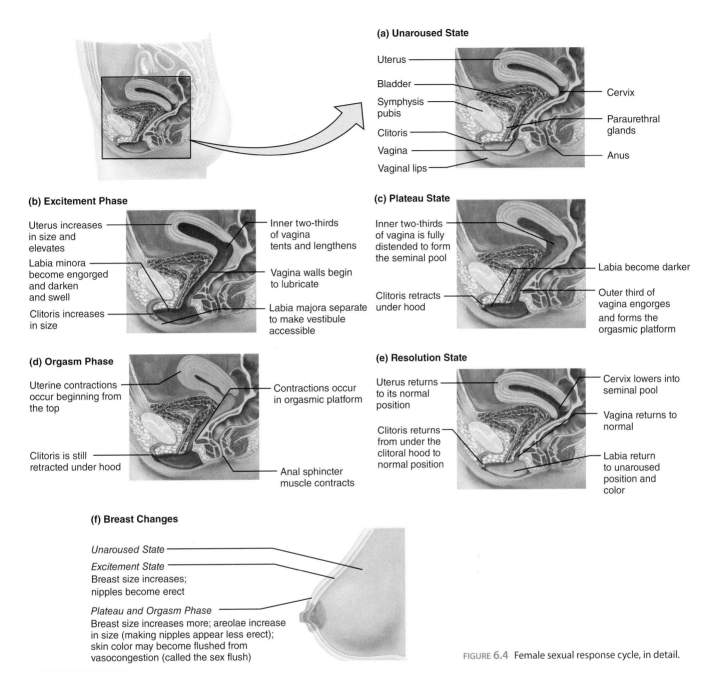

FIGURE 6.4 Female sexual response cycle, in detail.

As with Kaplan's model, Zilbergeld and Ellison's model allows for sexual dysfunctions that pertain to desire although other responses may be normal. Consequently, this component can be isolated from the other components for treatment by a sex therapist. One might describe the triphasic and five-component models as being more inclusive of the psychological aspects of the sexual response, whereas the Masters and Johnson model is more concerned with the physiological aspects.

Walen and Roth's Model
The contribution of Walen and Roth (1987) relates to the inclusion of perception as the beginning of the

sexual response. They argue that without perceiving a potential stimulus as sexually exciting, no sexual response is elicited. Further, they state that a stimulus that is sexually arousing in one situation may not be in another situation. For example, having one's genitals fondled in private may be arousing, but having one's genitals fondled in public may only be embarrassing.

Further, Walen and Roth's model of sexual response includes people evaluating the situation and their response to it to determine if everything is going according to plan. They might evaluate the amount of vaginal lubrication, the presence of penile erection, or heavy breathing. Expecting these to occur and finding that they have occurred validates that the encounter is progressing as expected. The partners can then relax and enjoy the situation, thereby becoming more sexually aroused. However, determining things aren't going as planned can interfere with the sexual response as we try to decide what the problem is and how to solve it. The result might be an inability to have an orgasm, or even to just enjoy the sexual encounter. Recognizing that evaluating one's performance or the situation too critically can interfere with sexual arousal, Walen and Roth advise not placing too high an expectation on performance, not spending too much time observing what is occurring, and relaxing and being fully involved in a manner that will enhance sexual arousal and the enjoyment of the sexual encounter.

Thayton's Model

Wiliam Thayton (2002) is a Baptist minister, and the model of sexual arousal he developed, understandably, has a spiritual and theological perspective. Thayton acknowledges that sex is pleasurable. He proposes that God intended for humans to respond to sex with pleasure and to enjoy the blessing of sexual arousal. Thayton offers evidence of this view by stating that Jesus never preached that sexual pleasure was sinful or to be avoided, in spite of advocating self-denial in other areas of life. Therefore, Thayton concludes that spirituality, sexuality, and love are bound together in God's creation of people who are sexual by nature. As a result, when one is sexual, one is also spiritual. However, love is an important component in this mix for Thayton. Love is the glue that binds sexuality, spirituality, and pleasure. After all, he argues, love allows us to be one with the universe and what is more spiritual than that?

Lastly, Thayton considers sex researchers as sexual guides, just as clergy and theologians are spiritual and religious guides. They all study their area of expertise to understand it better, and then communicate their findings and recommendations to the public at large.

Basson's Model

Basson (2000) is a sex therapist and, as such, her model of sexual response stems from her experience in treating sexual disorders. Basson has no argument with the models offered by Masters and Johnson or Kaplan. However, like Walen and Roth, she believes that how one perceives and interprets a situation is an important component of sexual response. Basson states that feeling positive toward one's partner is necessary for sexual arousal to occur. If one hates one's partner or doesn't trust one's partner, sexual arousal will not occur.

Basson also believes there is a difference in sexual response between males and females. In females, she argues, emotions and intimacy are important precursors of sexual response. Whereas sexual response begins with desire or arousal in males, Basson believes it begins with intimacy in females. In other words, women desire being close to their partners, whereas men desire a physical release of sexual tension. Once women feel intimate toward their partners, desire and arousal are then possible. In fact, Basson believes that intimacy leads to arousal, which in turn leads to desire. Desire creates greater intimacy, which then results in even more arousal and desire. All along the way, though, there are interpretations and evaluations of what is occurring, similar to the recognition of perceptions in the Walen and Roth model. These interpretations and evaluations affect intimacy, arousal, and desire.

Orgasm is a possible result of this cycle, but not a necessary one for women to feel sexually satisfied, which is the key for Basson. Some people may experience orgasm but not feel the sexual encounter was satisfying. Others may not experience orgasm but feel the encounter was extremely satisfying. Basson believes that should be the goal of the encounter—being satisfied, not orgasm.

Erotic Stimulus Pathway

An important contribution to our knowledge of sexual response is that of the Erotic Stimulus Pathway (ESP) theory of David M. Reed (Haffner & Stayton, 1998). The ESP theory enhances our understanding and ability to treat sexual dysfunctions. Reed divides the sexual response cycle into four phases that correspond to those of Kaplan and Masters and Johnson. For many people, these phases are learned developmentally. Figure 6.5 compares the Masters and Johnson model with the Reed model.

In the *seduction phase* a person learns how to get aroused sexually and how to attract someone else sexually. Seduction translates into memories and rituals. For example, adolescents may spend much time on personal appearance, choice of clothes, and mannerisms, all of which can enhance positive self-esteem if the adolescents like the way they feel. If the adolescents feel good about the way they look and feel, then attracting another person will be much easier. As the adolescents get older, these positive feelings are translated into sexual desire and arousal. These seductive techniques are stored in memory and can be activated later on in life.

In the *sensations phase*, the different senses can enhance sexual excitement and ideally prolong the plateau phase. The early experiences of touch (holding hands, putting arms around a loved one) become very important. The sense of vision (staring at a loved one, holding an image of him or her when absent)

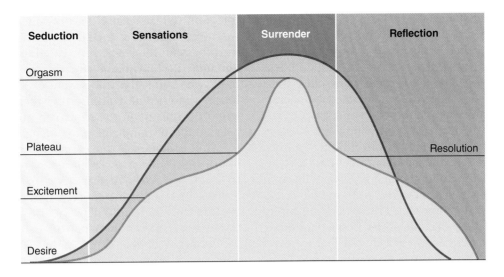

FIGURE 6.5 Sexual response curve.
Source: Data from Masters, W. H., & Johnson, V. E. *Human sexual response.* Boston: Little Brown, 1966; Kaplan, H. S. *Disorders of sexual desire.* New York: Simon & Schuster, 1979.

Many senses can evoke a sexual response. The soft touch, kiss, sight, or smell of a partner can be quite sexually stimulating.

is a way of maintaining interest and arousal. Hearing the loved one in intimate conversation or over the telephone becomes very important. Hearing the sounds of a partner responding to sexual stimulation can be titillating. The smell of the loved one, either a particular scent he or she wears or the sexual smell, produces additional excitement. Finally, the taste of a food or drink or the taste of the loved one becomes important to memory and fantasy. All these senses extend the excitement into a plateau phase, which makes one want to continue the pleasurable moment over a longer period. These seduction and sensation experiences are the psychological input to the physiology of sexual response. They are the precursors to sexual climax and orgasm.

In the *surrender phase*, orgasm is a "psycho-physiological surprise." The psychodynamic issues surrounding orgasm are power and control. Persons with orgasmic dysfunction may be in a power struggle with themselves or with their partners or with the messages received about sex. Overcontrol or undercontrol can affect orgasmic potential and the ability to allow all of the passion to be expressed.

In the *reflection phase*, meaning is given to the experience. Whether the sexual experience is interpreted as positive or negative may determine the desire for subsequent sexual activity—at least with that sexual partner, under those circumstances, or with those behaviors. Recognize, though, that not every sexual experience can be, or should be, a "10." As the authors have heard it expressed, "Sometimes sex is a four-course gourmet meal, and sometimes it's like having cereal for dinner. Most of the time it's like having hamburgers or chicken. When it's cereal, you have to remember that there are better times ahead."

Aphrodisiacs: Seeking the Ultimate in Sexual Pleasure

An *aphrodisiac*, named after the Greek goddess Aphrodite, the goddess of love, is any substance that arouses sexual desire and/or enhances sexual response. For centuries people have searched for a safe and effective aphrodisiac without much luck. This search has led to "Spanish fly" (*cantharidin*), which results in irritation of the urinary tract. Now, is that sexually arousing? It has led to substances to make one "horny," such as ground-up rhinoceros horns or elephant tusks, which just do not work. Oysters, clams, and even the testicles of bulls ("prairie oysters") have been tried without the desired effect.

Even toxic substances have been ingested in the hope of enhancing sexual desire and response; *amyl nitrate* is one of these substances. Amyl nitrate is designed for use by heart patients to reduce chest pain. Its container is "popped" open when chest pain occurs; thus the containers are often called "poppers." Amyl nitrate became popular among some gay men as an aphrodisiac because it facilitated anal intercourse by relaxing the anal sphincter muscle. Although it does dilate blood vessels in the brain and genitals, resulting in warmth in the abdomen and pelvis, facilitating erection, and possibly prolonging orgasm, it is also associated with disturbing side effects. For example, amyl nitrate can cause dizziness, headaches, and fainting, and can even result in death in extreme cases.

Bupropion (acquired under the brand name Wellbutrin) and L-dopa are other substances that have been ingested for their aphrodisiac effects. Bupropion is an antidepressant drug, and L-dopa is a drug used for treating patients with Parkinson's disease. Both of these drugs act on the brain receptors that produce dopamine and so can increase libido. However, unsupervised use of a drug that affects the brain is dangerous; it must be monitored by a physician and prescribed for a specific medical purpose.

Alcohol and *marijuana* have also been ascribed aphrodisiaclike qualities. However, if they work at all, they diminish judgment and make people feel less stress about sex. That may be good, or that may be bad. A decrease in inhibitions may result in high-risk sexual behaviors (such as vaginal or anal intercourse without a condom) that may transmit a sexually transmitted

infection (STI) or cause an unwanted pregnancy. Furthermore, alcohol is a central nervous system depressant that can interfere with sexual arousal rather than enhance it. Marijuana can distort perceptions and make one think that the sexual experience continued longer than it really did. Both of these substances can lead to problems in the short run and over prolonged use; in addition, marijuana is illegal in most states.

One substance that appears to have potential as an aphrodisiac is *yohimbine hydrochloride*, from the sap of a West African tree, the yohimbine tree. Yohimbine has been reported to aid some men with erectile dysfunction to achieve and maintain an erection for a long-enough period to engage in sexual intercourse (Senbel & Mostafa, 2008). However, it does not work for all men with erectile dysfunction, and whether it enhances the sexual response of other men is unknown.

Even drugs that inhibit sexual desire have been the focus of researchers for many years. These drugs are called *anaphrodisiacs*. For years, rumor has had it that one of these substances, *potassium nitrate*, known as *saltpeter*, is used by the military to diminish the sexual desire of soldiers and is used in summer camps to control the "raging urges" of teenagers. However, all that potassium nitrate does is increase the need to urinate; some people obviously think that is enough to interfere with sex.

Yet some drugs do interfere with sexual response. These tend to be central nervous system depressants such as opiates (for example, heroin), tranquilizers, antihypertensive medications, antipsychotic and antidepressant drugs (such as Prozac), and, surprisingly to many people, nicotine, which constricts blood vessels and decreases vasocongestion in the genitals.

■ Orgasm

Our nonsexual lives tend to be goal oriented. We may have goals to graduate from college, to become established in a good career, or to live in a large house. It should be no surprise that goal orientation has invaded our sexual lives as well. For too many of us, orgasm becomes the goal of almost all of our sexual behavior. We forget about the pleasure that can be derived from sexual activity that does not lead to orgasm, and we forget that the communication and the quality of our relationships can be enhanced through sexual activity that does not result in orgasm. The question "Did you come?" tends to be as much a part of the sexual experience as removing one's clothes.

Orgasmic Sensation

The feelings that accompany orgasm are quite different from the physiological responses and may even

Yohimbine hydrochloride is the one substance that may act as an aphrodisiac. Most other substances thought to have aphrodisiac effects actually do not.

Global
DIMENSIONS

Aphrodisiacs and Tigers: A Strange Mix

Some of the most expensive aphrodisiacs in the world are made from parts of male tigers. The most prized and valuable aphrodisiacs are made from the tiger's penis—often made into a soup! Less expensive "love potions" are made from everything else down to the tiger's crushed bone. Such aphrodisiacs are extremely popular, predominantly in Asian countries.

The net result is that the last several thousand of the world's tigers are endangered—and all for naught.

As with many other aphrodisiacs, no physiological sexual response results from ingesting tiger parts.

Do you think that such an "aphrodisiac" might have positive psychological effects in countries where there is a long-standing cultural belief that it works? Might the ability to pay lots of money for such an aphrodisiac have a psychological boosting effect? What would you say to a friend who told you that parts from the tiger's penis could be a great aphrodisiac? Explain your answers.

©dptro/Shutterstock

contradict what we know is occurring physiologically. For example, women may experience a physiologically intense orgasm (a dozen or so measurable muscular contractions) but report the orgasm to be of mild intensity, or they may experience a mild orgasm physiologically (four muscular contractions) but report the sensation of an intense orgasm. The reason for this discrepancy lies in the understanding that sexual experience is interpreted by the mind as well as the body. When the relationship is a healthy one, sexual partners may experience a great deal of pleasure from a mild orgasm because the experience was shared and made them feel closer. Other factors such as mood, expectations, and the setting can also affect one's subjective judgment regarding the intensity of the orgasm.

Generally, sensations from orgasms are experienced similarly by males and females, but there are exceptions (Fogel, 2014; Silverberg, 2008). In women, there is a highly pleasurable feeling that usually begins

at the clitoris but quickly spreads to the whole pelvic area. The genitals often feel warm and tingly, and then a sensation of throbbing in the lower pelvis may be noticed. In men, the experience is also highly pleasurable. They usually experience warmth, pressure, and sometimes a throbbing during the moment when they have reached the "point of no return" (that is, ejaculatory inevitability), at which point men cannot prevent ejaculation. In many men, ejaculation itself is experienced as a sensation of pumping.

The similarity of male and female orgasms was vividly demonstrated many years ago by two studies involving college students (Proctor, Wagner, & Butler, 1974; Wiest, 1977). In these studies, students wrote descriptions of their orgasms, and these descriptions were analyzed by a group of experts. The experts could not distinguish between the male and female descriptions, and the researchers concluded that males and females experience similar sensations as a result of orgasm. Although males and females do

Researchers (Rubenstein, 1991) asked 5,000 readers of *American Health* magazine, admittedly a biased sample, what they might do to feel more sexually attractive and to respond better sexually. Just over half the women (58%) and almost half the men (49%) surveyed said they would be willing to exercise 1 hour a day to be better lovers, but relatively few of either the women (9%) or the men (12%) would take an aphrodisiac. To enhance their sexual response, 61% of the women and 55% of the men listened to music while engaged in sexual intercourse at some time during the month before the survey, and 19% of the women and 23% of the men watched an X-rated videotape during coitus. What

was surprising is that 38% of the women and 34% of the men watched television during intercourse.

In a study of 1,000 readers of *Women's Health* magazine (Kylstra, 2014), 57% of women said that during sex they are wondering if their partner was enjoying it—enjoying her, really. Although men often worry about what women think during sexual intercourse, only 4% of women are critical of their partners' penis size, only 12% are critical of the sounds their partners make, and only 11% object to their partners' facial expressions during sex.

Source: Kylstra, C. Her secret sex thoughts. *MH Lists*, 2014. Available: http://www.menshealth.com/mhlists/secret-sex-thoughts/index.php.

not generally differ in the sensations they report accompanying orgasm, orgasms *do* differ. That is, an individual may experience an orgasm today that is either more or less intense than one yesterday, and one person may experience orgasms generally more intensely than another person. These differences are not a function of gender; rather, a less pleasurable experience may be a result of guilt, shame, embarrassment, an uncomfortable setting, frustrations with the sexual partner, hostility, distrust, low self-esteem, or other factors.

Controversies About Orgasm

Several controversies surround the topic of orgasm.

Types of Orgasm

First, experts disagree about the types of orgasms that exist. In the early 1900s, Freud theorized there were two different types of female orgasm: the clitoral and the vaginal. He viewed the clitoral orgasm as an immature sexual response that women outgrew. Because he considered the clitoris to be a stunted penis, Freud believed the clitoral orgasm was an expression of masculine sexuality rather than feminine sexuality. If at adolescence the woman had not transferred her erotic focus from the clitoris to the vagina, Freud believed

that psychotherapy was in order. When Freud's theory was operationalized, surgical removal of the clitoris (**clitoridectomy**) was actually performed on girls who were too clitorally focused, as determined by their masturbating by stimulating the clitoris.

Masters and Johnson's (1966) research identified but one type of orgasm. Regardless of the point of stimulation—clitoris or vagina—and regardless of the method of stimulation—penile insertion or vibrator—Masters and Johnson reported the same physiological occurrences during orgasm. However, Masters and Johnson did report a difference in the sensations of orgasm that depended on whether they were a result of coital or noncoital activities. They found orgasms from coitus to be less intense than orgasms from noncoital means. This finding was validated by Hite (1976), who found the clitorally stimulated orgasm to be more intense than the orgasm from coitus. Hite also found the coital orgasm to be more diffused throughout the body than was the locally intense clitoral orgasm.

To complicate matters further, other researchers (Singer & Singer, 1972) have reported three distinct types of orgasms: vulval, uterine, and blended. Singer and Singer included emotional satisfaction as a consideration in their research. **Vulval orgasm** is the same as the orgasm described by Masters and Johnson and includes contractions of the orgasmic platform; however, the vulval orgasm is not sexually satiating, and therefore another orgasm can be experienced immediately. A **uterine orgasm** can occur only in the presence of vaginal penetration and involves a woman's holding her breath just before orgasm and then exhaling when the climax occurs. In contrast to the vulval orgasm, the uterine orgasm is sexually satiating and is therefore usually followed by

clitoridectomy Surgical removal of the clitoris.

vulval orgasm An orgasm in a female that includes the contractions of the orgasmic platform, which is not sexually satisfying and, as a result, allows another orgasm to occur almost immediately.

uterine orgasm An orgasm in a female that can occur only in the presence of penile penetration and that involves a woman's holding her breath just before orgasm and then exhaling when the climax occurs.

Communication
DIMENSIONS

Discussing Sexual Desires

Communicating sexual desires is embarrassing for many people. After all, sex is not something we are taught to talk about openly. The irony for many of us is that we are taught at a very young age that sex is so "dirty" that we should save it for someone we love. Does not make much sense, does it? Of course, sex is not dirty, although it may make sense to refrain from certain sexual activities altogether and to engage in others only when you are ready. When the time is right, if we could share what we find sexually arousing with a partner, we would be that much more satisfied. To help you along in this process, we have prepared the following guidelines. We recognize, though, that not all of you have chosen to engage in sexual activities with a partner. Still, these guidelines will be useful if and when you decide the time is right for you to do so.

- Speak about what you like sexually at times in which you are not engaged in sexual activity. This allows for a conversation that can be more rational than one carried on while emotions are running high.
- Be specific. State what you like and how you like it, what you dislike and why you dislike it.
- Ask your partner to do the same. Let your partner know that you want to please him or her as well as yourself. If your partner realizes you are concerned

about his or her pleasure, he or she will be more likely to be concerned about your pleasure.
- During sex, let your partner know how you feel about what he or she is doing. Reinforce the behaviors you like by letting him or her know they are pleasing.
- Do not hesitate to refrain from any sexual activity you find unpleasant, uncomfortable, or distasteful. When doing so, explain your reasons to your partner.

Remember, you can have a more satisfying sexual relationship, when you are ready to do so, by being able to communicate freely about sex and what you find pleasurable and what you find displeasing.

a refractory period. The **blended orgasm** is a combination of these two; that is, there are contractions of the outer third of the vagina as well as breath holding. These researchers make it clear that no one form of orgasm is better than another, just different.

How many forms of orgasm are there? As with other areas of human sexuality, there is disagreement. The important point is that orgasm can be conceptualized as merely a physiological reaction to sexual stimulation or as a complex of interactions between partners (the setting, the mood, and a host of other variables). To consider an orgasm as solely a bodily reaction is to ignore the interactive nature of the human mind and the human body and the impossibility of separating them. Without a mind to realize that sexual stimulation is, in fact, stimulating, there is no orgasm.

Recognizing Orgasms
At the beginning of the sexuality classes we teach, we ask students to write questions they would like

answered before the semester ends. A common question asks how a man can recognize when his female partner is faking an orgasm. The women in the class are astute enough to know that when their male partners ejaculate, they experience orgasm. What they do not usually know is that sometimes orgasm can occur without an ejaculate—for example, in men with disease of the prostate or in prepubescent boys. Men, however, want to know how to recognize that their partners are sexually satisfied. In a recent study of young adult males and females (Salisbury & Fisher, 2014), participants agreed that men have the physical responsibility to stimulate their female partner to orgasm, while women have the psychological responsibility of being mentally prepared to

blended orgasm An orgasm in a female in which there are contractions of the muscles in the outer third of the vagina as well as breath holding; a combination of the vulval and uterine orgasms.

Myth vs Fact

Myth: It is easy to tell when a male has an orgasm because the ejaculate gives it away.

Fact: Although it is usually true that a male will ejaculate during orgasm, this is not always the case. Males may have an orgasm without ejaculating.

Myth: During the plateau phase of the Masters and Johnson sexual response cycle, conditions remain pretty much the same.

Fact: Although Masters and Johnson chose to call the second phase of the sexual response cycle the *plateau phase*, changes do occur. What occurred during the excitement phase is intensified during the plateau phase.

Myth: Whereas women can be multiorgasmic, men cannot.

Fact: Although it occurs relatively infrequently, some men do report needing very little time before being able to have another orgasm.

Myth: Males and females differ tremendously in their responses to sexual excitation.

Fact: There certainly are many differences between males and females in their responses to sexual excitement. Still, there are many similarities as well.

Myth: The clitoris can be stimulated easily during sexual intercourse.

Fact: Relatively early in the sexual response of women, the clitoris retracts under the clitoral hood. Therefore, it is not easily accessible to touch and/or stimulation unless the clitoral hood is purposefully pulled back.

experience the orgasm—and hence the question, "Did you come?"

This question has several implications that deserve some attention. First, it expresses a concern for the woman's sexual satisfaction. On the surface, that appears to be healthy; however, it is our experience that when asked by men, this question is more related to a man's ego than to a woman's satisfaction. That is, if the male can "give" the woman an orgasm, he must be a good lover. Another interpretation of this question could be that men are afraid their female sexual partners might fake orgasms. A woman may fake an orgasm to meet her partner's expectation, to feed her partner's ego, to end the sexual encounter, to present herself as "normal," or to meet the "goal."

Beyond the fact that faking an orgasm is dishonest and deceitful, it may lead your partner to think that something unsatisfying to you was great and should be repeated the next time. However, if what a partner does is pleasurable but does not result in a climax, that might be enough. If so, why not tell your partner? Sexual activity can be enjoyed for itself without being directed toward the goal of orgasm.

Men are also prone to faking orgasms if they are unable to achieve one. When a man has been drinking alcoholic beverages, for example, and cannot reach the orgasmic phase, he might feel threatened

Ethical DIMENSIONS

Should Sexual Enhancements Be Used to Increase Sexual Arousal?

How far should people be allowed, or encouraged, to go in their search for sexual satisfaction and sexual arousal? Some people argue that anything that does not negatively affect another person is appropriate to enhance sexual arousal. They believe the use of X-rated videos, sexually explicit written material, and erotic clothing is within the bounds of acceptability. They also suggest that engaging in sexual relations with a number of different people can provide the experience necessary to reach one's sexual potential. Further, any physical barriers to sexual arousal should be eliminated at any cost. So if a man has blockage of the penile arteries, he should undergo bypass surgery to provide the penis with the blood it needs to become erect. And if there is damage to the penis as a result of an accident, options should include Viagra, artificial penises, surgery to implant rods in the penis to provide an erection, or penis transplantation

(from someone who has recently died—similar to heart, kidney, and other organ transplantation).

Others believe that enhancing sexual arousal is appropriate, but only within certain limits. They argue that sexually explicit material is pornographic and/or obscene. Its use is unacceptable for any reason, and it should be outlawed. Furthermore, altering the body "merely" for sexual purposes goes against nature, is therefore "unnatural," and should not be tolerated. Sexual arousal should be enhanced through improving the relationship between the couple, and that can be accomplished only in a marriage, and one in which the spouses remain sexually faithful to each other. Only then, advocates of this view argue, can the couple engage in "lovemaking" as opposed to "sex-making," because sex without love can never achieve the level of arousal that sex with love can.

What do you think? What is appropriate and what is inappropriate when trying to enhance sexual arousal?

by how this may be interpreted by his partner. Will his partner think he is less than a real man? Will his partner think he is sexually dysfunctional? Will his partner think he does not find him or her sexually attractive? Some men believe it is easier to fake an orgasm than to allay these fears.

Whether a man or woman fakes orgasm regularly, the person would be well advised to discuss the situation candidly with his or her partner. Such a discussion can often result in a closer relationship and the understanding that setting up sexual performance goals is self-defeating. Some women do not reach orgasm, some have an orgasm once during intercourse, and some are multiorgasmic. Some men do not reach orgasm, some have an orgasm once during intercourse, and some are multiorgasmic (although some recovery time between orgasms is necessary). For people of either gender who do not reach orgasm, pleasure from coitus can still

be attained. Rather than asking, "Did you come?" we should ask, "What did I do that you liked?" "How can I pleasure you more?" "How can we feel more intimate?" "How can we improve our relationship?"

Simultaneous Orgasm

Another question students often ask is how they and their partners can achieve an orgasm together. Unfortunately, some couples have as an ideal a choreographed orgasmic release, timed so that it occurs at the same time for both partners. Not only is this difficult to achieve, but concentrating on this goal detracts from the enjoyment of the coital experience. As long as each person is satisfied, the exact timing of the orgasm is of no particular importance. Although simultaneous orgasm is an undeniably exciting event, it is only one of a wide range of satisfying sexual patterns.

DIMENSIONS

Age of First Intercourse

The average age at first sexual intercourse varies considerably by country (see the table below), as does the percentage of people reporting unprotected sex. Given that the World Health Organization reports more than 1 million people acquire a sexually transmitted infection every day, that each year an estimated 500 million people become ill with one of four STIs (chlamydia, gonorrhea, syphilis, and trichomoniasis), that more than 530 million people have the virus that causes genital herpes (HSV2), and that more than 290 million women have a human papillomavirus (HPV) infection, the statistics on average age at first intercourse and the percentage of people engaging in unprotected sex are alarming (World Health Organization, 2015).

Average Age at First Sexual Intercourse

Country	Age	Country	Age	Country	Age
Malaysia	23.0	Taiwan	18.9	Croatia	17.3
India	22.9	Switzerland	18.2	Austria	17.3
Singapore	22.8	Canada	18.1	Czech Republic	17.2
China	22.1	Netherlands	18.1	Chile	17.2
Thailand	20.5	Greece	18.1	Belgium	17.2
Hong Kong	20.2	United States	18.0	Portugal	16.9
Vietnam	19.7	Australia	17.9	Bulgaria	16.9
Nigeria	19.7	Turkey	17.8	Israel	16.7
Japan	19.4	New Zealand	17.8	Finland	16.5
Spain	19.2	Slovakia	17.8	Norway	16.5
Indonesia	19.1	Germany	17.6	Sweden	16.2
Poland	19.0	Brazil	17.4	Denmark	16.1
Italy	18.9	Ireland	17.3	Iceland	15.6

Source: Average age at first sex by country. *ChartsBin*, 2015. Available: http://chartsbin.com/view/xxj.

(continues)

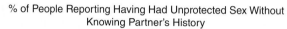

DIMENSIONS

Age of First Intercourse (continued)

Alarmingly, a large percentage of people around the world are engaging in unprotected sexual intercourse even though they do not know their partners' sexual histories. Not surprisingly, the countries with the highest percentages of unprotected sexual intercourse experience the highest percentage of STIs.

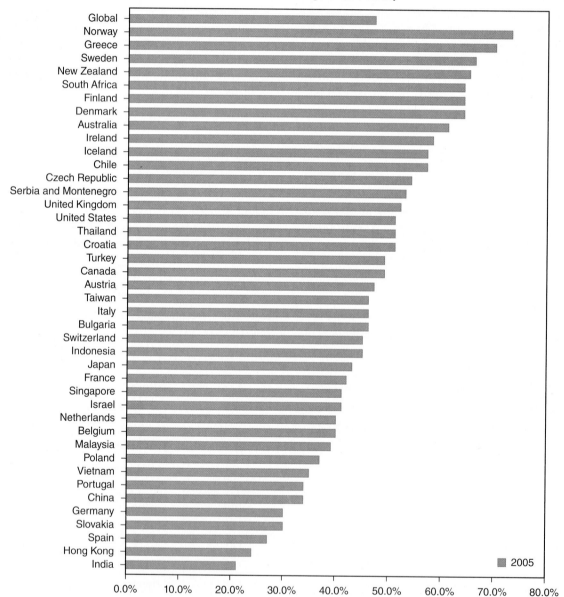

% of People Reporting Having Had Unprotected Sex Without Knowing Partner's History

Source: Data from Data360.org. 2005. Available at: http://www.data360.org/dsg.aspx?Data_Set_Group_Id=1101

Did You Know . . .

An ancient Indian philosophy rebelled against the tenets of organized religion that restricted sexual practices. *Tantra* taught that sexuality was a doorway to the divine and that earthly pleasures were sacred acts. Becoming more popular in Western culture, *tantric sex* seeks to teach means of pleasuring one's lover and connecting with him or her fully, rather than simply to achieve an orgasm. It is seen as a dance with no beginning or end, and the goal is to be in the present moment. One of the outcomes of tantric sex, however, is to extend orgasm and to enjoy multiple orgasms. Among the tantric sex techniques are these (Painter, 2009; Peterson, 2010; Tantra Tantric Sex, 2012; WEWOMEN, 2013):

• Create an inviting atmosphere. Light candles, have flowers strewn around, and use scent such as jasmine, ylang-ylang, or rose.

• Sync with your partner by harmonizing your breathing. Straddle your partner's lap (called the yab-yom position) and inhale while your partner exhales, and vice versa.

• Take it slowly and let the erotic tension build. This can be done by touching, bathing, or bodily contact.

• Maintain a deep level of intimacy by intently and purposefully looking into your partner's eyes for several minutes.

• Use erotic and sensual touch and other means to stimulate the senses. This can include blindfolding and then using a variety of sensory stimulants: cinnamon or vanilla for smell; music or reading a love poem for sound; feeding berries, chocolate, or honey licked off a finger for taste; and caressing the body with silk, feathers, or rose petals for touch.

• Using a variety of sexual positions that stimulate the clitoris and the G-spot (called the "sacred spot" in tantra).

©Karen Moskowitz/Getty Images

Did You Know . . .

Did you know that women who experience vaginal orgasms can be identified by how they walk? When women were videotaped walking on the street, trained sexologists were 85% accurate in judging whether they were vaginally orgasmic or anorgasmic (Nicholas et al., 2008). They were not, however, able to identify women who were clitorally orgasmic. The observational keys were greater pelvic and vertebral rotation and stride length. In addition, vaginally orgasmic women's gaits were fluid, energetic, sensual, free, and absent of locked muscles.

Exploring the Dimensions of Human Sexuality

Although the human sexual response cycle is a physiological pattern, many factors influence the ways individuals actually experience the stages. Physical differences, including age, illness, injuries, and disabilities, may alter the response. Illicit drugs, alcohol, and aphrodisiacs also may alter the physical sensation we experience. Some drugs, such as Viagra, may enhance the response cycle.

The stimuli that we react to differ with culture and ethnic group, media exposure, even hygiene. Education and religious beliefs may also have an effect; a person who feels guilty about sexuality may have a more repressed reaction.

Finally, our self-image and our feelings about our partner greatly influence sexual response and arousal. Many people believe that happy times—experiencing a loving relationship, being successful professionally, and so on—make for better sex.

Biological Factors

- Sexual arousal and response are physiological reactions to sexual stimuli.
- Masters and Johnson showed that some aspects of the human sexual response cycle are similar in men and women; however, differences exist.
- The body releases hormones when a person is sexually stimulated.
- Physical disabilities, injuries, or illness may alter the ability to respond to sexual stimuli.
- Male testosterone levels decline with age, affecting sexual response.
- Drugs, alcohol, and some aphrodisiacs may alter sexual response.

Sociocultural Factors

- Biological factors are influenced by sociocultural and psychological factors. For example, some people are turned on by pornography; others are turned off.
- Religious beliefs influence our feelings about sexuality in general.
- Culture and ethnic heritage influence what we find sensual or attractive.
- Media and ads influence the types of sexual stimulation to which we react.
- Family, neighbors, and friends provide information about and influence our sexuality.
- Ethical decisions must be made regarding how far you and your partner are willing to go to achieve sexual arousal.

Psychological Factors

- Our feelings toward our partner influence the sexual response derived.
- Our level of experience influences our response to sexual stimuli.
- Learned attitudes and behaviors include discovering the stimuli to which we respond.
- Body image influences our self-concept. The better we feel about ourselves, the sexier an image we portray to others.

Summary

- When a sexual stimulus is encountered, a message is sent via nerves to the brain. Upon reaching the brain, the message passes through the reticular activating system either from or to the limbic system and the thalamus.

- During sexual arousal, the autonomic nervous system is responsible for sending signals through nerves that result in blood vessels in the penis and clitoris dilating. The effect of the dilation is that these structures become engorged with blood and, consequently, become erect.

- Sexual hormones are produced in the testes and ovaries and affect many different sexually related functions. For example, testosterone affects sexual interest, also known as libido.

- Masters and Johnson described the human sexual response cycle as consisting of four phases: excitement, plateau, orgasm, and resolution. Kaplan described the human sexual response cycle as being triphasic: desire, excitement, and resolution.

- The female sexual response cycle is more varied than the male sexual response cycle. Females sometimes experience a sexual response cycle similar to males except they are more capable of having multiple orgasms without having to pass through a refractory period. In addition, females can move from the excitement phase to the plateau phase and, without having an orgasm, return to resolution; they can also experience rapid escalation from excitement to orgasm without passing through a plateau phase.

- Orgasm is the release of sexual tension resulting in muscular contractions and, at least in males, ejaculation. In most males, orgasm is followed by a refractory (recovery) period in which orgasm is not possible. In many females, orgasm can occur without a refractory period.

- Orgasm in females is preceded by the uterus increasing in size and elevating, the inner two-thirds of the vagina lengthening and expanding, lubrication of the vaginal walls, engorgement of blood in the outer third of the vagina, and retraction of the clitoris under the clitoral hood.

- In males, orgasm is a two-stage process: emission and expulsion. Emission involves contractions of the vas deferens, seminal vesicles, prostate, and external and internal urethral sphincters. Expulsion consists of relaxation of the external urethral sphincter, contractions of the urethra and muscles at the base of the penis and the anus, and the expulsion of the ejaculate from the penis.

Discussion Questions

1. Describe the reaction of the mind and the body when one is aroused by a sensual stimulation. How might artificial hormones or aphrodisiacs alter the response cycle? How would alcohol or other mood-altering drugs affect the cycle?

2. Compare and contrast the Masters and Johnson human response cycle with the models proposed by Kaplan, Zilbergeld and Ellison, and Reed. Why does the Masters and Johnson model continue to attract the most attention?

3. Explain how understanding types of orgasms and recognizing orgasms could lead to a better sexual relationship.

Application Questions

Reread the story that opens the chapter and answer the following questions.

1. Assuming that Brian and Tanya start dating, which visible signs of sexual arousal (aside from erection) might Tanya detect in Brian? Which signs might Brian detect in Tanya?

2. Do you think Brian's feelings about Tanya might differ if he met her after gym class and she reeked of sweat? Explain.

Critical Thinking Questions

1. Laurie Cabot, a well-known practicing witch, often suggests that love potions or spells do work. She writes that a "spell is a thought, a projection, or a prayer." Thus Cabot implies that the psychological effort that you put into a spell can produce a physiological response. Given this idea, would a love potion work? Put another way, would the extra attention you lavish on someone make that person more attracted to you?

2. The drugs Viagra and Cialis positively affect sexual response, especially in older men. However, increased sexual response is accompanied by higher blood pressure and a faster heartbeat—which has resulted in heart attacks and some deaths. Explain why 30 million U.S. males have been willing to take this risk, albeit a small one. Also consider why their partners would want them to risk their health for sexual pleasure.

3. Sexy soap operas are some of the most-viewed TV shows in the world, with more than 1 billion viewers per week. Apply what you learned in the chapter to explain why.

Critical Thinking Case

It has been argued that too much emphasis is placed on orgasm and not enough on the total sexual experience, including talking and nongenital touch. Because sexual intercourse is a way of expressing love for another, the argument proceeds, the emphasis during the experience should be on the total relationship, the love expressed, whole-body sensations, and the feeling of closeness. Concentrating exclusively or primarily on the orgasm is self-defeating and narrows one's experience of sexuality.

In contrast, some people believe that sexual intercourse (or mutual masturbation or oral–genital sex) certainly includes all of the above but, in addition, has a culmination—orgasm. This culmination is so satisfying and, given effective sexual therapy, so available that it should be sought. Although sexual intercourse and other modes of sexual expression can be satisfying without orgasm, an orgasmic conclusion certainly adds to the experience and satisfaction.

What do you think? Why?

Exploring Personal Dimensions

Sexual Stimuli

Once the senses encounter sexual stimuli, the brain takes over, deciding how to respond. You become sexually aroused, although you may decide, for many reasons, not to act on that sexual arousal. Which of the following sexual stimuli do you find arousing? If you have a partner, which does your partner find arousing? More importantly, with which stimuli do you share sexual arousal?

What other sexual stimuli can you think of?

SIGHT	YOU		YOUR PARTNER	
Sexually explicit movies	Y	N	Y	N
Sexually explicit magazines	Y	N	Y	N
Romantic movies	Y	N	Y	N
Books	Y	N	Y	N
Lingerie	Y	N	Y	N
Skin	Y	N	Y	N
TOUCH				
Satin sheets	Y	N	Y	N
Leather	Y	N	Y	N
Massage	Y	N	Y	N
Scratching	Y	N	Y	N
SMELL				
Perfume (or cologne)	Y	N	Y	N
Flowers	Y	N	Y	N
Scented candles	Y	N	Y	N
TASTE				
Kissing	Y	N	Y	N
Oral sexual activities	Y	N	Y	N
Whipped cream	Y	N	Y	N
SOUND				
Whispering	Y	N	Y	N
Moaning (or groaning)	Y	N	Y	N
Music	Y	N	Y	N
Silence	Y	N	Y	N

Suggested Readings

Berman, L. *Loving sex: The book of joy and passion.* New York: DK Publishing, 2011.

Bodansky, V. *To bed or not to bed: What men want, what women want, how great sex happens.* Alameda, CA: Hunter House, 2005.

Clunis, M., & Green, D. *Lesbian couples: A guide to creating healthy relationships.* Berkeley, CA: Seal Press, 2004.

Corwin, G. *Sexual intimacy for women: A guide for same-sex couples.* Berkeley, CA: Seal Press, 2010.

Guerrero, L. K., Andersen, P. A., & Afifi, W. A. *Close encounters: Communication in relationships.* Thousand Oaks, CA: Sage, 2013.

Hathaway, C. *Erotic massage: Sensual touch for deep pleasure and extended arousal.* Chanhassen, MN: Quiver, 2007.

Herbenick, D. *Because it feels good: A woman's guide to sexual pleasure and satisfaction.* Emmaus, PA: Rodale Books, 2009.

Kerner, I. Passionista: *The empowered woman's guide to pleasuring a man.* New York: HarperCollins, 2013.

Kerner, I. *She comes first: The thinking man's guide to pleasuring a woman.* New York: HarperCollins, 2009.

Klein, M. *Sexual intelligence: What we really want from sex—and how to get it.* New York: HarperOne, 2012.

Lacroix, N. *Tantric sex and lovemaking.* London, UK: Lorenz Books, 2008.

McCarthy, B. W., & McCarthy, E. *Discovering your couple sexual style: Sharing desire, pleasure, and satisfaction.* New York: Routledge, 2009.

Taylor, S. *101 sex positions: Steamy new positions from mild to wild.* Berkeley, CA: Amorata Press, 2008.

Winston, S. *Women's anatomy of arousal: Secret maps to buried pleasure.* Kingston, NY: Mango Garden Press, 2010.

Web Resources

SexTutor.com
www.sextutor.com

Sex Tutor offers accurate, clearly written, helpful sex advice on such topics as anal sex, cunnilingus, fellatio, female ejaculation, female masturbation, male masturbation, kissing, sex positions, prolonging sex, adult toys, and others.

Sex Life Guide
http://sexlifeguide.com/

Introduces and illustrates numerous sexual intercourse positions. The benefits of each position are discussed as well as other sexual issues.

About.com: Sexual Arousal
http://sexuality.about.com/od/glossary/g/Sexual-Arousal.htm

Discusses topics related to sexual activity and sexual arousal, including better-sex tips and techniques, sex toys, sex and disability, sexual arousal, and sexual positions.

Health Central: Sex Tips and Advice
http://www.healthcentral.com/sexual-health/sextechniques.html

Discusses topics related to enhancing readers' sex lives, including five ways to feel sexier, speaking up for a better sex life, five steps to a healthy sex life, salvaging so-so sex, and multiple orgasms.

The Science of Sexual Arousal
www.apa.org/monitor/apr03/arousal.aspx

A site of the American Psychological Association that describes what research has found regarding the cognitive, physiological, and subjective aspects of sexual arousal.

References

Basson, R. The female sexual response: A different model. *Journal of Marital Therapy, 26* (2000), 51–65.

Fogel, A. Body sense: Male and female orgasm: Not so different? The experience of orgasm for men and women is very similar. *Psychology Today,* 2014. Available: http://www.psychologytoday.com/blog/body-sense/201004/male-and-female-orgasm-not-so-different.

Greenberg, J. S. *Comprehensive stress management,* 13th ed. New York: McGraw-Hill Higher Education, 2013.

Haffner, D. W., & Stayton, W. R. Sexuality and reproductive health, in *Contraceptive technology,* 7th revised ed., Hatcher, R. A., et al. New York: Ardent Media, 1998.

Hite, S. *The Hite report.* New York: Macmillan, 1976.

Kaplan, H. S. *The new sex therapy: Active treatment of sexual dysfunction.* New York: Brunner/Mazel, 1974.

Kaplan, H. S. *Disorders of sexual desire.* New York: Simon & Schuster, 1979.

Kylstra, C. Her secret sex thoughts. *MH Lists,* 2014. Available: http://www.menshealth.com/mhlists/secret-sex-thoughts/index.php.

Masters, W. H., & Johnson, V. E. *Human sexual response.* Boston: Little, Brown, 1966.

Nicholas, A., Brody, S., de Sutter, P., & de Carufel, F. A woman's history of vaginal orgasm is discernible from her walk. *Journal of Sexual Medicine, 5* (2008), 2119–2124.

Painter, A. *Tantric sex techniques to reinvigorate lovemaking.* Discovery Health. Sexual Health Center: Tantric Sex, 2009. Available: http://health.discovery.com/centers/sex/tantric/tantricsex.html.

Peterson, V. *Tantric sex for beginners: 4 easy tips!* 2010. Available at: http://www.care2.com/greenliving/tantric-sex-for-beginners-4-easy-tips.html.

Population Reference Bureau. *The world's youth 2000.* Washington, DC: Author, 2000.

Proctor, F., Wagner, N., & Butler, J. The differentiation of male and female orgasm: An experimental study, in *Perspectives on human sexuality,* Wagner, N., ed. New York: Behavioral Publications, 1974.

Salisbury, C. M. & Fisher, W. A. "Did you come?": A qualitative exploration of gender differences in beliefs, experiences, and concerns regarding female orgasm occurrence during heterosexual sexual interactions. *Journal of Sex Research, 51* (2014), 616–631.

Senbel, A. M., & Mostafa, T. Yohimbine enhances the effect of sildenafil on erectile process in rats. *International Journal of Impotence Research, 20* (2008), 409–417.

Silverberg, C. Are male and female orgasms different? *About.com: Sexuality,* 2008. Available: http://sexuality.about.com/od/sexualhealthqanda/f/sex_question41.htm.

Singer, J., & Singer, I. Types of female orgasms. *Journal of Sex Research 8* (1972), 255–267.

Tantra Tantric Sex. *Tantric sex technique: The 3 basic tantra tantric sex technique categories,* 2012. Available: http://at-tantra-tantric-sex.com/different-types-of-tantra.htm.

Thayton, W. R. A theology of sexual pleasure. *SIECUS Report, 30* (2002), 393–400.

Walen, S. R., & Roth, D. A cognitive approach to sex therapy, in *Theories of human sexuality,* Geer, J. H., & O'Donohue, W. T., eds. New York: Plenum, 1987.

WEWOMEN.com. *5 tantric sex tips for OMG orgasms,* 2013. Available: http://www.wewomen.com/sex-sexuality/5-tantric-sex-tips-for-orgasms-d51138.html.

Wiest, W. Semantic differential profiles of orgasm and other experiences among men and women. *Sex Roles, 3* (1977), 399–403.

Zilbergard, B., & Ellison, C. R. Desire discrepancies and arousal problems in sex therapy, in *Principles and practices of sex therapy,* Lieblum, S. R., & Pervin, L. A., eds. New York: Guilford, 1980.

CHAPTER

7

Contraception

© Gayvoronskaya Yana/Shutterstock

CHAPTER OBJECTIVES

1 Discuss the reasons to use contraceptives, ways to choose a contraceptive, and the difference between perfect use and typical use.

2 Evaluate the nonprescription methods of contraception, including the effectiveness, the reversibility, and the advantages and disadvantages of each. Explain why some have higher rates of user effectiveness than others.

3 Evaluate the prescription methods of contraception, including the effectiveness, the reversibility, and the advantages and disadvantages of each. Explain why some have higher rates of user effectiveness than others.

4 Discuss the viability of future contraceptive methods. Consider the impact of gender issues, pharmaceutical industry costs for litigation, federal regulation compliance, and FDA approval.

INTRODUCTION

*T*hroughout life, people's use of and need for contraceptives change. The case history of Susan presents a typical contraceptive user. During her first sexual encounter at age 18 years, Susan's high school boyfriend used withdrawal.

During her freshman year at college, Susan began a steady sexual relationship with Jack. Because she was in a monogamous relationship and believed she did not have to worry about sexually transmitted infection (STI) transmission, Susan began to use oral contraceptives (the pill). After she had difficulty remembering to take her pill every day, Susan switched to injectable medroxyprogesterone acetate (Depo-Provera). Every 3 months she would receive her birth control shot at a clinic.

After she and Jack broke up, Susan was abstinent for a year—the most foolproof method of contraception available. She graduated from college and was fitted with a diaphragm; she also used condoms with her two partners.

By age 25 years, Susan married Stephen and had etonogestrel (Implanon) inserted into her upper arm. Implanon releases a steady stream of contraceptive into the reproductive system and is effective for up to 3 years. When she was starting to think about having a child, at her doctor's suggestion, she switched to a non–hormone-based contraceptive (foam and condoms) for 3 months before trying to conceive a child.

After the birth of her first child, Susan was fitted with an intrauterine device (IUD). Two years later, it was removed when she planned to conceive a second child. After the birth of their second child, Stephen had a vasectomy. After several follow-up tests to assure that no sperm were left in his ejaculate, Susan and Stephen enjoyed monogamous, unprotected sex.

Five years later, Susan and Stephen divorced. As one of her first acts as a newly divorced woman, Susan had a laparoscopy—a method of female sterilization. Although she could not become pregnant, she also began to practice safer sex and insisted that her partners wear latex condoms.

In other words, it is possible for a woman to use nearly every contraceptive method available during her more than 30 years of fertility. The method may change, depending on where she is in the life cycle.

This chapter reviews the currently available methods of contraception, their effectiveness, and their advantages and disadvantages.

▪ Contraception

Contraception is the prevention of conception. You may already have thought hard about the consequences of such decisions as whether to become pregnant, have an abortion, or adopt a child. If you have considered or do consider such matters, you will understand how significant contraception can be to your life. Many babies are born each year to mothers who are too young or too emotionally immature to raise them well, or to mothers whose eggs are too old and have a high probability of developing into a fetus with a birth defect. Many pregnant teenagers and their sexual partners never finish their schooling because of the need to support and care for their child. Some couples who marry in response to pregnancy are soon divorced. Married couples who have already raised children may find yet another pregnancy a threat to their economic and psychological health; managing this financial burden, as well as dealing with the time and energy necessary to care for an infant, can be as harmful to them—though perhaps in different ways—as to teenagers. But clearly the economic burden a child entails can present problems for people in various age groups and income levels.

Contraceptive and condom use should be routine for sexually active young people and adults unless they are seeking pregnancy, preferably in a mutually monogamous relationship. Yet, too many people use contraception inconsistently or ineffectively. The result is that the United States has a higher rate of unintended pregnancies than all other developed countries. Currently, more than half of all pregnancies in the United States are unintended—meaning

that they are mistimed or unwanted; thus, every year, about 1 in 20 American women of reproductive age has an unintended pregnancy (Guttmacher Institute, 2013). Researchers know that many factors increase one's motivation to use contraception, including the following:

- Ability to communicate with a partner
- Cost and convenience of a method
- Frequency of sexual intercourse
- Motivation to avoid pregnancy
- STI concerns and risks
- Contraceptive's side effects (including effect on menses)
- Beliefs of their religion, family, and peers
- One's attitudes and openness about sexuality (Zieman & Hatcher, 2012)

Ask yourself these questions as you read this chapter: Am I ready to have sexual intercourse? Am I committed to avoiding pregnancy myself or preventing a partner's pregnancy at this time? Am I committed to avoiding passing on a sexually transmitted infection? Am I committed to using a contraceptive method every time I have intercourse? Is my partner? If the answer to any of these questions is no, ask yourself another question: What will I do when a pregnancy occurs? Remember, almost 9 in 10 heterosexual couples who do not use a contraceptive method become pregnant within a year.

Contraceptive Effectiveness

We begin our discussion of contraception methods with a warning: The effectiveness of each method is

---

contraception Means of preventing pregnancy.

difficult to determine precisely, so you should consider the rates cited as *approximations only.* For each method we provide both the percentage of women experiencing an unintended pregnancy during the first year of contraceptive method use when used perfectly (consistently and correctly) and the percentage when used typically (Trussell, 2011).

With typical use, mistakes are often made—for example, a condom may be put on incorrectly or the pill is taken late. Consequently, **typical use** is always less effective than **perfect use**. Use is measured by the number of women in 100 who will become pregnant during the first year of use of the particular method. A good contraceptive method is one that limits the gap between the way it is prescribed to be used and the way it is actually used. Table 7.1 shows the effectiveness of varied methods of contraception, and, as can be seen, there is usually a vast difference between these two measures of contraceptive effectiveness.

Contraception Versus Safer Sex

Opposite-sex couples need to discuss how they will prevent both pregnancy and transmission of STIs. The most effective methods of preventing pregnancies—oral contraceptives, hormonal implants, intrauterine devices (IUDs), sterilization—provide *no* protection against STIs. The male condom provides the best protection available against STIs but has a lower rate of effectiveness against pregnancy. There are two ways to achieve maximal effectiveness against both STIs and pregnancies relative to penile–vaginal sex: abstain from penile–vaginal sex or use a condom and a hormonal contraceptive together. Because STIs pose a threat to the future fertility and health of college students, and because emergency contraception (EC) and abortion are available, some experts recommend that if only one method is used, it should be a condom.

Nonprescription Methods

Abstinence

People define **abstinence** in different ways: For some, it means no sexual contact of any kind; for others, it means no **penetrative behaviors**, including vaginal sex, oral sex, or anal sex. Many adolescents, young adults, and adults choose to abstain. People choose abstinence for a variety of reasons:

- Their religion teaches that penetrative behaviors are appropriate only in marriage.

- They are not in a loving, committed relationship.

- They do not have a partner.

- They want to avoid the risk of pregnancy or STI.

- The relationship they are in is not ready for the intimacy of penetrative behaviors.

- They are not ready to experience vaginal, oral, or anal sex.

- They are ill or their partner is ill.

- They or a partner have been exposed to an STI.

- They feel that a sexual relationship would complicate their life.

Choosing abstinence does not necessarily mean forgoing sexual pleasure. There are many ways to give and receive sexual pleasure without the risks of sexual intercourse. These include deep kissing, massages, fondling, dancing, masturbating alone, masturbating together, and showering together. However, for these activities not to end in oral, vaginal, or anal sex, couples must communicate their desire not to engage in such behaviors and must agree to stick to sexual limits.

Effectiveness

Abstinence is the only 100% effective method of fertility control and STI prevention—if the couple or individual is truly committed to refraining from oral, vaginal, and anal sex, and if contact with genitals is also limited. Actual user effectiveness rates are unknown. A popular saying is that "vows of abstinence fail more frequently than condoms"—that is, people say that they are practicing abstinence but have sex in spite of their intention. Communication and commitment are essential. Because abstinence has never had the scientific scrutiny given other methods to determine typical use effectiveness, there are no data to make a fair comparison between abstinence effectiveness and other methods. Proponents of abstinence may cite typical use of various contraceptive methods to demonstrate their risk of failure and yet claim the typical use effectiveness rate of abstinence as 100%.

Such a comparison is inappropriate from a public health perspective unless perfect use effectiveness

---

typical use The ability of a method of contraception to prevent pregnancy as actually used at home by people not being monitored.

perfect use The ability of a method of contraception to prevent pregnancy as measured by consistent and correct use.

abstinence Avoidance of any type of sexual intercourse.

penetrative behaviors Any behavior whereby penetration occurs—for example, penile–vaginal sex, oral sex, or anal sex.

TABLE 7.1

Contraceptive Effective: Rates of Unintended Pregnancies per 100 Women During First Year of Use

Method	Consistent and Correct (Perfect Use) in United States	As Commonly Used (Typical Use) in United States	As Commonly Used (Typical Use) in Developing Countries
Implants (Implanon)	0.05	0.05	—
Male sterilization (vasectomy)	0.10	0.15	—
Levonorgestrel IU (Mirena IUD)	0.2	0.2	—
Female sterilization	0.5	0.5	—
Copper-bearing IUD (ParaGard)	0.6	0.8	2
Progestin-only injectable (Depo-Provera)	0.2	6	2
Combined oral contraceptive pills	0.3	9	7
Progestin-only contraceptive pills	1	9	—
Combined patch (Ortho Evra)	0.3	9	—
Combined vaginal ring (NuvaRing)	0.3	9	—
Diaphragm with spermicide	6	12	
Cervical cap			
Never given birth	5	9.5	
Have given birth	5	20.5	
Sponge			
Never given birth	9	12	
Have given birth	20	24	
Condom[1]			—
Male	2	18	—
Female	5	21	—
Fertility awareness-based methods[2]		24	—
Symptothermal method	0.4	—	—
Ovulation method	3	—	—
Standard days method	5	—	—
Withdrawal	4	22	
Spermicides[3]	18	28	—
No method[4]	85	85	—

Most effective methods	Moderately effective methods	Less effective methods

Notes: LAM (lactational amenorrhea method) is a highly effective, *temporary* method of contraception. However, to maintain effective protection against pregnancy, another method of contraception must be used as soon as menstruation resumes, the frequency or duration of breastfeeding is reduced, bottle feeding is introduced, or the baby reaches 6 months of age. Prospective studies have shown pregnancy rates of 0.5% to 1.5% for 6-month perfect use with LAM (Kennedy & Trussell, 2011).

1. Without spermicides.
2. The ovulation method evaluates cervical mucus. The standard days method avoids intercourse on cycle days 8 through 19. The symptothermal method evaluates cervical mucus to determine the first fertile day and considers cervical mucus and temperature to determine the last fertile day.
3. Foams, creams, gels, vaginal suppositories, and vaginal film.
4. Based on data from populations where contraception is not used and from women who stop using contraception to become pregnant. Among such populations, approximately 89% become pregnant within 1 year. This estimate was lowered to 85% to represent the percentage who would become pregnant within 1 year among women now relying on reversible methods of contraception if they stopped using contraception altogether.

Sources: U.S. data (first two columns): Cates, W., & Harwood, B. Vaginal barriers and spermicides. In R. A. Hatcher et al., eds. *Contraceptive technology.* 20th ed. New York: Ardent Media, 2011, 391–408; Centers for Disease Control and Prevention. *Contraception,* 2015. Available: http://www.cdc.gov/reproductivehealth/UnintendedPregnancy/Contraception.htm#; Trussell, J. Contraceptive efficacy. In R. A. Hatcher et al., eds. *Contraceptive technology.* 20th ed. New York: Ardent Media, 2011, 779–864. Developing country data: Cleland, J., & Ali, M. M. Reproductive consequences of contraceptive failure in 19 developing countries. *Obstetrics and Gynecology, 104* (2004), 314–320.

rates are used for the other methods (for example, male condom, 98%; withdrawal, 96%) (Dailard, 2003).

Reversibility

Abstinence does not affect fertility.

Advantages and Disadvantages

Abstinence is an excellent method of fertility control and STI prevention. It is free, you always have it with you, and there are no side effects. It is 100% effective—but only if you use it every time, and only if your partner is equally committed to its use. Just as with any method, one should occasionally reconsider whether it is still the method of choice. Research demonstrates how difficult it is to practice abstinence consistently over time. One study showed that 60% of college students who pledged to maintain virginity had broken their vow to remain abstinent until marriage. Such a high risk of failure would be concern enough, but another study showed that teens who promised to abstain from sex until marriage were more likely to have unprotected sex when they broke their pledge than those who never made such a promise. It is essential for anyone using abstinence as a contraceptive method to choose a different method *before* they stop using abstinence.

Ethical DIMENSIONS

Sexuality Education in the United States

For more than three decades, "abstinence-only until marriage" was the government-sanctioned approach to reducing U.S. rates of teen pregnancy and STIs. More than $1.7 billion has been spent on federal and mandated state matching grants supporting sexuality education that restricts or ignores the effectiveness of contraceptives and safer-sex behaviors (Sexuality Information and Education Council of the United States [SIECUS], 2014).

Several studies have indicated that these programs are ineffective. Rosenbaum (2009) found that teens signing virginity pledges are just as likely to engage in sexual behavior as those who do not sign such pledges. Moreover, they are less likely to use contraception, are less likely to get tested for STIs, and may have STIs for longer periods of time when they do break their pledges. Trenholm and colleagues (2007) in the Mathematica study and Kirby (2007) demonstrated that the evaluated abstinence education programs have no statistically significant beneficial impact on the sexual behavior of young people. Only one abstinence-only program—targeted at middle school students—has been shown to delay sexual initiation. However, this program focuses on delaying sexual activity "until a later time in life when the adolescent is more prepared to handle the consequences" and not specifically marriage. In addition, facilitators of this program were instructed to correct misinformation about condoms and were not allowed to criticize the benefits of condoms, factors that differ from most other abstinence-only programs (SIECUS, 2010).

Given these findings, it is not surprising that many leading health professional groups have raised serious ethical concerns about U.S. support for abstinence-only sexuality education programs. As a result, funding for these programs has decreased. In addition, several forms of medically accurate sexuality education are now being funded by the federal government: Teen Pregnancy Prevention Initiative, Personal Responsibility Education Program and school-based programs through the Division of Adolescent and School Health (DASH) (SIECUS, 2014).

This change in direction matches what Americans say they want for their children. Surveys of parents have demonstrated strong support for comprehensive sexuality education (favored by 82% of those polled); 68% favored instruction on how to use a condom, whereas only 36% supported abstinence-only education (Bleakley, Hennessy, & Fishbein, 2006).The goal underlying this fundamental change is to make sure that young people have the information and skills they will need to make healthy choices about sexual behavior. If adolescents are sexually active, or will be shortly, they need information to protect themselves.

Think about the sexuality education that you received as an adolescent in middle or high school. Was it abstinence-only until marriage? Did it provide information about contraception or safer sex? Is it ethical to deny accurate information to individuals? How did the type of sexuality education and information you received affect your sexual decision making and behaviors? Do you wish that you would have received something different in terms of sexuality education? After you consider how sexuality education influenced you, think about which type of sexuality future generations (i.e., your children) should have.

© Jones and Bartlett Publishers. Photographed by Christine McKeen

A wide variety of condoms are available in various colors, sizes, and even flavors. Latex, polyurethane, and polyisoprene have been shown to prevent transmission of STIs, including HIV. Animal skin or natural skin condoms only reduce the risk of pregnancy; they provide no protection from STIs. When practiced incorrectly, the rate of efficacy decreases to 22 pregnancies per 100 per year (Trussell, 2011).

Withdrawal

Withdrawal is probably the oldest contraceptive method on record. In the Bible, Onan practices withdrawal, or **coitus interruptus**, so as not to impregnate his brother's widow. To practice withdrawal, the couple has penile–vaginal sex until the man feels that he is about to ejaculate. He withdraws his penis and ejaculates away from the woman's vulva.

Effectiveness

Many people assume that withdrawal is an ineffective method of contraception. However, some contraceptive experts believe that withdrawal is an underrated method. With perfect use, it is about as effective as most barrier methods, with an efficacy rate of 4 pregnancies per 100 per year.

Many people have been taught that pre-ejaculate fluid might contain sperm. However, pre-ejaculate fluid is actually a neutralizing solution produced by the Cowper's glands. The results of studies examining sperm levels in the pre-ejaculate vary. Some have shown no sperm (Zukerman & Orvieto, 2007; Zuckerman, Weiss, & Orvieto, 2003), whereas others have detected enough motile sperm to potentially impregnate a partner (Killick et al., 2011).

While there are many other more effective means of preventing pregnancy, if there are no other options available, withdrawal can reduce the risk of pregnancy and is better than ejaculating into a partner. However, if the man does not withdraw in time and/or the woman is at a fertile point in her cycle, emergency contraception should be considered (covered later in this chapter).

Advantages and Disadvantages

Withdrawal is free, always available, and relatively easy to use. It has no medical side effects, and it encourages male involvement.

The major disadvantage to withdrawal is that some men—particularly young men—do not recognize impending ejaculation and thus ejaculate inside their partner, putting her at risk of pregnancy. Withdrawal has a relatively high failure rate among typical users and does not protect against all STIs, although it may reduce the risk of fluid-borne infection. Some couples report that withdrawal reduces the sexual pleasure of the woman and intensity of orgasm of the man. It requires the man to think about what is happening during intercourse.

Male Condom

Condoms are one of the oldest contraceptive methods (Maatouk & Moutran, 2013). Today most condoms are made of **latex**, a synthetic form of rubber. About 5% of condoms are made from the intestines of lambs; these are known as *lambskin* or *natural condoms*. Lambskin condoms, because they are more porous than latex condoms, do not provide protection against many STIs and are not recommended for that purpose.

While lambskin and latex condoms have been available for centuries, two other types of condom material—polyurethane and polyisoprene—have been introduced in the United States. In 1997, the U.S. Food and Drug Administration (FDA) approved the first condom made of **polyurethane**, a type of plastic. Studies comparing polyurethane and latex condoms indicate that non-latex condoms have higher breakage rates, but there are no reported differences in typical effectiveness rates (Gallo, Grimes, & Schulz, 2003). Polyisoprene condoms were approved in 2008; polyisoprene is a synthetic rubber that allows those allergic to latex to use them without concern. These condoms are said to stretch more and be more comfortable than polyurethane condoms (GoAskAlice, 2009).

Individuals who use condoms to prevent unwanted pregnancies and STIs must understand the meaning of *consistent* and *correct* condom use. To practice *consistent* and *correct* condom use, follow these guidelines:

withdrawal Removing the penis from the vagina before ejaculation.

coitus interruptus The Latin term for *withdrawal*, which means "interrupted intercourse."

condom A sheath that covers the penis.

latex A synthetic rubber.

polyurethane A type of plastic.

CONSISTENT USE

- Use a condom every time, from start to finish, for penile–vaginal sex, oral sex on a male, and anal sex. A new condom must be used for each sex act.

CORRECT USE

- Store condoms in a cool place out of direct sunlight (not in wallets or glove compartments). Latex will become brittle as a result of changes in temperature, rough handling, and age. Do not use damaged, discolored, brittle, or sticky condoms.

- Check the date on the condom. If it is an expiration date, do not use the condom beyond that date. If it is a date of production, the condom may be used for several years beyond that date (2 years for spermicidal condoms, 5 years for nonspermicidal latex condoms) (Zieman & Hatcher, 2012).

- Carefully open the condom package—teeth or fingernails can tear the condom.

- Use a new condom for every act of oral, penile–vaginal, and anal sex. If engaging in oral sex first, use a new condom for penile–vaginal sex. If using penetrative sex toys, use a new condom between partners.

- Put on the condom after the penis is erect and before it touches any part of a partner's body. A man who is uncircumcised must pull back the foreskin before putting on the condom.

- Put on the condom by pinching the reservoir tip and unrolling it all the way down the shaft of the penis from head to base (see Figure 7.1). If the condom does not have a reservoir tip, pinch it to leave a half-inch space at the head of the penis in which semen can collect after ejaculation.

- Withdraw the penis immediately if the condom breaks, and put on a new condom before resuming. When a condom breaks, access emergency contraception at a drug store or supermarket.

- Use only water-based or silicone-based lubrication with latex or polyisoprene

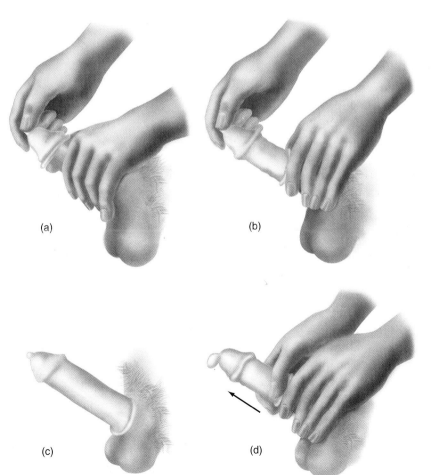

(a)

(b)

(c)

(d)

FIGURE **7.1** If you have never used a condom, you should practice before the first time you use one during sex activity with a partner. To put a condom on: (a) Put on the condom by pinching the reservoir tip and unrolling it all the way down the shaft of the penis. (b) Be sure that there are no air bubbles, which could cause the condom to break. (c) The condom should have extra rubber at the top and should be unrolled to the very base of the penis. (d) After ejaculation, hold the rim of the condom so that it does not accidentally slip off or leak and withdraw the penis.

condoms. Oil-based lubricants can be used with polyurethane condoms but avoid using common household oils such as cooking/vegetable oil, baby oil, hand lotion, or petroleum jelly as they are not designed to be inserted into the body. Spermicidal condoms are no longer recommended; although spermicides do not damage latex, many people are irritated by spermicides, which can increase discomfort and risk of infection.

- Immediately after ejaculation, while the penis is still erect, grasp the rim of the condom between the fingers, and slowly withdraw the penis (with the condom still on) so that no semen is spilled.

- Check for breakage; dispose of condom (Zieman & Hatcher, 2012).

Effectiveness
Condoms are very effective. Only 2% of couples using a condom correctly and for every act of intercourse become pregnant in the first year of use; however, this method is only 82% effective in typical users. The major reason condoms fail is that people forget to

Communication
DIMENSIONS

Condom Use and Consistency: Talking About Condom Use

Except for withdrawal, condoms have the greatest gap between perfect use (98% effectiveness) and typical use (82% effectiveness) of all the contraceptive methods (see Table 7.1). Because this method is popular and is one of the few contraceptive methods that provides protection against STIs, understanding factors associated with its use and consistency is important. Among teens, high rates of both STIs and unintended pregnancy could be reduced with condom use. A study examining condom use patterns among sexually experienced male adolescents, age 15–19, found multiple domains of influence. Those who had formal sex education, had positive attitudes about condoms, were younger, had a partner close in age, and were committed to a relationship had greater odds of correct and consistent condom use. Recommendations include providing programs with targeted services that address condom use attitudes and that help teens negotiate condom use decision making with sexual partners (Sonenstein, 2008).

The following scenario could be helpful with decision making:

You are on your third date in a nice restaurant with a new friend. You are attracted to each other; on the last date, you spent a pretty hot half-hour kissing and touching each other. You are pretty sure that you are ready to have sex and are hoping that your new friend feels the same way. But how do you know? And how do you bring up condom use or other safer sex techniques?

The waiter just delivered dessert. Dinner is coming to an end. Your date says, "Hmmm, do you want to come back to my place?" You say, "I think there are a few things we need to talk about first."

Here's how a successful discussion about condoms with a new partner might go:

Chris: I really like you. I've been fantasizing a lot since our last date about us having sex.

Pat: Me, too. But, it's important to me that we use condoms and practice safe sex.

Chris: Of course. I always use condoms. And because I was hoping you were interested, too, I bought some today.

Pat: I bought some today, too! How about we skip dessert?

Of course, it is not always that easy (although it should be). Chris might have said, "I hate condoms." Here are some ways that Pat might answer:

1. "Not with me you won't. I've learned how to make condom use really fun. I hope you want me to show you."
2. "I'm really sorry to hear that. I would never have sex with someone unless we use a condom."
3. "Tell me which condoms you've used. Maybe we can try a different brand or type."
4. "Well, it looks as if we have an important decision to make. We can agree not to have any kind of sex and just mess around. Or, we can just be friends. But I won't have sex with you without a condom."

Condom use with a new partner is essential until you have both been tested for STIs and have decided to have sex only with each other. Remember, "A man who doesn't want to use a condom with you probably didn't use one with his last partner either" (Haffner & Schwartz, 1998).

use them for each act of intercourse (Trussell, 2011). Breakage, slippage, or leakage can also reduce effectiveness. Condom fit may be a factor. If adding more lubricant inside a condom to increase sensation, be sure that the amount added is less than dime-size. Also make sure that the condom is the correct size—one that is too large may slip off. If the condom is too small, breakage or reduced sensation may be a problem. Condoms are also highly effective at preventing the spread of HIV, gonorrhea, chlamydia, and trichomoniasis (Zieman & Hatcher, 2012).

Advantages and Disadvantages

Advantages of condoms include the following: They are relatively inexpensive, they are easy to obtain, they do not require a visit to the doctor, they may help a man control ejaculation, they provide protection from STIs, and they have none of the side effects associated with hormonal methods of contraception. Finally, condom use is one of the few methods that involves men directly in the practice of birth control and prevention of pregnancy.

The major disadvantage of male condoms is that many men complain that condoms reduce sensitivity and spontaneity. Trying different brands can improve

Courtesy of Health Education Resource Organization

Smart sportswear for the active man.

Introducing the latest in evening wear for the man-on-the-go; Condoms.
Available in a wide variety of styles, colors, textures—even flavors. At finer drugstores, pharmacies and creative outlets everywhere. One size fits all. Condoms also stop AIDS.

So don't be caught dead wearing anything less.

Use condoms.
There's living proof they stop AIDS.

HERO
Health Education Resource Organization

945-AIDS • 251-1164 • 1-800-638-6252

sensation, and putting the condom on as foreplay can make it more fun. Another potential problem is a latex allergy or reaction to spermicide. Discontinue spermicide use first. If that does not help, try polyurethane or polyisoprene condoms.

Female Condom

One vaginal barrier is the **female condom** (Figure 7.2). The female condom appeared on the market in the United States in 1993 (FDA, 1993). Originally it was a loose-fitting sheath made of polyurethane with rings on both ends. One ring covers the cervix; the other ring remains outside the vagina and partially covers the vulva. A new version of the female condom, the FC2, was approved by the FDA in March 2009. Although it looks similar to its predecessor, it is made from synthetic rubber, making it cheaper to produce. The FC2 is also less noisy during use. In addition to cost, complaints about squeaky noises were among the factors that slowed acceptance of the original version. The price of one female condom is about 60 cents compared to less than 4 cents for mass-distributed male condoms, a difference that is an issue in the developing world (Crary, 2009).

The female condom is like the male condom in that it can be used only for one act of intercourse. It is unlike the male condom because it can be inserted up to 8 hours before intercourse, although it may not be comfortable for everyday wear. Female and male condoms should *not* be used together because it increases the risk of one or both condoms breaking.

Effectiveness

The effectiveness rates for the female condom are based on the original version. No studies have been conducted on FC2. For perfect use, it is 95% effective in preventing pregnancies. In typical use, studies have found it to be 79% effective. Although it is not as effective as the male condom, the female condom is a valuable option to empower women who want to prevent STIs and unintended pregnancy. The only other contraception that prevents both STIs and pregnancy is the male condom.

Advantages and Disadvantages

The female condom is available without prescription, is controlled by the woman, can be inserted in advance of intercourse, and is a safe alternative for people with latex allergy or sensitivity. For some women, the outer ring may rub against the external clitoris, which could increase pleasure. Its

female condom A polyurethane or synthetic rubber sheath with flexible inner and outer rings worn inside the vagina.

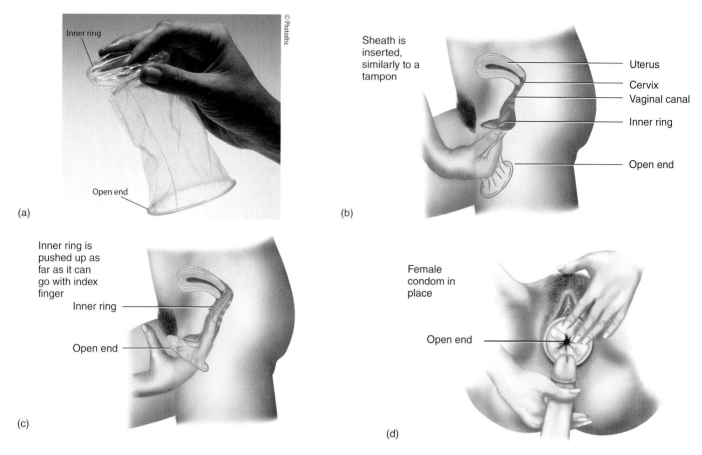

© Photodisc

(a)

(b)

Sheath is
inserted,
similarly to a
tampon

Uterus
Cervix
Vaginal canal
Inner ring

Open end

Inner ring is
pushed up as
far as it can
go with index
finger

Inner ring

Open end

(c)

Female
condom in
place

Open end

(d)

FIGURE **7.2** Inserting a female condom. (a) Photo of a female condom. (b) The inner ring is squeezed for insertion and the sheath inserted into the vagina similarly to a tampon. (c) With the index finger, push the inside of the inner ring as far as it will go. Make sure the sheath is not twisted during insertion. The outer ring should remain outside the vagina. (d) Hold the outer ring in place while inserting the penis, making sure the penis is inserted into the condom and not next to it. Be careful when removing the condom to ensure semen does not spill out.

disadvantages include somewhat difficult insertion requiring practice for new users. The FC2 version should be less noisy, but if still troublesome, the noise can be reduced with use of additional lubricant.

Contraceptive Sponges

The Today contraceptive sponge is made of polyurethane foam (latex-free) and is prefilled with nonoxynol 9 spermicide (discussed in the next section), which is continuously released into the vagina during use. The sponge acts both as a mechanical barrier to sperm migration into the cervical canal and as a chemical agent by applying spermicide directly to the cervix. It is not reusable. The sponge is sold over the counter, without the need for a prescription (three sponges for around $15). When used as a primary method, this barrier method should be coupled with counseling to have emergency contraceptive (EC) pills on hand at home.

This contraceptive method was originally introduced in 1983. The manufacturer stopped distributing the product over a dispute not related to its quality or efficacy. In spring 2009, the new, exclusive distributor of the Today Vaginal Contraceptive Sponge for the United States, Canada, and European Union relaunched the sponge in the United States (Mayer Laboratories, 2009).

Effectiveness
When the sponge was introduced originally, its perfect-use failure rate in the first year of use was 8%; the typical-use failure rate in the first year was not much different at 13% (Edelman & North, 1987). Table 7.1 reports that the sponge is twice as effective for women who have never given birth (nulliparous women: perfect use 9% and typical use 12%) as for those who have given birth (parous women: 20% perfect use and 24% typical use).

Advantages and Disadvantages
The contraceptive sponge method is controlled by the woman, is active immediately after placement, can be inserted several hours before sexual intercourse to

Multicultural DIMENSIONS

Ethnic and Age Differences in Access to Emergency Contraception

Background Information

Emergency contraception (EC) includes any method used after intercourse to prevent pregnancy. None of the current methods is an abortifacient and none disturbs an implanted pregnancy. Currently, three methods are in widespread use worldwide:

- Hormonal contraceptive pills (e.g., Plan B One-Step, Next Choice One Dose)
- Progesterone receptor modulator (ella)
- Copper-T IUD insertion (ParaGard)

While the hormonal methods and the progesterone receptor modulator are more commonly utilized in the United States, a growing number of practitioners are recommending insertion of the copper-T IUD because it is more effective as an emergency contraception, all women (regardless of body mass index [BMI] or weight) can use it, and it provides continued pregnancy protection for up to 12 years.

Women are becoming more aware of EC; a 2013 survey showed that 86% of women had heard of EC, although teens were less aware of this option compared to older women (Kaiser Family Foundation, 2014). Awareness, however, has not translated into greater use. Approximately 11% of women reported using EC between 2006 and 2010 (up from 4% in 2002), with approximately 5% reporting use in the previous 12 months (Kaiser Family Foundation, 2014).

Research Findings

- Studies have found women getting EC in advance are not more likely to have unprotected sex or to use EC repeatedly.
- Increased access to EC enhanced use but did not decrease pregnancy rates.
- EC is an appropriate backup option for adolescents. Having EC available does *not* make teens less likely to use regular contraception or more likely to have unprotected sex.

Accessibility

Starting in February 2014, generic versions of hormonal EC became available over the counter without prescription or age restrictions. While the labeling indicates that medication is intended for people older than age 17, no ID is required to purchase the medication. A prescription is still required for ella, which is more effective for obese or overweight women.

The Affordable Care Act requires the coverage of the cost of prescribed contraception, including ella, but over-the-counter EC is not covered and its cost must be paid out of pocket. Some states allow pharmacists to write prescriptions; in those areas, individuals may be able to receive hormonal EC and have it covered by their insurance.

At the same time, states differ in how they assist with or restrict accessibility. Some states have required emergency services to provide EC-related services for women who have been sexually assaulted. Theoretically, some types of EC should be available without interaction with the pharmacy, but in some instances that is not the case; EC is still locked in cabinets or requires access through the pharmacy, increasing barriers to its use, especially for adolescents who may be reluctant to ask for EC.

Equal Access?

Timely access to this method of contraception is critical to reduce the rate of unintended pregnancy among adolescents. One study was designed to explore barriers adolescents might face and differences in access to EC by age, ethnicity, and region. At the time of the study (2005–2006), EC was available to females younger than 18 years of age through pharmacy access. Researchers posing as English- and Spanish-speaking females—who either said they were 15 and had had unprotected intercourse last night or that they were 18 and had had unprotected sex 4 days ago—called 115 pharmacies in California. Each pharmacy received one call using each scenario; a call was considered successful if the caller was told she could come in to obtain the method. Statistical measures were

(*continues*)

Multicultural DIMENSIONS

Ethnic and Age Differences in Access to Emergency Contraception (Continued)

used to assess differences between subgroups. In-depth interviews with 22 providers and pharmacists were also conducted, and emergent themes were identified.

Thirty-six percent of all calls were successful. Spanish speakers were less successful than English speakers (24% versus 48%), and callers to rural pharmacies were less successful than callers to urban ones (27% versus 44%). Although rural pharmacies were more likely to offer Spanish-language services, Spanish-speaking callers to these pharmacies were the least successful of all callers (17%). Spanish speakers were also less successful than English speakers when calling urban pharmacies (30% versus 57%).

Interviews suggested that little cooperation existed between pharmacists and clinicians and that dispensing the EC method at clinics was a favorable option for adolescents. Adolescents face significant barriers to obtaining emergency contraception, but the expansion of Spanish-language services at pharmacies and greater collaboration between providers and pharmacists could improve access (Sampson et al., 2009). If this study were conducted today, with the new laws intended to increase access and more awareness about the benefits of EC, ideally the results would be different.

Courtesy of Allendale Pharmaceuticals, Inc.

The contraceptive sponge is a one-time use method combining a barrier that prevents sperm from entering the cervix with a chemical spermicide.

permit spontaneity, can remain in place for multiple acts of intercourse up to 24 hours, and is entirely reversible.

Some disadvantages are that the sponge requires placement prior to genital contact, which may reduce spontaneity of sex; some women do not like placing their fingers or an object into their vagina; the sponge does not provide protection against HIV and some STIs; failure rates are higher than with hormonal contraception; odor may develop if the sponge is left in place too long; and severe obesity or arthritis may make insertion or removal of the sponge difficult. No cases of toxic shock syndrome have been reported, but theoretically the risk may be increased if this method is left in too long or used during menses. An increase in uterine tract infections is another possible complication (Zieman & Hatcher, 2012).

Spermicides

A **spermicide** kills and/or immobilizes sperm on contact and acts as a cervical barrier, thereby preventing their movement toward an egg (Figure 7.3). Spermicides are available as vaginal creams, films, foams, gels, suppositories, and sponges.

Foams and creams are placed against the cervix by means of a plastic applicator. Spermicidal films (small squares coated with spermicides) and suppositories are inserted manually, high into the vagina. Most spermicides must be inserted within 1 hour of intercourse, and some are not effective for the first 10 to 15 minutes after insertion. Users should read the packet insert instructions carefully.

Effectiveness

The perfect-use effectiveness rate of spermicides is 82%, meaning that 18% of women using spermicides perfectly would become pregnant in 1 year. However, the typical user effectiveness rate is only 72%. Just as with condoms, spermicides' ineffectiveness is

spermicide Chemical detergent compound that immobilizes or kills sperm on contact; as a barrier, prevents sperm from entering the uterus through the cervical os.

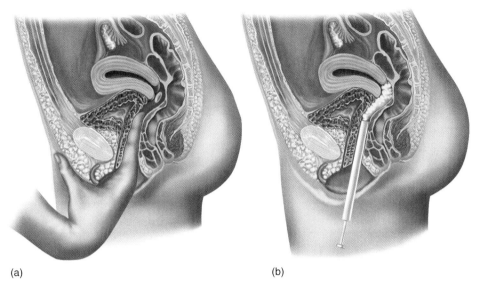

(a)   (b)

FIGURE **7.3** (a) Read the instructions for use of suppositories carefully and follow them. Be sure to wait the proper time for the suppository to dissolve. (b) Insert the plastic applicator into the vagina as far as possible to make sure that the foam covers the cervical opening, and press the plunger.

probably due to inconsistent use of the spermicide with every act of penile–vaginal sex or incorrect use (for example, putting it in too soon or too late). By using condoms and spermicide together, effectiveness rates almost equal those of oral contraceptives. Unfortunately, few couples use both methods simultaneously.

Reversibility
Spermicide use has no effect on future fertility.

Advantages and Disadvantages
There are many advantages to spermicide use. Spermicides are easy to use, are available at drug stores and supermarkets without a prescription, and do not require partner involvement.

The major disadvantages of spermicides are the relatively high failure rates for both perfect and typical use and the reversal in recommendations involving **nonoxynol 9 (N-9)**, the major spermicidal ingredient sold over the counter in the United States. Other spermicides that are used in products available in Canada and in Europe are not available in the United States.

Women are advised to avoid products with N-9 because several studies have shown vaginal irritation due to this spermicide can actually increase the possibility of acquiring HIV and other STIs from an infected partner. Although a potentially effective contraceptive method, use during anal sex or repeated use during penile–vaginal sex in one day should be avoided.

Fertility-Awareness Methods

Natural family planning (NFP) is also known as **fertility-awareness methods (FAMs)**, or the *rhythm method*. There are several FAMs: the *calendar method*, the *ovulation method*, and the *symptothermal method*. Each of these methods is based on the identification of the days in the woman's menstrual cycle when she is most likely to be fertile and the avoidance of penile–vaginal sex during those days (natural family planning) or use of a barrier method or withdrawal during those days.

FAMs are more effective for women who have regular menstrual cycles (i.e., cycles that are about the same number of days apart). These methods are based on the knowledge that there are only about 5 to 7 days in a cycle during which a woman can become pregnant. The ovum lives less than 1 day; sperm can live up to 6 days inside the woman's genital tract (Zieman & Hatcher, 2012).

People interested in using these methods need education to help them learn to observe, chart, and recognize the woman's fertility signs and patterns. While one school of thought is that it requires 4 to 6 hours over two or three menstrual cycles to learn

nonoxynol 9 (N-9) The major spermicidal ingredient in U.S.-made products.

natural family planning (NFP) Calculation of a woman's fertile times and abstention from penile–vaginal sex on fertile days.

fertility-awareness methods (FAMs) Methods used to determine fertile days.

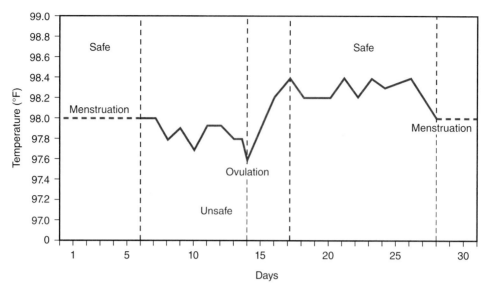

FIGURE **7.4** The basal body temperature method of contraception involves charting a woman's body temperature each morning to determine when unprotected sexual intercourse is safe. Once the basal body temperature has risen for three consecutive days, she can assume that ovulation has taken place and that the remaining days in that menstrual cycle are safe for unprotected intercourse.

FAMs, another is that it takes less than 20 minutes for a woman to understand that she should consider herself fertile on days 8–19 of her menstrual cycle (Jennings & Burke, 2011). Researchers have recently developed comprehensive web-based education to increase awareness and knowledge of FAM, with moderate success (Fehring, Schneider, Raviele, et al., 2013).

Couples using the **calendar method**, first developed in the 1930s, keep track of the woman's menstrual cycles for several months and then, with the help of a trained person, determine which days she is most likely to ovulate. The calendar method is the least effective of the fertility-awareness methods; even with perfect use, there is a 5% chance of becoming pregnant.

Ovulation methods are much more effective. Women can chart their **basal body temperature** or their cervical secretions, or both. Basal body temperature is a person's temperature upon awakening. Temperatures usually drop immediately before ovulation and then rise sharply during and after ovulation (Figure 7.4). Thus a woman takes her temperature by using a specially calibrated **basal body thermometer** before she gets up each morning. The temperature is then charted on a monthly graph, and after 3 days of elevated temperature, it is considered safe to have intercourse without the risk of pregnancy.

Cervical secretions can also be monitored and charted. After menstruation, cervical secretions are scant. As estrogen levels increase, cervical mucus

calendar method Charting of the length of a woman's periods for several months to determine the days she is most likely to be fertile.

ovulation methods Observation of signs of ovulation to calculate fertile days.

basal body temperature A woman's body temperature immediately upon waking.

basal body thermometer A special thermometer used to measure changes in basal body temperature.

cervical secretions Normal fluids from the cervix that change consistency during the month.

CycleBeads are used as part of the calendar method. Using a string of 33 colored beads, women keep track of their cycle. When used correctly, the efficacy rate is 5 pregnancies per 100 per year.

Gender DIMENSIONS

Gender Equality in Contraception Use

During most of human history, contraception was a male responsibility. The only methods available were the condom and withdrawal. When oral contraceptives became available in 1961, many women were elated. They could now control contraceptive use and, therefore, their risk of becoming pregnant. The pill was effective, was easy to use, and did not require partner participation. Many men who came of age during the 1960s and 1970s never thought much about contraception.

In the 1990s, the HIV/AIDS epidemic and the epidemic of STIs once again shifted the responsibility. Men who are not in monogamous committed relationships now have to use condoms on a regular basis. Many women, however, are unwilling to rely on condoms for pregnancy prevention because they are only 82% effective in preventing pregnancies in typical users. Some men are unwilling to use condoms once they find out that their partner is using the pill. And many men do not like to use condoms, claiming that they reduce sensitivity and sensation.

Heterosexual couples today need to negotiate how they will prevent an unwanted pregnancy *and* how they will protect themselves against STIs. Couples need to discuss who has primary responsibility for contraception. They need to address such questions as the following: Who will buy the condoms? Who will pay for contraception? Should the man accompany the woman to the clinic visit? And, perhaps most important, what will they do if an unplanned pregnancy occurs?

There are ways that couples can share the responsibility for contraceptive and condom use. Men can remind their partners to take their pills or check their IUD strings. They can learn to insert the diaphragm or female condom as part of foreplay. Women can learn to place the condom on the man's penis as part of foreplay. Contraceptive use and safer sex practices can truly be a shared responsibility.

---

becomes thick and cloudy. When estrogen peaks at midcycle, the secretions become clearer, stretchy, and slippery. In fact, at ovulation, the mucus can be stretched 2 to 3 inches between the thumb and forefinger. After ovulation, the secretions become thick again, and some women may notice a cervical mucus plug. At this point, it is considered safe to have intercourse without worrying about pregnancy.

The **symptothermal method** involves checking both basal body temperatures and cervical secretions and charting them to identify fertile periods (which begin as soon as cervical secretions are noticed) and nonfertile times (beginning the fourth day after the last day of wet, clear, slippery mucus—post ovulation). When this method is used perfectly, fewer than 1% of women become pregnant, making it almost as effective as the most effective prescription forms of contraception (Trussell, 2011).

Individuals can also use an electronic hormonal fertility monitor to track changes in hormones (specifically, luteinizing hormone). Often these monitors are used by individuals who want to become pregnant, but they can also be used to prevent pregnancy and may be more effective than some traditional FAMs (e.g., cervical mucus monitoring) (Fehring, Schneider, Raviele, et al., 2013). In general, FAMs do not have many costs, but purchasing such a monitor would increase expenses by several hundred dollars.

Effectiveness

Natural family-planning methods can be highly effective methods of contraception. If they are used perfectly, only 0.4% to 5% of women using these methods in a year have an unintended pregnancy. The symptothermal method is the most effective natural family-planning method; using a calendar alone is only 87% effective in typical use. However, many of the studies have design flaws, so true effectiveness is difficult to determine (Jennings & Burke, 2011). FAMs can also be used effectively to help couples become pregnant.

Reversibility

Natural family-planning methods stop preventing pregnancies as soon as they are discontinued.

Advantages and Disadvantages

FAMs have many advantages. They are an excellent way for men and women to learn about their own fertility. They require both partners' involvement, they are free, and they may alert women to

symptothermal method A combination of natural family-planning methods, in which both temperature and signs of ovulation are observed and charted.

the need for some kind of medical attention. Their primary disadvantage is that they provide no protection against STIs, cervical mucus techniques may be complicated by vaginal infections and different stages of life (e.g., perimenopause), and the couple must be vigorously committed to abstaining from intercourse during fertile times. When both partners are more motivated to avoid pregnancy, FAM is more effective (Fehring, Schneider, Barron, & Pruszynski, 2013). If the couple is not rigorous about following the methods or has intercourse during fertile periods, pregnancy is likely to occur.

▮ Prescription Methods

Oral Contraceptives

Although many methods of contraception are available to U.S. women, **oral contraceptives (OCs)**, which are pills taken daily to prevent pregnancy, have been one of the most commonly used methods in the United States since 1982 (Daniels, Mosher, & Jones, 2013). OCs can be categorized as monophasic formulations, in which all the active pills contain the same amount of hormone, and multiphasic formulations, in which the active pills throughout the cycle contain varying amounts of progestin and/or estrogen (Nelson & Cwiak, 2011).

The **combined pill** or **combined oral contraceptive (COC)**, used since the 1960s, contains both estrogen and progestin (synthetic progesterone). To use the COC, a woman ingests the first pill in the packet and takes a pill each succeeding day. Most packets contain 28 pills, but some contain only 21. Most 28-pill packets contain 7 pills that have no benefit other than convenience. The woman does not stop taking her pills and then have to remember to resume taking them 7 days later—as is required if using the 21-day packets. Usually menstruation occurs on the 23rd or 24th day (2 or 3 days after the last pill containing a hormone is ingested). Newer formulations have different numbers of hormonal and placebo pills; for example, some have only 5 reminder pills. In 2003, the FDA approved an extended version of the COC called Seasonale. It has 84 consecutive hormone-containing pills followed by 7 placebo pills, resulting in only 4 menstrual periods per year rather than the monthly periods associated with traditional pill cycles. Newer formulations of extended-version OCs follow a similar pattern but appear to control side effects better.

The COC's estrogen signals the brain's hypothalamus to prevent the pituitary gland from producing follicle-stimulating hormone (FSH) and luteinizing hormone (LH); the progesterone also inhibits LH production. Ovulation is suppressed. This suppression mimics the changes that occur in pregnancy.

The progestin-only pill was introduced in 1972. In spite of its lack of estrogen (high dosages of which were found to be related to physical complications), the **minipill (POP)** never achieved a great deal of popularity, and the percentage of women using it remains relatively low. To use this type of OC, a woman takes a pill on the first day of menstruation and every day thereafter. Because progestin is included in every pill, the hormone is ingested daily. With POPs, ovulation is suppressed in approximately 50% of the cycles (Zieman & Hatcher, 2012). However, the main mechanism of action is the thickening of cervical mucus, which inhibits the sperm from entering the uterus. In addition, the endometrium is thinned, which prevents implantation. Sperm motility is also affected. POPs are appropriate for women who cannot use estrogen.

The chemical composition of OCs has changed over the years in response to research on their effects and side effects. In early birth control pills, the typical amount of estrogen was 0.15 milligrams (mg) and 10 mg of progestin. In 1968, fewer than 1% of retail prescriptions for OCs contained less than 0.05 mg of estrogen. In 1988, approximately 82% of retail prescriptions contained less than 0.05 mg of estrogen. In the 1970s, it was found that use of the higher-dosage pills (more than 0.05 mg) was related to cardiovascular complications. Today those higher-dosage pills are still available and are used by women with specific medical problems such as uterine bleeding and endometriosis. However, most OCs using estrogen now contain between 0.02 and 0.035 mg and 1.0 mg to 1.2 mg of progestin.

Regardless of which pill is used, a backup method of contraception should be employed for the first 7 days of pill use and as a precaution if a pill is forgotten for 2 or more days in a row. If a pill is forgotten on one day, that pill should be taken immediately and the next pill taken as regularly scheduled.

Some medications interfere with the effectiveness of OCs. Women should check with their healthcare provider before taking any medication. Previously, some antibiotics were thought to affect pill function, but further research has shown that pregnancy risk is not affected by broad-spectrum antibiotics; only grisiofulvin and rifampicin appear to affect COC effectiveness (Zieman & Hatcher, 2012). There is no medical reason

---

oral contraceptive (OC) A daily pill taken to prevent pregnancy.

combined pill or combined oral contraceptive (COC) Oral contraceptive containing estrogen and progestin.

minipill (POP) A progestin-only birth control pill.

for a woman to "take a break" from pill use (Zieman & Hatcher, 2012).

In the United States, OCs require a visit to a healthcare provider—which typically includes a pelvic exam and possibly other screening—and a prescription. A follow-up exam is often required 3 or 6 months after starting OCs, with annual visits thereafter. To increase access to contraceptives, there is a growing interest in making OCs available over the counter—an idea supported by some physician groups (American Academy of Family Physicians, 2014; American College of Obstetricians and Gynecologists, 2012). While this notion may seem radical, only about one-third of other countries require a prescription to obtain oral contraception, with many requiring no health screening at all (Grindlay, Burns, & Grossman, 2013). A survey of U.S. women showed that almost one-third were strongly in favor of OCs being sold over the counter, with an additional one-third being somewhat in favor. Women who were younger, were single, were living in the South, and had private insurance or no insurance were more likely to report support of over-the-counter OCs (Grossman et al., 2013).

Effectiveness

Oral contraceptives provide one of the most effective means of preventing pregnancy. Only 3 in 1,000 women using OCs become pregnant in 1 year of perfect use. Among typical users—for example, some who forget to take their pills as directed—as many as 9% become pregnant in the first year (Trussell, 2011).

It cannot be overemphasized that OCs provide *no* protection from STIs. Unless one is in a 100% monogamous relationship with a partner who has

Gender DIMENSIONS

Margaret H. Sanger: A Woman of Influence

In 1931, the futurist H. G. Wells said Margaret H. Sanger (1879–1966) started the most influential movement of all time (Lehfeldt, 1967). In 1998, she was recognized among the 100 most important people of the 20th century by *Time* magazine. In the 21st century, her life concerns—health disparities due to poverty, the burdens of unintended pregnancy, and women's access to safe methods of birth control—are still problems, but are now recognized public health priorities. In her lifetime, Margaret Sanger was a catalyst for contraceptive research, an emancipator of women, and a practicing nurse among the marginalized and poor who eventually became known as the woman who established the American birth-control movement.

Margaret H. Sanger was born in 1879, the sixth child of a working-class, Irish Catholic family in New York. As a young nurse tending to the poor on the Lower East Side, Sanger witnessed the severe illness and even death that women suffered when attempting self-induced abortions (Hymowitz & Weissman, 1978). Seeing such tragedy combined with "revolting conditions," where extreme poverty and child labor added to the misery, moved Sanger to find the "secret" of preventing unwanted pregnancies (Lehfeldt, 1967).

The barriers she faced were huge. At first, Sanger began in earnest by writing her radical journal *The Woman Rebel* as well as the *Family Limitation* pamphlet.

Even though she did not give instructions regarding specific methods for contraception, the Comstock Laws' definition of "obscene, lewd, lascivious" matter was cited to have her arrested and eventually jailed (Jensen, 1981). Sanger temporarily fled to Europe, where she was introduced to the various contraceptive technologies currently available, as well as several European benefactors and professionals who championed her cause, including British sexologist Havelock Ellis. Based on these experiences, Sanger believed that the diaphragm, along with spermicidal jellies, were the secrets to having a simple, cheap, harmless contraceptive that could be used throughout the world (Lehfeldt, 1967).

In the latter part of Sanger's career, she concentrated on the development of new contraceptive technologies—specifically oral contraceptives. Through the Planned Parenthood Foundation, she arranged for the first grant supporting investigation of progestinal compounds for the purpose of contraception. She obtained additional funding for the scientists who would later be recognized as the inventors of the oral contraceptive (Lehfeldt, 1967). Although she received neither the Nobel Peace Prize nor the Presidential Freedom Award for which she was nominated, she was successful in searching for safe, effective forms of birth control, offering the leading voice in the development of oral contraceptives, as well as providing the foundations for Planned Parenthood.

CONTRACEPTIVE TIMELINE

Ancient Practices—Coitus interruptus (the withdrawal method) was first mentioned in the Biblical Book of Genesis (Genesis 38:8).

1564—The earliest published description of the "condom" was by the Italian anatomist Gabriel Fallopius in 1564. The term "condom" was likely derived from the Latin word *condus*, meaning "receptacle" (Birth control, 2009).

1873—State and federal legislation, collectively referred to as the Comstock Laws, prohibited the importation or mailing of obscene matter. Obscene matter included contraceptive products as well as information about those products.

1350 b.c.—As one of the earliest forms of the condom, Egyptian men may have placed linen sheaths on the penis before intercourse. It is difficult to determine the accuracy of this claim; this time period covers prehistorical events, and evidence suggests that Egyptians worshipped the god of fertility (Youssef, 1993).

1840 through 1870s—Paralleling Charles Goodyear's vulcanization of rubber in the first half of the 19th century, the rubber condom became a popular choice of contraception. Other rubber-made contraceptive products, such as the earliest intrauterine devices, douching syringes, and diaphragms, were referred to as "womb veils" (Birth control, 2009; *Timeline*, 2002).

1879—Margaret H. Sanger was born Maggie Louise Higgins (*Timeline*, 2002).

1881—Surgical occlusion of the fallopian tubes (e.g., the first female sterilization) was performed by an Ohio surgeon (Birth control, 2009).

1957–1972—Hormonal contraceptives became the new face for birth control. Although approved early on by the U.S. FDA, oral contraceptives were not legally available to all women (e.g., married and unmarried) in every state until 1972 (Birth control, 2009; *Timeline*, 2002).

1967—12.5 million women used "the pill" worldwide (*Timeline*, 2002).

1984—Between 50 million and 80 million women used "the pill" worldwide (*Timeline*, 2002).

1998—Margaret Sanger was named to *Time* magazine's list of 100 Most Important People of the 20th Century.

1963—2.3 million American women used some type of oral contraceptive (*Timeline*, 2002).

1973—The landmark U.S. Supreme Court decision in *Roe v. Wade* effectively legalized abortion in the United States. A woman's right to an abortion became protected by her constitutional right to privacy (Hock, 2007).

1993—The FDA approved the first female condom under the brand name Reality (FDA, 1993).

20th Century—*Hormones*, from the Greek *hormaô*, meaning "stir up" or "incite," were isolated (e.g., estrogen). This development opened the door for the hormonally based methods of contraception in the latter half of the 20th century (Birth control, 2009).

1916—Sanger opened the first birth control clinic in the United States. Ten days after the opening, the clinic was raided, all birth control devices were confiscated, and Sanger was arrested and jailed (Hock, 2007).

1950s and 1960s—Strong arguments were made for the acceptance and use of oral contraceptives. Factors included advancements in hormonal/synthetic research, growth in pro-contraceptive sociopolitical movements, and federal government policy decisions supporting an individual's right to personal privacy.

1914—Pioneer Margaret Sanger published the first major statement on birth control and contraception in her pamphlet *Family Limitations* (Jensen, 1981). She coined the term "birth control" and challenged women to use the term from the pages of her radical journal *The Woman Rebel* (*Timeline*, 2002).

1923—Sanger opened the first legal birth control clinic in the United States (*Timeline*, 2002).

1936—In the *United States v. One Package of Japanese Pessaries*, the court ruled that contraceptives could be sent through the mail if they were to be intelligently employed by conscientious physicians for (1) the purpose of saving life or (2) promoting the well-being of their patients (Birth control, 2009). This decision marked a reversal of one of the last surviving Comstock Laws (Hock, 2007).

1951—The Roman Catholic Church sanctioned the use of the rhythm method, but remained opposed to any other form of birth control, including "the pill." Pope Paul VI issued the encyclical *Humanae Vitae* ("Of Human Life") in 1968 as the authoritative guide for birth regulation among many Catholics (Catholic Church, 1968).

1999—The FDA approved the emergency contraceptive Plan B by prescription only. Although emergency contraceptives had been available since the 1970s, Plan B found a new generation of consumers.

2002–2004—New forms of hormonal contraceptives (extended-use pills, implants, patch, vaginal ring) were introduced. Many of these methods either reduce or eliminate a woman's menstrual cycle.

2009—Plan B becomes available over the counter to women 17 and older, but those under 17 must acquire a prescription. A one-pill version of Plan B (Plan B One Step) is approved by the FDA.

2013—FDA approves Plan B One Step for over-the-counter use without age restriction.

2008—Four federally funded longitudinal studies showed abstinence-only sex education is associated with (1) no significant impact on teen sexual activity, (2) no differences in rates of unprotected sex, and (3) some impacts on knowledge of STIs and perceived effectiveness of condoms and birth control pills (Trenholm et al., 2007).

2010—ella, a single dose EC pill is approved by the FDA.

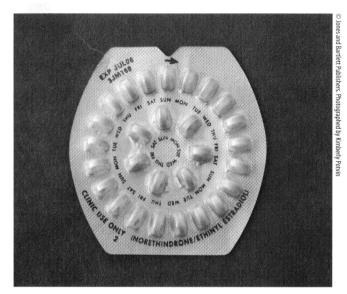

Although oral contraceptives are effective in preventing pregnancy, they offer no protection against STIs or HIV. For protection against pregnancy and STIs, combine the use of oral contraceptives and latex condoms.

been tested for STIs and HIV, a condom must be used for each act of intercourse.

Reversibility

Discontinuation of OCs provides an immediate return of fertility. For most women, there may be a delay of 1 to 2 weeks for ovulation to occur. Some women may experience amenorrhea (absence of menses), although this phenomenon is more common in women with a history of irregular periods (Zieman & Hatcher, 2012).

Advantages and Disadvantages

Birth control pills have been reported as being 92% effective as actually used and 99.7% effective if used correctly all the time (Trussell, 2011). In addition to being effective, the pill does not necessitate interrupting sexual activity. An added benefit for some women is that it helps to regulate the menstrual cycle. Other side effects can include increased breast size, reduction in acne, elimination of mittelschmerz (a sensation of abdominal pain that sometimes occurs during ovulation), and reduction of menstrual cramps. For estrogen-related problems with the combination pill, the progestin-only pill is recommended both because it contains no estrogen and because its low progestin dosage is thought to reduce adverse effects that progestin might otherwise cause.

COCs are very safe. In addition to protecting a woman against pregnancy, they lower a woman's risk of ovarian cancer, endometrial cancer, breast masses, and ovarian cysts. They also lessen menstrual blood loss, cramps, and acne. Their primary disadvantage for sexually active college students is that they provide *no* protection against STIs, including HIV.

Symptoms indicating a severe problem with OCs usually develop within 3 to 6 months of starting the pill, but they can develop later. Abdominal pain, chest pain, shortness of breath, headaches, eye problems such as blurred vision, and severe leg pain are examples of such symptoms. If a woman experiences any of these symptoms, she should call the doctor. The most severe health risk associated with COCs is a greater risk of circulatory system diseases, including heart attacks and strokes. If a woman is obese, diabetic, or hypertensive, the risk of circulatory system diseases is greatly increased; women with any of these risk factors should use a different method (Nelson & Cwiak, 2011). Smoking is also a risk factor, especially for heavy smokers and smokers older than 35 years. In addition, women with liver function problems, hypertension, circulatory problems, heart disease, breast cancer, asthma, varicose veins, or migraine headaches should avoid using COCs (Nelson & Cwiak, 2011).

There has been considerable debate over the years about whether OC use can lead to breast cancer. After more than 50 studies and 50 years, most experts believe that low-dose COCs have little—if any—effect on the risk of developing breast cancer. Multiple studies have found no increased risk for breast cancer among women currently using OCs, with use of OCs by women with a family history of breast cancer, or with initiation of OCs use at a young age (Nelson & Cwiak, 2011). Breast cancers diagnosed in women currently using OCs or women who have taken OCs in the past are more likely to be localized (less likely to be metastatic). By the age of 55, the risk of having had breast cancer diagnosed is the same for women who have used OCs and those who have not. While there may be some unanswered questions about OCs and breast cancer, today the overall conclusion is that OCs do not cause breast cancer (Zieman & Hatcher, 2012).

Emergency Contraception

Condoms sometimes slip or break; women forget more than two contraceptive pills in a row; the man ejaculates too close to the vulva even though he withdraws; a couple vowing abstinence has intercourse anyway. For all these cases, **emergency contraception (EC)** is available. In addition, EC is available

emergency contraception (EC) The use of oral contraception or insertion of an IUD after unprotected sex has occurred at midcycle.

Myth **vs** Fact

Myth: Birth control pills cause cancer.

Fact: Birth control pills are very safe. Women who have taken birth control pills have a 25% reduction in risk for benign breast disease. Furthermore, the pill is protective against other cancers such as ovarian and endometrial cancer as well as death from colon cancer. Thus, women using the pill are less likely to contract cancer than women who have never been on the pill.

Myth: You need to take a break from the pill.

Fact: Women can stay on oral contraceptives as long as medical side effects do not develop. There is no need to take a break.

Myth: All condoms protect against STIs.

Fact: Only latex, polyurethane, and polyisoprene condoms protect against STIs. Animal skin condoms provide no protection against STIs.

Myth: Condoms protect against all STIs.

Fact: Condoms are highly effective at preventing the spread of such infections transmitted through fluids, such as HIV infection, chlamydia, and gonorrhea. While they reduce the risk of STIs that are transmitted through skin-to-skin or genital contact—such as genital warts, herpes, syphilis, and crabs (pubic lice)—they are not completely effective in providing protection against them, as pubic hair and other parts of the genitals are not covered by the condom.

Myth: Withdrawal is not a method of birth control.

Fact: Withdrawal is about as effective as barrier methods. It is much better than using nothing.

Myth: Once a person has had penile–vaginal sex, he or she can no longer practice abstinence.

Fact: Abstinence is always a choice. Many teens, college students, and adults choose abstinence even though they have already had oral, penile–vaginal, or anal sex.

Two types of emergency contraceptive pills are available in the United States. The first type, a progestin-only one-pill dose, is available over-the-counter to individuals regardless of age. The second type, ella, is also a one-pill formulation. It is a progesterone receptor moderator and is available with a prescription.

in cases of rape or incest. There are three main types of EC: hormonal pills, a pill containing ulipristal acetate, and a copper-T intrauterine device (IUD).

COCs can also be used, and have been since the 1960s, as EC. However, the estrogen in the COC formulations often causes nausea, so antinausea medication is needed. The dosages in COCs used for EC are four to five times the daily dosage and require taking two doses 12 hours apart.

Today, hormonal pills are available that are specifically designed for use as EC. These progestin-only formulations consist of one pill that should be taken within 72 hours of unprotected intercourse to be most effective. If taken within this window, the EC will decrease the risk of pregnancy by 81% to 90% (Kaiser Family Foundation, 2014). Some recent studies indicate that the progestin-only pills may not be as effective in overweight and obese women. For women with a body mass index (BMI) greater than 25, use of progestin-only EC is not recommended.

Another single-dose pill for use as EC is ella, which contains 30 mg of ulipristal acetate, a progesterone receptor modulator. It is available by prescription only and is approved by the FDA for use up to 120 hours after unprotected penile–vaginal sex. Some studies have shown ella to be less effective in obese women, so it is not recommended for women with a BMI greater than 35.

Regardless of the type of EC used, the sooner the pills are taken, the greater the chance that pregnancy will be avoided. If a woman is already pregnant or becomes pregnant following the use of EC, there are no documented negative impacts on fetal development.

The most effective method of EC is insertion of a copper-T IUD, which reduces the pregnancy risk by 99%. Women can have the device inserted up to 120 hours after unprotected sex, and it can be left in place to provide continuous contraception for up to 12 years. Unlike pill-based EC, there are no efficacy concerns related to weight with the insertion of the copper-T IUD. While all women are not equally good candidates for IUD use (Trussell & Raymond, 2011), more clinicians and researchers are recommending IUDs as an emergency contraception option for more women because of the increased effectiveness and the continued pregnancy prevention (Cleland et al., 2012).

How EC prevents pregnancy depends on the day of the menstrual cycle on which the pills are taken. Several mechanisms are possible—inhibition of ovulation, prevention of fertilization, or interference with implantation. It is important to differentiate that EC is not an **abortifacient**, meaning that it does not disrupt an implanted fertilized ovum (Zieman & Hatcher, 2012).

Knowledge and access are critical barriers that keep EC from being widely used, yet research has clearly demonstrated that access does not increase sexual behavior, nor does it diminish use of other methods of contraception (Zieman & Hatcher, 2012). Some university clinics offer EC as part of their reproductive health services. If they do not, a good resource to learn more about EC and ways to access it in the United States and other countries is http://ec.princeton.edu and its companion hotline 888-NOT-2-LATE.

Effectiveness
To be most effective, EC should be used before ovulation. Taking the pills as soon as possible after an unprotected act of penile–vaginal sex will also increase the effectiveness. Studies indicate that using COCs for EC can reduce pregnancy risk by 75%, with progestin-only EC pills being more effective (81–90%) within 72 hours after unprotected penile–vaginal sex. Studies have indicated that the medication can be moderately effective if taken between 72 and 120 hours, but this is not ideal. Ella is the most effective pill option, especially on days 4 and 5 after the unprotected coitus. However, because it is available through prescription only and has a higher cost, gaining access to this medication may not be as easy as with the other options. The most effective method is the insertion of a copper-T IUD, which prevents pregnancy 99.9% of the time (Trussell & Raymond, 2011).

Advantages and Disadvantages
The advantage to EC is that it is the only method available if unprotected intercourse has occurred when fertility is likely. EC should not be used as a regular method of contraception. It is significantly less effective than other methods, and its long-term use has not been studied. It also provides no protection against STIs. Because EC has no impact on existing pregnancies, there is no need to test for pregnancy before taking it. However, if menses do not occur within 21 days, a pregnancy test should be done. After using EC, it is critical that another regular method of contraception be established to prevent future "emergencies."

The Combined Contraceptive Patch

The first contraceptive patch, Ortho Evra, became available in the United States in March 2003. Similar to the nicotine patch, the contraceptive patch releases a steady dose of medication through the skin—in this case, the hormones estrogen and progestin. Users wear the patch, which is approximately the size of a matchbook, on the lower abdomen, buttocks, upper arm, or upper torso (but not breasts). Each patch is used for 7 days, but contains sufficient hormone for 9 days; then it is removed and discarded. Patches are worn for 3 weeks, followed by a patch-free week to allow menstruation to occur. The patch delivers a higher dosage of hormones compared to other combined hormonal methods—approximately 60% more than most COCs and 3 times more than the vaginal ring (Zieman & Hatcher, 2012). Studies are investigating the effectiveness of contraceptive patches that provide lower doses of hormones, but these products remain in clinical trials (Kaunitz, Mishell, & Foegh, 2012; Kaunitz et al., 2015; Wiegratz et al., 2014).

Effectiveness
The patch is approximately as effective as COCs. It is 99.7% effective when used perfectly; for typical use, it has a 91% user effectiveness rate. Some clinicians recommend using a different method if the patient weighs more than 198 pounds. The patch prevents pregnancy by the same mechanisms as COCs—that is, by preventing ovulation, thickening the cervical mucus, and suppressing endometrial growth (Zieman & Hatcher, 2012).

Advantages and Disadvantages
This method is comparable to COCs in menstrual advantages. It adheres well to the skin. The Ortho Evra patch is light colored; women with darker skin tones may not be comfortable wearing it. Although weight is a restricting factor, age is not, and compliance among teens is good. Disadvantages include breakthrough bleeding and spotting in early use, lack of STI protection, and visibility on the skin. The primary side effects of the patch are similar to those associated with COCs, such as headache and nausea, although some individuals report skin reactions at the application site (Nada, 2011).

Injectables

Combined injectables—that is, injectable contraceptives that contain both a progestin and an

---

abortifacient A medical method that causes an embryo or fetus to die.

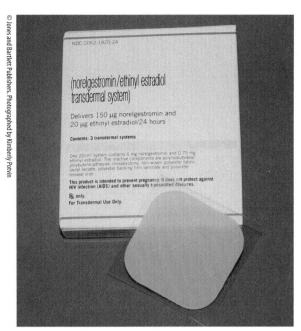

Ortho Evra, the birth control patch, contains hormones similar to those in combined oral contraceptives. However, the patch needs to be changed only once a week, minimizing the margin of error and the subsequent decreased effectiveness that is often observed with oral contraceptives.

estrogen—are gaining new attention among family planning clients and providers. Combined formulations are generally injected once a month, compared with once every 2 or 3 months for progestin-only injectables such as norethindrone enanthate (NET-EN) and depot-medroxyprogesterone acetate (DMPA; Depo-Provera). Compared with progestin-only injectables, combined injectables disturb vaginal bleeding patterns less and allow earlier return to ovulation after women discontinue use. Although combined injectable contraception has been available worldwide for years, no such options are currently available in the United States. (The FDA approved Lunelle in 2000, but it is no longer available.) Worldwide, the combined injectable contraceptives are supported by the Word Health Organization (WHO) and other organizations (WHO & Johns Hopkins University, 2011).

Depo-Provera is another form of a progestin-only contraception method. It is an injection that is given every 12 weeks. Depo-Provera suppresses ovulation by inhibiting production of FSH and LH.

Effectiveness

Depo-Provera is even more effective than the pill. In 1 year, only 0.2% of women using Depo-Provera become pregnant. Also, because it is an injection, there is no chance that a typical user can use it incorrectly, unless she does not return in 3 months for her next shot. Many couples prefer Depo-Provera because its use does not affect the spontaneity of sexual activity.

Reversibility

For Depo-Provera users, fertility may resume immediately after 13 weeks have passed since the last injection. However, studies show that women generally do not conceive for an average of 10 months after the date of the last injection (Zieman & Hatcher, 2012). In contrast, women who stop using combined injectables can become pregnant as soon as 6 weeks after their last injection (WHO & Johns Hopkins University, 2011).

Advantages and Disadvantages

Depo-Provera is easy for a woman to use, simply requiring that she return to the clinic every 3 months. It does not interrupt sexual activity, and it is one of the most effective methods of preventing pregnancies.

Depo-Provera has few practical disadvantages. Women do need to have injections every 3 months, which may be difficult for some to schedule. Significant weight gain is a common side effect, with an average gain of 5 pounds reported in the first year. Obese adolescents who use Depo-Provera have significantly more weight gain than those starting COCs (Zieman & Hatcher, 2012). Many women report changes in their periods; some have no periods on Depo-Provera, while others have frequent bleeding. Spotting between periods is common in the first months of use. Temporary and reversible bone density

Depo-Provera (DMPA) An injectable progestin-only contraceptive.

FIGURE **7.5** The IUD is inserted past the cervix into the uterus. Before insertion, the length of the uterus is measured with an instrument called a *sound*. Upon insertion, the arms of the IUD gradually unfold. Once the inserter is removed, the threads attached to the IUD are clipped to extend into the vagina through the cervical opening.

loss is also associated with Depo-Provera, so calcium supplements are often recommended for users. After discontinuing the medication, bone density returns to normal levels. A major disadvantage to Depo-Provera is that it provides no protection against STIs.

Implants

Implants are small plastic rods or capsules containing progestin that are inserted into the nondominant upper arm of a woman by her healthcare provider. The rod or capsule releases progestin, which prevents pregnancy by (1) thickening the cervical mucus, which blocks the sperm from meeting the egg, and (2) disrupting the menstrual cycle and preventing ovulation (WHO & Johns Hopkins University, 2011). Depending on the brand, implants last anywhere from 3 to 7 years. They may be replaced immediately following the end of life of the previous implant.

Implants are available under the brand names Implanon, Norplant, Jadelle (Norplant II), and Sino-Implant (II). Currently, Implanon and Nexplanon, which are both effective for 3 years, are the only implants available in the United States. These implants are almost identical, at 4 cm long and 2 mm in diameter, and they release the same amount of hormone. Nexplanon, however, has a coating that allows it to be seen via X ray and a preloaded applicator to make insertion easier.

Effectiveness
The efficacy rate for implants is fewer than 1 pregnancy per 100 users per year (5 pregnancies per 10,000 women). However, some evidence suggests that the effectiveness of some implants decreases for women who weigh more than 150–176 pounds (WHO & Johns Hopkins University, 2011), although other experts do not consider the implants to have decreased efficacy in overweight women (Zieman & Hatcher, 2012). As with all implants, the risk of pregnancy increases slightly after the first year of use and continues during its lifespan (WHO & Johns Hopkins University, 2011).

Reversibility
Implants are considered a reversible form of birth control, as the woman returns to normal fertility once the implant is removed.

Advantages and Disadvantages
Implants are safe for nearly all women, including women who cannot take estrogen. Irregular bleeding (e.g., between 6 and 12 months) is the primary side effect but is not harmful. Once the implant is in place, very little maintenance by the user is required. The disadvantages include unpredictable or irregular menstrual bleeding, hormonal side effects (of which headache is most common), and lack of STI protection (WHO & Johns Hopkins University, 2011).

Intrauterine Devices

Intrauterine devices (IUDs) are reversible methods of contraception. Four types of IUDs are currently available in the United States: ParaGard Copper-T, Mirena, Skyla, and Liletta. All are T-shaped plastic devices that are inserted through the vagina and cervix into the uterus to prevent pregnancy (Figure 7.5). A spherical ball-shaped IUD is currently being studied but is not yet available for use outside clinical trials (Baram, Weinstein, & Trussell, 2014; Ilan, Ariel, & Seidman Daniel, 2014).

intrauterine device (IUD) Synthetic device that is inserted into the uterus to prevent the sperm from fertilizing the ovum.

The ParaGard Copper-T is also labeled for use as an EC and can remain in place for 12 years. During that time, women experience regular menstrual cycles that may involve heavier flow or more cramping than prior to insertion of the IUD. Mirena, Skyla, and Liletta release a progestin hormone (levonorgestrel); Mirena is effective for 5 years and Skyla and Liletta are effective for 3 years. Skyla is sometimes referred to as "Mirena's little sister" because it is similar to Mirena in mechanism and shape but is smaller in size and releases less hormone. Skyla has specifically been approved by the FDA for use in women who have not had a child, and because of its reduced size may cause less discomfort when being inserted. Liletta, approved by the FDA in 2015, is being marketed as a low-cost but equally effective IUD for women with and without children. Use of hormonal IUDs reduces or may eliminate menstrual flow over time, although some initial irregular spotting or breakthrough bleeding may occur after insertion of the device. This effect is less noticeable with Skyla than with Mirena (National Campaign to Prevent Teen and Unplanned Pregnancy, 2015).

The intrauterine copper contraceptive works primarily as a spermicide, immobilizing sperm so they rarely reach the fallopian tube, thereby preventing fertilization. Evidence suggests that copper IUDs do not work after fertilization has already occurred. The hormone levonorgestrel in the other IUDs operates differently; it causes cervical mucus to thicken so sperm cannot enter the upper reproductive tract to reach an ovum. Changes in uterotubal fluid also restrict sperm movement. Finally, the endometrium is altered to prevent implantation. In the first years of use, IUDs with hormones inhibit ovulation as well (Zieman & Hatcher, 2012).

IUDs are a highly effective method of birth control and the copper-T IUD is a good alternative to hormone-based methods. Worldwide, IUDs are the most commonly used reversible contraceptive (Zieman & Hatcher, 2012); however, the rate of IUD use in the United States is not comparable to that in other regions. Many misperceptions about the IUD exist, such as that use causes increased risk of pelvic inflammatory disease (PID) and infertility and that IUDs are only for women who have had children or do not want more children. Several studies have confirmed the safety and efficacy of IUDs for the great majority of women (Doyle et al., 2008; Kaneshiro & Aeby, 2010), demonstrated that former IUD users are no more likely than other women to be infertile (WHO & Johns Hopkins University, 2011), and shown that women conceive within 1 year of IUD removal at rates similar to those who have never used contraception (Ramchandran & Salem, 2008).

Effectiveness
The IUD is one of the most effective contraceptive methods. Because compliance is not an issue, its typical use efficacy and perfect-use efficacy are nearly the same. For the copper-T IUD, the pregnancy rate has been fewer than 1 pregnancy per 100 women each year. Mirena, Skylar, and Liletta effectiveness rates are comparable to those for female sterilization (0.01%, 0.04%, and 0.05%, respectively). Women are advised to check the strings to assure the IUD is still in place; failure to do so accounts for the minor difference in effectiveness rates.

Reversibility
Once the IUD is removed, fertility resumes immediately. Compared to possible detrimental effects of other hormonal contraceptives (COCs, implants, injectables) on subsequent fertility, the use of Mirena does not affect the conception rate; all users in one study conceived within 1 month of discontinuation (Backman et al., 2004). Additionally, 72% to 96% of women conceived within 1 year of having their IUD removed; this rate is comparable to levels among women who have never used contraception (85%) (Ramchandran & Salem, 2008).

Advantages and Disadvantages
The IUD is an excellent contraceptive method for most women. In addition to being highly effective, it is easy to use and has no systemic side effects. A major advantage of the IUD is that once inserted it remains in place, so planning before intercourse is unnecessary. (When it is in place, a string attached to the IUD emerges through the cervix. The woman feels for the string to make sure the IUD is present, because it is possible for it to pass out of the uterus with the menstrual flow or at other times. The device can also be removed by a physician by means of this string.) Other advantages of the IUD include probable protection against endometrial cancer and possible protection against cervical cancer. The copper version has additional advantages as an option for women who cannot use hormonal methods, the length of effectiveness (12 years), and use as an EC. All types of IUDs offer a rapid return to fertility, reduce the woman's risk of ectopic pregnancy, offer convenience as a single insertion that provides 3 to 12 years of protection depending on the type, provide cost-effectiveness in terms of the greatest net benefit of any contraceptive if used for more than 2 years, and are associated with a high level of user satisfaction.

In terms of disadvantages, the copper-T IUD may cause increased monthly blood loss (menorrhagia) and possibly anemia due to lowered hemoglobin levels in some users. Conversely, Mirena actually increases hemoglobin levels over the years of usage

Myth vs Fact

by reducing or eliminating menstrual flow (amenorrhea). IUDs also require an office procedure for their insertion and removal; both procedures can be uncomfortable. Some protocols recommend a chlamydia/gonorrhea check before insertion, as these STIs could lead to the development of PID as a consequence of the insertion process. This contraceptive method offers no protection from HIV or other STIs. Expulsion of the IUD, either obviously with cramping or bleeding, or silently without the user's awareness, places the woman at risk for pregnancy (Zieman & Hatcher, 2012). The likelihood of expulsion declines over time, but women who have expelled one IUD have about a one in three chance of expelling another (Zieman & Hatcher, 2012).

While the IUD has some disadvantages, more clinicians are recommending it as one type of long-acting reversible contraception (LARC). Given the high rates of unplanned pregnancy in the United States, the need for more consistent and correct use of birth control is a priority. Using LARC—specifically, IUDs and implants—requires less user involvement, so the risk of pregnancy is also decreased.

Diaphragm

When in place, the **diaphragm** prevents sperm from traveling through the uterus and up the fallopian tubes to fertilize an egg, and it holds spermicide against the cervix (Figure 7.6). The diaphragm is a shallow rubber (or synthetic rubber) cap surrounding a flexible metal ring that covers the cervix.

Diaphragms are available in several sizes and styles. Because the diaphragm's purpose is to prevent sperm from going beyond the vagina, its size and shape are very important. If the diaphragm does not fit exactly right, a chance exists that sperm can bypass this barrier. Clearly, using someone else's diaphragm is a poor idea. Diaphragms are fitted by a clinician and refitted after women give birth or gain or lose a significant amount of weight. Fit should also be checked during the yearly gynecological exam, and the diaphragm should be replaced every 2 years or with any signs of wear or damage.

The diaphragm must remain in place for at least 6 hours after intercourse, and spermicide must be added for *each* act of intercourse. This combination of requirements, besides increasing effectiveness, allows the male and female to share the responsibility for contraception. Diaphragms should be removed at least once every 24 hours to reduce the risk of toxic shock syndrome.

Effectiveness

When inserted properly and used with spermicide, the diaphragm is theoretically 94% effective and 88% effective as actually used. The contraceptive effectiveness of diaphragms without a spermicide containing N-9 has been insufficiently studied. However, this combination should be assumed to decrease effectiveness. Women infected with or at high risk for HIV, however, should *not* use spermicides containing N-9 (WHO & Johns Hopkins University, 2011).

© Jones and Bartlett Publishers. Photographed by Kimberly Potvin

A diaphragm is a barrier method of contraception that can be used repeatedly with spermicidal cream or jelly. It requires a physician to fit the diaphragm initially.

diaphragm Shallow rubber cap that covers the cervix and prevents sperm from entering the uterus.

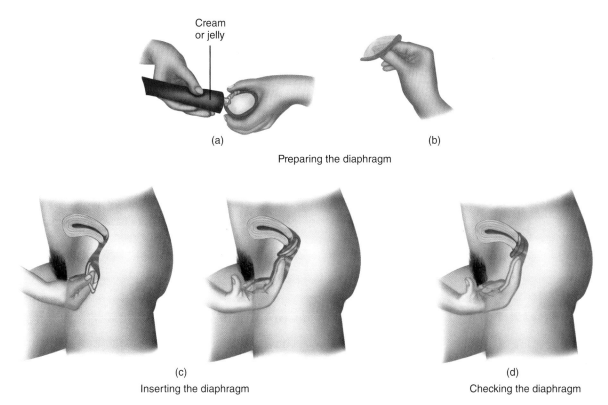

Cream
or jelly

(a)　　　　　　　　　　　　　　　　(b)

Preparing the diaphragm

(c)　　　　　　　　　　　　　　　　　　　　　(d)

Inserting the diaphragm　　　　　　　　　　　Checking the diaphragm

FIGURE **7.6** Procedure for inserting a diaphragm: (a) Before inserting the diaphragm, coat the rim and cup with a spermicidal cream or jelly. (b) Squeeze the rim of the diaphragm together between your thumb and index finger. (c) Insert the diaphragm into the vagina with the rim facing up and push it toward the small of your back. As you let go of the diaphragm, it will spring open. Continue to guide it to your cervix with the tips of your fingers. (d) Be sure to check that the diaphragm completely covers the cervix.

Reversibility
The diaphragm does not affect fertility (except when it is in place).

Advantages and Disadvantages
The major advantages of the diaphragm are that it is highly effective if used correctly and consistently, is easy to learn to use, and has no systemic side effects unless latex allergy or spermicide irritation is present. Some couples make diaphragm insertion part of foreplay. The man can insert it into the woman's vagina before penile–vaginal sex.

One disadvantage of the diaphragm is that it must be inserted properly and before penile–vaginal sex, requiring the woman or couple to plan ahead. Some women are not comfortable touching their genitals and therefore find diaphragm use uncomfortable. Diaphragms provide very limited protection against certain STIs, so condoms must also be used to prevent STI transmission. In addition, some users may experience an increased risk of urinary tract infections. Oil-based lubricants should not be used with diaphragms as they erode the rubber. Odor and risk of toxic shock syndrome may develop if the diaphragm is left in place for more than 24 hours. Severe arthritis or obesity may make insertion or removal difficult. A reaction to latex or superficial cervical erosion may cause vaginal spotting or discomfort in some women (Zieman & Hatcher, 2012).

Cervical Cap

The **cervical cap** is a silicone rubber, latex-free, dome-shaped device that covers the cervix and holds spermicidal cream or jelly. It is similar to, but smaller than, the diaphragm; is meant to stay in place longer; and is slightly less effective than the diaphragm (Figure 7.7). The first cervical cap was approved for use in the United States in 1988; currently, the FemCap is the only cervical cap available in the United States.

The cervical cap can be left in place for 48 hours. However, it must be removed during menstruation to allow the menstrual flow to leave the body. Although the cap is available in three different sizes, not all women can use it because of the variation in shapes and sizes of cervixes.

cervical cap Shallow silicone rubber device, smaller than a diaphragm, that covers the cervix to prevent sperm from entering the uterus.

The FemCap is available in three sizes based on pregnancy and birthing history.

FIGURE **7.7** It is important that the cervical cap is always inserted correctly. You should practice inserting before using the cap during penile–vaginal sex.

Effectiveness
Overall, the cervical cap and the diaphragm have similar rates of effectiveness. Theoretical effectiveness of the cervical cap ranges from 91% to 74%. The cap is much more effective in women who have never been pregnant (nulliparous women). Typical effectiveness for the cap is 84% for nulliparous women, compared to only 68% in women who have been pregnant. In nonmonogamous couples, condoms should also be used to prevent STI transmission. The same precautions and uncertainties regarding the use of N-9 apply to cervical caps.

Reversibility
The cap does not affect fertility (except when it is in place).

Advantages and Disadvantages
The cap is easy to use and has no systemic side effects unless spermicide sensitivity is present. Many women like the fact that it can be kept in place for up to 48 hours and that spermicide use for additional acts of intercourse is optional.

Disadvantages associated with cap use may include occasional irritation of the cervix, an unpleasant odor or vaginal dryness, and the potential for the cap to become dislodged during vaginal–penile sex. The cap can also cause toxic shock syndrome if it is not removed regularly.

Combined Vaginal Ring

The NuvaRing provides protection from pregnancy by releasing low doses of estrogen and progestin daily for 21 days. By comparison, low-dose estrogen contraceptive pills contain slightly more estrogen, and other contraceptive pills contain almost twice as much estrogen. Additionally, with COCs, there is a daily spike in hormone levels when the pill is swallowed, followed by a gradual drop in those levels throughout the day. In contrast, the ring provides a steady rate of hormone release. Whereas the diaphragm and the cervical cap must be positioned correctly to provide maximum protection, the NuvaRing cannot be inserted incorrectly because position does not matter; it releases hormones and does not provide a barrier for sperm.

NuvaRing costs approximately the same as a cycle of pills in pharmacies and requires a prescription to be purchased.

NuvaRing is a flexible, transparent, odorless ring that is about as big as a silver dollar and is inserted into the vagina, where it continuously releases low doses of estrogen and progestin that prevent pregnancy.

Effectiveness

NuvaRing is an effective hormonal contraceptive with a theoretical or perfect-use effectiveness rate of 99.7%. Because once it is in place there is nothing else to do, its effectiveness is greatly enhanced. User effectiveness is not yet established but is expected to be approximately 91% (Trussell, 2011).

Reversibility

Fertility is not affected after NuvaRing is removed.

Advantages and Disadvantages

NuvaRing contains the lowest serum levels of estrogen and progestin in any combined hormonal method, thereby decreasing the risks associated with synthetic estrogens. In addition, the ring does not require any daily action, such as taking a pill each day as is the case for COCs. All that is required is replacement of the ring after 21 days or 1 month. Some women may consider this method more private than others because there is no visible patch or need to take a daily pill. Furthermore, most women cannot feel the ring when it is in place and report being satisfied with this method of contraception.

As with all methods of contraception, there are also disadvantages associated with NuvaRing. The risk of synthetic estrogen is not eliminated; it is merely reduced with the lower dose. Therefore, as is true with other hormonal methods that contain both estrogen and progestin, smokers and those susceptible to blood clots should not use the ring. Other side effects, such as nausea and headache, are similar to the effects noted with COCs. Vaginal discomfort and vaginitis may also occur. Partners may feel the ring during penetration, although most reported they did not perceive that to be a problem. If necessary, it can be removed for up to 3 hours without losing its effectiveness. Women must be comfortable touching their genitals; if they are not, they should consider another contraceptive method because vaginal insertion is required. In addition, NuvaRing does not offer any protection against STIs (Zieman & Hatcher, 2012).

The preceding discussion has focused on the combined vaginal ring, but there is also a progesterone-only vaginal ring currently available in some countries (but not in the United States). This method is designed to extend lactational amenorrhea among breastfeeding women. The ring is inserted in the vagina for continuous use for up to 3 months. If breastfeeding is continued and extended contraception is desired, women insert a new ring and use this method continuously for up to 1 year. Because of the type of hormone used, this method is safe for both mother and infant and is the first type of contraception designed specifically to be used during breastfeeding (Brache, Payán, & Faundes, 2013).

Permanent Methods

Sterilization

Sterilization is a form of contraception that renders a person biologically incapable of reproducing. Men and women both may choose to be sterilized—made infertile—because they have all the children they want or because they do not want to have children. Sterilization is selected as a contraceptive method by older individuals much more frequently than it is chosen by younger women. By age 35, more women rely on sterilization than OCs: 27.5% of women are either sterilized or have a partner who has been sterilized compared to 17.7% of women the same age who using OCs (Jones. Mosher, & Daniels, 2012).

Effectiveness

Male and female sterilization is highly effective. In the first year after sterilization, only 1 woman out of every 1,000 sterilized becomes pregnant, and only 1 in every 2,000 sterilized men causes a pregnancy.

Reversibility

Both men and women should consider sterilization procedures as permanent and irreversible. Thoughtful consideration should be given before undergoing any sterilization procedure. Even with counseling, some individuals may experience regret due to a change in life circumstances or other reason. Microsurgical techniques can be used to reverse male and female sterilization procedures with varying levels of success. For men, a **vasovasectomy** can result in a return of sperm to ejaculate in 75% to 100% of men, but the pregnancy rate ranges from 35% to 89%. Reversibility rates decrease as time since the procedure increases, especially after 10 years. Other factors affecting reversal are the skill of the microsurgeon, the presence of antisperm antibodies in the man, and the type of vasectomy performed (Roncari & Hou, 2011).

More recently, microsurgery has been used to reverse laparoscopy (female sterilization). The original studies showed wide ranges of success with this procedure, but more recent studies report a pregnancy rate of around 70%, with one study having an ongoing pregnancy rate of 59% and another having a birth rate of 62%. In all cases, the female's age played a critical role in the ability to become pregnant

sterilization A procedure that makes a person biologically incapable of reproducing.

vasovasectomy Reversal of a vasectomy, so that sperm can be ejaculated.

FIGURE **7.8** Vasectomy.

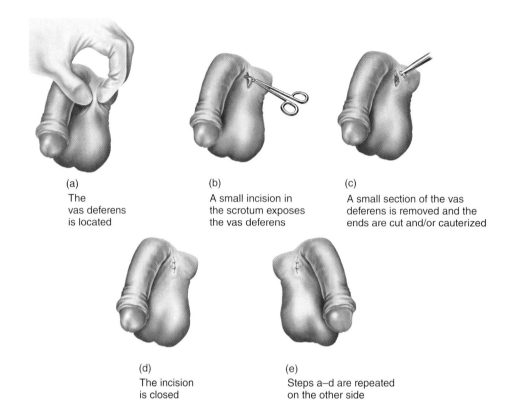

(a)
The
vas deferens
is located

(b)
A small incision in
the scrotum exposes
the vas deferens

(c)
A small section of the vas
deferens is removed and the
ends are cut and/or cauterized

(d)
The incision
is closed

(e)
Steps a–d are repeated
on the other side

(Caillet et al., 2010; Gordts et al., 2009; Schepens et al., 2011).

Advantages and Disadvantages

Sterilization is only for people who are certain that they do not want more (or any) children and who are fertile. Both female and male sterilizations have the same advantages. They are permanent, highly effective (99.9%), and cost-effective; lack side effects; do not interfere with sex; and are very safe. Their primary disadvantage is they provide no protection against STIs.

Male Sterilization

In men, sterilization entails interruption of the vas deferens in a procedure called a **vasectomy** (Figure 7.8). The vasectomy became popular as a method of contraception in the late 1960s and early 1970s. The interest in vasectomy was a result of several factors, including concern about the health hazards of OCs and extensive promotion by several national organizations (Association for Voluntary Sterilization, Planned Parenthood Federation of America, and Zero Population Growth). In addition, the medical community announced its support for vasectomy as a contraceptive method that was safe and effective.

Despite acceptance among the medical community, vasectomy continues to be an underused method. Only about 500,000 vasectomies are performed annually in the United States (Eisenberg et al., 2009). Low-income and minority men are less likely to receive a vasectomy. By recognizing these underserved groups, providers may be able to reduce the large difference in utilization, which could help close the gap between male and female sterilization rates (Eisenberg et al., 2009).

Vasectomy is a simple, minor surgical procedure that takes about 30 minutes. A small opening is made in the scrotum, and the vas deferens is severed. This severing blocks sperm from entering the ejaculate, because it has no route out of the testes. Clips and plugs can also be used to interfere with the vas deferens passageway; the most widely used technique involves cutting the vas and sealing off its ends (by suturing or cauterization). Vasectomies are done under local anesthesia and require minimal care afterward. Vasectomized men are instructed to avoid hard labor or strenuous exercise for several days, to wear a scrotal support for a week, and to apply ice and take mild painkillers for postoperative discomfort. As soon as the man feels ready, he may resume sexual intercourse.

Unlike female sterilization, a vasectomy does not provide immediate infertility. Sperm may still

vasectomy Cutting or cauterizing of the vas deferens to prevent sperm from being ejaculated; a means of sterilization.

be stored in the urethra or elsewhere in the reproductive tract and may not be expelled for 10 weeks or more. The amount of time required to expel this sperm depends partly on the frequency of ejaculation. For this reason, men are asked to return to the physician after the vasectomy with a semen specimen to be tested for the presence of motile sperm. This may require more than one visit. Until the absence of sperm is verified, another method of contraception is required to prevent conception.

Female Sterilization

Female sterilization takes several forms. The goal is to prevent the egg from moving down the fallopian tube to be fertilized by a sperm. Currently, most female sterilization procedures involve tubal ligation, in which the woman's fallopian tubes are surgically cut or blocked by applying clips, rings, or heat. The two most common surgical approaches are the minilaparotomy and laparoscopy. These approaches require skilled medical professionals and sterile conditions. Local or general anesthesia is also required.

There are newer, transcervical approaches to sterilization that do not involve surgery. One such approach is called Essure. This nonsurgical method uses a springlike device (microcoil) inserted through the cervix and uterus into each fallopian tube. This causes gradual tubal blockage over a 3-month period by encouraging local scar tissue growth with polyester (PET) fibers. At 5 years, the effectiveness of this approach is 99.74%. While becoming more acceptable in the United States, Essure is unlikely to be introduced in developing countries soon because of the high cost and complexity of the insertion instruments (WHO & Johns Hopkins University, 2011).

Minilaparotomy
A **minilaparotomy**, sometimes called a *minilap*, requires a small incision just above the pubic hairline. An instrument is then inserted into the cervix to move the uterus and pull each fallopian tube into the incision. Part of the tube is taken out of the incision, where it is blocked by **ligation**, clips, or rings, and then replaced in the abdomen. This procedure takes about 20 minutes, and the woman can usually leave the medical setting in 2 or 3 hours. Because the incision is very small (about 3 cm), few complications develop.

Laparoscopy
A **laparoscopy** involves inserting a narrow stainless steel tube with fiber-optic cylinders that transmit light into the abdomen (Figure 7.9). This tube is called a *laparoscope*. Two types of laparoscopes can be used. With one, the physician can insert forceps and other instruments through the tube itself;

therefore, only one incision is necessary. With the other type of laparoscope, two incisions are required because the tube does not permit other instruments to be inserted through it. Ligation by electrocoagulation (high-frequency electrical current) or application of clips or rings can take place during this procedure to prevent the passage of the egg.

Transcervical Methods
Transcervical techniques permanently prevent pregnancy by blocking the fallopian tubes via insertion of materials through the vagina and the uterus. In addition to Essure, another nonsurgical method is the Adiana procedure, which involves implanting a porous plastic matrix into a superficial lesion in each fallopian tube to block the tube. Both Adiana and Essure require skilled use of an expensive hysteroscope for insertion and follow-up imaging 3 months after insertion. Unlike the other female sterilization procedures, they are not immediately effective (Zieman & Hatcher, 2012).

Reversibility
Like male sterilization, female sterilization should generally be considered irreversible. As previously discussed, surgical techniques can be successful in opening up the fallopian tubes, but highly skilled surgeons and modern microsurgical equipment are required and such procedures are very costly. Therefore, women seeking sterilization must expect it to be permanent because reversal is costly and failure rates are high. For women who want to become pregnant after being sterilized, in vitro fertilization may be possible, but many cannot afford this procedure and it is not always successful (Zieman & Hatcher, 2012).

▦ The Future of Contraceptives

Research to find better methods of contraception continues. The perfect method of contraception, which will probably never exist, would meet the following criteria:

1. Be 100% effective
2. Be very inexpensive (or even free)
3. Have no side effects

---

minilaparotomy Female sterilization procedure that involves a small incision in the abdomen through which the fallopian tubes are pulled so they can be blocked.

ligation The tying of the fallopian tubes to prevent the sperm–egg union.

laparoscopy Female sterilization procedure that involves inserting a narrow viewing instrument—a laparoscope—through an incision in the abdomen and then performing ligation or applying clips or rings to block the fallopian tubes.

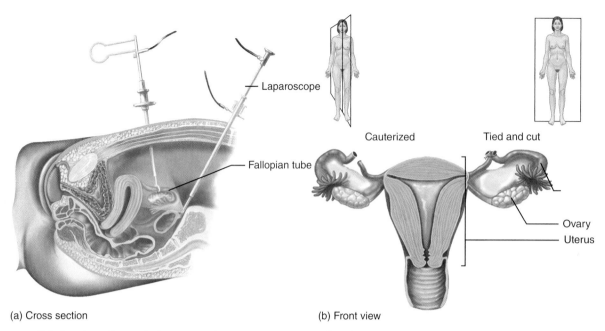

Laparoscope

Fallopian tube

Cauterized

Tied and cut

Ovary

Uterus

(a) Cross section

(b) Front view

FIGURE **7.9** Female sterilization by laparoscopic ligation. (a) Cross section: The tubes are located using a laparoscope and cut, tied, or cauterized through a second incision. (b) Front view: The tubes after ligation.

4. Be reversible

5. Involve no remembering to do something

6. Be convenient (not messy)

7. Prevent STIs

8. Be religiously and morally acceptable

9. Not interrupt sexual behaviors

During the 2000s, several new methods were approved for use in the United States. These included two different nonlatex male condoms, an improved female condom, implants, the patch, the vaginal ring, long-lasting emergency contraceptive pills, extended OCs, and new methods of female sterilization. However, some new methods and some of the old standbys were removed from the market. It seems the driving influence behind business decisions to withdraw a product are based on costs—profit and loss—rather than a product's safety and efficacy. It would be ideal if there was a way for useful methods to still be made available after a manufacturer decides they are no longer a profit maker.

The contraceptive methods now being researched include the options discussed here.

Male Contraceptive Methods

Exploration of new male conceptive methods has occurred since early 1970s without success. Every few years, the media claims "a new breakthrough" in male contraceptive research that will result in "a new method available soon!" While we are cautiously optimistic, previous experience suggests that it may be a while before a new male method is finally available. Having said that, it is valuable to consider the most recent research on male contraception.

Hormonal contraception is the most studied type of new method for males. These methods affect the development of the sperm by suppressing gonadotropin-releasing hormone (GnRH), luteinizing hormone, and FSH, and as a result testosterone produced by the body. Delivery methods include injections, implants, and transdermal delivery systems (Kogan & Wald, 2014). Some researchers are examining synthetic steroids that resemble testosterone but that protect the prostate; the largest successful study used one such product, testosterone undecanoate, as a monthly injection. Though this product was considered successful, the frequency of the injections was considered burdensome (Nieschlag, 2011).

Nonhormonal male contraceptive methods, which focus on sperm development or sperm–egg interactions, are appealing because they would not have the systemic side effects of hormonal methods and may have a more rapid onset (Chao, Page, & Anderson, 2014). Unfortunately, less development in this area has occurred and most formulations have been plagued by side effects, reversibility, and efficacy issues, leading to few phase 2 or 3 studies (Kogan & Wald, 2014).

Development of male contraceptive methods is not supported by the pharmaceutical companies; most current research funding comes from non-profit agencies and the U.S. Department of Health and Human Services' National Institutes of Health (Kogan & Wald, 2014; Murdoch & Goldberg, 2014; Sitruk-Ware, Nath, & Mishell, 2013). Some believe that without the support of pharmaceutical companies, new methods will not be developed quickly.

New Versions of Existing Methods

Researchers are trying to improve on several existing methods. As already mentioned, contraceptive patches with lower hormone doses (Kaunitz et al., 2012; Kaunitz et al., 2015; Wiegratz et al., 2014), one of which is transparent (Dorflinger, 2013), and a newly shaped IUD (Baram et al., 2014; Ilan et al., 2014) are being tested. Researchers are also investigating new versions of vaginal rings. One newer vaginal ring offers pregnancy protection for an extended period of time—up to a year (Dorflinger, 2013) and others act as dual-protection systems, protecting against sexually transmitted HIV in addition to pregnancy (Population Council, 2015a). Other research on hormonal methods focuses on formulations that reduce the cardiovascular risks and effects of androgens on women (Sitruk-Ware et al., 2013).

New versions of two barrier methods are also being researched. One is a new female condom with the pouch contained in a dissolving capsule (designed to improve insertion) with foam dots on the outer surface (designed to improve connection to the vaginal walls to reduce slipping). The other is a new diaphragm design that does not require a clinician fitting (Dorflinger, 2013).

Transdermal Sprays and Gels

Recent efforts expand transdermal (through the skin) hormone delivery. In Australia, a spray-on system (Metered Dose Transdermal System) has been tested. The spray-on approach is a new technique for transferring a preset dose of fast-drying hormones onto the skin, where it is almost instantly absorbed. The hormones slowly diffuse into the bloodstream over several hours, reaching their peaking levels 20 hours after application and plateauing after 4 or 5 days of daily application (Bahamondes & Bahamondes, 2014). Another transdermal method delivers a progestin called Nesterone in the form of a gel.

Spray-on contraception is a new way to supply a preset dose of hormones.

One formulation also contains estradiol, a form of estrogen; it has produced anovulation in most of subjects and also allows regular bleeding patterns (Bahamondes & Bahamondes, 2014; Population Council, 2015b).

"On-Demand" Contraception

For women who have sex only occasionally, a highly effective "on-demand" method may be of interest. Researchers are investigating a progestin-only pill that women could take before sex that would prevent pregnancy. Initial small studies were promising, and the World Health Organization is conducting a larger study with women who have sex up to 6 times per month (Bahamondes & Bahamondes, 2014).

Unmet Need for Contraception

What is "unmet need"?

A woman has an unmet need for contraception if she is sexually active, is able to become pregnant, does not want a child in the next 2 years or wants to stop childbearing, but is not using any method of contraception.

How extensive is unmet need?

- Approximately 225 million women in the world want to avoid pregnancy but are not using a modern method of contraception (Guttmacher Institute, 2015).
- There has been some improvement in unmet contraceptive needs. Worldwide, contraceptive prevalence among married or cohabiting women rose from 36% in 1970 to 63% in 2010, and unmet need fell in the same period from 22% to 12% (United Nations [UN], 2013a).
- While these improvements are impressive, the absolute number of women with unmet need has increased (from 127 million to 142 million) because of population growth (Cleland, Harbison, & Shah, 2014).

Are there different rates when comparing regions?

- When considering regions and looking at total numbers, Asia, because of its large population, has the most women with an unmet need (84 million), followed by sub-Saharan Africa with 32 million (Cleland et al., 2014).
- Overall, sub-Saharan Africa continues to be the region with the lowest level of contraceptive use (24%) and highest level of unmet need (25%). These rates are similar to the levels recorded in Asia and Latin America 40 years ago. Among the 35 countries in sub-Saharan Africa, 24 have unmet need of more than 20%, and in 7 of these the rate is more than 30% (UN, 2013b). By comparison, in Europe and Asia, the contraceptive use rate is almost 70% (Cleland et al., 2014).
- Because some regions prohibit premarital sex, the unmet contraceptive need among sexually active single or formerly married women is often higher. In developing countries, the rate of unmet need for contraception is 21.9% for unmarried women compared to 12.4% for married women (Cleland et al., 2014).
- When comparing married and unmarried women, the largest difference can be found in Eastern Asia, where 28% of unmarried women experience an unmet contraceptive need compared to 2.5% of married women (Cleland et al., 2014).
- Many women with an unmet need have discontinued a contraceptive method (38%)—a rate that increases to 50% when examining developing countries (Jain, Obare, & RamaRao, 2013).

Why do women not use or discontinue using contraceptives?

- While access is often cited as a cause for unmet need, little evidence supports this claim (Cleland et al., 2014).
- Research suggests that informational and social barriers constitute major contributors to unmet need. These can include, but are certainly not limited to, attitudes toward sex, childbearing, and contraception; perceived ability to act; spousal communication; and quality of sex education.
- In one study, young women's premarital awareness of sexual and reproductive matters including contraceptive methods and services determined their use of contraceptives to delay first pregnancy (Jeejeebhoy, Santhya, & Zavier, 2014).
- Other factors include medical and health concerns and personal experiences with negative side effects (Cleland et al., 2014; Sedgh & Hussain, 2014).

Recommendations for Meeting Unmet Need

- While we need to focus on places where the gap between fertility desires and contraceptive practice is greatest—which include many countries in sub-Saharan Africa—other areas should not ignored.
- Bongaarts (2014) stresses the need for substantial information, education, and communication in well-organized family planning programs; such programs can, on average, reduce unmet need by 10% and raise contraceptive use by 22%. This approach may be particularly relevant for low-use, high-unmet-need countries.
- It is critical to ensure that as many options are available as possible and to help women match their method with their needs (Sedgh & Hussain, 2014).
- Promoting societal receptivity to contraceptive use would help women overcome cultural and social barriers to achieving their desired family size.
- Family planning should be integrated with other related health services, as the latter can be "missed opportunities" to address an unmet need for contraception (Malarcher & Polis, 2014).
- Healthcare providers need to help women anticipate and tolerate side effects. There has been little to no progress in understanding the lack of willingness of women to endure side effects. More understanding and mechanisms to help women prepare for and continue a contraceptive method in spite of side effects would likely increase continuation of methods (Cleland et al., 2014).

Case Study

When choosing a method of contraception, you must consider the effectiveness, side effects, convenience, cost, and protection from STIs and HIV. However, your partner's willingness to use the same method also comes into play, because contraceptives are ineffective if not used properly.

Many factors influence your contraceptive use. Legally, the federal government regulates which contraceptives you can buy in the United States. Socioeconomic status may also be a factor. While all insurance plans are required to cover contraception, the actual coverage provided may vary. In general, people of higher socioeconomic status have greater access to prescription contraceptive methods and are more likely to receive education about contraceptive methods.

Religion also plays a role in contraceptive choice, because some religions officially sanction only natural family-planning methods. Communication skills also are involved as you negotiate your contraceptive use with a partner.

Biological Factors

- Gender may affect contraceptive decision making. Males have only the options of condoms, vasectomy and withdrawal; women have to deal with the fact that only they can become pregnant.
- STIs and HIV can be prevented only through strict use of latex, polyurethane, or polyisoprene condoms; abstinence; or 100% monogamy with an uninfected partner.
- Natural family planning relies on using physiological cycles and changes to monitor ovulation.
- Hormones such as estrogen and progesterone prevent the pituitary gland from producing FSH, which prevents ovulation.

Sociocultural Factors

- Socioeconomic status affects contraceptive availability and use.
- Laws and government regulations limit contraceptive approval and availability.
- Religion affects contraceptive decisions, limiting some couples to natural family planning.
- Media and ad information can affect both contraceptive choice and brand choice.

Psychological Factors

- Experience may determine the contraceptive you choose.
- Emotions often get in the way of practicing contraception and safer sex.
- Learned attitudes and behaviors affect your willingness to negotiate contraceptive use and practice safer sex.
- Your self-concept may influence whether you negotiate contraceptive use with your partner or simply accept what your partner desires.

Summary

- Contraception is used to avoid unplanned pregnancy. User motivation accounts for much of the variability in the effectiveness of different methods.

- Perfect use of a contraceptive method reflects the number of pregnancies likely to occur among 100 women in a year's time if the method is always used consistently and correctly. Often typical use effectiveness is less because of human error.

- Except for abstaining from oral, penile–vaginal, and anal sex, condom use (male or female) is the only readily available and widely used contraceptive method that protects against sexually transmitted infections (STIs).

- Of the nonprescription methods, both abstinence and withdrawal are free, always available, and theoretically easy to use with no side effects. However, in practice, both methods have lower effectiveness because intentions and practice do not always match.

- More than 100 brands of male condoms are available. All materials protect against pregnancy if condoms are used consistently and correctly; latex, polyurethane, and polyisoprene protect against many STIs, but lambskin condoms do not. Female condoms, made of synthetic rubber, are more costly.

- The vaginal contraceptive sponge and spermicides in the form of gels, foams, films, and inserts all use nonoxynol 9. The use of this spermicide does not protect against HIV or other STIs and can cause irritation, which may actually increase risk of STI transmission if these products are used multiple times daily.

- Fertility awareness methods depend on tracking a woman's fertile time using the calendar, basal body temperature, cervical secretions, cycle beads, or some combination of these methods; effectiveness can be high but requires careful record keeping.

- Prescription contraceptive methods are for females only; they include combined oral contraceptive pills containing both estrogen and progestin to suppress ovulation, progestin-only pills, and other mechanisms to deliver hormones such as the patch, injections, implants, and vaginal rings.

- Progestin-only emergency contraceptive (EC) pills may be used effectively (up to 72 hours) after intercourse to prevent pregnancy. None of the current methods is an abortifacient, and none disturbs an implanted pregnancy. The EC pills are available in the United States without prescription; ella is available with prescription and can be used 120 hours after unprotected vaginal–penile sex.

- Intrauterine devices are highly effective and reversible contraceptive methods. The copper-T IUD can be used for EC and then can remain in place for up to 12 years; the Mirena IUD delivers a hormone that reduces or eliminates menstrual flow and is effective for up to 5 years; Skyla delivers hormones but is smaller than Mirena and lasts up to 3 years, and Liletta also contains hormones and last for 3 years.

- Long-acting reversible contraceptives (LARCs), such as IUDs and implants, are becoming increasingly recommended for women. Because these methods have very high effectiveness rates with typical use and last for years, they are excellent choices for decreasing pregnancy rates.

- Diaphragms and cervical caps are barrier methods that are clinically fitted to cover a woman's cervix and used in combination with a spermicide to prevent sperm from entering the uterus.

- Sterilization for males and females is a permanent method of contraception that is almost 100% effective and widely used among adults older than age 35 who are certain they do not want children or more children.

Discussion Questions

1. List six key considerations in choosing a contraceptive method, and rank their relative importance. What method did you use to rank their importance?

2. Describe the nonprescription methods of contraception. Discuss the relationship issues that affect the choice of these methods.

3. Describe the methods of contraception requiring prescriptions. Which types of information should be disclosed to a doctor when making a selection?

4. What are LARCs? What are the benefits and disadvantages of these methods? Do you think clinicians should be promoting these methods? Why or why not?

5. Discuss the varied methods of female and male sterilization. Should the possibility of reversibility be part of the decision process?

Application Questions

Reread the chapter-opening story and answer the following questions.

1. Discuss how Susan altered her contraception use in light of her changing lifestyle. Which other contraceptive methods could she have used at each point? Which suggestions would you have for her?

2. If Susan had a family history of diabetes, high blood pressure, or breast cancer, how would her choices of contraceptive be altered?

3. Consider Stephen's decision to have a vasectomy. Although it might have seemed the perfect method for him at the time—married, monogamous, finished with childbearing—it also leaves him without the ability to father more children, should he remarry. In light of this, should men routinely postpone sterilization until a later age—just in case? Or should they have sperm frozen for the future?

Critical Thinking Questions

1. Assume that you began a relationship with a partner who wanted to use natural family planning because of religious convictions. Which advantages and disadvantages would that hold for you from a contraceptive and safer sex standpoint? Answer this question from both male and female viewpoints.

2. The prescription methods of birth control are all female based. What role, if any, should the male partner have in the decision to use these methods?

Critical Thinking Case

Ben and Allie, both age 25 years, had been dating for 6 months and using latex condoms as their contraception method. Because their relationship was monogamous and increasingly dedicated, they had talked about switching to a different method but had never taken the time to discuss the options and how they would fit their lifestyle.

Then one evening, a condom broke. Allie pulled out the calendar on which she mapped her period, and the news was bad. It was right around the time of ovulation. Although committed to one another, they were not prepared to face the possibility of parenthood.

First consider what Allie and Ben should do immediately. Then outline some options for the couple's future, so that they do not face this situation again.

Exploring Personal Dimensions

Choosing a Contraceptive

There is no such thing as a 100% safe, 100% convenient, 100% easy-to-use contraceptive. Every contraceptive has advantages and disadvantages. People need to weigh these advantages and disadvantages for themselves.

Some questions that people need to ask themselves are as follows:

1. *Effectiveness.* What are the typical effectiveness rates for each method considered? How important is it to prevent pregnancy now? Is using abortion as a backup acceptable to you and your partner, or is an unplanned pregnancy acceptable at this time?

2. *Side effects.* Are you a good candidate for this method? Will you experience adverse side effects? Do you have a medical condition that should prevent you from using this method?

3. *Convenience.* Is this method easy for you to get? Is it easy to use? Will you use it every time?

4. *Cost.* Can you afford it? Does your campus health center provide it? Does your insurance cover it?

5. *STI protection.* Are you in a monogamous relationship? Are you sure? Do you have more than one partner? Do you know your partner's HIV status? Are you willing and committed to using a condom in addition to this method?

6. *Partner.* What does your partner think about this method? Will he or she want to use it every time? Do you want contraception to be a shared responsibility, or is it yours alone?

Suggested Readings

Boston Women's Health Book Collective & Norsigian, J. *Our bodies, ourselves: Informing and inspiring women across generations.* New York: Touchstone/Simon & Schuster, 2011.

Eig, J. *The birth of the pill: How four crusaders reinvented sex and launched a revolution.* New York: W. W. Norton, 2014.

Foster, A. M., & Wynn, L. L., eds. *Emergency contraception: The story of a global reproductive health technology.* New York: Palgrave MacMillan, 2012.

Guttmacher Institute. *Perspectives on sexual and reproductive health,* 2015. Available: http://www.guttmacher.org/archive/PSRH.jsp.

Web Resources

The Emergency Contraception Website: NOT-2-LATE.com
http://ec.princeton.edu/questions/dose.html

This website is operated by the Office of Population Research at Princeton University and by the Association of Reproductive Health Professionals. Funding is provided by the Educational Foundation of America. It provides accurate information about emergency contraception derived from the medical literature. It has no connection whatsoever with companies that manufacture or sell emergency contraceptives.

Bedsider
http://bedsider.org/

Bedsider is an online birth control support network for individuals 18–29 years old. The website is operated by the National Campaign to Prevent Teen and Unplanned Pregnancy, a private nonprofit organization concerned about unintended pregnancy in the United States. In addition to comprehensive information about each method, Bedsider provides personal stories about the method. Additionally, individuals can sign up for reminders for appointments or to use their birth control (think remembering to take the pill every day!).

Guttmacher Institute: Contraception
www.guttmacher.org/sections/contraception.php

The Guttmacher Institute helps advance sexual and reproductive health worldwide through research, policy analysis, and public education. Its website takes a comprehensive look at contraception in the United States and abroad. As such, it provides access to media kits, fact sheets, state policies, policy articles, research articles, reports, statistics, slide shows, and audio clips.

Planned Parenthood: Birth Control
www.plannedparenthood.org/health-info/birth-control
www.youtube.com/user/plannedparenthood

The Planned Parenthood website provides a broad, up-to-date list of safe and effective methods of birth control for both women and men. Covering all methods, the website describes how the contraceptive works, what the advantages and disadvantages of using the method are, and what research says about its effectiveness, safety, and reversibility. The Planned Parenthood YouTube channel contains videos that provide a brief overview of individual contraceptive methods; these videos are available in both Spanish and English.

Association of Reproductive Health Professionals: Method Match
www.arhp.org/methodmatch/

This simple and interactive tool allows individuals to identify their preferences about contraception and selects possible methods to consider. The site also has the capability of comparing various methods to help visitors decide what method is best for them.

References

American Academy of Family Physicians. *Over-the-counter oral contraceptives,* 2014. Available: http://www.aafp.org/about/policies/all/otc-oral-contraceptives.html.

American College of Obstetricians and Gynecologists, Over-the-counter access to oral contraceptives: Committee Opinion No 544. *Obstetrics and Gynecology, 120* (2012), 1527–1531.

Backman, T., Raumaro, I., Huhtala, S., & Koskenvuo. Pregnancy during the use of levonorgestrel intrauterine system. *American Journal of Obstetrics and Gynecology, 190* (2004), 50–54.

Bahamondes, L., & Bahamondes, M. V. New and emerging contraceptives: a state-of-the-art review. *International Journal of Women's Health, 6* (2014), 221–234. doi: 10.2147/IJWH.S46811.

Baram, I., Weinstein, A., & Trussell, J. The IUB, a newly invented IUD: a brief report. *Contraception, 89* (2014), 139–141.

Bleakley. A., Hennessy. M., & Fishbein, M. Public opinion on sex education in US schools. *Archives of Pediatrics and Adolescent Medicine, 160* (2006), 1151–1156.

Bongaarts, J. The impact of family planning programs on unmet need for contraception, *Studies in Family Planning, 45* (2014), 247–262.

Brache, V., Payán, L. J., & Faundes, A. Current status of contraceptive vaginal rings. *Contraception, 87* (2013), 264–272.

Caillet, M., Vandromme, J., Rozenberg, S., Paesmans, M., Ger-maya, O., & Degueldre, M. Robotically assisted laparoscopic microsurgical tubal reanastomosis: A retrospective study. *Fertility and Sterility, 94* (2010), 1844–1847.

Chao, J., Page, S. T., & Anderson, R. A. Male contraception. *Best Practice & Research Clinical Obstetrics & Gynaecology.* 28 (2014), 845–857 doi: 10.1016/j.bpobgyn.2014.05.008.

Cleland, J., Harbison, S., & Shah, I. H. Unmet need for contraception: issues and challenges. *Studies in Family Planning, 45* (2014), 105–122.

Cleland, K., Zhu, H., Goldstuck, N., Cheng, L., & Trussell, J. The efficacy of intrauterine devices for emergency contraception: a systematic review of 35 years of experience. *Human Reproduction, 27,* 7, (2012), 1994–2000. doi: 10.1093/humrep/des140.

Crary, D. Health advocates tout new model of female condom. *Associated Press* (April 16, 2009).

Dailard, C. Understanding "abstinence": Implications for individuals, programs and policies. *The Guttmacher Report, 6, no. 5* (December 2003).

Daniels, K., Mosher, W. D., & Jones, J. Contraceptive methods women have ever used: United States, 1982–2010. *National Health Statistics Reports,* no 62. Hyattsville, MD: National Center for Health Statistics, 2013.

Dorflinger, L. J. New developments in contraception for US women. *Contraception, 87* (2013), 343–346.

Doyle, J., Stern, L., Hagan, M., Hao, J., & Gricar, J. Advances in contraception: IUDs from a managed care perspective. *Journal of Women's Health, 17,* (2008), 987–992.

Edelman, D. A., & North, B. B. Updated pregnancy rates for the Today contraceptive sponge. *American Journal of Obstetrics and Gynecology,* 157 (1987), 1164–1165.

Eisenberg, M. L., Henderson, J. T., Amory, J. K., Smith, J. F., & Walsh, T. J. Racial differences in vasectomy utilization in the United States: Data from the National Survey of Family Growth. *Urology,* 74 (2009), 1020–1024.

Fehring, R. J., Schneider, M., Barron, M. L., & Pruszynski, J. Influence of motivation on the efficacy of natural family planning. *MCN: The American Journal of Maternal/Child Nursing,* 38 (2013), 352–358.

Fehring, R. J., Schneider, M., Raviele, K., Rodriguez, D., & Pruszynski, J. Randomized comparison of two Internet-supported fertility-awareness–based methods of family planning. *Contraception, 88* (2013), 24–30.

Food and Drug Administration (FDA). *Female condom,* 1993. Available: http://www.fda.gov/ForConsumers/ByAudience/ForPatientAdvocates/HIVandAIDSActivities/ucm126373.htm.

Gallo, M. F., Grimes, D. A., & Schulz, K. F. Nonlatex vs. latex male condoms for contraception: A systematic review of randomized controlled trials. *Contraception, 68* (2003), 319–326.

GoAskAlice. *Five kinds of condoms: A guide for consumers,* 2009. Available: http://www.goaskalice.columbia.edu/1835.html.

Gordts, S., Campo, R., Puttemans, P., & Gordts, S. Clinical factors determining pregnancy outcome after microsurgical tubal reanastomosis. *Fertility and Sterility, 92* (2009), 1198–1202.

Grindlay, K., Burns, B., & Grossman, D. Prescription requirements and over-the-counter access to oral contraceptives: A global review. *Contraception, 88* (2013), 91–96.

Grossman, D., Grindlay, K., Li, R., Potter, J. E., Trussell, J., & Blanchard, K. Interest in over-the-counter access to oral contraceptives among women in the United States. *Contraception, 88* (2013), 544–552.

Guttmacher Institute. *Investing in sexual and reproductive health in the developing world* [Video]. 2015. Available: http://www.guttmacher.org/pubs/AddingItUp2014-vid.html.

Guttmacher Institute. *Unintended pregnancy in the United States,* 2013. Available: http://www.guttmacher.org/pubs/FB-Unintended-Pregnancy-US.pdf.

Haffner, D. W., & Schwartz, P. *What I've learned about sex.* New York: Perigee Books, 1998.

Hock, R. R. *Human sexuality.,* 2nd ed. New York: Prentice Hall, 2007.

Hymowitz, C., & Weissman, M. *A history of women in America: From the founding mothers to feminists—how women shaped the life and culture of America.* New York: Bantam Books, 1978.

Ilan, B., Ariel, W., & Seidman Daniel, S. A Three-dimensional way to prevent pregnancy: The IUB intrauterine ball—a newly introduced IUD in clinical trials. *The Journal of Obstetrics and Gynecology of India, 64* (2014),152–154. doi: 10.1007/s13224-014-0539-y.

Jain, A. K., Obare, F., & RamaRao, S. Reducing unmet need by supporting women with met need. *International Perspectives on Sexual and Reproductive Health, 39* (2013), 133–141.

Jejeebhoy, S. J., Santhya, K. G., & Zavier, A. G. F. Demand for contraception to delay first pregnancy among young married women in India. *Studies in Family Planning, 45* (2014), 183–201.

Jennings, V. H., & Burke, A. E. Fertility awareness–based methods. In R. A. Hatcher et al., eds. *Contraceptive technology.* 20th ed. New York: Ardent Media, 2011, 417–434.

Jensen, J. M. The evolution of Margaret Sanger's *Family Limitation* pamphlet, 1914–1921. *Journal of Women in Culture and Society, 6,* 3 (Spring 1981), 548–567.

Jones, J., Mosher, W., & Daniels, K. Current contraceptive use in the United States, 2006–2010, and changes in patterns of use since 1995. *National Health Statistics Reports,* no 60. Hyattsville, MD: National Center for Health Statistics. 2012.

Kaiser Family Foundation. *Emergency contraception,* 2014. Available: http://kff.org/womens-health-policy/fact-sheet/emergency-contraception/.

Kaneshiro, B., & Aeby, T. Long-term safety, efficacy, and patient acceptability of the intrauterine copper T-380A contraceptive device. *International Journal of Women's Health, 2* (2010), 211–220.

Kaunitz, A. M., Mishell, D. R., & Foegh, M. *Comparative phase 3 study of AG200-15, a low-dose estrogen and levonorgestrel contraceptive patch.* Poster presented at the American College of Obstetricians and Gynecologists (ACOG) annual clinical meeting, May 2012.

Kaunitz, A. M., Portman, D., Westhoff, C. L., Archer, D. F., Mishell, D. R., & Foegh, M. Self-reported and verified compliance in a phase 3 clinical trial of a novel low-dose contraceptive patch and pill. *Contraception 91*(2015), 204–210. doi: 10.1016/j.contraception.2014.11.011.

Kennedy, K. I., & Trussell, J. Postpartum contraception & lactation. In R. A. Hatcher et al., eds. *Contraceptive technology*, 20th ed. New York: Ardent Media, 2011, 483–512.

Killick, S. R., Leary C., Trussell, J., & Guthrie, K. A. Sperm content of pre-ejaculatory fluid. *Human Fertility, 14* (2011), 48–52.

Kirby, D. *Emerging answers 2007: Research findings on programs to reduce teen pregnancy and sexually transmitted diseases.* Washington, DC: National Campaign to Prevent Teen and Unplanned Pregnancy, 2007.

Kogan, P., & Wald, M. Male contraception: History and development. *Urologic Clinics of North America, 41* (2014), 145–161.

Lehfeldt, H. Margaret Sanger and the modern contraceptive techniques. *Journal of Sex Research, 3, 4* (November 1967), 253–255.

Maatouk, I., & Moutran, R. The origins of the condom. *Sexual Health, 10* (2013), 287–287. doi: 10.1071/SH12183.

Malarcher, S., & Polis, C. B. Using measurements of unmet need to inform program investments for health service integration. *Studies in Family Planning, 45* (2014), 263–275.

Mayer Laboratories. *Mayer Labs acquires Today sponge distribution rights*, April 6, 2009. Available: http://www.mayerlabs.com/images/pdf/today-media-kit.pdf.

Murdoch, F. E., & Goldberg, E. Male contraception: Another holy grail. *Bioorganic & Medicinal Chemistry Letters, 24* (2014), 419–424.

Nanda, K. Contraceptive patch and vaginal contraceptive ring. In R. A. Hatcher et al., *Contraceptive technology.* 20th ed. New York: Ardent Media, 2011, 343–370.

National Campaign to Prevent Teen and Unplanned Pregnancy. *Bedsider: IUD*, 2015. Available: http://bedsider.org/methods/iud#details_tab.

Nelson, A. L., & Cwiak, C. Combined oral contraceptives. In R. A. Hatcher et al., *Contraceptive technology.* 20th ed. New York: Ardent Media, 2011, 249–342.

Nieschlag, E. The struggle for male hormonal contraception. *Best Practice and Research Clinical Endocrinology & Metabolism, 25* (2011), 369–375.

Population Council, Inc. *Developing ARV-based microbicide and microbicide/contraceptive vaginal rings,* 2015a. Available: http://www.popcouncil.org/research/developing-arv-based-microbicide-and-microbicide-contraceptive-vaginal-ring.

Population Council, Inc. *Nestorone®/estradiol transdermal gel contraception,* 2015b. Available: http://www.popcouncil.org/research/nestorone-estradiol-transdermal-gel-contraception.

Ramchandran, D., & Salem, R. M. New findings on contraceptives. *Population Reports, Series M (20).* Baltimore, MD: INFO Project, Johns Hopkins Bloomberg School of Public Health, June 2008.

Roncari, D., & Hou, M. Y. Female and male sterilization. In R. A. Hatcher et al., *Contraceptive technology.* 20th ed. New York: Ardent Media, 2011, 435–482.

Rosenbaum, J. E. Patient teenagers? A comparison of the sexual behavior of virginity pledgers and matched nonpledgers. *Pediatrics, 123,* (2009), e110–e120.

Sampson, O., Navarro, S. K., Khan, A., Hearst, N., Raine, T. R., Gold, M., Miller, S., & Thiel de Bocanegra, H. Barriers to adolescents' getting emergency contraception through pharmacy access in California: Differences by language and region. *Perspectives on Sexual and Reproductive Health, 41,* (2009), 110–118.

Schepens, J., Mol, B., Wiegernick, M., Houterman, S., & Koks, C. Pregnancy outcomes and prognostic factors from tubal sterilization reversal by sutureless laparoscopical reanastomosis: A retrospective cohort study. *Human Reproduction, 26* (2011), 354–359.

Sedgh, G., & Hussain, R. Reasons for contraceptive nonuse among women having unmet need for contraception in developing countries. *Studies in Family Planning, 45* (2014), 151–169.

Sexuality Information and Education Council of the United States (SIECUS). *New abstinence program shows some results, shortcomings,* 2010. Available: http://www.siecus.org/index.cfm?fuseaction=Feature.showFeature&featureID=1856.

Sexuality Information and Education Council of the United States (SIECUS). *Support federal adolescent sexual health education & promotion programs,* 2014. Available: http://siecus.org/_data/n_0001/resources/live/ProgramFactsheet.pdf.

Sitruk-Ware, R., Nath, A., & Mishell, D. R. Contraception technology: Past, present and future. *Contraception, 87* (2013), 319–330.

Sonenstein, F. L. Can we afford to be complacent about teens' use of condoms. *Journal of Adolescent Health, 43* (October 2008), 313–314.

Timeline—the pill. The American Experience. PBS, 2002. Available: http://www.pbs.org/wgbh/amex/pill/timeline/index.html.

Trenholm, C., Devaney, B., Fortson, K., Quay, L., Wheeler, J., & Clark, M. *Impacts of four Title V, Section 510 abstinence education programs, final report.* Princeton, NJ: Mathematica Policy Research, 2007. Available: http://aspe.hhs.gov/hsp/abstinence07/report.pdf.

Trussell, J. Contraceptive failure in the United States. *Contraception, 83* (2011), 397–404.

Trussell, J., & Raymond, E. G. *Emergency contraception: A last chance to prevent unintended pregnancy,* 2011. Available: http://ec.princeton.edu/questions/ee_review.pdf.

United Nations (UN), Department of Economic and Social Affairs, Population Division. Model-based estimates and projections of family planning indicators, 2013 revision. 2013a.

United Nations (UN), Department of Economic and Social Affairs, Population Division. 2013b. World contraceptive patterns 2013.Wall chart. 2013b.

Wiegratz, I., Bassol, S., Weisberg, E., Mellinger, U., & Merz, M. Effect of a low-dose contraceptive patch on efficacy, bleeding pattern, and safety: A 1-year, multicenter, open-label, uncontrolled study. *Reproductive Sciences, 21* (2014), 1518–1525. doi: 10.1177/1933719114532840.

World Health Organization (WHO), Department of Reproductive Health and Research, & Johns Hopkins Bloomberg School of Public Health/Center for Communication Programs (CCP), INFO Project. *Family planning: A global handbook for providers (2011 update).* Baltimore & Geneva: CCP & WHO, 2011.

Youssef, H. The history of the condom. *Journal of the Royal Society of Medicine, 86* (April 1993), 266–228.

Zieman, Z., & Hatcher, R. A., *Managing contraception on the go 2012–2014.* Tiger, GA: Bridging the Gap Foundation, 2012.

Zukerman, Z., & Orvieto, R. Letter to the editor. *Journal of Andrology, 28,* 5 (2007), 635. doi: 10.2164/jandrol.107.003434.

Zuckerman, Z., Weiss, D. B., & Orvieto, R. Does preejaculatory penile secretions originating from the Cowper's gland contain sperm? *Journal of Assisted Reproduction and Genetics, 20* (2003), 157–159.

CHAPTER 8

Conception, Pregnancy, and Birth

FEATURES

Global Dimensions
The Couvade Syndrome

Communication Dimensions
Communicating About Pregnancy

Gender Dimensions
Fathers and Childbirth

Multicultural Dimensions
Differences in Infant Mortality

Ethical Dimensions
Surrogate Mothers

CHAPTER OBJECTIVES

1 Explain what happens during the process of conception and implantation.

2 Explain what happens developmentally to the mother and embryo and fetus during the three trimesters of a pregnancy.

3 Describe the concept of prenatal care and discuss the options for birth attendants and place of birthing.

4 Explain the many factors that can affect pregnancy outcomes, including use of drugs, diseases, and Rh incompatibility.

5 Identify maternal health problems that may be experienced during pregnancy.

6 Describe the physical and emotional reactions common during the three stages of giving birth.

7 Cite the causes of infertility, and describe various methods of treating it.

INTRODUCTION

Mary was in her early 40s when she married her husband, Rich. Rich had a son from a previous marriage whom they were raising together, and the couple decided not to have biological children together. Mary had been using birth control pills for years, and the pair decided to continue with that method to prevent further pregnancies.

About 6 months after their wedding, Mary noticed she was extremely tired and felt like she had food poisoning—except that the condition did not go away. When she went to her doctor, he asked if she could be pregnant; Mary said that she was on the pill. After listening to her symptoms, the doctor decided to do a pregnancy test just to be sure. To Mary's surprise, the test came back positive. When talking with the doctor about how the pregnancy could have happened, he reminded her that there is a small chance of getting pregnant on the pill. Mary was not sure how she felt about the pregnancy; she knew about the increased risks for older women of having a child with a genetic disorder. When she told Rich about the pregnancy, he was also anxious. They decided to visit an obstetrician to get more information about the pregnancy and the risks involved.

At the obstetrician's office, the clinician conducted a vaginal sonogram to examine the fetal heartbeat. After looking at the screen for a little bit, the clinician said, "I hope you like kids, because you are having two!" Upon hearing this news, both Mary and Rich were shocked and felt a bit numb. After going home and discussing the issue, even though this was not a planned pregnancy and there were risks for both mother and children, they decided to continue with the pregnancy.

Unfortunately, Mary's nausea continued throughout most of the pregnancy, and she developed pregnancy complications. The boys' development was restricted and they were not growing in length and weight appropriate for their gestational age. At week 27 of her pregnancy, Mary was put on bed rest so that all of her energy (e.g., calories) could be used to help the boys growth. The doctors were concerned that if the boys did get any larger before they were delivered, they would not be able to survive outside the uterus. Finally at 33 weeks' gestation, the doctor decided that the boys' growth was not improving and a cesarean section should be done the following week. When Mary asked about the possibility of a vaginal delivery, the doctor said he was concerned about an extended labor that could be stressful to the baby who would come out second. Reluctantly, Mary agreed to the cesarean delivery.

The babies were born at 34 weeks' gestation and weighed 4 pounds 2 ounces and 3 pounds 11 ounces, respectively. Immediately after the surgery, the boys were taken to the neonatal intensive care unit (NICU) so they could be examined and receive any treatment needed. Unfortunately, both of the boys had breathing and eating problems that required interventions for an extended period of time. This experience was very stressful for Rich and Mary. Both knew about the importance of touch and bonding with infants, and they wished they could just be at home with their babies, but they also realized that the boys would likely not survive without this highly specialized care. About 4 weeks after their birth, the boys were able to go home with Mary and Rich.

Although Mary and Rich's experience has some aspects common to others' experiences—for example, the pregnancy was unplanned— other aspects, such as having twins delivered prematurely, make their experience unique. In this chapter, we discuss the usual and the unusual aspects of conception, pregnancy, and birth.

■ Creating a New Life

After the man ejaculates during penile–vaginal sex, the sperm move through the cervical mucus into the woman's uterus, reaching the fallopian tube within about 5 minutes. Propelling movements of the uterus and fallopian tubes help the sperm to move. Also, prostaglandin, a hormone found in semen, may intensify uterine contractions—not felt by the woman— and shorten the sperm's travel time. Sperm stay alive in the female reproductive tract for 72 to 120 hours. During the first 24 hours after ejaculation, they are at a peak level of health and fertility. The egg's peak fertile period lasts 8 to 12 hours, although an egg can be fertilized for up to 24 hours after ovulation.

Most frequently, the millions of sperm in the ejaculate meet an egg in one of the fallopian tubes. For egg and sperm to unite, one sperm must penetrate the transparent outer layer of the egg. The sperm secretes an enzyme, hyaluronidase, that dissolves this outer layer, allowing the sperm to enter and fertilize the egg. The union of the egg and the sperm is called **conception**, and the product of that union is called a **conceptus**. At this point, the sex of the

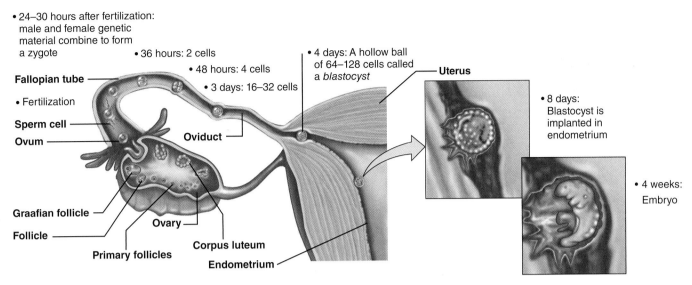

- 24–30 hours after fertilization: male and female genetic material combine to form a zygote
- Fertilization
- 36 hours: 2 cells
- 48 hours: 4 cells
- 3 days: 16–32 cells
- 4 days: A hollow ball of 64–128 cells called a *blastocyst*
- 8 days: Blastocyst is implanted in endometrium
- 4 weeks: Embryo

Fallopian tube
Sperm cell
Ovum
Oviduct
Uterus
Graafian follicle
Follicle
Primary follicles
Ovary
Corpus luteum
Endometrium

FIGURE 8.1 Following the ovum from ovulation through fertilization and implantation. After being ruptured from the ovary, the ovum is fertilized within the fallopian tube. It then travels to the uterus, where, as a blastocyst, it implants on the endometrium (lining) of the uterus.

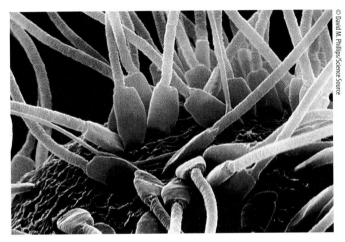

© David M. Phillips/Science Source

Although many sperm cells may reach the egg cell, usually only one will fertilize it.

potential offspring has already been determined by the absence or presence of a Y chromosome in the sperm. It is also possible, though not certain, that the number of offspring has been determined (more than one conceptus may have been conceived).

Implantation

Once the egg is fertilized, the conceptus is known as a **zygote**. The one cell of the zygote begins to divide as it travels down the fallopian tube on its way to implant itself in the uterus. One cell divides into two cells, the two become four, and so cell division continues. One week after conception, the zygote is a hollow ball of 100 cells. At this point it is termed a *blastocyst*. Now two layers of cells begin to form.

The inner layer of cells will become the **embryo**; the embryo is the zygote from the time of implantation through the first 8 weeks of development. The outer layer of cells, called *trophoblasts*, secretes enzymes that erode the uterine lining so that the blastocyst can attach itself to the endometrium 7 or 8 days after fertilization (Figure 8.1). After implantation, these trophoblasts and other cells proliferate and eventually form the placenta, the umbilical cord, and the amniotic sac. The amniotic sac is a membrane filled with **amniotic fluid**; it surrounds the developing fetus and embryo by the end of the eighth week and absorbs shocks (Shier, Butler, & Lewis, 2003).

Immediately after implantation, the embryo begins receiving nourishment from the endometrial tissue of the mother. Progesterone acts on this tissue to produce the necessary nutrients—glycogen, proteins, lipids, and some minerals. The embryo is nourished from this source for 8 to 10 weeks until the placenta has developed sufficiently to take over.

The **placenta** is a disc-shaped organ that attaches to the uterine wall and is connected to the fetus by

conception The union of the sperm and ovum; also called *fertilization*.

conceptus The fertilized ovum; the product of conception

zygote A fertilized egg.

embryo The developing fetus during the 2 months after conception.

amniotic fluid The fluid inside the amniotic sac in which the fetus floats; it acts as a shock absorber, maintains the fetus at a constant temperature, and serves as a nutrient.

placenta An organ of interchange between mother and fetus; oxygen, nutrients, and waste are exchanged through its cells.

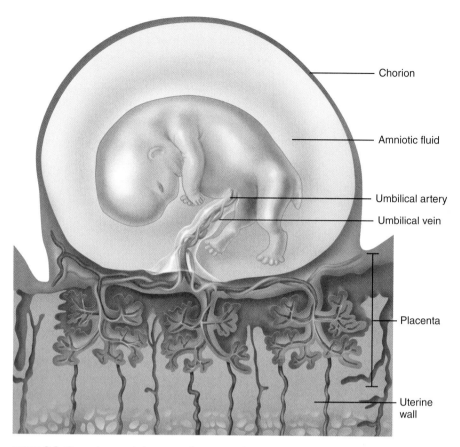

Chorion

Amniotic fluid

Umbilical artery

Umbilical vein

Placenta

Uterine wall

FIGURE 8.2 The embryo and placenta as they appear during the seventh week of development.

the **umbilical cord**. Together the placenta and the umbilical cord (which is attached to the baby at the navel and to the mother at the placenta) form the lifeline between the mother and the fetus. Nutrients, oxygen, and chemicals pass through the walls of the placenta to the fetus. Waste from the fetus is returned to the mother's blood for elimination through her body. The placenta, which by the end of the pregnancy will reach a diameter of 8 inches (about 20 centimeters), contains two sets of blood vessels (Figure 8.2). Fetal circulation occurs within the fetus and the inner part of the placenta, while the mother's circulation flows in the walls of the uterus and the uterine side of the placenta. The fetus's blood flows through two umbilical arteries to the placenta and back from the placenta to the fetus by one vein.

One important function of the placenta is to keep the blood systems of the mother and child separated from each other. It does this even though the placenta has *permeability*—that is, it allows some substances to pass between mother and fetus. Throughout the pregnancy, besides allowing nourishment and waste to pass between mother and child, the placenta helps to keep bacteria away from the fetus and allows antibodies (disease fighters) to cross to the fetus. These antibodies make the baby immune to diseases to which the mother is immune for approximately 6 months after birth; after that time, the infant makes its own antibodies.

As the embryo develops, the placenta secretes the hormone **human chorionic gonadotropin (HCG)**. This hormone is detectable through blood tests 8 days after fertilization, just as the blastocyst is implanting, and its presence confirms pregnancy. HCG reaches its maximal level 7 weeks after fertilization and its lowest level about 9 weeks later (16 weeks after fertilization). The function of HCG is to keep the corpus luteum of the ovum alive so that it can continue to secrete estrogen and progesterone. Estrogen and progesterone maintain the uterine endometrium,

umbilical cord The lifeline between mother and fetus, which contains two arteries and one vein. Food, oxygen, and chemicals are transported to the child through the arteries, and waste is returned to the mother through the vein.

human chorionic gonadotropin (HCG) The hormone that appears in the blood and urine, providing evidence that a pregnancy has occurred.

which nourishes the early pregnancy. By about the 11th week of pregnancy, the placenta itself secretes enough progesterone and estrogen to maintain the pregnancy, and the corpus luteum dies.

Pregnancy

In the preceding section we focused on the developing zygote almost as if it were a separate being. In reality, the development of a new person involves physiological changes in two human beings: the forming fetus and the mother. Let us back up now to account for the changes in a woman after an egg is fertilized within her body.

After the fertilized egg becomes implanted in her uterus, a woman is in a state of pregnancy, which lasts for the time the fetus takes to develop. This period can vary, but the time span from the last menstrual period to the birth of the baby is usually 9 calendar months (10 lunar months, 40 weeks, or 280 days). Most women deliver their babies within 2 weeks of the predicted date, sometimes called the **expected date of confinement (EDC)**. Approximately 4% deliver on the exact date. The EDC is calculated by a formula called *Nägele's rule:* establish the first day of the last normal menstrual period, add 7 days, and subtract 3 months from this date. The result is the EDC. Nägele's rule is based on a 28-day cycle, however, and not all women have this cycle. Therefore, a medical practitioner will calculate each patient's EDC to the best of his or her ability, adapting the rule as necessary. At the point at which the fetus has the optimal chance for survival outside the uterus, the pregnancy has reached term, or completion.

Ectopic Pregnancy

An **ectopic pregnancy** is characterized by implantation of the blastocyst in a site other than the uterus. Most often these occur in the fallopian tubes, although ectopic pregnancies can develop in other body parts. Blockage in the fallopian tubes prevents the fertilized egg from traveling down the fallopian tube; this blockage is often caused by a previous ectopic pregnancy, past infection in the fallopian tubes (such as **pelvic inflammatory disease**), or surgery of the fallopian tubes (such as tubal sterilization) (Sherieh, Cottrell, & Mancuso, 2014).

In the United States, the rate of ectopic pregnancy is 1% to 2% of all pregnancies, with approximately 100,000 ectopic pregnancies occurring each year; however, this rate has been increasing (Sherieh et al., 2014). Other factors, such as being older than 35 years of age, having many sexual partners, having surgery to reverse a tubal sterilization, smoking, becoming pregnant while using an IUD, and using

Myth (vs) Fact

Myth: The peak period for sperm and egg to be fertilized is 1 week after they are released.
Fact: The peak period for sperm is about 24 hours after ejaculated, and the peak period for the egg is approximately 12 hours after release.

Myth: The egg is fertilized by the sperm in the uterus.
Fact: The egg–sperm union occurs in the fallopian tube.

Myth: Obstetricians are very accurate at predicting the date of delivery.
Fact: Only 4% of women actually deliver on the expected date of confinement, although most women deliver within 2 weeks of their predicted due date.

Myth: To protect the fetus, pregnant women should refrain from exercising during their pregnancy.
Fact: Pregnant women can exercise without causing harm to the fetus. However, they should follow the exercise guidelines of the American College of Obstetrics and Gynecology and speak with their clinician if they have any special circumstances in their pregnancy.

Myth: As long as drugs are available over-the-counter, a pregnant woman can feel safe taking them.
Fact: All drugs have the potential to cause harm to fetuses. Therefore, pregnant women should refrain from taking all medications and supplements (including herbal alternatives) without discussing those medications with their clinician.

assisted reproductive technologies, may also increase the risk of an ectopic pregnancy (Sherieh et al., 2014).

It is essential that an ectopic pregnancy be diagnosed quickly. Ectopic pregnancies account for approximately 6% of pregnancy-related deaths in women (Sherieh et al., 2014). If a woman experiences symptoms of an ectopic pregnancy, such as abnormal vaginal bleeding, amenorrhea, breast tenderness, low back pain, mild cramping on one side of the pelvis, nausea, or pain in the lower abdomen or pelvic area, she should seek medical treatment. Unfortunately, about half of women with an ectopic pregnancy do not experience these symptoms (Sherieh et al., 2014). Ultrasound can confirm the presence of an ectopic pregnancy by 6 weeks' gestation, allowing for treatment that is less destructive and costly. The precise treatment will depend on the gestation time and whether the area of pregnancy has ruptured. In some cases, medication to expel the pregnancy may

expected date of confinement (EDC) Due date for normal pregnancy that is usually estimated by Nägele's rule.

ectopic pregnancy The development of the zygote in a location other than the uterus.

pelvic inflammatory disease (PID) Infection of the reproductive organs, particularly the uterus, fallopian tubes, and pelvic cavity.

be used; in other cases, surgery may be required (Capmas, Bouyer, & Fernandez, 2014).

Confirming Pregnancy

The signs of pregnancy—which were known long before current methods of testing became available—are divided into three categories: presumptive, probable, and positive. Because many of the signs and symptoms of pregnancy may also be attributed to other conditions, medical practitioners proceed with caution to avoid a wrong conclusion. Emotional, endocrine, or systemic conditions can cause symptoms identical to the early signs of pregnancy.

Presumptive symptoms are those that may indicate pregnancy but can also occur when a woman is not pregnant. These include missed menstrual periods, nausea and vomiting, a tingling feeling in the breast (*mastodynia*), increased urinary frequency, some weight gain, fatigue, a rise in the basal body temperature, some skin changes, slight abdominal enlargement, and some vaginal discoloration and discharge. Not all pregnant women experience all these symptoms. Probable signs and symptoms include the presumptive symptoms plus enlargement of the abdomen and the uterus, some painless uterine

contractions, *ballottement* (at 16 to 20 weeks, bimanual examination gives the physician an impression that a floating object is in the uterus), and *uterine soufflé* (a rushing sound, which the physician hears through a stethoscope placed on the woman's abdomen). Uterine soufflé in pregnant women is caused by blood filling placental blood vessels and spaces. Most conventional positive signs of pregnancy are not present until the 17th week after conception: fetal heartbeat, which can be monitored at 17 to 18 weeks; active fetal movement, at about the 5th month or between the 20th and 24th weeks; and palpation of the abdomen, by which the practitioner can detect the fetus.

Women today do not need to wait months to confirm a pregnancy; indeed, for the health of both the woman and the developing fetus it is best not to do so. Echography or ultrasonography (which measures sound waves as they pass through tissues of various densities, each returning its own echo) can be done as early as 4 weeks, and laboratory tests can now be done as early as 8 days after conception.

Pregnancy Tests

Pregnancy is confirmed by the presence of the hormone human chorionic gonadotropin, which is found

Global DIMENSIONS

The Couvade Syndrome

Around the globe, some men whose partners are pregnant experience pregnancy symptoms. Called *couvade syndrome*, cases have been reported across cultures, continents, and centuries (Frey, 2011). Symptoms include indigestion, increased or decreased appetite, weight gain, diarrhea or constipation, headache, nausea, and bloating. Symptoms typically occur during the late stages of the first trimester, with an increase during the late stage of the third trimester. They generally resolve with childbirth (Frey, 2011). Prevalence estimates range from fewer than 20% to 80% of expectant fathers (Frey, 2011); however, the exact cause of modern couvade is unknown. One challenge in determining the cause is that researchers—and their studies—often define couvade differently (Wynne-Edwards, 2006).

In spite of this challenge, possible social and biological causes have been hypothesized: a psychiatric disorder in which the males experience jealousy of the woman's ability to give birth, or guilt for impregnating their partner (Frey, 2011); lifestyle changes that the couple experiences together during pregnancy; social attachment (fathers who have strong empathy for their partner are more likely to demonstrate symptoms) (Kazmierczak et al., 2013); and hormonal changes in the father. Men with higher levels of prolactin, the hormone that causes lactation in women, report more couvade symptoms. In men, the prolactin causes a decrease in testosterone and sperm production; prolactin levels peak just before delivery (Berg & Wynne-Edwards, 2001; Storey et al., 2000). The conclusion of researchers is that men experience hormonal changes similar to changes experienced by their pregnant partners, though it is unknown if these hormonal changes are a cause-and-effect phenomenon or simply a correlation (Wynne-Edwards, 2006).

Because many men have mild symptoms, they may not seek help for the condition. For those who are bothered, having a clinician explain the condition and confirm that it is not uncommon typically alleviates any concerns. In almost all cases, symptoms disappear after the baby is born (Frey, 2011).

in the blood and urine if a pregnancy exists. Tests typically measure the level of or detect the presence of HCG. The most sensitive blood tests can detect HCG in a blood sample and can confirm pregnancy about 8 days after conception occurs.

Home pregnancy tests are slightly different than laboratory blood testing. These commercial test kits detect the presence of HCG in urine and can be used as early as the day menstruation should have started. When used according to directions, they are considered to be quite accurate. However, not all tests have the same sensitivity, and user error can affect the accuracy of the test results. Even with tests claiming the ability to test "early," waiting until the day after the menstrual cycle is expected will decrease the likelihood of obtaining a false-negative result. Reading and following the directions carefully will reduce possible user-related mistakes, but sometimes nervousness or anxiety will increase one's concern about the test. Often people feel the tests should be repeated, which may increase the cost to the user without increasing the likelihood of accurate findings.

If one has the time and ability to access a clinic, a professional laboratory procedure, done by a private health facility, clinic, or hospital, may be a better option to obtain an accurate result. However, it is important to choose a pregnancy testing facility carefully. Some "crisis pregnancy centers" offer free pregnancy testing but do not provide balanced information about pregnancy options.

Due Date and Delivery Date

As mentioned earlier, to determine the approximate due date, obstetricians use what is called Nägele's rule. They identify the first day of the last period, count back 3 months, and then add 7 days. For example, if the first day of the last missed period was January 1, 2016, the approximate due date would be October 8, 2016. If the pregnancy exceeds 40 weeks—and more urgently after 41 weeks—concern for the health of the fetus may necessitate inducing labor. Pregnancies of that length are associated with a higher risk of infant mortality and injury to the mother and baby (Bruckner, Cheng, & Caughey, 2008; Kaimal et al., 2011; Oros et al., 2012). In addition, induction may be recommended if there is a maternal illness such as high blood pressure, diabetes, or uterine infection.

Labor can be induced in several ways. One method involves the intravenous administration of Pitocin, an artificial version of the hormone oxytocin. Generally, the amount is increased every 15 to 30 minutes until a good contraction pattern is achieved. Induction can also occur by the administration of prostaglandin gels or suppositories. These are used when the cervix is not favorable, meaning that it has not dilated very much, is hard, posterior, not effaced, or barely effaced, or some combination of these characteristics making a vaginal delivery unlikely (ACOG District XI and The Texas Collaborative for Healthy Mothers and Babies, 2009). Another method of inducing labor is to artificially rupture the membrane ("breaking the bag of waters"). Lastly, some midwives or other holistic providers practice *natural induction*, which may include use of herbs, castor oil, or other agents to stimulate or advance a stalled labor. While medical induction is more common, approximately 30% of women used some form of nonmedical induction in 2005. Unfortunately, effectiveness of these natural methods is unknown and needs to be examined more (Kozhimannil, Johnson, et al., 2013).

Fetal Development

Prenatal development is commonly regarded as having two stages: the **embryonic stage** (from the Greek *embryo*, "to swell"), which lasts 2 months, and the **fetal stage** (from the Latin *fetus*, "the young one"), which lasts from the beginning of the third month to birth (Figure 8.3). The 9-month pregnancy, however, is commonly viewed as consisting of three 3-month developmental periods called **trimesters**.

© Petit Format/Nestle/Science Source

By the beginning of the eighth week of development, the embryonic body has recognizable human features.

embryonic stage The stage of prenatal development that includes the first 8 weeks of pregnancy.

fetal stage Period from the ninth week of pregnancy to birth.

trimester A 3-month period of the 9-month pregnancy, which is typically divided into three trimesters.

FIGURE 8.3 Major changes in fetal development from the third week after conception through the 10th week.

FIGURE 8.3 Major changes in fetal development from the third week after conception through the 10th week. (Continued)

The First Trimester

During the first trimester, weeks 1 through 12, most of the embryo's physiological systems and body parts begin to form. At the end of the first month, the embryo is about 0.25 inch (0.6 centimeter) long. By this time, three cell layers have formed: the *ectoderm* (outer layer), from which the skin, sense organs, and the nervous system will grow; the *mesoderm* (middle layer), from which the muscular, circulatory, and excretory systems will form; and the *endoderm* (inner layer), from which the digestive system, glandular systems, and lungs will develop.

At the end of the second month, the embryo is about 1¼ inches (3 centimeters) long and weighs 1/30 ounce (0.9 gram). The head represents almost half the embryo's total bulk. Facial features such as eyes, ears, nose, lips, and tongue are visible, and the forehead is prominent because of the brain size (Figure 8.4).

When the third month begins, as mentioned, the developing child is called a **fetus**. At the third month the fetus, afloat in the amniotic fluid, is 3 inches (7.6 centimeters) long and 1 ounce (2.8 grams) in weight. It can move, but its motions are not yet felt by the mother. The fingers and toes have nails, and the genitals can be seen as male or female. By the end of the first trimester, the fetus is a miniature human. During the next two trimesters, organs mature and general growth occurs.

The Second Trimester

During the fourth month, the first month of the second trimester, the greatest amount of fetal growth occurs. The fetus is now 6 inches (15 centimeters) long, the lower body is growing increasingly larger, and the head is now one-third the length of the body. The fetus moves and can suck, and its motion, called **quickening**, is felt by the mother. During the fifth month, the halfway point of the pregnancy, the fetus weighs about 1 pound (454 grams) and is about 12 inches (30 centimeters) long. It sleeps and wakes and has a preferred body position. During the sixth month the fetus grows about 2 inches (5 centimeters) and gains another pound. By this point the fetus's eyes are formed, it is sensitive to light, and it can hear uterine sounds. The skin is wrinkled and covered with fine hair. Although development is well under way, a baby born at this stage may not survive. Several months of care in a neonatal intensive care unit (NICU) would likely be required, depending on its development.

The Third Trimester

During the period of the third trimester, the fetus positions itself for birth. The most common fetal position, or *presentation*, is head down (Figure 8.5).

As a fat layer is built underneath the skin, the fetus takes on a more babylike form. By the end of the seventh month, the baby can live outside the uterus, although it may still need to spend time in a NICU after birth. By the end of the eighth month, the fetus weighs about 5 pounds 4 ounces (2,384 grams) and is about 20 inches (51 centimeters) long. During the eighth and ninth months, skin redness lessens and wrinkles begin to disappear as the fetus begins to gain about 1½ pound (227 grams) per week. The nails reach the end of the fingers and toes, and the fetus's actions become limited because of its tight fit in the uterus. As birth becomes imminent, in the 38th to 40th weeks, the head is 60% of its full size, the fine body hair has almost disappeared, and the skin becomes smoother and is now covered with a waxy protective substance called the *vernix caseosa*.

During this last trimester, the fetus will have reached a weight and size that prepare it to live independently of the mother. The baby is ready for delivery and birth.

◼ Bearing a Healthy Infant: Prenatal Choices

Staying as healthy as possible is the pregnant woman's chief responsibility to her developing child. Pregnancy is a time of great change. Both physical and psychological factors affect the health and well-being of an expectant mother and her developing child. Many choices must be made by expectant parents, including who to seek out for advice during pregnancy, where the birth will take place, and which health-enhancing lifestyle modifications they can make throughout the pregnancy. In the sections that follow, we discuss the many decisions facing today's expectant parents.

Birth Attendant Options

Even though pregnancy is a normal physiological event, there is no question that a woman's general health affects not only her own experience of pregnancy but also the health of her developing child. The best advice for a healthy pregnancy is supervision by a health practitioner trained to give prenatal

---

fetus The developing child from the ninth week after conception until birth.

quickening Movements of the fetus felt by the mother; usually occurs about the fourth month of pregnancy.

Actual size

4 weeks

5 weeks

6 weeks

7 weeks

FIGURE **8.4** In the fifth through seventh weeks of development, the embryonic body and face start to develop a humanlike appearance.

Uterus

Pelvic bones

Vaginal canal

Head down with baby's chin on chest

Head extended, face presentation

Head down, brow presentation

Frank breech, baby's legs over abdomen (most common breech presentation)

Incomplete foot presentation

Transverse, with shoulder presentation

Full breech, baby cross-legged in mother (most infrequent presentation)

FIGURE **8.5** Fetal positions.

 Communication DIMENSIONS

Communicating About Pregnancy Although it is not routinely discussed, most women do not have an easy time with pregnancy. Morning sickness, continual tiredness, and new physical sensations may bring about momentary feelings of "Did I do the right thing?" This is balanced against society's view of happy pregnant women, who work until the last days of pregnancy and always smile.

From our experience, pregnant women who talk to other women who have been pregnant gain a great sense of relief. They find that their experience is not unique. Few women go through a "perfect" pregnancy. Perhaps surprisingly, women who have been pregnant usually wait for the pregnant woman to discuss an issue before opening up about their experience.

In contrast, pregnant women who talk to those who have not had children (a group that includes men) are often chided for their complaining. One pregnant woman recently said that after she had morning sickness at work—every day for weeks on end—most colleagues would smile and remind her of how "lucky" she was. Any complaining during lunch or breaks was met with reproachful glares—how dare she have a negative thought about the fetus inside her! She soon learned to keep her feelings to herself.

Why do you think people have such a hard time talking about pregnancy? Is it because pregnancy is the result of sexual activity? Because of the special roles that young children play in our society? Or some other reason?

(prebirth) care. Thus, the selection of a health professional who will advise the woman during her pregnancy and serve as the birth attendant during labor and delivery is an important decision that should be made by the expectant parents early in the pregnancy.

In the United States, all physicians are trained in medical school in the procedures involved in pregnancy and birth. Nevertheless, the family-practice specialist (a newer term for general practitioner) and the **obstetrician** are typically the primary providers of pregnancy care. The obstetrician has had specialized advanced training in this area and is trained to provide medical care for high-risk pregnancies. Many women physicians specialize in obstetrics, and a considerable number of pregnant women purposely seek out women obstetricians. Some women believe that a female physician is more empathetic and understanding of the variety of body changes that occur during pregnancy and delivery. There is also the possibility that the female physician has experienced parturition (the process of giving birth), and many pregnant women find this reassuring and relaxing.

Midwifery has also been used in the United States. Historically, American midwives were laypeople who helped with birth deliveries. Today, most midwives are trained as nurses; nurse–midwives are registered nurses (RNs) and certified nurse–midwives (CNMs) who receive advanced training in childbirth processes. Midwives work with women who have low-risk pregnancies; if a pregnancy is high risk, then typically a midwife would refer the woman to an obstetrician. Midwives often approach pregnancy, prenatal care, and delivery with a more natural approach than physicians. As with a physician, prenatal visits are essential; with a midwife, these visits may take longer as there may be more questions and discussion than with a physician. During delivery, a "wait and see" approach is the norm, with interventions not being used unless there is a medical need for them. Midwives are not trained to perform cesarean sections.

Nurse–midwifery is often chosen by families who consider birthing to be a natural process and not a medical event that requires highly technological interventions. Nurse–midwives routinely practice in freestanding birth centers and in hospitals. Some nurse–midwives work with an obstetrician present at the delivery; others work alone but have an affiliation with an obstetrician who is on call for problem deliveries. Some nurse–midwives assist in home deliveries with a physician present or on call.

Many states require nurse–midwives to pass a national certification exam given by the American Midwifery Certification Board (AMCB) to be licensed. In those states that do not require certification, some individuals may work as midwives without nursing

training or certification. While many of these practitioners have valuable experience, some research indicates that screening procedures for low-risk home births may not be followed as consistently by midwives without AMCB certification (Grünebaum, McCullough, Brent et al., 2015)

Midwife-attended births in the United States steadily increased from less than 1% in 1975 to 8% in 2004, but the rate has remained relatively stable since then. In 2012, 8.7% of all births in the United States were attended by midwives—91.7% of whom were CNMs (Martin et al., 2013). Because midwives are not typically involved in surgery (such as cesarean sections), the percentage of midwife-attended births changes when considering vaginal births only. For example, in 2009, 12.1% (i.e., more than 1 in 8) of vaginal births were attended by a midwife (Declercq, 2012). In the United States, most midwife-attended births occur in hospitals (88.6%) (Martin et al., 2013).

Although rates of midwives as birth attendees are low in the United States, the practice and approach of midwifery is recognized as one that may be better suited to most women both in the United States and globally. The strategy of considering the whole mother–child system in the pregnancy, instead of just focusing on the identification of problems and issues, may be better equipped to reach more women and may potentially reduce global infant mortality by as much as 80% (Horton & Astudillo, 2014). A 2014 series in *The Lancet*, a renowned British medical journal, outlines the benefits of midwifery and suggest ways to increase its utilization.

Some women also elect to involve a *doula* in their pregnancy and delivery plans. A doula is a nonmedical attendant who assists a pregnant woman and her family before, during, and after delivery of her child, offering both emotional support and physical assistance as needed. Continuous labor support is associated with many positive outcomes for childbirth—such as reduced cesarean delivery rates, shorter length of labor, less need for pain medications, fewer operative vaginal deliveries, and better overall assessed health of newborn—and these effects are more positive when the person providing the support is not a medical person or part of the woman's family or social support network and the person has

obstetrician A physician who specializes in the care of pregnant women and the process of childbirth. Because these physicians are also gynecologists, they are often referred to as obstetrician–gynecologists (OB-GYNs).

midwifery The practice by nonphysicians of assisting in the process of pregnancy and childbirth. Lay midwives may have training but are not considered healthcare professionals; nurse–midwives are registered nurses who have received advanced training and often certification in the techniques of the birthing process.

received training (Hodnett et al., 2012). Postpartum, involvement of a doula has shown to increase rates of breastfeeding among low-income diverse women (Kozhimannil, Attanasio et al., 2013), improve parenting of young mothers (Hans et al., 2013) and offer a possible route for educating new parents about postpartum depression (McComish, Groh, & Moldenhauer, 2013). Doulas are most often thought of in terms of their involvement and assistance during the delivery and postpartum period, but in many cases the role of the doula starts well before delivery, as the doula aids the woman and her family in the process of preparing for childbirth and the baby's arrival, typically in the second trimester.

Increasingly, women and couples are planning their deliveries, making decisions that suit them, and choosing birth attendants and facilities to match their needs. Some postulate that understanding how the woman perceives childbirth—that is, as a natural event versus a medical event—and choosing a practitioner with similar beliefs will enhance the birth experience (Gibson, 2014).

Birthing Alternatives

To receive the kind of care they want before, during, and after delivery, future parents should investigate the birthing alternatives available in their area as early as possible. Often the choice of a birth attendant is tied to the setting in which that birth attendant chooses to (or is allowed to) practice. Currently in the United States there are three major settings where labor and delivery typically occur: hospitals, the home, and freestanding birth centers. Each setting has advantages and disadvantages that should be considered by prospective parents.

Hospital Birth

Not many years ago, most babies were born in hospital delivery rooms, with the mother heavily drugged and the father barred from participating. Nowadays, expectant parents often have a wide range of choices regarding the kind of delivery they will experience in the hospital setting.

Perhaps the most marked change is the increased participation of fathers and same-sex partners in the birth of their children. In traditional births and some cesarean section procedures, fathers and partners are now allowed to be present in the delivery and operating rooms of many hospitals. In some cases, fathers

Many hospitals encourage fathers to participate in the birth of their children. Some allow the father to hold the newborn as it emerges from the birth canal, or to help cut the umbilical cord.

and partners are active participants, perhaps by helping to hold the newborn as it emerges from the birth canal or by cutting the umbilical cord (under guidance, of course).

This inclusion reflects an appreciation specifically for the role of fathers in child rearing. Although long considered "women's work," childbearing and raising children are increasingly being recognized as joint undertakings, involving both parents equally. The benefit of this trend is that fathers share openly not only in the work and responsibility of parenting, but also in the joys and satisfactions. Many believe that this form of "male liberation" results in sounder father–child relationships and that strong father–infant bonds begin, as do mother–child bonds, at the moment of birth. Some hospitals offer consultation specifically for fathers about ways that they can increase their connection to the infant—for example, via "kangaroo care," a technique that allows infants to experience skin-to-skin contact.

Most traditional hospital maternity facilities consist of separate rooms for labor, delivery, and recovery. Physicians, usually obstetricians, serve as the primary birth attendant, with assistance from nurses. Emergency equipment and trained personnel are quickly accessible should the need arise. **Analgesics** and **anesthetics** are options typically available only in this setting. High-risk pregnancies especially benefit from technological advances found in the hospital setting. Some hospitals may be connected to midwife groups that allow the use of midwives as primary birth attendants. This setup allows the woman to enjoy the benefit of the midwife experience, but

analgesics Substances that decrease pain locally, such as topical creams.

anesthetics Substances that elicit unconsciousness and thereby relieve pain.

(a) (b)

Many hospitals offer a birthing room alternative (a) in addition to the traditional hospital delivery room (b).

with hospital emergency services being readily available if complications arise.

Although traditional labor and delivery rooms are still the standard in many hospitals, many hospitals provide the option of a more homelike birth setting for their clients. Typically this takes the form of a **birthing room**, which is attached to a labor and delivery suite and is often run by nurses and

Many hospitals have built plush birthing centers to attract patients to this highly profitable area. Birthing centers, like the one pictured here, typically offer a more homelike atmosphere for delivering a child. Unfortunately, these types of centers do not exist in all areas. Consumers should review options available to them and ask people they know for referrals before making a final decision about their preferred birthing location.

nurse–midwives. The birthing room may be decorated in a homelike style, often including soft lighting, wallpaper, a rocking chair, and a private bath. Mothers labor, deliver, and recover in one room with a support person, such as a partner or other family member, present. Regulations regarding the use of a birthing room vary among hospitals, and birthing rooms are generally used only for low-risk pregnancies. Couples interested in using a hospital birthing room need to find out whether this option is available at local hospitals and whether they are candidates for its use.

Home Birth

For healthy women with low risk pregnancies, home birth is another option. Typically, the birth attendant at home births is a nurse–midwife, who is trained to screen out women who might be at risk of complications during labor and delivery. Home birth candidates are watched closely during pregnancy for signs of possible risk. In addition, individuals need to consider which services are available nearby should complications arise during delivery. One large observational study found that approximately 11% of women who had planned a home birth at the start of labor needed to be transferred to a medical facility, with the most common reason for the transfer being failure of the delivery to progress (Cheyney et al., 2014).

If a couple chooses the home birth option, the midwife or physician—although relatively few physicians support home birth—goes to the couple's home and helps deliver the baby in a previously selected room. Children and other family members may be present. In 2012, only 0.89% of women in the United

birthing room A homelike birth setting available in some hospitals.

States had their babies at home (Martin et al., 2013). While this rate is quite low, it has increased more than 40% since 2004. White women choose home births more than women of other ethnicities, with about 1 in 74 births to white, non-Hispanic women occurring in the home compared to 1 in 325 for black and Hispanic women (Martin et al., 2013).

Although home births are quite common in several European countries, they are not considered best practice by two prominent medical organizations in the United States: Both the American College of Obstetricians and Gynecologists (ACOG, 2013) and the American Academy of Pediatrics (AAP, 2013) recognize hospitals and birthing centers as the safest places for delivery. For low-risk women, several studies have found home birth to be as safe as hospital delivery (de Jonge et al., 2009; Janssen et al., 2009; Johnson & Daviss, 2005); however, other research has determined that, although the absolute risk may be low, there is an increased risk for neonatal death for home births (Grünebaum, McCullough, Sapra et al., 2014; Wax et al., 2010). One of the key factors in safety related to the home birth experience may be the type of midwife selected as a birth attendant. One study indicates higher risk factors for home births attended by midwives not certified by American Midwifery Certification Board compared to AMCB-certified midwives (Grünebaum, McCullough, Brent et al., 2015).

Freestanding Birth Centers

The birth center is a birthing alternative available to prospective parents that represents a compromise between the traditional hospital delivery and the option of home birth. Birth centers are facilities that offer a homelike birth experience outside a hospital setting. Most birth centers are licensed by the state, and many are run by nurse–midwives. Typically, birth centers limit their clientele to low-risk pregnancies. Women are monitored throughout the pregnancy by a nurse–midwife and may be referred to a hospital for delivery if complications arise during the prenatal period. Some emergency equipment is available in birth centers, and most birth centers are located in close proximity to a hospital for ready access if medical care is needed.

Both prenatal care and postnatal care are provided by the birth center's staff, and this continuity of care is a major benefit of birth centers. Freestanding birth centers are family oriented, encouraging family participation throughout the prenatal period.

Couples are active participants in designing their personal birth plan, and family members are allowed to stay near the mother during labor and delivery. Additionally, the infant remains with the mother after delivery.

Although birth centers have increased in popularity and availability, they are not available in every city or even every state. Couples who wish to use a birth center must investigate the availability of this alternative in their community.

Nowadays it is acknowledged that childbirth is an emotional experience as well as a physical one—not just for the mother and child, but for the father or partner as well. The many birthing options available reflect this perspective and responsible decision-making by expectant parents is increasingly important. If a birthing center option is chosen, a center that is accredited by the Commission for the Accreditation of Birth Centers (CABC) should be selected. In addition, some states regulate birth centers; therefore, only those facilities sanctioned by the state should be considered.

Prenatal Care

Traditionally, **prenatal care** consists of monitoring fetal development, screening for high-risk pregnancy, and educating those involved about pregnancy and childbirth. For most normal pregnancies, 10 to 12 prenatal care visits, beginning at about the sixth week of pregnancy, are optimal. For a high-risk pregnancy, more frequent visits may be necessary. Studies show that the risk of very low-birth-weight babies increases when women do not receive comprehensive prenatal care.

The prenatal evaluation begins, as most medical visits do, with the taking of a personal health history, relevant social and emotional factors, employment of the parents, conditions of their work environment, and the stability of their relationship. The practitioner is usually interested in knowing what sort of support system the woman and her new child will have, because many factors—both medical and nonmedical—can affect the well-being of a pregnant woman and her child. Additionally, a series of laboratory tests is usually completed at the first prenatal examination. These normally include examination for hemoglobin levels, glucose or protein in the urine, evidence of a current syphilis infection, antibodies for rubella (German measles), and blood type and Rh determination (discussed shortly). An examination of the cervix is also done at this time.

A family history is taken. Is the woman on her own—and therefore possibly facing greater levels of stress and financial anxiety—or does she live with a partner? Is the father involved in the pregnancy? Is

prenatal care Care given to an expectant mother before the birth of her child that typically consists of monitoring fetal development, screening for high-risk pregnancy, and providing education for pregnancy and childbirth.

Staying as healthy as possible is the pregnant woman's chief responsibility to her developing child. Many choices must be made by expectant parents, including which health-enhancing lifestyle modifications, such as following a healthy diet, they can make throughout the pregnancy.

the baby wanted or unwanted? Was the pregnancy planned or unexpected? All of these factors can place stress on the mother, so they have a bearing on her prenatal care. The medical practitioner overseeing her care will—or should—take an interest in these matters from the start. On the basis of this medical and social history, the practitioner will also determine how much information the expectant parents lack, which sort of guidance they need to adapt to the pregnancy, and, of course, which sort of delivery they favor. When pregnancy is the issue of concern, the practitioner–client relationship is unique. If the couple, and particularly the mother, feel misgivings about their first choice, seeking another practitioner early in the pregnancy is highly advisable.

Nutrition and Weight Gain

Maternal nutrition directly affects fetal growth and development. The developing fetus depends on the mother for nutrition and can deplete her supply of necessary nutrients. The food intake of the mother fuels the development of the baby and directly influences the baby's weight gain. Even if they eat healthfully, women may miss out on key nutrients. A daily prenatal vitamin, ideally starting 3 months before conception, can compensate for any missed nutritional needs. Healthcare providers may also recommend special supplements for women who follow a strict vegetarian or vegan diet or who have chronic health conditions.

Among the most important nutrients to obtain during pregnancy is folate (a B vitamin), which helps prevent serious abnormalities of the fetal brain and spinal cord. Lack of folate also may increase the risk of preterm delivery, low birth weight, and poor fetal growth. Folate obtained through vitamin supplements is called folic acid.

There are also some foods that pregnant women should avoid; among the most commonly discussed are foods containing mercury. All fish contain mercury—and although fish is considered a healthy food, too much mercury can affect the development of the fetus's nervous system. Some fish (e.g., shark, swordfish, king mackerel, and tilefish) contain higher levels of mercury, so pregnant women should avoid these types of fish. Others (such as albacore tuna) contain moderate amounts, so their consumption should be limited. Talking with a healthcare provider or consulting with a dietician can help the pregnant woman and her partner understand other specific recommendations or restrictions.

In the past, it was common practice in prenatal care to place pregnant women on strict regimens to prevent them from gaining more than about 20 pounds. Obese patients were even put on weight-reduction programs. Current attitudes suggest that dieting during pregnancy can be harmful in that breakdown of fat produces toxic substances (called *ketones*) that can impair the mental and physical development of the fetus. Current recommendations for a healthy weight gain during pregnancy vary with the pre-pregnancy weight of the mother (National Research Council, 2013). Those mothers who were considered by their physician to be at a normal weight before conception should gain between 25 and 35 pounds. Those women who were underweight should gain slightly more (28 to 40 pounds); those who were overweight before pregnancy should gain less weight (15 to 25 pounds). Women identified as obese before pregnancy should gain 11 to 20 pounds during the pregnancy. This weight gain includes a variety of components for both the mother and the fetus (Figure 8.6). As noted earlier, extra nutrients are needed in pregnancy, and a wide variety of foods is needed to provide them. If a woman is planning to become pregnant, having a healthy weight before the pregnancy is best for both the mother and baby, both during and after pregnancy.

Exercise During Pregnancy

In the past, the safety of aerobic exercise during pregnancy was questioned. More recently, however,

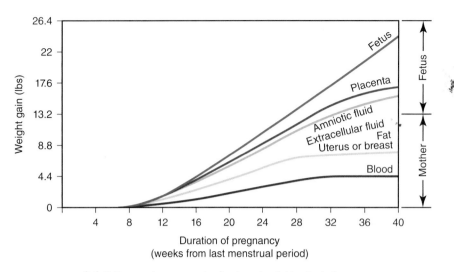

FIGURE **8.6** Pattern and components of maternal weight gain during pregnancy.

studies have shown that exercise is safe for both the pregnant woman and the fetus and that it offers both psychological and physiological benefits (ACOG, 2011b; Kader & Naim-Shuchana, 2014; Nascimento, Surita, & Cecatti, 2012). For example, the physical discomforts of pregnancy, such as backaches, bloating, constipation, and swelling, are reduced with exercise. Risk for gestational diabetes and treatment of the condition can also be lowered with regular exercise. Energy and mood are both elevated. In addition to benefits during pregnancy, because individuals who exercise regularly are more fit, they can often handle the physical efforts of labor and have an easier labor (ACOG, 2011b).

To ensure the safety of both the mother and the developing infant, pregnant women should follow the exercise guidelines of the American College of Obstetrics and Gynecology (ACOG, 2011b). ACOG recommends that pregnant women engage in 30 minutes or more of moderate exercise on most, if not all, days of the week. The exceptions to this recommendation include proscriptions against scuba diving (due to the risk of fetal decompression sickness), contact activities that carry a risk of abdominal injury (e.g., hockey, basketball, and soccer), and activities that have a risk of falling (e.g., gymnastics, skiing, and horseback riding).

Before exercising during pregnancy, a woman should consult her physician or nurse–midwife. Certain conditions, such as cardiac disease, a history of three or more spontaneous abortions (miscarriages), or abnormal bleeding, are contraindications to exercise during pregnancy. Thus, such a consultation

There is no reason that pregnant women should not maintain an exercise regimen. In fact, the American College of Obstetrics and Gynecology recommends pregnant women engage in 30 minutes or more of moderate exercise on most days.

is especially important for women with high-risk pregnancies. If a woman has been sedentary before her pregnancy, she should not attempt to take up a strenuous aerobic exercise program. Walking and swimming are appropriate activities for pregnant women who are beginning to exercise. Runners can continue to run, although their program may need to be modified (ACOG, 2011b). If a woman experiences fatigue, shortness of breath, dizziness, nausea, uterine contractions, pain, vaginal bleeding, or decreased fetal movement during exercise, she should stop exercising immediately and call her physician or nurse–midwife. Pregnant women who honestly share their exercise habits with their healthcare provider and follow their guidelines improve their chances of experiencing a satisfying pregnancy and delivering a healthy baby.

Threats to Having a Healthy Infant

Parents-to-be often worry about whether their baby will be born healthy. In our highly technological society, we are exposed to a larger number of risks to healthy pregnancy than ever before. Exposure to chemicals and radiation at the work site and in the home, lifestyle factors such as cigarette smoking and other drug use and abuse, and exposure to infectious agents are just some of the factors currently posing a risk to bearing healthy children. Although the great majority of infants are born healthy, both public health professionals and parents-to-be have legitimate concerns about infant morbidity and mortality.

In 2013, the National Center for Health Statistics reported an infant death rate of 5.8 deaths per 1,000 births in the United States (Centers for Disease Control and Prevention [CDC], 2014f). This is the rate of infants who die before their first birthday, and for the United States, the 2013 rate represents a significant decrease from the 1988 rate of 10.1 deaths per 1,000 births. Even so, compared with other countries, the United States fares poorly on this score; in 2014, 55 other countries were estimated to have a lower infant mortality rate than the United States (Central Intelligence Agency, 2014). Additionally, the U.S. infant death rate is more than twice as high for African Americans as for whites (CDC, 2014d).

Birth defects are the leading cause of infant mortality in the United States. Approximately 120,000 children are born every year with a birth defect (March of Dimes, 2014a), and while many of these babies will die during the first year, the majority must cope with a range of defects throughout their lives. A pregnant women can take some steps to reduce the chance of a birth defect, but approximately 70% of the causes of birth defects remain unknown (March of Dimes, 2014a). **Teratology** is the branch of research that searches for causes of birth defects. Some known causes include chromosomal defects, mutant genes, and environmental causes, such as exposure to harmful chemicals and drugs. Education can decrease risk of birth defects by environmental factors.

Birth defects are one of the important causes of infant death in the United States; another leading cause is low birth weight, often associated with premature birth (Lau et al., 2013). Low birth weight (a birth weight of less than 5 pounds 8 ounces) and very low birth weight (less than 3 pounds 4 ounces) substantially increase an infant's chances of dying during the first year of life. This is especially true for African Americans, for whom low birth weight is the leading cause of infant death in the United States.

There are two types of low birth weight. The first involves infants who are born preterm or prematurely (before 37 weeks' gestation) and therefore are underweight. A second type of low birth weight is known as *fetal growth restriction*. These infants are born full term, but they are underweight. Some of these babies are healthy, whereas others have low birth weight because something slowed or halted their growth in utero. Risk factors associated with low birth weight include smoking, alcohol and other substance use, chronic health problems in the mother, infections in the mother or fetus, problems with the placenta, having a low-birth-weight baby in a previous pregnancy, low pregnancy weight gain, and socioeconomic factors such as low income, low educational levels, maternal age younger than 17 or older than 35, or being black (March of Dimes, 2014c).

Research into the causes and prevention of birth defects and low birth weight continues to be needed. We already know a great deal about preventing these conditions, so reducing these risk factors is the focus of our attention here.

Drugs and Other Substances

Any drug taken by a pregnant woman can potentially pass through the placenta to the fetus. If the drug (whether medically prescribed or self-prescribed) affects the mother in some way, it will also affect the developing baby. A danger of taking drugs during pregnancy is that an adult dose can be an overdose for a fetus. The liver of the fetus cannot metabolize drugs as can the adult liver, and the unchanged drug can affect the fetus differently from the mother. Furthermore, drugs can alter the metabolism of the

---

teratology The study of causative factors of birth defects.

mother, influence hormones in the bloodstream, and affect placenta functioning.

Over-the-Counter Drugs

Many Americans are polydrug users. Over-the-counter (OTC) drugs, which can be sold legally without a prescription, are widely used for self-medication purposes. The use of many OTC drugs causes special concerns for pregnant women. Because of the extensive number of OTC drugs available, it is beyond the scope of this chapter to provide a complete review. The safest course of action for pregnant women is to avoid self-medication and OTC drugs unless their use is approved by the clinician providing prenatal care.

Cigarette Smoking

Smoking during pregnancy has been identified as the most preventable cause of illness and death among infants; unquestionably it is harmful to the unborn baby. One study showed that approximately 10% of U.S. women in 2011 still smoked during pregnancy (CDC, 2014h). In general, smoking during pregnancy is associated with ectopic pregnancy, higher rates of spontaneous abortion, lower birth weight, structural changes in and decreased functioning of the placenta, and cleft lip or palate in the child (CDC, 2014h). After birth, babies whose mothers smoked during pregnancy are more susceptible to childhood illnesses, especially development of respiratory problems such as asthma (Midodzi et al., 2010), and are more likely to die of sudden infant death syndrome (SIDS) (CDC, 2014h). Studies have also indicated a link between smoking and the development of attention-deficit/hyperactivity disorder (ADHD) in children (Knopik, 2009; Pinkhardt et al., 2009) and other mental health conditions, and smoking as adults (Biederman et al., 2014). However, more recent research has indicated that smoking itself may not have physiological effects in utero; rather, some of these conditions are likely caused by other genetic or family factors (Langley et al., 2012; Skoglund et al., 2014).

Marijuana

Tetrahydrocannabinol (THC), the primary psychoactive agent in marijuana and other cannabinoids, can pass through the placental barrier and affect the ability of the placenta to function. For pregnant women with heavy marijuana use (typically defined as use of 5 or more times per week), most research indicates an increased risk of slow fetal growth and premature

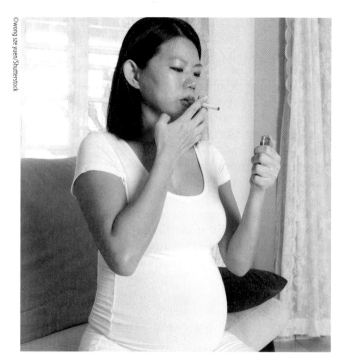
©wong sze yuen/Shutterstock

Cigarette smoke is one of the most toxic substances for fetuses and newborns. Smoking before birth exposes the fetus to a range of health risks, including low birth weight and birth defects. Smoking after birth exposes the infant to breathing problems and other health risks.

birth (Brown & Graves, 2013; Hill & Reed, 2013), although there are some exceptions (Desai, Mark, & Terplan, 2014). Other studies have linked marijuana use in pregnancy to visuoperceptual ability, reasoning, and attention issues in older children (Brown & Graves, 2013; Hill & Reed, 2013) and to use of marijuana as an adolescent (Day, Goldschmidt, & Thomas, 2006). Many marijuana users are polydrug users, so separating out the specific effects of marijuana has been a challenge for researchers (Hill & Reed, 2013). One recent modeling study indicated that marijuana does have a negative effect on birth weight by itself, but that tobacco use is the greatest predictor of low birth weight (Janisse et al., 2014).

With legalization of recreational marijuana use occurring in several U.S. states, pregnant women need to carefully consider the potential risks of marijuana use. Most medical organizations recommend pregnant women refrain from using marijuana to ensure as healthy a pregnancy as possible.

Alcohol

Many women realize that consuming large quantities of alcohol during pregnancy is a risk to the developing fetus. **Fetal alcohol spectrum disorders (FASD)**, formerly called **fetal alcohol syndrome (FAS)**,

fetal alcohol spectrum disorders (FASD) The full spectrum of birth defects that are caused by prenatal alcohol exposure.

fetal alcohol syndrome (FAS) Impaired psychological and physical characteristics common in infants born to alcoholic women.

comprise a range of problems and abnormalities that can appear as a result of heavy alcohol consumption during pregnancy. The prevalence of FASD is difficult to determine. While governmental studies of FAS have demonstrated rates of 0.5 to 1.5 per 1,000 births in the United States (CDC, 2014b), a recent community-based study of first graders indicted much high rates of FASD—in the range of 2.4% to 4.8% (May et al., 2014).

Infants suffering from FASD may have unusual facial features, such as small eye slits, deep epicanthic folds (a fold of skin from the eyelid to the inner corner of the eye, giving it a slanted effect), an upturned nose and a thin flattened upper lip, and a flattened or decreased groove in the upper lip. They may also have heart defects, dysfunctions of the central nervous system, or growth deficiency. Most often, some level of mental challenges exists; these issues can include problems with learning, remembering, understanding and following directions, controlling emotions, communicating, and socializing. In severe cases, mental retardation and difficulty completing life skills, such as feeding and bathing, can exist (U.S. National Library of Medicine, 2014).

There is some debate about the safety of low or moderate amounts of alcohol consumption during pregnancy, with some media reports and pregnancy books stating that small amounts of alcohol are safe. Almost all U.S. health organizations (for example, the U.S. Surgeon General, ACOG, and the March of Dimes) recommend no alcohol be consumed if someone is trying to become pregnant, might become pregnant unintentionally, or is pregnant. Alcohol crosses the placental barrier and can affect fetal cells and tissues. At least one review study showed effects on socioemotional and cognitive development in children with low to moderate alcohol consumption (Swedish National Institute of Public Health, 2009).

Cocaine

In the early months of a pregnancy, cocaine use has been associated with miscarriages. In later months, cocaine use can trigger preterm labor (labor that occurs before a completed pregnancy of 37 weeks). Placenta problems—such as placenta abruption, in which the placenta disconnects from the uterine wall—can also occur and cause life-threatening complications (March of Dimes, 2013). Of all other outcomes, preterm birth is consistently related to cocaine use (Gouin et al., 2011; Janisse et al., 2014), although the associated low birth weight and developmental issues are often not distinguished.

In addition to infant concerns, prenatal cocaine exposure has been associated with a number of long-term health issues: impaired motor development (Bigsby et al., 2001; Richardson et al., 2008);

less ability to self-regulate one's behavior (Ackerman, Riggins, & Black, 2010); impaired language development and processing (Beeghly et al., 2006); attention deficits in preschool and elementary school (Ackerman et al., 2010); and increased likelihood of being in a special education program (Levine et al., 2008). The long-term effects of prenatal cocaine use may be difficult to separate from other environmental factors, such as poverty, low caregiver intelligence, lower-quality home environment, malnutrition, and other substance use (Lambert & Bauer, 2012).

Heroin and Other Narcotics

Today several types of narcotic drugs are used on a prescription basis, including morphine, codeine, paregoric, hydromorphone hydrochloride, laudanum, meperidine, methadone, and others. Pregnant women should not take these drugs without the consent and approval of their healthcare provider. Another type of narcotic—heroin, an illegal street drug—will be the focus of this section.

Use of and addiction to heroin and other opiates in a pregnant woman can result in a fetus who must go through withdrawal after birth; the effect on the fetus is called neonatal abstinence syndrome (NAS). Signs and symptoms of NAS vary. Most appear within 72 hours of birth, but some can appear within a few weeks of birth. NAS symptoms can include tremors, seizures, and twitching; excessive crying or having a high-pitched cry; issues with feeding, including poor sucking or slow weight gain; fast breathing; fever, sweating, or blotchy skin; difficulty sleeping and lots of yawning; diarrhea; vomiting; and stuffy nose or sneezing (March of Dimes, 2014b).

There are also risks if the woman attempts withdrawal from heroin while pregnant. Rapid withdrawal of the mother during the first trimester may result in miscarriage and during the third-trimester may result in life-threatening fetal distress. Pregnant women using heroin should consult with their healthcare provider about potential treatment plans during pregnancy.

In addition to NAS, heroin use during pregnancy is associated with poor fetal growth (about half of all babies of heroin users have low birth weight), premature birth, and stillbirth. Some research suggests that prenatal heroin exposure also affects language and cognition development (Beckwith & Burke, 2015). Although the research in this area is limited, potential effects on socialization, drug use, and mental health problems have been documented in adults who were exposed prenatally to heroin (Herranz et al., 2014).

Methamphetamine

Compared to other drug use, there is less research on the effects of methamphetamine use during pregnancy and on the fetus (Abar et al., 2013). As with the use of other substances, distinguishing the effects of methamphetamine from the effects of other factors is difficult (Lindsay & Burnett, 2013). Research indicates increased pregnancy risks associated with methamphetamine use, inlcuding hypertension, postpartum hemorrhage, and admittance to the intensive care unit. Fetal and newborn risks include preterm birth, intrauterine growth restriction, low birth weight, birth defects, and increased neonatal death. Like fetuses exposed to heroin, fetuses exposed to methamphetamine are at high risk of suffering from NAS (Lindsey & Burnett, 2013). In addition, studies document that both behavioral and emotional control and executive function continue to be affected in elementary school children who were exposed to methamphetamine prenatally (Abar et al., 2013).

Steroids
Steroids are prescribed drugs such as sex hormones and other specific chemicals (cortisol and prednisone) used to treat kidney inflammations, joint inflammation, and tissue damage caused by rheumatic fever and other serious diseases. They can cross the placenta and cause fetal distress.

Diethylstilbestrol
Diethylstilbestrol (DES) is a synthetic nonsteroid estrogen first prescribed in the 1950s to prevent miscarriage. In 1971, it was discovered that DES caused a specific vaginal cancer in some female offspring of women who took the hormone during their pregnancy before 19 weeks' gestation. Additionally, approximately 35% of exposed women exhibit benign vaginal epithelial cell changes. There is also a risk of problems with fertility and pregnancy. Male offspring are possibly vulnerable to infertility and prostatic problems.

Diseases

Certain diseases can be passed from mother to fetus, but their significance varies with the stage of pregnancy. No matter how severe or how innocuous a disease might be in the pregnant woman, the effect on the fetus depends on the stage of fetal development. Discussion of common diseases that can be transmitted to the fetus with harmful consequences is included here.

German Measles (Rubella)
The disease rubella is most harmful to the fetus in the first trimester (the effect is almost nil after the third or fourth month). As many as 85% of babies born to women who contract rubella in the first 3 months of pregnancy will be born with a birth

defect (CDC, 2014g). Common effects on the infant include hearing loss or deafness, eye defects, mental retardation, and liver and spleen damage. Death sometimes occurs shortly before or after birth.

To prevent rubella and its effects, it is recommended that women who have not had rubella be vaccinated well before they decide to conceive. Additionally, vaccines should be given to children at 12 to 15 months of age, because children are the major sources of rubella infection of pregnant women.

Diabetes
Diabetes is an insulin deficiency that affects sugar metabolism and can influence fetal weight and complicate delivery. Infants of diabetic women may have a high birth weight (10 pounds or more) and a higher than average mortality rate.

Human Immunodeficiency Virus
A fetus can become infected with the human immunodeficiency virus (HIV) when the virus crosses the placenta of an infected woman or during the birth process, when the infant might have contact with the mother's infected blood during delivery. Breastfeeding after birth can also transmit the virus to the infant. Worldwide, without treatment, 15% to 45% of infants born to HIV-positive women will also be HIV positive and may contract acquired immunodeficiency syndrome (AIDS) (World Health Organization [WHO], 2014). AIDS is a viral disease characterized by depression of the immune system and the presence of certain opportunistic infections. When appropriate interventions are given, however, the rate of transmission drops to 5% worldwide. With systematic HIV testing of pregnant women, antiretroviral medications given to the female during pregnancy and labor and to the infant in the first weeks of life, plus a complete avoidance of breastfeeding, the risk of mother-to-child transmission has been reduced to 1% in the United States (CDC, 2014c).

Syphilis
Syphilis, a sexually transmitted infection (STI), is a common cause of stillbirth and can infect a fetus when the spirochetes cross the placenta. The infected fetus may show signs of syphilis at birth or may appear normal until adolescence, when signs of late syphilis appear. The fetus will not be affected by this disease if the mother receives penicillin before the 4th month of her pregnancy.

Gonorrhea
This STI affects the eyes as the baby passes through the vagina and can, by transmission through the placenta, eventually cause a form of arthritis.

Genital Herpes

Genital herpes is an STI caused by the herpes simplex virus (HSV). If lesions are present on the genitals of the mother at the time of delivery, the virus can be absorbed by the baby, causing encephalitis, inflammation of the brain, and possibly death. A woman with a history of genital herpes will be followed closely from 32 weeks' gestation until delivery. If herpes lesions are present on her genitals, delivery will likely be by cesarean section.

Chlamydia

The STI chlamydia is caused by the intracellular parasite *Chlamydia trachomatis*. Infants born to mothers with chlamydia infections have a chance of acquiring either inclusion conjunctivitis (an eye infection) or chlamydial pneumonia during delivery. All pregnant women should be screened for chlamydia at their first prenatal visit. The infection is easily treated with antibiotics.

Genital Warts

Genital warts, another STI, are caused by the human papillomavirus (HPV). Infected mothers may transmit HPV to the fetus in utero or during the birth process, but transmission during birth is rare. If transfer of HPV does occur, it is most commonly associated with respiratory papillomatosis, which causes hoarseness and respiratory distress in the infant. If a pregnant woman has genital warts that are large, they may interfere with the birth process, requiring a cesarean delivery; however, this is uncommon.

Rh Incompatibility

The **Rh factor** is a substance found in the blood of approximately 85% of the population. If the Rh factor is present, the person's blood type is Rh positive (Rh+); if it is not present, the blood type is Rh negative (Rh−).

A problem in pregnancy exists when an Rh− mother is pregnant with an Rh+ child, a child who has inherited the positive factor from the Rh+ father. The mother's body develops anti-Rh agglutinins—antibodies to the presence of the Rh+, which are similar to the antibodies that fight disease. These anti-Rh antibodies enter the fetus and cause its red blood cells to clump together—that is, agglutinate. During the first such pregnancy, the mother's body does not develop many agglutinins. However, in subsequent pregnancies, her body develops the anti-Rh agglutinins rapidly, and the babies of these pregnancies may be born anemic and jaundiced, with red blood cells and hemoglobin below normal. This condition can be prevented if the woman is given an injection of Rh immunoglobulin (RhIg), which prevents the sensitization of the Rh factor. RhIg is used during pregnancy and after delivery, which includes any miscarriage, ectopic pregnancy, or induced abortion. If the preventive treatment is not given to the mother, the newborn infant will receive a blood transfusion (Medline Plus, 2011).

Testing for Disorders

Many different tests can be performed during a pregnancy. Some of these tests are virtually risk free and as simple as a blood test. Others are more invasive and carry more risk to the pregnancy.

A blood test that can be used as early as 7 weeks' gestation can screen for sex-related disorders without invasive testing. This cell-free fetal DNA testing looks for the Y chromosome; the results can help parents who may be worrying about male-only genetic disorders such as hemophilia or a specific type of muscular dystrophy (Devaney et al., 2011).

Because this test is relatively new, and is typically used only in individuals older than age 35, many insurance companies do not cover its cost. Studies have provided evidence of benefits from using this test more widely (Bianchi et al., 2014), and the test may decrease the need for more invasive testing (Pettit et al., 2014). Thus, if the costs of cell-free fetal DNA testing can be decreased, it is likely to become the standard of care for pregnant women.

Another, more common prenatal blood screening test is the maternal serum alpha-fetoprotein (MSAFP). This test is part of a blood panel performed at 16 to 18 weeks' gestation to detect neural tube defects such as spina bifida (an open spine) and anencephaly (lack of higher brain structures). Abnormal levels of MSAFP could indicate several other conditions, such as twin pregnancy, ventral wall (heart) defects, Down syndrome, and fetal demise.

Both MSAFP and cell-free fetal DNA testing are screening tests that detect *potential* problems; they are not *diagnostic* tests that can confirm these conditions with certainty. Abnormal results are an indication that a diagnostic test such as amniocentesis should be performed. If high-risk pregnant women, such as women older than age 35, receive results indicating a low risk for fetal abnormalities, such testing could spare them from having another procedure like amniocentesis, which carries an inherent risk of miscarriage.

Rh factor The presence of Rh agglutinogens (antigens) in the blood, which indicates that a person is Rh positive, whereas its absence designates the person as Rh negative.

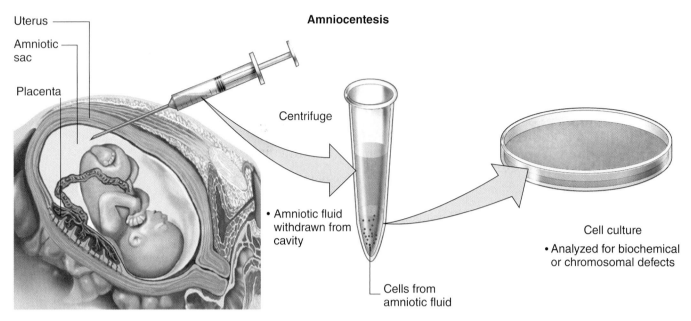

FIGURE **8.7** Amniocentesis is a test for fetal abnormalities that involves withdrawing amniotic fluid and inspecting the cells contained within it.

Another almost risk-free procedure is the ultrasound, or **sonogram**. During this procedure, high-frequency sound waves are directed at the pregnant woman's uterus. The echo from the waves is transformed into a visual representation of the uterus and fetus, including the internal structures of the fetus. This technique can provide indication of the sex of the fetus, the number of fetuses, and some abnormalities. If the ultrasound shows a possible abnormality, fetal magnetic resonance imaging (MRI) might be used to provide a more detailed and clearer image (Obebauer & Maestre, 2008). Fetal MRI relies on the same techniques as brain imaging and can better detect some internal abnormalities, such as those found in the central nervous system, gastrointestinal tract, genital area, and chest (Baysinger, 2010; Weston, 2010).

Another technique for prenatal detection of genetic defects, **chorionic villi sampling (CVS)**, is performed ideally at 8 to 10 weeks' gestation. The chorion is the outermost protective covering of the growing embryo. The villi are threadlike, vascular (containing blood) protrusions growing on the outer surface of the chorion. In the CVS procedure, a plastic catheter is passed through the vagina into the uterus to these villi. Ultrasound is used to guide the insertion of this catheter. Approximately 30 milligrams (0.001 ounce) of tissue is suctioned and then studied. If an abortion might be considered, CVS has the advantage of providing information several weeks earlier in a pregnancy than an amniocentesis. A first-trimester abortion is less risky to the mother than an abortion done in the second trimester. However, certain defects, such as neural tube defects, cannot be detected by CVS. If such a problem is suspected, amniocentesis must be performed. CVS carries about double the risk of miscarriage associated with amniocentesis—0.22% versus 0.11%, respectively (Akolekar et al., 2014).

Amniocentesis is the drawing of fluid from the amniotic sac for the purpose of diagnosing fetal abnormalities (Figure 8.7). The procedure cannot be safely performed until the 16th week of pregnancy. A sonogram picture is taken to show the outline of the fetus so that the needle used will not touch the baby. Under sterile conditions and using a local anesthetic, a physician inserts a long needle through the abdominal and uterine walls into the amniotic sac and withdraws up to 20 milliliters (⅔ ounce) of fluid. The fluid, which contains cells sloughed off by the fetus, is analyzed for a variety of fetal abnormalities. The test analysis are usually complete in two weeks but can take longer. Chromosomal disorders, genetically induced metabolic disorders, sex-linked diseases, and genetics-linked inherited conditions can be determined by this procedure. Maternal age older than 35 years carries a higher risk of chromosomal

sonogram A diagnostic picture revealing the fetal outline. In ultrasonography, sound waves are bounced off the fetus. With a scanner, the image is then projected onto a computer screen, revealing whether certain defects are present.

chorionic villi sampling (CVS) A technique for prenatal detection of genetic defects that involves removal of some of the villi growing on the outer surface of the chorion and examining their chromosomes.

amniocentesis Withdrawal by syringe of amniotic fluid to determine the presence of fetal abnormalities.

disorders (such as Down syndrome), and amniocentesis may be recommended for these pregnant women depending on the results of other, less invasive tests, such as blood tests. The sex and exact age of the fetus can be determined by means of amniocentesis, although it is rarely performed for these reasons alone because it always entails some risk to the fetus. Even though the procedure is performed under sterile conditions, there is always the risk of introducing infection into the uterine environment, inducing miscarriage, or damaging the fetus.

Maternal Health Problems During Pregnancy

More than 20% of all pregnant women and their babies are described as "at risk." When a practitioner deems a pregnancy to be a high-risk one, this label indicates that the mother and/or child could suffer some adverse effects during pregnancy, labor, or delivery. The mother's health, economic status, and access to medical care, as well as the genetic history of both parents, influence the risk status of the pregnancy. The mother's age, too, has a major effect. Those women younger than 18 years and older than 35 years are at greatest risk of high-risk pregnancy. The most common causes of maternal deaths in pregnancy and childbirth in the United States are hemorrhage, infection, preeclampsia, eclampsia, and convulsions.

Hypertension

Hypertension is the condition in which blood pressure is above normal while the heart is contracted or relaxed, or both. Women who have a history of hypertension or who become hypertensive in pregnancy need attentive medical supervision, but their condition by no means precludes a successful pregnancy.

Hypertensive conditions induced by a pregnancy have been traditionally called **toxemias of pregnancy**. Despite the term, these conditions are not caused by toxins—poisons—circulating in the blood, as some people believe. Toxemias are also called *preeclampsia* and *eclampsia*. **Preeclampsia** is pregnancy-induced hypertension accompanied by swelling of the face, neck, and upper extremities. These body parts swell when tissues retain too much fluid. Proteinuria, an abnormal amount of protein in the urine, is another symptom of preeclampsia. The term **eclampsia** refers to the preeclampsia events, plus convulsions or coma, which can be fatal. At present, the causes of preeclampsia and eclampsia are unknown.

It is important to recognize that edema—swelling of the tissues—does not always indicate an abnormal condition in pregnancy. In fact, it is quite common among pregnant women. There is more than one type and cause of edema in pregnancy.

Nausea and Vomiting

Although the exact cause is unknown, the nausea and vomiting common to early pregnancy are thought to be caused by hormonal changes. **Morning sickness** is the usual term applied to these conditions, because the nausea often occurs early in the day and dissipates relatively quickly. Small meals, avoidance of strongly flavored foods, and eating toast and jelly before moving around in the morning are suggested. As the body adjusts to the pregnancy, the nausea and vomiting typically disappear. Some alternative methods may be used to address morning sickness (such as acupuncture or ginger), but their effectiveness has not been consistently validated through studies (Matthews et al., 2014).

Severe, continuous vomiting in pregnancy (*hyperemesis gravidarum*) can be serious. Dehydration, loss of electrolytes, and dietary insufficiency can result and threaten the pregnancy. Bed rest and sedation are frequently necessary, and, in extreme cases, hospitalization and intravenous feeding are required. The treatment usually includes a search for the physiological or psychological causes, because most practitioners favor limiting the use of medication in pregnancy.

Hemorrhoids

Hemorrhoids are varicose veins of the anal area. They are caused by the same pressures that create varicose veins in the legs. The increased flow of blood to the pelvic area during pregnancy results in added pressure of blood flow, which stresses the inelastic veins. In an effort to accommodate the increased blood flow, the veins become stressed, resulting in swelling, pain, and bleeding. The usual treatment employs sitz baths (a bath in which only the hip area

toxemias of pregnancy Hypertensive conditions, subdivided into preeclampsia and eclampsia.

preeclampsia Pregnancy-induced hypertension; symptoms include swelling of the face, neck, and upper extremities; and excess levels of protein in the urine.

eclampsia Pregnancy-induced hypertension accompanied by swelling of the face, neck, and upper extremities, plus convulsions or coma, which may be fatal.

morning sickness The condition of nausea and vomiting that is common in early pregnancy; thought to be caused by hormonal changes.

is immersed) and topical creams. A pregnant woman who has hemorrhoids should tell her practitioner and allow him or her to prescribe treatment.

Other Conditions

A number of conditions frequently associated with pregnancy, although not serious, are often irritating. **Chloasma**, or the "mask of pregnancy," is a usually yellow to brown patch of skin pigmentation that appears on the faces of white women. The mask is thought to be caused by hormonal action that increases the number of pigment cells. Estrogen and progesterone can also produce these skin changes, as can ultraviolet light. When the pregnancy ends, the chloasma disappears.

Stretch marks, which are also more common in white women than in others, are visible white streaks in the skin of the abdomen and breasts, which become enlarged during pregnancy. They are thought to be caused by a weakening of fibers in the tissue under the skin. It is believed that some people have a predisposition to this condition. In most instances, stretch marks do not disappear after childbirth, although they may fade or lighten in time.

Hair loss sometimes occurs because of an increase in hormone production. It is temporary when it does occur, and as long as no significant health problems exist, normal growth recurs within 6 months after delivery.

Reddish branchlike vascular "spiders" in the neck, chest, face, and arms are due to high estrogen levels and vascular weakness. Small capillaries under the skin surface break, and uneven streaks become visible on the surface. These streaks also fade, but in some women they do not disappear completely.

During the last few months of a pregnancy, weak and slow contractions of the uterus occur. Known as **Braxton-Hicks contractions**, these contractions become more frequent as the pregnancy proceeds. Some researchers consider this a means through which the uterus practices for labor.

Childbirth

Parturition, derived from a Latin term meaning "to produce," is the process of giving birth. It begins with **labor**—contractions of the uterus, a gradual opening of the cervix, and purposeful bearing down by the woman—and ends in **delivery**—the expulsion of a child and the placenta. Sometimes women experience what is called *false labor*. False labor, which is common in late pregnancy, is characterized by brief uterine **contractions**, sometimes accompanied by mild back and abdominal pain and involving no changes in the cervix. **True labor** is characterized by (1) regularly spaced contractions of the uterus that gradually gain intensity, (2) thinning and **dilation** (gradual opening) of the cervix, and (3) descent of the presenting part of the fetus into the vagina (Figure 8.8). The presenting part of the fetus is that part of its body that can be felt through the cervix during a vaginal examination. Usually the cervix begins to soften and dilate a few days to a few weeks before the actual delivery time.

Labor

Labor takes place in three distinct stages—at least from an obstetrician's point of view. Stage I is the period from the onset of labor to the point at which the cervix is fully dilated—that is, when the cervix is opened to 4 inches (10 centimeters) across. The average length of the first stage in a first pregnancy is 8 to 12 hours, but it often lasts up to 20 hours. Stage II is the period from full cervical dilation through the birth of the child. This stage can last from a few minutes to 2 hours in a normal delivery, though the longer time is most common. Stage III is the period from the infant's birth to delivery of the placenta, or **afterbirth** (usually taking up to 30 minutes).

Contractions indicate the beginning of labor and will continue throughout the first stage. Often the contractions are irregular at first and of unequal length; once the woman is in true labor, they eventually occur in a settled pattern—for example, contractions of 30 to 40 seconds occurring every 2 to 3 minutes. Along with the onset of contractions, a **bloody show** occurs—the disintegration of the

---

chloasma A yellow to brown patch of skin pigmentation that may appear on the faces of pregnant white women; sometimes referred to as the "mask of pregnancy."

Braxton-Hicks contractions Weak and slow uterine contractions that occur during the last few months of pregnancy.

parturition The process of giving birth.

labor The process of expelling a child by uterine contractions, dilation of the cervix, and bearing-down pressure.

delivery The stage of childbirth characterized by the expulsion of the infant and the placenta.

contraction The shortening or tension of uterine muscles during labor.

true labor Characterized by regularly spaced contractions of the uterus, thinning and dilation of the cervix, and a descending of the presenting part of the fetus into the vagina.

dilation In childbirth, the gradual opening of the cervix during labor.

afterbirth Delivery of the placenta.

bloody show Expelling of the mucus plug (often streaked with blood) that has closed off the cervix during pregnancy.

(a) Early first-stage labor

(b) Later first-stage labor: the transition

(c) Early second-stage labor

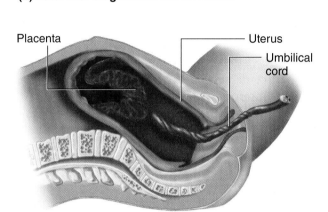

(d) Third-stage labor: delivery of afterbirth

FIGURE **8.8** Childbirth: The stages of labor. (a) First stage: The cervix is dilating. (b) Late first stage (transition stage): The cervix is fully dilated, and the amniotic sac has ruptured, releasing amniotic fluid. (c) Second stage: The birth of the infant. (d) Third stage: Delivery of the placenta (afterbirth).

mucus plug at the cervix. Usually the **amniotic sac** (the "bag of waters") ruptures spontaneously near the beginning of labor, experienced as either a rush or trickle of fluid through the vagina. Sometimes, however, contractions increase, but the amniotic sac remains unruptured; in such cases, the birth attendant breaks the sac. As mentioned earlier, in some situations in which labor is overdue or dilation is progressing poorly, the drug oxytocin (Pitocin) is used to start labor or to increase the frequency of the contractions.

The medical attendants monitor the heartbeat of the fetus regularly by placing a stethoscope on the mother's abdomen, and they perform vaginal examinations periodically. If the woman is giving birth in a hospital, an **electronic fetal monitor** is also used to assess fetal heart rate. The nurse attaches an electrode to the woman's abdomen, and electrocardiographic impulses are transmitted to paper, giving a tracing (a reading) of the fetal heartbeat. Fetal heart rate can be influenced by such conditions as uterine contractions, problems with the placenta, and problems with the umbilical cord.

If anesthesia is used to reduce or eliminate the pain of contractions, it is administered late in the first stage or in the second stage. We discuss some of the choices women have regarding anesthesia later in the chapter.

Delivery

The physician or midwife may try to control the delivery to prevent a too sudden or too forceful ejection of the baby. The goal is to prevent injury to the central nervous system of the baby or injury to the mother's perineum, the area between the vulva and the anus.

Sometimes there is a need to enlarge the vaginal opening to permit the baby to pass through and to

amniotic sac A fluid-filled membrane that surrounds the developing infant in the uterus.

electronic fetal monitoring A technique used during labor whereby a physician places an electrode on the woman's abdomen to monitor the fetal heart rate for signs of fetal distress.

Gender
DIMENSIONS

Fathers and Childbirth

One of us vividly remembers driving his wife to the hospital when she went into labor and being met by a very accommodating nurse. She took us immediately into the labor room, an area in which women could scream and shout and kick. The comfort I was able to offer my wife was not immediately acknowledged—she had other things on her mind—but was nonetheless helpful and appreciated in retrospect. Yet, when it came time for her to deliver our son, my wife was wheeled into the delivery room and I was escorted to the waiting room. That was how it was done in those days.

Since then, more and more fathers are accompanying the mothers of their babies into the delivery room and observing the birth. Some even view the birth through a camera lens as they try to capture the moment for posterity. In this way they feel involved in all phases of childbirth and, some research indicates, develop a greater sense of closeness—bonding—with their children as well as with their partners.

Although this trend may be welcomed by most men, it places a burden on others. Akin to the pressure on women to work outside the home or to have a "natural childbirth delivery," the one-model-fits-all approach ignores those men who prefer not to be in the delivery room. Some men may feel squeamish about medical procedures and fear fainting during the delivery, and others may feel uncomfortable observing their partners in pain.

Which types of accommodations could a hospital or birthing center provide for fathers who do not feel comfortable attending a delivery?

prevent the mother's tissue from tearing. In this event an incision is made into the perineum, a procedure called an **episiotomy**. Although in the past episiotomy was performed routinely in all hospital births, physicians and midwives have been challenging the need for routine episiotomies, making the incision only when absolutely necessary (ACOG, 2006).

The usual delivery is divided into three phases: delivery of the head, of the shoulders, and of the body and legs. **Crowning** is the presentation of the baby's head at the vaginal opening. In a **breech delivery**, the baby presents the hip, body, shoulder, and head, in that order. A breech delivery can be hazardous to the mother or baby, or both, for several reasons. The membranes can rupture prematurely, predisposing the mother to infection; because the buttocks of the baby do not conform to the contours of the lower uterus, labor can be prolonged; manipulation of the baby is more involved than in a head presentation; and lacerations may occur in the cervix, vagina, and perineum, possibly causing infection or hemorrhage. A breech delivery can be hazardous to the baby in that the umbilical cord may separate or

be compressed between the baby and the inner wall of the uterus, depriving the baby of oxygen; intracranial hemorrhage can occur because of stress on the head as it is delivered last; and injuries to the head, neck, and upper arms can occur during manipulations of delivery. These complications are rare with appropriate monitoring and care. Each breech delivery is managed according to its need, and in some circumstances a cesarean section may be required.

Under certain conditions in which resistance inhibits the normal delivery mechanism, a forceps delivery may be necessary. Such conditions include the mother's exhaustion, cardiac or pulmonary problems, or illness; fetal distress; or certain obstetrical conditions (such as certain positions of the baby's head). The forceps is a tool designed to deliver the baby's head and is used to gain traction and to rotate the baby. Forceps must be used carefully, however, because they exert force and can cause fetal damage. Delivery with forceps is a relatively uncommon practice; forceps were used in only 0.61% of births in 2012 (Martin et al., 2013). After delivery of the baby, the umbilical cord is clamped and cut.

Delivery of Placenta

The third stage, delivery of the placenta and the membranes, usually occurs about 5 minutes after the baby is born. When the placenta emerges—again through contractions of the uterus—the doctor or midwife examines it carefully to be sure it is completely smooth.

episiotomy Incision between the vulva and anus to enlarge the vaginal opening at the time of birth.

crowning The presentation of the baby's head at the vaginal opening.

breech delivery A delivery in which the infant is born with another body part first, rather than head first. This form of delivery can be hazardous for both mother and infant.

(a) In stage I of labor, the mother and baby are monitored electronically and helped by the attending staff. (b) During stage II of labor, the child is born, with the head appearing first. (c) The baby, 1 minute old, with umbilical cord. (d) After delivery and checking over of the baby, the parents begin to bond with their newborn child.

If the placenta is not smooth, it is likely that some placental tissue has remained in the uterus. Any tissue left behind may cause uterine bleeding or infection. If contractions stop before the placenta is expelled, manual techniques or injection of medication is used to facilitate its delivery. If an episiotomy has been performed, it is repaired after the placenta is delivered.

Drugs Used in Childbirth

Expectant parents must grapple with the question of whether drugs will be used during delivery. Decisions about drugs in childbirth require some homework, because many kinds of drugs are available, all having different effects. Anesthetics inhibit perception, not just of pain but of touch and all other sensations, in the mother. General anesthetics not only affect the mother but also cross the placental barrier and reach the fetus. Most are central nervous system depressants and can act as such on the fetus. Some general anesthetics are used in pain-reducing concentrations, in which case they are less powerful depressants. These drugs, which are usually inhaled, include continuous nitrous oxide and enflurane.

Whereas general anesthetics put the individual to sleep, local anesthetics and local and regional analgesics (reducers of pain perception) inhibit feelings and sensations in specific parts of the body. They can be used to reduce pain without placing the fetus in jeopardy. This type of anesthetic is generally administered during the latter part of the first stage of labor and during all of the second stage. Single or multiple injections are administered via a catheter into the spinal area. Drugs commonly used for local pain relief include tetracaine, lidocaine, and bupivacaine. Different areas of the pelvic region are anesthetized by different procedures. **Saddle blocks**, or **epidural blocks**, anesthetize the area of the buttocks, perineum, and inner thigh (the area that literally sits on a saddle). In a **paracervical block**, injections are given at positions around the cervix.

Drugs have been used successfully and safely during labor for many years. However, as with all drugs, there are potential, though minimal, risks with their use during labor. Spinal anesthesia, for example, can cause headache, nausea and vomiting, and a drop in blood pressure. A reduction in blood pressure can reduce the oxygen supply to the baby and can change the fetal heartbeat. Due to these potential complications, some individuals prefer to use **obstetrical analgesia**, or a nondrug pain reliever, like hypnosis.

Because pregnancy is a 9-month experience, expectant parents have plenty of time to discuss alternatives. Talks with the physician or midwife, with friends who have used different methods, and, most important, with each other will yield a well-thought-out decision.

Natural Childbirth

Drug-free childbirth gained support in the latter part of the 20th century, particularly as the adverse effects of some drugs on the newborn were discovered. This mode of giving birth is called **natural childbirth**—or sometimes prepared childbirth, because it involves education and practice. Electing to have a natural delivery often means that both parents are more involved in the pregnancy than they would be in a more traditional approach.

The natural childbirth movement began early in the 1930s with Dr. Grantly Dick-Read, an English

Natural, or prepared, childbirth involves prospective parents being educated in techniques—exercise and breathing techniques among them—to decrease the likelihood that anesthetics will be required during childbirth.

physician. He developed a method of childbirth with no anesthetics or analgesics and published his approach in *Childbirth Without Fear*. At the heart of his method were techniques for relaxing tension to reduce the pain of labor. In 1950, a Russian scientist named Velvoski published a work on his theory of psychoprophylaxis, which was taken up in France by Fernand Lamaze. Psychoprophylaxis is based on the premise that with the aid of a supportive coach (usually a partner, though it could be a doula or any concerned, interested adult friend), a woman who has a positive attitude can reduce the stress and tension of parturition and relax the pelvic muscles. The objective is to reduce the pain of labor to the point where painkilling drugs become unnecessary. Exercise and breathing techniques are integral to what has come to be called the **Lamaze method**. The woman and her coach attend classes together once a week for approximately 6 to 8 weeks before the expected delivery date. Both adults participate in the birth process, with the coach guiding the mother in performing the exercises appropriate to the stage of labor.

With the Lamaze method, the woman receives both emotional support and coaching, particularly during the delivery. This method allows the father or same-sex partner to increase his or her involvement in the delivery process. Because some people may feel frightened or uncomfortable at the prospect of being present at a birth, a couple must discuss this option thoroughly. Does the partner eagerly look forward to participating? Is the woman willing to undergo a natural birth without her partner present and perhaps with another coach? Like most other aspects of reproductive behavior, the natural childbirth option requires free and open communication between partners.

saddle (epidural) block An anesthetic used during childbirth that blocks pain sensations in the buttocks, perineum, and inner thigh.

paracervical block An anesthetic used during childbirth that blocks pain sensations in the pelvic area, in which injections are given at positions around the cervix.

obstetrical analgesia A nondrug pain reliever used in delivery (e.g., hypnosis).

natural childbirth Drug-free childbirth; sometimes called *prepared childbirth*.

Lamaze method An approach to childbirth in which exercise and breath control are central to reducing anxiety and discomfort.

Did You Know . . .

Some women choose to give birth immersed in a pool of water as a way to relax, alleviate pain, and minimize the need for medications during childbirth (Nutter et al., 2014). The baby receives oxygen via blood passing through the placenta, so the fact that birth occurs under water is not a cause of concern. A healthy baby—that is, one not in distress—will take a breath only as soon as it feels cold air on its nose and mouth. Therefore, it is imperative that the woman's hips and pelvis be fully submerged to ensure that the baby is not exposed to any cold air as it arrives. The child is immediately brought out of the water by an attendant, usually seconds after birth. To ensure safety, water births should be attended by a nurse–midwife or other healthcare provider who is trained in water births. Some water births occur at home, whereas others occur in a birthing center or hospital setting.

As with any delivery procedure, a number of aspects need to be considered with this method. The temperature of the water needs to be close to 98 degrees Fahrenheit (37 degrees Celsius) to mimic human body temperature. Water that is too hot or too cold can cause stress to the baby (Oregon Health and Science University, 2014). Many professionals recommend that women be dilated by at least 4 centimeters before entering the water, because this practice seems to speed labor. Entering the water too early may actually extend and slow labor (Oregon Health and Science University, 2014). Some individuals are concerned about infection (because of fecal matter released from the mother into the water during labor),

but at least one study showed that infection risk to the infant is no greater than with a conventional vaginal delivery (Thoni, Mussner, & Ploner, 2010).

Although more research is needed, studies have shown water births to provide some potential benefits. For example, women having water births had significantly shorter labor duration (Qiu & Liu, 2008; Zanetti-Dallenbach et al., 2007), were less likely to need an episiotomy (Jin et al., 2009; Thoni et al., 2010; Zanetti-Dallenbach et al., 2007), and experienced less pain and/or were less likely to request pain relievers (Jin et al., 2009; Thoni et al., 2010; Zanetti-Dallenbach et al., 2007). Overall, when the procedure is used for low-risk pregnancies and attended by a trained health professional, risk to mother and fetus have not been demonstrated (Young & Kruske, 2013).

That is not to say that water births are not without debate (Phillips, 2014). The American College of Obstetricians and Gynecologists (2014) considers water birth to be an experimental procedure and does not support water births even in hospital settings. However, medical organizations in other countries believe that the practice can be beneficial (Royal College of Midwives, 2012) and strongly disagree with ACOG's statement on this method (Royal College of Midwives, 2014). As with any aspect of pregnancy and delivery, learning more about water birth procedures and their risks, and considering how this delivery method matches the desired birthing experience, are critical.

Although natural childbirth can be extremely satisfying, it is important to realize that natural methods are not suited to every pregnancy. The mother's health, as well as her pain threshold, will influence the decision. It is particularly important for expectant parents to realize that even when they have made the decision to have a drug-free delivery, the woman may decide during labor that she needs something for pain. In such a case, the mother may be given a mild tranquilizer. Women ought not to feel guilty about asking for drugs in labor. Natural childbirth is not a contest!

Cesarean Section

Cesarean section (C-section) is the delivery of the fetus and placenta through an incision in the walls of the abdomen and uterus. This procedure is performed

when a delivery through the vagina would be risky to the mother or baby. Possible reasons for a C-section include fetal distress, failure of labor to progress, or problems with the umbilical cord or placenta. Sometimes reasons for a C-section may be identified in advance, such as a breech presentation, a multiple pregnancy (especially for three or more fetuses), a baby that is 9 or 10 pounds, maternal infection, other maternal health condition (such as high blood pressure), or a previous C-section. C-sections are also performed if the mother has an STI that can be transmitted to the baby during a vaginal delivery, if the baby is too large to pass easily through the

cesarean section (C-section) Surgical intervention to deliver the fetus, placenta, and membranes through an incision in the walls of the abdomen and uterus.

vaginal canal and opening, and if a vaginal delivery will cause potential harm to the mother because of certain illnesses (such as diabetes).

In 2013, C-sections accounted for 32.7% of all deliveries in the United States (Osterman & Martin, 2014). This rate was only slightly lower than the 2012 rate of 32.8% of total U.S. deliveries, and nearly a 2% increase from 2007. There is much debate about the high rates of C-sections in the United States and other parts of the world. According to WHO, there is no reason for any country to have rates higher than 10% to 15%. A WHO study of 137 countries showed only 14 countries in that range, with 69 countries above that range, accounting for 6.2 million medically unnecessary procedures (Gibbons et al., 2010).

ACOG has advocated for a reduction in the number of non-medically indicated cesarean deliveries and inductions of labor prior to 39 weeks' gestation, with an emphasis on changing hospital policies to disallow elective delivery prior to 39 weeks' gestation (ACOG, 2011c; Clark et al., 2010). Queenan (2011) also outlined several strategies to decrease the cesarean rate. These suggestions include increasing the number of vaginal birth after cesarean delivery (VBAC) procedures, compensating clinicians equally for vaginal deliveries and cesarean section deliveries (but more for VBAC procedures), increasing education and training with regard to breech vaginal deliveries, changing litigation practices so that clinicians do not resort to cesarean deliveries as protection from possible lawsuits, increasing the use of midwives in the birthing process, and educating patients about the risks of the surgical procedure. As a result of these efforts, there has been a decline in the number of low-risk cesarean deliveries in the United States since 2010 for all full-term (37 or more weeks) deliveries, all maternal age groups, and all ethnicities. The largest percentage decreases occurred in women who were at 38 weeks into their pregnancy (9%), women younger than age 40 (6–8%) and white women (6%) (Osterman & Martin, 2014).

There are several disadvantages to having a C-section. The procedure is expensive; the mother needs a recuperative period that may interfere with her caring for her baby; there is scarring of the uterus; and there is the possibility—though slight—of hemorrhage or infection. Nevertheless, many babies and mothers would die without surgical intervention. The same WHO study previously mentioned also showed that worldwide 3.18 million cesarean section procedures were needed but did not happen, causing severe complications and death for those involved

Although it has declined in recent years, the cesarean section rate in the United States is higher than in most other developed countries. Some argue that this difference reflects a fear of lawsuits and a desire for convenience on the part of obstetricians. Others believe C-section is less traumatic for the mother than the strains of natural childbirth and is best for the newborn. Most experts agree that the U.S. rate is too high and strategies need to be implemented to reduce the frequency of this surgery.

(Gibbons et al., 2010). Cesarean intervention is an alternative delivery method to be considered in certain complicated situations.

Premature Birth

A child born before the normal gestation period is completed is considered **premature or preterm**. In 2012, 11.6% of all babies born in the United States were preterm (Martin et al., 2013). A preterm infant is usually between 28 and 36 weeks' gestation, although some are as young as 24 weeks' gestation. Delivery at an earlier gestational age is associated with low birth weight, and 39.4% of these preterm infants weigh less than 5.8 pounds (2,500 grams), with approximately 10.2% weighing less than 3.3 pounds (1,500 grams). This weight average drops dramatically when looking at births at less than 28 weeks' gestation. More than 90% of such newborns have a very low birth weight (less than 1,500 grams), and 96% have a low birth weight (less than 2,500 grams), (Martin et al., 2013).

Preterm births are caused by many factors. One common cause is a maternal age younger than 17 years or older than 35 years. Other causes include maternal malnutrition, cigarette smoking and alcohol consumption, inadequate prenatal care, more than one fetus, and a history of a previous premature delivery.

The preterm baby is born before some of its body systems can perform adequately. The respiratory

premature or preterm birth Infants born that have not reached 37 completed weeks of gestation.

system in particular is immature in these babies. They may forget to breathe and may have difficulty in moving the air through the respiratory tract. Sometimes their lung surfaces are unable to work with the necessary amounts of oxygen needed for survival because of immaturity of the lungs. These infants are usually placed in incubators, which are special cribs with controls to monitor temperature and oxygen levels. Because oxygen is necessary to sustain life, on the one hand, and because an excess of oxygen can cause eye damage (retrolental fibroplasia [RLF]), on the other hand, oxygen levels must be carefully controlled. A device has been developed that, when put on the baby's skin, can measure blood oxygen levels continuously.

Preterm infants often have difficulty swallowing and digesting food, so they may require special intravenous feedings. Small amounts of breast milk are fed to the baby as he or she begins to mature, both for nutrition and for the antibodies provided by the milk. Chemical tests that can detect some metabolic problems are used in the monitoring techniques.

Neonatal intensive care is the name given to the medical specialty of preterm infant care. It is costly because it requires the talents of trained specialists and special equipment. Given this care, however, many preterm babies—especially those born closer to 37 weeks' gestation—develop normally and catch up to their peers somewhere between the end of the first year and the third year of life. The investment to child, family, and ultimately society certainly justifies the time and costs involved.

◼ Psychological and Physical Adjustment After Childbirth

Psychological reactions after childbirth can occur. One of these reactions is depression, called *postpartum depression*. It is not unusual for women to have the "blues" after childbirth, in which they experience mood swings; feel sad, anxious, or overwhelmed; or have crying spells, loss of appetite, or trouble sleeping. These symptoms usually go away after a few weeks. When they persist or include thoughts of hurting the baby or oneself, or the mother demonstrates no interest in the baby, postpartum depression may exist. Approximately 14% of women experience postpartum depression (Wisner et al., 2013). Because of the life changes involved with having a child, research also shows that approximately 4% of fathers experience a major depressive episode during the child's first year of life (Davé et al., 2010).

For mothers, there is also a biological component to their postpartum adjustment. Hormonal changes may trigger symptoms of postpartum depression.

During pregnancy, levels of the hormones estrogen and progesterone increase greatly. In the first 24 hours after childbirth, these hormones' levels quickly return to normal. Researchers think continued fluctuations in hormone levels may lead to postpartum depression for certain women (O'Hara & McCabe, 2013).

Certain factors may increase a woman's risk of developing postpartum depression. These include a personal history of depression or another mental illness, a family history of depression or another mental illness, lack of support from family and friends, anxiety or negative feelings about raising the child, problems with a previous pregnancy or birth, relationship or money problems, stressful life events, young age, and substance abuse. Women who are depressed during pregnancy have a greater risk of depression after giving birth.

The most common types of treatment for depression consist of counseling and medication. Counseling involves talking to a therapist, a psychologist, a social worker, or perhaps a nurse specifically trained in postpartum depression to learn to change how depression makes one think, feel, and act. Medication includes a variety of antidepressant drugs that appear to be safe for breastfeeding women (O'Hara & McCabe, 2013). Some research has indicated that regular exercise may also help in treating postpartum depression (Daley, Macarthur, & Winter, 2007). The interaction between partners may play a role in postpartum depression; one study indicated that when fathers are highly supportive, the mother is less likely to develop postpartum depression (Smith & Howard, 2008).

Physical changes also occur after childbirth (U.S. Department of Health and Human Services, 2010). For example, women will have a discharge of blood, called *lochia*. This shedding of the uterine lining will begin as bright red, but then become lighter and eventually stop before the 6-week postpartum checkup.

Pain in the perineum (the area between the vaginal opening and the rectum) may also occur because of stretching, tearing, or episiotomy (if one was performed during delivery). Although uncomfortable, damage to this area should heal quickly, even if an episiotomy was performed.

Uterine contractions, sometimes called *afterpains*, may occur in some women. This is a normal part of involution, the process by which the uterus returns to its pre-pregnancy state. After birth, the uterus weighs 2 or 3 pounds; by 5 or 6 weeks after birth, it weighs only 2 to 4 ounces.

neonatal intensive care *A medical specialty that focuses on the care of premature infants.*

Changes in the breast will also occur. Breast milk comes in 3 to 6 days after delivery. Even if a woman is not breastfeeding, milk can leak from nipples and the breasts might feel full, tender, or uncomfortable. Breastfeeding regularly is the best strategy to address engorgement; cold compresses and a supportive bra can also help.

In addition to these and other changes, one of the most critical physical issues is sleep—or lack thereof (Gunderson et al., 2008). Fatigue can contribute to a woman's poor self-concept and confidence in her abilities as a mother (Runquist, 2007).

Breastfeeding

To ready the breasts for producing milk (**lactation**), glandular tissue and ducts proliferate during pregnancy as a result of the placenta's secretion of estrogen, progesterone, and **lactogen**. These developments account for the increase in breast size in pregnancy. Large amounts of estrogen and progesterone secreted by the placenta prevent milk production before birth, but after the placenta is delivered, both estrogen and progesterone levels drop significantly, and the level of the pituitary hormone prolactin rises. Prolactin secretion then activates the breast cells to produce milk. A second pituitary hormone, **oxytocin**, acts as a stimulant for the breasts to eject milk.

Twenty-eight to 48 hours after delivery, the lactation process begins. For the first 3 or 4 days, a thin, yellowish liquid called **colostrum** is secreted by the breasts. Colostrum is a high-protein substance containing many antibodies. Actual milk production begins between the fourth and seventh days after delivery, and by the seventh day mature milk production begins.

The infant's sucking stimulates nerve cells in the nipples; the mother's brain receives the message and stimulates the pituitary to secrete oxytocin, which in turn stimulates ejection of milk from the breasts. When the milk is forced out, the mother feels a tingling sensation known as **letdown** approximately 30 to 60 seconds after suckling begins. This feeling is produced by a neurogenic reflex that is necessary for

Breastfeeding conveys many benefits to both the newborn and the breastfeeding mother. Breastfeeding provides newborns with uncontaminated nutrients and antibodies against infection. It also helps the mother's uterus return to its nonpregnant shape and postpones the return of menstruation.

adequate milk supply to reach the infant. Continued milk supply is dependent on sucking. The infant's demand regulates the breasts' supply. When the baby sucks longer, the breasts produce more milk to meet the increased demand. When the baby sucks less, milk production decreases.

Breastfeeding benefits the baby by providing a diet of balanced, uncontaminated nutrients and antibodies against disease. It has also been shown to have a variety of protective benefits for the child, including reduced risk of ear infections, gastroenteritis, and severe lower respiratory infections and lower rates of sudden infant death syndrome, childhood obesity, type 2 diabetes, and leukemia (U.S. Department of Health and Human Services, 2011). The breastfeeding mother benefits, too. Nursing helps the uterus to return to its nonpregnant shape and postpones the return of menstruation (although it is not a sufficient contraceptive by itself). In addition, women who breastfeed have lower rates of breast cancer (Akbari et al., 2011), ovarian cancer (Stuebe & Schwarz, 2010), and a small reduction in the risk of type 2 diabetes (Stuebe & Schwarz, 2010). Other studies have indicated that women with a lifetime history of

lactation Production of breast milk.

lactogen A hormone that stimulates the production of milk, the principal one being prolactin.

oxytocin A pituitary hormone that stimulates the breasts to eject milk so that breastfeeding may occur after childbirth.

colostrum The yellow fluid secreted by the breasts just before and after childbirth until milk production begins.

letdown The tingling sensation in the breasts when milk is forced out about 30 to 60 seconds after the infant begins to suckle.

Multicultural
DIMENSIONS

**Differences in
Infant Mortality**

Infant mortality comprises deaths occurring within the first year of life. The good news is that the infant mortality rate continues to decline. In 1983, the U.S. infant mortality rate was 10.9 deaths per 1,000 live births, but by 2013 this rate had declined to 5.96 deaths per 1,000 live births (CDC, 2014f; Mathews, MacDorman, & Thoma, 2015).

The bad news is that the infant mortality rate for African Americans is still much higher compared to other subgroups in the U.S. population. In 2013, the white infant mortality rate was 5.06 deaths per 1,000 live births, but the black infant mortality rate was 11.1 deaths per 1,000 live births (Mathews et al., 2015). The main factor associated with infant mortality among black infants is related to premature birth: Approximately 17% of black infants are born preterm (before 37 weeks' gestation) compared to 10.9% of white babies (Mathews et al., 2015).

The reasons for the high rate of premature birth and subsequent infant mortality among African Americans are many and varied; poverty is the foremost among them. Poverty rates are disproportionately higher among Black Americans than among whites. Consequently,

many African Americans cannot as readily afford health care, proper nutrition, and other services and behaviors that are conducive to birth of healthy babies. For example, whereas 78.8% of white mothers began prenatal care during the first trimester, only 63.4% of African American mothers did so (U.S. Department of Health and Human Services, 2013). If all women were able to access prenatal care earlier, then a decrease in black, non-Hispanic infant mortality might occur.

To respond to the infant mortality rate gap between African Americans and white Americans, communities have instituted educational campaigns encouraging early prenatal care, particularly targeted at Black American populations. Some of these programs rely on public service advertisements in newspapers, on signs on buses, or as messages over radio or television. Other programs employ women who live in the targeted communities to identify pregnant women, meet with them, and encourage them to see a healthcare provider. Still other programs employ a combination of these and other methods in conjunction with free or low-cost health care to help pregnant mothers be healthier and deliver healthier children.

---

breastfeeding of at least 12 months have a decreased risk of developing hypertension, diabetes, high serum cholesterol, or cardiovascular disease (Gunderson et al., 2010; Schwarz et al., 2009). But probably most important, breastfeeding encourages the close attachment, or **bonding**, of infant and mother. Perhaps not incidentally, breast milk is less expensive than formula milk. Because of these multiple benefits, the American Academy of Pediatrics and the U.S. federal government recommend breastfeeding over formula feeding.

A woman's right to breastfeed in public is protected by law in the United States, and the Patient Protection and Affordable Care Act provides protection for pumping and storing breast milk at work for up to the first year after birth. In addition, support through organizations such as La Leche League can help women with the practical, how-to aspects of breastfeeding. Many times a woman will use a breast pump to extract milk that is stored for use by fathers and other caregivers during bottle feeding.

While breastfeeding is recommended for the first year of the baby's life, with exclusive breastfeeding recommended for 6 months of life, most women

do not follow this recommendation. Almost 79% of women start breastfeeding, but only 49% are still breastfeeding at 6 months, with only 19% of those using breast milk exclusively; the others supplement with formula (CDC, 2014a).

Women may not breastfeed initially or continue to breastfeed for a variety of reasons. For example, some women may not produce sufficient milk to breastfeed; this may be true for women who have multiple infants. Others may experience pain or discomfort during breastfeeding. For those women, bonding can be experienced by holding an infant close during bottle feeding.

◼ Sexual Activity During Pregnancy and After Delivery

Some—perhaps many—pregnant couples are afraid to engage in sexual activity for fear of hurting the fetus. The frequency and kinds of sexual activity that

---

bonding A sense of close emotional attachment.

FIGURE **8.9** Pregnancy need not mean the end of sexual intercourse.

are safe during and after pregnancy are determined both by personal preference and by health. A woman with no medical problems can continue to have the kind of sexual and sensual life she had before pregnancy (Figure 8.9). Even for healthy women, though, changes in body size and sense of comfort might dictate alterations in sexual habits. In advanced pregnancy, some heterosexual couples tend to replace vaginal–penile penetration with manual stimulation.

When certain physical conditions are present, however, coitus might add risk to the pregnancy. For example, when spotting, bleeding, pain, or past history of spontaneous abortion is present, a medical practitioner should decide whether intercourse is permissible. In healthy women, orgasmic contractions are not harmful to the fetus and will not initiate labor.

Sexual feelings can change during pregnancy. A woman's desire may be influenced by her personal involvement with the baby late in pregnancy, her individual personality, her attitudes toward sexuality, her feelings about her physical appearance, and so on. Here again, the necessity for honest sexual communication, in a safe and trusting environment, cannot be stressed enough.

Penile–vaginal sex or other vaginal penetration after delivery depends on many factors: whether there were complications during and after delivery, whether a cesarean section was performed, and, of course, whether the woman is comfortable, particularly after a difficult delivery. Most obstetricians prefer that couples delay vaginal penetration until after the first postdelivery examination, which usually takes place 4 to 6 weeks after delivery. This delay is to intended to ensure that the vulva has healed if there was a tear or an episiotomy and to allow time to discuss the choice of a method of birth control.

Couples should resume contraception use before penile–vaginal sex after childbirth. Despite the fact that breastfeeding delays the return of menstruation, that method alone is not a dependable form of birth control.

■ Hormonal Influences on Prenatal Development: Becoming Male or Female

The process of becoming a male or a female is a complicated one, involving chromosomes and hormones. As mentioned elsewhere in this text, a key influence on sex determination is the presence or absence of a Y chromosome.

Typical Sexual Differentiation

Sexual differentiation, or the process of gonad and duct development, does not start until the seventh week of fetal development (Figure 8.10). In the uterus, the fertilized egg always develops as if it were going to be female unless the Y chromosome is present. The Y chromosome contains the SRY gene. This gene gives instructions for the development of the testes; specifically, it tells the indifferent gonads (neither male nor female) to develop testis-determining factor (TDF). The TDF causes the indifferent gonads to develop into testes. Because there is no SRY gene in females, no TDF is produced, and consequently ovaries develop (Hospital for Sick Children, 2014).

A similar process occurs for the development of the urogenital ducts. Before the seventh week of fetal development, embryos have two sets of urogenital

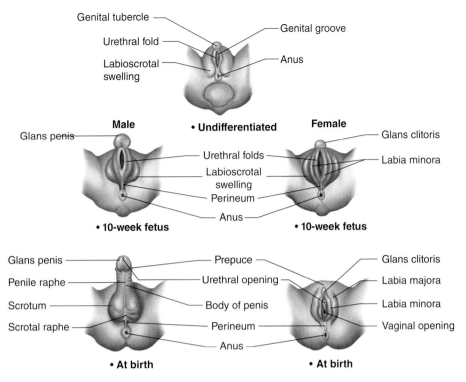

FIGURE **8.10** Prenatal development of external genitalia.

ducts, called Müllerian and Wolffan ducts. Once the gonads have formed, they influence duct development. In a male fetus, the testes make two hormones, Müllerian inhibiting substance (MIS) and testosterone. MIS makes the Müllerian ducts disappear by week 10, and testosterone causes the Wolffan ducts to develop into spermatic ducts by week 12. In a female fetus, in the absence of testosterone, the Wolffan ducts disappear around week 10, and by week 20 the Müllerian ducts have developed into the uterus, fallopian tubes, and vagina (Hospital for Sick Children, 2014).

The presence or absence of male hormones determines whether a particular piece of tissue becomes a penis or a clitoris, a prostate gland or a Skene's gland, a Cowper's gland or a Bartholin's gland, or a scrotum or a labia majora. Structures that develop from the same tissue in this way are called **homologous** structures (see Table 8.1).

The differentiation of the male and female brain is called *brain dimorphism*. Brain differentiation may extend into the first few days or weeks after birth. Interestingly, it appears that brain differentiation allows for the coexistence of both masculine and feminine nuclei and pathways in some, if not all, parts of the brain. Some researchers, in fact, postulate that differentiation between males and females in many areas of the brain is not that great (Joel, 2011). While many continue to be believe that males and females differ greatly, this research shows how men and women may be more alike than previously thought.

TABLE 8.1

Homologous Structures

Female	Male
Clitoral glans	Penile glans
Clitoral shaft	Penile shaft
Clitoral hood	Penile foreskin
Labia majora	Scrotum
Labia minora	Bottom of penile shaft
Ovaries	Testes
Bartholin's gland	Cowper's gland
Skene's gland	Prostate gland

homologous Organs that differ but that developed from the same tissue—for example, the glans penis and clitoris.

Variance of Sexual Differentiation

The description of sexual differentiation assumes that everything goes according to plan, and it usually does. However, once in a while, development does not follow the typical path. In fact, it is possible for the genetic sex, or *genotype* (the chromosomes); the gonadal sex, or *phenotype* (testes or ovaries); and the internal sexual structures (uterus, fallopian tubes, prostate gland, and vas deferens) to differ. For example, a person could be born with two X chromosomes, have a penis, an empty scrotum (without testes), two ovaries, a uterus, and a fallopian tube. Another individual may have male chromosomes (XY), male gonads (testes), and female external genitalia, as in complete androgen insensitivity syndrome.

Androgen insensitivity syndrome (AIS) is a condition in which individuals with XY chromosomes do not respond to androgens, or male hormones, in a typical way. People with complete AIS (CAIS) do not respond to androgens at all. They have testes and typical female external genitals. People with partial AIS (PAIS) do respond to androgens, but only partially and to varying degrees. They have testes and can have a range of different body types. Their genitals may not look exactly like typical female or typical male genitals.

These conditions are examples of **disorders of sexual development (DSD)**, referring to anomalies of the sex chromosomes, the gonads, the reproductive ducts, and the genitalia. This term was introduced at an international consensus conference (Hughes et al., 2006). Previously the term *intersex* was used to describe individuals who had chromosomal or anatomic differences that made them not clearly either male or female. (Before that, the term *hermaphrodite* was also used.) Today, many organizations use DSD because of the lack of precision with the term *intersex* (Accord Alliance, 2008). However, others—especially many international groups—still use *intersex* because of dislike for the "disorder" component of DSD (Diamond, 2009) and a variety of other concerns with the term (e.g., not inclusive for adults living with these conditions; does not translate clearly to other languages).

Within DSD, there is much variation. Some individuals have typical male or female chromosome structure but exhibit physical differences. Examples of these include (1) *46, XY, micropenis*, in which an individual has male chromosome makeup but an extremely small penis; (2) *clitoromegaly*, in which an individual has an enlarged clitoris; and (3) *MRKH syndrome*, in which ovaries are present but the uterus is absent, misshapen, or small (Accord Alliance, 2008).

Other examples of DSD can be traced to the chromosomes. For example, in a condition called *Turner's syndrome*, which is caused by the presence of only one X chromosome (instead of two), the female may be infertile, have short stature, and be at risk for some cardiac or renal anomalies. In *Klinefelter's syndrome*, a condition caused by an XXY genetic makeup, boys appear normal until puberty but then do not develop the normal secondary sex characteristics and may develop breasts at that time. Individuals with Klinefelter's syndrome may also have low levels of sperm.

Accord Alliance (formerly known as the Intersex Society of North American) is one organization helping educate families and clinicians about treatment options and psychological needs of children with DSD. In the past, genital surgery was often performed for cosmetic reasons, resulting in physical and emotional damage. Today, more informed decisions about gender assignment are made with the hope of lessening the emotional toll. Likewise, non-medically needed surgeries may be delayed until the individual with DSD can consent. Hormonal therapy may also be part of the treatment; counseling for the child with DSD and the family is recommended.

Another condition associated with sexual differentiation is *inguinal hernia*. The testes descend into the scrotum through a structure called the *inguinal canal*. This normally occurs by the seventh month of fetal development. If the inguinal canal does not close properly after the testes descend or if it opens up afterward, it is possible for the intestine to move down the canal and enter the scrotum. An inguinal hernia can be corrected surgically.

If the testes do not descend down the inguinal canal, as occurs in approximately 2% of male newborns, the condition is called *cryptorchidism* (more commonly called *undescended testes*). Usually the testes will descend during early childhood or by puberty. If they do not, either surgery or hormonal therapy is necessary for two reasons: (1) Testes in the abdomen are at too high a temperature to produce viable sperm, and if they are left undescended, infertility is likely to result; and (2) there is a greater risk of testicular cancer if testes are left undescended.

◼ Infertility

Infertility, or the inability to reproduce, can cause great emotional anguish for people who want children. This unhappiness, accompanied by tension, frustration, and even resentment, can damage the health and the relationships of infertile couples. The situation may be further complicated by an inability

---

disorders of sexual development Anomalies of the sex chromosomes, the gonads, the reproductive ducts, and the genitalia.

infertility The inability to reproduce.

or unwillingness to adopt a child. Of course, while adoption may relieve the stress of wanting to raise children, it may not eliminate the stress related to infertility.

More than 6.7 million people of childbearing age experience impaired fertility in the United States. It is estimated that 6% of married women in the country experience infertility (Chandra, Copen, & Stephen, 2013). Some studies distinguish between primary infertility, meaning the inability to conceive despite having unprotected intercourse for at least 1 year or 6 months if older than age 35, and secondary infertility, referring to the inability to conceive despite having unprotected intercourse for at least 1 year and having previously conceived. International rates of primary and secondary infertility are estimated to be 1.5% and 0.5%, respectively (Mascarenhas et al., 2013)

Women and men can both contribute to infertility. Infertility related to sperm and other male problems is indicated in one-third of cases; issues related to female functioning are suspected in an additional one-third of situations. In the remaining one-third of situations, a combination of male and female factors is the cause. In approximately 20% of cases, however, the precise cause cannot be determined (American Society for Reproductive Medicine [ARSM], 2014a).

Causes of Infertility

In women, the most common cause of infertility is related to problems with ovulation, resulting in no eggs to fertilize (ARSM, 2014a). In women older than 35, this issue may be age related: Older women may encounter problems with diminished ovarian reserve, meaning that their remaining eggs are few in number and/or of poor quality. Other conditions leading to infertility in women can include blocked fallopian tubes due to pelvic inflammatory disease, endometriosis, or surgery for an ectopic pregnancy; physical anomalies with the uterus; and uterine fibroids (non-cancerous buildup of tissue and muscle on the walls of the uterus). PID can be caused by untreated chlamydia or gonorrhea infections. Sexually active college students can reduce their risk of future infertility by using condoms, practicing safer sex behaviors, and getting regularly tested for STIs.

STIs are not the only diseases that affect fertility. Some health problems in women cause hormonal changes (e.g., polycystic ovarian syndrome) and as a result, an increased risk of infertility. In men, mumps, kidney disease, or hormone problems can be related to infertility issues. People with sickle-cell disease have higher infertility rates. In both males and females, radiation and chemotherapy treatment related to cancer can affect fertility. Several drugs may inhibit sperm production or sperm function,

including antimalarial drugs, antihypertensive agents, and calcium-channel blockers.

One of the major factors affecting infertility is age. Women are most fertile in their mid-20s; after age 30, fertility potential gradually declines. Similarly, men older than age 40 may be less fertile than younger men.

Substance use is another component of infertility; if either partner smokes, the chance of pregnancy decreases, and tobacco use also reduces the benefit of any fertility treatment. Miscarriages are also more frequent in women who smoke. For women, moderate to heavy levels of alcohol use make it more difficult to become pregnant.

For women, weight—either being overweight or underweight—affects ovulation function and consequently, fertility in about 12% of cases (ARSM, 2014c). Environmental and occupational exposure to chemicals such as pesticides, herbicides, and some insecticides can affect both male and female reproductive functioning (Rolland et al., 2013). Although infertility can cause stress, there is no conclusive evidence that stress can cause infertility (ASRM, 2014b).

Finally, in some couples, a lack of knowledge about anatomy, physiology, and reproduction leads to infertility. These couples may not know when conception is most likely to occur, they may not have penile–vaginal sex frequently enough to conceive, and they may not know how to time intercourse. The ovum is alive for less than 1 day; sperm can live as long as 5 days inside the woman. Couples must have penile–vaginal sex before ovulation to maximize the possibility of pregnancy.

Testing and Treatment for Infertility

As couples increasingly focus on education, careers, and other aspects of life, delayed parenthood is becoming more common—and with that, the risk of infertility is growing. While media reports often focus on specific reproductive technologies in isolation, the path to addressing infertility can be quite long for many couples.

Some individuals prefer to try "natural" ways to enhance their fertility. Unfortunately, research has shown that there is very little related to the act of sex that changes the likelihood of conceiving. Specific timing of sex, positioning during sex, or having the female rest on her back after sex have no significant impact on fertility (ASRM, 2008). Penile–vaginal sex every 1 to 2 days yields the highest pregnancy rates, but having sex only 2 or 3 times per week is associated with nearly the same rates. For those who have penile–vaginal sex less frequently, devices that help identify when ovulation occurs may be helpful. In reality, age, lifestyle factors, and frequency of sex are the most important ways to influence fertility (ASRM, 2008).

If a couple has been trying to conceive for more than 12 months without success (or more than 6 months if the woman is 35 years or older), they should consult with a clinician about testing. In many cases, infertility can be successfully treated. In fact, most infertility cases—85% to 90%—are treated with conventional medicine, such as medication and surgical repair of the reproductive organs (ASRM, 2014a). In all cases, the first step is to determine why a couple is unable to conceive. Several basic infertility screening procedures may be used in this examination phase:

1. *Semen analysis.* The man is asked to masturbate and collect the ejaculate in a container. The ejaculate is then examined to determine the number of sperm present, the sperm's motility, and the amount of fructose (nourishment for the sperm) in the semen.

2. *Basal body temperature (BBT) recordings.* The woman is required to record her body temperature (with an oral or BBT thermometer) daily. The decrease in estrogen production as ovulation nears causes the basal temperature to drop about 0.3 degree Fahrenheit (0.17 degree Celsius). When ovulation occurs, basal temperature rises about 0.6 degree Fahrenheit (0.34 degree Celsius) as a result of the corpus luteum's production of the hormone progesterone. Thus a physician can determine whether ovulation is occurring normally by monitoring the basal temperature.

3. *Endometrial biopsy.* A biopsy (microscopic examination of excised body tissue) of the endometrium is performed. This procedure helps identify uterine abnormalities.

4. *Tubal patency tests.* Dye is projected through the fallopian tubes and observed by X ray to detect any blockage; this test is also called a *hysterosalpingogram.*

5. *Postcoital examination.* Two to 4 hours after the couple has had penile–vaginal sex, the cervical mucus is examined microscopically. The physician checks for several conditions of the cervical mucus that can be fatal to sperm (e.g., too much viscosity or too little salt). The sperm are counted and their ability to travel determined, because the more motile the sperm, the greater the likelihood of conception.

6. *Hormone monitoring.* Several ovulation prediction kits are currently sold over the counter. These kits measure the level of luteinizing hormone (LH), the hormone causing ovulation midway through the menstrual cycle. Urine tests can also be used to measure the amount of progesterone during various phases of the cycle. Other hormones (such as prolactin, thyroid hormones, and follicle-stimulating hormone [FSH]) can be monitored as well.

7. *Cervical mucus evaluation.* The cervical mucus can be evaluated for its elasticity, its nature just before ovulation (it should be thin, watery, salty, and stretchy), and the presence of cells, debris, and proper pH level (degree of acidity or alkalinity).

8. *Ultrasonography.* High-frequency sound waves are transmitted and reflected by internal organs and structures. From the resulting pattern, detailed outlines of the reproductive system can be obtained.

9. *Hysteroscopy.* The uterus is expanded with carbon dioxide gas or liquid and is observed through a hysteroscope—a long, narrow, illuminated instrument that is inserted through the cervix into the uterus. Abnormalities such as polyps, fibroids, and adhesions can be identified in this manner.

10. *Laparoscopy.* In this minor surgery, a small incision is made in the lower abdomen and a laparoscope (small tool with a light) is inserted. The ovaries, fallopian tubes, and uterus can be checked for disease and physical problems, such as scarring or endometriosis.

© AbleStock

In spite of their love for one another, their understanding of the menstrual cycle and ovulation, and their ability to effectively engage in sexual intercourse, some couples are not able to conceive. There are several reasons for such infertility, and several screening tests are available to help determine the reason for any particular couple. Once the reason is uncovered, treatment can begin to increase the likelihood of conception.

Depending on the couple's medical history, personal factors, and other available medical information, a couple may be asked to undergo some (but usually not all) of these screening procedures. Generally, male semen analysis is almost always done to determine any male factors. Once the cause or causes of the infertility are determined, treatment can be prescribed. Cessation of ovulation can be restarted by administering hormone therapy or by increasing or decreasing body fat through nutritional therapy. Blocked fallopian tubes can be cleared through microsurgical techniques. In some cases, more complicated and advanced procedures are required. Depending on the woman's age, the reason for infertility, and other medical factors, a doctor may recommend **intrauterine insemination (IUI)** and/or assisted reproductive technologies, such as in vitro fertilization.

In IUI, specially prepared sperm are injected into a women's uterus. Sometimes in this procedure the woman uses medication to stimulate ovulation, although this practice can increase the number of eggs released. IUI is often used to treat mild male factor infertility, cervical mucus problems in females, and couples with unexplained infertility. For men who produce no sperm (a condition called *azoospermia*) or who have a sperm count too low to ensure fertilization (*oligospermia*) or for females without male partners, a donor could also be used for the sperm.

If the woman does use medications to increase the number of follicles maturing and the potential number of eggs, it is not possible to control the number of eggs that will be fertilized. Therefore, IUI increases the chance for a pregnancy of multiple fetuses. As the number of fetuses increases, concern about health issues for the mother and the fetuses also increases. Babies born as part of a multiple pregnancy are more likely to be born premature and with low or very low birth weights. In some cases, a woman may opt for selective abortion, in which one or more fetuses are aborted to give the remaining fetuses a better chance to develop.

Procedures in which the clinician handles both the sperm and the egg are collectively called **assisted reproductive technologies (ART)**. In these methods, eggs are removed from a woman's body, fertilized with sperm, and allowed to develop into embryos in a laboratory. The embryos are then put back in the woman's body (CDC, 2014i). Common methods of ART include the following:

- In vitro fertilization (IVF) is often used when a woman's fallopian tubes are blocked or when a man produces too few sperm. The woman takes medication that causes the ovaries to produce multiple eggs. Once mature, the eggs are removed from the woman and put in a dish in the lab along with sperm for fertilization. After 3 to 5 days, if healthy embryos have been produced, they are implanted in the woman's uterus. Recommendations for the number of embryos to transfer have been established (ASRM & Society for Assisted Reproductive Technology, 2013). These guidelines are based on the woman's age, the maturity of the embryo, and other medical factors, but in most cases implanting fewer than four embryos is recommended. There is increasing emphasis to limit transfers to one embryo because of the increased risk of a multiple pregnancy. IVF is the most successful ART and is also the most common.

- Zygote intrafallopian transfer (ZIFT) or tubal embryo transfer is similar to IVF. Fertilization occurs in the laboratory; however, a very young embryo is transferred to the fallopian tube instead of the uterus.

- Gamete intrafallopian transfer (GIFT) involves transferring eggs and sperm into the woman's fallopian tube. In this case, fertilization occurs in the woman's body. Because of the lower success rates associated with this technique, few clinics provide GIFT as a procedure.

- Intracytoplasmic sperm injection (ICSI) is often used when there are serious problems with the sperm or if there are genetic disorders that an individual does not want to pass on to a child. ICSI may also be used for older couples or for those with failed IVF attempts. In ICSI, a single sperm is injected into a mature egg. The embryo is then transferred to the uterus or fallopian tube.

In 2012, 44% of ART transfer procedures using nondonor eggs resulted in a pregnancy, and 36% led to delivery of one or more live-born infants; this equates to approximately 1% of U.S. infants. However, the success rate declines with the age of the eggs. For women using their own eggs, the rate of success with a live birth is 47% in women younger than 35 years, 37.5% in women aged 35–37 years, 28.4% in women aged 38–40 years, 16.1% in women aged 41–42 years, 6.7% in women aged 43–44 years, and 3.1% in those women older than 44 years (CDC,

intrauterine insemination (IUI) Introduction of semen into the uterus by noncoital means.

assisted reproductive technologies (ART) Procedures in which the clinician handles both the sperm and the egg.

ASRM, & Society for Assisted Reproductive Technology, 2014). The age of the eggs is so critical that if everything else was equivalent, a 38-year-old woman using her own eggs would likely have less success with IVF than a 42-year-old woman using the eggs from a 25-year-old egg donor.

While many women are able to successfully conceive with ART, these technologies are not without risk. Studies show that preterm deliveries and low/very low birth weight are increased with ART, largely because of the increased risk of a multiple pregnancy. A multiple pregnancy can place additional strain on the mother, such as increasing her risk for complications during pregnancy and delivery. In addition, adverse prenatal and postpartum outcomes are more common among singleton ART infants than among naturally conceived singletons (Hansen & Bower, 2014), although how much risk is directly connected to use of ART versus other issues related to infertility is up for debate. Research studies tend to use different criteria (e.g., definitions of anomalies) and ART procedures differ between studies, both of which make drawing definitive conclusions challenging (Simpson, 2014).

With any of the ART procedures, individuals could use donor eggs (eggs from another woman), donor sperm, or previously frozen donor embryos. Individuals may choose these paths because of health conditions, such as not being able to produce sperm or eggs themselves, or when one partner has a genetic condition that can be passed to the child. Donor embryos are either created by couples who were already undergoing infertility treatment or created from donor sperm and donor eggs. The donor embryos may then be transferred into the uterus. Procedures are in place to screen sperm and egg donors for communicable infections; egg donors also receive a genetic screening both via a detailed family history and specific blood tests that are determined by ethnic/racial background (CDC, 2013).

Other individuals who desire to become parents may consider surrogacy. In this situation, a woman agrees to become pregnant using sperm from a male and her own egg. After birth, the surrogate gives up the baby for adoption by the parents. Some same-sex male couples may also choose this option. While similar, using a gestational carrier may be an option for a woman with ovaries but no uterus, with a uterus that cannot support a pregnancy, or who should not become pregnant because of a serious health problem. In this situation, a woman's own egg is fertilized by the man's sperm and the embryo is placed inside the carrier's uterus. The carrier then gives the baby to the parents at birth. In everyday language, the term *surrogate* is sometimes used to refer to both situations, although they are actually quite different.

All of these scenarios can include legal and potentially ethical issues. In many clinics, more eggs

Ethical DIMENSIONS

Surrogate Mothers Some couples who attempt to conceive children cannot. In some cases, the cause is a lack of viable sperm. In other cases, the problem is a blockage of the fallopian tubes, which prevents the sperm–ovum union. In still other cases, the woman does not produce an ovum to be fertilized or, because of some medical condition, cannot carry a fetus in her uterus until delivery. In the latter circumstance, the woman's ovum can be fertilized by her partner's sperm outside the womb and implanted in the uterus of another woman, known as a *surrogate womb* or gestational carrier. When a woman does not produce ova for fertilization, sometimes another woman's egg is fertilized by her partner and develops in that other woman's uterus. Upon delivery, the baby becomes the child of the father and his partner rather than of the father and the woman whose eggs and uterus were used for 9 months or so. The woman whose eggs and uterus were used is the biological mother, referred to as a *surrogate mother*.

When surrogate motherhood occurs without complications, it provides for everyone's needs. However, every once in a while, circumstances requiring creative solutions develop. For example, what do you think should happen if the surrogate mother does not want to give up the child after delivery? (Maybe she develops an attachment to the baby, or her situation has changed and she now wants a child of her own.) What should happen if the father and his partner do not want to accept the baby? (Maybe the baby has a birth defect, the couple has separated or divorced, or they just changed their minds about wanting children.) Each of these situations has actually occurred. What is your opinion?

are harvested and fertilized than the number needed for a single cycle. These embryos are then frozen so they can be used for future IVF procedures. However, in some cases couples have divorced before the transfer of the embryos, and couples have fought over these embryos as part of a divorce settlement. In a few widely publicized cases, embryos have been implanted after the man has died. Is the child in that case born to a married couple or to a single mother?

Some clinics are taking steps to minimize such legal issues. Having couples decide in advance of any procedures if embryo use requires the consent of both partners, what happens to stored eggs, and what decision-making process should be followed if one partner dies are some examples of decisions clinics are asking patients to consider.

Another ethical issue is if insurance companies and Medicaid should pay for IUI and ART? A basic IVF procedure (without special circumstances such as genetic testing or use of donors) costs $12,000 to $15,000 per cycle. Fewer than half all U.S. states require ART to be covered by insurance. Most clinics offer financial aid and payment plans, but in reality, the costs are out of reach for many couples. Some clinics are establishing shared risk programs in which couples pay a flat rate for a set number of cycles; if none of them works, the couple gets a full refund. With this approach, if the woman gets pregnant on the first or second attempt, the couple ends up paying more money than if they had paid individually per cycle, but many couples like the "guarantee" factor.

A national plan to address some of these issues at the population level—that is, causes of infertility, access to safe treatments—has recently been developed (CDC, 2014e). In reality, it is has been only a little more than 30 years (1981) since the first baby was conceived by IVF in the United States. We are just beginning to understand the potential of these technologies and the complications they bring.

Exploring the Dimensions of Human Sexuality

© Gayvoronskaya Yana/Shutterstock

Case Study

Pregnancy is a time of wonder and joy. For first-time parents, the world is forever changed after their infant is born. But even the degree of responsibility and emotional attachment to the child are influenced by many dimensions.

Biological age of the mother plays a factor. Teen pregnancies tend to have more medical complications for both mother and child. Risk of Down syndrome increases with age, from 1 in 1,300 births at age 25 years, to 1 in 900 births at age 30 years, to 1 in 350 births at age 35 years, to 1 in 55 births at age 42 years, to 1 in 25 births at age 49 years (Eunice Kennedy Shriver National Institute of Child Health and Human Development, 2014).

Socioeconomic status plays a role in the health care of children. Parents on the lower end of the socioeconomic scale may lack resources for parental and infant care, as well as the education and resources needed to raise healthy children.

Social pressure about child rearing is exerted by grandparents as well. When disposable diapers were introduced, Pampers advertised them as "easier." But grandparent pressure—"What was wrong with the diapers we used on you?"—caused many parents to return to cloth diapers. Pampers had to change its marketing strategy from emphasizing "being easier" to "being better for the baby."

Working parents tend to rely on a far-flung network of day care providers, friends, family, and peer parents for emotional and practical advice. Without such support, the emotional impact of raising a child can be overwhelming.

Biological Factors

- Hormones create sex differentiation during the second month of prenatal development.
- Physiological cycles and changes in the fetus take place at an extremely fast pace.
- Physical appearance of the mother changes (for example, clearer skin) as hormonal changes occur.
- Parents' genetic characteristics determine many attributes of their children, such as height and hair color.

Sociocultural Factors

- Socioeconomic status influences infant and maternal health, because poor people have less access to prenatal care than well-off people do.
- Laws restrict access to abortions during the third trimester.
- Religion, culture, and ethnic heritage influence many beliefs about pregnancy, childbirth, and parenting.
- Media and ads may influence the choice of where to have a child or whether to use the services of a midwife or a physician.
- Family, neighbors, and friends who have children can provide invaluable advice and assistance to new parents.

Psychological Factors

- A pregnant woman's emotions can swing wildly because of hormonal shifts. The postpartum period can be associated with the "baby blues" or more severe depression.
- Experience counts in pregnancy; subsequent infants go through labor faster and breastfeed more readily.
- Self-concept during pregnancy usually increases as a result of the responsibility of caring for another person.
- Learned attitudes and behaviors are often exhibited by pregnant couples.
- A woman's body image can suffer if she views herself as "getting fat" rather than as "carrying a child."

Summary

- Conception occurs in the fallopian tube. Sperm stay alive in the female reproductive tract for 72 to 120 hours. The ovum's peak fertile period is 8 to 12 hours, although an egg can be fertilized for as long as 24 hours after ovulation.

- The conceptus is known as a zygote until 8 weeks of development, when it becomes known as an embryo. At the beginning of the third month of development, the conceptus is known as a fetus. The embryo develops in the amniotic sac cushioned with amniotic fluid.

- Sometimes an ectopic pregnancy occurs in which the blastocyst becomes implanted in a site other than the uterus. Ectopic pregnancies are a large cause of maternal morbidity and mortality in the first trimester.

- Childbirth can occur under the supervision of a physician or a nurse–midwife. It can take place in a hospital, in a free-standing birthing center, or at home.

- Among the threats to a normal birth delivery are the use of over-the-counter drugs and alcohol, cigarettes, marijuana, cocaine, heroin, and other narcotics. Diseases such as diabetes, HIV infection, and other STIs are additional concerns.

- The pregnant woman may experience hypertension, nausea and vomiting, hemorrhoids, and other conditions.

- Labor occurs in three stages. Stage I is the period from the onset of labor to the point at which the cervix is fully dilated. Stage II is the period from full cervical dilation through the birth of the child. Stage III is the period from the infant's birth to the delivery of the placenta, or afterbirth.

- Sex differentiation occurs during the second month of pregnancy. If development does not follow typical male/female patterns, a child may be born intersex, with a disorder of sexual development.

- Infertility, or the inability to reproduce, can be caused by occlusion of the fallopian tubes, blocked sperm ducts, low sperm production, or poor semen quality. Infertility can be treated by intrauterine insemination (IUI), in vitro fertilization (IVF), or other assisted reproductive technologies.

Discussion Questions

1. Explain the process by which life begins, providing as much detail as possible.

2. What are the characteristics of fetal development that differentiate the three trimesters?

3. What can a pregnant woman do to increase her chance of having a healthy pregnancy and child?

4. Describe how various drugs and diseases can threaten infant health.

5. Which maternal problems may occur during pregnancy? What can be done to alleviate some of these problems?

6. Differentiate the three phases of labor and methods of reducing the pain of labor.

7. Describe the benefits of breastfeeding an infant.

8. Is sex safe during pregnancy? Explain the situations in which it is or is not safe.

9. Compare and contrast the prenatal undifferentiated and sex-differentiated external genitalia, including the hormones that create the sexes.

10. Explain the most common causes of infertility and the methods to treat such problems.

Application Questions

Reread the chapter-opening story and answer the following questions.

1. The Rich and Mary story underscores how the many dimensions of human sexuality play into our decision making. Although Mary believed in the social and ethical right of women to have abortions, her personal convictions led her to continue her pregnancy in spite of the pregnancy not being intended or wanted. What would you have done in Rich and Mary's situation? Which of the dimensions of human sexuality mentioned here would influence you?

2. The Rich and Mary story presents the fact that there are increased risks with multiple births. If you had been in their situation, which information would you want to know about twin births? Where could you find more information on how to handle and prepare for a twin pregnancy, delivery, and child rearing?

Critical Thinking Questions

1. A premature baby born at 24 weeks' gestation (5½ months), weighing about 1 pound, can be saved—at a cost of more than $300,000. But that is just the start. Many "preemie" children continue to have problems in infancy, as a toddler and in school, possibly requiring the services of special-education programs. Choose a side and debate for or against saving children born more premature than 32 weeks' gestation. (*Note:* This question was submitted by a parent of two premature babies to provoke discussion.)

2. Hospitals have found that birthing centers are enormously profitable ventures. In major cities, hospitals compete for patients by having birthing rooms designed to look like homes with extra amenities and "freebies" (such as a champagne breakfast the morning after). Yet to maintain profits, patients are sent home as soon as state laws allow—usually 24 to 48 hours after birth. Do patients benefit from such an arrangement—or is it simply a business deal for the hospitals?

Critical Thinking Case

For many years, there had been concern that too many cesarean birth deliveries were being performed in the United States. In 2012, the U.S. cesarean rate of nearly 32.8% of all births was higher than that of other industrialized nations. Interestingly, the data indicated that the increase in the cesarean rate did not contribute to the decline in the infant mortality rate. Making matters worse, maternal morbidity and mortality rates are higher in cesarean deliveries than in routine vaginal deliveries. One of the *Healthy People 2010* national health objectives was to decrease the rate of cesarean deliveries in women giving birth the first time to 15% of live births and to 63% of women giving birth who had a prior cesarean. The continued increase in C-section rates eliminated the possibility of reaching that goal. The *Healthy People 2020* objectives aim for a 10% decrease in the cesarean section rates by 2020, with a new goal of 23.9% for first-time births and 81.9% for women with a prior cesarean section (U.S. Department of Health and Human Services, 2012).

In the past, it had been thought unwise and unhealthy for women who had a previous cesarean delivery to attempt a vaginal birth. The concerns cited were for tearing of the tissue and possible infection for the baby. The standard practice was "Once a cesarean, always a cesarean." However, it was found that, barring complications, many women who had a cesarean delivery could deliver vaginally the next

time without endangering their own or their baby's health.

Think about these questions:

Are the high rates of C-sections the result of the current hyper-legal climate in the United States, which causes physicians to perform C-sections more often to protect themselves against a lawsuit?

Is the fact that C-sections earn the obstetrician more money a factor in the decision to perform them?

Given the increased risk to the mother of a cesarean delivery, and the evidence that it has little effect on the infant mortality rate, is the relatively high rate of cesarean deliveries ethical?

Exploring Personal Dimensions

How Much Do You Know About Pregnancy and Birth?

For each of the statements that follow, indicate whether you think the statement is true or false. The correct answers and explanations appear after the questions.

True____False____ 1. Pregnant women should stop exercising as soon as they discover they are pregnant.

True____False____ 2. Once a woman has had a C-section, she should have C-sections for subsequent deliveries to prevent tearing of the abdominal tissue.

True____False____ 3. The use of midwives has decreased in recent years.

True____False____ 4. Breastfeeding is covered by the Patient Protection and Affordable Care Act, which guarantees that working women may breastfeed.

True____False____ 5. Teen birth rates have steadily increased and are of significant concern.

True____False____ 6. In terms of a newborn baby's health, the length of time before its mother becomes pregnant again does not matter.

Answers and Explanations

Each of these statements is false.

1. Pregnant women are encouraged to continue exercising if they exercised before becoming pregnant. Some studies have suggested that exercise during pregnancy helps make the labor and delivery easier and shorter, promotes

earlier recovery after delivery, and reduces the chance of C-sections. However, women who have not maintained an exercise regimen before becoming pregnant should not begin one after becoming pregnant. Rather, they should exercise by adopting a mild walking or swimming program or by consulting an expert on exercise and pregnancy for other activities that will be beneficial for them and their fetuses.

2. There is no reason why, as a matter of routine, women who have had one C-section need to have C-sections for subsequent pregnancies. C-sections need be performed only if the woman has an STI that can be transmitted during childbirth, if the baby is too large to pass through the vaginal opening, or if the stress of the delivery has the potential to cause harm to the mother.

3. Contrary to popular belief, the proportion of women who use a nurse–midwife rather than an obstetrician to deliver their babies has remained constant; approximately 8% of births are attended by a midwife.

4. Many women have been fired or discriminated against for breastfeeding at work. The Patient Protection and Affordability Care Act, coupled with increased support for breastfeeding, provides clear guidelines for employees about their rights regarding breastfeeding at work. It also provides clear guidelines for employers about the actions and policies they are required to follow.

5. The birth rate for teenagers decreased in 2012 to 29.4 births per 1,000 females aged 15–19 years. This rate is a historic low for the United States and represents a 6% decrease in the rate from 2011 (Martin et al., 2013). While the recent decline is impressive, U.S. teen birth rates vary by race/ethnicity and geographical region. For example, the birth rate ranges from 13.8 births per 1,000 teenaged females in New Hampshire to 47.5 births per 1,000 teenaged females in New Mexico. In general, teen birth rates were lowest in the Northeast and highest across the South and Southwest (Martin et al., 2013).

6. Research has shown that either a short interpregnancy interval (less than 18 months) or a long interval (more than 59 months) is a risk factor for mother and child. Short or long pregnancy spacing is associated with increased risk for infant mortality; low birth weight; being small for one's gestational age; and, less consistently, preterm birth (Conde-Agudelo, Rosas-Bermudez, & Kafury-Goeta,

2006; de Weger et al., 2011; Thompson & Clark, 2011). Possible explanations for the negative consequences of short pregnancy spacing include physiological factors (e.g., nutritional—especially folate—depletion in the mother, uterine abnormalities including incomplete healing from a previous cesarean section, and cervical insufficiency) and family interaction factors (such transmission of infections from mother to child or among siblings, poor lactation related to breastfeeding–pregnancy overlap, sibling competition). For the cause of negative effects when considering longer pregnancy spacing, the woman's physiological regression is the only hypothesis that has been supported (Conde-Agudelo et al., 2012).

Suggested Readings

American Academy of Pediatrics (AAP). *Caring for your baby and young child: Birth to age 5.* 6th ed. New York: Bantam, 2014.

American College of Obstetricians and Gynecologists. *Your pregnancy and child birth.* 5th ed. Atlanta, GA: American College of Obstetricians and Gynecologists, 2010.

Brott, A. A., & Ash, J. *The expectant father.* 4th ed. New York: Abbeville Press, 2015.

Sher, G., Davis, V. M., & Stoess, J. *In vitro fertilization: The A.R.T. of making babies.* 4th ed. New York: Skyhorse Publishing, 2013.

Simkin, P. *The birth partner: A complete guide to childbirth for dads, doulas, and all other labor companions.* 4th ed. Boston, MA: Harvard Common Press, 2013.

Tsigdinos, PM. *Silent sorority: A barren woman gets busy, angry, lost, and found,* 2nd ed. Charleston, SC: BookSurge Publishing, 2010.

Web Resources

Accord Alliance
www.accordalliance.org

As the focus of the organization narrowed to helping clinicians and families address issues of disorders of sexual development, the Intersex Society of North America transitioned into Accord Alliance. The website contains guidelines for clinicians and documents for families that are living with a child with DSD. The ISNA website (www.isna.org) is still available as a historical document for those who may be interested.

RESOLVE: The National Infertility Association
www.resolve.org

Established in 1974, this nonprofit organization is a national network mandated to promote reproductive health and to ensure equal access to all family building options for men and women experiencing infertility or other reproductive disorders. The website includes current information and support for people who are experiencing infertility. RESOLVE also works to increase awareness of infertility issues through public education, such as National Infertility Awareness Week, and advocacy.

Maternal and Child Health Bureau
www.mchb.hrsa.gov

A bureau of the Health Resources and Services Administration of the U.S. Department of Health and Human Services, this site provides links to information pertaining to issues dealing with the health of mothers and their children. Included are links to programs, funding opportunities, data, and resources and publications.

National Campaign to Prevent Teen and Unplanned Pregnancy
www.thenationalcampaign.org

This organization has an extensive repository of information related to unplanned pregnancy and programs that have been successful in preventing pregnancy in teens and young adults. There is also information provided about acquiring materials to support a National Day to Prevent Teen Pregnancy.

Association of Reproductive Health Professionals
www.arhp.org

Provides information and resources pertaining to many aspects of reproduction. Among the topics about which information is provided are abortion, contraception, emergency contraception, menopause, politics and reproductive health news, international reproductive health news and issues, and patient education materials.

National Center for Fathering
www.fathers.com

Seeks to inspire and equip men to be the involved fathers, grandfathers, and father figures their children need. The center provides practical, research-based training and resources, and reaches more than 1 million fathers annually through seminars, small-group training, the WATCH D.O.G.S. (Dads of Great Students) program, a daily radio program, and weekly email.

References

Abar, B., LaGasse, L. L., Derauf, C., Newman, E., Shah, R., Smith, L. M. et al. Examining the relationships between prenatal methamphetamine exposure, early adversity, and child neurobehavioral disinhibition. *Psychology of Addictive Behaviors, 27* (2013), 662–673. doi: 10.1037/a0030157.

Accord Alliance. *Clinical guidelines for the management of disorders of sex development in childhood,* 2008. Available: http://www.accordalliance.org/dsd-guidelines.html.

Ackerman, J. P., Riggins, T., & Black, M. M. A review of the effects of prenatal cocaine exposure among school-aged children. *Pediatrics, 125* (2010), 554–565.

Akbari, A., Razzaghi, Z., Homaee, F., Khayamzadeh, M., Movahedi, M., & Akbari, M. E. Parity and breastfeeding are preventive measures against breast cancer in Iranian women. *Breast Cancer, 18* (2011), 51–55.

Akolekar, R., Beta. J., Picciarelli, G., Ogilvie, C., & D'Antonio, F. Procedure-related risk of miscarriage following amniocentesis and chorionic villus sampling: A systematic review and meta-analysis. *Ultrasound in Obstetrics and Gynecology,* 2014. [Epub ahead of print]. doi: 10.1002/uog.14636.

American Academy of Pediatrics (AAP). Policy statement: Planned home birth. *Pediatrics, 131* (2013), 1016–1020. doi: 10.1542/peds.2013-0575.

American College of Obstetricians and Gynecologists (ACOG). *ACOG recommends restricted use of episiotomies,* 2006. Available: http://www.acog.org/from_home/publications/press_releases/nr03-31-06-2.cfm.

American College of Obstetricians and Gynecologists (ACOG). *Frequently asked questions: Exercise during pregnancy,* 2011b. Available: http://www.acog.org/publications/faq/faq119.pdf.

American College of Obstetricians and Gynecologists (ACOG). Patient safety checklist no. 5: Scheduling induction of labor. *Obstetrics & Gynecology, 118* (2011c), 1473–1474.

American College of Obstetricians and Gynecologists (ACOG). *Committee opinion #476: Planned home birth,* 2013. Available: http://www.acog.org/Resources-And-Publications/Committee-Opinions/Committee-on-Obstetric-Practice/Planned-Home-Birth.

American College of Obstetricians and Gynecologists (ACOG) District XI and The Texas Collaborative for Healthy Mothers and Babies. Induction of Labor Toolkit, 2009. Available: http://www.acog.org/-/media/Districts/District-XI/Induction-of-labor-Toolkit.pdf?dmc=1&ts=201509 20T2311469187.

American College of Obstetricians and Gynecologists (ACOG). Immersion in water during labor and delivery: Committee opinion no. 594. *Obstetrics & Gynecology, 123* (2014), 912–915.

American Society for Reproductive Medicine (ASRM). Optimizing natural fertility. *Fertility and Sterility, 90* (2008), S1–S6.

American Society for Reproductive Medicine (ASRM). *Frequently asked questions about infertility,* 2014a. Available: http://reproductivefacts.org/awards/index.aspx?id=3012.

American Society for Reproductive Medicine (ASRM). *Stress and infertility,* 2014b. Available: http://www.reproductivefacts.org/FACTSHEET_Stress_and_Infertility/.

American Society for Reproductive Medicine (ASRM). *Weight*, 2014c. Available: http://www.reproductivefacts.org/topics/detail.aspx?id=1763.

American Society for Reproductive Medicine (ASRM) & Society for Assisted Reproductive Technology. Criteria for number of embryos to transfer: A committee opinion. *Fertility and Sterility, 99* (2013), 44–46.

Baysinger, C. L. Imaging during pregnancy. *Anesthesia & Analgesia, 110* (2010), 863–867.

Beckwith, A. M., & Burke, S. A. Identification of early developmental deficits in infants with prenatal heroin, methadone, and other opioid exposure. *Clinical Pediatrics, 54* (2015), 328–335. doi: 10.1177/0009922814549545.

Beeghly, M., Martin, B., Rose-Jacobs, R., Cabral, H., Heeren, T., Augustyn, M., ... & Frank, D. A. Prenatal cocaine exposure and children's language functioning at 6 and 9.5 years: moderating effects of child age, birthweight, and gender. *Journal of Pediatric Psychology, 31*(1) (2006), 98–115.

Berg, S. J., & Wynne-Edwards, K. Changes in testosterone, cortisol, and estradiol levels in men becoming fathers. *Mayo Clinic Proceedings, 76,* 6 (2001), 582–592.

Bianchi, D. W., Parker, R. L., Wentworth, J., Madankumar, R., Saffer, C., Das, A. F., et al. DNA sequencing versus standard prenatal aneuploidy screening. *New England Journal of Medicine, 370* (2014), 799–808. doi: 10.1056/NEJMoa1311037.

Biederman, J., Martelon, M., Woodworth, K. Y., Spencer, T. J., & Faraone, S. V. Is maternal smoking during pregnancy a risk factor for cigarette smoking in offspring? A longitudinal controlled study of ADHD children grown up. *Journal of Attention Disorders,* 2014. [Epub ahead of print]. doi: 10.1177/1087054714557357.

Bigsby, R., LaGasse, L. L., Lester, B., Shankaran, S., Bada, H., Bauer, C., & Liu, J. Prenatal cocaine exposure and motor performance at 4 months. *American Journal of Occupational Therapy, 65,* 5 (2001), e60–e68.

Brown, H. L., & Graves, C. R. Smoking and marijuana use in pregnancy. *Clinical Obstetrics and Gynecology, 56* (2013), 107–113.

Bruckner, T. A., Cheng, Y. W., & Caughey, A. B. Increased neonatal mortality among normal-weight births beyond 41 weeks of gestation in California. *American Journal of Obstetrics and Gynecology, 199* (2008), 421.e1–421.e7. doi: 10.1016/j.ajog.2008.05.015.

Capmas, P., Bouyer, J., & Fernandez, H. Treatment of ectopic pregnancies in 2014: New answers to some old questions. *Fertility and Sterility, 101* (2014), 615–620.

Centers for Diseases Control and Prevention (CDC). *Reproductive health: Infertility FAQs,* 2013. Available: http://www.cdc.gov/reproductivehealth/Infertility/index.htm.

Centers for Disease Control and Prevention (CDC). *Breastfeeding among U.S. children born 2001–2011: CDC National Immunization Survey,* 2014a. Available: http://www.cdc.gov/breastfeeding/data/NIS_data/.

Centers for Disease Control and Prevention (CDC). *Fetal alcohol spectrum disorders (FASDs): Data and statistics,* 2014b. Available: http://www.cdc.gov/ncbddd/fasd/data.html.

Centers for Disease Control and Prevention (CDC). *HIV among pregnant women, infants, and children,* 2014c. Available: http://www.cdc.gov/hiv/risk/gender/pregnantwomen/facts/index.html.

Centers for Disease Control and Prevention (CDC). *Infant mortality,* 2014d. Available: http://www.cdc.gov/reproductivehealth/MaternalInfantHealth/InfantMortality.htm

Centers for Disease Control and Prevention (CDC). *National public health action plan for the detection, prevention, and management of infertility.* Atlanta, Georgia: CDC, June 2014e.

Centers for Disease Control and Prevention (CDC). *Provisional monthly and 12-month ending number of live births, deaths, and infant deaths and rates: United States, January 2013–June 2014,* 2014f. Available: http://www.cdc.gov/nchs/data/dvs/provisional_tables/Provisional_Table01_2014Jun.pdf.

Centers for Disease Control and Prevention (CDC). *Rubella and the vaccine (shot) to prevent it,* 2014g. Available: http://www.cdc.gov/vaccines/vpd-vac/rubella/downloads/PL-dis-rubella-bw-office.pdf.

Centers for Disease Control and Prevention (CDC). *Tobacco use and pregnancy.* 2014h. Available: http://www.cdc.gov/reproductivehealth/tobaccoUsePregnancy/index.htm.

Centers for Diseases Control and Prevention (CDC). *What is assisted reproductive technology?* 2014i. Available: http://www.cdc.gov/ART/.

Centers for Disease Control and Prevention (CDC). *2011 mortality multiple cause micro-data files,* n.d. Available: http://www.cdc.gov/nchs/data/nvsr/nvsr63/nvsr63_03.pdf.

Centers for Disease Control and Prevention (CDC), American Society for Reproductive Medicine (ASRM), & Society for Assisted Reproductive Technology. *2012 assisted reproductive technology fertility clinic success rates report.* Atlanta, GA: U.S. Department of Health and Human Services, 2014.

Central Intelligence Agency. Country comparison: Infant mortality rate. *The World Factbook,* 2014. Available: https://www.cia.gov/library/publications/the-world-factbook/rankorder/2091rank.html.

Chandra, A., Copen, C. E., & Stephen, E. H. Infertility and impaired fecundity in the United States, 1982–2010: Data from the National Survey of Family Growth. *National Health Statistics Reports;* no 67. Hyattsville, MD: National Center for Health Statistics, 2013.

Cheyney, M., Bovbjerg, M., Everson, C., Gordon, W., Hannibal, D., & Vedam, S. Outcomes of care for 16,924 planned home births in the United States: The Midwives Alliance of North America Statistics Project, 2004 to 2009. *Journal of Midwifery & Women's Health, 59* (2014), 17–27. doi: 10.1111/jmwh.12172.

Clark, S. L., Frye, D. R., Meyers, J. A., Belfort, M. A., Dildy, G. A., Kofford, S., et al. Reduction in elective delivery < 39 weeks of gestation: Comparative effectiveness of 3 approaches to change and the impact on neonatal intensive care admission and stillbirth. *American Journal of Obstetrics and Gynecology, 203* (2010), 449.e1–449.e6.

Conde-Agudelo, A., Rosas-Bermudez, A., Castaño, F., & Norton, M. H. Effects of birth spacing on maternal, perinatal, infant, and child health: A systematic review of causal mechanisms. *Studies in Family Planning 43* (2012), 93–114.

Conde-Agudelo, A., Rosas-Bermudez, A., & Kafury-Goeta, A. C. Birth spacing and risk of adverse perinatal outcomes: A meta-analysis. *Journal of the American Medical Association 295* (2006), 1809–1823.

Daley, A. J., Macarthur, C., & Winter, H. The role of exercise in the treatment of postpartum depression: A review of the literature. *Journal of Midwifery and Women's Health, 52* (2007), 56–62.

Davé, S., Petersen, I., Sherr, L., & Nazareth, I. Incidence of maternal and paternal depression in primary care a cohort study using a primary care database. *Archives of Pediatrics and Adolescent Medicine, 164* (2010), 1038–1044.

Day, N. L., Goldschmidt, L., & Thomas, C. A. Prenatal marijuana exposure contributes to the prediction of marijuana use at age 14. *Addiction, 101* (2006), 1313–1322.

Declercq, E. Trends in midwife-attended births in the United States, 1989–2009. *Journal of Midwifery & Women's Health, 57* (2012), 321–326. doi:10.1111/j.1542-2011.2012.00198.x.

de Jonge, A., van der Goes, B., Ravelli, A., Amelink-Verburg, M., Mol, B., Nijhuis, J., et al. Perinatal mortality and morbidity in a nationwide cohort of 529,688 low-risk planned home and hospital births. *BJOG, 116, 9* (2009), 1177–1184.

Desai, A., Mark, K., & Terplan, M. Marijuana use and pregnancy prevalence, associated behaviors, and birth outcomes. *Obstetrics & Gynecology, 123* (2014), suppl 1:46S. [Published presentation abstract]. doi: 10.1097/01. AOG.0000447331.83496.71.

Devaney, S. A., Polamaki, G. G., Scott, J. A., & Bianchi, D. W. Noninvasive fetal sex determination using cell-free DNA systematic review and meta-analysis. *Journal of the American Medical Association, 306, 6* (2011), 627–636.

de Weger, F. J., Hukkelhoven, C., Serroyen, J., te Velde, E. R., & Smits, L. J. Advanced maternal age, short interpregnancy interval, and perinatal outcome. *American Journal of Obstetrics and Gynecology, 204, 5* (2011), 421.e1–421.e9.

Diamond, M. Human intersexuality: Difference or disorder? *Archives of Sexual Behavior, 38, 2* (2009), 172–173.

Eunice Kennedy Shriver National Institute of Child Health and Human Development. *How many people are affected by or at risk for Down syndrome?* 2014. Available: http://www .nichd.nih.gov/health/topics/down/conditioninfo/Pages/risk .aspx.

Frey, R. Couvade syndrome. In L. J. Fundukian (Ed.), *Gale encyclopedia of medicine.* 4th ed. (Vol.2, pp. 1203–1205), Detroit, MI: Cengage Learning, 2011.

Gibbons, L., Belizan, J. M., Lauer, J. A., Betran, A. P., Merialdi, M., & Althabe, F. The global numbers and costs of additionally needed and unnecessary caesarean sections performed per year: Overuse as a barrier to universal coverage. *World Health Report, Background Paper, 30* (2010). Available: http://www.who/int/healthsystems/topics /financing/healthreport/30C-sectioncosts.pdf.

Gibson, E. Women, birth practitioners, and models of pregnancy and birth: Does consensus exist? *Health Care for Women International, 35* (2014), 149–174. doi: 10.1080/07399332.2013.810219.

Gouin, K., Murphy, K., Shah, P. S., et al. Effects of cocaine use during pregnancy on low birthweight and preterm birth: Systematic review and meta-analyses. *American Journal of Obstetrics and Gynecology, 204, 4* (2011), e1–e12.

Grünebaum, A., McCullough, L. B., Brent, R. L., Arabin, B., Levene, M. I., & Chervenak, F. A. (2015). Perinatal risks of planned home births in the United States. *American Journal of Obstetrics and Gynecology, 212*(3), 350-e1. doi: 10.1016/j.ajog.2014.10.021.

Grünebaum, A., McCullough, L. B., Sapra, K. J., Brent, R. L., Levene, M. I., Arabin, B., & Chervenak, F. A Early and total neonatal mortality in relation to birth setting in the United States, 2006–2009. *American Journal of Obstetrics and Gynecology, 211* (2014), 390.e1–390.e7.

Gunderson, E. P., Jacobs, D. R., Chiang, V., Lewis, C. E., Feng, J., Quesenberry, C. P., & Sidney, S. Duration of lactation and incidence of the metabolic syndrome on women of reproductive age according to gestational diabetes mellitus status: A 20-year prospective study in CARDIA (Coronary Artery Risk Development in Young Adults). *Diabetes, 59, 2* (2010), 495–504.

Gunderson, E. P., Rifas-Shiman, S. L., Oken, E., Rich-Edwards, J. W., Kleinman, K. P., Taveras, E. M., & Gillman, M. W. Association of fewer hours of sleep at 6 month postpartum with substantial weight retention at 1 year postpartum. *American Journal of Epidemiology, 167* (2008), 178–187.

Hans, S. L., Thullen, M., Henson, L. G., Lee, H., Edwards, R. C., & Bernstein, V. J. Promoting positive mother–infant relationships: A randomized trial of community doula support for young mothers. *Infant Mental Health Journal, 34* (2013), 446–457. doi: 10.1002/imhj.21400.

Hansen, M., & Bower, C. The impact of assisted reproductive technologies on intra-uterine growth and birth defects in singletons. *Seminars in Fetal and Neonatal Medicine, 19* (2014), 228–233. doi: 10.1016/j.siny.2014.03.002.

Herranz, G. S., Vílchez, M. A. L., Ledo, J. D., & Sierra, A. M. Children born to heroin-addicted mothers: What's the outcome 25 years later? *Journal of Addiction Research and Therapy, 5* (2014), 2. Available: http://dx.doi .org/10.4172/2155–6105.1000180.

Hill, M., & Reed, K. Pregnancy, breast-feeding, and marijuana: A review article. *Obstetrical and Gynecological Survey, 68* (2013), 710–718.

Hodnett, E. D., Gates, S., Hofmeyr, G. J., & Sakala, C. Continuous support for women during childbirth. *Cochrane Database of Systematic Reviews, 10* (2012), CD003766. doi: 10.1002/14651858.CD003766.pub4.

Horton, R., & Astudillo, O. The power of midwifery. *Lancet, 384* (2014), 1075–1076. doi: 10.1016/S0140-6736(14)60855-2.

Hospital for Sick Children. *Sexual differentiation,* 2014. Available: http://www.aboutkidshealth.ca/En/HowTheBodyWorks /SexDevelopmentAnOverview/SexualDifferentiation.

Hughes, I. A., Houk, C. P., Ahmed, S. F., Lee, P. A., & International Consensus Conference on Intersex organized by the Lawson Wilkins Pediatric Endocrine Society and the European Society for Paediatric Endocrinology. Consensus statement on management of intersex disorders. *Archives of Disease in Childhood, 91, 7* (2006), 554–563.

Janisse, J. J., Bailey, B. A., Ager, J., & Sokol, R. J. Alcohol, tobacco, cocaine, and marijuana use: Relative contributions to preterm delivery and fetal growth restriction. *Substance Abuse, 35* (2014), 60–67. doi: 10.1080/08897077.2013.804483.

Janssen, P. A., Saxell, L., Page, L. A., Klein, M. C., Liston, R. M., & Lee, S. K., Outcomes of planned home birth with registered midwife versus planned hospital birth with midwife or physician. *Canadian Medical Association Journal, 181, 6–7* (2009), 377–383.

Jin, W., He, X., & Liu, P. Maternal and neonatal outcomes in water birth. *Journal of Practical Obstetrics and Gynecology, 11* (2009). [Abstract retrieved from http://en.cnki.com.cn /Article_en/CJFDTOTAL-SFCZ200911016.htm].

Joel, D. Male or female? Brains are intersex. *Frontiers in Integrative Neuroscience, 5, 57* (2011), 1–5.

Johnson, K. C., & Daviss, B., Outcomes of home births with certified professional midwives: Large prospective study in North America. *BMJ, 330* (2005), 1416.

Kader, M., & Naim-Shuchana, S. Physical activity and exercise during pregnancy. *European Journal of Physiotherapy, 16* (2014), 2–9.

Kaimal, A. J., Little, S. E., Odibo, A. O., Stamilio, D. M., Grobman, W. A., Long, E. F., et al. Cost-effectiveness of elective induction of labor at 41 weeks in nulliparous women. *American Journal of Obstetrics and Gynecology, 204* (2011), 137.e1–137.e9. doi: 10.1016/j.ajog.2010.08.012.

Kazmierczak, M., Kielbratowska, B., Pastwa-Wojciechowska, B., & Preis, K. Couvade syndrome among Polish expectant fathers. *Medical Science Monitor, 19* (2013), 132–138. doi: 10.12659/MSM.883791.

Knopik, V. S. Maternal smoking during pregnancy and child outcomes: Real or spurious effect? *Developmental Neuropsychology, 34* (2009), 1–36.

Kozhimannil, K. B., Attanasio, L. B., Hardeman, R. R., & O'Brien, M. Doula care supports near-universal breastfeeding initiation among diverse, low-income women. *Journal of Midwifery & Women's Health, 58* (2013), 378–382. doi: 10.1111/jmwh.12065.

Kozhimannil, K. B., Johnson, P. J., Attanasio, L. B., Gjerdingen, D. K., & McGovern, P. M. Use of nonmedical methods of labor induction and pain management among U.S. women. *Birth, 40* (2013), 227–236.

Lambert, B. L., & Bauer, C. R. Developmental and behavioral consequences of prenatal cocaine exposure: A review. *Journal of Perinatology, 32* (2012), 819–828.

Langley, K., Heron, J., Smith, G. D., & Thapar, A. Maternal and paternal smoking during pregnancy and risk of ADHD symptoms in offspring: Testing for intrauterine effects. *American Journal of Epidemiology, 176* (2012), 261–268. doi: 10.1093/aje/kwr510.

Lau, C., Ambalavanan, N., Chakraborty, H., Wingate, M. S., & Carlo, W. A. Extremely low birth weight and infant mortality rates in the United States. *Pediatrics, 131* (2013), 855–860. doi: 10.1542/peds.2012-2471.

Levine, T. P., Liu, J., Das, A., Leter, B., Lagasse, L., Shakarna, S., et al. Effects of prenatal cocaine exposure on special education in school aged children. *Pediatrics, 122* (2008), e83–e91.

Lindsay, M. K., & Burnett, E. The use of narcotics and street drugs during pregnancy. *Clinical Obstetrics and Gynecology, 56* (2013), 133–141.

March of Dimes. *Cocaine and pregnancy*, 2013. Available: http://www.marchofdimes.org/pregnancy/cocaine.aspx.

March of Dimes. *Birth defect research*, 2014a. Available: http://www.marchofdimes.org/research/birth-defects-research.aspx.

March of Dimes. *Neonatal abstinence syndrome*, 2014b. Available: http://www.marchofdimes.org/baby/neonatal-abstinence-syndrome-(nas).aspx.

March of Dimes. *Your premature baby: Low birth weight*, 2014c. Available: http://www.marchofdimes.org/baby/low-birthweight.aspx.

Martin, J. A., Hamilton, B. E., Sutton, P. D., Osterman, M., Curtin, S. C. & Mathews, T. J. Births: Final data for 2012. *National Vital Statistics Reports, 62, 9* (2013). Available: http://www.cdc.gov/nchs/data/nvsr/nvsr62/nvsr62_09.pdf.

Mascarenhas, M. N., Flaxman, S. R., Boerma, T., Vanderpoel, S., Mathers, C. D., & Stevens, G. A. Trends in primary and secondary infertility prevalence since 1990: A systematic analysis of demographic and reproductive health surveys. *Lancet, 381* (2013), S90. doi: http://dx.doi.org/10.1016/S0140-6736(13)61344-6.

Mathews, T. J., MacDorman, M. F., & Thoma, M. E. Infant mortality statistics from the 2013 period linked birth/infant death data set. *National Vital Statistics Report, 64 9* (2015). Hyattsville, MD: National Center for Health Statistics.

Matthews, A., Haas, D. M., O'Mathúna, D. P., Dowswell, T., & Doyle, M. Interventions for nausea and vomiting in early pregnancy. *Cochrane Database of Systematic Reviews, 3* (2014), CD007575. doi: 10.1002/14651858.CD007575.pub3.

May, P. A., Baete, A., Russo, J., Elliott, A. J., Blankenship, J., Kalberg, W. O., et al. Prevalence and characteristics of fetal alcohol spectrum disorders . *Pediatrics, 134* (2014), 855–866. doi: 10.1542/peds.2013-3319.

McComish, J. F., Groh, C. J., & Moldenhauer, J. A. development of a doula intervention for postpartum depressive symptoms: Participants' recommendations. *Journal of Child and Adolescent Psychiatric Nursing, 26* (2013), 3–15. doi: 10.1111/jcap.12019.

Medline Plus. *Rh incompatibility*, 2011. Available: http://www.nlm.nih.gov/medlineplus/ency/article/001600.htm.

Midodzi, W. K., Rowe, B. H., Majaesic, S. M., Saunders, L. D., & Senthilselvan, A. Early life factors associated with incidence of physician-diagnosed asthma in preschool children: Results from the Canadian Early Family Childhood Development cohort study. *Journal of Asthma, 47, 1* (2010), 7–13.

Nascimento, S. L., Surita, F. G., & Cecatti, J. G. Physical exercise during pregnancy: A systematic review. *Current Opinion in Obstetrics & Gynecology, 24* (2012), 387–394. doi: 10.1097/GCO.0b013e328359f131.

National Research Council. *Implementing guidelines on weight gain and pregnancy (bundle of 10)*. Washington, DC: National Academies Press, 2013.

Nutter, E., Meyer, S., Shaw-Battista, J., & Marowitz, A. Waterbirth: An integrative analysis of peer-reviewed literature. *Journal of Midwifery & Women's Health, 59* (2014), 286–319. doi: 10.1111/jmwh.12194.

Obebauer, S., & Maestre, L. Fetal MRI of lung hypoplasia: Imaging findings. *Clinical Imaging, 32* (2008), 48–50.

O'Hara, M. W., & McCabe, J. E. Postpartum depression: Current status and future directions. *Annual Review of Clinical Psychology, 9* (2013), 379–407. doi: 10.1146/annurev -clinpsy-050212-185612.

Oregon Health and Science University. *Risks and safety concerns,* 2014. Available: http://www.ohsu.edu/xd/health/services /women/services/midwifery/our-services/waterbirth/risks .cfm.

Oros, D., Bejarano, M. P., Cardiel, M. R., Oros-Espinosa, D., Gonzalez de Agüero, R., & Fabre, E. Low-risk pregnancy at 41 weeks: When should we induce labor? *Journal of Maternal–Fetal and Neonatal Medicine, 25,* 6 (2012), 728–731. doi: 10.3109/14767058.2011.599079.

Osterman, M. J. K., & Martin, J. A. Trends in low-risk cesarean delivery in the United States, 1990–2013. *National Vital Statistics Reports, 63,* 6. Hyattsville, MD: National Center for Health Statistics. 2014.

Pettit, K. E., Hull, A. D., Korty, L., Jones, M. C., & Pretorius, D. H. The utilization of circulating cell-free fetal DNA testing and decrease in invasive diagnostic procedures: An institutional experience. *Journal of Perinatology, 34* (2014), 750–753. doi: 10.1038/jp.2014.102.

Phillips, K. Is the evidence on waterbirth watertight? *British Journal of Midwifery, 22* (2014), 776–780.

Pinkhardt, E. H., Kassubek, J., Brummer, D., Koelch, M., Ludolph, A. C., Feget, J. M., & Ludolph, A. G. Intensified testing for attention-deficit hyperactivity disorder (ADHD) in girls should reduce depression and smoking in adult females and the prevalence of ADHD in the long term, *Medical Hypothesis, 72,* 4 (2009), 409–412.

Qiu, J., & Liu, X. A clinical study on 280 cases of water birth. *Chinese Journal of Woman and Child Health Research, 5* (2008). [Abstract retrieved from http://en.cnki.com.cn /Article_en/CJFDTOTAL-SANE2008805021.htm].

Queenan, J. T. How to stop the relentless rise in cesarean deliveries. *Obstetrics and Gynecology, 118* (2011), 199–200.

Richardson, G. A., Goldschmidt, L., & Willford, J. The effects of prenatal cocaine use on infant development. *Neurotoxicology and Teratology, 30* (2008), 96–108.

Rolland, M., Le, Moal, J., Wagner, V., Royère, D., & De Mouzon, J. Decline in semen concentration and morphology in a sample of 26,609 men close to general population between 1989 and 2005 in France. *Human Reproduction, 28* (2013), 462–470. doi: 10.1093/humrep/des415.

Royal College of Midwives. *Evidence based guidelines for midwifery-led care in labour. Immersion in water for labour and birth.* London: Royal College of Midwives, 2012.

Royal College of Midwives. *Response to joint American College of Obstetricians and Gynecologists(ACOG), and American Academy of Pediatrics (AAP) Committee's opinion regarding birthing pool use during labour and waterbirth.* London: Royal College of Midwives, 2014.

Runquist, J. Persevering through postpartum fatigue. *Journal of Obstetric, Gynecologic, and Neonatal Nursing, 36* (2007), 28–37.

Schwarz, E. B., Ray, R. M., Stuebe, A. M., Allison, M. A., Ness, R. B., Freiberg, M. S., & Cauley, J. A. Duration of lactation and risk factors for maternal cardiovascular disease. *Obstetrics and Gynecology, 113* (2009), 974.

Sherieh, M., Cottrell, D. B., & Mancuso, P. Medical management of ectopic pregnancy: Early diagnosis is key. *Clinician Reviews, 24* (2014), 29–38.

Shier, D., Butler, J., & Lewis, R. *Hole's essentials of human anatomy and physiology.* New York: McGraw-Hill, 2003.

Simpson, J. L. Birth defects and assisted reproductive technologies. *Seminars in Fetal and Neonatal Medicine, 19* (2014), 177–182. doi: 10.1016/j.siny.2014.01.001.

Skoglund, C., Chen, Q., D'Onofrio, B. M., Lichtenstein, P., & Larsson, H. Familial confounding of the association between maternal smoking during pregnancy and ADHD in offspring. *Journal of Child Psychology and Psychiatry, 55* (2014), 61–68. doi: 10.1111/jcpp.12124.

Smith, L. E., & Howard, K. S. Continuity of paternal social support and depressive symptoms among new mothers. *Journal of Family Psychology, 22* (2008), 763–773.

Storey, A. E., Walsh, C. J., Quintone, R. L., & Wynne-Edwards, K. E. Hormonal correlates of paternal responsiveness in new and expectant fathers. *Evolution and Human Behavior, 21,* 2 (2000), 79–95.

Stuebe, A. M., & Schwarz, E. B. The risks and benefits of infant feeding practices for women and their children. *Journal of Perinatology, 30* (2010), 155–162.

Swedish National Institute of Public Health. *Low-dose alcohol exposure during pregnancy: Does it harm?* 2009. Available: http://www/fhi.se/PageFiles/7261/R2009-14-low-dose- alcohol-exposure-pregnancy.pdf.

Thompson, D. R., & Clark, C. L. *Short birth intervals: Associated maternal factors and subsequent risk of adverse birth outcomes.* Florida Department of Health, Division of Family Services, 2011. Available: http://doh.state.fl.us /family/mch/docs/birthintervalpaper09-29-11-final.pdf.

Thoni, A., Mussner, K., & Ploner, F. Water birthing: Retrospective review of 2625 water births: Contamination of birth pool water and risk of microbial cross-infection. *Minerva Ginicologica, 62,* 3 (2010), 203–211.

U.S. Department of Health and Human Services. *Pregnancy: Recovering from birth,* 2010. Available: http://www .womenshealth.gov/pregnancy/childbirth-beyond/recovering- from-birth.cfm.

U.S. Department of Health and Human Services. *The Surgeon General's call to action to support breastfeeding.* Washington, DC: U.S. Department of Health and Human Services, 2011.

U.S. Department of Health and Human Services, Health Resources and Services Administration, Maternal and Child Health Bureau. *Child Health USA 2013.* Rockville, MD: U.S. Department of Health and Human Services, 2013.

U.S. Department of Health and Human Services, Office of Disease Prevention and Health Promotion. *Healthy people 2020: Maternal, infant, and child health objectives.* Washington, DC: U.S. Department of Health and Human Services. Available: http://www.healthypeople.gov/2020/topicsobjects2020/pdfs/MaternalChildHealth.pdf.

U.S. National Library of Medicine. *Fetal alcohol spectrum disorders,* 2014. Available: http://www.nlm.nih.gov/medlineplus/fetalalcoholspectrumdisorders.html.

Wax, J. R., Lucas, F. L., Lamont, N., Pinette, M. G., Cartin, A., & Blackstone, J. Maternal and newborn outcomes in planned home birth vs. planned hospital births: A metaanalysis. *American Journal of Obstetrics and Gynecology, 203, 3* (2010), e1–e8.

Weiss, R. E. Couvade syndrome: Sympathetic pregnancy. *About. com,* 2009. Available: http://pregnancy.about.com/cs/forfathersonly/a/couvade.htm.

Weston, M. J. Magnetic resonance imaging in fetal medicine: A pivotal review of the current and developing indications. *Postgraduate Medicine Journal, 86* (2010), 42–51.

Wisner, K. L., Sit, D. K., McShea, M. C., Rizzo, D. M., Zoretich, R. A., Hughes, C. L. et al. Onset timing, thoughts of self-harm, and diagnoses in postpartum women with screen-positive depression findings. *JAMA Psychiatry, 70* (2013), 490–498. doi: 10.1001/jamapsychiatry.2013.87.

World Health Organization (WHO). *HIV/AIDS: Mother to child transmission of HIV,* 2014. Available: http://www.who.int/hiv/topics/mtct/en/.

Wynne-Edwards, K. Ask the brains: Why do some expectant fathers experience pregnancy symptoms such as vomiting and nausea? *Scientific American Mind, 17, 3* (2006), 84.

Young, K., & Kruske, S. How valid are the common concerns raised against water birth? A focused review of the literature. *Women and Birth, 26* (2013), 105–109.

Zanetti-Dallenbach, R., Lapaire, O., Maertens, A., Holzgreve, W., & Hösli, I. Water birth: More than a trendy alternative: A prospective, observational study. *Obstetrical & Gynecological Survey, 62, 4* (2007), 222–223.

CHAPTER 9

Unexpected Pregnancy Outcomes

© Gayvoronskaya Yana/Shutterstock

FEATURES

Ethical Dimensions
Should Intact Dilation and Evacuation Be Banned?

Ethical Dimensions
Crisis Pregnancy Centers: Are They "Fake" Clinics?

Communication Dimensions
Debating the Abortion Issue

Global Dimensions
A Worldwide Preference for Boys

Gender Dimensions
Baby "Richard"

Multicultural Dimensions
International Adoptions

CHAPTER OBJECTIVES

1 Discuss abortion procedures.

2 Provide an overview of legal history and current laws related to abortion.

3 Describe current attitudes toward abortion in the United States.

4 Describe the various types of adoptions: closed and open adoptions, and agency adoptions and non-agency adoptions.

5 Provide an overview of laws related to adoption.

INTRODUCTION

*T*oo many pregnancies are unplanned and unwanted. The dilemma this causes for some men and women is eloquently described by the author Anna Quindlen (1988, 209–212).

It was always the look on their faces that told me first. I was the freshman dormitory counselor and they were freshmen at a women's college where everyone was smart. One of them would come into my room, a golden girl, a valedictorian, an 800 verbal score on the SATs, and her eyes would be empty, seeing only a busted future, the devastation of her life as she knew it. She had failed biology, messed up the math; she was pregnant. That was when I became prochoice.

Quindlen then describes the birth of her own son.

It was the look in his eyes that I will always remember, too. They were as black as the bottom of a well, and in them for a few minutes I thought I saw myself the way I had always wished to be—clear, simple, elemental, at peace. My child looked at me and I looked back at him in the delivery room, and I realized that out of a sea of infinite possibilities it had come down to this: a specific person, born on the hottest day of the year, conceived on a Christmas Eve, made by his father and me miraculously from scratch.

Once I believed that there was a little blob of formless protoplasm in there and a gynecologist went in there with a surgical instrument, and that was that. Then I got pregnant myself—eagerly, intentionally, by the right man, at the right time—and I began to doubt. My abdomen still flat, my stomach roiling with morning sickness, I felt not that I had protoplasm inside, but, instead, a complete human being in miniature to whom I could talk, sing, make promises. Neither of these views was accurate; instead, I think, the reality is something in the middle. And that is where I find myself now, in the middle—hating the idea of abortions, hating the idea of having them outlawed.

For I know it is the right thing in some times and places. I remember sitting in a shabby clinic far uptown with one of those freshmen, only three months after the Supreme Court had made what we were doing possible, and watching with wonder as the lovely first love she had had with a nice boy unraveled over the space of an hour as they waited for her to be called, degenerating into sniping and silences. I remember a year or two later seeing them pass on campus and not even acknowledge each other because their conjoining had caused them so much pain, and I shuddered to think of them married, with a small psyche in their unready and unwilling hands....

I don't feel all one way about abortion anymore, and I don't think it serves a just cause to pretend that many of us do. For years I believed that a woman's right to choose was absolute, but now I wonder. Do I, with a stable home and marriage and sufficient stamina and money, have the freedom to choose abortion because a pregnancy is inconvenient just now? Legally I do have the right; legally I wanted always to have that right. It is the morality of exercising it under those circumstances that makes me wonder....

I have taped on my VCR a public television program in which somehow, inexplicably, a film is shown of a fetus in utero scratching its face, seemingly putting up a tiny hand to shield itself from the camera's eye. It would make a potent weapon in the arsenal of the antiabortionists. I grow sentimental about it as it floats in the salt water, part fish, part human being. It is almost living, but not quite. It has almost turned my heart around, but not quite my head.*

Many people are surprised to learn that about half of all pregnancies in the United States are unintended. Yet, that is the case. When an unintended pregnancy occurs, decisions are required. Should the pregnancy be terminated? If so, which method of abortion should be used? What are the legal, moral, and health implications of this decision? Should the fetus be brought to term and a baby born? If so, should the child be raised by the biological parents? Do both parents want to be involved? Should the child be placed for adoption? If placed for adoption, should adoption be arranged through an agency or through a relative? What are the legal and moral implications of this decision?

This chapter explores two of the alternatives presented to people who experience an unintended pregnancy: abortion and adoption.

*Reproduced from *Living Out Loud*, by Anna Quindlen, © 1994 by Anna Quindlen. Used by permission of Random House, Inc.

Abortion

For unplanned pregnancies, the first decision to be made is whether to continue the pregnancy. Sometimes the woman or the couple decides to allow the pregnancy to continue, but something goes wrong and the fetus stops developing. Such natural cessations of the pregnancy are called **spontaneous abortions**, or miscarriages. Abortions requiring intervention to end the pregnancy are technically called **induced abortions**, though that terminology is rarely used in everyday conversation.

Abortion is safest in the earliest weeks of pregnancy. If a woman thinks she is pregnant and does not want to continue the pregnancy, she should perform a home pregnancy test or go to a clinic as soon as she misses a period. In the United States, approximately 89% of abortions are performed in the first 12 weeks of pregnancy, with about 1.2% occurring after 21 weeks (Guttmacher Institute, 2014). For all abortion procedures, women should receive counseling before the procedure to ensure that they have carefully considered all of their options, that they do indeed want an abortion, and that they are not being coerced into the decision.

Abortion Procedures

Medical Abortions

Medical abortions are procedures that use drugs to induce abortion during an early pregnancy. These

---

spontaneous abortion (miscarriage) The natural termination of a pregnancy.

induced abortion Purposeful termination of a pregnancy.

medical abortion A procedure that uses drugs to induce abortion.

medications include **mifepristone** or **methotrexate** in combination with **misoprostol**.

Mifepristone was discovered by a French pharmaceutical company in 1978 and was originally known as RU 486. (*RU* refers to Roussel Uclaf, the French pharmaceutical company.) In 2000, the U.S. Food and Drug Administration (FDA) approved mifepristone; this medication blocks progesterone, a hormone needed to maintain a pregnancy. The FDA-approved protocol for medical abortions requires two clinic visits. In the first visit, mifepristone is administered to the woman, who must be no more than 49 days past her last menstrual period (LMP). The woman then returns to the clinic 2 days later and takes misoprostol, a prostaglandin that causes uterine contractions to expel the contents of uterus. This protocol successfully terminates the pregnancy approximately 92% of the time.

Because two clinic visits can be burdensome, many clinics utilize other evidence-based practices. For example, a lower dose of mifepristone—200 milligrams orally—followed by 800 micrograms of misoprostol taken vaginally at home can be equally effective through 70 days past the LMP, has fewer side effects, and allows women more privacy. Other evidence-based methods use 200 milligrams of mifepristone orally followed by 800 micrograms of misoprostol buccally (between the gum and the cheek), or 200 milligrams of mifepristone orally followed by 400 micrograms of misoprostol under the tongue (National Abortion Federation [NAF], 2013). Some have advocated for a misoprostol regimen alone because of its lower cost (mifepristone is quite expensive) and easier access, especially in developing countries. However, using misoprostol alone is significantly less effective: Only three-fourths of abortions are successfully completed with this approach, compared to more than 90% of abortions when using both mifepristone and misoprostol (Blum et al. 2012; Ngoc et al., 2011). In the United States, 98% of medical abortions use mifepristone and misoprostol (Jones & Jerman, 2014).

Methotrexate works differently than mifepristone; methotrexate blocks rapid cell division. While some studies have examined the use of methotrexate in women who are 63 days past their LMP, most follow guidelines that a woman should be no more than 49 days past her LMP (Bryant, Regan, & Stuart, 2014). Various delivery mechanisms for the methotrexate have been used (intramuscular versus oral), at different doses (ranging from 25 mg to 75 mg), with varying timing and routes for the administration of misoprostol after the methotrexate. Because the methotrexate–misoprostol combination is less effective than the mifepristone–misoprostol combination, it not commonly used in the United States (Bryant et al., 2014).

Currently, in the United States, methotrexate medical abortions are available only on an "off-label" basis (NAF, 2014). When drugs are approved by the FDA, their safety and efficacy are judged to warrant their use for specific conditions. Often, however, physicians discover other uses for those drugs and prescribe them for these other purposes. This practice, termed *off-label use*, is perfectly legal. Methotrexate is currently approved by the FDA for use by physicians for psoriasis and for rheumatoid arthritis but is used off-label by physicians for medical abortions. Because of the teratogenicity of methotrexate (MacDonald, Norman, & Popescu, 2013), it can cause severe side effects if the pregnancy is not terminated. For all women having medical abortion procedures, but especially for those whose procedures use methotrexate, follow-up appointments to ensure termination and completion of the abortion (i.e., all is material expelled from the uterus) are critical.

While most abortions in the United States are performed surgically, the percentage of medical abortions is increasing (Jones & Jerman, 2014). Many women prefer the privacy of being at home when they undergo a medical abortion. A study examining the experience of medical abortion showed that most (81%) of the women stated that bleeding was either "as expected" or "not as bad as expected," and 58% of the women stated that the pain was "as expected" or "not as bad as expected." The majority (84%) of the women said that they would recommend this method to a friend (Cameron et al., 2010), and an international study has shown high rates of satisfaction both immediately after the procedure and at a 2-week follow-up (Rodriguez et al., 2012). Another study indicated that the pain associated with medical abortion was correlated with the pain during menstruation (Suhonena et al., 2011), and the authors recommended that clinicians and women seeking an abortion consider this factor when choosing between a medical or surgical procedure.

Vacuum Aspiration

Most abortions in the United States are performed during the first trimester of pregnancy using a surgical procedure called **vacuum aspiration**. This procedure

---

mifepristone A drug that blocks the hormone progesterone, which is needed to maintain a pregnancy.

methotrexate A drug that blocks the hormone progesterone, which is needed to maintain a pregnancy.

misoprostol A prostaglandin that causes uterine contractions.

vacuum aspiration Surgical procedure that uses a suction tube to evacuate the contents of the uterus, which can be used through the first weeks of the second trimester.

uses suction equipment to evacuate the contents of the uterus. It can also be used in the first weeks of the second trimester, until about 16 weeks past the LMP. **Manual vacuum aspiration (MVA)** is a variation of vacuum aspiration that can be used from the detection of pregnancy to up to 12 weeks since the LMP. In contrast to traditional vacuum aspiration procedures, it uses nonelectric suction instruments. The procedure takes 5 to 15 minutes, and the woman usually leaves the clinic within 2 hours.

Dilation and Evacuation

During the second trimester of pregnancy, typically after 16 weeks past the LMP, **dilation and evacuation (D&E)** is the abortion procedure used. It involves dilating the cervix, scraping the walls of the uterus, and removing the endometrial lining with suction. Women receive antibiotics to reduce the chance of infection and pain medication. In later second-trimester abortions, women may need medication through injection to stop the fetus's heart before the procedure begins. While the D&E procedure takes only 10 to 20 minutes, more time is needed to prepare the cervix. Because of this factor, pre-procedure consultation and recovery time, a woman can expect to spend several hours at the clinic.

As previously mentioned, almost 90% of all abortions are performed during the first trimester and only about 1.2% are performed at 21 weeks or more (Guttmacher Institute, 2014). Third-trimester abortions are very rare, but occasionally a clinician might perform an intact D&E, also called dilation and extraction (D&X), which has been dubbed by opponents of legal abortion as a "partial-birth abortion." The procedure is similar to a D&E in that dilation of the cervix is required; however, dilation to a greater point is required because the fetus passes through the cervical opening partially intact. This procedure is required when the fetus is too large for other abortion procedures to be performed safely and effectively (see the box "Ethical Dimensions: Should Dilation and Extraction Be Banned?").

The Law and the Debate

Because abortion is an issue debated by citizens, ruled on by the judiciary, and legislated by elected representatives—not to mention it being a major decision for people who become directly involved in unplanned pregnancies—it is a topic that needs the fullest possible study and consideration.

For more than four decades, abortion has been vehemently debated in the political sector. Although in vitro fertilization, contraception, and sterilization all have their controversial aspects, none of them generates the political, religious, and emotional heat that abortion does. Some people believe induced abortion to be murder of a baby, whereas others see it as a medical intervention into a biological process. Some people feel that the question of when life begins is central to this debate: Is it at conception, at some point when the fetus could (with help) exist outside the uterus, or at birth? But a person's view of when life begins is only one factor in shaping his or her attitudes on whether induced abortion is morally acceptable. Another central issue is whether the individual woman has the right to make a decision so basic to her own life or whether the government has that right and power. Other attitudes also enter into the debate—for instance, attitudes regarding world population, religious issues, women's "place," political power, poverty, public and private child care, and the degree of responsibility people should assume for their sexual behavior.

Today, pro-life political groups are actively supporting candidates who are totally opposed to abortion. Their goal is to pass legislation making abortion illegal or even to pass a constitutional amendment prohibiting abortion in the United States. Groups labeled pro-choice, however, believe that women should have the right to decide for themselves what they will do with their bodies. Consequently, they oppose legislative restrictions on the availability of abortion to women who choose that option, and they wish to uphold the Supreme Court decision of 1973, which established the current legal status of abortion in the United States. The Court ruled (in *Roe v. Wade*) that abortion should be available to women during the first trimester (the first 3 months) of pregnancy. The decision is made by the pregnant woman and her physician. With regard to abortion during the second trimester, the Court ruled that the states can develop the regulations they deem necessary to maintain the pregnant woman's health. In the third trimester, the states can limit or prohibit abortions if the mother's health is not in jeopardy.

In 1983, the Supreme Court reaffirmed its 1973 decision and stated that the government could not interfere with abortion unless such interference was clearly justified by "accepted medical practice." In effect, this ruling prohibited governmental interference even into the second trimester and invalidated state laws that required abortions during the second trimester to be performed in a hospital.

manual vacuum aspiration (MVA) A variation of vacuum aspiration that uses nonelectric suction instruments and can be used from the time of detection of pregnancy through 12 weeks.

dilation and evacuation (D&E) Surgical procedure that involves dilating the cervix, scraping the walls of the uterus, and removing the endometrial lining with suction.

DIMENSIONS

Should Dilation and Extraction Be Banned?

Dilation and extraction (D&X; also called intact dilation and evacuation) is performed late in the second trimester when, in the judgment of the physician, it is deemed the best means of abortion—that is, the most effective and safest. Some reasons for this type of abortion are concern for the health of the pregnant woman, late determination of birth defects in the fetus, or the woman's delay in seeking abortion as a result of fear of letting others know that she is pregnant. Objections have been raised to this method of abortion because it is performed at or near viability of the fetus. Those opposed to abortion at any time in any form are understandably opposed to D&X. However, even some Americans supportive of a woman's right to abortion during the first trimester and through the second trimester until the fetus could live outside the womb are disturbed by abortions occurring so late in the pregnancy. In their desire to secure support for their position, opponents have dubbed D&X "partial-birth abortion," attempting to have D&X viewed as the interference with the birth of a live baby, rather than the termination of a pregnancy.

Those opposed to placing restrictions on the type of abortion allowed argue that the most qualified person to make this decision is the physician. Therefore, they believe a ban on any type of abortion procedure would limit physicians' options at a time when performing it would be most effective and safest. Opponents to restrictions also believe that once restrictions are allowed, "right to life" supporters will use them as a wedge to introduce more restrictions, eventually eroding a woman's right to abortion.

In 1997, Congress passed a law banning D&X procedures. President Bill Clinton vetoed that law, however, and Congress could not muster the votes required to override his veto. The following year, Congress again passed a similar law, but it was again vetoed by President Clinton. However, this time the House of Representatives overrode the veto. Once the bill arrived back in the Senate, the veto was sustained, thereby preventing the legislation from becoming law.

In June 2000, the U.S. Supreme Court ruled in *Stenberg v. Carhart* that bans on D&X abortions were unconstitutional. Nevertheless, in 2007, the Supreme Court, in *Gonzales v. Carhart*, upheld the federal Partial-Birth Abortion Ban Act of 2003, which prohibits this type of abortion without any exemptions (that is, regardless of concerns for the woman's health). As a result, dilation and extraction abortions are banned by the federal government. Confusion still exists, because the federal law does not provide a precise description of what is banned. Consequently, states have proposed their own laws. As of 2015, 32 states had enacted bans on "partial-birth" abortions (13 of which were blocked by a court and are not in effect); all of them include some sort of exemption if the woman's health is jeopardized by the pregnancy (Guttmacher Institute, 2015a).

Do you believe D&X should be banned as an abortion procedure? Why do you believe as you do?

In 1989, a Supreme Court made more conservative by new presidential appointments revisited this issue. The justices decided in *Webster v. Reproductive Health Services* that a Minnesota law requiring physicians to test fetuses to determine whether they could survive outside the womb before performing abortions was constitutional. That opened up the possibility that other regulations of abortion would be reviewed positively by the Court. Subsequently, two other cases were taken before the Supreme Court and decided in 1990. In *Hodgson v. Minnesota*, the Court rejected a law requiring a physician to notify both parents of a minor before an abortion could be performed. The rationale for this ruling was that some minors either do not live with both parents or have abusive or otherwise uncaring parents. The Court made it clear that if this law included a judicial bypass (in which a judge could approve the abortion if the parents were not the ones most appropriately notified), this law would be considered constitutional. In fact, in *Ohio v. Akron Center for Reproductive Health*, the Court held that a similar law that required notification of one parent and that did include a judicial bypass was constitutional.

In 1992, the Supreme Court reaffirmed the constitutionality of states attaching regulations to abortions, although it also reaffirmed the right of a woman to have an abortion if she chooses. In *Planned Parenthood of Southeastern Pennsylvania v. Casey*, the Court ruled that Pennsylvania could require a woman seeking an abortion to receive counseling; to wait 24 hours before an abortion could be performed; and, if a minor younger than 18 years, to obtain a parent's informed consent or a judge's approval. The

Both sides of the abortion issue attempt to show their strength in numbers with annual marches in Washington, D.C., coinciding with the anniversary of *Roe v. Wade*. The marches do not happen on the same day, to minimize conflict as well as to accommodate the huge influx of people to Washington.

Ethical DIMENSIONS

Crisis Pregnancy Centers: Are They "Fake" Clinics?

While there are many legitimate and medically driven services for pregnant woman, some "pregnancy centers" are not truly designed to help pregnant woman. Often called crisis pregnancy centers (CPCs), the intention of these facilities is to guilt, scare, or otherwise manipulate women into having their child.

A 2015 investigation of 25% of the CPCs in California revealed that these organizations provided extensive misinformation, demonstrated little medical knowledge, and failed to provide information or referrals—a failure that could potentially be dangerous to a woman's health (NARAL, 2015). In 91% of the visits, workers stated that abortion was linked to an increased risk of breast cancer, infertility, miscarriage, and/or severe post-abortion depression resulting in suicide. All of these claims are blatant lies.

In other visits, when CPC workers conducted ultrasounds on the investigators, none was concerned or referred the investigator to a physician when no fetal heartbeat was detected. In one case, the CPC worker identified the investigator's IUD on the ultrasound and said it was "her baby." Much of the paper literature collected during the CPC visits provided inaccurate information about birth control. Likewise, CPC workers emphasized abstinence with statements such as "To not get pregnant, it would be best to stop whoring around" and "Everybody should just stop using birth control because it's not healthy for your body; it's not good for you."

When investigators presented with symptoms indicating high-risk pregnancies, none was referred to a physician for additional examination, even when the symptoms presented would indicate severe health issues. In other visits, when investigators presented with abusive situations, none was asked about safety plans or provided with referral information to local resources that assist with interpersonal violence.

Many people believe that visiting a place that provides only one option in a fear-based and shaming way and that is "supported" by inaccurate information does not truly help a pregnant woman with her decision. Others believe that "saving the unborn" child justifies the means.

What do you think? Does a pregnant woman have to have accurate information about abortion as she is making her decision about the pregnancy? How would you feel if you or your partner visited such a clinic in search of information, only to realize it was using such a biased approach?

Source: NARAL. *Crisis pregnancy centers lie: The insidious threat to reproductive freedom*, 2015. Available: http://www.prochoiceamerica.org/assets/download-files/cpc-report-2015.pdf.

Court also ruled that a physician had to keep detailed records of abortions and reasons for performing late-term abortions. However, the Court refused to overturn *Roe v. Wade*, as many opposed to abortion had hoped a conservative Court would do.

In June 2000, the Supreme Court returned its most significant abortion ruling since the *Casey* case (NARAL, 2015). In *Stenberg v. Carhart*, the Court ruled that bans on D&X procedures (referred to as partial-birth abortions) were unconstitutional because they did not take into account the health of the pregnant woman. Still, in 2003, the federal government passed the Partial-Birth Abortion Ban Act, which prohibited D&X abortions. In 2007, the Supreme Court upheld the constitutionality of that law.

While not directly affecting *Roe v. Wade*, a Supreme Court decision made in 1980 profoundly affected the availability of legal abortions. In this case, the Court ruled that the federal government could refuse to fund abortions for the poor, even though it funded other health care (Hyde Amendment). The consequence of this action has been to prohibit poor women from obtaining safe abortions—the same abortions that middle- and upper-class women can receive by paying for them—with Medicaid funds. People who oppose abortion acknowledge that an inequity exists between poor and affluent women regarding the availability of abortion, but they view this circumstance as leaving the fetuses of more wealthy women unprotected by law. Some states have taken on the financial costs of abortion for poor women who are denied federal assistance by the Hyde Amendment.

Current Laws on Abortion Services

People who oppose legalized abortion have unsuccessfully tried to outlaw abortion services completely. However, they have been successful at limiting the availability of abortion under many circumstances.

The federal government has restricted access to abortion by denying abortion coverage to military personnel and their families, women receiving care from Indian Health Services, and people on disability insurance. In fact, military health insurance does not cover abortion in cases of rape or incest, and personnel stationed overseas are not permitted to use personal funds to pay for abortions at overseas military facilities; this means that servicewomen must use local services (but potentially incur safety issues and language barriers) or take vacation leave to fly back to the United States to get an abortion.

In addition, many states have passed laws limiting abortion services. These include limiting funding for abortion, parental consent laws, waiting periods, and bans on certain procedures (see Tables 9.1 and 9.2 for state laws regarding parental consent and waiting period laws). Interestingly, one study has shown that in areas of the United States with more restrictive abortion policies and less access to abortion, the rates of searching for abortion information on the Internet are higher compared to areas with fewer restrictions and greater access (Reis & Brownstein, 2010). The Alan Guttmacher Institute (www.guttmacher.org) is a good resource for updated information about state policies.

Communication DIMENSIONS

Debating the Abortion Issue

Because of the intense emotions associated with abortion, as well as the moral and ethical implications, pro-choicers and pro-lifers tend to talk past one another. Often, this is because they are using different ethical principles as a basis for their beliefs. Many pro-life individuals use nonmaleficence (do no harm) as a guide that abortion should not be allowed at all. Pro-choice proponents often cite autonomy and liberty as the principles that factor most prominently and therefore allow women to make their own decisions. These different principles can be in conflict however. Approximately half (52%) of all U.S. adults believe abortion should be legal under certain, but not all, circumstances (Gallup, 2013).

The vocal minority—on both sides—attracts media attention and often takes extreme positions. For example, extreme pro-lifers emphasize late-term abortions, even though these abortions represent only approximately 1% of all abortions. Conversely, extreme pro-choicers oppose any restrictions on abortion through all three trimesters of pregnancy.

The result is a figurative—and too often a literal—shouting match rather than a conversation, and this form of communication can unfortunately lead to extreme actions. The National Abortion Federation reports that between 1977 and 2013, there were 6,849 attacks on abortion providers (NAF, n.d.).

Is this an effective way of communicating? Is this the way to resolve an ethical dilemma? How might groups such as clergy, citizens, or politicians work together to employ communication techniques that require listening as well as speaking?

TABLE 9.1

Parental Involvement in Minors' Abortions

State	Parental Involvement			Judicial Bypass				Exceptions	
	Consent Only	Notification and Consent	Notification Only	Available	Specific Criteria	"Clear and Convincing" Evidence	Other Adult Relatives	Medical Emergency	Abuse, Assault, Incest or Neglect
Alabama	X			X				X	
Alaska			X	X					X
Arizona	X*			X	X	X		X	X
Arkansas	X*			X	◆	◆		X	X
California	▶								
Colorado			X	X		X		X	X
Delaware‡			X†	X†			X‡	X‡	
Florida			X	X	X	X		X	
Georgia			X	X				X	
Idaho	X			X		X		X	X
Illinois			X	X			X	X	X
Indiana	X			X				X	
Iowa			X	X			X	X	X
Kansas	Both parents*			X	X	X		X	
Kentucky	X			X	X			X	
Louisiana	X*			X		X		X	
Maryland			X†						X†
Massachusetts	X			X				X	
Michigan	X			X				X	
Minnesota		Both parents		X				X	
Mississippi	Both parents			X		X		X	X
Missouri	X			X					
Montana	§		§						
Nebraska	X*			X		X		X	X

State									
Nevada	▶								
New Hampshire		X		X				X	X
New Jersey	▶			X					
New Mexico	▶								
North Carolina	X			X			X	X	X
North Dakota	Both parents			X		X		X	X
Ohio	X		X	X	X	X		X	
Oklahoma	X*		X	X	X	X		X	X
Pennsylvania	X			X		X		X	
Rhode Island	X			X		X		X	
South Carolina‡	X†		X‡	X‡		X‡	X‡	X‡	X‡
South Dakota		X		X		X		X	
Tennessee	X			X		X		X	X
Texas	X*		◆	X		◆	◆	X	X
Utah	X			XΩ		X		X	X§
Virginia	X*			X			X	X	X
West Virginia	X†			X*		X*		X	
Wisconsin	X†			X*		X*		X	X
Wyoming	X			X		X		X	
Total	**21**	**5**	**12**	**37**	**5**	**13**	**7**	**35**	**16**

Note: Except where indicated, policies require the involvement of one parent.

▶ Enforcement permanently enjoined by court order; policy not in effect.
§ Enforcement temporarily enjoined by court order; policy not in effect.
◆ New laws scheduled to take effect in early 2016.
* Requires parental consent documentation to be notarized.
† Allows specified health professionals to waive parental involvement in limited circumstances.
‡ The laws in Delaware applies to women younger than 16 and South Carolina's law to those younger than 17.
Ω The provision applies only to parental consent requirements.
ξ The provision applies only to the parental notice requirements.

Source: Reproduced from Guttmacher Institute, *Parental Involvement in Minors' Abortions, State Policies in Brief,* New York: Guttmacher, 2015, http://www.guttmacher.org/statecenter/spibs/spib_PIMA.pdf, accessed April 14, 2015.

TABLE 9.2

Abortion Counseling and Waiting Periods

States with Detailed Abortion-Specific Information Consent Requirements (29 states)

State	Length of Waiting Period (in hours)	In-Person Counseling Necessitates Two Trips to Clinic	Writing Materials Given or Offered	Woman Informed that Abortion Cannot Be Coerced	Description of Procedure		Fetal Development		Ability of a Fetus to Feel Pain	Personhood Begins at Conception
					Specific	All Common	Gestational Age of Fetus	Throughout Pregnancy		
Alabama	48		Given	V,W	V	W	V	W		
Alaska			Offered		V	W	V	W	W*	
Arizona	24	X	Offered	V,W	V	W	V	W		
Arkansas	48		Offered	V,W		W	V	W	V†,W	
Florida	24	X	Offered		V		V	W		
Georgia	24		Offered			W	V	W	W	
Idaho	24		Given	W	V	W	V	W		
Indiana	18	X	Given		V	W	V	W	V‡	V,W
Kansas	24		Given	W	V	W	V	W	V,W	W
Kentucky	24		Offered		V		V	W		
Louisiana	24	X	Given	W	V	W	V	W	V,W	
Massachusetts	▶									
Michigan	24		Given		V,W	W	V,W	W		
Minnesota	24		Offered			W	V	W	V‡,W	
Mississippi	24	X	Offered		V		V	W		
Missouri	72	X	Given	W	V	W	V	W	W†	W
Montana	▶									
Nebraska	24		Offered			W	V	W		
North Carolina	72		Offered	V	V	W	V	W		
North Dakota	24		Offered	W		W	V	W		V
Ohio	24	X	Given		V		V	W		
Oklahoma	24◆		Offered			W	V	W	V‡,W	◆

State	Hours		Materials							
Pennsylvania	24		Offered	W		V		W		W
South Carolina	24		Offered		V	V		W		W
South Dakota	72^Ω	X	Given	V		W	V	W*		W
Texas	24	X^ξ	Offered	W*	V	W*	V	W*		
Utah	72	X^Э	Given	W	V	W	V			V‡, W
Virginia	24		Offered		V	W	V			W
West Virginia	24		Offered	W*		W	V			W
Wisconsin	24	X	Offered	V,W		W	V			W
States with Customary Informed Consent Provisions (8 states)										
California						V				
Connecticut					V	V				
Delaware		▶				V				
Maine						V				
Nevada					V	V				
Rhode Island					V	V				
Tennessee^Ψ	48	X				V				
Total	**28**	**14**	**28**	**14**	**25**	**23**	**28**	**33**	**12**	**5**

All states waive mandatory waiting period requirements in a medical emergency or when the woman's life or health is threatened. In Utah, the counseling is waived if the pregnancy is the result of rape or incest or the patient is younger than 15. In Alabama, the counseling requirement is waived in cases of ectopic pregnancy or severe fetal impairment and in Georgia and Rhode Island it is waived in cases of medical emergency.

▶ Enforcement permanently enjoined by court order; policy not in effect.

§ Enforcement temporarily enjoined by court order; policy not in effect.

◆ New law scheduled to take effect later in 2015.

V = verbal counseling; W = written materials.

* Included in written counseling materials although not specifically mandated by state law.

† Information given only to women who are at 20 weeks of pregnancy or more; in Missouri the law applies at 22 weeks of pregnancy and in Utah a physician may waive the requirement if the abortion is because of rape, incest, life endangerment, a severe health problem or if the fetus has a lethal condition.

‡ In Indiana, the provision is not enforced against Planned Parenthood of Indiana due to a court case.

Ω The law prohibits the inclusion of weekends and annual state holidays as part of the waiting period.

Ψ Enforcement of a provision of the Tennessee law requiring that a woman be told that an abortion constitutes major surgery is enjoined.

ξ In person counseling is not required for women who live more than 100 miles from an abortion provider.

Э Counseling must be conducted "face-to-face" at "any location in the state."

Continues

TABLE 9.2

Abortion Counseling and Waiting Periods (Continued)

State	Inaccurate Information on Stopping Medication Abortion	Future Fertility — Accurately Portrays Risk	Future Fertility — Inaccurately Portrays Risk	Breast Cancer — Correctly Reports No Link	Breast Cancer — Inaccurately Asserts Possible Link	Mental Health — Correctly Reports Range of Emotional Responses	Mental Health — Describes Negative Emotional Responses	Counseling on Health Risks of Pregnancy
States with Detailed Abortion-Specific Informed Consent Requirements (29 states)								
Alabama						W†		W
Alaska		W†			W†	W		W
Arizona	§		W			W		V
Arkansas	W	W†				W		V,W
Florida								V
Georgia		W†				W		V,W
Idaho		V				W†		V,W†
Indiana		V,W		W				V
Kansas			W†		V,W		W	V,W
Kentucky								V
Louisiana		W†					W	V,W
Massachusetts								
Michigan		W					W	V,W
Minnesota		V,W†		V,W†		W		V,W
Mississippi		V,W		V	W†			V,W
Missouri		V				V,W		
Montana								
Nebraska		V,W†					W	V,W

State							
North Carolina	V					W	V
North Dakota	V					V	V
Ohio	V					V	V
Oklahoma	W†		W	W†			V,W
Pennsylvania	W†		W				V,W
South Carolina	W†		W				W
South Dakota	V	W†		W†		W†	V,W†
Texas	V	W	W		V	W†	V,W
Utah	W		V,W			V,W	V,W
Virginia	W			W		W	W
West Virginia	V		W			W	V,W
Wisconsin	V,W		V,W				V,W
States with Customary Informed Consent Provisions (8 states)							
California							
Connecticut							
Delaware							
Maine							V
Nevada			Φ				
Rhode Island							
Tennessee							V
Total	**21**	**4**	**13**	**5**	**1**	**9**	**29**

V = verbal counseling; W = written materials.

§ Enforcement temporarily enjoined by court order; policy not in effect.

◆ Policy scheduled to take effect later in 2015.

† Included in written counseling materials although not specified by state law.

‡ Law specifically requires the provider to inform in writing a woman seeking an abortion that depression and suicide ideation are risks of the abortion.

Φ Law requires discussion of emotional impact of abortion.

Who Has Abortions?

In 2011 (the latest data available at the time of this writing), an estimated 1.06 million abortions were performed in the United States, down from 1.31 million in 2000. The 2011 rate was the lowest rate since 1973. Overall, 21 abortion procedures occur for every 100 pregnancies (not including miscarriages) (Jones & Jerman, 2014). At current rates, each year approximately 1.7% of women ages 15–44 will have an abortion (Jones & Jerman, 2014). Also—and surprising to most people—half of them have had at least one previous abortion (Jones, Finer, & Singh, 2010). Based on these same rates, it is estimated that nearly 1 in 10 U.S. women will have an abortion by age 20, one-fourth by age 30, and nearly one-third by age 45 (Jones & Kooistra, 2011).

The Alan Guttmacher Institute monitors abortion laws and the characteristics of those having abortions. It reports that approximately half (51%) of all pregnancies of U.S. women are unplanned and that 40% of these are terminated by abortion (Finer & Zolna, 2014). What surprises some people is that of these women, 61% already have one or more children (Jones et al., 2010).

Fifty-one percent of abortions are performed in women younger than 25 years. One-third of abortions are performed in women aged 20 to 24 years, and teenagers have 18% of all abortions (Jones et al., 2010).

Of the women who have abortions, 30% are black, 36% are white, 25% are Hispanic, and 9% are other races. Income is another characteristic that varies greatly among women seeking abortion; 42% of women obtaining abortions in 2008 reported income levels that would classify them as poor, which is a significant increase from the 27% rate identified in 2000. In addition to this general increase, poor women have five times the abortion rate of women who are considered "better off" with incomes at 200% or more of the poverty level (Jones et al., 2010). One factor in the difference in abortion rates is the difference in unintended pregnancy rates among women of different incomes. The overall rate of unintended pregnancy in the United States has remained around 50%; however, the unintended pregnancy rate for poor women is more than five times that for women at the highest income level. Black and Hispanic women have higher unintended pregnancy rates compared to White women regardless of income level (Finer & Zolna, 2014).

Religion plays a role as well. Unintended pregnancy rates are highest among women who report no religious affiliation, but they are similar for women identifying as Catholic or Protestant. When comparing those who identify a religious affiliation, more unplanned pregnancies among Catholic women ended in abortion compared to women identifying other religious affiliations (Finer & Zolna, 2014).

Marital status is another variable associated with unintended pregnancy and abortion. While the proportion of unintended pregnancies among married women was less than half that of unmarried women, cohabiting women had the highest rate—almost four times that of non-cohabiting or married women (Finer & Zolna, 2014). Interestingly, the proportion of abortions occurring among cohabiting women has drastically declined—from 53% of unintended pregnancies resulting in abortion in 2001 to 39% in 2008 (Finer & Zolna, 2014).

There are three primary reasons women give for seeking an abortion (Guttmacher Institute, 2014). Three-fourths say that having a baby would interfere with their work, education, or other responsibilities. Approximately three-fourths say they cannot afford a child. Finally, half say they do not want to be a single parent or are having problems with their husband or partner. In addition, some abortions are performed for health-related reasons.

The Safety of Abortion

Abortion is an extremely safe procedure. With first-trimester procedures, fewer than 0.05% of abortion patients experience a major complication that would require hospitalization (Weitz et al., 2013). The primary risks are pelvic infection, hemorrhage, or unintended major surgery. For abortions performed during the first 8 weeks of pregnancy, 1 death occurs per 1 million abortions. The risk rises as the pregnancy progresses, rising to 1 death per 29,000 abortions during gestational weeks 16 to 20, and 1 death per 11,000 abortions after 20 weeks' gestation (Guttmacher Institute, 2014). In comparison, the risk of death associated with childbirth is 12 times greater than that associated with abortion (Grimes, 2006). Furthermore, there is no effect on subsequent pregnancies or births in women who have a first-trimester abortion procedure. There is also no connection between such procedures and breast cancer or any other form of cancer.

Although concerns have been raised about the psychological health of women as a result of experiencing an abortion, little evidence indicates that women are negatively affected. A 2009 review of existing studies found that the majority of adult women who terminate a pregnancy do not experience mental health problems and that there is no evidence to support the claim that mental health problems are caused by abortion (Major et al., 2009). A similar study on adolescents showed that abortion does not cause either depression or low self-esteem among young women in the short term or up to 5 years after the abortion (Warren, Harvey, & Henderson, 2010). Likewise, a rigorous research study in Denmark with more than 84,000 participants found no evidence of increased risk of mental disorders after a first-trimester abortion (Munk-Olsen et al., 2011). This study has been heralded as the most methodologically sound research study to date. Although collectively these studies show that most do not experience mental health issues, there is great variation among women, and it is important to remember that some women do experience issues after an abortion even if the abortion is not the sole factor for their distress (Major et al., 2009).

Availability of Legal Abortion

Although abortion is technically still legal, it is becoming increasingly difficult for a woman to have an abortion in the United States. The number of abortion providers has declined since the early 1980s; as of 2011, there were 1,720 abortion providers in the country. In addition, 89% of all U.S. counties lacked an abortion provider in 2011, with 38% of U.S. women living in those counties (Jones & Jerman, 2014). These data are not surprising considering that one study found 40% of medical schools do not offer formal education on abortion in the preclinical years, and 25% do not offer it for third-year students doing clinical rotations in obstetrics and gynecology (Espry

et al., 2005). In reality, gynecologists and obstetricians need to have the opportunity to receive this training. In one study, 97% of practicing gynecologists and obstetricians had encountered patients seeking abortions, but the same survey revealed that only 14% provided that service (Stulberg et al., 2011). Another study found that regardless of intention to provide abortion before residency, the availability of abortion training is positively correlated with providing abortions in the future practice of obstetricians and gynecologists (Steinauer et al., 2008).

Furthermore, most abortion clinics are harassed by pro-life advocates; in 2011, 84% of clinics experienced some type of harassment, with picketing being the most common (80%), followed by phone calls (47%) (Jerman & Jones, 2014). Instances of obstruction—defined as causing or attempting to cause a delay in the conduct of business or to prevent persons from entering or leaving an area—appear to be increasing (NAF, n.d.). In many cities, college students volunteer as escorts at local abortion clinics to assure that women can use the clinic without interference. Only 16 states have specific laws protecting abortion clinics (Guttmacher Institute, 2015b); see Table 9.3 for details.

More extreme forms of violence have also plagued abortion clinics and abortion providers. Between 1977 and 2013, there were 42 bombings, 181 arsons, 99 attempted bombings and arsons, and 661 bomb

A Worldwide Preference for Boys Around the world, on average, there are 105 boys born for every 100 girls born. Yet in some countries—such as India—there are many more boys born than girls; in India's case, 1,000 boys are born for every 914 girls (PBS NewsHour, 2013). Why does this happen? Because in most countries, boys are preferred over girls.

Throughout the world, especially in densely populated countries, there are many reasons that boy babies are preferred, most based on long-term gender bias. In India, boys perform the last rites at their parents' funerals; they carry the family name and also bring a dowry into the family when they marry (even though dowries have been illegal for more than 50 years). Daughters, in contrast, are often seen as a financial liability.

So the preference is for boy babies, but what is done to ensure that more boys will be born than girls? If

medical care is available, abortion based on sex selection is a common response. In India, it is illegal to abort a fetus based on sex, but few charges have been brought against those facilitating the procedure or those undergoing it. A new pregnancy blood test can determine the sex of the fetus as early as 7 weeks after conception. Some are concerned that this new test will increase abortions based on sex.

Looking at the practice of aborting female fetuses through the eyes of Western culture, experts have concluded that until gender equality is achieved around the world, these practices will be difficult to eradicate. Along with female genital mutilation, this practice may be culturally based. Some people believe that Western culture should refrain from interfering with the practices of other cultures. Others believe that in this case interference is warranted.

What do you believe?

TABLE 9.3

Protecting Access to Clinics

State	Specific Prohibited Actions					Protected "Bubble Zone"
	Obstruction	Threat	Damage	Telephone Harassment	Other	
California*	X	X	X		Online harassment	
Colorado						8-ft. zone within 100 ft. of door
Dist. of Columbia	X	X		X	Noise, Trespassing	
Kansas	X					
Maine	X			X	Noise, Odor	
Maryland	X					
Massachusetts	X	X				25 feet if ordered by police
Michigan		X				
Minnesota	X					
Montana	X					8-ft. zone within 36 ft. of door
Nevada	X					
New Hampshire						♦
New York	X	X	X			
North Carolina	X	X			Weapon	
Oregon	X		X			
Washington	X	X		X	Noise, Trespassing	
Wisconsin					Trespassing	
Total	**12 + DC**	**6 + DC**	**3**	**2 + DC**	**5 + DC**	**3**

* Requires the collection and analysis of data by state attorney general's office and training for law enforcement officers by experts on clinic violence.
♦ New law scheduled to take effect later in 2015.

Source: Reproduced from Guttmacher Institute, Protecting Access to Clinics, State Policies in Brief, New York: Guttmacher, 2015, http://www.guttmacher.org/statecenter/spibs/spib_PAC.pdf, accessed April 14, 2015.

threats directed at abortion providers (NAF, n.d.). Abortion providers have been murdered at the clinics where they worked in Florida and Massachusetts. In 2009, Dr. George Tiller was murdered while attending church services because he provided abortions. Table 9.4 summarizes the incidents of abortion-related violence over the past four decades.

In addition to the lack of providers and clinic violence, many states are attempting to restrict access through state laws and policies that make obtaining an abortion challenging, if not impossible. From 2010 to 2014, 231 new abortion restrictions were adopted across the country. Today, more than half of U.S. women (57%) live in a state that is considered either hostile or extremely hostile to abortion rights, with hostile states having four to five major restrictions and extremely hostile states having six to ten major restrictions related to abortion. These percentages are up from 31% of women living in a hostile

state and none living in an extremely hostile state in 2000 (Nash et al., 2015). Many of the abortion limitations instituted in hostile and extremely hostile states are considered superfluous from a medical standpoint; they include excessive and unnecessary regulations on abortion clinics, mandated counseling that is designed to discourage a woman from obtaining an abortion (see Table 9.2), a required waiting period, required parental involvement for minors seeking an abortion (see Table 9.1), and the prohibition of state Medicaid funds to pay for medically necessary abortions.

In addition to the restriction of state Medicaid funds, the cost of an abortion can affect access. In 2011–2012, the average cost of a medical abortion before 10 weeks' gestation was $504, and $480 for nonhospital surgical abortion at 10 weeks' gestation (Jerman & Jones, 2014). For poor or low-income women, public funds may not be available to assist

TABLE 9.4

Incidents of Violence and Disruption Against Abortion Providers in the United States and Canada

Violence	1977–1994	1995	1996	1997	1998	1999	2000	2001	2002	2003	2004	2005	2006	2007	2008	2009	2010	2011	2012	2013	Total
Murder[1]	5	0	0	0	2	0	0	0	0	0	0	0	0	0	0	1	0	0	0	0	8
Attempted Murder[1]	11	1	1	2	1	0	1	0	0	0	0	0	0	0	0	0	0	0	0	0	17
Bombing[1]	29	1	2	6	1	1	0	1	0	0	0	0	0	0	0	0	0	1	0	0	42
Arson[1]	124	14	3	8	4	8	2	2	1	3	2	2	0	2	0	0	0	1	5	0	181
Attempted Bomb/Arson[1]	64	1	4	2	5	1	3	2	0	0	1	6	4	2	1	1	1	1	0	0	99
Invasion	347	4	0	7	5	3	4	2	1	0	0	0	4	7	6	1	0	0	0	8	399
Vandalism	585	31	29	105	46	63	56	58	60	48	49	83	72	59	45	40	22	27	12	5	1,495
Trespassing	0	0	0	0	0	193	81	144	163	66	67	633	336	122	148	104	45	69	47	264	2,482
Butyric Acid Attacks	80	0	1	0	19	0	0	0	0	0	0	0	0	0	0	0	0	0	0	0	100
Anthrax Bioterrorism Threats	0	0	0	0	12	35	30	554	23	0	1	0	0	1	3	2	1	1	0	0	663
Assault & Battery	95	2	1	9	4	2	7	2	1	7	8	8	11	12	6	9	4	3	7	0	198
Death Threats	225	41	13	11	25	13	9	14	3	7	4	10	10	13	2	16	2	2	6	2	428
Kidnapping	2	0	0	0	1	0	0	0	0	0	0	0	1	0	0	0	0	0	0	0	4
Burglary	34	3	6	6	6	4	5	6	1	9	5	11	30	12	7	12	13	8	5	0	183
Stalking[2]	200	61	52	67	13	13	17	10	12	3	15	8	6	19	19	1	7	1	6	20	550
TOTAL	1,801	159	112	223	144	336	215	795	265	143	152	761	474	249	237	187	95	114	88	299	6,849

Continues

TABLE 9.4

Incidents of Violence and Disruption Against Abortion Providers in the United States and Canada (Continued)

Violence	1977–1994	1995	1996	1997	1998	1999	2000	2001	2002	2003	2004	2005	2006	2007	2008	2009	2010	2011	2012	2013	Total
Disruption																					
Hate Mail/ Harassing Calls	1,833	255	605	2,829	915	1,646	1,011	404	230	432	453	515	548	522	396	1,699	404	365	452	420	15,062
Email/Internet Harassment	0	0	0	0	0	0	0	0	24	70	51	77	25	38	44	16	44	17	41	88	535
Hoax Device/ Susp. Package	0	0	0	0	0	0	0	0	41	13	9	16	17	23	24	17	8	2	7	2	179
Bomb Threats	311	41	13	79	31	39	20	31	7	17	13	11	7	6	13	4	12	1	1	4	661
Picketing[4]	7,768	1,356	3,932	7,518	8,402	8,727	8,478	9,969	10,241	11,348	11,640	13,415	13,505	11,113	12,503	8,388	6,347	4,780	5,706	5,574	170,710
Obstruction[5]																			79	396	475
Total	9,912	1,652	4,550	10,426	9,348	10,412	9,509	10,404	10,543	11,880	12,166	14,034	14,102	11,702	12,980	10,124	6,815	5,165	6,286	6,484	188,494
Clinic Blockades																					
Number of Incidents	634	5	7	25	2	3	4	2	4	10	34	4	13	7	8	1	1	5	6	3	778
Number of Arrests[3]	33,661	54	65	29	16	5	0	0	0	0	0	0	0	3	1	0	0	0	4	1	33,839

All numbers represent incidents reported to or obtained by NAF. Actual incidents are likely much higher. Tabulation of trespassing began in 1999 and tabulation of email harassment and hoax devices began in 2002.

1. Incidents recorded are those classified as such by the appropriate law enforcement agency. Incidents that were ruled inconclusive or accidental are not included.

2. Stalking is defined as the persistent following, threatening, and harassing of an abortion provider, staff member, or patient away from the clinic. Tabulation of stalking incidents began in 1993.

3. The "number of arrests" represents the total number of arrests, not the total number of persons arrested. Many blockaders are arrested multiple times.

4. NAF changed its method for collecting this data in 2011.

5. Tabulation of Obstruction began in 2012. Obstruction is defined as the act of causing a delay or an attempt to cause a delau in the conduct of buisness or prevent persons from entering or exiting an area. This would apply to violations of the FACE Act.

Source: Reproduced from National Abortion Federation, *Incidents of violence and disruption against abortion providers in the United States and Canada*, n. d., http://prochoice.org/wp-content/uploads/Stats_Table2.pdf.

Did You Know . . .

On January 22, 2001, President George W. Bush reinstated the Global Gag Rule (also called the Mexico City Policy). This policy restricts foreign nongovernmental agencies that receive funds from the U.S. Agency for International Development from

- Providing legal abortions, except in the case of rape, incest, or endangerment of the woman's life
- Lobbying their governments to legalize abortion or to decriminalize abortion
- Providing advice or information regarding the availability of abortion and referring women to another clinic that offers abortion services
- Conducting educational campaigns regarding abortion

Consequently, healthcare organizations had to decide whether to give up needed funds for family planning and other reproductive services or to give up their rights of free speech and to provide their patients with complete and accurate medical information.

In 2009, President Barack Obama rescinded the Gag Rule. Depending on the results of 2016 election, the policy could be reinstated.

Do you think this rule is wise policy? If so, why? If not, why not?

---

them in paying these fees. The patchwork of state laws concerning public funding for abortion services is complex. As a result of the Hyde Amendment, the use of federal Medicaid funds for abortion is prohibited except in cases in which the woman's life is in danger. The amendment was expanded in 1993 to include situations in which the pregnancy resulted from rape or incest. Each state establishes its own abortion funding policy related to state revenues. In 2015, the Guttmacher Institute reported that 17 states funded abortion in their state medical assistance programs in all or most circumstances (Guttmacher Institute, 2015d), but several states restrict insurance coverage for abortion unless women pay an extra premium or the situation involves life endangerment for the woman (Guttmacher Institute, 2015c).

Attitudes About Abortion: Changing and Unchanging

This chapter has discussed the legal history of abortion and the current climate of legal abortion in the United States. But what do Americans really think about abortions? Since the Supreme Court's decision in *Roe v. Wade*, attitudes toward abortion have been evolving, and many studies have attempted to clarify Americans' attitudes. Many of the studies and polls are limited by study methods and sampling procedures, so it is important to consider survey results as general approximations and not exact percentages. This perspective is important because abortion beliefs greatly depending on how the question is asked—that is, whether it is perceived as dealing with access, women's rights, or self-labels.

The general trend since the mid-1990s, when the United States generally had a more pro-choice

Myth vs Fact

Myth: Most abortions are performed late in the pregnancy.
Fact: Almost 90% of all abortions are performed during the first trimester. These abortions are usually performed by vacuum aspiration, but an increasing number are medical abortions.

Myth: Abortion is a dangerous procedure.
Fact: The risk of death during childbirth is 12 times greater than it is during abortion procedures. Furthermore, fewer than 0.05% of first-trimester abortion patients experience a major complication.

Myth: Late-term abortions result in partial birth of the baby.
Fact: Opponents of abortion have labeled late-term abortion "partial-birth abortion." This is a political tactic rather than an accurate description of late-term abortions. The correct term for these abortions is dilation and extraction (D&X) or intact dilation and evacuation.

Myth: Adoptions must be coordinated through an adoption agency.
Fact: Adoptions can be arranged independently, although these adoptions require court approval. In addition, adoptions can be arranged with relatives, although, again, they require court approval.

Myth: The withholding of the names of the birth parents (confidentiality and anonymity) is guaranteed by agencies and courts that arrange adoptions.
Fact: There is a debate taking place in our society regarding the rights of the birth parents versus the rights of the child. Several states have passed or are considering legislation to unseal adoption records.

viewpoint on the issue, is toward an increase in the number of individuals who believe in restricting abortion in at least some way. A 2012 study specifically looking at abortion approval found that most individuals approve of abortion when the woman's health is in jeopardy (87%), when a woman has been raped (78.3%), or when the fetus has a serious defect (77.1%). Other situations did not garner the same levels of approval: 45% of respondents approved of abortion when the family is too poor to afford another child, 42.1% when a married woman does not want more children, 42.0% when an unmarried woman does not want to marry the father, and 38.5% when the woman wants an abortion for "any reason" (Smith & Son, 2013).

A 2013 national Gallup poll showed an almost equal division between individuals calling themselves pro-choice (45%) or pro-life (48%). When asked whether abortion should be legal, 26% of the respondents wanted abortion legal in all circumstances, and 20% wanted it illegal in all circumstances. The highest percentage indicated a middle-ground philosophy, with 52% of U.S. adults saying abortion should be legal under certain circumstances (Gallup, 2013).

A 2015 poll asked individuals to choose a pro-life or pro-choice label and 39% of respondents did not identify with either label exclusively: 21% said "neither" and 18% said "both." Interestingly, this survey also found that how questions were worded affected individuals' responses: When questions were framed as dealing with women's access to abortion versus as a legal discussion, individuals were more likely to support abortions by almost 10%. Additionally, 70% or more of respondents agreed that each of the following factors should be included in a woman's abortion experience—informed by medically accurate information, nonjudgmental, without pressure, comfortable, affordable, and without added burdens (Kliff, 2015).

As we consider the political spectacle and media coverage on abortion, it often appears to be an issue that polarizes the nation. In reality, people—as individuals—may be able to find agreement about what abortion should or should not be in the United States.

Adoption

Another response to an unwanted pregnancy is delivery of the baby followed by adoption placement. Women who are unwed and choose not to raise a baby or who do not have the financial resources necessary to raise a baby often select adoption as an alternative for providing a good life for their babies. In some cases, married women may also choose this option based on financial considerations or other life circumstances.

Types of Adoptions

There are two basic types of adoption. *Closed adoptions* are confidential; there is no contact between the birth parents and the adoptive parents. The identities of the birth parents and adoptive parents are

kept secret. *Open adoptions* allow contact between the birth parents and the adoptive parents. In fact, the birth parents may even select the adoptive parents. Contact can occur regularly or intermittently throughout the child's upbringing.

Although there have been some highly publicized cases of birth parents seeking to reverse them, adoptions are legally binding and irreversible after a limited period. Birth parents sign "relinquishment papers" after the baby is born, and, unless both birth parents have not signed these papers, the courts have refused to reverse adoptions.

Domestic adoptions (adoptions within the United States) can be facilitated through a state health and human services department, an agency licensed by the state, or an agency meeting certain state criteria. Adoptions can also be a nonagency placement; these types of adoptions are often called private or independent adoptions. These can include direct placement of a child in an adoptive family by the birth parents and adoptions facilitated by intermediaries, usually attorneys. Each state regulates adoption, so who can place a child for adoption and who may adopt a child vary from state to state (Child Welfare Information Gateway, 2012c).

Public agencies mainly handle the adoption of children in a state's foster care system; these children can range in age from infants to teens. In a licensed agency adoption, the birth parents relinquish their parental rights to the agency, and adoptive parents then work with the agency to adopt. These agencies are licensed by the state government and may offer a number of services. They provide counseling, handle legal matters, make hospital arrangements for the birth, select adoptive parents, and refer the mother

For many reasons individuals or couples may choose to adopt. International adoptions are among many options available.

to agencies if financial assistance is needed. Usually, though not always, adoptions arranged through agencies are open adoptions. Adoption agencies can be located through contacting most religious organizations; several national organizations can also be good resources, such as the National Council for Adoption (www.adoptioncouncil.org) and Independent Adoption Center (www.adoptionhelp.org).

In a private adoption facilitated by attorneys, families adopting independently identify the expectant parents (or pregnant woman) without an agency's help. Private adoptions are usually open adoptions, and attorneys who facilitate the adoptions must adhere to the standards of the American Bar Association. Some attorneys who specialize in adoption are members of the American Academy of Adoption Attorneys, a professional membership organization with standards of ethical practice. Not all states allow private adoptions (Child Welfare Information Gateway, 2012b), and the services offered by lawyers in private adoptions also vary by state (American Academy of Adoption Attorneys, 2015). It is recommended that prospective parents and birth parents have separate legal representation to ensure that no one is exploited. Because of negative outcomes and attempts by individuals to exploit either birth parents or adoptive parents, most states (41) have developed specific guidelines for what facilitators can and cannot do related to the adoption process and which types of fees they can claim; in fact, 17 of those states do not allow any use of facilitators (Child Welfare Information Gateway, 2012b). For those individuals in unregulated states, the use of adoptive services offered by facilitators can be risky, as there is no supervision or oversight of the process. Families who work with facilitators often have little recourse if the plan does not work out as they had hoped.

In an independent adoption, the adoptive parents typically agree to pay the medical costs associated with the pregnancy and may even agree to pay for the woman's living expenses during that time. However, fees and other payments during the adoption process are governed by state law; in some states, living expenses are not allowed.

Sometimes the birth parents want the child to stay in the family, in which case the baby may be adopted by relatives. Even so, these adoptions must follow the same process as applies to other adoptive parents to ensure that the relatives have the ability to provide care for the child. Once the adoption is approved, the birth parents have no more rights pertaining to the child than they would in any other form of adoption.

Regardless of the type of adoption process, almost all families must undergo a home study prior to a placement of an adopted child into the home. The main purpose of a home study is to ensure that a child is placed in a suitable home with a good match between the child and the family. Home studies also help to ensure that prospective homes comply with state and local laws for placement of adoptive children, and that parents and families are educated about adoption and have the information they need to make the best decisions for their families about adoption (Child Welfare Information Gateway, n.d.).

Contemplating Adoption

Adopting a child is a decision that requires a great deal of consideration, as does the decision to give a child up for adoption. While this option is often touted as alternative to abortion, few women in the United States opt to relinquish their child for adoption; in fact, only about 1% of infants born to unmarried women are relinquished for adoption during the first month of life (Centers for Disease Control and Prevention [CDC], 2015). Most women who have an unintended pregnancy choose—at least initially—to raise the child themselves.

If someone is considering adoption, it is important to be familiar with the particular state's adoption laws. States vary in how long after birth or signing relinquishment papers a birth parent can revoke this decision—a critical piece of information to know. In addition, anyone considering relinquishing their parental rights should ask these questions:

1. Can you accept your child living with someone else?

2. For the birth mother, will going through pregnancy and delivery change your mind? For the partner, will watching the birth mother go through a pregnancy and childbirth change your mind?

3. Are you willing to get good prenatal care?

4. Does adoption feel like what you *should* do, not what you *want* to do?

5. Will you be able to cope with any feelings of loss?

6. Will the child's father approve of adoption?

7. Is anyone pressuring you to choose adoption?

8. Are you confident your child will be treated well?

9. How will you handle any feelings of jealousy toward the adoptive parents?

10. Do you respect women who place their children for adoption?

11. How important are other people's opinions of your decision?

Gender DIMENSIONS

Baby "Richard"   In June 1990, Daniella Janikova and Otakar Kirchner, both immigrants from what is now Slovakia, conceived baby "Richard" (his name has been changed to protect his identity). However, before Richard's birth, Otakar returned to his country with a former girlfriend, leaving Daniella in the United States. Prior to the delivery, Daniella arranged to place Richard for adoption. Daniella was then introduced to the "Warburtons," a pseudonym for a family interested in adopting Daniella's baby. Daniella signed the necessary forms to arrange for the Warburtons to adopt Richard. However, under Illinois law, the father has to agree to an adoption. When Daniella was asked for the name and address of the father, she refused to give it, falsely stating that he had abused her. Richard was born on March 16, 1991.

A few days after Richard's birth, Otakar received a call informing him that Richard had died. One month later, however, he learned that the baby was alive, and soon he returned to Daniella. Otakar then hired an attorney, who started legal proceedings for the return of his child. Subsequently, he and Daniella were married.

The Warburtons contested the return of Richard, and a Cook County Circuit Court judge ruled the adoption valid, declaring Otakar unfit largely because he had not filed a petition within 30 days of the birth (as required in Illinois) and because the prior testimony of Daniella alleged that he was abusive. When this decision was appealed, the Illinois Supreme Court in June 1994—after Richard had been living with the Warburtons for more than 3 years—overturned the adoption, stating that Otakar was led to believe that Richard had died and therefore could not have been expected to pursue his parental rights in a timely fashion.

After several appeals to the U.S. Supreme Court proved unsuccessful, Otakar and Daniella took custody of Richard on April 30, 1995. At the time of the wrenching transfer Richard appealed to his adoptive mother, "I'll be good. Don't make me leave. I'll be good."

This case, tragic as it was for all parties, was decided on the rights of the father to agree to adoption of his biological offspring. In the mid-1990s, father's rights were often not protected. Because of this case and others, there is a stronger foundation and more awareness about the rights of biological fathers. Each state has different laws regarding the rights of biological fathers, and it is important for all involved in an adoption process to be aware of those rights to prevent heartbreaking stories like this one.

Someone contemplating placing a child for adoption may want to discuss these questions with a partner, clergy, professional counselor, or a trusted relative or friend.

Foster Care and Adoption

For parents who are not ready to decide between placing a child for adoption and parenting, many cities and counties provide temporary residences for their children. This arrangement is termed *foster care*. To arrange for this option, the birth parents must sign a legal foster care agreement that allows another family to care for the child. Often, foster care agreements specify the frequency of visits between the child and birth parents that will be allowed, the duration of stay with the foster care family, the amount of money the birth parents will have to provide the foster care parents for caring for their child, and the number and frequency of visits to a professional counselor (usually a social worker). Although foster care arrangements and regulations vary from state to state, if the foster care agreement is violated, the birth parents can lose the child permanently.

Foster care is also provided for children who are taken from their birth parents for abuse, neglect, or other behavior that precludes them from being able to raise their children and places their children at risk. Children placed in foster care permanently are eligible for adoption—in fact, that outcome is the goal of state agencies that supervise foster care arrangements.

The U.S. foster care system includes more than 402,000 children, of whom 25% are eligible for adoption (Administration on Children, Youth and Families, Children's Bureau, 2014). Fortunately, more and more of these children are being adopted. In 2013, 50,608 children in the foster care system were adopted. In 1997, the U.S. Congress passed the Adoption and Safe Families Act, designed to speed up adoption of children in the foster care system. That legislation provided bonuses of $4,000 to states for every child in the child protective system for whom they arranged adoption. For particularly difficult cases—such as older children or those with disabilities—states were provided $6,000 for each adoption. To further the goal of arranging for adoptions of children in foster care, AdoptUsKids (www.adoptuskids.org) was created in

Multicultural
DIMENSIONS

International Adoptions

Previously, many children from other countries were adopted by Americans. These adoptions may be the result of humanitarian concern of people who see children orphaned by war or widespread disease, or difficulty in locating the type of American child they wish to adopt. Given that only 1% of unmarried women in the United States relinquish their child in the first month of birth, the number of people who would like to adopt an infant and the number who can are not equivalent.

International adoptions can involve other challenges. Notably, they can be very costly. Some countries require one or more visits for parents to become eligible for adoption. Others require a short-term residency. There are also additional fees to be paid to the agencies involved.

In addition, there is controversy about how international adoptions are facilitated. In the past, there have been several examples of Americans adopting children from other countries and not being provided correct information—either knowingly by the adoption facilitators or perhaps unknowingly. For example, in 2010, a Tennessee woman placed a 7-year-old boy she had adopted from Russia alone on a one-way flight back to Moscow with a note saying he was violent and had severe psychological problems. The adoptive mother claimed that she was lied to about his mental state; Russian officials said that she had not been lied to and demanded that the U.S. government take action against the woman and considered blocking all future adoptions to the United States. In another situation, in 2011, a 6-year-old girl adopted from Guatemala by a U.S. couple was identified as a child kidnapped from her biological mother when she was 2 years old. The U.S. couple had no knowledge of the kidnapping, and the child entered the United States through a valid immigration process and presumably became a U.S. citizen at that time. A Guatemalan judge issued a court decision that the child should be returned to Guatemala and her biological family; this was the first time that the return of an adopted child by a country of origin has been ordered. However, in May 2012, the U.S. State Department stated that it did not have jurisdiction to help return the girl to Guatemala because the Hague Convention on the Protection of Children and Cooperation in Respect of Inter-Country Adoption (Hague Convention) had not been signed at the time of the adoption.

The Hague Convention went into effect in 2008 in the United States and provides more stringent regulation and supervision of international adoption. However, these restrictions apply only to other countries that have also adopted the Hague Convention. Many people adopt from countries that are not part of this agreement. Indeed, when considering children adopted internationally in 2014 by U.S. adults, two of the top five countries from which children were adopted were not part of the Hague Convention (Bureau of Consular Affairs, 2015).

Interestingly, there has been a decline in the number of international adoptions. Since the peak of 22,991 adoptions in 2004, the number of annual international adoptions has decreased significantly—by more than 70% in 2014 (6,441 adoptions). The reasons for this trend are complex and, for many countries, include an increased emphasis on domestic adoptions. The challenging examples presented earlier also have had an impact. For more than 10 years, Russia was one of the top five countries from which Americans adopted children. However, in 2014, only two children were adopted from Russia. In addition, many individuals want to help when natural disasters, such as the 2010 earthquake in Haiti, leave children without families. For both 2013 and 2014, Haiti was in the top five countries from which Americans adopted children. Over the period 2008–2012, the top five countries were China, Ethiopia (non-Hague Convention), Russia, South Korea (non-Hague Convention), and Ukraine.

The media also play a role in the perception of international adoptions. Most international adoptions are portrayed negatively in the media, although there are differences between countries (e.g., Russia often receives more negative media focus than China). Such perceptions also influence parents' adoption decisions (Jacobson, 2014).

Given that there are many older American children waiting to be adopted, should the federal government discourage international adoptions? If so, what will happen to children orphaned by war? To children abused or neglected in other countries? Should people who want to adopt children be supported wherever those children come from?

2002 by the U.S. Children's Bureau to raise public awareness about the need for foster and adoptive families and to assist states, territories, and tribes in their efforts to find families for children in foster care. In addition, most states maintain websites to facilitate adoption of children in the foster care system in their state and/or provide information to private agencies that maintain such websites.

Finding the Birth Parent

Because they are curious, want to have more complete knowledge of their origins, or have some other reason, many adults who were adopted seek to identify their birth parents. There is a good deal of disagreement as to whether and how this process should be facilitated. Some experts believe that contacting the birth parents might make them feel guilty about the adoption. Also, the birth parents might reject the adopted person, who might then have an unhealthy reaction to that rejection.

Before World War II, it was common practice for adoption records to be open. However, after the war, the combination of an increase in out-of-wedlock pregnancies and a conservative mood in the country resulted in adoption going "into the closet." Adoption records became sealed so that secrecy could be maintained. Since then, several states have passed legislation to open these records.

When an adoption is finalized, a new birth certificate for the child is usually issued to the adoptive parents. The original birth certificate is sealed and kept confidential by the state. In the past, nearly all states required adopted persons to obtain a court order to gain access to their original birth certificates, and as of 2012 that was still the case in 25 states and the District of Columbia. Other states have changed their laws to allow easier access. Some laws allow access to original birth certificates through the following means: a court order when all parties have consented; at the request of the adopted person when he or she becomes an adult; at the request of the adopted person unless the birth parent has filed an affidavit denying the release; when eligibility to receive identifying information has been established with a state adoption registry, or when consent forms from the birth parents to release identifying information are on file (Child Welfare Information Gateway, 2012a).

To facilitate access to records that require consent, many states (about 31 in 2012) offer a mutual consent registry. A mutual consent registry is a means for individuals directly involved in adoptions to indicate their willingness or unwillingness to have their identifying information disclosed. Procedures for mutual consent registries vary significantly from state to state, but most registries require consent of at least one birth parent and an adopted person older than the age of 18 or 21, or consent of the adoptive parents if the adopted person is a minor. Some states without established registries use alternative methods for disclosing identifying information. In some cases, search and consent procedures authorize an agency to assist an individual in locating birth family members to determine if they consent to the release of information. Other states use a system in which an individual—called a confidential intermediary—is certified by the court to access sealed adoption records with the intent of using that information to aid in the search for birth family members to obtain their consent for contact (Child Welfare Information Gateway, 2012a). The Child Welfare Information Gateway is a resource with updated information about each state's policies.

Exploring the Dimensions of Human Sexuality

Case Study

Pregnant women (ideally in consultation with their partners) have the burden of deciding which action to take regarding the pregnancy. Outsiders, however, often feel justified in criticizing the decision or in taking steps to limit their options. The issue of an unplanned pregnancy is complex from both an individual's perspective and a societal perspective.

Births resulting from unplanned pregnancies have an impact on society as a whole. Teens and women in their twenties who have an unplanned pregnancy are less likely to complete their education, have a lower income, and are unlikely to maintain the relationship with the child's father. Children born to women in their teens and twenties from unplanned births have lower academic success, are more likely to be teen parents themselves, and if male, are more likely to experience juvenile detention. In 2010, the impact of births to teens cost U.S. taxpayers $9.4 billion, with most of those costs related to negative consequences including increased costs for health care, foster care, incarceration, and lost tax revenues.

Rates of teen pregnancy are at an all-time low, but the overall percentage of pregnancies that are unplanned has remained stable, indicating that the mother's age for these pregnancies has shifted but they are still unplanned. As we—as a society—search for ways to decrease abortion, reducing the percentage of unplanned pregnancies through increased access to contraception, especially long-acting reversible contraceptive methods, and education about how to use methods correctly and consistently will prevent others from having to make this difficult decision.

Biological Factors

- A woman who experiences an unintended pregnancy and decides to relinquish the child to adoption or raise the child herself needs to seek prenatal care.
- Abortions earlier in a pregnancy are safer, less complex procedures.
- Waiting to make a decision may limit options because the fetus may be viable and abortion may no longer be an option in some states.
- Termination may be chosen because of health reasons related to the pregnant woman or the fetus.

Sociocultural Factors

- Attitudes toward unplanned pregnancies, abortion, and adoption are influenced religion, education, and culture.
- Cultural attitudes toward family also affect attitudes toward unplanned pregnancy.
- Laws restrict access to abortion, especially third-trimester procedures.
- Emphasis on a woman's place in society can affect perspectives on unplanned pregnancy.
- The role of men in deciding the outcome of an unplanned pregnancy varies.

Psychological Factors

- Women who experience an unintended pregnancy and decide to relinquish the child to adoption may struggle with this decision as they carry the pregnancy to term.
- The importance placed on different ethical principles—nonmaleficence (do no harm), beneficence (do good), and autonomy (the individual's right to choose)—can affect one's view of abortion.
- The effects on males regarding decisions about unplanned pregnancy are rarely discussed and acknowledged.
- The ability to actualize one's goals and dreams for the future can affect decisions regarding an unplanned pregnancy.

Summary

- Abortions can be spontaneous (miscarriages) or induced. Induced abortions can be performed by medical abortion, vacuum aspiration, manual vacuum aspiration, or dilation and evacuation.

- The U.S. Supreme Court legalized abortion in the *Roe v. Wade* ruling in 1973. Since then, several restrictions have been placed on abortions by the states and declared constitutional by the Supreme Court. In 2007, the Supreme Court upheld the constitutionality of the 2003 Partial-Birth Abortion Ban Act, which banned intact dilation and extraction for late-term abortions.

- Approximately half of all pregnancies are unplanned in the United States, and approximately 40% of these pregnancies are terminated by abortion.

- Fifty-one percent of abortions are performed in women younger than 25, one-third in women aged 20 to 24 years of age, and 18% in teenagers. Women who report no religious affiliation are more likely to obtain an abortion compared to other women, and cohabiting women are more likely than married women or non-cohabiting women to receive an abortion.

- Abortion is a safe procedure, with only 0.05% of abortion patients experiencing a major complication. Abortions are safest when performed during the first 8 weeks of pregnancy.

- Many Americans (52%) believe that abortions should be legal under certain circumstances, while 26% believe abortion ought to be legal under all circumstances and 20% believe it ought to be illegal under all circumstances.

- Adoptions can be closed—confidential with no contact between the birth parents and the adoptive parents—or open—allowing contact between birth parents and adoptive parents.

- Adoptions can be through an agency, including state departments of health and human services, which handle adoptions for children in the foster care system, or private agencies, in which case the parents release the baby to the adoption agency.

- Non-agency adoptions can also occur. These include direct placement of a child in an adoptive family by the birth parents and adoptions facilitated by intermediaries, usually attorneys.

- Although sealed in the past, adoption records have been opened in several states. Other states make records available if birth parents have not filed an objection.

Discussion Questions

1. What are the methods of abortion, and in which situations are they used?

2. Create a personal chart showing your own dimensions of human sexuality that relate to the abortion issue. After seeing all the issues involved, have you altered your position on abortion?

3. Explain the types of adoption available and the way each works.

Application Questions

Reread the chapter-opening story and answer the following questions.

1. The author Anna Quindlen appears to take a situational view of abortion: She thought abortion was acceptable for a bright college student but had second thoughts about an older and financially secure adult (herself). Does the situation matter? In which situations is it acceptable to get an abortion? In which situations is it unacceptable?

2. The chapter also mentions the possibility of adoption. Should Quindlen have counseled her freshman client by providing information about adoption? Explain why or why not.

Critical Thinking Questions

1. When the issue of abortion versus adoption is discussed, the father rarely enters into the discussion. Should the father have control over whether a woman can have an abortion or give a child up for adoption?

2. When do you believe that life begins? At conception? At a certain point in fetal development? At about 24 weeks, when the fetus can survive outside the womb (albeit with neonatal intensive care)? At about 35 weeks, when most babies can sustain life without medical intervention? Explain your answer.

3. Because many infertile couples want to adopt a child, why are there not more incentives for women to place children of unexpected pregnancies up for adoption? What could be done to motivate such a practice? Should the federal government be involved in such an effort?

Critical Thinking Case

In the late 1970s, Dr. Milfred Jefferson, an African American surgeon and chairperson of the national Right to Life organization, stated that abortion was genocide. She believed that a federally funded abortion program was aimed at eliminating the poor, African American population of the United States. Dr. Jefferson cited statistics showing that 30% of all abortions funded by Medicaid were performed on African Americans (while African Americans made up approximately 11% of the population). Said Dr. Jefferson, "Abortion is accomplishing what 200 years of slavery and 300 years of lynching didn't."

Opponents argued that the disproportionate number of Medicaid-funded abortions performed on African American women resulted from higher representation of African Americans among the poor in the United States; hence, they would have more need of financial support for abortions. Along these lines, people of lower socioeconomic status have less access to sex education, birth control information, and prescription birth control.

Abortion rates are still disproportionately high for African Americans. In 2008, the abortion rate for whites was 11.5 per 1,000 live births, the abortion rate for Hispanics was 28.7 per 1,000 live

births, and the abortion rate for African Americans was 40.2 per 1,000 live births—almost four times the rate for whites (Jones & Kavanaugh, 2011).

What are your thoughts about these different rates? What other factors could be involved?

Exploring Personal Dimensions

What are your feelings about abortion? Place an A, B, C, D, or E in the blank to the left of each of the following items, using the provided scale:

A. I *strongly agree* with the statement.

B. I *tend to agree* with the statement (some reservation).

C. I am *undecided* (uncertain about my feelings or have no feelings one way or the other).

D. I *tend to disagree* with the statement (some reservation).

E. I *strongly disagree* with the statement.

_____ 1. Abortion penalizes the unborn [child] for the mother's mistake.

_____ 2. Abortion places human life at a very low point on a scale of values.

_____ 3. A woman's desire to have an abortion should be considered sufficient reason to do so.

_____ 4. I approve of the legalization of abortion so that a woman can obtain one with proper medical attention.

_____ 5. Abortion ought to be prohibited because it is an unnatural act.

_____ 6. Having an abortion is not something to be ashamed of.

_____ 7. Abortion is a threat to our society.

_____ 8. Abortion is the destruction of one life to serve the convenience of another.

_____ 9. A woman should have no regrets if she eliminates the burden of an unwanted child with an abortion.

_____10. The unborn [child] should be legally protected against abortion because it cannot protect itself.

_____11. Abortion should be an alternative when there is contraceptive failure.

_____12. Abortions should be allowed because the unborn [child] is only a potential human being, not an actual human being.

_____13. Any person who has an abortion is probably selfish and unconcerned about others.

_____14. Abortion should be available as a method of improving community socioeconomic conditions.

_____15. Many more people would favor abortion if they knew more about it.

_____16. A woman should have an illegitimate child rather than an abortion.

_____17. Liberalization of abortion laws should be viewed positively.

_____18. Abortion should be illegal, because the Fourteenth Amendment in the Constitution holds that no state shall "deprive any person of life, liberty, or property without due process of law."

_____19. The unborn [child] should never be aborted no matter how detrimental the possible effects on the family.

_____20. The social evils involved in forcing a pregnant woman to have a child are worse than any evils in destroying the unborn child.

_____21. Decency forbids having an abortion.

_____22. A pregnancy that is not wanted and not planned for should not be considered a pregnancy, but merely a condition for which there is a medical cure, abortion.

_____23. Abortion is the equivalent of murder.

_____24. Easily accessible abortions will probably cause people to become unconcerned and careless with their contraceptive practices.

_____25. Abortion ought to be considered a legitimate health measure.

_____26. The unborn child ought to have the same rights as the potential mother.

_____27. Any outlawing of abortion is oppressive to women.

_____28. Abortion should be accepted as a method of population control.

_____29. Abortion violates the fundamental right to life.

_____30. If a woman feels that a child might ruin her life, she should have an abortion.

To score this instrument, use the following point values for items 3, 4, 6, 9, 11, 12, 14, 15, 17, 20, 22, 25, 27, 28, and 30 only: A = 5, B = 4, C = 3, D = 2, E = 1.

For items 1, 2, 5, 7, 8, 10, 13, 16, 18, 19, 21, 23, 24, 26, and 29, use the following scale: A = 1, B = 2, C = 3, D = 4, E = 5.

Now add your points; the score should fall between 30 and 150. A score of 30 represents an unfavorable attitude, a score of 90 represents a neutral attitude, and a score of 150 represents a favorable attitude toward abortion.

Source: Reproduced from Snegroff, S. _Manual and guide for the abortion attitude scale and knowledge inventory._ Saluda, NC: Family Life Publications, 1978.

Suggested Readings

Brabender, V. M., & Fallon, A. E. _Working with adoptive parents: Research, theory and therapeutic interventions._ Hoboken, NJ: John Wiley & Sons, 2013

Cohen, D. S., & Connon, K. _Living in the crosshairs: The untold stories of anti-abortion terrorism._ New York: Oxford University Press, 2015.

Seek, A. _God and jetfire: Confessions of a birth mother._ New York: Farrar, Straus & Giroux, 2015.

Seligmann, L. _Broken links, enduring ties: American adoption across race, class and nation._ Stanford, CA: Stanford University Press, 2013.

Ziegler, M. _After Roe: The lost history of the abortion debate._ Cambridge, MA: Harvard University Press, 2015.

Web Resources

Alan Guttmacher Institute
www.guttmacher.org

The Alan Guttmacher Institute is a nonprofit organization focused on sexual and reproductive health research, policy analysis, and public education. Its website contains links to the Guttmacher Institute publications: *Perspectives on Sexual and Reproductive Health, International Family Planning Perspectives, The Guttmacher Report on Public Policy*, and special reports on topics pertaining to sexual and reproductive health and rights. The Guttmacher Institute's mission is to protect the reproductive choices of women and men in the United States and throughout the world. It supports individuals' ability to obtain the information and services needed to achieve their full human rights, safeguard their health, and exercise their individual responsibilities in regard to sexual behavior and relationships, reproduction, and family formation.

National Abortion and Reproductive Rights Action League
www.naral.org

NARAL is committed to protecting the right to choose abortion and electing candidates who will promote policies to prevent unintended pregnancy. The latest laws and political issues pertaining to a woman's right to choose abortion are available on the NARAL website, as well as information on related issues such as emergency contraception.

Child Welfare Information Gateway
www.childwelfare.gov

Child Welfare Information Gateway connects child welfare and related professionals to comprehensive information and resources to help protect children and strengthen families. Its website includes updated information on a variety of topics, including establishing permanent homes for children, child abuse and neglect, foster care, and adoption.

National Adoption Center
www.adopt.org

Devoted to increasing the number of children adopted, the National Adoption Center works to expand adoption opportunities for children living in foster care throughout the United States and is a resource to families and to agencies who seek the permanency of caring homes for children. Included on the website are information on how to adopt, resources and matching programs for prospective parents and adoption agencies, and photo listings of children waiting to be adopted.

References

Administration on Children, Youth and Families, Children's Bureau. *The AFCARS report, preliminary FY 2013 estimates*, 2014. Available: http://www.acf.hhs.gov/sites/default/files/cb/afcarsreport21.pdf.

American Academy of Adoption Attorneys. *Adopting parents*, 2015. Available: http://www.adoptionattorneys.org/aaaa/adopting-parents/adopting-parents.

Blum, J., Raghavan, S., Dabash, R., Chelli, H., Hajri, S., Conkling, K., & Winikoff, B. Comparison of misoprostol-only and combined mifepristone–misoprostol regimens for home-based early medical abortion in Tunisia and Vietnam. *International Journal of Gynecology & Obstetrics, 118* (2012), 166–171.

Bureau of Consular Affairs. *FY 2014 annual report on intercountry adoption*, 2015. Available: http://travel.state.gov/content/dam/aa/pdfs/fy2014_annual_report.pdf.

Bryant, A. G., Regan, E., & Stuart, G. An overview of medical abortion for clinical practice. *Obstetrical & Gynecological Survey, 69* (2014), 39–45.

Cameron, S. Glasier, A., Dewart, H., & Johnstone, A. Women's experiences of the final state of early medical abortion at home: results of a pilot survey. *Journal of Family Planning and Reproductive Health Care, 36* (2010), 213–216.

Centers for Disease Control and Prevention (CDC). *Fast stats: Adoption*, 2015. Available: http://www.cdc.gov/nchs/fastats/adoption.htm.

Child Welfare Information Gateway. *Access to adoption records*, 2012a. Available: https://www.childwelfare.gov/pubPDFs/infoaccessap.pdf#page=5&view=Original Birth Certificate.

Child Welfare Information Gateway. *Use of advertising and facilitators in adoptive placements*, 2012b. Available: http://www.childwelfare.gov/pubPDFs/advertising.pdf.

Child Welfare Information Gateway. *Who may adopt, be adopted, or place a child for adoption?*, 2012c. Available: https://www.childwelfare.gov/pubPDFs/parties.pdf#page=1&view=Introduction.

Child Welfare Information Gateway. *Home study*, n.d. Available: https://www.childwelfare.gov/topics/adoption/adoptive/home-study/.

Espey, E., Ogburn, T., Chavez, A., Qualls, C., & Leyba, M. Abortion education in medical schools: A national survey. *American Journal of Obstetrics and Gynecology, 192* (2005), 640–643.

Finer, L. B., & Zolna, M. R. Shifts in intended and unintended pregnancies in the United States, 2001–2008. *American Journal of Public Health, 23* (2014), e1–e9.

Gallup, Inc. *Americans' abortion views steady amid Gosnell trial,* 2013. Available: http://www.gallup.com/poll/162374 /americans-abortion-views-steady-amid-gosnell-trial.aspx.

Grimes, D. A. Estimation of pregnancy-related mortality risk by pregnancy outcome, United States 1991 to 1999. *American Journal of Obstetrics and Gynecology, 184* (2006), 92–94.

Guttmacher Institute. *Induced abortion in the United States,* 2014. Available: http://www.guttmacher.org/pubs /fb_induced_abortion.html.

Guttmacher Institute. *Bans on "partial-birth" abortion,* 2015a. Available: http://www.guttmacher.org/statecenter/spibs /spib_BPBA.pdf.

Guttmacher Institute. *Protecting access to clinics,* 2015b. Available: http://www.guttmacher.org/statecenter/spibs /spib_PAC.pdf.

Guttmacher Institute. *Restricting insurance coverage of abortion,* 2015c. Available: http://www.guttmacher.org/statecenter /spibs/spib_RICA.pdf.

Guttmacher Institute. *State funding of abortion under Medicaid,* 2015d. Available: http://www.guttmacher.org/statecenter /spibs/spib_SFAM.pdf.

Jacobson, H. (2014). Framing adoption the media and parental decision making. *Journal of Family Issues, 35* (5), 654–676.

Jerman, J., & Jones, R. K. Secondary measures of access to abortion services in the US, 2011–2012: Gestational age limits, cost, and harassment, *Women's Health Issues, 24* (2014), e419–e424.

Jones, R. K., Finer, L. B., & Singh, S. (2010). *Characteristics of U.S. abortion patients,* 2008. Available: http://www .guttmacher.org/pubs/US-Abortion-Patients.pdf.

Jones, R. K., & Jerman, J. Abortion incidence and service availability in the United States, 2011. *Perspectives on Sexual and Reproductive Health, 46* (2014), 3–14.

Jones, R. K., & Kavanaugh, M. L. Changes in abortion rates between 2000 and 2008 and lifetime incidence of abortion. *Obstetrics and Gynecology, 117* (2011), 1358–1366.

Jones, R. K., & Kooistra, K. Abortion incidence and access to services in the United States, 2008. *Perspectives on Sexual and Reproductive Health, 43* (2011), 41–50.

Kliff, S. *What Americans think of abortion: It's not so black and white,* 2015. Available: http://www.vox.com/a/abortion- decision-statistics-opinions.

MacDonald, K., Norman, W. V., & Popescu, O. New anomalies due to methotrexate and misoprostol exposure in early pregnancy. *International Journal of Gynecology & Obstetrics, 122* (2013), 267–268.

Major, B., Appelbaum, M., Beckman, L., Dutton, M. A., Russo, N. F., & West, C. Abortion and mental health: Evaluating the evidence. *American Psychologist, 64* (2009), 863–890.

Munk-Olsen, T., Laursen, T. M., Pedersen, C. B., Lidegaard, O., & Motensen, P. B. Induced first-trimester abortion and risk of mental disorder. *New England Journal of Medicine, 364* (2011), 332–339.

NARAL. Roe v. Wade *and the right to choose,* 2015. Available: http://prochoiceamerica.org/media/fact-sheets/government- federal-courts-scotus-roe.pdf.

Nash, E., Gold, R. B., Rathbun, G., & Vierboom, Y. *Laws affecting reproductive health and rights: 2014 state policy review,* 2015. Available: http://www.guttmacher.org /statecenter/updates/2014/statetrends42014.html.

National Abortion Federation (NAF). *Educational resources,* 2014. Available: http://prochoice.org/health-care-professionals /educational-resources/.

National Abortion Federation (NAF). *NAF protocol for mifepristone/misoprostol in early abortion in the U.S.*, 2013. Available: http://prochoice.org/wp-content/uploads/Mifeprotocol2013.pdf.

National Abortion Federation (NAF). *NAF violence and disruption statistics*, n.d. Available: http://prochoice.org/wp-content/uploads/Stats_Table2.pdf.

Ngoc, N. T., Blum, J., Raghavan, S., Nga, N. T., Dabash, R., Diop, A., & Winikoff, B. Comparing two early medical abortion regimens: mifepristone+misoprostol vs. misoprostol alone. *Contraception, 83*, 5 (2011), 410–417.

PBS NewsHour. *Pervasive preference for baby boys over girls prevails among parents in India*, 2013. Available: http://travel.state.gov/content/adoptionsabroad/en/about-us/statistics.html,

Quindlen, A. *Thinking out loud*. New York: Random House, 1988.

Reis, B. Y., & Brownstein, J. S. Measuring the impact of health policies using Internet search patterns: The case of abortion. *BMC Public Health, 10* (2010), 514.

Rodriguez, M. I., Seuc, A., Kapp, N., et al. Acceptability of misoprostol only medical termination of pregnancy compared with vacuum aspiration: An international, multicentre trial. *BJOG: An International Journal of Obstetrics & Gynaecology, 119* (2012), 817–823.

Smith, T. W., & Son, J. *General social survey 2012 final report: Trends in public attitudes towards abortion*, 2013. Available: http://www.norc.org/PDFs/GSS%20Reports/Trends%20in%20Attitudes%20About%20Abortion_Final.pdf,

Steinauer, J., Landy, U., Filippone, H., et al. Predictors of abortion provision among practicing obstetrician-gynecologists: A national survey. *American Journal of Obstetrics and Gynecology, 198* (2008), 39.

Stulberg, D. B., Dude, A. M., Dahlquist, I., & Curlin, F. A. Abortion provision among practicing obstetrician–gynecologists. *Obstetrics and Gynecology, 118* (2011), 609.

Suhonena, S., Tikkaa, M., Kivinena, S., & Kauppilab, T. Pain during medical abortion: Predicting factors from gynecologic history and medical staff evaluation of severity. *Contraception, 83* (2011), 357–361.

Warren, J. T., Harvey, S. M., & Henderson, J. T. Do depression and low self-esteem follow abortion among adolescents? Evidence from a national survey. *Perspectives on Sexual and Reproductive Health, 42* (2010), 230–235.

Weitz, T. A., Taylor, D., Desai, S., Upadhyay, U. D., Waldman, J., Battistelli, M. F., & Drey, E. A. Safety of aspiration abortion performed by nurse practitioners, certified nurse midwives, and physician assistants under a California legal waiver. *American Journal of Public Health, 103* (2013), 454–461.

CHAPTER 10

Gender Dimensions

© Gayvoronskaya Yana/Shutterstock

FEATURES

 Multicultural Dimensions
Examples of Gender Equity Promoting Programs

 Communication Dimensions
Men Are from Mars; Women Are from Venus

 Gender Dimensions
Terminology Related to Gender

 Global Dimensions
The Oppression of Women

 Multicultural Dimensions
International Gender Equality Comparisons

 Gender Dimensions
Gender Equality on the College Campus

 Ethical Dimensions
Extreme Gender Roles—The Price of Honor

 Ethical Dimensions
Should Dad Dress as a Woman?

 Multicultural Dimensions
Has the Women's Movement in France Caught Up?

 Gender Dimensions
Is There Gender Equality in College Sports?

CHAPTER OBJECTIVES

1 Describe the biological, psychological, and sociocultural differences between males and females.

2 Explain the effects of gender identity, gender roles, and gender stereotypes on sexuality.

3 Analyze how the women's movement has affected both females and males.

INTRODUCTION

When Mark attended college, he thought all the talk about gender differences was bunk. Men and women appeared to share equal places in classrooms and in faculty positions. Women appeared to have the same opportunities as men in the outside work world. He and his classmates believed that the wage gap and glass ceiling were things that past generations dealt with. Those were the days.

But Mark still remembers one college guest speaker—a distinguished American composer. During his speech, the aging composer asserted that women were not good composers because their social upbringing left them devoid of technical skills. He told the stunned audience—among whom sat several prominent female composers—that boys take things apart and put things together, while girls play with dolls. Therefore, boys grow up with more technical abilities, which to him included the ability to orchestrate music. It seemed that everyone in attendance wrote off his comments as those of an elderly man from another era.

But as Mark joined the workforce, married, and had children, he began to witness more and more gender differences and biases. As the years passed by, the number of female friends who had experienced sexism in the workplace grew from none to all of them. It became clear that women and men did communicate differently, manage differently, work differently, play differently.

In Mark's marriage, gender roles have been reversed—because of work situations, not a deliberate decision. While his spouse works a managerial "nine-to-five job" (read, 7:00 A.M. to 6:00 P.M.), Mark writes and edits out of his home. He is responsible for raising two young children and for doing most household jobs. Because children cannot be ignored, he often has to put off work until they are in bed.

Mark has become keenly aware of the gender differences among parents. At his son's independent school, where most students' mothers do not have a job, he is one of the few fathers who take the child to school, go to parent–teacher conferences, and volunteer for various events. This creates quite a dilemma in friendships: While playing both the mother and father roles, he really does not fit into either group. Mark also notes that teachers react differently to him: When several mothers voiced a complaint to a teacher, the teacher spoke to them directly; however, the teacher would only communicate with Mark in the presence of a senior administrator.

Suprisingly, gender biases exist even among medical professionals. At his son's first pediatric appointment, the male doctor's first question was a stern "Where is the child's mother?" Some years later, during a hospital emergency room visit, the doctors and nurses clearly listened to every small comment his spouse made—yet brushed off Mark's input as insignificant.

As Mark's experience shows, gender plays a role in many aspects of our lives—at home, at work, and in our social activities. We develop a sexual identity, which is the outgrowth of the interaction of biology— being male or female—and social learning. Society's expectations for the behavior of men and women are conveyed to the individual by a process called socialization, which has a dominant influence on gender roles. As children model adults' behaviors, these gender roles are perpetuated, although traditional gender roles are changing as a broader range of behaviors is accepted by society.

If someone asked you whether you were a woman or a man, your first thought would probably be, What a ridiculous question! You know what gender I am. Still, that question might lead you to ask other questions about gender, such as, How did I learn to act as a man or woman? To what extent is my masculinity or femininity natural, and to what extent is it learned? Are my personal characteristics determined or influenced by my gender? In this chapter we explore some of the forces that influence our conceptions of gender, including **masculinity** *and* **femininity**.

▪ Gender Differences

When gender differences and similarities are considered, discussions often center on "nature versus nurture." Those who argue from a nature perspective attribute most characteristics to biological differences or similarities. Those who argue more for nurture believe that we become the way we are mostly as a result of social factors and learning. There are persuasive arguments on each side, and some people believe that a combination of nature and nurture makes us the way we are.

People learn attitudes and values and have their personal experiences in a "gendered world." Gender issues are dealt with differently in different societies. For example, there may be more or less gendered examples in spheres such as occupational roles, child care, clothing styles, and some social and recreational activities.

In this chapter, we discuss some gender differences related to attitude and behavior. Caution is needed when considering such differences, however, because many variations in these attitudes and behaviors exist. Overgeneralization can result in inappropriate stereotypes. At the same time, however, many argue that different genders have their own important characteristics.

Developmental Differences

There is no question that males and females differ biologically in more than their physical structure and biological function. Developmentally, girls are more advanced than boys at birth—that is, their central nervous system is more mature. Boys tend to weigh more when born, but girls have fewer physical defects and a higher survival rate. More male children are conceived, but the miscarriage rate for males is greater than for females, and more males die in the first 12 months of life. The female's two X chromosomes, compared with the XY chromosomes of the male, may be a biological advantage. The X chromosomes are larger than Ys and can supply the female with a greater variety of genetic material. Even if one of the female's X chromosomes is a carrier of genetic defects, the second one can have normal genes that offset any genetic defect.

In infancy and early childhood, growth in boys and girls is similar. The development of language, the growth of body organs and the nervous system, and perceptual and motor development proceed in sequence. The female is more developed prenatally, but the male develops more rapidly postnatally. Until age 8 years the male is heavier and taller than the female, but he reaches puberty more slowly. The onset of puberty occurs approximately 2 years earlier in the female. In the preadolescent period the female, having greater physical maturity, can perform physical and athletic tasks better than the male. With menarche, estrogen influences the increase of **adipose** (fat) tissues and enlargement of the female pelvis. Eventually the estrogen prevents growth in the skeletal long bones, and height stabilizes for girls at about age 17 years.

When the male reaches puberty, androgen increases his muscle mass and skeletal development, and thus the adolescent boy has more body mass but less fat than the girl. This androgenic effect on male development gives him more strength and more speed. Furthermore, the male's greater lung and heart

According to one study, men and women also differ in their reaction to holiday shopping. All 36 male subjects showed a dramatic increase in blood pressure when confronted with crowds and lines. But one in four females showed increased blood pressure. What physiological, psychological, and social factors would cause such a result?

capacity and greater capacity for oxygen transport to tissues, combined with his predisposition toward being taller and heavier than the female, give him more power.

Many researchers have studied the brains of males and females. Although most researchers agree that men's brains are about 10% bigger than women's, women's brains seem to have more connections between the two brain hemispheres. In some regions, the female brain is more densely packed with neurons. Women tend to use more parts of their brain to accomplish certain tasks. This might help explain why they often recover better from a stroke, because the healthy parts of the brain may more easily compensate for the injured regions. Even though men and women have different brain architectures, we really don't know yet what that might mean (Ripley, 2005).

Gender and Abilities

There are various opinions about similarities and differences in abilities between males and females. Although it is always possible to find someone who disagrees, most experts agree that until about

masculinity Those qualities characteristic of and suitable for boys and men according to the rules and expectations of a society.

femininity Those qualities characteristic of and suitable for girls and women according to the rules and expectations of a society.

adipose Pertaining to fat tissue in the body.

age 11 or 12 males and females have similar verbal abilities. Around age 11 or 12, females have greater abilities in language and verbal tasks, but males perform better on visual–spatial tasks. This difference seems to persist into adulthood (see Figure 10.1). In addition, girls seem to speak sooner than boys. On average, women show more verbal skills than men.

(a) Problem-Solving Tasks Favoring Women

Women tend to perform better than men on tests of perceptual speed, in which subjects must rapidly identify matching items—for example, pairing the house on the far left with its twin:

In addition, women remember whether an object, or a series of objects, has been displaced:

On some tests of ideational fluency, such as those in which subjects must list objects that are the same color, and on tests of verbal fluency, in which participants must list words that begin with the same letter, women also outperform men:

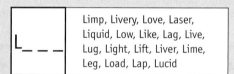

Women do better on precision manual tasks—that is, those involving fine-motor coordination—such as placing the pegs in holes on a board:

And women do better than men on mathematical calculation tests:

| 77 | $14 \times 3 - 17 + 52$ |
| 43 | $2(15 + 3) + 12 - \frac{15}{3}$ |

(b) Problem-Solving Tasks Favoring Men

Men tend to perform better than women on certain spatial tasks. They do well on tests that involve mentally rotating an object or manipulating it in some fashion, such as imagining turning this three-dimensional object:

or determining where the holes punched in a folded piece of paper will fall when the paper is unfolded:

Men also are more accurate than women in target-directed motor skills, such as guiding or intercepting projectiles:

They also do better on disembedding tests, in which they have to find a simple shape, such as the one on the left, once it is hidden within a more complex figure:

And men tend to do better than women on tests of mathematical reasoning:

| 1,100 | If only 60% of seedlings will survive, how many must be planted to obtain 660 trees? |

FIGURE **10.1** Problem-solving tasks for women and men. Research suggests that some problem-solving tasks may demonstrate gender-related performance differentiation.
Source: © Jared Schneidman

Whether boys have better mathematical abilities than girls is still debated. Historically, math was seen as a masculine area of study in which girls were not expected or encouraged to excel. Because many females were raised thinking they should not succeed in math, their performance on math measures tended not to be high. Several decades ago, however, females' perceptions of their ability to do well in math showed signs of change.

Interestingly, math scores on national tests for fourth-graders have been improving for both genders, with no statistically significant differences between boys and girls. However, girls score about 7% lower than boys on the math part of the SAT. It has been suggested that one reason for this might be that more girls than boys from lower-income families take the test.

Looking at a different type of ability, Horgan et al. (2004) found that women more accurately recalled information concerning the appearance of other people, such as physical features, clothing, and postures. Both men and women did better at remembering the appearance of women than remembering how men looked.

Does this mean that biology is destiny when it comes to these abilities? No, because even though each gender seems to have specific abilities, there are also cultural explanations for these differences. These include teachers' assumptions and their treatment of students, parents' attitudes toward their children, the perception of society that math has been for males, each gender's self-perception and ambitions, and social pressures on adolescents—just to name some possibilities.

Gender and Aggression

Some experts believe that boys are more physically and verbally aggressive than girls, beginning at preschool age. Given that this seems to be true in many cultures, there may be some biological basis for this difference. Males probably remain more aggressive into their college years, but as they mature the trait diminishes. There is some evidence that boys are punished more than girls for aggression.

Intimate-partner violence continues to be a major problem in the United States. Many forms of violence have decreased in recent years, but intimate-partner violence has increased. While traditionally it was thought to be only a male-to-female activity because usually males are bigger and stronger than females, acts of violence against both women and men have increased within intimate relationships.

Tavris (2002) provided an interesting view related to female aggression. She pointed out that many authors have written about hidden and formerly

Boys seem to be more aggressive than most girls.

secret female aggressiveness. She said that girls are not sweeter than boys, but just as bad, sexual, and aggressive—maybe even meaner, given the ruthless and sneaky ways they control one another. For example, our culture refuses girls access to open conflict, and it forces their aggression into nonphysical, indirect, and covert forms. Girls use backbiting, exclusion, rumors, name calling, and manipulation to inflict psychological pain on targeted victims. Boys, in short, resort to physical aggression; girls, to "relational" aggression.

Orpinas et al. (2014) shed additional light on this issue. They followed 620 randomly selected sixth graders for 6 years and had the students complete yearly surveys. They found that boys were more likely to engage in relationally aggressive behaviors (malicious rumors, social exclusion, and refection, for example) compared to girls. It had long been believed that girls were the ones more likely to engage in these types of behaviors. The boys were also more physically aggressive than the girls.

Anger and aggression are learned behaviors and are characteristic of humans. Traditionally they have been viewed as more appropriate for males than for females. However, as we move toward humanism and less-defined parameters of what is male and what is female, we must reevaluate our cultural acceptance of these behaviors.

Gender and Health

While there is not unanimous agreement on this point, there seem to be differences in males' and females' health attitudes and behavior. Examples include women being more likely to take action to prevent health problems, men tending to rely on spouses for social support related to their health, and

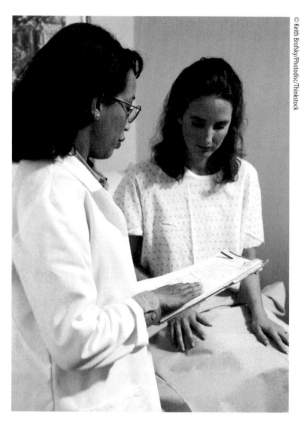

Women seem to prefer a female medical care provider in general practice and in gynecology.

women being more likely to turn to friends and their children for assistance in this area. Women also seem to experience more health problems and make more extensive use of health services.

When it comes to health care, there are also some interesting comparisons between males and females. While women show a preference for a female physician in the fields of general practice and gynecology (probably due to the intimate nature of the clinical intervention), beyond that most people do not have a strong preference for a healthcare provider of a particular sex.

Men are more likely to avoid regular health care than are women (Galdas, Chaeter, & Marshall, 2005). They often say they feel fine and do not need to consult physicians. Because of their needs related to reproductive health, women find it more difficult to avoid the health care system regardless of how well they may feel. Men and women seem to have similar experiences of daily symptoms, but women are more likely to seek medical care for these symptoms. Men also seem to have more trouble adopting the patient role than do women.

Another gender issue related to health is that some health insurance plans provide coverage for prescription drugs, but exclude coverage for prescription contraceptives. This can result in an extra financial burden on women and also make it more likely that some will use less-effective contraceptive methods—making unwanted pregnancy more likely.

Another issue related to health insurance is the practice of having different rates based on sex. Some have argued that split rates are justified because younger women typically seek healthcare services more often than men. Some women have been paying as much as 20% more than men for the same individual coverage. Federal law prohibits employers that offer health plans from charging different rates based on sex, and some states have similar laws.

On an international level, power imbalance can increase HIV risk. For example, in many societies there is a culture of silence surrounding sexuality that dictates that "good" women are expected to be ignorant about sexual behavior and passive in sexual interactions. This makes it difficult for women to be informed about HIV risk reduction and, even if informed, to be proactive in negotiating safer sexual activity. In addition, the traditional norm of virginity for unmarried females increases young women's risk of infection, because it restricts their ability to ask for information about sexuality because of fear that they will be thought to be sexually active. In cultures in which virginity is highly valued, some young women practice alternative sexual behaviors, such as anal intercourse, to preserve their virginity. These behaviors may place them at increased risk of HIV. Accessing treatment services for STIs can be highly stigmatizing for women. Finally, using barrier methods as safer options for sexual activity can be a dilemma for women in societies in which motherhood is considered to be a feminine ideal.

Other international examples were given by Billowitz and Kukke (2004). They pointed out that sex roles can have direct implications for health outcomes. For example, in many countries female infants die at a significantly higher rate than boys because they are not as highly valued. Boys are more likely to be immunized, have better nutrition, and receive medical care more promptly. These authors estimated that more than 1 million girls die each year from malnutrition, neglect, and abuse who would not have died had they been male. Sex-selective abortion is also still practiced in some countries where males are more highly valued.

Billowitz and Kukke (2004) also indicated other effects of sex roles. Norms may keep males from asking vital questions about sexuality. Men are supposed to demonstrate a bravado that makes it impossible to admit they don't know something about sexuality. In some cultures masturbation is believed to negatively affect a man's "manliness." This leads males to seek casual or commercial sexual activity when they have a desire to ejaculate, resulting in pressure to engage

Multicultural DIMENSIONS

Examples of Gender Equity Promoting Programs

Nigeria

In Nigeria, girls are traditionally taught to be subservient to their male family members. The Girls' Power Initiative provides girls with information on sexuality, human rights, sexual and reproductive health and rights, leadership, self-esteem, and life skills. The girls are trained to speak out against inequities. There is a counterpart program that works with young men to change attitudes toward sex roles and issues.

Kenya

Maendeleo Ya Wanawake Organization, a grassroots women's organization, was the first group in Kenya to advocate for the elimination of female genital cutting (FGC). The Organization goals included raising awareness about the harmful effects of FGC, devising ways to provide a positive image of uncircumcised girls, and developing an alternative rite of passage for girls that would replace initiation by cutting. As a result, the prevalence of FGC dropped among girls ages 14 to 19, and the number of women in favor of discontinuing the practice grew substantially.

Brazil

Project H is a training project based on research into the factors necessary for young men to be "gender equitable." Activities focus on themes of sexuality and sexual/reproductive health, paternity and care, violence prevention, mental health, and HIV/AIDS prevention and care. The project aims to reduce gender-based violence and generally improve health indicators. As a result, young men's attitudes have improved, and fewer young men are agreeing with statements such as "Men need sex more than women" and "I would be outraged if my wife asked me to use a condom." There was also a drop in STI symptoms and an increase in condom use.

India

The Better Life Options Program in India uses an empowerment approach to train low-income girls ages 12 to 20 (married and single) in family life education, literacy and vocational skills, and general and reproductive health. The project stresses leadership and social mobilization through advocacy and community involvement. Goals include building girls' self-esteem and self-confidence, as well as expanding their choices related to marriage, fertility, health, vocation, and civic participation. Girls completing the program were more likely to be literate, have completed secondary education, be employed, have learned a vocational skill, have traveled outside their village or visited the health center alone in the last 6 months, and to make autonomous decisions about going to the market, spending what they earned, and deciding when to marry.

Sweden

In Sweden, there has been a push for gender equity, but some believe it is really gender neutrality. For example, in a preschool, dolls might have no distinguishable sex. There are other efforts to do away with gender distinctions, including referring to people by a gender-neutral pronoun. Intended as an alternative to the Swedish words *han* (he) and *hon* (she), *hen* was proposed for this purpose in Sweden decades ago, but became very popular when it was used in a popular children's book. Now many major newspapers routinely employ the pronoun in place of the phrase *he or she*. Some Swedes feel that the push for gender neutrality is a noble project, while others feel it is an example of political correctness gone overboard.

Source: Data from Billowitz, M., & Kukke, S. Doing gender the 'rights' way. *SIECUS Report, 32, no. 3* (Summer 2004), 5–10; Abend, L. Boys won't be boys. *Time, 182, 25* (December 16, 2013), 38–44.

in frequent sexual activity with multiple partners, often without using a condom. Poor females who go to clinics may be intimidated by clinic personnel who show their attitudes about what women should do and not do. Also, in many countries economic inequities leave women few options for their livelihood, which may lead them to engage in transactional sexual activity or formal sex work, making them vulnerable to negative health consequences.

Some people think healthcare delivery and research benefit men at the expense of women. They believe that heart disease has been studied more in men and that women have been excluded from major national clinical studies. Others believe that women have benefited from medical research, as shown by improvements in breast cancer research as well as developments in laparoscopic surgery and ultrasound that were initially used on women's bodies.

Kluger (2003) reported that twice as many women as men suffer from depression and twice as many men suffer from alcoholism. Similarly, women tend to be more prone to anxiety disorders, and men are more likely to have conditions stemming from impulsiveness and violence.

In recent decades it was found that men with a history of heart disease were two to four times more likely than females to die later of sudden cardiac death. However, now female heart attack survivors are becoming almost as likely as men to succumb to sudden cardiac death. This gap has narrowed a great deal.

Some have pointed out a need for more gender-based medicine because of some differences between males and females. For example, major illnesses like heart disease and lung cancer are influenced by sex, and treatment for women may need to be slightly different from the approach used for men. Lung cancer, not breast cancer, is the number one cancer killer among women. The American Heart Association has developed heart disease prevention guidelines tailored for women. Also, heart attacks in women frequently don't involve chest pain; rather they may exhibit as more vague, flu-like symptoms. Women who do not smoke appear to be more susceptible to lung cancer than nonsmoking men. Women are less likely than men to get oral cancer, and more prone to autoimmune diseases including lupus, rheumatoid arthritis, and multiple sclerosis.

Males report more withdrawal and physical symptoms of depression than females.

Kulkarni et al. (2011) reported that men are increasing their life expectancy at a higher rate than women. Between 1987 and 2007, life expectancy in the United States increased nationwide from 71.3 years to 75.6 years for men and from 78.4 to 80.8 years for women. Possible reasons given for this include the fact that women are increasing their smoking more than men in general, the obesity epidemic in women

Communication
DIMENSIONS

Men Are from Mars; Women Are from Venus

John Gray, the author of the bestseller *Men Are from Mars, Women Are from Venus*, explains one reason why men and women may sometimes be frustrated in communicating with each other. He says women expand, and men contract. By this he means that women are likely to expand a topic, whereas men want them to get to the point. For example, he says that generally when a man speaks he has already silently mulled over his thought until he knows the main idea he wants to communicate. Then he speaks. A woman, in contrast (according to Gray), does not necessarily speak to make a point; speaking assists her in discovering her point. When she explores her thoughts and feelings out loud, she figures out where she wants to go.

For example, a man may want to pull away and take a little time to mull over his thoughts so he knows what he wants to say. However, a woman may find greater clarity by expanding and sharing. When she begins sharing, she is not necessarily aware of where it will take her, but she is confident it will take her where she needs to go. For her, this is a process of self-discovery.

There have been mixed feelings about Gray's book. Some feel it is inaccurate and biased, while others feel that while it may have some good points, Gray does not offer enough solutions. For example, Hamson (2004) feels that the book is completely useless as a "fix," but its popularity is invaluable for what it tells us about ourselves as a society. She points out that boys and girls/men and women share more traits than society is willing to admit. She further indicates that while we all have differences as human beings, biases and stereotypes based on sex must be understood to be not only groundless but just as divisive and nonproductive as racial prejudice.

Source: Data from Gray, J. *Men, women and relationships.* New York: Harper Paperbacks, 1996.

is greater, and reducing high blood pressures has been emphasized much more in men than women. Despite this increase, Americans still lag more than 3 years behind the 10 longest-living nations, including Japan, Australia, Singapore, and Sweden. In addition, the researchers pointed out that many women still do not understand that they will be affected by heart disease. They are also more stoic, have a higher pain threshold than men, and often do not say they are in pain.

An interesting gender twist related to nutrition has occurred. Supermarket aisles contain nutrient-rich female-friendly treats. For example, one nutrition bar was decorated with silhouetted dancing girls and packed with ingredients women are supposed to need. At least a few cereals are supposed to have nutrients that benefit women in particular. Manufacturers try to appeal as much to women's emotional needs as to their dietary ones, but in reality the basic laws of nutrition still apply to both men and women.

It has often been thought that men have higher self-esteem than women do. However, studies have shown that there is no significant difference between men's and women's self-esteem during adolescence or young adulthood. False beliefs in sex differences, however, may carry substantial costs. For example, parents, teachers, and counselors may overlook self-esteem problems in males because of the widespread belief that males have higher self-esteem than females. They need to give attention to both males and females if there appear to be self-esteem difficulties (Erol & Orth, 2011).

One final example related to health and sex focuses on college students. A survey of more than 1,400 college students in the Northeast showed that more than 83% reported having had sexual intercourse, with slightly higher rates for females (86%) than males

Many people seem to enjoy watching the romantic relationships of celebrities.

(78%). Females (86%) were more likely than males (79%) to have had sexual intercourse without a condom. Yet, when asked if they would have sexual intercourse with a partner who refused to use a condom, significantly fewer females (8%) than males (24%) reported they would have sexual intercourse without a condom in this situation. Males (53%) were significantly more likely to report frequent condom use than females (44%) (Bontempi et al., 2009).

Sex and Dating

Some experts think there are male/female issues related to dating. For example, some have indicated that females assume males will try to deceive them, but males don't seem to feel females will try to deceive them. Two issues related to sexual behavior and dating are frequency of sexual behavior and

Did You Know . . .

In 2011 the White House issued the first federal report since 1963 on the welfare of women (Women in America, 2011). Among the findings: Although more women than men have college degrees, women still earn only 29% of total household incomes in the United States. Other findings include:

- Women are having children later. The percentage of women in their thirties giving birth for the first time in 1970 was 4%, but in 2007 it was 22%.
- The average age at which women first gave birth in 2007 was 25, compared to 21 in 1970.

- Both men and women are marrying later. Between 1970 and 2010, the average age at first marriage increased from 20.8 to 26.1 years for women and from 23.2 to 28.2 years for men.
- More women than men are enrolled in college. The 2008 college enrollment was 57% women and 43% men.
- Women are less likely than men to be unemployed. In 2010 about 8.5% of women were unemployed, as compared to about 10% of men.
- A pay gap still exists. In 2009 women earned 75% of the salaries earned by men.

number of partners. Common sense would indicate that, on average, heterosexual men and women would have about equal numbers of sexual partners. However, males consistently report more partners than females do. Does this discrepancy arise because men are inclined to exaggerate sexual experience, and women to minimize it? Or is it because people have faulty memories? Or do women and men view sexual behavior differently?

Some think that the nature of intimacy is also a factor in male–female relationships. Many women derive intimacy from talking and may be disappointed if men do not verbally share their problems, express their emotions, or listen to their feelings. In contrast, men may feel emotional closeness by working or playing side by side.

When the topic of "dating" is discussed with many contemporary college students, talk soon turns to "hanging out" and "hooking up." For some college students, dating is an outdated concept. Instead, they prefer to attend activities in groups or simply "hang out" with one or more people. Interestingly, in a number of sexuality classes one of your authors has asked college students to define "hanging out" and "hooking up." In each of these conversations the conclusion was that college students do not agree on the definition of either of these terms, even though the terms are commonly used.

Other Gender Issues

Various experts have studied what males and females talk about with their friends. It is common to hear that men often discuss work issues, sports, and future goals. For women, the top three topics seem to be children, personal problems and self-doubts, and work issues. People believe that women's speech is more emotional than men's, although that stereotype has decreased in recent years. People also think women are more likely to show sympathy and communicate their support in problem situations. However, it is not unusual to see studies in which few differences appear between men's and women's communication styles.

There are also some stereotypical behaviors that seem to bother males and females about the other sex. Women often report being disturbed about men making sexual demands (making them feel sexually used or trying to force sexual behavior), making them feel inferior or stupid, and emotional constriction (hiding his emotions) and excess (drinking or smoking too much). Men commonly report being disturbed about women's sexual rejection (being unresponsive to sexual advances, being a sexual tease), moodiness, and self-absorption (fussing over appearance or spending too much on clothes).

The division of household labor has long been an interest area for gender researchers because who does the various tasks reveals information about power and equity in relationships. For decades, research has indicated that even when women are employed outside the home, they still do the majority of housework and child care chores. Even though the differences are not as great today as they were in past years, women still perform about twice as much household work and child care as men do. Interestingly, gay couples seem more likely to split tasks, with each partner performing a set of chores. Lesbian couples seem more likely to alternate in sharing tasks, taking turns in performing the same chores (Sayer, 2005).

Other gender differences have been mentioned as well. For instance, men are described as wanting to cut straight to the point and not get sidetracked by other issues. Women may have a more contextual view of the world and see issues as part of a larger whole. Also, young males often take more risks than young females do. It is thought that this behavior may be linked to different levels of a chemical in the brain. In addition, it seems that females are more likely than males to bear grudges, sometimes for a long time.

Peplau (2003) states that a large body of research documents four important gender differences related to sexuality. First, in many ways, men show greater sexual desire than do women. Second, compared to men, women place greater emphasis on committed relationships as a context for sexuality. Third, aggression is more strongly linked to sexuality for men than for women. Fourth, women's sexuality tends to be more malleable and capable of change over time. Obviously, not all of these differences are absolutes because men and women can vary a great deal. In general, however, these differences affect thoughts, feelings, and behavior. Also, they characterize not only heterosexuals but lesbians and gay men as well.

Gender and the Workplace

Do men and women approach things differently in the workplace? Are women being treated fairly in the workplace? Are salaries and benefits the same for males and females? These, and other interesting issues, have long provided hot topics for research and discussion.

An extensive study showed that women scored higher on orientation to production and getting results, and men scored higher on strategic planning and organizational vision. Women were seen as operating with more energy, intensity, and emotional expression; men were seen as more low-key and quiet through the control of emotional expression. Women were rated higher on people-oriented leadership skills, whereas men were rated higher on business-oriented leadership skills by bosses and peers (Do men and women lead differently?, 2000).

Eagly (2003) analyzed 45 studies of leadership styles and concluded that women in management positions were actually better leaders than men in equivalent positions. Women were more likely than men to be "transformational" leaders, or leaders who try to inspire workers and develop their skills and creativity. They serve as role models, mentor and empower workers, and encourage innovation even when the organization they lead is generally successful. Other kinds of leaders include transactional leaders, who lead by rewarding and punishing, and laissez-faire leaders, who take a hands-off approach. Previous studies indicate that transformational leaders create the most productive and satisfying work environments. Women also scored higher than men on one measure of transactional leadership—rewarding employees for good performance. One reason why women may favor transformational leadership is that such a leader operates more like an excellent teacher than a traditional boss.

Stoker et al. (2011) examined whether the sex of an employee, the sex of the manager, and the management–sex ratio in an organization were related to employees' managerial stereotypes. They found that although the general stereotype of a manager is masculine, and although most employees prefer a man as a manager, female employees, employees with a female manager, and employees working in an organization with a high percentage of female managers have a stronger preference for feminine characteristics of managers and for female managers.

It is often assumed that women would rather work with and be supervised by other women, but some studies indicate that women can be each other's worst enemies on the job. According to such studies, women often betray and undermine one another; they damage other women's career aspirations; and they often fail to support other women—even actively undermining their authority and credibility. One theory is that for two women to forge a positive relationship, their self-esteem and power must be kept "dead even." When one woman gets more power, it sets off tensions and leads to hostility and sniping. In practice, many women say they would prefer a male boss.

Relatedly, Meese (2009) reported out that at least 40% of the bullies in the workplace are women. They choose other women as targets more than 70% of the time. Men seem to bully men and women pretty much equally. Reasons given for women's bullying include women believing they need to be aggressive to be promoted, women sabotaging other women because they believe helping female coworkers

Employment opportunities for males and females have changed in recent years.

could jeopardize their own careers, women withholding information such as promotional information from other women to help themselves, and other women supposedly being easier to bully than men because they are less tough than men. Many women have learned they are supposed to be nurturers and supporters, but bullying behavior is antithetical to the way they are supposed to be.

Sheppard and Aquino (2013) showed how the negative stereotyping related to "catfights" carries over into work situations. In their study, participants were asked to assess one of three workplace conflict scenarios, all identical except for the names of the individuals involved: Adam and Steven, Adam and Sarah, or Sarah and Anna. Participants rated those involved in all-female conflicts as being less likely to repair a frayed relationship and more likely to let the argument negatively influence job satisfaction than male–female or male–male quarrelers. Female participants were just as likely as males to see the all-female conflict as more negative.

Namie (2010) indicated that 35% of the U.S. workforce report being bullied at work, and an additional

15% witness it. Men make up 62% of the bullies, and 58% of the targets are women. Women bullies target women in 80% of the cases. Bullying is four times more prevalent than illegal harassment, and the majority (68%) of bullying is same-sex bullying. In the study, bullying was defined as "repeated mistreatment: sabotage by others that prevented work from getting done, verbal abuse, threatening conduct, intimidation, and humiliation."

Because more than half the women with babies younger than 1 year are in the workforce, increasing numbers of them want to breastfeed their infants. In response, more companies are meeting this need by setting up a private room and a work schedule so mothers can pump their breast milk. Some companies provide a private room, a hospital-grade pump, a carrying case for discreet transport of the pumping paraphernalia and expressed milk, plus bottles and access to a refrigerator. One company, Cigna, in which 80% of the workforce is female, saved about $240,000 per year in healthcare expenses for breast-feeding mothers and their children and another $60,000 through reduced absenteeism. This does not include the incalculable goodwill of happy new parents.

The relationship between salaries of men and salaries of women has long been a subject of interest. In 2009, the National Organization for Women indicated that for full-time, year-round workers, women are paid, on average, only 78% of what men are paid, and the gap is significantly wider for women of color. This gap remains despite the passage of the 1963 Equal Pay Act and a variety of legislation prohibiting employment discrimination (On Equal Pay Day NOW calls attention to persistent gender wage gap, 2009). The Bureau of Labor Statistics (2011) reported that women who usually worked full time had median earnings 82.4% of the median for men.

In 2012, the U.S. Census Bureau provided data showing women's earnings as a percentage of men's earnings from 1980 to 2010. These data indicate that overall women earned 63% of what men earned in 1980, 72% of what men earned in 1990, 75% of what men earned in 2000, and 81% of what men earned in 2010. A number of other sources also indicate the pay gap is in the range of 78% to 82%.

It is difficult to interpret the meaning of these data accurately without knowing more about years of experience, academic preparation, levels of responsibility, and other variables that may influence salary levels. One effort to look at these other variables (Do men really earn more than women, 2014) resulted in some interesting information. For example, when pay for men and women who were similarly qualified was compared, the differences ranged from 1% to

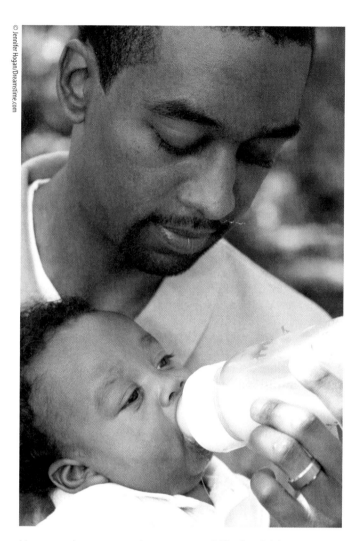

Many men have assumed more responsibility for child rearing.

4%. It is also interesting to consider why men earn more than women. A major part of this difference stems from the fact that men and women tend to gravitate toward different careers. The most popular choices for men tend to offer better pay than the most popular choices for women. Also, women's pay growth tends to slow around age 30, which is when college-educated woman typically start having children.

In 2008, the Center for Women's Business Research reported that women owned 20% of U.S. businesses with revenues exceeding $1 million per year. A total of 10.1 million firms were owned by women, employing 13 million people and generating $1.9 trillion in revenues. Women business owners who exceed the $1 million revenue mark typically are "gutsy," action-oriented women, have a solutions orientation, believe that larger business provides more freedom; are energized by the "business of growing a business," create their own rules; focus on internal business culture, and are lifelong learners (New study shows women own 20% of businesses with revenues exceeding $1 million, 2008).

An interesting study was reported by McKeen (2005). She surveyed 214 Canadian and 160 Chinese business students regarding their future spouses' employment and family roles relative to their own. Results showed that a large proportion from both countries hoped for equality between the spouses, especially in the distribution of domestic tasks. However, significant discrepancies existed between their ideal hopes and their expectations of what will actually happen. Many men and women of both countries expected that the wives would do more of the domestic work and have less prestigious jobs and lower earnings than their husbands.

Catalyst is a nonprofit organization working globally with businesses and the professions to build inclusive workplaces and expand opportunities for women and business. In 2009, several of its reports provided information on related issues. For example, in 2008 women's representation as corporate officers rose to 16.9%, an increase of 1.8% since 2006 (Jenner & Ferguson, 2009). Because men dominate executive positions, the flow of information from senior leaders tends to perpetuate gender gaps in senior leadership. In addition, gender bias inhibits the establishment of inclusive and effective talent management programs (Warren, 2009). Clearly, men have a critical role to play in inclusion and diversity efforts. Men who are more aware of gender bias are more likely to say that it is important to them to achieve gender equality. Three key barriers that undermine men's support for initiatives to end gender bias are apathy, fear, and ignorance about gender issues. Men must be helped to understand their critical role in gender initiatives (Prime & Moss-Racusin, 2009).

In today's marketplace, the female management style is distinctly different, but it is essential. Women manage more cautiously than men; they focus on the long term. Men thrive on risk, especially when they are surrounded by other men. Women are less competitive, in a good way: They are consensus builders, conciliators, and collaborators (Shipman & Kay, 2009).

Although women have not held a high percentage of leadership positions in industry, in May 2009 a historical event occurred when Ursula Burns became the first African American female to head a Fortune 500 company (Xerox). That made her one of about 15 women leading Fortune 500 companies. Her ascension marked the first female-to-female transition.

In February 2014, another significant event occurred related to females being leaders in industry.

Mary Barra was named chief executive officer of General Motors (GM). In her previous roles, she was responsible for the design, engineering, program management, and quality of GM vehicles around the world. In 2014, Barra was named to the *Time* 100 (the 100 most influential people in the world), *Forbes* magazine named her one of the "World's 100 Most Powerful Women," and *Fortune* magazine placed her first on its list of the "50 Most Powerful Women in Business."

As you can see, some of the facts and observations already mentioned can relate to money and power. Some experts feel that as female economic power grows, it is changing how men and women work, play, shop, share, court, and even love each other (Mundy, 2012). Related information and examples include:

- In dual-earner couples, women now contribute an average of 44% of the family income, up from 39% in 1997.

- In the majority of U.S. metro areas, single, childless women in their 20s make more per dollar than their male peers (from $1.09 in Los Angeles to $1.14 in Atlanta to $1.18 in Dallas).

- In 2012 women earned 57% of the bachelor's, 60% of the master's, and 52% of the doctoral degrees conferred.

- Less than 1 in 5 married-couple families are supported by the husband alone.

- In households where the male brings in more income, buying decisions are made equally, but in households where the female earns more, she typically makes twice as many buying decisions as the male.

- It is predicted that within a generation a majority of working wives will outearn their husbands.

While much attention is being given to opportunities for females in the workplace and to comparative salaries between males and females, some females find climbing the career ladder to be less of a concern than finding a position that offers paid sick leave, flexible scheduling, or the opportunity to work fewer hours. While women may want rewarding careers, more than that they want *flexible* ones—part of their quest to find ways to get a career to accommodate family life, rather than the other way around. That ranking of priorities is not always the one described in best-selling books advising women to seek out leadership positions, throw themselves at their careers, find a partner who helps with child care and supports their ambition, and negotiate for raises and promotions (Rampell, 2013).

Another issue related to flexibility in the workplace is paternity leave. Although the Family and Medical Leave Act of 1993 required companies with more than 50 employees to provide 12 weeks of unpaid leave for new parents, it requires no paid leave. The 14% of companies that do offer such pay do so by choice. Twenty percent of companies that are supposed to comply with the law still do not offer paternity leave, and half the workers in the United States work at smaller companies that are not required to offer any leave at all. Even when the organization has a formal policy on the books, unwritten workplace norms can discourage men from taking leave. There still is some stigma about men who say, "My kids are more important than my work." In some areas, paternity leave—which increasingly is called partner or primary caregiver leave—is already the norm, partly because of some companies' efforts to accommodate same-sex and adoptive parents. At the same time, the percentage of companies that offer paternity leave dropped 5 percentage points from 2010 to 2014, highlighting the fact that employers do not always see leave as beneficial to the company (Miller, 2014).

Sex Roles and the Media

Advertising has long contributed to thinking about sex roles. Stereotypical examples include females with beautiful bodies often dressed in skimpy clothing being the object of another's gaze much more than their male counterparts. The authoritative male voice is still used in many commercials. It seems that through the years there has been a change in the images of women in commercials—but not the images of men. Today women are shown more often representing managerial and professional occupations. They are shown in more diverse occupations than in the past, whereas images of men have changed little. There is probably only a small increase in images of men parenting and doing housework.

Preidt (2008) has indicated that the way men and women are portrayed in TV commercials can have a major impact on how they behave in their daily lives. Men, in particular, are influenced by commercials that more often depict them in a career setting than doing domestic chores. TV advertisements help to socially construct gender and influence how people think about their own gender as well as other genders. Most commercials featuring women focus on selling home products, such as food, cleaners, personal care items, and furniture. Men are most likely to be engaged in work behavior in commercials, whereas women are least likely to be depicted

working outside the home. Only some 2% of commercials show men doing domestic chores, such as cooking, cleaning, or caring for children.

Monk-Turner et al. (2008) looked at how sexual themes are used in magazine ads. Most ads did not use a sexual theme to sell a product. If used, however, this theme was more likely to appear in an ad aimed at a male audience.

Zimmerman and Dahlberg (2008) looked at attitudes of young women toward sexually objectified advertising and compared their results to findings from earlier studies. Respondents agreed that females were portrayed as sex objects in advertisements, but were less offended by these portrayals than were female respondents in earlier years. Respondents also indicated that attitudes toward the advertisement have little influence on whether they intend to purchase the products.

As the preceding information shows, there have probably been some improvements in the way ads treat sex-role issues, but a number of these issues remain. For example, Andersen (2009) indicated that ads admonish women to be afraid—afraid of aging, afraid of food, afraid of being alone, or afraid of having a bust that is too small or too big. They promise that with the right products, a woman can

Myth vs Fact

Myth: Females lack achievement motivation compared to males.
Fact: There are no differences here. Females have just as much achievement motivation as males.

Myth: Females have lower self-esteem.
Fact: Self-esteem is influenced by many factors. A person's gender, however, has no effect on self-esteem.

Myth: Females are better at learning roles and simple repetitive tasks.
Fact: The ability to learn roles and simple repetitive tasks is not influenced by sex.

Myth: Males are more analytical.
Fact: There is no difference in analytical skills between males and females.

Myth: All men think about women the same way. (Or all women think about men the same way.)

Fact: It is incorrect to conclude that all people of a certain sex think the same way about anything.

Myth: Females are more social than males.
Fact: The interest in being social, or the ability to be social, does not vary by sex even though it certainly can vary from one individual to another.

Myth: Females are more affected by heredity than males.
Fact: We are all influenced by our heredity, but our sex makes no difference in this situation (except that a few diseases are specific to one sex or the other).

Myth: Males are more affected by environment than females.
Fact: Everyone is influenced by the environment, but we are not affected more or less because of our sex.

be seductive, change how she looks, and wear the right scent and be more attractive in general for one major purpose—to attract a partner. These are powerful messages that many take seriously. In fact, the impact of these messages is so strong that the American Psychological Association (2007) concluded that "throughout U.S. culture, and particularly in mainstream media, women and girls are depicted in a sexualizing manner. These representations can be seen in virtually every medium."

Taylor and Setters (2011) looked at the impact of media representations of film stars on sex role expectations for women. They found that college students perceived more attractive film leads as better role models than the less attractive leads. Their findings suggested that both men and women expect women to fulfill both feminine and masculine roles, that women generally have higher expectations of women than men, and that watching attractive, aggressive heroines exaggerates these expectations.

Screen star Geena Davis became concerned about the portrayal of females in the media. She observed that male characters largely outnumbered female characters, that female characters hardly ever had powerful roles, and that females were almost always portrayed in skimpy or overly sexualized clothes. She then established the Geena Davis Institute on Gender in the Media. The Institute sponsored the largest study ever done on G-rated movies and on TV shows for kids 11 and younger. Results confirmed her observations. Male characters outnumbered females 3 to 1. In scenes featuring groups, the ratio increased to 5 to 1. In addition, aspirations and occupations of female characters were very limited. The female characters had very narrow stereotypes. Almost the only aspiration for female characters was to find romance. Hypersexualization was common. The female characters in G-rated films wore about the same amount of sexually revealing clothing as the female characters in R-rated movies. Realizing that there was a clear message that girls and women are less important than boys and men to our society, Davis worked with the National Institute of Health to establish a research agenda designed to promote better ways to establish more positive stereotypes and expectations for girls and women in the media (Garnett, 2011).

Smith et al. (2013) reported that gender imbalance is alive and well in the media. This is illustrated by the relatively small percentages of speaking characters who are female in family films (28.3%), prime time television programs (38.9%), and children's shows (30.8%). In addition, females are stereotyped and sexualized in popular entertainment. Females are far more likely than males to be depicted wearing sexy attire showing some exposed skin and referenced by another character as physically attractive

or desirable. In addition, males (66.6%) are more likely than females (45.3%) to be shown working, and only a small number of females are shown as holding higher-level positions in family films. In prime time TV, things are a little better, with females being shown as 14% of corporate executives, 27.8% of high-level politicians, 29.6% of doctors/hospital managers, and 38.5% of academic administrators.

According to Lister (2014), actress Reese Witherspoon created her own production company with a clear feminist goal—making more interesting film roles for women. Just 30% of all speaking roles and 15% of major characters belong to women, and only 13% of the top 100 films of all time featured an equal number of male and female characters. Men get double the screen time of women—an imbalance that may be attributable to the fact that women account for just 16% of all directors, producers, writers, cinematographers, and editors.

Myths About Male–Female Differences

Socialization determines a great deal of what many people choose to see as "naturally" masculine or feminine. People look at the ways many women and men and girls and boys *do* behave and conclude that those are the only ways in which females and males *can* behave. Countless myths explain real or apparent differences in male–female feelings, attitudes, aptitudes, and behavior. (See examples of such myths in the box on the previous page.)

▥ Gender Identity, Roles, and Stereotypes

When a baby is delivered and "It's a boy!" or "It's a girl!" rings out, social influences go to work to form the baby's gender identity and mold his or her future role. Each society has a set of rules for how its males and females should behave. Boys and girls learn early to conform to these established behavior standards and take on their accepted roles. Psychologists have tried to explain how children do this in terms of psychoanalytical, social-learning, cognitive-developmental, and gender-schema theories.

According to psychoanalytical theory (explained by Sigmund Freud), appropriate gender typing means that boys grow to identify with their fathers and girls with their mothers. Identification is completed as children resolve the **Oedipus complex** (sometimes

---

Oedipus complex A development stage in which the boy wants to possess his mother sexually and sees the father as a rival (similar to the female *Electra complex*).

Gender DIMENSIONS

Terminology Related to Gender

Terms related to gender can be confusing because some meanings change over time, and some meanings might be used differently by different people. Following are definitions of many gender-associated terms, but do not be surprised if you see or hear definitions for some of these terms elsewhere that differ somewhat from these.

- *Gender:* A socially constructed system of classification that ascribes qualities of masculinity and femininity. Gender characteristics can change over time and vary between cultures (*Definition of terms*, 2014).
- *Gender diverse:* A person who either by nature or by choice does not conform to gender-based expectations of society (e.g., transgender, transsexual, intersex, genderqueer) (*Definition of terms*, 2014).
- *Gender expression:* The way a person communicates gender identity to others through behavior, clothing, hairstyles, voice, or body characteristics (American Psychological Association, 2015).
- *Gender fluid:* A person whose gender identification and presentation shifts, either within or outside of societal gender-based expectations (*Definition of terms*, 2014).
- *Gender identity:* A person's internal sense of being male, female, or something else (American Psychological Association, 2015).
- *Genderqueer:* A person whose gender identity is neither man nor woman, is between or beyond genders, or is some combination of genders. This identity is usually related to or in reaction to the social construction of gender, gender stereotypes, and the gender binary system. Some genderqueer people identify under the transgender umbrella, and some do not (*Definition of terms*, 2014).
- *Intersex:* A person whose sexual anatomy or chromosomes do not fit with the traditional markers of "female" and "male"—for example, people born with both female and male anatomy or with XXY chromosomes (*LGBT terms and definitions*, 2015).

- *Pansexual:* A person who is romantically and/or sexually attracted to both men and women (*Definition of terms*, 2014). A person who experiences sexual, romantic, physical, and/or spiritual attraction for members of all gender identities/expressions, not just people who fit into the standard gender binary (i.e., men and women) (*LGBT terms and definitions*, 2015).
- *Queer:* A term that has different meanings to different people, which usually falls into four categories: (1) an umbrella term referring to all LGBTIQ (lesbian, gay, bisexual, transsexual, intersex, queer) people; (2) a political statement, as well as a sexual orientation, which advocates breaking binary thinking and seeing both sexual orientation and gender identity as potentially fluid; (3) a simple label to explain a complex set of behaviors and desires—for example, a person who is attracted to multiple genders may identify as queer; (4) to many older LGBT people, a word that has been hatefully used against them and that they are reluctant to embrace it (*Definition of terms*, 2014).
- *Questioning:* The process of exploring and discovering one's own sexual orientation, gender identity, or gender expression (*LGBT terms and definitions*, 2015).
- *Transsexual:* A person who experiences a mismatch of the sex the individual was born with and the sex the person identifies as. A transsexual sometimes undergoes medical treatment to change his/her physical sex to match his/her sex identity through hormone treatments and/or surgically. Not all transsexuals can have or desire surgery (*Definition of terms*, 2014).

Sources: Definition of terms. UC Berkeley Gender Equity Resource Center, 2014. Available: http://geneq.berkeley.edu/lgbt_resources_definiton_of_terms; American Psychological Association. *Answers to your questions about transgender people, gender identity, and gender expression*, 2015. Available: http://www.apa.org/topics/lgbt/transgender.aspx; *LGBT terms and definitions*. University of Michigan, International Spectrum, 2015. Available: http://internationalspectrum.umich.edu/life/definitions.

called the *Electra complex* in girls). From roughly age 3 to 5 years, children supposedly develop incestuous wishes for the parent of the other sex and see the parent of the same sex as a rival. This is resolved when the child eventually identifies with the same-sex parent and develops behaviors typically associated with that sex. Today the psychoanalytical theory of gender-role development is not widely accepted.

In social-learning theory, the development of gender-typed behavior is explained in terms of processes such as observational learning, identification, and **socialization**. Children learn what is deemed masculine or feminine by observing, experimenting, and being rewarded for certain behaviors.

In cognitive-developmental theory, children form concepts about gender and then make their behavior conform to their gender concepts. This is called **gender typing**. By about age 7 to 8 years, **gender constancy** develops in most children. They realize that gender does not change even if the appearance and actions of people change. When children learn that gender is permanent, they independently try to act the way boys or girls "should act," because of an internal need for their behaviors to be consistent with what they know.

Gender schema theory indicates that children develop a grouping of mental representations about male and female personality traits, physical qualities, and behaviors. Once they develop a gender schema, they begin to judge themselves according to traits considered relevant to their sex. By doing this, they blend their developing self-concepts with the gender schema of their culture. Many associations can be made between sex and other qualities, such as strength and affection. Traditionally, strength has been viewed as a masculine trait and affection as a feminine trait. Other gender distinctions may be viewed as important—such as men being sexually assertive and women being sexually passive, or men's being in leadership positions and women's being placed in lesser positions.

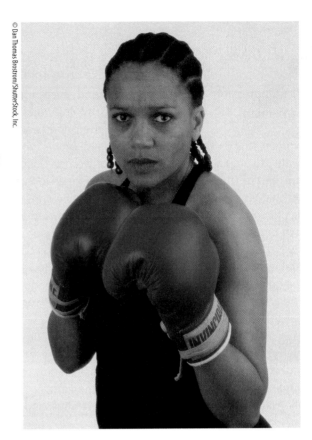

Gender roles and expectations may be defined differently by various people.

Gender Identity

Gender involves more than just a biological component; it also includes the biological, social, and cultural norms and something called **gender identity**. Gender identity is one's self-image as a female or a male; it is the attachment one has to one's role. Societal and cultural factors are thought to exert more influence on gender identity than the biological component. At the very least, gender identity should be considered a biopsychosocial process—it is a result of interaction of biological, psychological, and social factors.

Masculinity and femininity are not innate or instinctive. The masculinity or femininity of gender identity needs a healthy human brain in which to take root. However, the developing brain is shaped by the environment in which it grows and from which it takes its mental nourishment. In this way the biological foundation is shaped by psychological and sociological influences.

Because each society defines its roles for males and females and perpetuates behaviors through gender-role socialization, boys are given reinforcement for behaving in a "masculine" way, and girls receive reinforcement for exhibiting "feminine" behaviors. Should either gender engage in cross-sex conduct, such behavior is labeled gender-role-inappropriate; when each sex behaves as the society deems normal, that behavior is labeled gender-role-appropriate and is rewarded.

Sex roles differ markedly from society to society. Many societies discourage any deviation from the prescribed sex roles; others, such as ours, are now working toward flexibility and individualism in a wide variety of behaviors.

The expectation that people will exhibit certain characteristics and/or behaviors dictated by the

socialization The process of guiding people into socially acceptable behavior by providing information, rewards, and punishments.

gender typing The process whereby children develop behavior that is appropriate to their gender.

gender constancy The concept that people's gender does not change—even if they change their dress or behavior.

gender schema A grouping of mental representations about male and female physical qualities, behaviors, and personality traits.

gender identity The awareness and acceptance of one's gender.

DIMENSIONS

The Oppression of Women

In the past, and even today, there are many international examples of the oppression of women. In 2011 the government of Saudi Arabia moved swiftly to stop a protest movement of women claiming the right to drive. A woman was detained for up to 5 days on charges of disturbing public order and inciting public opinion by twice driving a car. She was arrested after two much-publicized drives to highlight Facebook and Twitter campaigns to encourage women across Saudi Arabia to participate in a collective protest. However, the government blocked the campaigns in the kingdom. The arrest was probably intended to give other women pause before participating in protests in a country where a woman's public reputation, including the ability to marry, can be badly damaged by an arrest. Whether or not women should drive in Saudi Arabia is a highly emotional issue in the kingdom, where women are also not allowed to vote, or even work without their husbands' or fathers' permission (MacFarquhar, 2011).

In 2011 more than 200 experts from five continents ranked countries on their overall perception of danger for women. On the top of the list was Afghanistan, with one of the highest maternal mortality rates in the world, minimal access to basic health care and education, and scarcely any economic rights for women and girls. Eighty-seven percent of Afghan women are illiterate, 1 in 11 dies in childbirth, and as many as 8 in 10 face forced marriages. The Congo was rated second because many threats prevail for women. The levels of sexual violence and rape there are the highest in the world, and a married woman cannot sign any legal documents without her husband's authorization. Pakistan was ranked third, based on religious traditions that are harmful to women. More than 1,000 women a year are victims of so-called honor killings, and many more are victims of acid attacks, child marriage, and abusive punishments, including stoning (Anderson, 2011).

In 2015, an Egyptian groom who knocked his bride out by fracturing her skull just after their wedding told police he did so at his mother's request to control his wife. He also told the police that his mother warned him that his brothers are all controlled by their wives because they did not listen to her advice to hit their brides. Police arrested the man on charges of causing serious injuries to his wife, who suffered from fractures in her skull and pelvis (Marwan, 2015a).

In Turkey, patriarchy runs deep. Shafak (2015) reported that a brutal rape and murder there galvanized women and drew attention to gender-related crime. The rape unleashed an unprecedented storm of protest throughout Turkey. The local bar association announced that none of the 1,600 lawyers licensed to work in the region would represent the murderer and his accomplices. Women went to work wearing black ribbons. The slain girl's funeral was attended by thousands of women. By tradition, Turkish women stay at the back of the funeral crowd and let the men carry the coffin and lead the prayers—but this time it was different. Despite repeated warnings, women refused to step back and said they were determined "no other man's hands would touch her again." Women carried her coffin, and women buried her. Domestic violence has increased drastically in Turkey, but Turkey's women are divided in how—and whether—to respond to it. The biggest rift is between those who defend silence and the status quo, and those who refuse to keep quiet in the face of growing gender violence.

As described by Marwan (2015b), a resident of the Chechen capital, Grozny, confessed to the killing of his daughter. He said he did it "to punish his daughter for amoral behavior." In another instance, a pregnant woman was stoned to death by her own family in front of a Pakistani high court for marrying the man she loved. These kinds of "honor killings" are driven by the position that women's bodies represent the repositories of family honor. Honor killings are done by family members because of a belief that the victim has brought dishonor to the family through her immoral conduct.

---

stereotyping The expectation that individuals will exhibit certain characteristics or behaviors.

gender-role stereotyping Expectation that individuals will behave in certain ways because they are male or female.

customs and traditions of the society is called **stereotyping**. Expecting individuals to behave in particular ways because they are male or female is referred to as **gender-role stereotyping**. There are still many rigid, unyielding traditional attitudes about gender-role behaviors that make it difficult for people to express

? Did You Know . . .

In 2014, two books gave support to both pessimistic and optimistic perspectives on the direction of gender relations and the prospects for more fairness and equity. One book used data from past economic studies to show how gender influences financial actions and relationships. In one set of experiments, women were found to be more generous than men. However, in a game in which each player received $10 and then decided how much to offer to a partner, both men and women made lower offers, on average, when the partner was female. Discrimination was worse coming from the women themselves.

Another economic test involved a game in which players would fare best collectively if they cooperated, yet individuals had an incentive to act more opportunistically for a higher payoff. Women were more likely to start off by cooperating,

then would learn through bitter experience that they would be taken advantage of if they continued to do so. Over time, the initially cooperative behavior of the women converged with the more opportunistic behavior shown by the men. Even so, the women's initial reluctance to use cutthroat strategies brought them losses.

In general, research shows that women are perceived as easier to take advantage of in a variety of economic settings. Nevertheless, the authors found that once women achieve a critical mass, their participation grows rapidly. Also, men tend to behave in a less stereotypically male way when more women are participating in an organization or activity.

Sources: Eswaran, M. *Why gender matters in economics.* Princeton, NJ: Princeton University Press, 2014; Karpowitz, C. F. *The silent sex: Gender, deliberation and institutions.* Princeton, NJ: Princeton University Press, 2014.

themselves and for society to implement change. Stereotypical images of people do not take into account individual differences. Until recently the stereotypical woman or wife in our society was passive, quiet, and concerned primarily with home, husband, and children; the stereotypical man was gruff, strong, unfeeling, and concerned mostly with work and money. The danger of such stereotypes is that people take them seriously and act on them, turning a blind eye to the qualities, capabilities, and interests of individuals—frequently denying even their own. People often believe that those who deviate from stereotypes are not as good as those who conform to them. Thus one who accepts as true the stereotypes described might look down on a woman who cared about work or a man who chose to stay home with his children. People become boxed in not only by social pressure to conform closely to the stereotype, but also by rigid customary practice (such as promoting men but not women in business and professions, hiring women but not men to nurse and teach small children, or paying men more than women, regardless of their responsibilities), as well as by law. The assumptions behind such stereotyped behavior are being challenged today, and laws are being changed as well, but popular assumptions and attitudes are slow to change and are still passed on.

Teaching Gender Roles and Stereotypes

Gender roles are taught throughout the life cycle, but parents probably have the greatest effect, especially when children are very young. Very early on,

parents reinforce the behaviors deemed acceptable to their child's sex with such remarks as "What a good, sweet girl!" or "What a big, strong boy!" accompanied by smiles and nods of approval. There is no doubt that most, if not all, of the forces of socialization in our culture—parents, teachers, peers, movies, television, the Internet, and books (targeted at children and adults)—encourage different behaviors in boys and girls. The resulting sets of traits are what we call *masculinity* and *femininity*. Let us look briefly at a few examples of how sex roles and stereotypes are taught.

The Influence of Schools

School personnel pass on social stereotypes in a number of ways. For example, if teachers feel that boys are naturally more aggressive or that girls are naturally more passive, how will this attitude influence the way they treat their students? If gender-role stereotyping exists in teachers' expectations, it can lead to biases in how they treat and evaluate their students.

Berk (2008) mentioned a number of ways teachers and the school environment might contribute to gender stereotyping. For example, younger girls often gather around the teacher, following directions, while boys are attracted to other areas of the classroom where teachers are minimally involved. Consequently, boys and girls engage in different social behaviors. Teachers also use more disapproval and controlling

---

gender role Complex groups of ways males and females are expected to behave in a given culture.

© AP Photos

During World War II, Rosie the Riveter was part of the U.S. government's public relations campaign to get women into the workforce. Rosie shows off a strong bicep but still has a perfect manicure.

discipline with boys. When girls misbehave, teachers tend to negotiate, coming up with a plan to improve behavior. Teachers seem to expect boys to misbehave more, a belief that seems based partly on boys' actual behavior and partly on gender stereotypes.

If teachers believe in stereotypes, they may expect one sex to excel more than the other in certain subjects, they may encourage one sex more than another, or they may favor one sex in terms of attention and/or extra help. They may even intentionally or unintentionally promote **sexism**, which is a prejudgment that because of gender a person will possess negative traits. In addition to these prejudgments, sexism can entail discrimination against someone because of sex. For example, not hiring a man for a day care job because it is believed that males cannot nurture children would be sexism. Teachers can help promote the healthy sexual development of children if they provide equal opportunities for girls and boys, do not impose gender stereotypes, and do not use sexist language. Although young children are busy establishing their own identities, and many may exhibit stereotypical behavior, it is the role of

the teacher to encourage learning and responsible behavior that does not discriminate.

School materials can also influence gender-role stereotyping. For example, in preschool picture books there has been a trend toward depiction of greater gender equality. At the same time, however, female characters are more likely to be shown as dependent or submissive, and males as independent and creative. Many subtle traditional expectations still exist.

Some people claim bias still exists in achievement tests. Language in the tests has often referred to males and their environments. Women were disproportionately shown to be homemakers, and men to be engaged in directive, leadership, achieving roles. Boys were described in action terms; girls were described in helping or more passive terms. A strong bias against nontraditional behavior in both sexes has been evident in many tests.

Sadker and Zittleman (2005) point out that gender bias lives for both sexes. It can be hard to detect because it affects boys and girls in different ways. For example, in school, the boys may be expected to "act out" and rebel at schoolwork, while the girls are expected to be docile. Both of these expectations reflect gender stereotyping, or bias. Other examples of challenges related to gender bias include:

- Boys and girls like and do well in math and science in elementary school, but girls become less positive and do less well in higher grades.

- Boys receive more math- and science-related toys than girls do.

- Girls receive higher report card grades throughout their schooling.

- Boys often regard reading and writing as "feminine" subjects, and report that reading threatens their masculinity.

- Current software products are likely to reinforce gender stereotypes and bias rather than reduce them.

- Teachers call on boys more often than girls, wait longer for boys' answers, and provide more precise feedback to boys.

- Girls are more likely to be quiet in class and praised for neatness.

Even at the college level, educators need to be sensitive to the influence of the classroom environment. It has been thought that female students participate less often and less assertively than male students in college classrooms and that the professors' discriminatory behaviors are partly responsible.

sexism The prejudgment that because of gender a person will possess negative traits.

Multicultural DIMENSIONS

International Gender Equality Comparisons

In recent years, the World Economic Forum has published a gender gap index that examines disparities between men and women in terms of political empowerment, economic opportunity, health, and education. Iceland came out the best in 2014, scoring 0.86 on an index in which 1 denotes perfect equality. The Nordic countries all did well, taking the top five positions among the 142 countries in the ranking. The United States was ranked 20th in the group,

with a score of 7.4. Some emerging countries also have high gender equality. Nicaragua ranked 6th, and Rwanda was 7th overall and first in sub-Saharan Africa, thanks to a particularly small gap between men and women in the political empowerment category. Germany was ranked 12th, Great Britain 26th, Italy 69th, Russia 75th, Mexico 80th, China 87th, Japan 104th, and India 114th.

Source: Gender equality. *The Economist*, 2014. Available: http://www.economist.com/news/economic-and-financial-indicators/21629478-gender-equality.

Teachers, books, and tests are powerful forces, but it is important to stress that gender stereotypes are perpetrated by other factors as well. Children take to the classroom notions of gender roles formed through the influence of parents and peers.

The Influence of Parents and Peers

In most cases, as soon as a child is born, interaction between parents and child begins—interaction that differs according to the sex of the child. Traditionally, a girl is thought to be fragile, to need protection, and to have needs that revolve around personal appearance and development. A boy is

seen as tough, physically active, and unemotional. Children perceive these expectations, which tend to define their reality. Because the mother is usually the primary caregiver, the female child finds it easier to learn her appropriate sex role than does the male child. The female internalizes feminine behavior and is rewarded for her identification. The male may be in a bind. He may not have a constant role model because his father may not be around as much as his mother. He frequently learns from the mother's telling him that boys "don't do" certain things. Thus boys may learn to be anxious about gender-role identity.

Gender DIMENSIONS

Gender Equality on the College Campus

In recent years, a great deal of attention has been given to gender equality on college campuses for both male and female faculty. It is common to see gender-equality goals such as the following:

1. Foster faculty and administrative accountability for gender equality in curriculum and pedagogy
2. Implement diversity initiatives
3. Promote family-friendly policies (affordable and available child care, flex time, and parental leave policies)
4. Encourage women's academic and career development
5. Establish and support strong women's centers
6. End sexual harassment of and violence against all employees

7. Correct inequities in hiring, promotion, tenure, compensation, and working conditions for women employees

Critics claim that these goals outline a plot by women's studies faculty and others to stifle academic freedom—that they will determine gender-equality standards and impose them on faculty and other employees. They worry that feminist "indoctrination" of students will lower academic standards and destroy academic debate. However, others believe that it is time to ensure that gender equality prevails throughout higher education. They point out that there are fewer women faculty overall and they are concentrated in lower ranks, less well-paid career tracks, and part-time and non-tenure positions.

Do you think that the goals presented here are needed at your college or university? How is your institution dealing with promoting gender equality? Do you feel that anything else needs to be done on your campus?

Some parents try to avoid teaching gender stereotypes.

It seems that increasing numbers of parents try to prevent teaching gender-role stereotypes to their children, but this can be hard to achieve. They may act differently toward a child, depending on the child's sex, even if they do not intend to do so. For example, if a boy is asked to participate in sports or help his father with outside chores while a girl is asked to wash dishes or clean her room, this pattern sends messages about expected sex roles.

What children observe at home in regard to sex roles also sends important messages. For example, even when both parents work outside the home in managerial or professional jobs, the redistribution of roles within the family has not yet clearly or completely occurred. American women—even those employed full time—continue to work more hours than do their husbands on household tasks, and there is little evidence that men's proportionate share of family work has changed much in recent years. Many social scientists feel parents are very influential in regard to establishing sex roles.

The question of whether we can, or want to, raise "gender-neutral" children has been debated. Some argue that it not only is possible, but also can result

Ethical DIMENSIONS

ETHICS

Extreme Gender Roles—The Price of Honor

News of an interesting ethical situation related to female sexual behavior was reported in Jordan. Sirhan, a 35-year-old man, was proud to say that he had murdered his younger sister. She had reported to the police that she had been raped. Sirhan said, "She committed a mistake, even if it was against her will. Anyway, it's better to have one person die than to have the whole family die from shame." To Sirhan, it was more ethical to kill his sister than to suffer from the shame that would have sullied his "male honor."

For centuries, Arab men have engaged in "honor killing"—the intrafamily killing of errant females. Honor killing has its roots in the crude Arabic expression "A man's honor lies between the legs of a woman." For Arab women, virginity before marriage and fidelity afterward are considered musts. Men are expected to control their female relatives. If a woman strays, it is widely believed, the dignity of the man can be restored only by killing her. In Jordan the 25 or so cases of honor killing documented every year make up a quarter of all homicides there.

Forbidden sexual activity is not always the issue. Marrying or divorcing against the family's wishes can also provoke murder. The law winks at honor killers.

If a man catches his wife or a close female relative in the act of adultery and kills her, he is exempt from punishment.

Running away is next to impossible for women, because Arab societies are close knit, and few women have the means to live alone. "Rafa," 20 years old, was locked up in prison to protect her after her uncles and brothers vowed to murder her for having a 3-day affair with a coworker. She said, "With the mistake I made, I deserve to die."

Honor killing has started to receive media attention, and a hotline has been created for women in distress. However, honor killings are hard to combat because of the extremely strong feelings related to male and female gender roles in Jordan.

The exact origins of honor killings are not known. Among northern Arabian tribes, the practice predates Islam in the seventh century. It is sometimes a problem even in the United States. For example, Faleh al-Maleki was convicted in Arizona of killing his daughter. He ran over her with his car. He was upset with her fondness for tight jeans and makeup and a reluctance to accede to his plans for her. The plans included an arranged marriage to a man in Iraq (Labi, 2011).

? Did You Know . . .

In 2014, Barbie turned 55. The doll debuted in 1959 as a teenage fashion model, but through the years Barbie has been many things. Barbie has been an astronaut, a medical student, an Olympic athlete, a member of the military, and a candidate for President. She has had more than 100 careers and represented many nationalities. Some have called her the first feminist.

Others, however, think that Barbie is not a good role model because of her emphasis on appearance. The doll is 11.5 inches tall and weighs 7.25 ounces. This translates into a woman who would be 5 feet 9 inches tall, weighing about 110 pounds. It has been argued that this is an unrealistic and unhealthy build that promotes negative stereotypes for both males and females.

Barbie is so small that, if she were human, she would have to walk on all fours because of her tiny feet, and she would have room for only half a liver. To counteract her appearance, Nickolay Lamm created the Lammily doll—what the Barbie would look like if she actually had the measurements of an average 19-year-old woman's body. There is also a sticker-extension pack available for approximately $6 that gives the doll's face acne, freckles, moles, and the ability to blush. Lamm also included scrapes, bruises, and scars because they are part of real life.

Some people believe that Barbie sales have dropped because unrealistic ideals are losing clout in both the toy and fashion worlds. They point out that trends in toy sales are fiscal evidence that children and their parents want natural, realistic beauty rather than unattainable ideals.

Do you think that Barbie has been and is a positive or negative role model? Is it better to use a Barbie doll or a Lammily doll with young children? Why do you think so? If you were in charge of making dolls, how would they compare with Barbie and the Lammily doll?

Sources: Stampler, L. The new "normal Barbie" comes with an average woman's proportions—and cellulite-sticker accessories. *Time.com*, 2014. Available: http://time.com/3593968/the-new-normal-barbie-comes-with-an-average-womans-proportions-and-cellulite-sticker-extension-packs/; Stampler, L. Bye, bye, Barbie: 2015 is the year we abandon unrealistic beauty ideals. *Time.com*, 2015. Available: http://time.com/3667580/mattel-barbie-earnings-plus-size-body-image/.

---

in more positive self-esteem. They say that children raised with gender-neutral expectations will have a more open, positive view of the world in general. Others argue that gender and gender-role expectations are tied very closely to familial and cultural expectations. They believe that gender-specific role fulfillment is vital to certain cultures, ensuring the survival of important cultural traditions (Can we raise "gender-neutral" children?, 2003).

Sanchez-Flores (2004) pointed out that young men are exposed to many messages from different sources that inform them about what it means to be a man. Ideals such as "boys don't play with dolls," or "boys don't wear pink" may seem outdated to many adults today, but social groups still successfully transfer messages like this from generation to generation. As a result, boys live in social networks and follow norms that determine both acceptable behaviors and the consequences for not behaving that way. Another message males hear is "boys will be boys." It is most often used to dismiss actions that are challenging or seem impossible to change. This gives the impression that gender excuses behavior.

The peer group is also an important influence in learning about sex roles. Even early in life, children choose members of their own sex as playmates most of the time. This segregation by sex continues into the school years and helps contribute to sex-typing in play activities that help prepare children for adult roles.

The influence of peers becomes increasingly important by late childhood and early adolescence. Conformity can be viewed as being very important, and behaving according to traditional roles promotes social acceptance by peers. Those who do not behave in ways accepted by the peer group are likely to be pressured and even ridiculed.

There is no question that biology is important. There are biological factors that tilt males and females in different directions related to their interests and behavior, but numerous social factors influence the way the biological tilts can be redirected. In other words, regarding the nature versus nurture debate, biology does matter; however, the way we are treated and what we learn can drastically influence our expression of gender roles.

As a final thought related to sexism, it has been pointed out that sexist attitudes are not always hostile. Glick and Fiske (2011) note that subjective affection can be seen as a form of prejudice—a concept they labeled as "benevolent sexism." In other words, there can be negative consequences of attitudes that idealize women as pure, moral, pedestal-worthy objects of men's adoration, protection, and provision. People

Danish-born Mianne Bagger, a successful amateur golfer, was barred from membership in the Australian Ladies Professional Golf Association because she was born male. Bagger's contention, like that of many transsexuals, was that she was, in fact, born female.

who endorse benevolent sexism feel positively toward women, but only when women conform to highly traditional ideals about how women "should be." While the path to benevolent sexism may be paved with good intentions, it reinforces the assumption that men possess greater competence than women, whom benevolent sexists view as wonderful, but weak and fragile. Cross-national comparisons show that hostile and benevolent sexism go hand in hand (nations that endorse hostile sexism also endorse benevolent sexism). These beliefs work together because benevolent sexism "rewards" women when they fulfill traditional roles, whereas hostile sexism punishes women who do not toe the line, thereby combining to maintain traditional relations.

Gender Identity Difficulty

Some people experience **gender dysphoria**—they believe they are trapped in the body of the wrong sex. They feel they are not really the gender indicated by their genitals. The term *gender dysphoria* is sometimes used interchangeably with the term **transsexual**. Sometimes the term *transsexual* is used to refer to people who wish to have, or have

---

gender dysphoria   Feeling trapped in the body of the "wrong" sex.

transsexual   A person whose gender identity does not match her or his biological sex; also a person who wishes to have, or has had, his or her gender surgically altered to conform to his or her gender identity.

transgender   A general term used when one's identity does not match one's physical/genetic sex. It includes such diverse categories as transsexualism and transvestism.

---

had, their genitals surgically altered to conform to their gender identity. Therefore, an anatomically male transsexual feels that he is a female but that some quirk of fate provided him with male genitals. He wants to be socially identified as the female he believes himself to be. He does not derive sexual excitement from cross-dressing, as is the case with a transvestite, but views himself as a female.

Sometimes the terminology used related to gender identity difficulty can be tricky. For example, in addition to the terms mentioned previously, in recent years the term **transgender** has become more common. According to the International Foundation for Gender Education (2005), gender is a person's innate sense of themselves as being male or female, which may differ from their biological sex. The terms "sex" and "gender" are often used interchangeably, but they are not the same. People whose sex and gender differ are known as transgender.

Transsexualism, which is a gender orientation, is not to be confused with homosexuality, a sexual orientation. Some transsexuals are homosexual, and some are heterosexual. Unless a transsexual chooses to tell another person, an observer will probably not know whether homosexual or heterosexual behavior is being practiced.

According to the American Psychological Association Task Force on Gender Identity and Gender Variance (2008), the prevalence of gender identity disorder in adults is estimated to be about 1 in 11,900 for male-to-female transsexuals and 1 in 30,400 for female-to-male transsexuals. Male-to-female transsexuality is 1.5 to 3 times more prevalent than female-to-male transsexuality.

Boylan (2003) wrote an interesting book on this subject entitled *She's Not There: A Life in Two Genders*. Even as a child, James Boylan felt that he was supposed to be a woman, but he thought everyone would reject him if he made the transition. So he lived as a man, married, and had children. In spite of his loving family, a successful career, and hobbies he loved, he eventually decided that he couldn't live with being a man. So he made the transition to living as a woman (Jenny Boylan). The book includes a portrait of a loving marriage—the love of James for his wife, Grace, and against all odds, the enduring love of Grace for the woman who became her "sister," Jenny. Jenny's wife, children, mother, and colleagues responded with love and acceptance. Her sister cut off contact. Boylan feels fortunate to have been given a rare gift in life—the gift of being able to see into the worlds of both men and women with clear eyes. Through it all, Boylan was a professor of English at Colby College in Maine.

When an employee switches genders, there can sometimes be difficult issues for employers (Armour,

2005). Issues can relate to how an employee informs coworkers about switching genders, how clients might react, how others will handle a transitioning employee using the restroom, and logistical issues such as changing security badges to reflect a new gender. In many states it is legal to fire employees because they are transgender. However, many companies have put policies in place to protect against discrimination of transgender employees. Major companies, such as Merrill Lynch, Chevron, BP, and Microsoft are among those with such policies.

In April of 2012 the Equal Employment Opportunity Commission ruled that a refusal to hire or otherwise discriminate on the basis of gender identity is by definition sex discrimination under federal law. This was a groundbreaking decision because it set a national standard of enforcement that offered employers clear guidance on the issue (Rowe & Woodard, 2012).

Wilson (2005) reported on an interesting case at the University of Nebraska where, in 2005, a popular professor named Wally Bacon returned for the fall semester as a female, W. Meredith Bacon. After 29 years in the political science department, and 37 years of marriage, Ms. Bacon decided to become what she thought she was since she was a young child. In an eight-page letter, the professor explained to colleagues the decision to become a woman. Students were told that she would be happy to answer their questions if they desired. Few asked her any questions. The university administration was supportive. This had not been the case in some other situations. In one small college in New Hampshire, one man was fired after he informed the administration that he planned to become a woman. In Indiana, a professor decided to leave after his decision to disclose his sex-change plans to the college's president backfired. He says the president voiced her support, but said that he would lose his job because of the potential loss of contributions from donors who might disapprove. Ms. Bacon's wife, Lynne, remained supportive and the couple stayed together. Lynne mourned the loss of Wally, but also enjoyed counseling her spouse on her new female look.

There have been issues related to transgender athletes. The first famous transgender athlete in the U.S. was a former Yale tennis captain named Richard Raskin who underwent surgery in 1975 and became Renee Richards. She won a landmark legal battle in 1977 that enabled her to play as a female at the U.S. Open. Yet, it is only recently that transgender athletes are gaining sustained recognition from sports' governing bodies. In 2004 the International Olympic Committee ruled that any trans athlete who wants to compete against those not of their birth gender must undergo sex reassignment surgery and two years of hormone therapy to go from male to female. However, in 2011 the National Collegiate Athletic Association (NCAA) took a different approach. It decided against requiring surgery which typically costs five figures and isn't covered by insurance. The NCAA also said that trans females need to undergo only one year of testosterone suppression before they can compete against women, and trans males can receive a medical exemption to take testosterone under a doctor's supervision but can no longer compete on a women's team. Some colleges have created their own transgender inclusion policies (Torre & Epstein, 2012). It will be interesting to see what happens in the future related to policies for transgender athletes.

Wilson (2005) also reported that psychiatrists estimate that 1 in 30,000 men suffer from transgendered feelings. However, groups representing transgendered people say that number of men and boys who experience "intense transsexualism" is closer to 1 in 300 to 500 with about 1 in 2,500 having undergone genital surgery. She further reported that businesses are more likely than colleges to protect employees from discrimination. According to the Human Rights Campaign, an advocacy group for gay, transgendered, and bisexual people, 73 *Fortune* 500 companies do so, compared to 37 universities.

According to the National Center for Transgender Equality, transgender and gender-nonconforming people face injustice at every turn. To get more information about this issue, they surveyed 6,450 transgender and gender-nonconforming study participants to determine the depth and breadth of injustice in their lives (Grant et al., 2011). The key findings included the following: 41% of respondents reported attempting suicide compared to 1.6% of the general population; 90% reported experiencing harassment, mistreatment, or discrimination on the job; 26% reported having lost a job due to being transgender or gender nonconforming; 19% reported having been refused a home or apartment and 11% reported being evicted because of their gender identity/expression; 21% had been able to update all of their IDs and records; and 19% reported being refused medical care due to their transgender or gender-nonconforming status.

The proportion of transgender people who attempt suicide (41%) does not necessarily factor in successful attempts. That is a statistic that the people behind Trans Lifeline (www.translifeline.org) want to see decreased. Trans Lifeline went live in late 2014. A major aim of this organization is to give people in crisis—whether that person is a suicidal, closeted teenager or the confused parent of a 6-year-old child—access to volunteers who can understand what they are going through right away and direct them to help in their area. Connecting with good resources could spare people a lot of pain (Steinmetz, 2014).

Light et al. (2014) found that some transgender individuals face increased barriers to healthcare services, including those related to reproductive health. These authors surveyed 41 transgender men who had given birth. Half of the participants received prenatal care from a physician, and 78% delivered in a hospital. In general, the subjects reported low levels of healthcare provider awareness and knowledge about the unique needs of pregnant transgender men as well as a desire for resources to support transgender men through their pregnancy. Developing transgender-appropriate services and interventions may improve the health and healthcare experiences of transgender men.

There is also a need for health plans to cover transgender care. In 2015, several health insurance carriers for federal employees started covering gender affirmation surgery and other transgender care. However, not all carriers were in agreement that they should do so (*Some health plans for federal employees to cover transgender care*, 2014).

Believing that it is time to initiate policies that reduce the burdens on an already marginalized and vulnerable population, an increasing number of colleges and universities have dropped barriers to enrolling transgender students. This step is usually just a matter of changing a few words in their guidelines. For example, at one college the wording now allows "any qualified student who is female or identifies as a woman" to be considered for admission (Misner, 2014).

One of the questions that typically arises for transgender persons is which bathroom they can use. In Maine, the family of a transgender high school student filed a lawsuit against a school district that forced the student to use a staff restroom rather than a facility reserved for pupils. The court ruled that the school district had violated the state's Human Rights Act. The court also awarded the family of the transgender teenager $75,000 and directed the school district to allow transgender students access "to school restrooms that are consistent with their gender identity." This marked the first time a state's highest court ruled that a transgender person has the right to use the restroom of the gender with which the individual identifies (Stout, 2014).

In recent years, two transgender individuals have become well known to the public. Laverne Cox is the first openly transgender person to be nominated for a Primetime Emmy Award in the acting category for her performances in the TV show *Orange Is the New Black*. She is also well known for her appearances in other TV shows and a number of films. Cox was the first openly transgender person to appear on the cover of *Time* magazine. She has been named woman of year by *Glamour* magazine, was an Anti-Violence Project Courage Award honoree, was on the *Ebony* Power 100 list, was on *People* magazine's "World's Most Beautiful Women" list, and was included in *Time* magazine's "Most Influential People" list, among other recognitions. Cox has been noted for being a trailblazer in the transgender community.

The second example is Caitlyn Jenner. Prior to coming out as a transgender woman in 2015, she was known as Bruce Jenner. Bruce was famous as the 1976 Olympic men's decathlon event champion and as an American television personality (*Keeping Up with the Kardashians* and other TV shows). He was married three times and has six children. In 2015, Jenner came out as a transwoman and began to refer to herself with feminine pronouns. Many news sources describe her as the most famous openly transgender person in the world. As you might expect, many people had varying opinions about Jenner coming out. Here are some examples of comments:

- "The strong love and devotion Caitlyn's family has for her was deeply moving."

- "It is annoying that the vast amount of media coverage was celebratory."

- "Don't call Caitlyn 'brave' when there are lots of people more deserving of that label."

- "Caitlyn has done a very brave thing and is a positive example to others."

- "Bruce Jenner's becoming Caitlyn was disrespectful to the way he was created in God's image."

- "People should be free to live as what they believe their correct gender is."

- "People who are transgender should keep that information to themselves and not be public about it or change the way they live."

In a recent experiment, a group of children were shown photos of both Bruce and Caitlyn Jenner. They described the photo of Bruce simply, commenting they could see a strong man who was running. They described the photo of Caitlyn with words like "happy," "confident," and "calm." They were surprised when they were told that the two photos were of the same person. One child said, "Who she wants to be is who she should be."

Do you agree with this child? How do you feel about the opinions expressed in the bulleted comments? Which of them do you agree with?

There is no clear understanding of either the causes or the nature of transsexualism. Some theorists believe the causes relate to early parent–child relationships related to gender roles of mothers and fathers and the ways that parents treated the child.

Ethical DIMENSIONS

Should Dad Dress as a Woman? Should Dad Participate in His Child's Field Trip while Dressed as a Woman?

Most of the kids on a fourth-grade field trip did not notice or did not care that a classmate's father was dressed as a woman, in jeans, a sweater, and nice shoes. Most of the teachers were equally untroubled. However, one parent spotted the "cross-dressing" dad and alerted some friends. As a result, one school board member proposed a new policy that would require parent chaperones to wear "gender-appropriate" clothing for school functions.

The father described had dressed as a woman at work for years, kept his hair long, worn slacks and blouses, and used a name that could be either male or female. He had actively participated in his daughters' education and in their schools while in women's attire with no previous problems.

Some people argue that it is ethical to require parents to wear "gender-appropriate" clothing at school functions. Others argue that it is not ethical to do this because it violates the parents' rights to dress as they please—particularly because to qualify for sex-change surgery individuals must first go through a prolonged period of transition when they present themselves in public as the gender they want to become.

What do you think?

Others focus on hormonal imbalances that influenced the brain during prenatal development; however, no one knows for sure.

Gender-Reassignment Surgery

The idea of gender reassignment is controversial, and psychotherapy has not been very useful for most transsexuals. Surgery is part of gender reassignment, but, because it is irreversible, professionals usually require that the transsexual live publicly as a member of the desired gender for a year before undergoing surgery. During this time it is easier for the person or the medical personnel to change their minds. Surgery is not something to be taken lightly, and it is usually done only after careful screening of the individual.

A lifetime of hormonal treatment is also necessary. Male-to-female transsexuals take estrogen. It causes fatty deposits to develop in the breasts and hips, inhibits beard growth, and softens the skin. Female-to-male transsexuals take androgens, which promote deepening of the voice, masculine hair distribution, larger muscles, and loss of fatty deposits in the breasts and hips. The clitoris may also grow larger.

It is not possible to construct internal genital organs or gonads, so gender-reassignment surgery is mostly cosmetic. Male-to-female surgery is usually more successful because it is easier to construct a vagina than a working penis. The vast majority of transsexuals who undergo surgery are happy with the outcome. Gender-reassignment surgery is done in only a few places in the United States, is very expensive, and is usually not covered by health insurance

policies. Indeed, only several thousand such operations have been performed in the United States since 1953. Clearly this is something to be done only with extensive counseling and medical support.

A special case of potential gender-reassignment surgery relates to the question of what should be done with intersex infants—those born with ambiguous or mixed genitalia and chromosomal structures. It is estimated that every year in the United States about 65,000 babies are born with ambiguous genitalia. Some people believe that feminizing surgery should be done at birth to ensure that the baby will be able to function later as an adult woman. Others feel that children should remain intact until they are older and decide for themselves what, if anything, to do about their ambiguous genitalia.

Some experts point out that gender depends on more than anatomy or hormones. They feel gender is essentially hard-wired into the brain before birth. A review of 94 intersex children found that over half of the genetic males "transitioned" to become boys despite being raised as girls and undergoing female sex assignment. More doctors seem to be putting off sex-assignment surgery until later, so as to be more certain about the person's gender. The Intersex Society of North America (www.isna.org) is a good place to learn more about personal stories (Surgery may be hasty for unclear gender, 2005).

The Influence of Gender Stereotypes on Sexuality

As you can see, gender-role stereotyping limits self-expression and personal growth and development,

Gender roles are learned in many ways and from many different people.

The pressure to conform to socialization has provoked in both sexes anxieties that we are only now beginning to discuss freely and reevaluate. The emphasis on the macho aspects of male performance tends to obliterate consideration of men as sensitive, gentle, nurturant, and intimate beings who can relate to adult partners on a variety of levels. The emphasis on the passivity of women has long neglected consideration and acknowledgment of them as full sexual beings with the same needs as men for expression and fulfillment.

Males and females need to be able to express feelings heretofore defined as either masculine or feminine. They need to be directive and sensitive to function effectively. Women need to make decisions in parenting, in controlling their careers, and in their sexual behavior. Men need to accept responsibility for parenting, be comfortable as receivers as well as givers, and accept that sharing intimacy and intimate acts does not mean loss of control.

Many people in our society still differ in their expectations for interpersonal relationships. Some women still expect assertive, in-command, successful men; some men still expect supportive, helpful, receiving women. Stereotypes of the dominant male and the submissive female continue to influence the interpersonal dynamics between the genders. All people have been socialized into these expectations, and socialization probably accounts for more of these distinctions than does biology.

Men have often learned to equate sexual activity with the fulfillment of their needs for support, tenderness, and the feeling of being loved. Women have often not been taught that receiving sexual pleasure has value. Mixed feelings about what they really feel and what society tells them they are supposed to feel can confuse everyone.

The popular press suggests that men and women may always have problems because they are so different. Examples often given are in communication (she wants more talk; he wants more action); intimacy (she needs to relax to participate in intimate sexual

and that limiting in turn affects sexuality. When individuals define masculinity and femininity for themselves, they express personal beliefs through gender-role behaviors. The traditional definitions are confining, emphasizing as they do conventional conformity to long-existing gender-role norms. We have referred particularly to males being socialized toward initiating, aggressive, and directive behaviors and females being socialized toward receiving, passive, and compliant behaviors. In descriptions of anatomical function, for example, the vagina has tended to be described as receiver, not for sexual pleasure but for reproduction. The penis is often described in terms of insertion based on need, dominance, and desire. Thus again, men initiate and women are passively receptive.

Did You Know . . .

A study of 150 undergraduate students examined how being visually "checked out" (an objectifying gaze) by a member of the other sex affected each student's performance on math problems. The gaze caused decreased math performance for women, but somewhat ironically the same women also wanted more interaction with the person who had objectified them. The men were unfazed when females stared at their chests. The researchers felt that one explanation for the math performance change is stereotype threat. Math performance may decrease because the gaze conveys that women's looks are valued over their other qualities. The objectifying gaze may trigger a vicious cycle in which women underperform but continue to interact with the people who led them to underperform in the first place (Gervais, 2011).

© Stephen Coburn/ShutterStock, Inc.

Male and female roles are often very similar.

behavior, but he needs to participate to relax); division of household labor and child care (she says she does more; he talks about how much he does); and money and careers (she says he does not value her job as much as his; he notes that he makes more money).

Related to communication, the following are some of the ways to close the gender gap:

- Get honest before you get angry: Something deeper than dry cleaning or dishwashing is probably bothering you.

- Establish systems for sharing chores and child care.

- Negotiate the division of labor and the division of love.

- Do not get locked into your role: Try swapping responsibilities on occasion.

- Express your emotional needs and expectations and really listen to your partner.

- Review the cultural messages of your childhood to help understand the conflicts inherent in your new roles.

- Give each other time to change: Do not monitor or criticize.

- Accept your differences and applaud each other's strengths.

- Protect your intimate time together.

There is increased thinking that similarities between men and women, particularly in the human struggle for intimacy, far outweigh differences. Healthy couples appear to transcend traditional gender roles, and the roles, such as pursuer and distancer, are interchangeable. There is no one definition of an intimate, healthy relationship. Love and respect are essential in a good relationship.

In terms of human sexual expression, both partners need the freedom to be self-disclosing, intimate, and communicative. Restrictive definitions of roles serve only to repress the joy, pleasure, and emotionally fulfilling responses of sexual intimacy. And perhaps equally important is the fact that gender-role stereotyping also restricts personal fulfillment in nonsexual relationships between men and women.

The Possibilities of Androgyny

According to legend, there once were three kinds of humans—the male, the female, and the androgyne. All humans had two sets of arms and legs. The males and females had two faces and two sets of genitalia of the same sex. The androgynes each had one masculine face and one feminine face, one set of female genitalia, and one set of male genitalia. This group of humans had tremendous strength and an arrogant nature, which offended the gods.

Zeus, to punish them, split the androgynes in half and remade them as hemipeople. Thus men and women have lost their other half and seek it in other people.

The word **androgynous** originated from the story of the androgynes. An androgynous person is one who has a combination of masculine and feminine characteristics—one who exhibits some traits of both masculinity and femininity as defined by the society. Thus an androgynous male might be nurturing in addition to providing, and an androgynous female might be assertive as well as soft-spoken. The idea of androgyny can serve as a means of doing away with gender-role stereotyping. Many people believe that they must conform absolutely to society's notions of maleness and femaleness, especially in the ways they acknowledge and express (or repress and deny) their feelings. In conforming, they lose the opportunity to express themselves as individuals. But if, as a society, we were to view people as androgynous, then

androgynous Exhibiting a combination of masculine and feminine traits as defined by the society.

Can you tell for sure which individuals in this picture are male and which are female?

all of us might consider the expression of a variety of emotions appropriate for everyone. A significant benefit would be that people who expressed their true feelings, unswayed by the demands of gender-role stereotypes, would experience a greater depth of sexual intimacy with their partners than would those concerned solely with how manly or womanly they appear.

The concept of androgyny has been around a long time. For example, in 1975 Sandra Bem, a noted proponent of androgyny, indicated that stereotypical gender roles were restrictive and unhealthy. She described androgynous people, by contrast, as flexible and healthy. She felt that rigidity in gender-role expectations was reflected in inflexible responses in real-life situations. To test her theory, Bem developed the Bem Sex Role Inventory. She gave a group of men and women a list of personality characteristics—some traditionally masculine (assertiveness, ambition, independence), some traditionally feminine (dependence, sensitivity, gentleness), and some neutral (friendliness, likability)—and asked the subjects to rate the accuracy of each term in describing them. Participants were then placed in situations that tested masculine and feminine behaviors such as nurturance, responsiveness to a troubled person, and conformity. Men who had described themselves as having masculine traits were not comfortable with "feminine" activities, and women who had described themselves as having feminine traits were not comfortable doing "masculine" tasks. But androgynous men and women were able to function in all situations.

It should be noted that not all studies are supportive of the androgyny concept. Yet many experts and numerous studies tend to agree that freedom from stereotypical gender roles allows for greater health and life satisfaction. People continue to do research related to androgyny. However, others criticize the concept and do not place much confidence in it.

The Women's Movement

In recent decades we have seen social upheaval that has changed our society in a variety of ways. Patterns of sexual behavior have been affected, for example, by contraceptive technology, abortion, and sterilization. Divorce has become more acceptable, and changes in leisure pursuits, delays in pregnancy, and the acceptance of intentional childlessness all offer women a greater diversity in lifestyle. But perhaps the single most important effect has been the women's movement. The ability of women to explore their potential has never been as great as at this time. Economic independence, control over reproduction, and choices in relationships and lifestyle have given women freedom from domination by men and the opportunity for self-direction as individuals. Statistics illustrate the increasing inroads into the labor force being made by women as they seek to achieve economic independence and/or to supplement the family's income.

There were at least four groups who converged in the 1960s to help create the modern women's movement. First, there were those, such as Eleanor Roosevelt, who used John F. Kennedy's Presidential Commission on the Status of Women to reveal

Eleanor Roosevelt helped raise people's awareness about sexism.

Did You Know . . .

Some people think that the women's movement started in the 1960s. There were actually many significant events prior to that time. Here is a list of selected important events related to the Women's Movement (National Women's History Project, 2015; http://www.nwhp.org/resources/womens-rights-movement/detailed-timeline/).

1769 American colonies based their laws on English common law. By marriage, husband and wife were considered one person under the law.

1777 All states passed laws taking away women's rights to vote.

1839 The first state (Mississippi) granted women the right to hold property in their own name, with their husbands' permission.

1869 The first woman suffrage law in the United States was passed in the territory of Wyoming.

1908 The first state (Wyoming) granted women the right to vote in all elections.

1916 Margaret Sanger tested New York's anticontraception law by establishing a clinic in Brooklyn. She helped establish a woman's right to control her own body.

1920 The Nineteenth Amendment to the U.S. Constitution, which states that the right to vote shall not be denied based on sex, was ratified.

1938 The Fair Labor Standards Act established a minimum wage without regard to sex.

1963 The Equal Pay Act promised equitable pay for the same work regardless of race, color, religion, national origin, or sex of the worker.

1968 Executive Order 11246 prohibited sex discrimination by government contractors and required affirmative action plans for hiring women.

1969 The Seventh Circuit Court of Appeals ruled that women meeting the physical requirements could work in many jobs that had been for men only.

California adopted the nation's first "no fault" divorce law, allowing divorce by mutual consent.

1972 Title IX prohibited sex discrimination in all aspects of education programs that receive federal support.

1973 The U.S. Supreme Court declared that the Constitution protects women's right to terminate an early pregnancy, thus making abortion legal in the United States (*Roe v. Wade*).

1974 Housing discrimination on the basis of sex and credit discrimination against women were outlawed by Congress.

1978 The Pregnancy Discrimination Act banned employment discrimination against pregnant women.

1984 Sex discrimination in membership policies of organizations such as the Jaycees, Kiwanis, and Rotary was forbidden by the Supreme Court.

1993 The U.S. Supreme Court ruled that the victim did not need to show that she suffered physical or serious psychological injury as a result of sexual harassment.

1994 Congress adopted the Gender Equity in Education Act to train teachers in gender equity, promote math and science learning for girls, counsel pregnant teens, and prevent sexual harassment.

1997 Elaborating on Title IX, the Supreme Court ruled that college athletic programs must actively involve roughly equal numbers of men and women to qualify for federal support.

1998 The Supreme Court ruled that employers are liable for sexual harassment even in instances when a supervisor's threats are not carried out. However, it also said the employer can defend itself by showing it took steps to prevent or promptly correct any sexually harassing behavior and the employee did not take advantage of available opportunities to stop the behavior or complain of the behavior.

1999 The U.S. Supreme Court ruled that a woman can sue for punitive damages for sex discrimination if the antidiscrimination law was violated with malice or indifference to the law, even if that conduct was not especially severe.

2003 The U.S. Supreme Court ruled that states can be sued in federal court for violations of the Family and Medical Leave Act.

2005 The U.S. Supreme Court ruled that Title IX, which prohibits discrimination based on sex, also inherently prohibits disciplining someone for complaining about sex-based discrimination.

(Continued)

2006 The U.S. Supreme Court upheld the ban on the "partial-birth" abortion procedure. It was the first ruling to ban a specific type of abortion procedure.

2009 President Obama signed the Lily Ledbetter Fair Pay Restoration Act, which allows victims of pay discrimination to file a complaint with the government against their employer within 180 days of their last paycheck. Previously, victims (mostly women) were allowed only 180 days from the date of the first unfair paycheck.

2010 The Patient Protection and Affordable Health Care Act is signed into law. Under this law, private health insurance companies must provide birth control without copayments or deductibles. The law requires private insurance companies to cover preventive services.

2013 The ban against women in military combat positions is removed.

2013 The Violence Against Women Act is reauthorized. The new bill extends coverage to women of Native American tribal lands who are attacked by non-tribal residents, as well as lesbians and immigrants.

2013 The U.S. Supreme Court decides that a key part of the Defense of Marriage Act, the law that restricts federal recognition of same-sex marriage, is unconstitutional because it violates the equal protection clause of the Constitution.

Multicultural DIMENSIONS

Has the Women's Movement in France Caught Up?

In 2011, the former International Monetary Fund chief, a Frenchman, was arrested in New York for the alleged sexual assault and attempted rape of a hotel housekeeper. Many key figures in France's intellectual and political elite converged to protect him. They minimized, cast doubt upon, or even ignored the plight of the single mother who had accused him. This angered a consortium of French feminist groups, which in response gathered thousands of signatures on a petition denouncing sexual violence against women, sexist remarks on the French airwaves, and the rise to the surface of sexist and reactionary remarks among leading French figures.

The show of anger by the feminist groups forced the political and media elite to quickly change their tune. Feminist commentary—some written by men—appeared in France's mainstream publications. Women reporters started to share their own stories of harassment and even assault by powerful men. There was talk about how feminist issues could play a prominent role in the election of the next French president. It was pointed out that all of this could mark the end of an era in which talking too forcefully about inequities between men and women was rejected as too old-school, too angry, too American.

Many French people believe that there has not been enough progress in the promotion of equality between men and women. Generous family policies aimed at promoting and allowing women to balance work and family have had the effect of reinforcing old gender stereotypes, as employers were unwilling to hire women of childbearing age on the grounds that they will take too many costly and disruptive maternity leaves. Many younger women and men were raised on the promise of equality, but have grown angry when reality has not met their expectations. For example, political parties are supposed to offer equal numbers of male and female candidates, but that hasn't happened. There have been repeated legislative efforts to promote pay equality, but wage inequality between men and women has persisted or even worsened in recent years. The trend towards workplace flexibility has tended to push women disproportionately into unstable and low-paid part-time positions.

In France, appearances have changed, but real life has not. It remains to be seen whether women's issues will remain front and center, but it seems that the dialogue about gender relations in France has been forever altered.

Source: Data from Warner, J. Cherchez les Femmes: Has the Women's Movement in France Finally Caught Up? *Time, 177, no. 23* (June 6, 2011): 38–39. Available at http://www.time.com/time/world/article/0,8599,2074070,00.html.

pervasive sexism in American society and law. Second, there were those who were from the civil rights movement, broadening the definition of equality to include women. The third group, working-class women, turned to feminism and the women's movement in their struggle for the Equal Pay Act of 1963. The fourth group was made up of white, middle-class suburban women, who found themselves stifled by gender stereotypes (Kerber, 1999).

The women's movement probably also is responsible for increased attention to victims of sexual assault and other forms of violence. A better understanding of aggressive behavior, improved services for assault victims, and greatly increased education on these topics are all evidence of this increased attention. In addition, the public discussion of sexual harassment throughout recent years must be at least partially attributed to the women's movement. There is also a growing body of literature about many issues related to gender.

With the change in the present and potential status of women, new pressures and anxieties about role redefinition and intimate relationships have arisen. Women are more informed about their physiology and their right not only to expect sexual fulfillment and satisfaction but also to initiate or refuse sexual behavior. For many, traditional values concerning virginity, self-sacrifice for children, lifelong commitment to marriage, and the support role of women are giving way to new modes of commitment. These changes can be seen as giving both women and men a chance to explore a number of alternatives.

Some people feel true female empowerment has been shown by women (notably some movie stars) who have chosen as partners men who are less successful than they are. Because many modern women work outside the home and are financially independent, they are empowered enough to make a choice among men based on their personality, as opposed to making a choice only among men who earn as much or more. His career is less important than hers, so when they go out she gets all the attention.

The Institute for Women's Policy Research reports that gains in education and income and an increased presence in politics helped women boost their economic and social status. Yet, even states rated highly in its report must progress for women to gain equality with men. The Institute looks at political participation, employment and earnings, economic autonomy, reproductive rights, and health and well-being in all states. Detailed results can be seen at the Institute's website at www.iwpr.org.

Since the enactment of Title IX in 1972, female high school athletic participation has increased by more than 900% and female college athletic participation has increased by almost 500%. An

Women have had more and varied opportunities in recent years.

unprecedented number of girls and women are playing sports and participating in activities that used to be perceived as primarily male (or at least dominated by males), including ice hockey, boxing, wrestling, and football, among others. However, there are still significantly fewer women than men in administrative and coaching positions. Even though many institutions are still not in compliance with Title IX, women continue to gain opportunities to participate and lead in sport. Some of them are thriving even in male-dominated sports and will no doubt continue to push the envelope.

The topic of women in the military has received increasing attention in recent years. In 1990, the National Board of the National Organization of Women (NOW) adopted a policy about women in the military. It said: "NOW demands equality for women in joining the military and in training, job assignments, and benefits in the military; and NOW actively supports elimination of statutory restrictions on women in the military" (Women in the military, 1990).

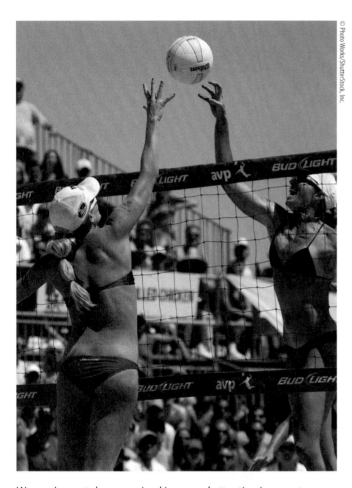

Women's sports have received increased attention in recent years.

Since 1995 a number of significant events have occurred related to women in the military (Chronology of significant legal and policy changes affecting women in the military: 1947–2003, 2005). For example, in 1995, the Marine Corps selected a woman for aviation training for the first time. Between 1996 and 2001, more than 15,000 American servicewomen served in Bosnia. In 1998, women aviators flew combat missions for the first time in Operation Desert Fox. In 1999, the Navy opened Coastal Mine Hunters and Mine Counter Measures ships to women. Also, women aviators participated in combat operations during the air war in Kosovo. In 2000, two women sailors were killed and several wounded in a terrorist attack on the USS *Cole*. In 2001, military women deployed to the Afghan theater as part of Operation Enduring Freedom, the war on terrorism. In 2002, the first woman Marine was killed in Afghanistan. In 2002, the Defense Authorizations Act required the Department of Defense to submit an annual report on the status of women in the services. In 2003, more than 25,400 women were deployed in support of Operation Iraqi Freedom. In 2013, CNN reported that more than 200,000 women were in the active-duty

military, including 69 generals and admirals. Women made up 14.5% of the active-duty force of nearly 1.4 million. This number includes 74,000 women in the Army, 53,000 in the Navy, 62,000 in the Air Force, and 14,000 in the Marine Corps. Nearly 167,000 women were in the enlisted ranks, making up 14.2% of that force. There were 36,000 women in the officer corps, or 16.6% (By the numbers: Women in the U.S. military, 2013). In 2015 the first women completed training as Army Rangers. Differences of opinion exist about how far equality should go for men and women in the military.

As more women began to serve in the military, a practical issue came up. Military gear was made with the male physique in mind. For women, this meant body armor that fit so poorly that it was tough to fire a weapon, combat uniforms with knee pads that hit around mid-shin, and flight suits that made it nearly impossible to urinate while in a plane. New combat uniforms and other equipment for women have been designed (Hefling, 2011).

Women's gains in educational attainment have significantly outpaced those of men since 1970 (Women in America, 2011). Since 1970, the percentage of women with at least a high school education rose from 59% (about the same as men) to about 87% (slightly more than men). In 1970, only about 8% of women and 14% of men were college graduates. Now, it is about 28% for each group. In 2008, for all racial and ethnic subgroups, a higher percentage of bachelor's and master's degrees were earned by women than men. Women earned about 57% of all college degrees in 2008, and constituted 57% of total undergraduate enrollment. Women age 25–34 are now more likely than men of that age group to have attained a college degree, reversing the norm from 1968. The percentage of women age 25–34 with 2 or more years of graduate school increased dramatically since the late 1970s to about 11%, while the percentage of men in that age group with 2 or more years of graduate school has remained around 8%. In 1998, more doctoral degrees were conferred to men than to women. A decade later, more doctoral degrees were conferred to women than men. Women account for about 59% of graduate school enrollment.

The Sexuality Education and Information Council of the United States (SIECUS) has issued the following position statement on gender equality and equity:

> SIECUS believes that gender equality and equity are fundamental human rights. Society must recognize how gender-based stereotyping, including prejudice toward transgender, transsexual, and intersex individuals, can result in harmful consequences, such as gender-based violence

Gender DIMENSIONS

Is There Gender Equality in College Sports?

Since 1972, Title IX of the Education Amendments has forbidden sex discrimination at institutions receiving federal funds. One important, and still controversial, part of this legislation relates to college sports. After over 40 years of living with Title IX, there are still many viewpoints about it. Some people believe that men have been penalized for having a higher interest in athletics than women. They point to the fact that in some cases men's sports have been cut to comply with Title IX. Others believe that Title IX has not hurt men's sports, and it has greatly helped women's athletic opportunities. Efforts continue among athletic officials, college administrators, and legislators to see how to deal best with Title IX and its implications.

and sexual, physical, and psychological abuse. Gender-based stereotyping must be eliminated, and the use of gender-inclusive language promoted. The legal system should guarantee the civil rights and protection of all people, regardless of gender, gender identity, or gender expression.

As we have pointed out throughout this chapter, some people have many different feelings about some gender issues. In 2008, the American Psychological Association (APA) adopted a policy statement related to transgender, gender identity, and gender expression nondiscrimination (American Psychological Association, 2008). Here is part of that statement:

Therefore be it resolved that APA opposes all public and private discrimination on the basis of actual or perceived gender identity and expression and urges the repeal of discriminatory laws and policies;

Therefore be it further resolved that APA supports the passage of laws and policies protecting the rights, legal benefits, and privileges of people of all gender identities and expressions;

Therefore be it further resolved that APA supports full access to employment, housing, and education regardless of gender identity and expression.

As a final note, some people have long felt that promoting gender equality for women was tantamount to reducing rights for males or even hating males. In 2014, Emma Watson, star of the *Harry Potter* films and goodwill ambassador for United Nations women, urged men around the world to join a campaign for gender equality called HeForShe. Said Watson, "Fighting for women's rights has too often become synonymous with man hating. This has to stop."

Exploring the Dimensions of Human Sexuality

© Gayvoronskaya Yana/Shutterstock

Case Study

Your gender plays a major role in how you perceive the world—and how the world perceives you. Gender plays a pervasive role in many areas that define our self-concept, including career opportunities. Men and women communicate in different styles, and they express emotions differently. Physiological differences play out in health—women do live longer, but are sick more often.

Gender roles are influenced by virtually all social and cultural aspects, including religion, ethnic heritage, family traditions, peers, and even the mass media.

In sexuality, a "double standard" still exists, as men are encouraged to be sexually aggressive and women are discouraged from being sexually active.

Biological Factors

- Chromosomes (XX or XY) determine biological gender.
- Primitive gonadal tissues differentiate into prenatal ovaries or testicles.
- At puberty, sex hormones cause emergence of primary and secondary sexual characteristics. Sex hormones continue to act throughout one's lifetime.
- Testosterone plays a role in aggression; estrogen has been linked to heart attack prevention.
- Most medical studies have been completed on men, and findings have been assumed to be the same for women, without taking into account sex differences in hormones and chemical makeup.

Sociocultural Factors

- Gender-role orientation begins at birth. Children are treated differently according to social standards for their sex.
- Family, neighbors, friends, and teachers influence our thinking about gender through their actions.
- Ethnic groups pass down sex specific heritages and gender roles.
- Mass media are often biased, portraying men and women in traditional, stereotypical roles.

Psychological Factors

- Expressiveness and communication style differ between sexes, as men withhold feelings and women express them openly.
- Women suffer more from self-esteem issues relating to body image, as they attempt to live up to the biologically impossible "Barbie" standard.
- In a society where men are presented with greater opportunities, motivation and possibility of achievement are more challenging for women.

Summary

- Discussions about gender similarities and differences often focus on "nature versus nurture." Some attribute most of these characteristics to biological factors; others attribute them to social factors and learning.

- Gender similarities and differences usually fall into certain categories, such as developmental differences, gender and abilities, gender and aggression, gender and health, and gender and dating.

- Many gender issues have emerged related to the workplace in recent years. Issues commonly discussed include different work styles and leadership styles of men and women, rights of males and females in the workplace, and arguments about the existence of a sex-based wage gap.

- There are many feelings about gender and advertising. Some people believe numerous ads promote gender stereotypes just to sell products; others see gender-based ads as nothing very important one way or the other.

- Gender identity, roles, and stereotypes are learned in many ways. They can differ markedly from society to society.

- Gender roles and stereotypes are taught in a number of ways in society. They are strongly influenced by teachers and the school environment, and by parents and peers.

- Some people experience gender identity difficulty. A transsexual is a person whose gender identity does not match his or her biological sex. Gender-reassignment surgery is usually done only after careful screening of the individual.

- Gender-role stereotyping limits sexuality in many ways. It can limit self-expression, personal growth and development, and healthy feelings about masculinity and femininity.

- The women's movement has had many influences on gender roles as well as social and legal issues.

- Today more women than men receive bachelor's, master's, and doctoral degrees. However, many different feelings about male and female roles still exist.

Discussion Questions

1. Of the many differences between the sexes, which do you believe are the most important nonbiological differences? Explain your answer. In your own college or university, are male and female students treated differently? Give specific examples.
2. Compare and contrast the feelings of males and females toward sexuality. Then discuss how the sexes can bridge those differences.
3. How can women achieve sexual equality with men without becoming competitive? Does such a change need to begin with women—or with men?

Application Questions

Reread the story that opens the chapter and answer the following questions.

1. Is the writer androgynous? Explain why or why not.
2. Which conflicts has the author experienced from his "reversed" gender role?
3. Is there any merit to the composer's comment that play during childhood influences abilities later in life? Which other factors probably influenced the development of women composers?
4. As a student, how do you view the future of gender roles? How will life experiences affect your view of gender roles?

Critical Thinking Questions

1. Consider the expression "Candy is dandy, but liquor is quicker." Explain the sex bias of the expression. Which type of tensions might such thinking create between the genders?
2. Is there a sex bias in the United States toward the male management style? What other reasons might explain the lack of women in high-level executive positions and on boards of directors?
3. Michael Jackson was often cited as an androgynous person. Why did the popular press believe this? Was it true?

Critical Thinking Case

Because of physiological differences, men and women often have slightly different medical symptoms. The same seems true for psychological problems. For example, school-aged boys who act out in class are often considered for the *DSM-IV* diagnosis of attention-deficit/hyperactivity disorder. Boys who receive treatment can learn to do quite well in school. However, girls have been socialized not to act out in class; they tend to have different symptoms and are less often diagnosed. That difference puts those young girls at a disadvantage, leading to poor scholastic achievement and low self-esteem.

In adulthood, depression is diagnosed in women nearly twice as often as in men. Research suggests that when men are faced with negative emotions, they distract themselves through drinking or sports. Women, in contrast, tend to focus attention on the negative mood. If such focus intensifies the negative mood, a woman would be more prone to a diagnosis of depression.

1. Should separate diagnostic manuals for psychiatric disorders be written for men and women? Explain your answer.

2. Should psychiatrists focus their training on one sex? Or should training be generic? Explain your answer.

Exploring Personal Dimensions

Female–Male Differences and Similarities

Females and males respond in similar ways to sexual stimulation. However, in some ways they also respond dissimilarly. To assess your knowledge of these similarities and differences, determine whether each of the following statements describes a response that is similar or dissimilar for females and males. Then place a check mark to indicate your answer. The correct answers appear at the conclusion of the statements.

Similar   Dissimilar

——   ——   1. Erection occurs.

——   ——   2. When a sexual fantasy occurs, hormones are secreted.

——   ——   3. Testosterone is produced by the body.

——   ——   4. During sexual excitement, the nipples become erect.

——   ——   5. Sex flush appears during the excitement phase of the sexual response cycle.

——   ——   6. Males and females can have multiple orgasms without requiring a rest period.

Correct Answers

1. Similar. Both the penis and the clitoris become engorged with blood and become erect.

2. Similar. Hormones in both genders activate various body parts in response to sexual stimulation.

3. Similar. Testosterone is produced in the interstitial cells of the testes in men and in the ovaries of women (although in a small amount).

4. Similar. Although nipple erection is more obvious in women, it occurs in men, too.

5. Dissimilar. In men, sex flush occurs during the plateau phase; in women, it occurs during the excitement phase.

6. Dissimilar. Whereas women have the capacity to be multiorgasmic, males generally need to experience a refractory period before subsequent orgasms.

Suggested Readings

"Boy or girl?" Gender a new challenge for schools. *Fox News*, May 28, 2013. Available: http://www.foxnews.com/health/2013/05/28/boy-or-girl-gender-new-challenge-for-schools/.

Brannon, L. *Gender: Psychological perspectives*, 5th ed. Boston: Pearson, 2008.

Educational attainment in the United States: 2013. U.S. Census Bureau. Available: http://www.census.gov/hhes/socdemo/education/Feminist Majority Foundation. *Campaign to expose fake clinics: 2015.* Feminist Campus. Available: http://www.feministcampus.org/campaigns/fake-clinics/.

Hirnstein, M., Andrews, L. C., & Hausmann, M. Gender-stereotyping and cognitive sex differences in mixed- and same-sex groups. *Archives of Sexual Behavior, 43*, 8 (2014), 1663–1673.

Lips, H. *Sex and gender*, 6th ed. New York: McGraw-Hill, 2007.

Matlin, M. W. *Psychology of women*, 7th ed. Belmont, CA: Waswsorth, 2011.

Overview of the status of women in the states. Institute for Women's Policy Research (2014). Available at: www.iwpr.org.

Steinmetz, K. America's transition. *Time, 183*, 22 (June 9, 2014), 38–46.

Garnett, C. Sharing the sandbox equally: screen star Davis urges gender balance in the media. *NIH Record, 63, no. 11* (2011). Available: http://nihrecord.od.nih.gov/newsletters /2011/05_27_2011/story1.htm.

Gervais, S. J., Vescio, T. K., & Allen, J. What you see is what you get: The objectifying gaze for women and men. *Psychology of Women Quarterly, no. 35* (March 2011), 5–17.

Glick, P., & Fiske, S. T. Ambivalent sexism revisited. *Psychology of Women Quarterly, 35* (2011), 530–535.

Grant, J. M., Mottet, L. A., Tanis, J., Harrison, J., Herman, J. L., & Keisling, M. *Injustice at Every Turn.* Washington, DC: National Center for Transgender Equality and National Gay and Lesbian Task Force, 2011.

Hafling, K. They're not guys: New gear to fit female soldiers. ABC News (April 22, 2011). Available: http://abcnews .go.com/US/wireStory?id=13433425.

Hamson, S. The passive/active divide: What the village is teaching our children about gender. *SIECUS Report, 32, no. 3* (Summer 2004), 14–16.

Horgan, T. G., Mast, M. S., & Hall, J. A. Gender differences in memory for the appearance of others. *Personality and Social Psychology Bulletin, 30, no. 2* (2004), 185–196.

Imbornoni, A. A women's rights movement in the U.S. Available: http://www.infoplease.com/spot /womenstimeline3 .html.

International Foundation for Gender Education (2005). Available: http://www.ifge.org/.

Jenner, L., & Ferguson, R. 2008 Catalyst census of women corporate officers and top earners of the FP500. Catalyst, March 2009. Available: http://www.catalyst.org /publication/295/2008-catalyst-census-of-women-corporate-officers-and-top-earners-of-the-fp500.

Kerber, L. K. Moving beyond stereotypes of feminism. *Chronicle of Higher Education, 45, no. 33* (April 23, 1999), B6–B8.

Kluger, J. What's sex got to do with it? *Time, 161, no. 3* (January 20, 2003), 35.

Kulkarni, S. C., Levin-rector, A., Ezzati, M., & Murray, C. J. L. Falling behind: Life expectancy in U.S. counties from 2000 to 2007 in an international context. *Population Health Metrics, 9, no. 16* (2011). Available: http://www .pophealthmetrics.com/content/pdf/1478-7954-9-16.pdf.

Labi, N. An American honor killing: One victim's story. *Time* (February 25, 2011). Available: http://www.time.com/time /nation/article/0,8599,2055445,00.html.

Light, D., Obedin-Maliver, J., Sevelius, J. M., & Kerns, J. L. Transgender men who experienced pregnancy after female-to-male transitioning. *Obstetrics & Gynecology, 124, 6* (2014), 1120–1127.

Lister, K. *Reese Witherspoon takes on Hollywood sexism,* November 24, 2014. Available: http://www.marieclaire .co.uk/news/547839/reese-witherspoon-takes-on-hollywood-sexism.html.

MacFarquhar, N. Saudis arrest women leading right-to-drive campaign. New York Times (May 23, 2011). Available: http://www.nytimes.com/2011/05/24/world /middleeast/24saudi.html.

Marwan, A. Groom beats bride at his mother's request. *Bulletin of the Oppression of Women,* 2015a. Available: http:// bulletinoftheoppressionofwomen.com/

Marwan, A. Honor killings in Chechnya and Pakistan. *Bulletin of the Oppression of Women,* 2015b. Available: http:// bulletinoftheoppressionofwomen.com/.

McKeen, C. A. Gender roles: An examination of the hopes and expectations of the next generation of managers in Canada and China. *Sex Roles, 52, nos. 7–8* (April 2005), 533–546.

Median usual weekly earnings of full-time wage and salary workers: 1980–2010. *Statistical abstracts of the United States.* U.S. Census Bureau, 2012. Available: http://www .censusgov/compendia/statab/2012/tables/12s0649.pdf.

Meese, M. Backlash: Women bullying women at work. *New York Times* (May 10, 2009). Available: http://www.nytimes .com/2009/05/10/business/10women.html.

Miller, C. Paternity leave: The rewards and the remaining stigma. *New York Times,* November 7, 2014. Available: http://www .nytimes.com/2014/11/09/upshot/paternity-leave-the-rewards-and-the-remaining-stigma.html?abt=0002&abg=1.

Misner, J. Women's colleges drop barriers to enrolling transgender students. *Chronicle of Higher Education, 51, 3* September 19, 2014), A13.

Monk-Turner, E., Wren, K., McGill, L., Matthiae, C., Brown, S., & Brooks, D. Who is gazing at whom? A look at how sex is used in magazine advertisements. *Journal of Gender Studies, 17, 3* (September 2008), 201–209.

Mundy, L. Women, Money and Power. *Time, 179, no 12* (March26, 2012), 26–34.

Namie, G. The WBI U.S. workplace bullying survey. Workplace Bullying Institute (2010). Available: http://www .workplacebullying.org/wbiresearch/2010-wbi-national-survey.

New study shows women own 20% of businesses with revenues exceeding $1 million. Center for Women's Business Research, December 3, 2008. Available: http://www .womensbusinessresearch.org.

On Equal Pay Day NOW calls attention to persistent gender wage gap. National Organization for Women, April 27, 2009. Available: http://www.now.org/press/04-09/04-27 .html.

Orpinas, P., McNicholas, C., & Nahapetyan, L. Gender differences in trajectories of relational aggression perpetration and victimization from middle to high school. *Aggressive Behavior,* November 17, 2014. doi: 10.1002 /AB.21563.

Overland, M. A. In Kashmir, militant group threatens to shoot female Muslim students who do not wear veil. *The Chronicle of Higher Education,* Today's News (September 17, 2001). Available: http://chronicle.com/daily/2001.

Overview of the status of women in the states. Washington, DC: IWPR, 2001. Available: http://www.iwpr.org/.

Peplau, L. A. Human sexuality: How do men and women differ? *Current Directions in Psychological Research, 12, no. 2* (April 2003), 37–40.

Preidt, R. TV commercials color gender choices for careers. *MedicineNet.com*, May 28, 2008. Available: http://www.medicinenet.com.

Prime, J., & Moss-Racusin, C. A. Engaging men in gender initiatives: What change agents need to know. Catalyst, May 2009. Available: http://www.catalyst.org/publication/323/engaging-men-in-gender-initiatives-what-change-agents-need-to-know.

Rampell, C. Coveting not a corner office, but time at home. *New York Times*, July 7, 2013. Available: http://www.nytimes.com/2013/07/08/business/coveting-not-a-corner-office-but-time-at-home.html?pagewanted=all&_r=0.

Ripley, A. Who says a woman can't be Einstein? *Time, 165, no. 10* (March 7, 2005), 51–60.

Rowe, S., A. & Woodard, D. L. National Law Review, May 22, 2012. Available: http://www.natlawreview.com/article/eeoc-rules-transgender-employees-are-covered-under-title-vii.

Sadker, D., & Zittleman, K. Gender bias lives, for both sexes. *Education Digest, 70, no. 8* (April 2005), 27–30.

Sanchez-Flores, H. Everything I do, a man does. *SIECUS Report 32, no. 3* (summer 2004), 17–20.

Sayer, L. C. Gender, time and inequality: Trends in women's and men's paid work, unpaid work and free time. *Social Forces, 84* (2005), 285–303.

Shafak, E. After years of silence, Turkey's women are going into battle against oppression. *The Guardian*, 2015. Available: http://www.theguardian.com/commentisfree/2015/feb/17/turkey-women-battle-oppression-protest.

Sheppard, L., & Aquino, K. "Catfight? Workplace conflicts between women get bad rap." *Academy of Management Perspectives 27, 1* (2013), 52–62.

Shipman, C., & Kay, K. Women will rule business. *Time, 173, 20* (May 25, 2009), 46–47.

Smith, S. L., Choueiti, M., Prescott, A., & Pieper, K. *Gender roles and occupations: A look at character attributes and job-related aspirations in film and television.* USC Annenberg School for Communication and Journalism, 2013. Available: http://seejane.org/wp-content/uploads/key-findings-gender-roles-2013.pdf.

Some health plans for federal employees to cover transgender care: Largest carrier will not include coverage. National Partnership for Women & Families, November 12, 2014. Available: http://go.nationalpartnership.org/site/News2?abbr=daily2_&id=46061&security=1201.

Statistics on women in the military. Women in Military Service for America Memorial Foundation, April 7, 2009. Available: http://www.womensmemorial.org/PDFs/StatsonWIM.pdf.

Steinmetz, K. New crisis line aims to help transgender people at risk of suicide. *Time.com*, November 20, 2014. Available: http://time.com/3598285/transgender-lifeline-help-line/.

Stoker, J. I., Van der Velde, M., & Lammers, J. Factors relating to managerial stereotypes: The role of gender of the employee and the manager and management gender ratio. *Journal of Business and Psychology* (March 19, 2011). Available: http://www/springerlink.com/content/y3458105hg318322/fulltext.pdf.

Stout, D. Transgender teen awarded $75,000in school restroom lawsuit. *Time.com*, December 3, 2014. Available: http://time.com/3615599/transgender-student-restroom-lawsuit-maine/.

Surgery may be hasty for unclear gender. *InteliHealth* (2005). Available: http://www.intelihealth.com/.

Tavris, C. Are girls really as mean as books say they are? *Chronicle of Higher Education, 48, no. 43* (July 5, 2002), B7–B9.

Taylor, L. D., & Setters, T., Watching aggressive, attractive, female protagonists shapes gender roles for women among male and female undergraduate viewers. *Sex Roles, 65, no. 1–2* (2011), 35–46.

The power of play. *Sports Illustrated* (May 7, 2012), 43–66.

Torre, P. S., & Epstein, D. The Transgender Athlete. *Sports Illustrated* (May 28, 2012), 66–73.

Warren, A. K. Cascading gender biases, compounding effects: An assessment of talent management systems. Catalyst, February 2009. Available: http://www.catalyst.org/publication/292/cascading-gender-biases-compounding-effects-an-assessment-of-talent-management-systems.

We want to live as humans. *Human Rights Watch, 14, no 11* (December 2002), 1–52.

Wilson, R. Second sex. *Chronicle of Higher Education, 52, no. 7* (October 10, 2005), A10–A12.

Women in American: Indicators of social and economic well-being. Washington, DC: White House Council on Women and Girls, 2011.

Zimmerman, A., & Dahlberg, J. The sexual objectification of women in advertising: A contemporary cultural perspective. *Journal of Advertising Research, 48, 1* (March 2008), 71–79.

CHAPTER

11

Body Image

© Gayvoronskaya Yana/Shutterstock

FEATURES

Gender Dimensions
Gender and Body Image

Multicultural Dimensions
Weight and Culture

Ethical Dimensions
To Train or Not to Train—That Is the Question

Gender Dimensions
Why Are Eating Disorders Mainly Found in Women?

CHAPTER OBJECTIVES

1 Discuss body image, its role in sexuality, and the way media have created impossible body-image ideals to emulate.

2 Describe how to improve one's self-image.

3 Describe the problems that poor body image causes for females and males, including eating disorders, muscle dysmorphia, steroid use, and cosmetic surgery.

INTRODUCTION

*I*f you had the privilege of knowing Marc Grabowski for some time, as one of your authors has, you would assume that he must have always been a confident young man. As a graduate of Boston University, with a double major in political science and philosophy, he worked as a trainer at a local gym while applying to law schools. Not only that: The month before he graduated, he placed fifth in the National Physique Committee's New England Body Building Competition as a heavyweight. Marc appears to be a pillar of strength and confidence.

But as with most people, Marc's confidence and bodily self-assurance have been built up over many years. In fact, Marc had very low self-esteem when he started high school. Smaller and lighter than his friends, he was picked on constantly (called "Ostrich Boy" because of his long neck). As his self-image sank, Marc decided to do something about it. He started lifting weights in his basement at age 14 years. By the time he was 16 years old, he had joined a gym. To Marc and his male friends, weight and size mattered. Their perception was that gaining any weight—fat, water weight, anything—was great.

It was not only his friends who pushed the weight issue. Marc would look at magazines like Flex and Muscle & Fitness and believe that he "could get like that": amazing abs or bulging biceps in 30 days! The articles focused on weight lifting but failed to mention nutrition, cardiovascular work, drugs (steroids), and muscle maturity. As Marc has learned, muscles take years to mature and grow dense in fibers so that they can stand out as hard as iron.

Yet those magazines continue to peddle false dreams. As Marc puts it, "They'll intentionally deceive the readers just to sell magazines." Worse than that: As many others do, Marc injured himself, rupturing the capillaries in his chest, by following the training routines in such magazines. And when the cover-boy results do not appear, that is a further blow to one's self-esteem.

Having a better body image has made Marc's social life easier. "Like it or not, the first thing people notice about you is your physical appearance. In social situations, that can be an advantage. But that is balanced against professional situations, where the negative connotations of a large size have to be overcome." Although he readily admits to "hiding behind the weight," Marc also says he enjoys life more. "It's nice to hear someone say, 'You've gotten in great shape.'"

By the time he reached Boston University, Marc set a goal to be in a bodybuilding show by the time he graduated. Although his studies always came first, Marc began the final preparations and dieting in his senior year.

The diet is what does most people in. During the off-season, Marc ate 10,000 calories or more a day. But as the contest drew nearer, he began to diet. By the last month, all Marc ate were 7 to 10 pounds of chicken and six potatoes a day! (And, of course, he drank water.) The diet takes a physical toll by depleting energy. Marc had trouble staying awake while studying for and taking exams.

The strict diet also has psychological effects. He felt "totally miserable" for the final 2 months of dieting. Marc deliberately tried to avoid social situations when he got cranky. He did not date during his final semester of college—and that, he ironically points out, somewhat defeated the original purpose of bodybuilding!

By the show, Marc was down to 206 pounds, with an incredibly low 2.7% body fat. Within 24 hours after the show, he had regained back 18 pounds (mostly water) and he gained an additional 10 pounds over the next 6 days. Marc lost the weight for a specific event but had no problem regaining it. Marc feels comfortable at an off-season weight of about 250 pounds and a body fat percentage of 10%.

As a personal trainer, Marc enjoys seeing the day-to-day growth of his clients—both in muscle and in confidence. The psychological effects of training are clear to Marc: Not only do clients have better body images, but their increased confidence is also seen in their becoming more outgoing. Clearly, a positive body image can improve your self-confidence.

As you will see in this chapter, obtaining your desired body image can be good for you both physically and psychologically. However, as Marc's story should show, it is important to keep your true goals in mind and, as you do so, respect your body and its needs.

Source: Interview with Marc T. Grabowski, June 9, 1999.

There's always a bigger fish in the water! A person in excellent shape for a young adult (bottom) can be dwarfed by a "professional" bodybuilder (top).

Body Image

Body image refers to the mental image we have of our own physical appearance. It is influenced by many factors—among them are weight, our weight distribution, our values about physical appearance, our concepts of a good physical appearance, our ethnic background, and what we see in others around us, what we hear through the media, and what we hear from others. We have previously discussed the importance of self-concept in relation to human sexuality. Self-concept is usually closely related to body image. A better body image contributes to a more confident individual; the better we feel about ourselves, the more likely we are to pursue a potential partner.

Body image also affects sexual behavior. People with a positive body image are more likely to be open to sexual expression that exposes the body. Those with a poor body image might be less likely to pursue sexual expressions that cause them to reveal themselves and make them feel uncomfortable. Therefore, body image is an important part of sexual health. People who feel comfortable in their bodies are more likely to make healthy sexual decisions, such as protecting their health by using condoms.

The way we feel about our bodies has a big influence on us every day, including on decisions we make. People who feel badly about their bodies sometimes make sexually unhealthy decisions. Conversely, the better one feels, the better the decisions one will make (*Body image and sexuality*, 2015). Many studies have shown that body image concern is higher in women, that negative body image is associated with a number of psychological and relationship problems, and that people with poorer body images are more likely to engage in sexual risk-taking. In addition, their sexual self-esteem seems to be lower, they engage in less regular sexual activity, and they have higher rates of sexual dysfunction. Although some conflicting evidence has been gathered on this point, body image seems to have a stronger relationship to sexual satisfaction than does a person's actual amount of body fat (Whitbourne, 2014). A number of research studies support the relationships between body image and sexual satisfaction. For example, Milhausen et al. (2014) found that body image concerns in men are very real, and can affect sexual functioning and happiness. However, for both men and women, the strongest predictor of sexual satisfaction is satisfaction with the overall relationship. Relatedly, but with a little different twist, Zhaoyang and Cooper (2013) found that an individual's satisfaction with his or her own body was not as important to the overall quality of sexual experience as the person's satisfaction with the partner's body or as the partner's satisfaction with the individual's body.

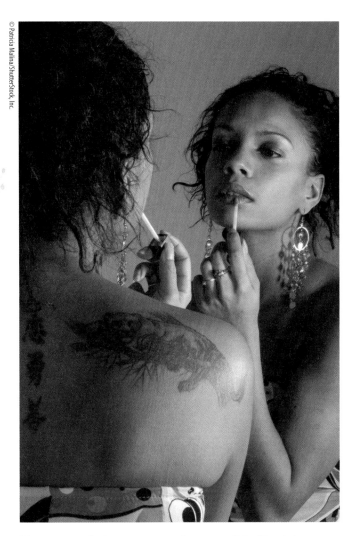

Many women feel pressure to conform to an "ideal" body image.

Many interesting points about body image were presented in the findings of *Psychology Today*'s 1997 body image survey (Garner, 1997). Despite the concerns of feminists and other observers, body image issues seem to be growing in importance. Body image influences much of our behavior and self-esteem. It governs whom we meet and whom we select as life partners, as well as our day-to-day interactions and our comfort level. Despite this importance, there is a growing gulf between actual and preferred shapes. As individuals, we are growing heavier, but our body preferences are growing thinner.

Results of the *Psychology Today* survey indicated that 89% of the women wanted to lose weight, and 22% of the men wanted to gain weight. Some women also reported avoiding pregnancy because

body image The mental image we have of our own physical appearance.

of a fear of what a pregnancy would do to their bodies. Sexual experiences affect our body image, and our body image affects our sexual experiences. For example, 40% of men and 36% of women said that unpleasant sexual experiences caused negative feelings about their body. However, 70% of men and 67% of women felt that good sexual experiences contributed to satisfactory feelings about their body. In addition, 23% of women considered sexual abuse very important in negatively shaping their body image. Finally, 93% of women and 89% of men wanted models in magazines to represent the natural range of body shapes.

It is not only college students and adults who have concerns about body image. For example, Grosick et al. (2013) investigated several attributes associated with body image among male and female middle school students. Their data indicated high levels of agreement among this sample (nearly 80%) that appearance is an important part of middle school students' personas. For many attributes, data for boys were parallel to the data for girls. For several attributes, girls had significantly higher levels of agreement and concern than boys. These attributes were dieting, depression over appearance, and an inclination toward risky eating behaviors.

A study of women at Duke University (Lipka, 2004) found that many undergraduate women felt relentless pressure to conform to an ideal. They described a social environment that supported the expectation that a woman would be "smart, accomplished, fit, beautiful, and popular." It was also found that people at other campuses said, "It's the same way at my college."

It is common for women attending college to have body image issues. Research at the Center for Appearance Research (2011) at the University of the West England found that 30% of college women would trade at least 1 year of their life to achieve their ideal body weight and shape. Ten percent would trade 2 to 5 years of their life, and another 2% would trade 6 to 10 years of their life. Seventy-nine percent of the women reported they would like to lose weight, despite the fact that the majority of them (78.4%) were within the underweight or "normal" weight ranges.

Leone et al. (2011) looked at how college students perceive their bodies and to what extent that perception affects their behavior. They found that there was a strong correlation between having lower levels of body image satisfaction and risky behavioral management strategies. For example, those who had lower levels of body image satisfaction were more likely to use more risky behavior management strategies such as excessive dieting, excessive exercise dependence, supplement use, and drug use.

In an ethnically diverse sample of U.S. female college students, Claudat and Warren (2014) found that body shame and body self-consciousness during sexual activity are negatively correlated with sexual satisfaction. Their study findings highlighted the negative consequences of body image for college women's sexual satisfaction.

Mumen et al. (2015) asked heterosexual women and men about their body type preferences for (hypothetical) romantic partners. Participants chose a particular silhouette value as ideal for a romantic partner, and rated how important it was for their partner to have this ideal body type. Men placed more importance on the body silhouette they chose for a partner than women did, and men's importance ratings were positively associated with the sexual permissiveness of their peer group and their media use. Accessing sports media and watching reality television were the best media predictors of men's judgments about women's bodies. Less variability was explained in terms of women's preference for men partners' bodies.

Body image may relate to various aspects of life in addition to self-image or partner preferences. For example, Chrisler et al. (2015) found that higher scores on body appreciation predicted more positive attitudes and beliefs about menstruation. They suggested that their findings might be useful in designing ways to increase women's comfort with their bodies and bodily functions. Blashill and Safren (2015) explored the influence of body dissatisfaction on condom use self-efficacy (strength of one's beliefs in one's own ability to complete tasks). They found that as body dissatisfaction increases, a person's self-efficacy regarding the use of condoms diminishes. Therefore, increasing body satisfaction may be a good way to increase condom use and thereby decrease the incidence of sexually transmitted infections.

A growing number of researchers say that many men are also suffering from body image problems—and they are often reluctant to seek help (Morgan, 2002). Some say that binge eating has become as prevalent for college men as binge drinking—about 40% of them do it. One group of researchers has named severe body-image problems in men "the Adonis complex." It can include eating disorders and a disorder called *muscle dysmorphia*, in which men perceive their bodies as perpetually puny. Some researchers argue that almost half of all college men are dissatisfied with their body.

Studies of men's body image have focused mainly on dimensions of adiposity and muscularity. Tiggemann et al. (2008), however, found that men were also dissatisfied with their head hair, body hair, height, and penis size. They were most concerned about their body weight, penis size, and height.

Research indicates that young men's body dissatisfaction increases when they see images of attractive muscular men. Those who are dissatisfied with their bodies are at risk for negative self-evaluations when exposed to idealized images, whereas those who are satisfied with their bodies seem to be protected against negative impacts from seeing such images (Blond, 2008). In addition, lower ratings of overall self-concept and higher levels of depression, anxiety, and interpersonal sensitivity are predictive of body image concerns in men (McFarland & Kaminski, 2009).

Research has shown that gay men's body-image concerns are generally similar to those of heterosexual men (Martins, Tiggemann, & Churchett, 2008). Also, an investigation of transsexuals who had gone through sex-change operations (both male-to-female and female-to-male) showed that their body image was much improved as compared to their body image prior to the surgery (Kraemer et al., 2008).

Body image can be a unique problem for physically challenged people, such as those who have any kind of physical difficulty, including changes in body contours due to accident or disease and changes in body functioning that might relate to sexuality. People with disabilities or disease may view themselves as flawed or unattractive.

Depending on the type of physical challenge, various areas of concern need attention, including the feelings of loss of control over one's bodily functions, the inability to care for personal needs, the fear of being less of a person, and the feeling of being unacceptable. Education and counseling about body image are important and ideally should also involve the partners of challenged persons.

For many people, thinking about body image and how they would like to look implies becoming thinner. In recent years, however, there has also been a movement to acknowledge that there is a great range of beauty and attractiveness. For example, in the 1990s Emme was a very successful plus-size model. She hosted a popular TV show and probably paved the way for other "plus size" models. When she was diagnosed with cancer in 2007, Emme left the spotlight to battle the disease. After dealing successfully with her illness, she returned to the fashion world to promote the design of more options in all types of clothes for plus-size women. In addition, a new doll called Emme was developed. On *Good Morning America*, Emme said, "We do have curves

 Did You Know . . .

For years, people have debated the pros and cons of Barbie dolls. Hains (2014) pointed out five good reasons to avoid Barbie altogether:

1. *Barbie's beauty is unhealthy and damaging.* The doll has an unrealistic body type and a rigid beauty ideal that studies show can be harmful to girls. For example, girls aged 5 to 6 years were more dissatisfied with their shape and wanted more extreme thinness after seeing Barbie dolls.

2. *Barbie products portray girls as unintelligent.* The Mattel book *I Can Be a Computer Engineer* featured Barbie as a computer science student—but also portrayed Barbie as incompetent and constantly in need of her male classmates' help.

3. *Barbie has a race problem.* Mattel struggles to present Barbies of color in ways that are equal to the iconic, Caucasian blonde Barbie. Kids know that there is only one "real" Barbie—and that Barbie is blonde and white.

4. *Barbie dolls are not age appropriate for young girls.* Barbie dolls were originally meant for girls 9 to 12 years old. However, to promote sales, Mattel now targets girls ages 3 to 7. These younger girls would be better served by dolls without the problems associated with Barbie dolls.

5. *Barbie buys its way into pro-girl spaces, appropriating girl empowerment to sell more dolls.* Mattel has a great deal of money that it uses as clout with girls to its own financial advantage. Examples of this practice are Barbie's 2010 sponsorship of "Take Our Daughters and Sons to Work Day" and Barbie's partnership with the Girl Scouts. Announced in 2014, the latter partnership involved the release of a Girl Scout–themed Barbie doll and a Barbie uniform patch for Girl Scouts to work to earn. It seems that Mattel is not actually promoting girls' empowerment—just Barbie.

According to Hains, when you are selecting gifts for the little girls in your life, you shouldn't give Barbie a second glance. With just a little time and care, you can find a perfectly fun, appealing, and healthy-image fashion doll that the child will love and cherish.

What do you think about Hains's point of view? Which of her five points do you agree with or disagree with? Why?

Source: Hains, R. 5 reasons NOT to buy Barbie for little girls: It's not just body image! *Parent–Child Discussion Guides*, December 15, 2014. Available: http://rebeccahains.com/2014/12/15/5-reasons-not-to-buy-barbie/.

Gender and Body Image

Stereotypically, people often think that only girls and women deal with issues relating to self-esteem and body image. In fact, boys and men deal with the same issues, although the specifics behind self-esteem and body image can vary by sex. For example, many people in the United States tend to value girls and women who are smaller and thinner and boys and men who are larger and muscular. In addition, girls and women are supposed to be the sexual gatekeepers in relationships with male partners, socialized to place limits and refuse sexual behaviors; as a result, girls and women who *want* to be in a sexual relationship may be labeled promiscuous. Conversely, boys and men may be socialized to always want to participate in sexual activity, and as a result, boys and men who want to wait to have sexual activity may be labeled cowards or told they are not real men.

on the doll, hips, and broad shoulders." She noted that it is a good idea for parents to provide their children with dolls that represent real people—they should have dolls of different hues and colors, and different shapes and sizes. Some believe that this doll may help promote a trend in the media of depicting more women and girls with normal (rather than super-skinny) body types.

For years the 11-inch-tall blonde, blue-eyed Barbie fashion doll (who celebrated her 55th birthday in 2014) represented the ideal American beauty—even though Barbie's stick-thin figure is impossible to achieve in real life. A new Barbie (the Lammily doll) with the measurements of an average 19-year-old girl was put on the market in 2014. Does the presence of that Barbie have any influence on how you feel about the points raised in the Did You Know? box related to the pros and cons of Barbie dolls?

There are varying opinions regarding why some people prefer certain body shapes. Research among adults has shown a preference for average-weight female figures with waist-to-hip ratios of 0.7, and average-weight male figures with waist-to-hip ratios of 0.9 (Connolly, Slaughter, & Mealey, 2004). In one study, more than 500 children from 6 to 17 years of age were asked to select drawings of males and females they thought looked the nicest or most attractive. The youngest children showed preferences for the underweight figures, changing to consistent preferences for the average weight figures in the teenage years.

Singh (2002) looked at cross-cultural feelings about attractiveness. He asked men and women from the Azores Islands, Guinea-Bissau, Indonesia, and the United States to judge the attractiveness of female figures differing in body weight and waist-to-hip ratio (WHR). There was a strong cross-cultural agreement for attractiveness. Figures with low WHR were judged to be more attractive than figures with high WHR within each weight category. Participants also judged attractive figures as less faithful than less-attractive figures. It was found that, compared to women with high WHRs, low-WHR women reported engaging in more flirting to make dates jealous, suggesting some truth to the attractiveness stereotype.

The AP–iVillage Poll (2009) suggested that there is a big disconnect between body image and true physical condition. Even though many women want to improve their body image, their behavior is often not consistent with that desire. Physical fitness is undervalued and absolute weight and appearance are overvalued. About 60% of Americans are overweight or obese. Half don't like their weight, but just a third don't like their physical condition, even though being overweight and sedentary are big risk factors for type 2 diabetes, heart disease, and other ailments. The Poll found women putting in a median of 80 minutes of exercise per week, meaning that half do even less. The average adult is supposed to get at least 2 ½ hours of exercise a week for good health. In addition, just 8% of women ate the minimum recommended servings of fruits and vegetables—five a day.

Stephen and Perea (2014) wanted to know if there was really a difference between judgments made by men and women regarding women's attractiveness. They had a group of 24 Asian participants manipulate the apparent body mass indices (BMIs) of full-length photographs of young Malaysian Chinese women to enhance their perceived healthiness and attractiveness. Results showed that both men and women differentiated attractiveness and health by preferring a lower BMI for attractiveness than for health. There was also consistency in the preferred ideal BMIs for attractiveness and appearance across both sexes. Results showed that BMI provides important clues to perceptions of attractive and healthy appearance.

As we have seen, many factors can influence body image. Even engaging in "fat talk"—the common negative conversations about one's own or others' bodies—can result in lower satisfaction with one's body and higher levels of depression. Arroyo and Harwood (2012) found that fat talk predicts changes in depression, body satisfaction, and perceived pressure to be thin. This was true for both males and females. The more often one engaged in fat talk, the lower that person's body satisfaction and the higher the level of depression was likely to be.

Self-esteem is how highly you regard yourself. One aspect of this is body image. Self-esteem is closely related to self-efficacy—that is, the belief that you are capable of accomplishing a task or goal. The better a person feels about her or his body, the better the decisions that individual will make relating to what she or he does with that body. For example, a person who feels unattractive may feel less discerning about who he has a sexual relationship with; a person who is insecure about her body may not insist that her partner practice safer sexual activity for fear that she will be rejected in favor of someone else. Self-esteem and body image are complex issues that have deep psychological roots, and both are important in sexual maturation. Self-esteem is a master key that can lead to positive psychosexual development, opening the door to the actualization of one's human sexuality potential (Bruess & Schroeder, 2014).

The Elusive Perfect Body

What does the perfect body look like? The answer to that question will probably depend on the purpose we have in mind. Taking a look at successful female athletes gives us some excellent examples. The best swimmers tend to be relatively tall and look like a capital *Y* from the front, with wide, flexible shoulders; long arms and hands; a narrow waist; and lightweight legs. Swimmers get by with more body fat than other athletes because it lets them ride higher in the water. Top speed skaters, in contrast, are shorter and look rather average from the waist up. Farther down, however, we see heavily muscled legs with rather short thighs. At the same time, the female gymnast probably has a lean, petite frame; a fine-boned face; small breasts; and long arms. A body that excels in one athletic context can be a hindrance in others.

Of course most of us are not training to be Olympic athletes, but there is a lesson here for all of us. The bodies closest to "perfect" are, to a large extent, born that way. We must take what we have and develop and use it as best we can. We can make the most of the genetic gifts we do have. In the end, the perfect body is the one that will allow you to do things you enjoy and allow you to live your life to the fullest—without compromising your health.

Why Models Look So Perfect

A quick glance at the covers of major fashion and sports magazines—or at the ads therein—seems to bolster the argument that "Some have it, some don't." These models, as well as many movie stars, seem too perfect to be real. Could these people look like that all the time? The answer is, of course, no. They may look that way only for the millisecond that the camera snaps. Some of the images may be completely computer generated. They might not even be real people! Some images of models actually consist of body parts from different people.

Getting "the look" begins long before the photo shoot takes place. Months before a movie begins production, the director (and/or art director) hires a specific personal trainer who will get "the look" that the director wants. Workouts and diet are structured to transform the actor or actress.

Still in preproduction, clothes, makeup, and lighting are chosen to enhance whatever qualities have been chosen. The day of shooting starts with hours of makeup application (sometimes over the entire body), hair styling, and clothes fitting. Ever wonder how clothes can fit so perfectly on some people? No problem: The clothes are literally pasted on!

Production is the time when the camera rolls (or snaps). The art director makes clear what is desired from the photographer, who in turn adjusts lighting and the camera lens to make it happen.

Then the fun begins. During postproduction, any alterations at all can be made to the pictures. You probably know that blemishes are covered, teeth are

Images we see may be carefully staged and even computer generated.

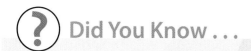

Did You Know . . .

In some places, super-skinny models have been banned. In 2006, models with a body mass index (BMI) of less than 18 were not allowed to participate in Madrid fashion shows. In 2009, the Australian Medical Association asked the government to work with the fashion industry to draw up a national code of conduct. In Milan, models with a BMI of less than 18.5 were banned from fashion shows.

BMI is the ratio of weight to the square of height. In Italy, for example, a 5 foot, 8 inch tall model weighing less than 122 pounds would be barred.

In 2013, Israeli lawmakers adopted legislation stipulating that fashion and commercial models should have a BMI of at least 18.5. It is also called the "Photoshop law" because it demands that computer-generated changes to make models appear thinner be noted along with the images.

Sources: Data from Cable News Network. Skinny models banned from catwalk. September 13, 2006. Available at: http://cnn.com/2006/WORLD/europe/09/13/spain.models/index.html; Miles, J. Call to ban skinny models. February 24, 2009. Available at: http://www.news.com.au/couriermail/story/0,23739,21324231-3102,00.html; Nota B. Israeli law bans skinny, BMI-challenged models. *ABC News*, January 3, 2013. Available at: http://abcnews.go.com/International/israeli-law-bans-skinny-bmi-challenged-models/story?id=18116291.

routinely whitened, wrinkles in clothes are deleted. But did you know that *Playboy* and *Penthouse* sometimes alter various body parts so they are more attractive to readers of the magazines? If photos are not approved, a postproduction team may put a more attractive body part on the model.

To increase the sex appeal of female models, it is not uncommon for art directors to "stretch" legs to give them a longer, thinner look. Just think, you could go from being short and stocky to having the body of Cameron Diaz with a few clicks of a computer mouse!

Eventually, the picture that is published is one that matches the art director's vision—not one that shows the person's real body. And that is not always good. To make the point that image retouching can go too far, the retouching artist Kathy Grove redid one of the most famous Depression-era photographs, Dorothea Lange's *Migrant Mother*. Grove's point is simple: Do not believe everything you see.

Some experts believe that the perfect models who grace magazine covers send powerful—and often negative—signals to figure-conscious adolescent girls. The website Mind on the Media (2009) provides some interesting related statistics: Roughly $12 billion is spent on advertising and marketing to young people every year; the average young person views more than 3,000 ads per day; the number one wish for girls ages 11–17 is to be thinner; females say the media is the most important source of pressure to be thin; and as early as age 13 approximately 53% of American girls are "unhappy with their bodies." In addition, advertisers admit that they sell more than products: They use images to affect the way we see ourselves.

Concerned about images that children and adolescents see in advertisements, the American Medical Association (AMA) adopted a policy encouraging advertising associations to develop guidelines for advertisements, especially those appearing in teen-oriented publications, that would discourage the altering of photographs in a manner that could promote unrealistic expectations of appropriate body image. In one image, a model's waist was slimmed so severely that her head appeared to be wider than her waist. An AMA spokesperson said, "We must stop exposing impressionable children and teenagers to advertisements portraying models with body types only attainable with the help of photo editing software" (AMA adopts new policies at annual meeting, 2011).

The Influence of the Media

For years, some people have criticized the Barbie doll for presenting children with standards for body size and appearance that are both unrealistic and unattainable for most females. Experts also have become concerned about the impact of the "GI Joe Extreme" action figure, which has a more muscular and defined body than past GI Joe figures. At issue is whether such dolls plant the concept of the ideal body in children's minds—a concept that usually cannot be achieved without using obsessive behaviors to lose weight and gain muscle.

Recently, some clothing manufacturers developed padded bras and bikinis for girls as young as age 7. As a result of pressure from some children's advocates, and concerns that such products sexualize children and encourage them to grow up too fast, in some instances the bras and bikinis have been removed from store shelves. These products also send messages to young girls about their body image.

Relatedly, beauty pageants are another way society defines its ideal of beauty, including weight and shape. Researchers computed the BMI (weight divided by the square of height) of winners of the Miss America Pageant from 1922 to 1999. There was a significant decline in the BMI over that time, placing an increasing number of winners in the range of undernutrition. Pageant winners' height increased less than 2%, but body weight decreased by 12%. (Rubinstein & Caballero, 2000).

Even *Playboy* centerfold models have changed over time (Voracek & Fisher, 2002). A review of *Playboy* centerfold models' body measurements over a 50-year period showed that over time bust size and hip size decreased, while waist size increased. BMI and bust-to-hip ratio decreased, while waist-to-hip ratio, waist-to-bust ratio, and androgyny index increased. The study's authors concluded that shapely body characteristics of centerfold models have given way to more androgynous ones.

Bryla (2002) explored the effects of media on female image and concluded that beyond media exposure, awareness and internalization of sociocultural ideals appear to be significant predictors of body image disturbance. In other words, looking at the effects of media on body image is not a simple matter.

Monro and Huon (2005) studied the effects of media-portrayed idealized images on female college students. They found that these images detrimentally affected the body image of the students.

Ashikali and Dittmar (2011) indicated that psychological research has consistently shown that women feel unhappy with their body after looking at images of thin, idealized models, which are typically represented in the media. However, they also found that materialism in the media is a further factor that makes women more vulnerable to negative body image.

While much of the media influence on body image focuses on women, men experience some similar influences and effects. In addition, we now have "men's shapewear," which are products designed to make men look better. For example, girdles have been specially designed to help men look better. There is also Spanx for Men—undershirts that fit and feel like a wetsuit. The cotton compression undershirt helps men to hide their love handles and beer bellies and gives them the look of having a sculpted chest.

There have been some attempts by advertisers to appeal to potential consumers of different sizes. One example in 2005 was the ad campaign for Dove beauty products. In the Dove ads, six women ranging from

When we see a photo of an attractive person, we can't be sure if the photo is really accurate or if it has been retouched. It is common for magazines to retouch photographs of models and celebrities, male and female. How do you think this practice affects the body image of young people?

size 6 to 14 were shown wearing only bras, panties, and big smiles. The Dove marketing director said, "It is our belief that beauty comes in different shapes, sizes, and ages. Our mission is to make more women feel beautiful every day by broadening the definition of beauty" (Babwin, 2005). Dove personnel reported that responses from women of various sizes seemed to indicate that the ads helped them develop a more positive body image.

Long (2005) pointed out that in *Seventeen, Teen People, CosmoGirl!*, and *Teen Vogue*, there are bathing suit sections partially illustrated by girls with less-than-perfect figures and tips on maximizing assets and minimizing defects. More average women and fewer models are being used to reflect changing body types and to help self-conscious teens see that not everyone is perfect. In 2004, *Glamour* broke a barrier of sorts by putting Queen Latifah on the cover. Compared to just a few years ago, there are now many efforts to use models of all shapes and sizes. Presenting a broader range of beauty, even under the guise of selling products, gives people more permission to believe they are attractive.

Even video games may have an influence on body image. Barlett and Harris (2008) conducted two studies to see whether playing video games that emphasized the body would increase negative body image. They found that participants in both studies had significantly lower body esteem after video game play. They concluded that video games have a negative influence on the body image of players.

Many people use social media even routinely. Fardouly and Vartanian (2015) examined the relationship between Facebook usage and body image concerns among female university students. They found that young women who spend more time on Facebook tend to feel more concerned about their body because they compare their appearance to others (especially to peers) seen in images on their Facebook pages.

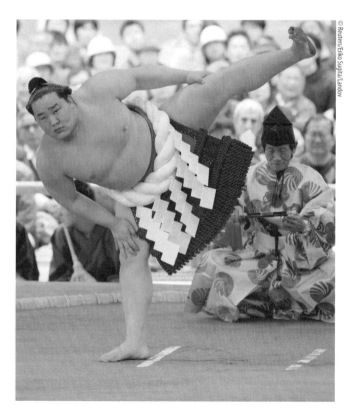

In Eastern cultures, the shape of a powerful body is that of a pyramid—with a strong base as the foundation. In Western culture the shape of a powerful body is that of an upside-down pyramid—broad shoulders and tapered waist.

The Internet in general has a role in reinforcing concepts of body image. The anonymity of the Internet has resulted in dating site users posting fake or outdated profile pictures due to fear of rejection. This practice is commonly known as "catfishing," a term inspired by the 2010 movie *Catfish*. A "catfish" is a person who pretends to be someone else on social media. This online identity is fabricated to trick people into emotional/romantic relationships over a long period of time. Possible motivations for this behavior include revenge, loneliness, curiosity, or boredom.

Warren (2014) points out that the goal of most mass-marketing campaigns and consumerism is to make us feel badly about ourselves. The worse we feel, the more we will buy—or so advertisers hope. After convincing us that we are less than ideal, the media offer us endless products that claim to fix our faults. Consequently, in addition to being one of the strongest predictors of eating disorder development, body dissatisfaction stimulates us to spend a great deal of resources—including time, money, and energy—trying to fix our perceived flaws. To counteract this, we need to become more critical consumers of the mass media. We need to think about the messages that we learn from a very early age about what makes us valuable or not valuable. Do we want to be a certain way because we think it is right, or because we were culturally conditioned to believe it is right?

Diversity and Body Image

In the past in the United States, the idea of beauty involved using the images of Barbie or Ken dolls or the like with the goal of creating some version of a white person. For example, it has been common for the winners of Latin American beauty contests to look "international": tall; not-too-dark hair; light skin; high, girlish bust; and long legs. Hispanic women often have to cope with the way the world would like to change them: if only the earrings were smaller, the makeup not so dramatic, the hair not so wild, the walk not so sexy, the hand gestures not so expressive, the emotions not so on-the-surface, and they were thinner.

Other examples related to diversity and body image are also apparent. A major problem for some African American women who seek psychological help is their skin color. Asian American women sometimes resort to eye surgery so they will look more like the stereotypical Caucasian ideal.

However, as the result of pressure from groups that emphasize the diversity of real life, products, methods, and goals relating to beauty have changed. Even plastic surgeons have learned a lot about working with people from diverse backgrounds.

Multicultural DIMENSIONS

Weight and Culture

The National Health and Nutrition Examination Survey (NHANES), which is conducted periodically by the U.S. Centers for Disease Control and Prevention (CDC), reported in 2011 that, after a quarter-century of increases, obesity prevalence did not measurably increase in recent years. But levels of obesity were still high—at 34% of U.S. adults aged 20 and older. Obesity means weighing at least 20% more than ideal weight. As noted by Fryar et al. (2014), the 2014 report indicated that 34.9% of U.S. adults aged 20 and older were obese. Data also suggested that the weight was not distributed equally among ethnic and cultural groups.

- There were large race–ethnic disparities in obesity prevalence among women.
- Approximately 57% of non-Hispanic black women, 49% of Mexican American women, and 44% of Hispanic women were obese, compared with 33% of non-Hispanic white women. The rate for non-Hispanic Asian women was 11%.
- For men, the disparities were not as great as for women. Approximately 37% of non-Hispanic black men, 44% of Mexican American men, and 40% of Hispanic men were obese, compared with 32% of non-Hispanic white men. The rate for non-Hispanic Asian men was 10%.

Other researchers have also looked at cultural differences in body weight and in body image. For example, Grammas and Schwartz (2009) found that more Asian males were dissatisfied with their muscles than were Caucasian, Hispanic, or African American males. Also, Thomas et al. (2008) reported on similarities and differences in black and white women's perceptions about obesity. Black women disagreed with the ideal of being thin and family members' dissatisfaction with their weight. White women were interested in losing weight, but desired support during weight loss from other obese individuals.

Building a Better Self-Image

Given that none of us will be perfect, and given that we all have imperfections in our appearance, we can still look better and improve our body image. It may not always be easy, but small efforts can also make a huge difference.

When we feel good about the way we look, we are happier and likely to feel better about others. Many actions can help you improve your body image. Here are some examples:

1. Do not feel a need to apologize about every blemish you might see in your appearance. Chances are, others do not notice them anyway. None of us is perfect.

2. Be careful about basing your body image on what you see and hear in advertisements. They are carefully produced to send certain messages to sell products. Few people look and act the way the people you see in the ads do.

3. Attractive people are often judged by others to be more warm, interesting, friendly, considerate, and strong than those who are less attractive. In spite of our defects, we can do things to feel more attractive. For example, clothes, styles, and personal hygiene all affect attractiveness. What can you do to feel more attractive?

4. You should be free to be yourself; however, the message you send about your appearance and the ones you receive from others may not always be the same. For example, a person might wear a certain outfit to be comfortable; another person might interpret that as a desire to be sexy. Which messages are you sending in the appearance you present?

5. The way you move your body (body language) can indicate the way you feel about yourself. Watch what others do when they are nervous, happy, or sad. Use this information to control some of your body movements so they send messages you want to send.

Here are some additional tips for a positive body image (Body image, 2009):

- Remember that health and appearance are two different things.

- Accept and value your genes—you probably inherited a lot of traits from your family members, so love those traits as you love your family.

People who feel good about themselves are more attractive to others.

- Keep a list of your positive qualities that have nothing to do with your appearance.

- Surround yourself with people who are supportive and who make you feel good about yourself.

- Treat your body with respect and kindness.

Powerful people use their bodies to convey authority. One high-power pose is sitting at a desk occupying as much space as possible—feet on the desk, fingers interlaced behind the head, and elbows straight out to the sides. Another high-power pose is standing straight and leaning forward on a table or desk while talking with people or listening. These poses are in contrast to low-power poses such as slouching in a chair or standing with arms wrapped around the body. Carney et al. (2010) found that using high-power poses causes hormonal and behavioral changes for both males and females. These changes can help people behave more positively and feel better about their body image. This is another example of the importance of positive body language.

Body image is important. People who feel good about themselves are more attractive to others than people who do not. Concentrate on your strengths. Do you have great hair? Eyes? Hands? Play them up. But remember your other strengths, too. Are you funny? Kind? Smart? You are more than just your looks.

There are excellent projects and information sources designed to help improve body image. One example is the Body Project at Bradley University (www.bradley.edu/thebodyproject/). It is intended for women and men of all ages, and provides information and programs of interest about body image and related issues. Another helpful source is emerge, the Body Image Project (www.emergebodyimage.com /BodyImageProject). A third source of information and programs is Mainely Girls (www.mainelygirls. org/). Since 1996, this site has administered numerous programs to make good things happen for girls.

Creating Your Optimal Body

Imagine that you are a personal trainer in a local fitness center. A center member gives you a magazine and says, "I want to look like the person in

Ethical DIMENSIONS

ETHICS

To Train or Not to Train: That Is the Question

A professionally prepared personal trainer knows how to help people develop the body to look the best it can. The trainer also knows that it is usually not possible to change the body type of a person drastically. So, what should a trainer who runs his or her own business and needs paying clients do when a person asks to look the way someone pictured in a magazine does? If the trainer agrees to help the person resemble the one in the picture, there will be false hopes created; however, you could argue that at least the person will improve his or her appearance and health—and probably body image as well. Or should the trainer tell the client that there is no way he or she can look like the picture and explain how unrealistic expectations can cause a waste of money if he or she tries to obtain objectives that cannot be reached?

this picture, and I need you to help me do it!" What should you do?

If you are the one who wants to resemble a person in a magazine picture, it might be wise to remember that you need to optimize your own body. It does us no good to strive to be someone else. There may be qualities of other people—physical as well as others—that we want to obtain, but we cannot be exactly like another person.

Genetics: Building on Your Strong Points

A person who is 5'4" tall may strive to be an Olympic basketball player, but his or her chance of success is not good; the 6'8", 225-pound man will probably not make a good competitive gymnast. Although these examples are extreme, we need to keep them in mind when we consider what is possible and best for each of us.

Many people are not happy with the appearance of their bodies. Al Sabbah et al. (2009) surveyed adolescents in 24 countries and regions in Europe, Canada, and the United States. They found that body weight dissatisfaction was highly prevalent but was more common in girls than boys, among overweight than non-overweight individuals, and among older adolescents than younger adolescents.

Your Body Weight
Most often when we think of body weight, we think about what the scale says when we stand on it. Although this is useful information, if you are serious about reaching your optimal body weight, it would be worthwhile to learn more about some topics beyond the scope of this book: **body mass index (BMI)** and **body composition**. Knowing about these will help you understand your body weight better and have more realistic goals.

What the scale says is not always the complete truth, and what we see is not always what we are. For example, sometimes overweight people see themselves as heavier than they really are. When they look in a mirror, they see a bigger abdomen, rear end, and thighs than they actually have. This body image may be hard to change, even if body weight decreases.

Other overweight people may see themselves as much slimmer than they really are. They often rationalize away their need to lose weight. However, some people see themselves as they really are. Those with realistic body images tend to have the greatest success with weight control.

Body weight can even continue to influence more established relationships. Meltzer et al. (2011) conducted a 4-year longitudinal study of newlywed couples. They found that husbands were more satisfied initially and wives were more satisfied over time to

the extent that wives had lower BMIs than their husbands. They concluded that marriages are more satisfying when wives are thinner than their husbands.

In recent years, approximately half of all U.S. states have passed legislation requiring BMI surveillance and screening programs in public schools. These programs have been the subject of ethical debates about confidentiality and privacy, school-to-parent communication, and safety and self-esteem issues for students. Ruggieri and Bass (2015) found that despite the controversies, such programs are valuable for all parties; such BMI screening programs are vital to the development of robust school-based obesity prevention programs and promotion of healthy lifestyles in schools.

Diet
The diet business is big business in the United States. Despite the interest in diet products and services, few people have long-term weight control success.

To have any hope of long-term success with weight loss, our approach to diets must change. A "diet" must mean permanent changes in eating habits. Do not waste time on dieting if you are not committed to maintaining a healthy weight throughout your life. If you want to change your eating habits, you must pay close attention to the kinds and amounts of foods you eat. There is no substitute for well-balanced diets and a reduction in intake of calories—especially when combined with proper exercise habits.

Exercise
Exercise plays an important role in losing pounds and keeping them off. Researchers have compared the effects of weight loss by diet only and by exercise only. They found that the group who were only exercising lost a higher percentage of fat and had more success keeping off the weight than the group who were only dieting.

Moderate exercise suppresses appetite, rather than increasing it, as many people think. You might want to exercise just before a meal to take advantage of that effect. Another benefit of exercise is that it strengthens muscle tissue. Muscle tissue requires more calories than fat tissue does to maintain itself, so as lean muscle tissue increases, more calories are burned. This is important, because our resting metabolic rate accounts for about 70% of the calories we burn.

The ultimate goal of any weight-loss program should be the loss of body fat, not just body weight.

body mass index (BMI) Weight in kilograms divided by the square of the height in meters.

body composition The percentage of fat versus lean tissue.

? Did You Know . . .

How can you tell if someone you love has an eating disorder?

Not all people with eating disorders experience symptoms, and there may be different combinations of symptoms. Someone does not have to have any or all of the following symptoms to have an eating disorder, but it is good to be alert for these symptoms:

1. Weight loss or weight fluctuation
2. Excessive exercise
3. Binging and/or purging
4. Caloric restriction
5. Picky eating
6. Misuse of laxatives or diet pills
7. Caffeine abuse
8. Misuse of ipecac or epsom salts
9. Females may quit menstruating
10. Hair loss
11. Anemia
12. Damaged teeth
13. Fingernails break easily
14. Growth of fine hair on face or body

Source: Data from How to recognize signs of an eating disorder. *International Business Times* (April 29, 2011). Available at: http://www.ibtimes.com/art/services/print.php?articleid=139835.

Those who combine diet and exercise lose more fat and are more likely to keep it off. Exercise and sound eating habits result in a steady weight loss that can be maintained on a permanent basis if you maintain your exercise and dietary changes.

▓ Issues Related to Trying to Be Perfect

Although we know it is impossible to be perfect, some people are so concerned about their body image that they run into problems, such as eating disorders, obsessive muscle dysmorphia, and complications of cosmetic surgery.

Eating Disorders

In the quest to be attractive and improve one's body image, some people are willing to pay a high price. It is common to want to look as good as we can, and many people attempt to control body weight by using various diets at some time during their lives. A fear of fat seems to drive some people to extreme forms of eating behaviors. Compulsive overeating (also called *binge eating*) and compulsive dieting are the behaviors known as *eating disorders*. Striegel-Moore et al. (2008) reported that women are more likely to have eating disorders than are men. Women are significantly more likely to participate in fasting, binge eating, and vomiting. Nevertheless, a substantial minority of men have eating disorder symptoms. In addition, many college athletes show disordered eating patterns, with the greatest prevalence occurring in gymnasts and swimmers.

While they probably mean well, sometimes athletic coaches and even parents might contribute to eating disorders. They could do this by encouraging young people to diet or by demeaning their bodies by telling them they are too fat or do not have the "correct" body proportions.

The exact causes of eating disorders are not known for sure, but they seem to be triggered by life's stressors, emotional trauma, tragic events, and the media. Common health problems associated with eating disorders include intestinal problems; decayed

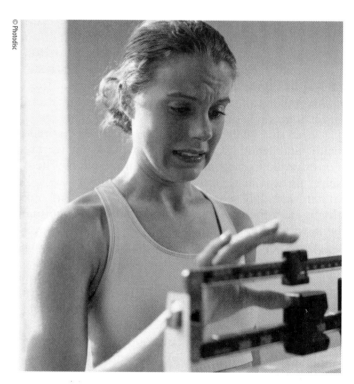

© Photodisc

We need to pay attention to our body composition as well as our body weight.

teeth; malnutrition; dehydration; stomach ruptures; esophagus tears; serious heart, kidney, and liver damage; and death.

Anorexia nervosa is a condition in which the individual severely limits calorie intake; it is sometimes described as self-induced starvation. The individual fears gaining weight even though he or she may already be underweight. There is also a disturbance in the way personal body weight or shape is viewed by the individual. Anorexia can be fatal. Most people with anorexia are white females younger than 25 years of age who are focused on a goal of extreme thinness and willingly starve themselves and overexercise to reach that goal.

Over the course of a lifetime, 0.5% to 3.7% of girls and women develop anorexia nervosa. Approximately 0.5% of the female population die each year as a result of their illness, making it one of the top psychiatric illnesses leading to death (Taylor et al., 2006). Although this condition affects females 95% of the time, it may be more common than previously thought among college males. Most males with anorexia are men who depend on their thin physique for employment—such as models. Anorexia results in death in about 10% of all cases in males and females.

Although the exact cause of anorexia is unknown, it seems to involve a combination of psychological and environmental factors. The female with anorexia might reject food in an attempt to avoid dealing with what she feels are society's demands that she become a superwoman. The severe weight loss can make the female resemble a young girl, in what some researchers feel is a conscious attempt to avoid dealing with issues related to intimacy and sexuality. People with anorexia might feel that their weight is the only factor they can control in a world where expectations of others seem difficult to fulfill. One of the most difficult to understand aspects of anorexia is self-perception. Regardless of how much weight has been lost, the person with anorexia still feels too heavy.

There are more than 500 websites that deal frankly, and sometimes approvingly, with anorexia and other eating disorders. On some websites, people with eating disorders gather for support and companionship, share tips for losing weight and hiding the signs of malnutrition, and provide "thinspiration," like photos of bony fashion models. No one knows for sure how many of the estimated 11 million Americans suffering from anorexia or bulimia visit the websites, but the developer of one of them claims to have had more than 85,000 hits in a period of about 18 months. Some are often referred to as "pro-ana forums" (ana being short for anorexia). Most adolescents tend to use the websites without their parents' knowledge, and the sites can be especially seductive. One girl said, "Now I can learn to be an anorexic

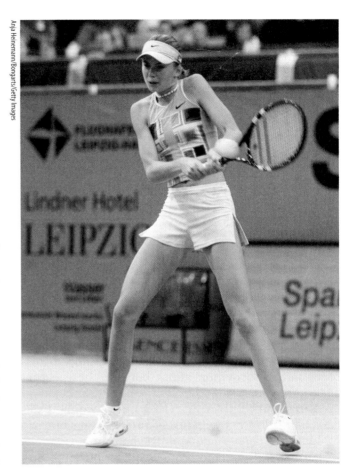

Many female athletes turn to some form of dieting to maintain an edge in competitions. As spectators having read this chapter, we may wonder what the female athletes have done to be as thin as they are.

from the Internet." The pro-ana sites are a world that is comforting to those with an eating disorder, and they provide a sense of belonging.

Bulimia nervosa is a condition in which the person periodically binges and purges, with an obsessive fear of becoming fat. Bulimia (insatiable appetite) has been confused with anorexia nervosa because periodic bingeing is common to both disorders; however, a number of the characteristics are different. People with bulimia are usually older than people with anorexia and may have been anorexic earlier. Whereas people with anorexia are obsessed with being thin, people with bulimia have an obsessive fear of becoming fat.

anorexia nervosa   A condition in which an individual severely limits caloric intake.

bulimia nervosa   A condition in which the individual periodically binges and purges, with an obsessive fear of becoming fat.

Approximately 2% to 3% of the U.S. population has bulimia. Some research indicates the rate is higher for college-age women—around 4%. The illness usually begins in late adolescence or early adult life. Only an estimated 5% to 15% of people with bulimia are male, but the incidence is increasing among males. Bulimia is often perceived to be an affliction of Caucasian girls and young women in middle and upper socioeconomic classes. However, increasing numbers of cases are being seen in men and women of all different ethnic and cultural groups. It is evident that bulimia occurs in all cultures (Schoenstadt, 2007; TieMeyer, 2007).

During their secretive eating binges, people with bulimia may consume many thousands of calories in only a few hours. Afterward, they try to purge the food through a variety of methods, including vomiting, laxatives, diuretics, and exercise. After bingeing and purging, the person with bulimia may feel discouraged about the behavior.

There is still a lot to be learned about both anorexia and bulimia. Researchers continue to discover new information about both of these eating disorders.

Binge-eating disorder (BED) is an eating disorder characterized by recurrent binge eating but not by inappropriate weight-control behaviors. Persons with BED do not regularly engage in purging, and the majority are obese. They also may be referred to as "compulsive overeaters."

Characteristics of binge eating include eating much more rapidly than normal, eating until feeling uncomfortably full, eating large amounts even though one is not hungry, eating alone because of embarrassment about eating habits, and feeling disgusted or guilty after overeating. There is usually a feeling that one cannot stop eating or control what or how much is being eaten.

Treating Eating Disorders
Many approaches are used in the treatment of anorexia, but the prognosis is not good. Drug therapy is used in about 25% of the cases, and behavior modification in about 45%. A combination of approaches is also used. Most specialists recommend a period of hospitalization to ensure weight gain, and families are often involved in the therapy. The prognosis for people with anorexia is worse than for people with bulimia.

Overcoming bulimia requires establishing a normal eating pattern that eliminates dieting. Although

It is important to be realistic about our eating practices.

people with bulimia can hide their disorder from others, they are more likely than people with anorexia to seek treatment; however, they might expect immediate results and become frustrated with therapy. Antidepressant drugs are used in the treatment of bulimia, as is psychological therapy. Antidepressant medication and psychological treatments can also reduce binge eating of BED patients.

Muscle Dysmorphia

Body image and goals related to it may change over time. Thus, as someone makes progress with weights, or in gymnastics or figure skating, the ideal of the perfect body image may become more "perfect." A perpetual chasing of the ideal can cause people to lose perspective about their actual body image. An example of this was given in the opening story of this chapter.

One disorder that afflicts bodybuilders is essentially the opposite of anorexia nervosa. Called **muscle dysmorphia (MD)**, also known as bigorexia and reverse anorexia, it involves bodybuilders who, despite their extremely muscular bodies and tip-top shape, consider themselves to be puny. Weight lifting, for some people, can become a dangerous obsession.

Dawes et al. (2009) provided an overview of the literature related to MD. They pointed out that MD is characterized by an overwhelming compulsion with accruing large amounts of lean mass. It occurs mainly in men, but women who are bodybuilders can also have MD. People with MD are preoccupied by

---

binge-eating disorder (BED) Eating disorder characterized by recurrent binge eating but not by inappropriate weight-control behaviors.

muscle dysmorphia A disorder whereby a bodybuilder in top shape considers himself or herself to be puny.

irrational thoughts regarding their perceived small musculature despite actually having high levels of muscular development. This preoccupation can lead to increased mood, social, and anxiety disorders. It is not uncommon for people with MD to miss important social, occupational, and/or recreational activities because of a compulsive need to maintain a specific workout and dietary schedule. They might even sever personal relationships and turn down professional opportunities and job promotions to devote more time to their time-consuming training regimes. Supplements and pharmacological interventions (especially steroids) are commonly used to attain greater levels of muscularity. It is hard to determine an exact cause of MD, but research indicates that continuous exposure to idealized male body images portrayed in the media and in male action figures may have a negative impact on male body image satisfaction. Some health risks associated with MD are musculoskeletal injuries from overtraining, increased risk of cardiovascular disease, kidney failure, steroid abuse, drug addiction, eating disorders, infections, disease from the use of dirty and/or shared needles, and even death.

Interestingly, in one study American and European college men were asked to pick a body type that they thought women would find attractive. The average pick had 20 to 30 more pounds of muscle than a normal man. When women were asked the same question, they chose the normal-sized man most of the time (Fahmy, 2004).

A simple test for bigorexia involves questions such as: (1) How often do you look at your body in the mirror? (2) Do you think your body needs to be leaner and more muscular? (3) Do you find yourself reading up on new training methods, diets, and supplements? (4) Do you eat special high-protein or low-fat diets or use food supplements to improve

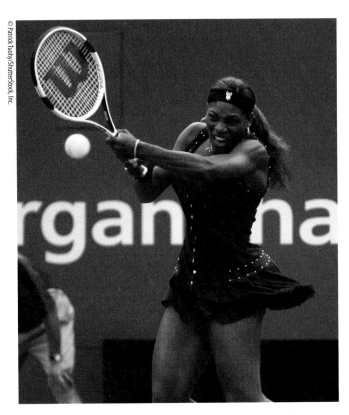

People have various opinions about which type of physique looks attractive.

muscularity? (5) Do you ever wear baggy clothes to hide the body you feel is too lean—or do you avoid situations where your body might be seen? (6) Do you still train when injured because you fear losing muscle mass? (7) Do you compare yourself to others and feel envious? (8) Do you ever think others are snickering at your puniness? (9) Would you rather spend time going to the gym than having sex, and has your libido taken a dive? (10) Have you turned

Gender DIMENSIONS

Why Are Eating Disorders Mainly Found in Women?

It seems clear that physical attractiveness is more important for women than men. This is because beauty is often a central aspect of femininity (girls learn early that being pretty draws attention to them), and women's self-worth is often tied to establishing and maintaining close relationships. They can improve their feeling of self-worth based on others' opinions and approval of them.

The ideal standard of physical attractiveness has become thinner over the past few decades. This makes

it even harder for women to meet the standard, so they are more likely to resort to extreme ways to control their weight—such as rigid dieting and purging.

Even when men take extreme measures to control their weight, it is usually done to improve their athletic performance (such as with jockeys and wrestlers). Their goal of losing weight is secondary to their goal of performing well. For women, however, dieting to achieve an ideal weight is related to their self-evaluation.

down social events, taken time off from work, or skipped family responsibilities so you can work out? Typically, people who have bigorexia will say "yes" to three or more of these questions (Mind over fatter, 2005).

Muscle dysmorphia does not usually involve the serious medical complications of anorexia, but it still can have significant effects. It is certainly normal for people who go to a gym to want to improve their physique and build larger muscles. The turning point from normal goals to muscle dysmorphia occurs when the quest for "massive" size takes over one's life, destroying career, relationships, and, ironically, self-esteem.

Sports and Dieting

Eating disorders may be the gravest health problem facing female athletes, affecting gymnasts, figure skaters, swimmers, distance runners, divers, and even tennis and volleyball players. Given the importance that sport attaches to weight—and, in subjectively judged sports, to appearance—it is not surprising that eating disorders are common among athletes.

But weight—and dieting—also play a major role in endurance sports. As an athlete's weight falls, his or her aerobic power increases. Put another way, it takes less energy to run if you weigh less; thus more energy can be expended on running faster. So runners and swimmers also succumb to the need to diet to win.

Steroid Use

Steroids are synthetic versions of the male hormone testosterone. Steroid abuse is fast becoming a very serious problem among adolescent males, both athletes and nonathletes, who take large doses in an attempt to achieve much greater body mass quickly. In addition to potential to halt growth and bone development, steroid use can cause testicular shrinkage, increased cholesterol levels, infertility, decreased sexual drive, prostate cancer, kidney disorders, liver malfunction, aggression and violence, suicidal tendencies, and extreme moodiness. Steroids can also be psychologically and physically addictive.

Steroid abuse is a problem among teenagers. Johnston et al. (2009) reported that there was a fairly sharp increase in the use of steroids by male teens in the late 1990s, with peak levels reached in 1999 among eighth-grade males, in 2000 among tenth-grade males, and in 2001 and 2002 among twelfth-grade males. Since those peak years, the annual prevalence rate has dropped by more than half among eighth- and

Many people look at eight-time Mr. Olympia Lee Haney only in terms of his muscles. But Haney keeps body image in perspective, placing God, family, and friends above business—and to Haney, bodybuilding was a business.

tenth-grade males (to 1.2% and 1.4%, respectively), and by one-third among twelfth-grade males (to 2.5% annual prevalence in 2008). Steroid use is not limited to males, however. While the prevalence rates tend to be much lower among females, the trend toward steroid use by females is much the same as for males.

People may go to unhealthy extremes simply to look good. The most common reason male bodybuilders give for using steroids is to enhance looks.

Women in endurance sports also take steroids. Steroids help a runner in two ways: A thin runner expends less energy in running; by speeding muscle recovery, a long-distance runner is able to recover faster, train more, and thus run faster.

The adverse effects of steroids in women include lowered voice, increased body and facial hair, male-pattern baldness, enlarged clitoris, decreased breast size, and changes in or cessation of menstruation. There are not sufficient studies of female steroid users to fully

steroids Synthetic versions of the male hormone testosterone that promote tissue growth.

understand the extent to which a woman's body may be damaged and whether the effects are permanent.

In addition to the many adverse effects of steroids listed, there is a risk of HIV transmission through shared needles. Finally, anabolic steroids are illegal in the United States; their use carries stiff fines and possible imprisonment.

Some feel that a "male body ideal" has caused increasing numbers of males to develop an "Adonis complex"—defined as a condition shared by millions of males who develop eating disorders, abuse steroids, work out compulsively, or otherwise obsess over their physical appearance. The taboo against overt male vanity inhibits men from seeking help for their disorders.

Makeovers and Cosmetic Surgery

If we pay attention to our favorite movie and TV stars, we see that they radically change their appearance from time to time. The makeover has become a powerful draw for many stars—they feel it can renew the spirit, save a career, and even mend the heart. Indeed, Hollywood may be in the grip of a redo revolution. Some stars like to re-create themselves, increase their confidence by showing that they can wear more than one style, and avoid being linked with a look created by a past role.

Sharp et al. (2014) examined the influence of media and peers on attitudes toward cosmetic surgery. They found that almost all the media and friend variables they used correlated with positive attitudes toward such surgery. Media exposure and friend conversations affected attitudes toward cosmetic surgery both directly and indirectly.

According to the American Society of Plastic Surgeons, the number of cosmetic procedures in the United States increased to more than 15.1 million in 2013, a 3% increase from 2012, and a 144% increase from 2000 (American Society of Plastic Surgeons, 2015). Some people feel this increase relates to a surge in reality cosmetic surgery television programming. Viewing reality cosmetic surgery shows can be related to more favorable cosmetic surgery attitudes, perceived pressure to have cosmetic surgery, past attainment of a cosmetic procedure, a decreased fear of surgery, and overall body dissatisfaction and disordered eating.

In our quest to create the perfect look, we may see the stars radically change theirs and decide we want to do it too. People today often view their body as increasingly malleable. Sometimes, they even want to use ways that look easy, such as liposuction, implants, and plastic surgery.

Liposuction is a technique for removing adipose (fat) tissue with a suction-pump device. A hollow suction tube, which is attached to a special vacuum,

According to the American Society of Plastic Surgeons, liposuction is the most popular cosmetic surgery procedure for men and women, after rhinoplasty. Comedian Kathy Griffin underwent liposuction in an attempt to drop from a size 4 to a size 2. Medical complications during and after the surgery, as she recounts in an article published by *Glamour* magazine, proved to be nearly fatal. Have you ever considered undergoing cosmetic surgery in pursuit of your ideal body? Do you think the benefits outweigh the risks?

is inserted into small incisions in the skin. It is used primarily to remove and reduce areas of fat around the abdomen, breast, legs, face, and upper arms. Liposuction can be helpful for the removal of fat in

liposuction A technique for removing adipose tissue with a suction-pump device.

particular areas, but it should not be viewed as a way to lose large amounts of fat or to change one's physique dramatically. Most people lose an average of only 3 pounds as a direct result of the procedure. According to the American Society of Plastic Surgeons (2014), liposuction was the fourth most common cosmetic procedure in 2013, with just over 199,000 such procedures performed. That was a 1% decrease since 2012 and a 44% decrease since 2000. The average physician fee was about $3,000.

Breast implants have been around for quite a few years. Silicone-gel–filled breast implants first went on the market in 1962. They were banned in 1992 by the Food and Drug Administration (FDA). The question of whether they should be used has been greatly debated. In April 2005, an FDA advisory committee voted to recommend allowing them back on the market under certain conditions—making sure women understand potential risk, having women get regular MRI exams, allowing only specially trained plastic surgeons to perform the insertions, and requiring continued research studies related to the implants. Women who wanted a return of the product say silicone-gel implants look and feel more natural than the saline-filled implants. The implants have been exonerated from concerns that they might cause serious or chronic illnesses such as cancer or lupus. Aside from the risk of breakage and pain, however, they can cause infection and development of painful scar tissue. Breast augmentation was the most common cosmetic surgical procedure in 2013, with just over 290,000 performed. This was a 1% increase over 2012 and a 37% increase over 2000. The average physician fee was about $3,400 (American Society of Plastic Surgeons, 2015).

Cosmetic surgery includes the procedures already mentioned, and there are also many other possibilities. Many people elect to have cosmetic surgery when a part of their body makes them self-conscious or uncomfortable. After surgery, many patients say they have a more positive self-image. Statistically, approximately 73% of all cosmetic operations are done on Caucasians (up 3% since 2012), 12% on Hispanics (up 6%), 8% on African Americans (up 5%), and 7% on Asian Americans (up 1%) (American Society of Plastic Surgeons, 2015).

Another common procedure is **rhinoplasty** (surgery done to change the shape of the nose). It usually takes 1 to 2 hours and costs an average of $4,500. It is not covered by insurance unless the nose structure impedes breathing. As with any surgery, there can be

© Reuters/Alex Grimm/Landov

Young girls emulate superstars, and some of these stars have had breast augmentation surgery. In fact, according to the American Society of Plastic and Reconstructive Surgeons, 8,200 girls age 19 and younger had the surgery in 2013. Breast augmentation surgery is the most common surgery procedure for women, with 290,000 operations performed in 2013—a 21% increase since 2000. Interestingly, many of the surgeries take place in California, Texas, and Florida. Why do you think this is the case?

undesirable results. The patient may not like the aesthetic result and want a revision, the newly formed nose may make breathing difficult, or fibrous scar tissue may form. In 2013 over 221,000 rhinoplasty procedures were performed. This was a drop of 9% from 2012 and 43% from 2000 (American Society of Plastic Surgeons, 2015).

Some men turn to implants to enhance their pectoral muscles. The average cost for putting in a pair of palm-size silicone discs is just over $4,500. This is a relatively new procedure. In 2013 342 pectoral implants were performed, a 2% increase over 2012. In 2013 more than 1.2 million men elected to

cosmetic surgery Surgery done for the sole purpose of improving the appearance.

rhinoplasty Surgery done to change the shape of the nose.

have cosmetic procedures, a 22% increase over 2000. Men accounted for 9% of all cosmetic procedures; 91% of all procedures were performed on women (13.1 million—a 1% increase over 2012) (American Society of Plastic Surgeons, 2015).

The top five surgical procedures may be listed differently depending upon the source. The American Society of Plastic Surgeons (2014) lists the top five for women as being breast augmentation (290,000), nose reshaping (164,000), liposuction (176,000), eyelid surgery (185,000), and face lift (121,000). The top five for men were nose reshaping (54,000), eyelid surgery (30,000), liposuction (23,000), breast reduction (23,000), and face lift (13,000).

Men's magazines and websites are filled with ads for pumps, pills, weights, exercises, and surgeries that are supposed to increase the length and/or the width of the penis. However, no scientific research supports the use of any nonsurgical method to enlarge the penis, and no reputable medical society endorses penis-enlargement surgery performed for purely cosmetic reasons. Many of these techniques can damage the penis and may even cause functional problems. Cosmetic surgeons have developed several enlargement techniques, but none of them are endorsed by medical organizations. Following various procedures, some men have had to undergo additional surgeries to correct deformities caused by the original procedure. Others have had scarring, shorter penises, hair on the base of the penis, low-hanging penis, loss of sensitivity, and bumps and lumps. Other complaints include loss of sexual function, urinary incompetence, and persistent pain. Surgery should only be an option for penises that have been amputated or damaged for some reason (Beware of penis enlargement scams, 2005).

Some women want breast implants; others want to have large, heavy breasts reduced in size. The latter procedure may not necessarily be considered cosmetic surgery, depending on the intention and the situation, because it may be performed to relieve physical ailments such as back and neck pain caused by large, heavy breasts. It involves removal of fat and breast tissue and may leave noticeable scars. The procedure may also affect the ability to breastfeed. It usually takes 2 to 4 hours and costs an average of $5,200. It may be covered by insurance if medical problems are associated with the size of the breasts. In 2013 about 123,000 breast reductions were performed on females, as compared with 48,000 in 1997 (American Society for Aesthetic Plastic Surgery, 2015).

Whereas liposuction only removes fat, the **tummy tuck (abdominoplasty)** is a more extensive surgical procedure that removes excess skin and fat from the lower abdomen and tightens the abdominal muscles. It usually requires a hip-to-hip lower-abdominal incision and takes 1 to 2 hours to complete if fat deposits are below the navel. If a more extensive procedure is needed, it can take 2 to 5 hours. It has an average total cost of $5,400, usually not covered by insurance (American Society of Aesthetic Plastic Surgery, 2015).

Other available procedures include face lifts, upper and lower eyelid reduction, and chin implantation. In short, we can have just about any part of our body altered if we are strongly motivated and have the means to pay for it. Because it is legal in most U.S. states for any physician to advertise himself or herself as a plastic or cosmetic surgeon, candidates for surgery must select a well-trained plastic surgeon for any type of cosmetic surgery.

Several trends indicate that cosmetic surgery will continue to be a growth industry. Younger people are getting more cosmetic procedures, people who have had cosmetic procedures tend to have others, men are becoming more "vain," the number getting surgery has increased rapidly, and the aging of the population is likely to result in more cosmetic surgery.

The top five nonsurgical cosmetic procedures in 2013 were Botox injection (3.8 million procedures); injection of hyaluronic acid (a jelly-like substance that softens facial lines and furrows) (1.9 million procedures); laser hair removal (901,000 procedures); microdermabrasion (mechanical scraping of the skin to soften sharp edges of surface irregularities) (480,000 procedures); and photorejuvenation (a skin treatment using lasers, intense pulsed light, or photodynamic therapy to treat skin conditions and remove wrinkles, spots, and textures) (457,000 procedures). People age 35 to 50 accounted for the largest proportion of the total number of procedures (4.7 million, 42% of the total). People age 19 to 34 accounted for 18%, people age 51 to 64 had 30%, people age 65 and older had 10%, and people age 18 and younger had 1% of the procedures (American Society for Aesthetic Plastic Surgery, 2015).

Finally, body piercing and tattoos have been used by some people to enhance their body image. No longer a practice carried out in back rooms, body piercing and tattoos have made their way into socially acceptable studios. Although many people have questioned the motivations behind body piercing, some feel it gives people a strong sense of self and a connection with others by marking relationship events in commitment ceremonies, by enhancing people's feelings about their body, by providing the rush of the piercing experience, and by giving people a way to rebel against mainstream society. The most common places for body piercing are the face or ears; some people pierce their tongues, nipples, abdomen, and genitals. This practice is not risk-free; it sometimes produces infection.

tummy tuck (abdominoplasty) Extensive surgical procedure that removes excess skin and fat from the abdomen.

Exploring the Dimensions of Human Sexuality

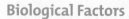

Body image refers to the mental image we have of our physical appearance. It is influenced by many factors. Our body image can influence our self-concept and our sexual behavior, and it is an important part of our sexual health.

There are few, if any, perfect bodies. What we see in the media, however, might make us think many others look great, but we don't. Photographers, cameras, and alterations made to pictures influence how we think we ought to look, but in real life very few people look like those depictions in the media. Many experts think there should be regulations preventing the alterations of photographs or other depictions that would promote unrealistic expectations of appropriate body image.

There are many ways to build a better body image. They include not feeling a need to apologize for every blemish you might have, being careful about basing body image on what is seen and heard in advertisements, and determining what you can do to feel more attractive (e.g., by choosing clothes, styles, personal hygiene, and the ways you move your body [body language]).

Some people are so concerned about their body image that they develop serious physical and psychological problems, such as eating disorders, obsessive muscle dysphoria, and complications of cosmetic surgery. Steroid use can also be a problem among some people trying to quickly achieve body mass.

Makeovers and cosmetic surgery have become more common in recent years. Popular procedures include liposuction and breast augmentation or reduction for females, and liposuction, breast reduction, and nose surgery (rhinoplasty) for men.

Body piercing and tattoos have been used as means to enhance body image. These procedures are not risk free; they sometimes produce infection. In addition, the effects of these procedures can be difficult to reverse if desired.

Biological Factors

- Increasing body satisfaction may help decrease sexually transmitted infections due to increased condom use during sexual activity.
- Many people in the United States tend to value females who are smaller and thinner and males who are larger and muscular.

Sociocultural Factors

- The media, including social media and the Internet, play a major role in influencing concepts of body image.
- People from different cultures may view body image very differently.
- Body image concerns seem to be higher in women, but many are also found in men.

Psychological Factors

- Body image refers to the mental image we have of our physical appearance.
- Some people are so concerned about their body image that they develop eating disorders.
- Body image influences sexual behavior, sexual self-esteem, and sexual satisfaction.
- We can do a lot to build a better body image.

Summary

- Body image refers to the mental image we have of our own physical appearance. It is influenced by many factors, and in turn, influences our attitudes and behaviors.

- The media play a major role in influencing people's body images. Many media images are unattainable in real life.

- People from different cultures may view body image very differently.

- We can do a lot to build a better body image by not apologizing for all our blemishes; not basing our body image on what we see in the media; dressing and acting in ways that make us feel more attractive; and paying attention to our body language.

- Diet and exercise can play major roles related to body image.

- Some people are so concerned about their body image that they develop eating disorders such as anorexia nervosa, bulimia nervosa, and binge-eating disorder.

- Using steroids in an attempt to develop one's body is a very dangerous thing to do. Steroids cause many serious health problems.

- Cosmetic surgery has become much more popular today than it was just 10 to 12 years ago. The most common procedures include liposuction, breast augmentation, eyelid surgery, tummy tuck, and nose reshaping.

Discussion questions

1. Explain how the media have created unrealistic body images for women and men.

2. Which strategies can be used to create a more positive body image?

3. Which problems, both physical and psychological, occur when people try to make themselves more "perfect"?

Application Questions

Reread the story that opens the chapter and answer the following questions:

1. As do many teens, Marc had a poor body image. Teased by his friends ("Ostrich Boy") and haunted by the images in men's magazines, he turned to lifting weights. If you had a chance to talk to a group of 14-year-old boys, what advice would you give them on how to handle body-image issues? What about a group of 14-year-old girls?

2. One of the problems about weight lifting to improve body image is that you can "never be too big." The more muscle you gain, the more you strive for. But as goals are set higher, workouts require more time in the gym, more sleep for recovery, and more time for eating properly. How is it possible to manage the desire for continued physical improvement without becoming obsessive?

3. Consider the changes in Marc's body image as he goes to law school, gets a job, gets married, has children, and so on. How might Marc's body image change across time? If he suddenly found himself divorced and single at age 40 years, should he hit the weights again?

Critical Thinking Questions

1. Because excessive weight has been linked to many health problems, why should we all not strive to be thin? Is it more harmful to diet excessively or to be obese?

2. You are an assistant college coach. An athlete returns from summer vacation, having put on 30 pounds of muscle. He says he spent the summer "lifting his ass off." You think he may have used steroids. Would you report him to the school's athletic director? (If he were found to have taken steroids, he could be expelled from school. However, if he continued to use steroids, he could suffer serious medical problems.)

3. Would your answer to question 2 be different if a female athlete returned in the fall with an additional 15 pounds of muscle? Explain your answer.

4. The noted eating-disorder psychologist G. Terence Wilson has stated that, biologically, women cannot be thin and have large breasts. Yet many women exercise and diet until they have low body fat and then have breast implants to compensate. Role models for the thin-yet-busty type include professional bodybuilders, many of the athletes on daytime TV exercise shows, and many actresses. How do such role models affect women?

Critical Thinking Case

Before attending college, your girlfriend Amanda ran cross-country and track. But with the pressures of college studies, part-time work, and your relationship, she has little time to exercise. She has started to worry more and more about the "freshman 15," the extra weight that many college freshmen gain. She often comments on how good the cover girls on fashion magazines look. That is not all: You have noticed she rarely eats when you go out. When you mention this, she says she is trying to help save money for a vacation. When you find over-the-counter diet pills hidden under her bed, she says, "Everyone takes them." When you tell her that someone heard her throwing up in the bathroom after meals, she flatly denies it. When you tell her she is looking "rather thin," she smiles and says, "Thank you."

You have read the information in this chapter and do not believe that she has an eating disorder. However, you are concerned about Amanda's physical health and psychological well-being. How could you help her to improve her body image?

Exploring Personal Dimensions

Body Image

How do you feel about the appearance of these regions of your body?

	Quite satisfied	Somewhat satisfied	Somewhat dissatisfied	Very dissatisfied
Hair	❏	❏	❏	❏
Arms	❏	❏	❏	❏
Hands	❏	❏	❏	❏
Feet	❏	❏	❏	❏
Waist	❏	❏	❏	❏
Buttocks	❏	❏	❏	❏
Hips	❏	❏	❏	❏
Legs and ankles	❏	❏	❏	❏
Thighs	❏	❏	❏	❏
Chest/ breasts	❏	❏	❏	❏
Posture	❏	❏	❏	❏
General attrac-tiveness	❏	❏	❏	❏

1. Which of your thoughts and actions enhance your body image?

2. Which of your thoughts and actions are detrimental to your body image?

3. Which societal forces (e.g., expectations of friends and parents, advertising, celebrities and professional athletes) influence your body image most strongly?

4. What could you do to become more satisfied with your body image?

Suggested Readings

Anderson, E., Siegel, E. H., Bliss-Moreau, E., & Barrett, L. F. The visual impact of gossip. *Science, 332, no. 6036* (June 2011), 1446–1448.

American Society of Asethetic Plastic Surgery. (2015). Available: http://www.surgery.org.

American Society of Plastic Surgeons. (2015). Available: http://www.plasticsurgery.org.

Benton, C., & Karazsia, B. T. The effect of thin and muscular images on women's body satisfaction. *Body Image, 13* (March 2015), 22–27.

Body image. *Psychology Today,* 2015. Available: http://www.psychologytoday.com/basics /body-image.

Johnson, S. K., Podratz, K. E., Dipboye, R. L., & Gibbons, E. Physical attractiveness biases in ratings of employment suitability: Tracking down the "beauty is beastly" effect. *Journal of Social Psychology, 150, no. 3* (May/June 2010), 301–318.

McCabe, M. P., Busija, L., Fuller-Tyszkiewicz, M., Ricciardelli, L., Mellor, D., & Mussap, A. Sociocultural influences on strategies to lose weight, gain weight, and increase muscles among ten cultural groups. *Body Image, 12* (January 2015), 108–114.

McLaughlin, E. A., Belon, K. E., Smith, J. E., & Erickson, S. J. Mothers' and daughters' beliefs about factors affecting preadolescent girls' body satisfaction. *Body Image, 13* (March 2015), 9–17.

Mumen, S. K., Poinsatte, K., Huntsman, K., Goldfarb, J., & Glaser, D. Body ideals for heterosexual romantic partners: Gender and sociocultural influences. *Body Image, 12* (January 2015), 22–31.

Web Resources

Eating Disorder Referral and Information Center
http://edreferral.com

Dedicated to the prevention and treatment of eating disorders. Information and treatment resources are given for all forms of eating disorders.

LiveWell Colorado
www.livewellcolorado.org

Committed to preventing and reducing obesity by promoting healthy eating and active living. LiveWell Colorado inspires and advances policy, environmental, and lifestyle changes that aim to provide access to healthy foods and opportunities for physical activity in the community.

National Eating Disorder Association
www.nationaleatingdisorders.org

Provides general information about eating disorders and body-image concerns along with possible referrals for treatment, educational materials, and opportunities to help through volunteering.

Teenshealth: Body Image and Self Esteem
http://kidshealth.org/teen/your_mind/body_image/body_image.html

Contains sections titled "Why Are Self-Esteem and Body Image Important?", "What Influences a Person's Self-Esteem?", "Healthy Self-Esteem," "Tips for Improving Body Image," and "Where Can I Go If I Need Help?"

Womenshealth.gov
www.womenshealth.gov/body-image/

A website of the Office of Women's Health, U.S. Department of Health and Human Services. It contains information about body image, cosmetic surgery, pregnancy and body image, body image and children, and eating disorders.

Women's Issues
www.womensissues.about.com

Contains information on many women's issues including stereotypes, body image, and self-improvement.

References

Al Sabbah, H., Vereecken, C., Elgar, F. J., Nansel, T., Aasvee, K., Abdeen, Z., Ojaia, K., Ahiuwalia, N., & Maes, L. Body weight dissatisfaction and communication with parents among adolescents in 24 countries: International cross-sectional survey. *BMC Public Health, 9, 1* (February 6, 2009), 52.

AMA adopts new policies at annual meeting. *AMA News*, June 21, 2011. Available: http://www.ama-assn.org/amam/pub/mews/news/a11-new-policies-page.

American Society for Aesthetic Plastic Surgery. *Statistics*, 2015. Available: https://s3.amazonaws.com/asaps/assets/stats/2013/ASAPS-2013-Stats.pdf.

American Society of Plastic Surgeons. Report of the 2013 plastic surgery statistics. 2015. Available: http://www.plasticsurgery.org.

AP–iVillage Poll, May 4, 2009. Available: http://www.msnbc.msn.com/id/30687221/ns/health_diet_and_nutrition/t/poll-women-value-weight-over-physical-health/.

Arroyo, A., & Harwood, J. Exploring the causes and consequences of engaging in fat talk. *Journal of Applied Communication Research, 40, no. 2* (May 2012), 167–187.

Ashikali, E., & Dittmar, H. The effect of priming materialism on women's responses to thin-idea media. *British Journal of Social Psychology*, 2011; DOI: 10.1111/j.2044-8309.2011.02020.x.

Babwin, Don. Dove ads featuring "real women" meant to be an inspiration. *The Birmingham News* (August 3, 2005), 1G, 5G.

Barlett C. P., & Harris, R. J. The impact of body emphasizing video games on body image concerns in men and women. *Sex Roles, 59, 7–8* (October 2008), 586–601.

Beware of penis-enlargement scams. MayoClinic.com (May 24, 2005). Available: http://www.mayoclinic.com/.

Blashill, A. J., & Safren, S. A. Body dissatisfaction and condom use self-efficacy: A meta-analysis. *Body Image, 12* (2015), 73–77.

Blond, A. Impacts of exposure to images of ideal bodies on male body dissatisfaction: A review. *Body Image, 5, 3* (September 2008), 244–250.

Body image and sexuality. Planned Parenthood, 2015. Available: http://www.ppnyc.org.

Bryla, K. Y. Effects of media on female body image: myth or reality? *Health Education Monograph Series, 19, no. 2* (2002), 13–16.

Carney, D. R., Cuddy, A. J. C., & Yap, A. J. Brief nonverbal displays affect neuroendocrine levels and risk tolerance. *Psychological Science, 21, no. 10* (October 2010), 1363–1368.

Centre for Appearance Research. 30% of women would trade at least one year of their life to achieve their ideal body weight and shape. *Science Daily*. March 2011. Available: http://www.sciencedaily.com/releases/2011/04/11040411812.htm.

Chrisler, J. C., Marvan, M. L., Gorman, J. A., & Rossini, M. Body appreciation and attitudes toward menstruation. *Body Image, 12* (2015), 78–81.

Claudat, K., & Warren, C. S. Self-objectification, body self-consciousness during sexual activities, and sexual satisfaction in college women. *Body Image, 11, 4* (2014), 509–515.

Connolly, J. M., Slaughter, V., & Mealey, L. The development of preferences for specific body shapes. *Journal of Sex Research, 41, no. 1* (Feb. 2004), 5–15.

Dawes, J., Roozen, M., & Spano, M. Muscle dysmorphia. National Strength and Conditioning Association, June 5, 2009. Available: http://www.nsca-lift.org/HotTopic/download/Muscle_Dysmporphia.pdf.

Fahmy, S. Males insecure over muscle mass. *The Spokane Spokesman Review*, (July 27, 2004), C6.

Fardouly, J., & Vartanian, L. R. Negative comparisons about one's appearance mediate the relationship between Facebook usage and body image concerns. *Body Image, 12* (2015), 82–88.

Fryar, C. D., Carroll, M. D., & Ogden, C. L. *Prevalence of overweight, obesity, and extreme obesity among adults: United States, 1960–1962 through 2011–2012.* Centers for Disease Control and Prevention, National Center for Health Statistics, National Health and Nutrition Examination Survey, 2014.

Garner, D. *The 1997 Psychology Today Body Image Survey.* Available: http://www.psychologytoday.com/print/25283.

Grammas, D., & Schwartz, J. Internalization of messages from society and perfectionism as predictors of male body image. *Body Image, 6, no. 1* (January 2009), 31–36.

Grosick, T. L., Talbert-Johnson, C., Myers, M. J., & Angelo, R. Assessing the landscape: Body image values and attitudes among middle school boys and girls. *American Journal of Health Education, 44* (2013), 41–52.

Johnston, L. D., O'Malley, P. M., Bachman, J. G., & Schulenberg, J. E. *Monitoring the Future national results on adolescent drug use: Overview of key findings, 2008.* Bethesda, MD: National Institute of Drug Abuse, 2009.

Kraemer, B., Delsignore, A., Schnyder, U., & Hepp, U. Body image and transsexualism. *Psychopathology, 41, 2* (December 2008), 96–100.

Leone, J. E., Partridge, J. A., & Maurer-Starks, S. Psychobehavioral attributes of body image in college freshman and seniors: Implications for long-term health. *The Health Educator, 43, no. 1* (Spring 2011), 13–20.

Lipka, S. Feminine critique. *Chronicle of Higher Education, 50, no. 37* (May 21, 2004), A35–36.

Long, C. Female magazines evolve to feature flabby. *Intelihealth.* Harvard Medical School's Consumer Health Information (2005). Available: http://www.intelihealth.com.

Martins, Y., Tiggemann, M., & Churchett, L. The shape of things to come: Gay men's satisfaction with specific body parts. *Psychology of Men and Masculinity, 9, 4* (October 2008), 248–256.

McFarland, M. B., & Kaminski, P. L. Men, muscles, and mood: The relationship between self-concept, dysphoria, and body image disturbances. *Eating Behavior, 10, 1* (January 10, 2009), 68–70.

Meltzer, A. L., McNulty, J. K., Novak, S. A., Butler, E. A., & Karney, B. R. Marriages are more satisfying when wives are thinner than their husbands. *Social Psychology and Personality Science, 2* (July 2011), 416–424.

Milhausen, R. R., Buchholz, A. C., Opperman, E. A., & Benson, L. E. Relationships between body image, body composition, sexual functioning, and sexual satisfaction among heterosexual young adults. *Archives of Sexual Behavior,* 2014. doi: 10.1007/s10508-014-0328-9.

Mind on the Media. Inspiring independent thinking and fostering critical analysis of media messages, 2009. Available: http://www.mindonthemedia.org/index.php?type=static&page=shocking.

Mind over fatter: The bulk of bigorexia (2005). Available: http://www.mindoverfatter.co.za/html/bigorexia.htm.

Monro, F., & Huon, G. Media-portrayed idealized images, body shame, and appearance anxiety. *International Journal of Eating Disorders, 38, 1* (July 2005), 85–90.

Morgan, R. The men in the mirror. *Chronicle of Higher Education, 49, no. 5* (September 27, 2002), A53–A54.

Mumen, S. K., Poinsatte, K., Huntsman, K., Goldfarb, J., & Glaser, D. Body ideals for heterosexual romantic partners: Gender and sociocultural influences. *Body Image, 12* (2015), 22–31.

People. Scoop. January 27, 2003. Available: http://www.people .com/people/article/0,,20139090,00.html.

Rubinstein, S., & Caballero, B. Is Miss America an undernourished role model? *Journal of the American Medical Association*, Research Letter, *283, no. 12* (March 22/29, 2000), 1569.

Ruggieri, D. G., & Bass, S. B. A comprehensive review of school-based body mass index screening programs and their implications for school health: Do the controversies accurately reflect the research? *Journal of School Health, 85, 1* (2015), 61–72.

Schoenstadt, A. Bulimia statistics. *MedTV*, January 29, 2007. Available: http://bulimia.emedtv.com/bulimia/bulimia-statistics.html.

Singh, D. Female mate value at a glance: Relationship of waist-to-hip ratio to health, fecundity, and attractiveness. *Human Ethology & Evolutionary Psychology, 23* (December 2002), 81–91.

Sharp, G., Tiggermann, M., & Mattiske, J. The role of media and peer influences in Australian women's attitudes toward cosmetic surgery. *Body Image, 11, 4* (2014), 412–425.

Stephen, I. D., & Perea, A. T. Judging the differences between women's attractiveness and health: Is there really a difference between judgments made by men and women? *Body Image, 11, 2* (2014), 183–186.

Striegel-Moore, R. H., Rosselli, F., Perrin, N., Debar, L., Wilson, G. T., May, A., & Kraemer, H. C. Gender differences in the prevalence of eating disorder symptoms. *International Journal of Eating Disorders* (December 23, 2008).

TieMeyer, M. Eating disorders: Bulimia statistics. *About.com Eating Disorders*, 2007. Available: http://eatingdisorders .about.com/od/whatisbulimianervosa/p/bulimiastats .htm?p=1.

Tiggemann, M., Martins, Y., & Churchett, L. Beyond muscles: Unexplored parts of men's body image. *Journal of Health Psychology, 13, 8* (November 2008), 1163–1172.

Voracek, M., & Fisher, M. L. Shapely centrefolds? Temporal changes in body measures: Trend analysis. *British Medical Journal, 325* (December 21, 2002), 1447–1448.

Warren, C. The mass media, body image, and self-deception. *Psychology Today*, 2014. Available: http://www .psychologytoday.com/blog/naked-truth/201406/the-mass-media-body-image-and-self-deception.

Whitbourne, S. K. Do you feel sexy? Your answer makes a big difference. *Psychology Today*, 2014. Available: http://www .psychologytoday.com/blog/fulfillment-any-age/201409 /do-you-feel-sexy-your-answer-makes-big-difference.

Zhaoyang, R., & Cooper, M. L. Body satisfaction and couple's daily sexual experience: A dyadic perspective. *Archives of Sexual Behavior*, 2013. doi: 10.1007/s10508-013-0082-4.

CHAPTER 12

Sexual Orientation, Identity, and Expression

© Gayvoronskaya Yana/Shutterstock

FEATURES

Multicultural Dimensions
Race and Ethnicity Identities Among LGBT Adults

Gender Dimensions
Gay–Straight Alliances and Gender Activism

Ethical Dimensions
Research on Causes of Homosexuality

Ethical Dimensions
Teaching About Gay History

Global Dimensions
Attitudes About Homosexuals in Various Countries

Communication Dimensions
Communication About Gay and Lesbian Athletes

Communication Dimensions
Coming Out

Multicultural Dimensions
LGBTQ in a Global Context

Ethical Dimensions
Should Gay Marriages Be Legal?

CHAPTER OBJECTIVES

1 Define sexual orientation, including the various orientations described in the chapter. Discuss the validity of the Kinsey continuum.

2 Compare and contrast the theories of sexual orientation, including biological, psychological, and sociocultural theories.

3 Discuss the challenges specific to LGBTQ people.

4 Discuss social issues that affect LGBTQ people.

INTRODUCTION

*B*y all appearances, Brad was an archetypal high school male: a
"good" student, a "really nice" guy with a willingness to help
out with school projects and panache in fixing cars. He dated
several girls. But his relationship with Peggy was extra special. They were
best friends, hanging out together and attending high school parties and
dances as a couple. They also engaged in a variety of sexual activities.

At first Brad could not quite understand why the idea of sexual
intercourse with Peggy did not appeal to him as much as it should.
Eventually Brad realized that he was gay. Peggy was hurt at first about
the abrupt end of their relationship, but she cared about Brad enough to
remain a close friend.

After high school, Brad attended a local college and continued to
hang out with his high school friends who had accepted his sexual
orientation, rather than venturing out to meet people who might not have
been so accepting. Gay bashing was common, and Brad had a legitimate
fear for his safety. During this time, he met Brian, whom he has been
with ever since.

Brad felt comfortable "coming out" to his friends, but he did not
tell his parents for fear of their reaction. This silence caused a bit of a
problem, because his parents (and relatives) were forever introducing him
to "nice girls" and wondering why nothing ever came of the dates Brad
claimed he had. About the time Brad turned 30 years old, over dinner
one evening, his father said to him, "You're gay, aren't you?" Although
Brad's parents may have initially been hurt or confused, or may have
questioned their own parenting, they continued to love and support Brad.

For Brad, as for many gays and lesbians, AIDS took a terrible toll. Many friends became sick and died. Many of Brad's friends learned about and began practicing safer sexual activities, no longer going to bathhouses or having quick, anonymous encounters. Brad attended rallies to promote governmental funding for AIDS research.

Brad was lucky: Both he and Brian tested negative for HIV. One thing that HIV did teach Brad, however, was that although he and Brian had been together for many years in a committed relationship, their situation was quite different from that of a legally married couple. When one of Brad's close friends died of AIDS, Brad's friend's parents, who did not want to believe their child was gay, demanded all his assets— which the deceased had intended to leave for his partner. Because the parents had the legal standing in the state in which the death occurred, the grieving partner lost everything. Even while his friend was dying, the parents were allowed to make all medical decisions and legally barred the partner from hospital visits.

In marriages, spouses automatically have each other's power of attorney, which means that if one spouse is incapacitated, the other has control over his or her affairs. A gay couple that is not married must go through lawyers to ensure that each partner has power of attorney for the other. Because Brian and Brad had purchased a home together and had made various other investments together, they realized it was imperative for them to complete the proper documentation to protect each other.

Brad's story illustrates many of the dimensions of sexual orientation. Sexual orientation takes time to develop and has an impact on many aspects of a person's life. In this chapter, we look at the ways that the many dimensions of human sexuality interact to determine sexual orientation, identity, and expression.

■ Sexual Orientation

Through the years, a variety of terms and labels have been used to apply to the information presented in this chapter. Much of the time there has not been— and often still is not—agreement among experts about the definitions of certain terms. Some terms can be very fluid—meaning they have been changing over time and may continue to change. It is impossible for many people to be in total agreement about the meaning of many terms related to this chapter. This can make it difficult to write about some of the information covered in this chapter, and may sometimes make it difficult for you to talk about these topics and be sure that you and others are referring to the same thing. Recognizing that there are no "perfect" definitions for many of the terms related to this chapter, some common definitions are shared here to help with your understanding of and conversation about some of the topics in this chapter. But don't be surprised if you hear others using the terms differently: It may sometimes be necessary to determine upfront if everyone is taking about the same thing. Self-identification can be a key. Sometimes we may simply have to ask the other person what he or she means when using a term, and sometimes we may have to define our definitions. Here are some starting points:

1. *Sexual orientation:* An enduring pattern of emotional, romantic, and/or sexual attraction to men, women, or both sexes. It ranges along a continuum from exclusive attraction to the other sex to exclusive attraction to the same sex. However, sexual orientation is usually discussed in three categories: heterosexual (having emotional, romantic, or sexual attractions to members of the other sex), gay/lesbian (having emotional, romantic, or sexual attractions to members of the same sex), and bisexual (having emotional, romantic, or sexual attractions to both men and women). In different cultures, different labels may be used to describe people who express these attractions (*Sexual orientation and homosexuality*, 2015).

2. *Gender identity:* One's internal sense of being male, female, or something else. Common words used to label gender identity include *straight, lesbian, gay, bisexual,* and *asexual* (*Answers to your questions about transgender people, gender identity, and gender expression*, 2015).

3. *Bisexual:* Person who is romantically and/or sexually attracted to both men and women (*Sexual orientation and homosexuality*, 2015).

4. *Pansexual:* A person who is fluid in sexual orientation and/or gender or sex identity (*Definition of terms*, 2014). People who identify as pansexual do so with purpose, to express that they are able to be attracted to various gender and sexual identities. Recognition of the existence of different genders and sexualities is a major aspect of pansexual identity (Prabhat, 2014).

5. *Intersex:* People who are born with "sex chromosomes," external genitalia, or internal reproductive systems that are not considered "standard" for either male or female (*Definition of terms*, 2014).

6. *Genderqueer:* A person whose gender identity is neither man nor woman, is between or beyond genders, or is some combination of genders. Some genderqueer people identify under the transgender umbrella, while others do not (*Definition of terms*, 2014).

7. *Queer:* A term that has different meanings to different people, which usually fall into four categories: (1) an umbrella term to refer to all LGBTIQ (lesbian, gay, bisexual, transsexual, intersex, queer) people; (2) a political statement, as well as a sexual orientation, which advocates breaking binary thinking and seeing both sexual orientation and gender identity as potentially fluid; (3) a simple label to explain a complex set of sexual behaviors and desires—for example, a person who is attracted to multiple genders may identify as queer; (4) a term that many older LGBT people feel has been hatefully used against them and are reluctant to embrace (*Definition of terms*, 2014).

8. *Questioning:* The process of exploring and discovering one's own sexual orientation, gender identity, or gender expression (*LGBT terms and definitions*, 2013).

9. *Transsexual:* People who experience a mismatch of the sex they were born with and the sex they identify as. A transsexual sometimes undergoes medical treatment to change his/her physical sex to match his/her sex identity through hormone treatments and/or surgically. Not all transsexuals can have or desire surgery (*Definition of terms*, 2014).

10. *MSM:* Men who have sexual activity with men. These men engage in same-sex behavior, but may not necessarily self-identify as gay or bisexual (Definition of terms, 2014).

11. *Gay:* Men attracted to men. More recently, "gay" has been used as an umbrella term to include all LGBTIQ people (*Definition of terms*, 2014).

12. *Lesbian:* Women attracted to women (*Definition of terms*, 2014).

"Sexual preference" is a term formerly used to describe sexual orientation. This term is now outdated because sexual orientation is no longer commonly considered to be one's conscious individual preference or choice; instead, it is thought to be formed by a complicated network of social, cultural, biological, economic, and political factors.

For our purposes, the term **gay** can apply to either males or females. The term **lesbian**, however, applies only to a female homosexual.

People have various feelings about sexual orientation—and even the topic of sexual orientation.

gay Male or female homosexual. (*Gay* used alone probably refers to a male, though it is acceptable to refer to a *gay female*.)

lesbian Female homosexual.

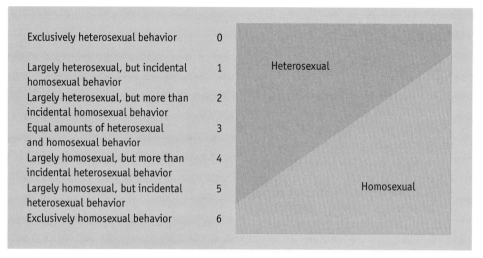

Exclusively heterosexual behavior	0
Largely heterosexual, but incidental homosexual behavior	1
Largely heterosexual, but more than incidental homosexual behavior	2
Equal amounts of heterosexual and homosexual behavior	3
Largely homosexual, but more than incidental heterosexual behavior	4
Largely homosexual, but incidental heterosexual behavior	5
Exclusively homosexual behavior	6

FIGURE **12.1** Kinsey sexual orientation continuum. The Kinsey continuum refers only to homosexual or heterosexual *behavior;* remember that it was developed in the 1950s. If such a continuum were developed today, it would likely refer to erotic, romantic, and affectional attraction, as do our definitions of sexual orientation. It would also probably recognize that a person's behavior and sexual orientation might differ. For example, a person can be heterosexually married, have sexual intercourse with a spouse, and still be gay or bisexual.

Source: Reproduced from Kinsey, A. *Sexual behavior in the human male.* Philadelphia: W.B. Saunders, 1948. With permission of The Kinsey Institute for Research in Sex, Gender, and Reproduction, Inc.

The Sexuality Information and Education Council of the United States (SIECUS) position statement on sexual orientation (2015) is as follows:

> *Siecus believes that individuals have the right to live in accordance with their sexual orientation, be they bisexual, heterosexual, gay, or lesbian. The legal system should guarantee the civil rights and protection of all people, regardless of sexual orientation. Prejudice and discrimination based on sexual orientation is unconscionable.*

The Kinsey Continuum

No clear-cut line separates homosexuality and heterosexuality; in fact, it is more accurate to think of these orientations as being on a continuum. Figure 12.1 shows a seven-point continuum of sexual orientation originally devised by Kinsey. Most of us probably experience varying degrees of sexual orientation; that is, most of us are attracted to both sexes, even though we may act in only one way sexually.

The notion of a continuum of sexual orientation helps explain not only differences among people but also a phenomenon known as **situational homosexuality**—that is, sexual behavior limited to specific circumstances in which members of the

same sex are generally deprived of contact with the other sex. Gay activity in a single-sex school or in a prison, for example, does not necessarily indicate that the individuals involved are primarily gay. They may never participate in gay activity in other situations, and their orientation may prefer sexual activity with the other sex. However, because people of the other sex are not available to them, and because they prefer sexual activity with another person to masturbation exclusively, they engage in sexual behavior with people of the same sex. You may have participated in sexual activity with someone of the same sex sometime in your life; however, unless you are sexually attracted to people of the same sex, fall in love with people of the same sex, have sexual behaviors with people of the same sex, and identify yourself as being gay, you are not classified as being gay.

The distinction we wish to make is between specific behavior and one's sexual orientation. A person's engaging in sexual activity with someone of the same sex does not indicate that person is gay; someone's not engaging in sexual activity with the same sex does not indicate that person is not gay. For example, a heterosexual person might engage in sexual behavior with a person of the same sex for the purpose of experimentation, or because of a situation such as being in prison or in a single-sex school. This does not mean the person is gay. Or, a gay person might engage in sexual behavior with a person of the other sex to appear more socially acceptable and/or to hide

situational homosexuality Homosexual behavior limited to circumstances in which members of the same gender are deprived of contact with the other gender.

Multicultural
DIMENSIONS

Race and Ethnicity Identities Among LGBT Adults

Four large national population-based surveys were used to consider the ways in which LGBT populations are demographically similar to or distinct from their non-LGBT counterparts in the United States. The surveys analyzed include the National Survey of Family Growth (NSFG), the General Social Survey (GSS), the National Health Interview Survey (NHIS), and the Gallup Daily Tracking Survey. It was found that LGBT populations generally share the racial and ethnic characteristics of non-LGBT individuals. The proportions in racial and ethnic identities among LGBT people age 18 to 44, by survey, are shown below (Gates, 2014):

	NSFG	NHIS	GSS	Gallup
White, non-Hispanic	65%	62%	59%	54%
African American non-Hispanic	12%	15%	17%	18%
Hispanic	13%	14%	19%	23%
Asian, non-Hispanic		6%		3%
American Indian/Alaska Native, non-Hispanic	NA	1%	NA	NA
Multiracial/other, non-Hispanic	9%	3%	6%	2%

true gay feelings. This does not mean that person is a heterosexual. Sexual orientation is not the same as sexual behavior.

Many of us take our sexual orientation for granted. However, a small percentage of junior and senior high school students may not be sure of theirs. Uncertainty about sexual orientation seems to decline with age.

Bisexuality

Bisexuality is enjoying and engaging in sexual activity with members of both sexes or recognizing the desire to do so. Our definition of bisexuality allows that someone who at one time engaged in bisexual behavior may not be a bisexual, and someone who has never participated in bisexual behavior could be a bisexual. For example, someone may fantasize about sexual relations with members of both sexes and find himself or herself attracted to people of both sexes but may never have engaged in sexual relations with a same-sex partner. This person may nevertheless be bisexual.

Bisexuals point to the variety that characterizes their sexual relationships. They are able to fully enjoy the sexual pleasures of both males and females and are open to the most erotic of activities. One of the disadvantages of bisexuality, though, is the suspicion

it provokes in both the heterosexual and LGBTQ communities. In one sense, bisexuals are both like and unlike these groups; however, it is often the "unlikeness" that is the focus. LGBTQ people might view bisexuals as being afraid to admit to their orientation. Some lesbians and gays reject sexual relations with bisexuals for this reason. It seems that lesbians are even more rejecting of bisexual women than are gay men of bisexual men. Some lesbians want bisexual women to declare openly their lesbianism and insist there is no such thing as a true bisexual.

On some college campuses, new student organizations for bisexuals who feel shunned by gay-student support groups are emerging. Interestingly, supporters of the new groups say many of the previous groups established for gay, lesbian, and bisexual students have exhibited the very kinds of intolerance and discrimination they were designed to fight. The name for this behavior is *biphobia*, or antipathy toward those who identify as bisexual. Supposedly, some gay students belittle bisexuality as a "cop-out" to avoid identification as gay. Others say that bisexuals are confused about their real sexual orientation.

There has been an increase in the number of research studies related to bisexuality. For example, Saewyc et al. (2009) found that bisexual adolescents had lower levels of most protective factors (family connectiveness, school connectiveness, and religious

We do not know a person's sexual orientation unless they tell us what it is.

involvement) than did heterosexual adolescents. They suggested that these factors help explain the higher prevalence of risky behavior among the bisexuals.

The Ontario Consultants on Religious Tolerance (2008) summarized the following points about bisexuality:

- Bisexuality may be a difficult concept to comprehend because we are often taught to look at things as a duality: male and female, light and dark, hot and cold, etc. In this case, at least three classifications (and perhaps more) are needed to represent sexual attractions and activities.

- A bisexual is attracted to both males and females, but not necessarily to the same degree.

- Bisexuality describes how people feel, not necessarily how they act.

- Misinformation about bisexuality is very prevalent.

- Although it has been said that only 2% of the population is bisexual, research indicated that almost 21% of men and 18% of women admitted to same-sex sexual attraction/behavior at some time in their lives.

- Some people believe that bisexuality is just a phase. While this may be true for some people, others regard themselves bisexual throughout their lives.

- It has been said that bisexuals are only satisfied if they have sexual partners of both sexes. This is not true because bisexuals do not necessarily act on their feelings of attraction.

Zivony and Lobel (2014) reported that some heterosexuals exhibit prejudicial attitudes toward bisexual men. Compared to heterosexual and gay men, bisexuals were evaluated as more confused, untrustworthy, open to new experiences, less inclined toward monogamous relationships, and not as able to maintain a long-term relationship. The authors pointed out that their two studies suggest that stereotypical beliefs regarding bisexual men are prevalent, but often are not acknowledged as stereotypes.

In 2014, the Movement Advancement Project (MAP) released a report indicating that while more than half of the LGBT community identifies as bisexual, bisexual people are vulnerable to poverty, discrimination, and poor physical and mental health—often at rates higher than their lesbian and gay peers. Further, the report indicated that despite being the largest population within the LGBT community, bisexual people are among the most invisible. The failure to account for bisexual lives and experiences compounds the lack of social support for these individuals and keeps bisexual people in the closet. The disparities that bisexual people experience include the following:

- *Poverty:* Approximately 25% of bisexual men and 30% of bisexual women live in poverty, compared to 15% and 21% of heterosexual men and women, respectively, and 20% and 23% of gay men and lesbians.

- *Employment:* While 20% of bisexuals report experiencing a negative employment decision based on their sexual orientation, almost 60% report hearing anti-bisexual jokes and comments on the job. Nearly half of bisexual people report that they are not out to any of their coworkers, compared to 24% of lesbian and gay people.

- *Violence:* Bisexual women experience significantly higher rates of violence—both overall and as intimate-partner violence—compared to lesbians and straight women: 46% of bisexual women have experienced rape, compared to 13% and 17% of lesbian and straight women, respectively. Bisexual men also report higher rates of sexual violence; nearly half of bisexual men report experiencing sexual violence other than rape in their lifetime.

- *Suicide:* Bisexuals are four times more likely, and lesbian and gay adults two times more likely, to report attempted suicide than straight adults.

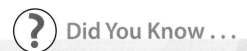

Did You Know . . .

In the past, Native Americans had interesting concepts of gender and sexual orientation. The two-spirited person is a native tradition that researchers have identified in some of the earliest discoveries of Native artifacts. Evidence indicates that Native people, at least prior to colonization, believed in the existence of cross-gender roles—that is, the male–female and the female–male—combined into what is now called the two-spirited person. People supposedly existed who were gifted among all beings because they carried two spirits. Women engaged in tribal warfare and married other women, and there were men who married other men. These individuals were looked upon as third and fourth genders in many cases, and they were usually honored and revered. Two-spirit people were often the visionaries—the healers, the medicine people, the caregivers.

Source: LaFramboise, S., & Anhorn, M. *Native American concepts of gender and sexual orientation.* Dancing to Eagle Spirit Society, 2008. Available: http://www.dancingtoeaglespiritsociety.org/twospirit.php.

Pansexuality

Pansexuality includes all kinds of sexual expression and sexual relationships that can exist in humans. It can involve sexual activity in many forms. A pansexual person can love not only the traditional male and female sexes, but also transgendered, transsexual, cross-dressing, androgynous, and gender-fluid people and all other variations of gender identification, including those who feel they do not have a gender. It is often confused with or included within the definition of bisexuality, but it is a more fluid and much broader form of sexual orientation in which the pansexual individual experiences sexual attraction towards members of all genders (not to be confused with sexes; a person's sex is purely physical, gender has to do with a person's psychological orientation).

While the term *pansexual* is relatively new, its roots date back to the early 20th century and the work of Sigmund Freud, who believed that all human behavior is motivated in one way or another by the "sex instinct." Freud was criticized by his peers for this theory, which they dubbed *pansexualism* (Palermo, 2013).

When thinking about sexual orientation in general, it is important to remember that terms, understandings, and labels can be very fluid. Self-identification is very important. That is, the person who can best indicate what his/her sexual orientation is must be the person himself/herself and not someone else. The use of particular labels does not seem to apply as well as it did in the past given this situation.

Asexuality

Asexuality has seldom been discussed, but more attention has been given to it in recent years. For example, the Asexual Visibility and Education Network (AVEN) was founded in 2001 with two distinct goals: creating public acceptance and discussion of asexuality, and facilitating the growth of an asexual community. It has thousands of members and can be reached at www.asexuality.org. According to the AVEN website, asexual people have the same emotional needs as anyone else. Many asexual people experience attraction, but feel no need to act out that attraction sexually. Because they don't see a lack of sexual arousal as a problem to be corrected, asexual people focus their energy on enjoying other types of arousal and pleasure.

Barnes (2005) summarized some interesting points about asexuals. He indicated that asexuality isn't celibacy—the refusal to act on attraction. It is the absence of sexual attraction. Asexuals insist that theirs is a valid fourth orientation, like straight, bisexual, and gay orientations. There is nothing wrong, they say; it is simply the way they were born and they are not interested in sexual activity. Many asexuals form deep emotional bonds that they define as "romantic"—resembling those commonly understood as coupledom, except for a lack of sexual behavior. As one asexual said: "In early high school all of my friends started talking about how they were attracted to people, who they had crushes on, and I just didn't understand why sexuality was such a big deal for everyone else."

Statistically speaking, according to Barnes, there may be as many as 4.5 million Americans who are asexual. A study in Britain indicated that more than 1% of the population agreed with the statement, "I have never felt sexually attracted to anyone at all." Many experts agree that motivation to engage in sexual intimacy is a dimension that runs from zero to extremely high; thus there are probably some people

pansexual One whose sexual orientation includes all kinds of sexual expression and sexual relationships that can exist in humans.

asexual One who does not experience sexual attraction. Some asexuals may experience attraction but feel no need to act out that attraction sexually.

You cannot tell a person's sexual orientation just by his or her appearance.

at that zero end. Asexuality seems to exist in the animal world as well.

Homosexuality in the Population

The U.S. Census Bureau first published reports of those who identified themselves as same-sex married couples in 2010. In 2011, data indicated there were 605,472 same-sex couples in the United States. This number included 214,773 male–male and 222,607 female–female unmarried partners, as well as 69,522 male–male and 98,570 female–female married partners (*Frequently asked questions about same-sex couple households*, 2013).

In 2015, U.S. Census Bureau data showed that in 2013 there were a total of 726,000 same-sex couples (352,624 male–male couples and 373,976 female–female couples) in the country. This compared to slightly more than 55.6 million married other-sex couples and more than 6.5 million unmarried other-sex couples. Male–male and female–female spousal relationships numbered 117,535 and 134,160, respectively. Unmarried same-sex partnerships included 474,905 total relationships, with 235,089 being male–male and 239,816 being female–female (U.S. Census Bureau, 2015).

In 2014, Ward et al. reported that 96.6% of U.S. adults identified as straight, 1.6% identified as gay or lesbian, and 0.7% identified as bisexual. The remaining 1.1% of adults identified as "something else," stated "I don't know the answer," or refused to provide an answer to questions about their orientation. The same researchers also found significant differences in health-related behaviors, health status, healthcare service utilization, and healthcare access among the various groups. Relative to most of these services and outcomes, sexual minorities tended to fare worse than their nonminority counterparts.

As noted by Gates (2014), the proportion of adults who identify as LGBT has varied across surveys from 2.2% to 4.0%. Researchers have consistently found that LGBT identity is more common among younger populations, LGBT populations generally share the racial and ethnic characteristics of non-LGBT individuals, and U.S. adults are more likely to identify as LGBT in the Northeast and West than in the South and Midwest. It is thought that the finding of higher levels of LGBT identity among younger populations is due, at least in part, to increased levels of social acceptance throughout the lives of younger LGBT individuals as compared to their older counterparts.

Here are some other interesting statistics. Generally, racial/ethnic minorities in same-sex couples are more likely to be raising children than white respondents in same-sex couples. Overall, individuals in same-sex couples are more likely to have completed a college degree than their counterparts in different-sex couples. Generally, individuals in same-sex couples are less likely to be covered by health insurance than their counterparts in different-sex couples. Unemployment rates are generally higher for individuals in same-sex couples. Regarding military status, in general men are much more likely than women to serve in the military. However, men in same-sex couples are less likely to report military service than those in different-sex couples. Women in same-sex couples are much more likely to report military service than those in different-sex couples. Individuals in same-sex couples generally report higher median incomes than their counterparts in different-sex couples. Females in both same-sex couples and different-sex couples report lower median incomes than males. Overall, individuals in same-sex couples are 2.2 times more likely to partner with individuals of another race/ethnicity compared to people in different-sex couples (Kastinas & Wilson, 2014).

Nearly one-fifth of same-sex couple households include children. Female–female couples more often have children present than male–male couples (27% versus 11%, respectively). Approximately 225,000 minor children were living in a same-sex couple household in 2013, and nearly three-fourths of these children were living with female same-sex couples. Same-sex couples living with minor children have—on average—1.8 minors in their households. Twenty-nine percent of children living in same-sex couple households are the only minor child residing in the household (Payne & Manning, 2015).

Heterosexuality in the Population

Regardless of the exact numbers of LGBTQ people in U.S. society, it is safe to assume that the sexual orientation of most people is heterosexual. As was seen in the statistics presented in the previous section, more than 90% of both males and females identify as being heterosexual. Because of this, some heterosexuals may have a difficult time understanding and supporting the need for equal rights and opportunities for people with different sexual orientations. Some heterosexuals may even be guilty of heterosexism, which means they think about human experience only in heterosexual terms and ignore or put down LGBTQ behaviors. They also may stereotype LGBTQ people in a negative manner and view them as dangerous to others.

While many people have wondered about the developmental process of those who do not identify themselves as heterosexuals, some researchers focused more on how heterosexuals develop their sexual orientation identities. For example, Worthington et al. (2002) indicated that heterosexual development encompasses the following six important dimensions to be accomplished over time:

1. Identification and awareness of one's sexual needs, as determined by sexual orientation.

2. Adoption of personal values related to sexual behavior and sexuality in general.

3. Awareness of which sexual activities are preferred.

4. Awareness of the specific characteristics that are preferred in sexual partners.

5. Awareness of preferred modes of sexual expression.

6. Recognition of one's sexual orientation and personal identification with that orientation.

People with a heterosexual orientation seem to go through some rather predictable developmental states as they integrate their sexual orientation into their personalities. Early in life, they realize their heterosexual orientation but have not yet acted on it sexually. This stage is termed *unexplored commitment* to being heterosexual. They may then enter into an *active exploration* phase, where they intentionally try out numerous sexual ideas and fantasies, and often engage in sexual activities with members of the other sex. This helps them clarify which activities and partners they prefer. Some people experience *diffusion*, which may involve sexual exploration, but with less intentionality and goal direction than active exploration. After some exploration along with maturation, heterosexuals enter into the stage of *deepening and commitment*, which is characterized by more intimacy and loving feelings in relationships. People can move through these stages at various times, but the final status of heterosexual identity is *synthesis*, in

which the various elements of identity, group membership, and attitudes toward sexual minorities have achieved congruence and meaning in the person, though this may be a difficult status to achieve. All of this helps to explain how heterosexual people gradually integrate their sexual orientation into their sense of self (Hoffman, 2004; Worthington et al., 2002).

Intersex

Intersex is a topic that can cross between a discussion of gender and a discussion of sexual orientation, identity, and expression. According to the American Psychological Association (APA), a variety of conditions may lead to atypical development of physical sex characteristics and are collectively referred to as *intersex conditions*. These conditions can involve abnormalities of the external genitals, internal reproductive organs, sex chromosomes, or sex-related chromosomes. Some examples include the following:

- External genitals that cannot be easily classified as male or female

- Incomplete or unusual development of the internal reproductive organs

- Inconsistency between the external genitals and the internal reproductive organs

- Abnormalities of the sex chromosomes or sex-related hormones (*Individuals with intersex conditions*, 2015)

Many experts and persons with intersex conditions have recommended adopting the term *disorders of sex development* (DSD) to describe these conditions. They believe this term is more accurate and less stigmatizing than the term "intersex." Some experts estimate that 1 in every 1,500 babies is born with genitals that cannot easily be classified as male or female. Nevertheless, intersex conditions are not always accurately diagnosed, experts sometimes disagree on what qualifies as an intersex condition, and government agencies do not collect statistics about intersex individuals. When a baby is born with ambiguous genitalia, doctors perform exams and tests to determine exactly which condition the baby has. A variety of factors go into the decision of sex assignment—for example, preserving fertility where possible, ensuring good bowel and bladder function, preserving genital sensation, and maximizing the likelihood that the baby will be satisfied with his or her assigned sex later in life. Most people with intersex conditions grow up to be heterosexual, but people with some intersex conditions seem to have an increased likelihood of growing up to be gay, lesbian, or bisexual adults (*Individuals with intersex conditions*, 2015).

The Intersex Society of North America (ISNA; www.isna.org) is devoted to systematic changes to end shame, secrecy, and unwanted genital surgeries for people born with an anatomy that has been arbitrarily decided is not standard for male or female. ISNA (2008) says that intersexuality is primarily a problem of stigma and trauma, not gender; parents' distress must not be treated by surgery on the child; professional mental health care is essential; honest, complete disclosure is good medicine; and, all children should be assigned as boy or girl without early surgery.

According to ISNA, the child should be assigned a gender after tests (hormonal, genetic, radiologic) have been done and the parents have consulted with the doctors on which gender the child is more likely to feel as she or he grows up. However, doctors and parents need to recognize that gender assignments of infants with intersex conditions are preliminary. Any child—intersex or not—may decide later in life that she or he was given the wrong gender assignment. This is a crucial reason why medically unnecessary surgeries should not be performed without the patient's consent; the child with an intersex condition may later want genitals (either the ones they were born with or surgically constructed anatomy) different than what the doctors would have chosen. Surgically constructed genitals are extremely difficult if not impossible to "undo," and children altered at birth or in infancy are largely stuck with what doctors give them (ISNA, 2008).

Intersex and the same-sex marriage debate have a lot to do with each other. People who are proponents of prohibitions against "same sex" marriage think it is easy to figure out who is "same sex" and who is not. As ISNA points out, this distinction is not always clear. In practice, where the category of "male" ends and "intersex" begins, or "intersex" ends and "female" begins, may be the subject of debate (ISNA, 2008).

Theories of Sexual Orientation

Although many studies have been done on the subject, no one knows exactly which factors shape sexual orientation. Some argue that biological factors account for sexual orientation. Others claim that psychological factors or learned behavior is responsible. Determining an accurate method for defining and identifying sexual orientation for the purpose of constructing representative samples of those of different sexual orientations is a goal of researchers. Different definitions and measures have been used to develop samples since the 1860s, when the topic of sexual orientation first attracted widespread research interest. If advances in the understanding of sexual orientations are to be made, it is critical that definitions and measures of sexual orientation be standardized.

Because the vast majority of people are heterosexuals, most theories about sexual orientation relate to other sexual orientations. It is as though heterosexuality is the "norm" and LGBTQ people are indications that something went wrong. These theories are described in the following paragraphs.

Biological Theories

The argument that biological factors account for sexual orientation may include a variety of biological factors such as genetics and hormones.

Genetics

Some experts believe that something in a person's genes causes that person to be sexually attracted to a member of the same sex. Researchers have studied twins, and some of these studies seem to indicate that the more genetically similar one twin is to his gay brother, the more likely he is to be gay as well. Of course, this outcome is more likely with identical twins because they share the same genetic material. But other questions remain: Which other factors might account for sexual orientation? What role do hormones and the environment play? Even if there is a possible genetic link, it is probably only part of the total picture.

Many researchers believe that the most promising support for a biological reason for sexual orientation comes from genetic studies. Several family and twin studies provide clear evidence to support a genetic component to both male and female sexual orientation.

Sexuality experts do caution that a specific gene linked to homosexuality has not been identified. Also, because of the complexity of sexual orientation, it is

Twins have been used in research to look at theories about the cause of sexual orientation.

Gender DIMENSIONS

Gay–Straight Alliances and Gender Activism

Gay–straight alliances have been formed in many places in communities and schools. Such groups can provide leadership and networking opportunities for youth. Activism focused on sexual identity and rights can be a controversial topic. Nevertheless, an increasing number of localities are passing antidiscrimination legislation protecting youth based on sexual identity and expression. Antidiscrimination policies necessitate grounded, comprehensive education and outreach strategies. The priority is to ensure that all youth remain safe from violence, harassment, and discrimination within schools. Many youth activists' efforts center on educating school communities toward a broader understanding of the diverse ways that all people live their gendered and sexual lives. They are focused on building a community based on difference rather than defining themselves and advocating based on a single group identity.

likely that a possible genetic link is only part of the picture.

Demir and Dickson (2005) reported on an interesting genetic study with fruit flies. They showed that a single gene in a fruit fly is sufficient to determine all aspects of the fly's sexual orientation and behavior. This means that instinctive behavior can be specified by genetic programs. However, it is not yet clear if there is a similar master gene for humans.

Burri et al. (2011) indicated that sexual orientation and "gender conformity" in women are both genetic traits. They followed a group of 4,000 British women who were one of a pair of twins. They found a connection between mental traits and how sexual orientation develops, with both factors being connected to genetics.

Hormones

The hormonal theory states that homosexuality is a result of hormonal imbalances that occur before or after birth. Because it is known that prenatal hormonal treatment in animals can lead to different male and female behavior patterns, some theorists have concluded that these same conditions might cause homosexuality.

For example, Levay (2011) has proposed that sex hormones affect brain development in a variety of ways. Differences between individuals in gendered traits such as sexual orientation could arise either because of differences in the levels of prenatal hormones themselves or because of differences in the brain mechanisms that respond to hormones.

As noted by Rice et al. (2012), as an embryo develops, sex-related genes are turned on and off in response to fluctuating levels of hormones in the womb, which are produced by both mother and child. This tug of war benefits the unborn child by keeping male and female development on a steady course even amid spikes in hormones. If these so-called epigenetic changes persist after the child is born and has children of its own, however, some of those offspring may be homosexual.

 Did You Know . . .

It is a myth that humans are the only species that practices gay behavior. In fact, same-sex pairings have been discovered in more than 10% of species throughout the world. For example, some penguins of the same sex engage in "mating rituals" such as entwining their necks and vocalizing to each other. In addition, male giraffes have been observed rubbing their necks against each other's body while ignoring the females. Yet another example is one genus of lizards that can copulate with both male and female mates. There can even be some benefits from gay/lesbian behavior. For example, one study of albatrosses showed that female–female pairing can increase the well-being of the offspring by taking advantage of the excess of females and the shortage of males in the population and provide superior care for offspring.

Source: Fereydooni, A. Do animals exhibit homosexuality? *Yale Scientific*, March 14, 2012. Available: http://www.yalescientific.org/2012/03/do-animals-exhibit-homosexuality/.

Savic et al. (2005) reported that gay men do not respond to the smell of bodily chemicals the same way that straight men do. Previously, they had isolated bodily chemicals from both males and females. When women smelled the male chemicals, their hypothalamuses "lit up," but they had no reactions to the female chemicals. In men, the results were exactly the opposite. Then the researchers included gay men in the study. When gay men were exposed to the smell of male chemicals, their hypothalamuses lit up just like a woman's. The smell of female chemicals did nothing for them. However, this study doesn't show that sexual orientation is biologically hardwired from birth. It could also be that the brains of gay men learn to respond to the smells over time and with experience.

As is the case with the genetic theories, there are problems in research on the hormonal causation of sexual orientation. There is no convincing evidence that sexual orientation is the result of either prenatal or postnatal hormonal imbalances, or that homosexuality causes these imbalances. However, research continues in this area.

Some experts argue that family relationships influence sexual orientation.

Fraternal Birth Order
It has been found that gay men have a greater number of older brothers than heterosexual men do. The estimated odds of being gay increase by approximately 33% with each older brother. Statistical modeling using epidemiological procedures suggest that about 1 in 7 gay men may owes his sexual orientation to this situation. The number of older sisters appears to be irrelevant to sexual orientation (Rahman, 2005).

Neural Circuitry
Some experts believe that neurodevelopmental mechanisms must wire neural circuits differently in those persons with same-sex attractions. However, little is known about this circuitry (Rahman, 2005).

Psychological Theories

Psychological theories of the development of sexual orientation consider psychoanalytical factors and the influence of learned behavior. Although these theories were historically believed, they have not been proved valid. Today many experts do not support these theories.

The Psychoanalytical Theory
Psychoanalytical theories of the cause of sexual orientation relate to parental and family characteristics. Sigmund Freud postulated that everyone is born with the potential to be bisexual. Whether someone becomes heterosexual or homosexual is, Freud believed, a result of circumstances that affect the child's psychosexual development. For example, if a young boy is unable to resolve the Oedipal complex (an attraction for his mother) satisfactorily and becomes "fixated" at this phase of psychosexual development, he may become homosexual; or if the boy continues to fear castration ("castration complex"), he may grow up to be homosexual.

Some theorists have suggested that gay men more often have overprotective and dominant mothers and weak, passive, and detached fathers than do heterosexual men. This environment supposedly makes men gay because they are fearful of interacting with women and unable to identify with their fathers. Of course, there are many heterosexuals who grew up in similar households but never became gay. Clearly this theory remains just that—a theory.

The Learned Behavior Theory
Some behaviorists believe that being LGB is the result of situations experienced in childhood and reinforced throughout one's life. For example, someone may experience an unsuccessful and unsatisfying heterosexual experience that leads him or her to experiment with LBG behavior, with which the person finds satisfaction. The attitude of many people is that "if they just had an effective lover, they would never be gay." Other people may believe that LGB people are unattractive to heterosexuals, so their sexual outlet is someone of the same sex. Still others believe that early childhood gay/lesbian experience "recruits" people to lesbian/gay behavior. Studies are not supportive of any of these viewpoints. As with other theories, the learned behavior theory demands further investigation before it can be supported.

Ethical DIMENSIONS

Research on Causes of Homosexuality

As shown in this chapter, many researchers are interested in what determines sexual orientation or, perhaps for some, what causes homosexuality. They would argue that it is important to know which factors determine sexual orientation because if causes are known, then sexual orientation could be influenced in whatever way might be desired.

Others argue that research into the cause(s) of homosexuality is unethical and should not be undertaken because it assumes more often than not that being gay or lesbian is a form of mental illness or an undesirable deviance from the heterosexual norm, which should be cured.

Do you think research about the causes of sexual orientation (or homosexuality) is ethical or unethical?

Integrated Theories

The integrated theory of the development of sexuality—homosexuality is just one form—argues that physical, psychological, and learned factors are involved. There is evidence presented by integrated theorists of the biological aspects of gay/lesbian behavior. Experiments on certain animals have shown that the brain can develop in contrast to the body's form and structure.

Integrationists, then, conclude that the prenatal influence on sexuality is important but that it plays out in a social context. Therefore, sexuality (heterosexuality and LGB) is a function of the interaction of all of these factors: biology, hormones, cultural expectations, learned behavior, and psychological variables.

No single scientific theory about what causes sexual orientation has been substantiated. Studies to associate orientation exclusively with genetic, hormonal, or environmental factors have so far been inconclusive.

Effect of School Environment

Something not always considered related to sexual orientation is the environment in educational institutions. How do teachers deal with the topic of sexual orientation or with students with various sexual orientations? How do heterosexual peers treat LGBTQ people?

LGBTQ adolescents face the same developmental challenges as their heterosexual counterparts, with the added burden of attempting to incorporate a stigmatized sexual identity with little support from school personnel. Teachers either avoid the topic of LGBTQ or, when discussing it, frequently present it in a negative manner.

Although the vast majority of LGBTQ youth become well-adjusted adults who lead satisfying, productive lives, their additional developmental challenges require a range of coping skills and adaptation. Unfortunately, unlike most of their heterosexual peers, they have no built-in support system. They must

Myth vs Fact

Myth: LGBTQ people can be easily recognized as being different from heterosexuals.
Fact: Only a small proportion of LGBTQ people are what can be termed "visible." The vast majority look and act just as everyone else does and differ only in their sexual orientation.

Myth: Gay men really want to be women and lesbians really desire to be men.

Fact: Most LGBTQ people are perfectly happy with their sex; they just prefer relationships with someone of the same sex.

Myth: Gays are effeminate and weak, and lesbians are masculine and physically strong.
Fact: Sexual orientation has nothing to do with one's body type or style of movement, nor does body type dictate sexual orientation.

LGBTQ students face extra adjustment challenges in schools.

learn to identify, explore, and ultimately integrate a positive adult identity despite persistent negative stereotypes of LGBTQ people. They also must learn to protect themselves from ridicule, verbal and physical abuse, and exposure. The social and emotional isolation experienced by LGBTQ youth is a unique stressor that increases risk for a range of health problems.

LGBTQ youth have more threats of violence as well as experiences of violence, have substance use and abuse rates well above the national average, and have a higher risk of thinking about and attempting suicide. Verbal, physical, and sexual harassment of LGBTQ students is widespread in U.S. schools and many teachers and administrators do not deal effectively with such incidents.

The individual consequences of living as an openly LGBTQ person can be profound—rejection by family and friends, physical violence and verbal abuse, insensitive health and social services, loss of jobs or housing, and lack of protection under the law. Gays are more likely than heterosexual boys to report poor body image, binge eating, and suicide attempts.

Frankowski (2004) and the Committee on Adolescence of the American Academy of Pediatrics pointed out that young people are recognizing their sexual orientation earlier than in the past. Nonheterosexual youth are at higher risk of dropping out of school, being kicked out of their homes, and turning to life on the streets for survival. Some of them engage in substance abuse, and they are more likely than their heterosexual peers to start using tobacco, alcohol, and illegal drugs at an earlier age. They are more likely to have had sexual intercourse, to have had more partners, and to have experienced sexual intercourse against their will. This puts them at increased risk of STIs, including HIV infection. They are also more likely to attempt suicide and be victimized. High levels of stress and lack of family support are also common.

Schools should be a child's primary place for learning, growing, and building a solid foundation for success in the world. Students should find their school environment to be supportive and caring, and under no circumstances should any child be afraid of being heterosexual, lesbian, gay, bisexual, transgender, or queer (LGBTQ) at school. However, many students who identify themselves as LGBTQ view the school environment as a space where they are institutionally ignored, silenced, and targeted for harassment (Payne & Smith, 2011). According to the 2013 National School Climate Survey, 55.5% of LGBTQ students felt unsafe at school because of their sexual orientation (Kosciw, Palmer & Boesen, 2014). This fear often arises from the negative attitudes toward LGBTQ students. For instance, it was reported that 74.1% of LGBTQ students were verbally

harassed, 36.2% were physically harassed, and 16.5% were physically assaulted in the past year because of their sexual orientation. As a result, many LGBTQ youth are at a greater risk for depression, substance use, and suicidal thoughts and behaviors (Centers for Disease Control and Prevention [CDC], 2014). Furthermore, many studies show that constant exposure to such negative behaviors can have adverse effects on the education and psychological health of these young students.

The victimization of LGBTQ students has been going on for decades, making school bullying a widespread public health problem (Russell et al., 2011). LGBTQ students are often subjected to homophobic teasing and slurs, which may then lead to mental health adjustments and negative psychological outcomes (Robinson & Esplage, 2011). According to Robinson and Esplage (2013), these stigmatizing messages create psychological distress (depression and anxiety) in LGBTQ students, regardless of the amount of bullying to which they are exposed. Hillard et al. (2014) report that these psychological issues are not just a result of their victimization and their sexual orientation, but also a reflection of these students' lack of social support within the school environment. Many schools fail to extend protection to LGBTQ students, do not represent LGBTQ individuals within the standard curriculum, and are generally unwelcoming and even prevent these students from attending school-sponsored functions (Poteat et al., 2012). It is not surprising, then, that these students are less likely to feel a part of their school community. In addition, Russell et al. (2011) have shown that there is a strong link between a history of victimization and later psychological adjustment for children and adolescents—especially for boys. According to these authors, the stakes for gender conformity are especially high for boys because much of the LGBTQ school victimization that is experienced by teens is also deeply rooted in a peer culture that demands conformity to masculine gender expectations.

In addition, there is a strong connection between the victimization of LGBTQ students in schools and these students' compromised academic achievement and school absenteeism. According to Russell et al. (2011), school victimization may result in school failure, poorer grades, and restricted life chances that limit future academic potential for students who identify as LGBTQ. The reported grade-point average of students who are more frequently harassed due to their sexual orientation or gender expression is almost half a grade lower than that of students who are harassed less often. The unnerving part of this trend is that these psychological outcomes and educational inequities are beginning earlier and earlier. According to Robinson and Esplage (2011), although

Ethical DIMENSIONS

Teaching About Gay History

As of January 2012, California became the first state to mandate that the contributions of gays and lesbians in the state and the country be included in social science instruction and in textbooks. The state already required schools to teach about the contributions of some other minority groups, including African Americans and women. Advocates for the legislation said they believed the shift would help make schools safer for gay and lesbian students. However, one lawmaker indicated that it is a sad day when the government essentially tells people what they should think. He said the law prohibited schools from presenting gays and lesbians "in other than a positive light, and I think that's censorship right there." State textbooks and curriculum will not be updated for several years. In the meantime, teachers will have to use supplemental materials in the curriculum.

Do you think this law is a good idea? Is it needed? Is it ethical to mandate that gay history be taught in schools? Is this any different than mandating other things that must be taught in schools?

Source: Data from Lovett, I. California to require gay history in schools. *The New York Times* (July 14 2011). Available: http:// www.nytimes .com/2011/07/15/us/15gay.html.

---

the risk of diminished school belongingness and unexcused absences is significant in high school, the gaps are significantly greater in middle school, suggesting heightened early risk for LGBTQ-identified students. Elementary-age students tend to have more flexibility around gendered expectations, yet pressures for children to outgrow gender transgression often intensifies as they get older and gender expectations become more rigid (Payne & Smith, 2012). In turn, a significantly larger number of LGBTQ students (22%) skip school due to fears of fighting or harassment (Hillard et al., 2014).

To address the extent of bullying and harassment of LGBTQ students, it is imperative that schools develop effective interventions aimed at eliminating negative educational and psychological outcomes. Russell et al. (2011) and Hillard et al. (2014) advocate for schools' development of antibullying and antiharassment policies that are aimed at reducing or eliminating the verbal and physical harassment of LGBTQ students, while Poteat et al. (2012) highlight the need for schools to incorporate community-based youth programs such as Gay–Straight Alliance (GSA) into their curriculum. In addition, Robinson and Esplage (2013) suggest that schools might benefit from faculty and staff in-service training on LGBTQ issues, as such training has been shown to increase knowledge, create more positive attitudes toward LGBTQ students, and improve school climate. Although these interventions have been effective in some schools, Payne and Smith (2011) argue for a broader worldview that uses a sociological framework as an alternative way of understanding the issues of LGBTQ harassment by focusing on school culture and gender policing. Focusing "safe school" efforts on the elimination of violent acts means that all the attention is being paid to individuals (bullies and victims) and their behavior, and none to the cultural systems that reproduce and sanction violence, intimidation, and harassment (Payne & Smith, 2011). Research demonstrates the need for change, but advocating for cultural change and sustainable change cannot occur without cultural awareness.

An additional relationship not often heard about is that LGB teens are at a higher risk of becoming pregnant or causing a pregnancy than their heterosexual peers. This is apparently because the discrimination, sexual abuse, and harassment these teens face prompt them to indulge in more sexually risky behavior, such as having sexual intercourse without using condoms, starting to have sexual intercourse before the age of 14, or having multiple sexual partners. Girls who describe themselves as lesbians or bisexuals are 2 to 2.5 times more likely to become pregnant at least once than are heterosexual girls. Males who describe themselves as bisexual or gay are 3 to 4 times more likely than heterosexual males to impregnate a girl. LGB teens may have sexual intercourse with members of the other sex for a variety of reasons. Some engage in this behavior to hide or to deflect the abuse they see inflicted on LGB teens. Others may have been told they are abnormal and wrong, so they may feel that "If I just have sexual intercourse with enough other-gender people, it will cure me" (Saewyc et al., 2008).

More and more universities are signaling to prospective students that they have gay-friendly campuses. Stanford University gives every freshman a CD highlighting the campus's gay and lesbian resources, including its community center. San Jose State University regularly features gay and lesbian people in its brochures. Several forces are driving the growing momentum to make gay students feel welcome. Students are coming out earlier and are searching for colleges where they will find social acceptance. As the gay population increases its visibility, students and scholars are demanding the same outreach efforts that ethnic groups and women fought for years ago. Also, school admissions staff are realizing that LGBTQ students represent an important demographic that should be reached in some way.

School personnel need to be familiar with legal matters related to sexual orientation. Here are some examples:

- Like all other students, lesbian, gay, bisexual, and transgender (LGBT) students are guaranteed equal protection under the Fourteenth Amendment to the Constitution and free speech and association under the First Amendment.

- The Equal Access Act requires schools to treat student clubs that address LGBT issues the same as other student groups.

- A school cannot refuse to allow a group such as a gay–straight alliance to meet because other students, teachers, administrators, parents, or community members object to the formation of the club.

- To be covered by the Equal Access Act, student clubs must be "student initiated." Outside community members may not direct, control, or regularly attend activities of student groups.

There have been attempts at helping homosexual students do better in schools by having a more positive environment for them. For example, in the San Francisco Unified School district there is a LGBTQ (lesbian, gay, bisexual, transgender, or questioning) liaison in place in every school that handles individual student concerns. The program helps to promote students' acceptance of one another. The Milwaukee high school called Alliance (started in 2005) and the Harvey Milk High School in New York City (started in 2003) are both intended specifically for LGBTQ students. Both schools were started to give these youths the chance to attend a public school populated by students like themselves and an environment in which their differences are welcomed. These schools provide much safer environments for the students, but they also reawaken the debate about school segregation (Calefati, 2009).

In 2010 a gay-friendly online high school was established in Maplewood, Minnesota. Supporters indicate that the online nature of the school allows

Myth (vs) Fact

Myth: LGBTQ people want to seduce children into a life of homosexuality.
Fact: Although some might seduce children, most sexual abuse of children is committed by heterosexuals. Both situations are intolerable, but to blame LGBTQ people alone for the sexual abuse of children is wrong.

Myth: LGBTQ people should not be teachers.
Fact: It would be clearly wrong for a teacher of any sexual orientation to seduce students or to encourage them to adopt a particular sexual lifestyle, but there is no reason to expect such behavior to be more or less prevalent among LGBTQ people.

Myth: LGBTQ people are suffering from a mental illness.
Fact: When LGBTQ people and heterosexuals are matched by age, IQ, and education, mental health experts cannot find differences in adjustment between the two groups.

Myth: LGBTQ people are poor security risks.
Fact: There may have been some foundation for this belief in the past because they were easy targets for blackmail; however, as society grows less homophobic and as many LGBTQ people identify themselves publicly, the supposed risk should evaporate.

it to reach young people wherever they have Internet access—especially in rural areas, where smaller populations make a physical version of the school impossible. They also say that it removes gay students from potentially hostile school environments and places them in a safe and welcoming educational community. Others feel that the online school is not a good idea because students might become further alienated. Students might stay isolated and feel uncared for. More information about the gay-friendly online school can be found at www.glbtqonlinehighschool.com.

Presgraves (2010) indicated potential positive interventions and support for LGBT students. All of them relate to more positive overall experiences for the students. They include having a gay–straight alliance in school, having supportive staff in school, and having an antibullying policy in the school.

There have been some interesting debates about population-specific services such as those mentioned previously. Some people argue that these services may meet acute needs and can be very helpful to some students. Others suggest that they may contribute to social isolation and seem to identify LGBTQ students as disabled or deviant. What do you think about these kinds of services?

It can be helpful for parents and teachers to talk about sexual orientation with school-age children. Here are some examples of important messages for young people of various ages.

Messages for young people age 5–8 include:

- Human beings can love people of the same sex and people of the other sex.

- There are men and women who are gay or lesbian, which means they can be attracted to and fall in love with someone of the same sex.

Messages for young people age 9–12 include:

- Sexual orientation is one part of who we are.

- LGBTQ people's relationships can be as fulfilling as heterosexual people's relationships.

Messages for young people age 12–15 include:

- People do not choose their sexual orientation.

- Having discussions about sexual orientation can be difficult for some people.

Messages for young people age 15–18 include:

- The understanding and identification of one's sexual orientation may change over the course of that person's lifetime.

- Civil rights for LGBTQ people are being debated in many places across the United States.

Sexual Orientation Issues

As we grow and develop, many challenges confront us regardless of our sexual orientation. Typically LGBTQ people are happy, well-balanced people just like anyone else. They basically enjoy the same activities as other people, have similar goals in life, and in recent years have been able to enjoy parenthood through adoption or, for some lesbians, through artificial insemination. This is not often the picture that heterosexuals get, however, because it is more commonly problematic behavior that is seen. For example, happy, healthy LGBTQ people do not seek psychotherapy more often than happy, healthy heterosexuals do; but we often tend to generalize about all LGBTQ people from those few who do seek help. If we did the same thing with heterosexuals, we would have a very skewed picture of what heterosexuals are really like.

Many LGBTQ peoples, however, are more likely to experience certain kinds of challenges than are heterosexuals. LGBTQ youth must cope with prejudiced, discriminatory, and violent behavior and messages in their families, schools, and communities. These often result in isolation, fear of stigmatization, and lack of peer or familial support.

An increasing number of gays seek marriage, even though these marriages are not always legally

recognized. Some lawmakers simply ignore the issue, and others have gone out of their way to institute laws prohibiting gay marriages. Sometimes LGBTQ people decide to have a marriage ceremony even though it may not be legally recognized. This can lead to other interesting issues. We will discuss more about this and other legal issues later in this chapter.

The Social Scene

In the United States the homosexual subculture centers on private clubs, gay bars, and LGBTQ organizations. These organizations are designed to help protect LGBTQ people, promote their rights, promote a positive image of their lifestyle, and help the general public better understand them. Clubs, bars, and organizations give LGBTQ people opportunities to fraternize with other gays and perhaps develop social and/or intimate relationships.

Although clubs, bars, and organizations are often safe places for LGBTQ people, there is a fear of police harassment and of possible discovery. In addition, some LGBTQ people desire to have more open and intimate relationships.

Like people in general who now use the Internet for various social reasons more than in previous years, those interested in same-sex relationships often choose this course. For example, there seems to be an association between online sexual activity seeking and risk for HIV infection among men who have sexual activity with men (MSM). Intention to go online seeking sexual activity has been found to predict more episodes of anal sexual activity. In addition, unprotected anal intercourse is a common activity with online-initiated liaisons. Therefore, MSM who go online to meet sexual partners are important targets for HIV interventions.

In a permanent relationship, living together seems to be more important to lesbians than to gay men. Many gays of both sexes believe that steady love relationships are quite meaningful and enjoy the warmth and understanding of such relationships.

Social Issues and LGBTQ People

Additional issues related to LGBTQ life are being considered all the time. For example, the issue of becoming parents has been controversial. Some people believe that LGBTQ people should have the same rights to be parents as others do. Other people believe that the inherent nature of same-sex attraction would prevent them from "properly raising" children.

Starting in 1994 the U.S. military adopted a "Don't ask; don't tell" policy. This meant that military officials were not supposed to ask about the sexual

Attitudes About Homosexuals in Various Countries

In 2011, the United Nations Human Rights Council passed a resolution supporting equal rights for all, regardless of sexual orientation. The resolution, introduced by South Africa, was the first-ever UN resolution on the human rights of LGBT persons. Although not everyone was in favor of it, supporters indicated that it sent a clear message that abuse based on sexual orientation and sex must end.

Below are some examples of LGBT rights by country.

Country	Same-Sex Sexual Activity	Recognition of Same-Sex Unions	Same-Sex Marriage	Adoption by Same-Sex Couples	LGB Allowed to Serve Openly in Military	Antidiscrimination Laws Concerning Sexual Orientation
Egypt	No penalty of up to 17 years in prison	No	No	No	No	No
Sierra Leone	No for males. Up to life in prison. Legal for females.	No	No	No	No	No
Canada	Legal since 1969	Yes	Legal since 2003	Yes	Yes, since 1992	Bans all discrimination, including hate speech
Mexico	Legal since 1872	Civil unions since 2007	Some states yes and some no	Some states yes and some no	No explicit ban, but LGBT persons have been discharged for "immorality"	Nationwide since 2003
United States	Legal since 2003	Yes, since 2015	Yes, since 2015	Varies by state	Yes, since 2011	Yes and no depending upon where employed
Brazil	Legal since 1831	"Stable unions" legal in some states since 2004	Legal in some states since 2011	Single gay persons since 1996—joint adoption since 2010	Since 1969	Yes and no—depends on state
Chile	Legal since 1999	Civil unions since 2015	Yes and no	Single gays may adopt, and joint custody is pending	Since 2012	Bans all antigay discrimination
Israel	Legal since 2003	Unregistered cohabitation	Cannot be done in country, but recognizes foreign same-sex marriages	Yes	Since 1993	Bans some antigay discrimination
China	Legal since 1997	No	No	No	?	No
Japan	Legal since 1880	No	No	No	Yes	No
Germany	Legal in West Berlin and West Germany since 1969	Registered life partnership since 2001	Pending	Yes and no—stepchild adoption is accepted	Yes	Bans some discrimination
Switzerland	Legal since 1942	Registered partnership since 2007	Pending	Gay individuals may adopt	Yes	Bans some antigay discrimination
Norway	Legal since 1972	Yes	Legal since 2009	Legal since 2009	Yes	Bans all discrimination
Sweden	Legal since 1944	Yes	Legal since 2009	Legal since 2009	Yes	Bans all discrimination
France	Legal since 1791	Yes	Legal since 2013	Legal since 2013	Yes	Bans all discrimination

Sources: Dougherty, J. U.N. Council passes gay rights resolution. *CNN World,* June 17, 2011. Available: http://www.cnn.com/2011/WORLD/europe/06/17/un.lgbt.rights/; LGBT rights by country or territory. *Wikipedia,* January 2015. Available: http://en.wikipedia.org/wiki/LGBT_rights_by_country_or_territory.

Gay bars cater to either females or males, but usually not to both.

Until 2011, more than 13,000 men and women were discharged from the military because there was a ban on openly gay troops. But this is no longer the case. In fact, in 2012 a woman became the first openly gay general in the U.S. Army.

orientation of members of the military, but that they were supposed to discharge openly gay troops. This policy was repealed late in 2010. Many other countries now also allow LGBTQ people to serve openly in the military.

In 1993 the American Medical Association (AMA) banned discrimination against gay, lesbian, and bisexual doctors by adding the words *sexual orientation* to the AMA nondiscrimination bylaws. In 2004 the American Academy of Pediatrics issued a report giving guidance to clinicians in rendering pediatric care. The Academy reaffirmed the physician's responsibility to provide comprehensive health care and guidance in a safe and supportive environment for all adolescents, including LGBTQ adolescents and young people struggling with issues of sexual orientation. The report outlined special needs of LGBTQ youth as well as special considerations for them. It emphasized the importance of trying to prevent the major physical and mental health problems that may confront LGBTQ youths in their transition to a healthy adulthood.

Evidence is accumulating that lesbians experience certain elevated health risks when compared to heterosexual women. These include increased risk of breast cancer, untreated STIs, and barriers to health care (Ellingson, 2002). The reasons for these risks are not totally clear. Although the prevalence of STIs is generally lower among lesbians than among heterosexual women, risk reduction behaviors also seem to be lower. Reasons given for relatively low frequency of early detection behaviors include low perceived need, fears of and experience of homophobic care providers, and lack of insurance.

Trebay (2004) pointed out that lesbians are a powerful presence in fashion, in both predictable and unexpected ways. While old stereotypes about lesbians have not faded, they have slipped into something decidedly "cool." Although lesbians wear a variety of

 Did You Know . . .

The Bear community exists as a subculture in reaction to the larger gay community. It rejects the idealized male beauty revered by mainstream gay men. Bears are more likely to be hairier, heavier, and shorter than mainstream gay men. They also want partners who are hairier and heavier. The sexual partners they reject are more likely to be young and weigh too little (i.e., not bearish). Bears are more likely than mainstream gay men to enact diverse sexual behaviors and are comparatively more masculine. Bears have lower self-esteem than mainstream gay men, but are no less hypermasculine

than non-bears. Bears are intensely sexual. They are probably viewed as less attractive than what is traditionally considered to be attractive. The partners they can attract may be limited and, in response to this, they may be attuned to seek out partners who will not reject them. Perhaps the Bear culture developed to ensure that even the heaviest, hairiest, and/or shortest individual can partner.

Source: Moskowitz, D. A., Turrubiates, J., Lozano, H., & Hajek, C. Physical, behavioral, and psychological traits of gay men identifying as Bears. *Archives of Sexual Behavior, 42* (2013), 775–784.

Communication
DIMENSIONS

Communication About Gay and Lesbian Athletes

Being accepted and being accepting can be issues for college athletes. Traditionally there is an assumption that male athletes are heterosexually virile and desirable. Female athletes can face a very different perception—that they are all lesbians or bisexual. Straight women can go to great lengths to avoid that stereotype, leaving their LGBTQ teammates out in the cold. After using a series of interviews with lesbian, bisexual, and heterosexual Women's National Basketball Association (WNBA) fans, Dolance (2005) argued that the (perceived) large lesbian attendance at WNBA games enables the construction of a lesbian community by lesbian and bisexual fans in a site very different from traditional locations of lesbian community. Because the WNBA is not an explicitly lesbian space, the process of speculating about which players, coaches, and fans are lesbians is a meaningful part of being a WNBA fan for many lesbian and bisexual fans. Fantasizing a large lesbian presence enables lesbian and bisexual fans to actively and interpretively create lesbian community at the games. The women socialize and connect with other lesbian and bisexual women. WNBA games are defined as a unique space that is different from lesbian bars and other traditional "gay-only" spaces.

In 2002 the Rice University football coach was quoted as saying that "while he would not necessarily kick a player off the team for being gay, he probably would think hard about doing so." Immediately, the president of Rice University indicated the need for the coach to affirm his commitment to the university's nondiscrimination policy and to apologize for "the damage done by his comments." The coach did so (Jacobson, 2002b).

In 2002, Esera Tuaolo, who had played defensive tackle in the National Football League for 9 years, revealed that he was gay. He said that he retired from pro football because of failing knees and shoulders, but also because of the discomfort he experienced hearing players make disparaging remarks about gays. One of his former teammates said, "Had other players known Tuaolo was gay, he would have been eaten alive" (Airing it out, 2002).

Thomas (2010) reported on the Oneonta College men's lacrosse team. When one of its captains announced in an online essay that he was gay, the team developed a new reputation as a model of tolerance. The gay player was embraced with open arms. Teammates came up to him and gave him handshakes. The team's coach was also very supportive of the player. He said, "If we had a roster of 30 players and 15 of them did not want to play on the team because you are gay, I would tell them to leave the team."

Bishop (2011) pointed out that dozens of gay leagues exist throughout the United States for most sports, from flag football to volleyball, with tens of thousands of participants. For example, the Gay Softball World Series attracts several hundred teams from around the country each year, and it has existed for over 35 years. In the interest of inclusion, some nongay athletes are usually allowed to play. The National Flag Football League sets the limit at 20% of each roster being heterosexual. The National American Gay Amateur Athletic Alliance limits the number of heterosexual players to two per team. But, questions remain. Is it enough to have an honor system where athletes simply indicate their sexual orientation? Should any "proof" of sexual orientation be required? Can bisexuals or those with other sexual orientations play? Rules have been challenged and discussions about appropriate rules and procedures continue.

In 2013, Jason Collins came out as the first openly gay man in one of the four major professional team sports (basketball). He then became the first openly gay male athlete to appear in a game in one of those leagues. Overall, he received a warm reception from most players, coaches, and fans. However, Collins also said society was not yet to the point where a gay couple could be totally open without having negative repercussions about being gay.

In 2014, Michael Sam, a football player at the University of Missouri told the world he was gay. He came out publicly shortly before the draft for the National Football League (NFL). He had brief stints with two NFL teams, but was not kept on either team for very long. He said he did not believe being gay kept him off an NFL roster, but still planned to work very hard to try to get a spot on an NFL team. In 2015, however, Sam announced he was leaving professional football.

In 2014, Martina Navratilova proposed to her long-time (6 years) girlfriend, a former Russian beauty queen, on the big screen at the U.S. Open. She did it in a TV suite between the two men's semifinal matches in New York City. Their engagement was broadcast on the arena's big screen as legions of tennis fans cheered the couple on.

Communication related to LGBTQ athletes remains an important social issue.

clothing types and styles just like anyone else, one fashion designer referred to a show where "a parade of models appeared in slashed jeans, flat shoes and mannish jackets that were hip and sexy-tough, vulnerable and imposing, just the sort of stuff one might expect a fashionable young lesbian to wear."

In 2005 MTV started a new gay cable TV channel called Logo. The prospect of a television channel entirely devoted to gay programs for gay people may strike some as unnecessary and others as a sign of immoral times, but media giant Viacom thought there was money in it. A spokesperson for Concerned Women for America, which describes itself as a conservative Evangelical group, said it was "a sad day for America." She said MTV was in a powerful position to influence youth and it was "unconscionable" to present in a positive view a promiscuous lifestyle that causes "illness and diseases." The general manager of Logo cited studies saying there were some 15 million openly gay people in America, an attractive demographic for advertisers, considering that many will have no children, meaning more disposable income.

In July 2005, Oprah Winfrey devoted a show to a lifestyle called living on the "down low." This is an expression to describe men who are married or have girlfriends, but are secretly sleeping with men. The main guest on the show, J. L. King, author of *On the Down Low: A Journey into the Lives of "Straight" Black Men Who Sleep with Men*, said the term applies only to blacks. He also said he doesn't consider himself gay. The behavior is not a social thing. Down low is just about sexual gratification and not a relationship. According to King, down low is on college campuses, too.

Examples of LGBTQ lifestyles in the media continue to grow. In 2005 a homosexual relationship was portrayed in a place that was probably unexpected—in a western film entitled *Brokeback Mountain*. The main characters, seen as very manly examples, participated in sexual encounters early in the film. Both went on to get married to females and even had children. However, after 4 years they got back together and their relationship flourished.

It has become much more common to see characters in the movies and on TV with various sexual orientations. While many people do not give this a second thought and accept it as part of normal life, others are bothered by the increasing presence of such characters. As stated earlier, the lives of those with different sexual orientations are, for the most part, very similar. The values people have in general, and the lives that they lead are very much the same, regardless of sexual orientation.

Another social issue is that people with disabilities who identify as LGB represent a population that has received little attention. Awareness of the unique needs and concerns of these individuals is crucial for optimizing their physical and mental well-being. This population is actually a double minority with some experiences similar to those of other minority groups.

It probably comes as no surprise that some social issues related to LGBTQ people seem to relate to the legal environment in which they live related to sexual orientation discrimination. For example, an LGBTQ social climate index, which measures the level of social acceptance of LGBTQ people, found that states with laws against discrimination based

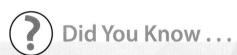

Did You Know...

The National Institutes of Health (NIH) asked the Institute of Medicine (IOM) to assess current knowledge of the health status of LGBT populations. In 2011 the IOM presented its findings in a report entitled *The Health of Lesbian, Gay, Bisexual, and Transgender People: Building a Foundation for Better Understanding*. It is available at www.iom.edu/Reports/2011/The-Health-of-Lesbian-Gay-Bisexual-and-Transgender-People.aspx.

The recommendations of the U.S. Department of Health and Human Services (HHS) based upon the report are available at www.hhs.gov/secretary/about/lgbthealth.html.

A number of actions resulted from the report. Here are a few examples:

• The HHS employment policies already prohibited discrimination based on sexual orientation, but they were updated to explicitly protect against unfair treatment of employees

and applicants for employment based on gender identity and genetic information.

• HHS was directed by the president to initiate rulemaking to ensure that hospitals receiving Medicare or Medicaid patients respect the rights of patients to designate visitors, regardless of sexual orientation, gender identity, or any other nonclinical factor.

• HHS was also directed to establish new guidelines allowing patients to designate who they want to make medical decisions on their behalf through advance directives.

• A national technical assistance resource center was funded to support organizations serving the needs of LGBT older adults.

• In cooperation with other federal agencies, the HHS established a national task force on bullying.

on sexual orientation offer a much friendlier climate for LGBTQ people than in those states without such laws. The average index scores were 70 in the state-law states and 52 in the no-state-law states. The South had a social climate index of 55, the lowest regional score in the United States. The states that best provide legal statewide protections against discrimination based on sexual orientation are largely clustered in the Northeast and Pacific regions of the United States, leaving most LGBTQ people in the Midwest, South, and Mountain states with more limited legal options to address experiences of discrimination based on sexual orientation (Hasenbush et al., 2014).

The Movement Advancement Project reported that in 2014, with wins ranging from the freedom to marry to Medicare's lifting of the exclusion of coverage for transgender-specific health care, LGBTQ Americans made gains on many fronts. However, despite those advances, deep disparities remained, including an overwhelming lack of employment non-discrimination protections, high rates of healthcare discrimination, poorer overall health, and poorer well-being (*Despite stunning marriage victories, LGBT Americans remain unequal*, 2014).

Do you think we need to make changes in society's views, or do you feel conditions are fine the way they are?

Issues Related to Religion/Morality

You are probably aware that many people have religious/moral concerns about sexual orientation. These concerns can vary among people and groups. However, there are some common themes. For example, some people believe that same-sex activity should be criminalized—that it is sinful and immoral, no matter what the relationship. Some people believe that LGBTQ behavior is hated by God, and that it is indicative of mental illness. Some believe it is a choice that people make—not just what they are. There are even still some people who think that LGBTQ behavior is changeable, even though there is no good evidence to support this contention. Finally, some people believe that LGBTQ behavior is abnormal and unnatural for everyone, and that it is an extreme danger to society.

The Religious Institute on Sexual Morality, Justice, and Healing offered advice to religious foundations on securing the freedom to marry for same-sex couples (An open letter to religious leaders on marriage equality, 2015). Religious leaders within the Institute felt that there are strong civil liberties arguments for ending the exclusion of same-sex couples from the legal institution of marriage. A list of the religious denominations supporting LGBTQ people is available at http://religiousinstitute.org.

Many religious denominations are debating about how to deal with LGBTQ issues in general, with LGBTQ religious leaders, and with same-sex marriages, among other issues. In 2005, The United Church of Christ became the first mainline Christian denomination to officially support same-sex marriages (Dewan, 2005). Its ruling body passed a resolution affirming "equal marriage rights for couples regardless of gender." Symbolically, the church passed the resolution on July 4.

In 2011 the Presbyterian Church (U.S.A.) voted to change its constitution and allow openly gay people in same-gender relationships to be ordained as ministers, elders, and deacons (Goodstein, 2011). This was a reversal of only 2 years earlier when a majority of the church's regions voted against ordaining openly gay candidates. This time the vote was 205 to 56. The church's stated clerk, its highest elected official, indicated that they had been having this conversation for 33 years. He said, "Some people are going to celebrate this day because they've worked for it for a long time, and some people will mourn this day because they think it's a totally different understanding of Scripture than they have."

Subsequently, in 2015, the Presbyterian Church (U.S.A.) voted to change the definition of marriage in the church's constitution to include same-sex marriage. The vote amended the constitution to broaden marriage from being between "a man and a woman" to "two people, traditionally a man and a woman." The church, with approximately 1.8 million members, is the largest of the U.S. Presbyterian denominations, but it had been losing congregations and individual members as it moved to the left theologically after the 2011 changes to its constitution. At the time the Presbyterian Church (U.S.A.) made its 2015 decision, other religious denominations that had officially decided to permit their clergy to perform same-sex marriages included the Episcopal Church, the United Church of Christ, the Quakers, the Unitarian Universalist Church, the Association of Churches, and, in Judaism, the reform and conservative movements. The Evangelical Lutheran Church in America left the matter open for individual ministers to decide. The United Methodist Church had been debating same-sex marriage for years, but it includes a growing membership in Africa, where there is little acceptance of gay relationships (Goodstein, 2015).

In 2014, the Vatican released a draft report in which Catholic bishops debated family issues. The original text contained an entire section, "Welcoming Homosexuals," that asked the church to provide gays with a "fraternal space." When the report came under criticism from conservative English-speaking bishops (Winfield, 2014), the Vatican released a revised version of the report 3 days later. The section initially entitled "Welcoming Homosexuals" was changed to

"Providing for Homosexual Persons," and the tone was significantly colder. The first version said homosexual unions can often constitute a "precious support in the life of the partners"; the revised report said gays' unions often constitute "valuable support in the life of these persons."

Sometimes changes related to how a religious group deals with LGBTQ issues occur in an individual church and not an entire denomination. One example of this in 2015 was at the EastLake Community Church in Seattle. The congregation had been quietly coming out as one of the first openly LGBT-affirming evangelical churches in the United States. A short welcome video that says, "Gay or straight here, there's no hate here," was played at the beginning of every service. The church's first gay wedding took place in 2015. According to the minister, "the message of Jesus was a message of wide inclusivity." It is not surprising that Seattle was an early adopter of this approach. It has a higher percentage of gay-couple households than San Francisco—1 in 17 couples living together in the city is gay.

As with many controversies, strong feelings can emerge supporting various positions. For many evangelicals, the debate about LGBTQ issues can be about the Bible itself. These persons believe that the words of the Bible are without error, and that the Apostle Paul called homosexuality a sin. After its embrace of the LGBTQ community, Seattle's EastLake church lost 22% of its income and 800 attendees over an 18-month period, and some believe those numbers will climb. The evangelical reformers, for their part, know that the fight is just beginning and that change can be very slow, but they seem to feel very strongly about their goals (Dias, 2015).

As you might expect, from time to time the official stands of religious groups related to LGBTQ rights and issues can change. The Religious Institute maintains up-to-date information about the official beliefs of most religious groups on issues related to sexuality—including LGBTQ issues. Its website (www.religiousinstitute.org/) provides those organizations' latest positions on these topics.

In "Brief Descriptions of the Six Belief Systems," Ontario Consultants on Religious Tolerance (2011) noted that most people can be divided into one of six groups, depending on their fundamental beliefs about homosexuality. Although these six groups are stereotypical, they illustrate the typical concepts shared by many adults. Of course, some people will fit neatly into a single viewpoint, whereas others will combine the beliefs of more than one point of view. Here are the six groups:

- *Abomination:* This is the most conservative position. Based on Biblical writings, homosexual behavior is to be condemned under all circumstances.

- *Change is expected:* This viewpoint teaches that homosexuality is a product of a sinful world. Gays and lesbians can be cured and converted to heterosexuality through prayer.

- *Celibacy is expected:* This position recognizes that adult sexual orientation is fixed and homosexuals cannot change. For them, God expects a celibate lifestyle, without loving partners with whom to share their lives.

- *Marginally acceptable:* Homosexuality is a psychosexual disability that victims must try to overcome. If they are unable to change and unable to be celibate, then the least horrendous option is a monogamous, long-term, same-gender relationship.

- *Equality:* Equal status and equal rights are the goal. Homosexuals are quite capable of entering into a loving, committed same-gender relationship that is the equal of an other-gender relationship. Morality of acts is judged exactly the same way as in heterosexual relationships.

- *Liberation:* This is the most liberal position. Homosexuality is seen to be equal to heterosexuality.

Homophobia

Although society's attitudes are gradually becoming more accepting, there are still many people who have strong negative feelings about LGBTQ people. **Homophobia** is an irrational fear of homosexuality in others, a fear of homosexual feelings within oneself, or an unhappiness with one's own homosexuality. Homophobia probably results from ignorance, a belief in the common myths about homosexuality, or even the tendency to judge homosexuals as immoral. People with strong negative feelings often reveal their homophobia by openly insulting LGBTQ people and even subjecting people suspected of being LGBTQ to verbal or physical assault. Also, homophobics are often careful to avoid behaving in ways that could be interpreted as LGBTQ, for example, by shunning certain kinds of clothing or physical activities.

Homophobia is an international problem. Every 2 or 3 days a person is killed in Brazil in violence connected with his or her sexual orientation. In Mexico, the reported figure is nearly two fatalies per week. Most of the victims are men who have sexual relations with other men (UNAIDS, 2009). It has been found that gay people in the United Kingdom

homophobia An irrational fear of homosexuality.

Rick Santorum, former senator and presidential candidate, was quoted by the Associated Press as comparing consensual homosexual activity to bigamy, polygamy, adultery, and incest. He later admitted to having a problem "with homosexual acts" and "acts outside of traditional heterosexual relationship." What message regarding the government's view of homosexuality did this send to the American public?

experience more extreme homophobia as young people than as adults. Two-thirds of young LGBTQ people experienced direct bullying in British schools, 92% of young people were subject to verbal abuse, and 41% were physically assaulted. In Latin America, a gay man was killed every 2 days because of his sexual orientation (Ruscombe-King, 2009).

It may be that homophobia is more pronounced in individuals with an unacknowledged attraction to the same sex and who grew up with authoritarian parents who forbade such desire. It seems that individuals who identify as straight, but in psychological tests show a strong attraction to the same sex, may be threatened by gays and lesbians because they remind them of similar tendencies within themselves (Weinstein, et al. 2012).

heterosexist An attitude that reinforces heterosexuality as the privileged and powerful norm.

come out Accept and make LGBTQ orientation public.

What can be done to tackle homophobia? Schools have an important role to play. LGBTQ students are more likely to feel positive about school if school personnel clearly state that homophobic behavior is against the rules. Also, it is likely that personal attitudes will become more accepting toward gay people if individuals are exposed to educational programs about LGBTQ people. Community-based organizations can also provide support to LGBTQ people who might feel isolated and, at the same time, campaign for tolerance toward LGBTQ behavior. Other bodies and agencies that could positively influence the way that LGBTQ people are treated are leaders of political parties, police forces, health services, broadcasters, and employers (Ruscombe-King, 2009).

We talked about school settings earlier; here it is appropriate again to mention teachers. A teacher can ask the following questions to create a more accepting classroom environment: (1) Do I make **heterosexist** (characterized by the belief that heterosexuality is the privileged and powerful norm) assumptions? (2) Do I ignore homophobic remarks? (3) Do I blame my audience for their own misinformation? (4) Do I use educational materials that assume that all my students are heterosexual?

Coming Out

The lifestyle of a gay person is greatly influenced by the extent to which he or she decides to remain in the closet—to keep his or her sexual orientation a secret—or to **come out**—accepting that orientation and making it public. Each choice can be made in varying degrees.

The decision to come out involves several stages: (1) acknowledging, (2) accepting, and (3) openly expressing one's sexual orientation. Some LGBTQ people never acknowledge their sexual orientation, even to themselves. The first step in coming out is usually to realize that one does not fit the heterosexual model. The second step is acceptance, a step that sometimes requires that the individual overcome a learned negative view of LGBTQ people that becomes a negative view of himself or herself.

Even when a LGBTQ person reaches the acceptance stage, he or she can still decide to remain in the closet. It is generally easier to pass as a heterosexual than to take the final step toward openness. However, a person who can live publicly within his or her true sexual orientation generally has a better chance of living a happier life than one who remains secretive. In some situations, however, such as being a parent, the pain of coming out may far outweigh that of staying in the closet.

Telling the family—whether parents, siblings, spouses, or children—can also be extremely difficult, and many people who would prefer an open LGBTQ life choose not to face this ordeal. In fact, parents are often the last to know if their son or daughter is a LGBTQ person.

It is no surprise that family support is an important factor when LGBTQ people decide to come out. LGBTQ young adults with higher levels of family rejection during adolescence are 8.4 times more likely to attempt suicide, 5.9 times more likely to report high levels of depression, 3.4 times more likely to use illegal drugs, and 3.4 times more likely to engage in unprotected sexual intercourse compared with peers from families with no or low levels of family rejection. There is a clear link between parental and caregiver rejecting behaviors and negative health problems for young LGBTQ adults. Family support is crucial for reducing risk and increasing well-being for these people (Ryan et al., 2009).

For most people, the process of deciding to come out begins during their school years. As students, few LGBTQ people choose to disclose their sexual orientation to principals, teachers, counselors, or friends. Reasons cited for nondisclosure include fear of the consequences and not wanting others to know. Most of those who do disclose their sexual orientation receive positive feedback for doing so, but both positive and negative consequences of coming out have been reported.

It is not possible to predict others' response to disclosure. This move can result in a student's experiencing everything from lack of support, isolation, rejection, and ostracism to unfair discipline, taunting, harassment, verbal slurs, persistent random acts of violence, and outright vicious beatings. Students must carefully consider the pros and cons of coming out and examine *why* they want to come out.

As indicated earlier, family support is very important to the well-being of LGBTQ youth. In fact,

Family support is very important to the well-being of LGBTQ youth.

the Substance Abuse and Mental Health Services Administration (SAMHSA) published *A Practitioner's Resource Guide: Helping Families to Support Their LGBT Children* (2014) dealing with these issues. This document indicates that adolescents self-identify as LGBTQ, on average, at age 13.4 years. Interestingly, some parents and families report children identifying as gay at earlier ages—between ages 7 and 12. Nevertheless, many families have strict cultural expectations about gender role behavior for males and females and have great difficulty tolerating gender nonconforming behavior in their children and adolescents.

Young people are disclosing their LGBTQ status more frequently today than in the past, and at younger ages. The average gay person comes out just before or just after graduating from high school. There are now many gay–straight alliances on high school campuses. Also, LGBTQ children can often watch TV shows with LGBTQ characters in them, get information about LGBTQ people and issues on the Internet, and subscribe to publications geared toward them such as *YGA Magazine* (YGA stands for "young, gay America").

The Point Foundation, the nation's largest scholarship granting organization for LGBTQ students of merit, wants to empower promising LGBTQ students to achieve their full academic and leadership potential—despite the obstacles often before them—so that they can make a significant impact on society. The Point Foundation promotes change through scholarship funding, mentorships, leadership development, and community service training. It seeks to provide a greater level of acceptance, respect, and tolerance for future generations for all persons, regardless of sexual orientation, gender expression, or gender identity (Point Foundation, 2015).

Recently the Internet has played a key role in the stages of coming out. Many young men initially come out into a virtual gay community, with online observation and connection with other gay or questioning people, well before making actual contact in the real world. This virtual coming out involves being able to watch and learn about the culture, language, and norms of gayness before actually moving into this new world. The Internet can serve as an important tool for psychological adaptation for LGBTQ youth, especially those who are geographically or psychologically isolated.

Unfortunately, it is difficult if not impossible to know what the reactions of people will be when a person comes out. For many reasons, the decision to come out remains difficult for most LGBTQ people.

The Gay Rights Movement

Gay and lesbian organizations can help gays deal with the stresses experienced as a result of their

Communication
DIMENSIONS

Coming Out   Each of us may be in a position to communicate with someone who is thinking about coming out. A few facts and a few communication suggestions may be helpful. First, the facts:

1. Coming out can be important as an affirmation of one's sexual orientation.
2. Coming out can jeopardize some relationships.
3. Coming out can promote a sense of pride in one's sexual orientation and, in the long run, actually improve relationships with both gay and straight people.
4. Coming out is usually a two-part process—first, coming out to oneself; second, coming out to others.
5. Coming out to oneself may involve gradually dealing with denial, putting matters into focus, and even dealing with personal homophobia.
6. Coming out to others probably involves stages— first involving a few very close friends or relatives, later more relatives, and then a larger public, such as employers, fellow students, and coworkers.
7. Some gays may be out only to a certain degree. For example, only families and very close friends may know about their sexual orientation.

Here are a few communication suggestions that can be helpful to all of us:

1. Coming out should be postponed until the person has a reasonably high sense of self-worth and a support network.
2. The person should be secure in his or her identity before coming out to others.
3. The person should be helped to weigh the pros and cons of coming out and to examine why he or she wants to come out.
4. People who are planning to come out, or who are coming out, usually need a great deal of support and encouragement from others.
5. It is not our responsibility to "make" the person straight or gay. It is our responsibility to help provide a supportive environment.
6. It is important to be ourselves and be sincere.
7. Confidentiality must be respected.
8. Communication should be done in a helpful way but not in a forceful way.
9. Use words that do not assume that everyone is or should be heterosexual. For example, substitute terms such as *partner* or *significant other* for *boyfriend* or *girlfriend*.
10. Role playing can be used to help someone who is going to come out to be prepared to handle a variety of situations.

sexual orientation. There are many different organizations that can provide the social support needed to manage such potentially stressful life situations as coming out or staying in the closet. The support of people who understand what you are experiencing and who can offer advice can be invaluable.

The gay rights movement has progressed, largely because of these organizations and their ability to mobilize their membership to march, to vote, and to boycott when necessary. The movement began in earnest after a raid by the New York City police on the Stonewall gay bar in June 1969. That raid led to a 2-day riot that forever changed the tolerance level of the gay community toward societal prejudice based on sexual orientation. As a result, gays have presented a united front in voting for political candidates who are willing to sponsor their causes. In cities such as San Francisco and Washington, D.C.,

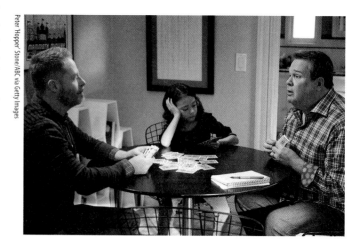

Peter 'Hopper' Stone/ABC via Getty Images

Not many years ago, it was almost unheard of to have LGBTQ characters in TV shows. Today, a number of openly LGBTQ people are cast in important roles in TV shows.

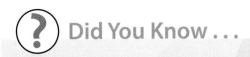

Did You Know...

Selected Significant Events in the Gay Rights Movement

December 10, 1924	The first recognized gay rights organization (Society for Human Rights) in the United States is founded in Chicago.
January 1, 1962	Illinois is the first state to eliminate its sodomy law.
June 28, 1969	Riots at the Stonewall Inn, in New York City.
June 28, 1970	First gay-pride parades (in New York, Chicago, and Los Angeles) to commemorate the one-year anniversary of the Stonewall riots.
January 1, 1974	Homosexuality is removed as a category of disorder from the American Psychiatric Association's *Diagnostic and Statistical Manual of Mental Disorders.*
November 2, 1976	Harvey Milk is elected to the San Francisco Board of Supervisors, proving that the gay community can be organized into an electoral constituency.
January 1, 1977	The rise of gay politics and activism is met by a massive counterrevolution. Singer Anita Bryant promises to lead a crusade to stop the establishment of the "legal right to propose to our children that theirs is an acceptable alternate way of life."
November 27, 1978	San Francisco Mayor George Moscone and Supervisor Harvey Milk are assassinated at San Francisco City Hall.
January 1, 1980	The Democratic National Convention announces its support for gay rights with the statement, "All groups must be protected from discrimination based on race, color, religion, national origin, language, age, sex or sexual orientation."
January 1, 1981	AIDS appears. Advances made toward great acceptance of gays are swept away by the hysteria surrounding the AIDS epidemic.
January 1, 1982	The *Village Voice* newspaper becomes the first business to offer domestic-partner benefits. The city of Berkeley, California, does so in 1984, becoming the first U.S. government body to reach this milestone.
December 21, 1993	The Department of Defense adopts "Don't ask; don't tell"—a policy allowing gay people to serve in the military without being able to divulge their sexual orientation on pain of dishonorable discharge.
September 21, 1996	President Bill Clinton signs the Defense of Marriage Act, which defines marriage as between one man and one woman.
April 16, 1997	Ellen DeGeneres comes out.
January 1, 1999	California establishes a domestic-partner registry and grants hospital visitation rights to same-sex couples for the first time.
July 1, 2000	Vermont becomes the first state to legalize civil unions for same-sex couples.
June 23, 2003	The U.S. Supreme Court strikes down state laws that criminalize sodomy.
May 17, 2004	Massachusetts becomes the first state to legalize same-sex marriage.
November 2, 2004	Eleven states pass constitutional amendments defining marriage as being one man and one woman.
March 5, 2006	*Brokeback Mountain* wins three Oscars.
May 15, 2008	California's gay marriage ban is ruled unconstitutional.
October 10, 2008	Connecticut legalizes gay marriage.
November 4, 2008	Voters approve Proposition 8 in California, which amends the state constitution to ban same-sex marriage.
April 7, 2009	Vermont legalizes gay marriage.
May 6, 2009	New Hampshire legalizes gay marriage.
December 15, 2009	Gay marriage is legalized in the District of Columbia.

(Continued)

June 24, 2011	Gay marriage is legalized in New York.
September 20, 2011	The "Don't ask; don't tell" policy is repealed.
September 30, 2011	The Department of Defense allows military chaplains to perform same-sex ceremonies.
May 9, 2012	President Barack Obama announces his support for marriage equality.
November 6, 2012	Gay marriage is legalized in Maine, Washington, and Maryland.
March 18, 2013	Hillary Clinton announces her support for same-sex marriage.
April 29, 2013	Jason Collins comes out as the first openly gay athlete in a major American team sport.
May 2, 2013	Rhode Island legalizes same-sex marriage.
May 7, 2013	Delaware becomes the 11th state with legal marriage for same-sex couples.
May 14, 2013	Minnesota becomes the 12th state with legal same-sex marriage.
May 23, 2013	The Boy Scouts of America votes to allow openly gay youth into their ranks, overturning a ban that had stood for more than 100 years.
June 16, 2013	The U.S. Supreme Court rules that legally married same-sex couples should get the same federal benefits as heterosexual couples.
November 12, 2013	Hawaii becomes the 15th state with legal same-sex marriage.
November 20, 2013	Illinois becomes the largest state in America's heartland to legalize gay marriage.
December 19, 2013	New Mexico approves gay marriage.
December 29, 2013	Robin Roberts, former athlete and television personality, comes out.
February 9, 2014	University of Missouri football player Michael Sam says that he is gay.
October 6, 2014	The U.S. Supreme Court turns away appeals from five states to limit same-sex marriages.
October 25, 2014	The U.S. Attorney General ruled that same-sex couples in six more states will receive federal benefits.
January 16, 2015	The U.S. Supreme Court agrees to review a previous court decision that upheld bans on same-sex marriage in Kentucky, Michigan, Tennessee, and Ohio.
June 26, 2015	The U.S. Supreme Court rules that couples of the same sex may not be deprived of the right to marry.

What else has happened even more recently that could be added to this list of significant events in the gay rights movement?

Source: Von Drehle, D. Why the Supreme Court is set to make history on gay marriage. *Time.com*, 2015. Available: http://time.com/3672582/supreme-court-gay-marriage-ruling/.

where there are significant numbers of homosexual citizens (voters), politicians are particularly sensitive to gay rights issues. In these cities, gays have made a difference in those elected to public office.

There is no way to know whether social activities, such as the gay rights movement, have influenced other aspects of society or whether aspects of society have influenced gay rights. There is no question that there is more openness about LGBTQ issues in today's society. A prime example of this was Ellen DeGeneres's decision to come out on her TV show in 1998. Another example is the way that films with LGBTQ themes have moved into the mainstream. In movies, LGBTQ people were first ignored, then scorned. By the early 1990s, with the AIDS epidemic,

LGBTQ people began to be pitied in films. Films about them tended to be about their sexual orientation and not about their overall lives. There are now more movies about LGBTQ people than ever, but these movies deal with overall issues and not just people's sexual orientation and generally appeal to viewers of all sexual orientations.

Legal Rights

Marriage in the United States is more than a public recognition of love. It is also a legally binding contract, providing the married couple with myriad tax and legal support benefits, from which LGBTQ people have often been excluded.

Multicultural
DIMENSIONS

LGBTQ in a Global Context

Sexuality and gender have different impacts on each culture's laws, attitudes, and organizations. More secular and "modernized" societies often have more favorable treatment of LGBTQ individuals than societies that value tradition. However, accurate generalizations are difficult to make. Even within the United States, attitudes toward LGBTQ individuals can vary from state to state.

Cultural differences in LGBTQ issues have wide-ranging effects. Other cultures may have different ways of expressing affection. For example, in India it is common for same-sex friends to hold hands without any assumption of a romantic connection. In parts of Latin America, a man is not considered gay if he engages in same-sex intercourse as the insertive partner. Thus, American English terms and conceptualizations of LGBTQ issues may not directly translate.

The visibility of LGBTQ individuals and organizations varies by culture. Some cultures have an underground LGBTQ scene where LGBTQ individuals are tolerated as long as they stay mainly closeted, whereas other cultures may have a more open and organized community of LGBTQ individuals. In addition, some cultures may provide legal protection for LGBTQ individuals and recognize their partnerships, whereas other cultures may criminalize same-sex intercourse. Finally, there may be major differences within the LGBTQ community in a specific culture; for example, in parts of southeastern Asia it is considered culturally acceptable for a man to have sexual activity with a feminine transgendered man, but there are no such provisions for women having sexual activity with transgendered women.

Source: LGBTQ in global context overview. International Spectrum, University of Michigan, 2015. Available: http://internationalspectrum .umich.edu/global/differentcultures.

Following are some of the legal benefits for married couples.

- *Income taxes*—In many instances, married couples receive a lower tax rate than would two individuals filing separately. (An exception to this, known as the "marriage penalty," occurs when both spouses earn relatively equal high incomes and consequently pay a higher rate than they would as individuals.)

- *Adoption*—Many states do not allow gay couples to adopt children. Even states that do allow it generally put married couples first in line.

- *Estate taxes*—Married couples do not have to pay any federal estate taxes (and usually only a limited amount of state estate tax) on the death of a first spouse. State laws provide (for people without wills) that property moves directly to the spouse (or spouse and children, depending on the state). Unless a gay couple has an updated will (and most people in the United States do not), the biological family of the deceased can claim all possessions.

- *Employment benefits*—Married couples share a variety of benefits from work (health, dental, and life insurance, to name some) that gay

partners do not. Many *Fortune* 500 companies have instituted policies in recent years to allow gay partners such rights, but there is no law requiring this. Some companies offer these benefits to recruit and retain high-quality talent. Whereas many large companies can afford to do this, many smaller companies are not so inclined.

- *Social Security survivorship benefits and pensions*—At death, the law provides that the surviving spouse receive continued benefits.

- *Disability decision making*—If a married person becomes seriously injured and needs medical care decisions made for him or her, the law provides that spouses can make those decisions. But in cases in which parents or siblings of a disabled gay person do not approve of his or her relationship, they can—and often do—challenge the domestic partner's decisions in court.

Related to many of these legal rights are financial issues. Bernard (2011) profiled a lesbian couple to determine how their costs compared to a similar without legal marriage status heterosexual married couple. Using a couple who made $140,000 per year, which is about average for a college-educated couple in the three states with the highest estimated gay populations—New York, California, and Florida—she

Increasingly, gay men and lesbians are choosing in vitro fertilization or adoption to start their own families. The issue of gay and lesbian adoption was widely discussed in the media after former talk-show host Rosie O'Donnell publicly criticized President George W. Bush's opposition to gay adoption. O'Donnell, who is openly gay, has three adopted children and says that her own experiences as a mother make her certain that gay people should have the right to be parents.

estimated that in a worst-case scenario the lifetime cost of being gay was over $467,000. In the best case for a couple with significantly better health insurance, plus lower taxes and other costs, it was about $42,000.

You can see from this list that there are many problems related to legal rights of gay couples. There is much to be done to ensure equal rights for all married couples.

In 2012 the Secretary of the Department of Health and Human Services indicated that the Affordable Care Act would give LGBTQ Americans improved access to health coverage. Insurers would no longer be able to turn someone away just because he or she was LGBTQ.

In 2010 a federal judge found that a law barring the federal government from recognizing same-sex marriage is unconstitutional, ruling that gay and lesbian couples deserve the same federal benefits as heterosexual couples (Goodnough & Schwartz, 2010).

Should same-sex couples be allowed to marry legally? Some people feel that same-sex couples should have the same human rights as others. They argue that when people work, pay taxes, enter into lifetime commitments, and raise children, there is no reason they should not be afforded the same social and legal benefits and status as heterosexual couples—including legal marriage. There are still quite varied opinions about the topic of same-sex marriage.

Herdt and Kertzner (2006) argued that depriving lesbians and gays of the right to marry restricts their citizenship and hinders their health and well-being. Even though research confirms the capacity

of gays and lesbians to form committed relationships and parent successfully, marriage denial continues to perpetuate an opportunity structure that disenfranchises gays and lesbians in the sociocultural, legal, economic, and political aspects of their lives. Herdt and Kertzmer point out that denial of marriage is an act of discrimination against both gays and lesbians.

As of 2015, 18 countries had granted freedom to marry for same-sex couples nationwide (Argentina, Belgium, Brazil, Canada, Denmark, Finland, France, Great Britain, Iceland, Luxembourg, the Netherlands, New Zealand, Norway, Portugal, South Africa, Spain, Sweden, and Uruguay). As of June 2015, the United States was added to this list. Mexico has established regional or court-directed provisions enabling same-sex couples to share in the freedom to marry. Many other countries provide some protection for LGBTQ couples (Freedom to Marry, 2015).

Some people believe that gay marriage bans have inspired a new wave of activists. For example, a group planned "A Day Without a Gay." The event organizers asked gay-rights supporters to avoid going to work by "calling in gay" and volunteering for the gay-rights movement instead. The burst of energy drew some comparisons to demonstrations during the early days of the AIDS crisis in the 1980s.

In 2011, a Gallup poll found that for the first time, a majority of Americans (53%) believed same-sex marriage should be legal, with such couples having the same rights as in other marriages (Newport, 2011). That year's 9-percentage-point increase in support for same-sex marriage was the largest year-to-year shift yet measured. The increase came exclusively among political independents and Democrats; Republican views did not change.

In a 2012 study, a majority of Americans (54%) said that same-sex marriage should be legally recognized, while 42% were opposed. There was a sharp partisan divide, with 70% of Democrats and 60% of

People disagree about the rights of homosexual couples.

Ethical DIMENSIONS

Should Gay Marriages Be Legal?

Given the many legal benefits enjoyed by married couples, there has been pressure to legalize gay marriages. Those individuals who believe gay marriages are not proper argue that gay marriages should not be legal. Those who believe there is an ethical responsibility to treat all people equally, and to recognize the rights of various groups, argue that gay marriages should be legal.

If you were a member of the U.S. Supreme Court that legalized gay marriage in all states in 2015, how would you have voted? Which of the following ethical points would have influenced your vote most?

Positive Points	Negative Points
The gay rights movement has stood for valuing all families—including those led by single parents, those with adopted children, and other configurations.	All the attention to gay marriages may take away from other important causes such as homeless youth, job discrimination, and transgender people, among others.
The right to marry is a fundamental right in the liberty of the person.	Some churches are increasing their anti-gay rhetoric.
There is dignity in the bond between two men or two women who seek to marry and in their autonomy to make such important choices.	Those who oppose same-sex marriage are free to decline to provide business services for same-sex weddings and other functions.
The children of same-sex parents benefit because their families have the same status as other families.	The court decision may pave the way for an all-out assault against the religious freedom rights of people who disagree.
When all Americans are treated equally, we are all free.	A number of religious groups continue to oppose same-sex marriage.
A solid and growing majority of Americans believe in marriage equality.	As more victories accumulate for gay rights, some gay institutions and rituals will disappear.
A number of religious groups support same-sex marriage.	There could be a loss of the specialness of being gay because the sense of community and sharing might be gone. It might be the end of gay culture.
It is right for gay couples to have equal dignity in the eyes of the law.	Many people believe being LGBT is a sin.
Having legal same-sex marriages may inspire the LGBT community to work for the greater good of all who are oppressed.	Perhaps religious organizations and other organizations that oppose same-sex marriages will have to change their policies related to hiring, firing, housing, and benefits.
Legal same-sex marriage is another step on the path to equality.	
It will make it easier for colleges and universities to support gay students and professors.	
There are potential employment benefits for same-sex employees who are married (e.g., sick days, retirement plans, vacation time).	
Statistics show that married same-sex couples are more economically secure than unmarried couples.	

independent voters saying it should be legal, but 72% of Republicans being opposed to same-sex marriage (Pruitt, 2012).

A 2015 Gallup poll reported several interesting statistics (Gay and lesbian rights, 2015). When asked whether they thought gay or lesbian relationships between consenting adults should or should not be legal, 66% of respondents said they should be legal (compared with 32% in 1986), and 30% said they should not be legal (compared with 57% in 1986). When asked if they thought marriages between same-sex couples should or should not be recognized by the law as valid, with the same rights as traditional marriages, 55% of respondents said they should (compared to 39% in 2006) and 42% said they should not be valid (compared to 58% in 2006).

McCarthy (2015) reported that 53% of Americans said they are satisfied with the level of acceptance of gays and lesbians in the United States. This percentage was up from approximately 35% in 2001. In contrast, 39% said they were not satisfied with the level of acceptance of gays and lesbians in the United States, down from approximately 57% in 2001. Sixteen percent wanted to see more acceptance, while 14% wanted less. Sixty percent of Democrats said they were satisfied with the level of acceptance of gays and lesbians, slightly more than independents (55%) and considerably more than Republicans (43%).

In 2012 it was found that a majority of Americans (54%) said that same sex marriage should be legally recognized, while 42% were opposed. There was a sharp partisan divide, with 70% of Democrats and 60% of independent voters saying it should be legal, but 72% of Republicans were opposed to same-sex marriage (Pruitt 2012).

Should lesbian and gay couples be allowed to adopt children? Some people start with the premise that LGBTQ behavior is wrong and believe that such a relationship is an inappropriate context in which to raise children. Because they fear that sexual orientation and behaviors can be learned, they fear that a child raised by a lesbian or gay couple would be more likely to become a lesbian or gay man. Others do not believe that sexual orientation determines one's ability to parent. They feel the most important requirements are the abilities to love, support, and care for a child. Most lesbians and gays were raised by heterosexual parents. Therefore, they believe being raised by a lesbian or gay couple will not create lesbian or gay children any more than being raised by a heterosexual married couple would guarantee heterosexuality. Interestingly, researchers in developmental psychology have concluded that no significant differences exist between children raised by lesbians and gay men and those raised by heterosexuals.

As lawmakers and courts expand the legal definition of the American family, some same-sex couples feel the same what-about-children pressure that heterosexual couples have long felt. Many gay men had resigned themselves to the idea that they would never be accepted by society as good and loving parents and assumed that they would never have children. However, parenting among same-sex couples is now more common and there can be pressure for same-sex couples to have childern. This raises related issues about whether to adopt or use a surrogate. At the same time, many people are uncomfortable with the idea of same-sex couples being parents. A

Pew Research Center survey found that for the first time a majority of people (52%) said that gay men and lesbians should be allowed to adopt children, up from 46% in 2008 and 38% in 1999 (Swarns, 2012).

Health and access to care are also often mentioned when discussing rights of the LGBTQ population. Ranji et el. (2014) indicated that LGBTQ people often face challenges and barriers to accessing needed health services and, as a result, can experience worse health outcomes. These challenges can include stigma, discrimination, violence, and rejection by families and communities, as well as other barriers, such as inequality in the workplace and health insurance sectors, the provision of substandard care, and outright denial of care because of sexual orientation or gender identity. In addition to experiencing many of the same health concerns as the general population, the LGBTQ population experiences certain health challenges at higher rates, as well as several unique health challenges. In particular, some subgroups of the LGBTQ community have more chronic conditions as well as higher prevalence and earlier onset of disabilities compared to heterosexuals. Other major health concerns include HIV/AIDS, mental illness, substance use, and sexual and physical violence. Some LGBTQ individuals are also more likely to experience challenges in obtaining health care. Barriers to such care include gaps in coverage, cost-related hurdles, and poor treatment from healthcare providers.

Some people might wonder where the proportion of LGBTQ people is the highest in the United States. Newport and Gates (2015) found that, of the 50 largest metropolitan areas, San Francisco had the highest percentage—6.2% of its total population. The cities with the next highest proportions were Portland–Vancouver–Hillsboro, Oregon and Washington (5.4%); Austin–Round Rock, Texas (5.3%); New Orleans–Metairie, Louisiana (5.1%); Seattle–Tacoma–Bellevue, Washington (4.8%); and Boston–Cambridge–Newton, Massachusetts (4.8%). The lowest LGBTQ percentage among the 50 largest cities was found in Birmingham–Hoover, Alabama (2.6), and the national average among the 50 cities was 3.6%.

Finally, it is interesting to note that in 2015 the United States appointed its first ever special envoy for LGBTQ rights (Regan, 2015). His job is to defend and promote the rights of LGBTQ people. This envoy will work to reduce violence and discrimination against LGBTQ people around the world, including those in some 75 countries where LGBTQ behavior and same-sex relationships are criminalized. In announcing this appointment, U.S. Secretary of State John Kerry said, "Defending and promoting the human rights of LGBTQ persons is at the core of our commitment to advancing human rights globally."

Exploring the Dimensions of Human Sexuality

Case Study

No single scientific theory about the biological causes of sexual orientation has been substantiated; neither have any psychological theories. It is likely that the biological, psychological, and sociocultural factors interact to influence our sexual orientation. Because the dimensions change over time, an individual's sexual orientation may change over time as well.

Culturally, not all societies view LGBTQ behavior in the same manner. In areas of the Pacific such as Papua New Guinea, boys regularly participate in gay activities until they reach the age of marriage (19 years). In Mexico, only a male who plays the receptive role in anal intercourse is considered gay.

Socially, gays and lesbians in the United States can feel stigmatized and socially isolated as a result of fear of disclosure. Those who disclose their orientation ("come out") face discrimination and possibly even violence. Further, family and friends may reject them.

Biological Factors

- Research into genetic factors affecting LGBTQ people has been inconclusive. No specific gene has been identified. Any genetic link would be only part of the picture for determining sexual orientation.
- Research into hormonal imbalances (either prenatal or postnatal) as a factor driving LGBTQ people has proved inconclusive. No specific hormonal factors have been identified. Any hormonal link would be only one aspect of determining sexual orientation.

Sociocultural Factors

- LGBTQ students often feel isolated and stigmatized.
- Family life can be disrupted by disclosure of LGBTQ status.
- Different cultures view LGBTQ people in different terms.
- Some states have laws making LGBTQ sexual activities illegal. Further, gay marriages sometimes do not have legal standing for state or federal benefits. Many large corporations have begun to offer employee benefits for domestic partners.

Psychological Factors

- Most theories suggesting that the influence of mothers or early sexual experiences lead to changes in sexual orientation have been discounted.
- Most LGBTQ people lead lives as fulfilling and satisfying as those of most heterosexuals.

Summary

- Sexual orientation can be viewed on a continuum, which Kinsey described as having seven points.

- Sexual orientations include a number of possibilites.

- There are many theories about what determines sexual orientation, including biological, psychological, and integrated theories. None of the theories is generally agreed upon.

- Both LGBTQ and heterosexual youths and adolescents face the same challenges related to growth and development, but LGBTQ youth face additional issues related to their acceptance.

- There are many examples of discrimination against people who have a sexual orientation other than heterosexual.

- In the United States, the LGBTQ subculture centers on private clubs, bars, and organizations. These groups are designed to protect LGBTQ people, promote their rights, promote a positive image of LGBTQ people, and help the general public better understand having them.

- Social issues related to sexual orientation include military policies, discrimination based on sexual orientation, and general understanding and support for people of various sexual orientations.

- There are many points of view about sexual orientation based on religion and morality.

- The gay-rights movement has helped many people better understand LGBTQ people and have more positive attitudes about them in general.

- Many legal issues remain related to sexual orientation, including the legal status of same-sex relationships of various types, the right of LGBTQ individuals to be parents, and legal rights concerning issues such as inheritance, health insurance coverage, income taxes, and employment benefits.

Discussion Questions

1. What defines a person's sexual orientation? Is sexual orientation constant throughout life, or can it change over time?

2. Describe the theories of the causes of sexual orientation, and indicate whether research supports their theoretical claims.

3. Compare and contrast LGBTQ activities with the heterosexual lifestyle.

4. What are the social issues surrounding LGBTQ people? How do such issues adversely affect them?

Application Questions

Reread the chapter-opening story and answer the following questions.

1. Explain why Brad was dating and engaging in sexual activities with Peggy if he thought he was gay.

2. Discuss the social and psychological effects on people who are unable to disclose their sexual orientation and introduce a lifetime partner to friends and family.

Critical Thinking Questions

1. If a genetic link were found for LGBTQ orientation, how might that affect those found to have the gene? Would society accept LGBTQ people as an inherited "defect"? Or would LGBTQ people encounter more discrimination in the workplace, in the military, and so on?

2. Assuming that studies claiming that only a small percentage of the population is gay are correct, why should efforts be made to accommodate such a small minority?

3. The "Don't ask; don't tell" policy of the U.S. military has been repealed. Should sexual orientation make a difference on the battlefield?

4. Given that many states ban same-sex sexual activity, is it ethical to vote admitted LGBTQ people into public office?

5. If LGBTQ behaviors had no social stigma, would there be more or fewer people living as LGBTQ people? Explain your answer.

Critical Thinking Case

When a filmmaker's son started kindergarten, she had more to worry about than the other parents. Her son thought that having two moms was great—but what would the other kids tell him?

The filmmaker and her female friend toured the country and filmed teachers in classrooms as they described gay and lesbian lifestyles to children.

Their goal was to show that the classroom could be a place where children are taught tolerance and acceptance of lifestyles different from those of their own families.

Originally, the film was used in school systems and colleges to educate teachers about the prejudice that exists among young children regarding LGBTQ people. But, the film caused quite a stir on the airwaves. After PBS turned it down for national distribution, San Francisco's KQED agreed to sponsor the film.

A number of public stations scheduled it, and others were on board or considering it. This caused some anger among the Christian Right and other conservative groups who did not believe the film should be broadcast where children might watch it without supervision, although the stations had scheduled it for nighttime airing. They also argued that the film did not take parents' rights into consideration.

What do you think? Should teachers be encouraged to educate elementary school children about the topic of LGBTQ people, or should this responsibility be left to parents? Should films about LGBTQ people be broadcast on national TV if the goal is to get people talking and thinking about educational issues?

Exploring Personal Dimensions

Take a few moments to measure the strength of your feelings about LGBTQ behavior and gender identity by using this values grid.

Place in the appropriate square of the grid the *italicized* key term in the questions following that shows how you feel about the question. Note that you will be identifying the *degree* of your feelings, not whether they are positive or negative. Fill in all 16 squares, placing only one key term in any one square. (You may change your mind as you go along if you discover other key words about which you feel more or less strongly.) After you complete the grid, look it over to see how strong your feelings are. If you can find a willing partner, compare your grids and discuss your responses.

	Very Strongly	Strongly	Mildly	No Reaction
1. How would you feel if your closest *friend* told you he or she was gay/lesbian?	❏	❏	❏	❏
2. How do you feel about *two girls* who greet each other with a kiss after a long summer vacation?	❏	❏	❏	❏
3. How do you feel about *two boys* greeting each other with a kiss after a long summer vacation?	❏	❏	❏	❏
4. How do you feel about a person who would *beat up* a gay person for fun?	❏	❏	❏	❏
5. How do you feel about two *girls holding hands* on the way to class?	❏	❏	❏	❏
6. How do you feel about girls wearing *boys' clothes*?	❏	❏	❏	❏
7. How do you feel about boys wearing *girls' clothes*?	❏	❏	❏	❏
8. How do you feel about two *boys holding hands* on the way to class?	❏	❏	❏	❏
9. How do you feel about *boys* who do not like sports?	❏	❏	❏	❏
10. How do you feel about *girls* who do like sports?	❏	❏	❏	❏
11. How do you feel about taking *group showers*?	❏	❏	❏	❏
12. How do you feel about a man taking over the household *chores*?	❏	❏	❏	❏
13. How do you feel about a male *hairdresser*?	❏	❏	❏	❏
14. How do you feel about a woman who becomes a *construction worker*?	❏	❏	❏	❏
15. How do you feel about going out only with persons of the *other sex*?	❏	❏	❏	❏
16. How do you feel about going out only with persons of the *same sex*?	❏	❏	❏	❏

How did you feel about these questions? Did any of them bother you for any reason? Why or why not? Do you have strong feelings about LGBTQ behavior?

Source: Bruess, C. E., & Greenberg, J. S. *Sexuality education: Theory and practice, 6th ed.* Sudbury, MA: Jones and Bartlett Publishers, 2014.

Suggested Readings

A resource guide to coming out. Human Rights Campaign, 2014. Available: http://www.hrc.org/resources/entry/resource-guide-to-coming-out.

Coming out as a supporter. Human Rights Campaign, 2014. Available: http://www.hrc.org/resources/entry/straight-guide-to-lgbt-americans.

Creating supportive environments for lesbian, gay, bisexual, and transgender youth. *The Prevention Researcher, 17, no. 4* (November, 2010) (Special Issue containing 5 related articles).

Journal of Bisexuality. Taylor & Francis Online. Available: www.tandfonline.com/toc/wjbi20/current.

Journal of Homosexuality. Taylor & Francis Online. Available: www.tandfonline.com/loi/wjhm20.

Just the facts about sexual orientation and youth. American Psychological Association, 2015. Available: http://www.hrc.org/resources/entry/transgender-visibility-guide

New Williams Institute data visualization: U.S. benefitting from $2.6 billion same-sex wedding spending boom. Williams Institute, 2014. Available: http://williamsinstitute.law.ucla.edu/press/press-releases/data-visualization-same-sex-spending-boom.

Russell, S. T., Ryan, C., Toomey, R. B., Diaz, R. M., & Sanchez, J. Lesbian, gay, bisexual, and transgender adolescent school victimization: Implications for young adult health and adjustment. *Journal of School Health, 81, no. 5* (May, 2011), 223–229.

Tracy, E. C., & Satariano, N. P. Differentiating between gay and heterosexual male speech. *Journal of the Acoustical Society of America, 129, no. 4* (2011), 2421.

Transgender visibility: A guide to being you. Human Rights Campaign, 2014. Available: http://www.hrc.org/resources/entry/transgender-visibility-guide.

Wilson, R. Gay academics find new paths to the top. *The Chronicle of Higher Education, 42, no. 30* (April 1, 2011), A1, A9–A10.

Web Resources

American Civil Liberties Union: Lesbian Gay Bisexual Transgender Project
www.aclu.org/lgbt-rights

Documentation of the ACLU's actions to fight discrimination and educate the public regarding LGBT rights.

American Psychological Association
www.apa.org/topics/lght/index.aspx

Provides answers to questions about sexual orientation and LGBTQ issues.

Hartford Institute for Religion Research: Homosexuality and Religion
www.hartfordinstitute.org/research/homosexuality_religion.html

Articles and research on the topic of LGBTQ issues and religion.

Lambda Legal
www.lambdalegal.org

Contains information about many legal issues including laws related to sexual orientation.

National Organization for Women: Information on LGBT Rights
http://now.org/issues/lesbian-rights/

Information on NOW's work on LGBT rights including support of same-sex unions.

Williams Institute
http://williamsinstitute.law.ucla.edu/

Conducts rigorous, independent research on sexual orientation and gender identity law and public policy.

References

Airing it out. *Time, 160, no. 19* (November 4, 2002), 84.

Answers to your questions about transgender people, gender identity, and gender expression. American Psychological Association, 2015. Available: http://www.apa.org/topics/lgbt/transgender.aspx.

Barnes, S. Individuals who don't follow the standard script of sex and romance find they are not alone. *Albany Times Union* (May 29, 2005), G1.

Bernard, T. S. The financial hurdles gay couples face. *The New York Times* (March 26, 2011). Available: http://bucks.blogs.nytimes.com/2011/03/26/the-financial-hurdles-gay-couples-face/.

Bishop, G. Three straights and you're out in gay softball league. *The New York Times* (June 29, 2011). Available: http://www.nytimes.com/2011/06/30/sports/softball-case-raises-question-who-qualifies-as-gay.html.

Burri, A., Cherkas, L., Spector, T., & Rahman, Q. Genetic and environmental influences on female sexual orientation, childhood gender typicality and adult gender identity. *PLoS ONE 6, no. 7* (2011), e21982. doi:10.1371/journal.pone.0021982.

Calefati, J. Gay high schools offer a haven from bullies. *U.S. News & World Report* (January 2, 2009). Available: http://www.usnews.com/articles/education/2008/12/31/gay-high-schools-offer-a-haven-from-bullies.

Census Bureau releases estimates of same-sex married couples. United States Census Bureau Newsroom (September 27, 2011). Available: http://www.census.gov/newsroom/releases/archives/2010_census/cb11-cn181.html.

Centers for Disease Control and Prevention (CDC). *LGBT youth*, 2014. Available: http://www.cdc.gov/lgbthealth/youth.htm.

Definition of terms. University of California, Berkeley, Gender Equity Resource Center, 2014. Available: http://geneq.berkeley.edu/lgbt_resources_definiton_of_terms#genderqueer

Demir, E., & Dickson, B. J. Fruitless splicing specifies male courtship behavior in Drosophila. *Cell, 121* (June 3, 2005), 785–794.

Despite stunning marriage victories, LGBT Americans remain unequal. Movement Advancement Project, 2014. Available: http://www.eriegaynews.com/news/article.php?recordid=201502mapreport.

Dias, E. A. Change of heart. *Time, 185, 2* (2015), 44–48.

Dolance, S. A whole stadium full: Lesbian community at Women's National Basketball Association games. *Journal of Sex Research, 42, no. 1* (February 2005), 74–83.

Ellingson, L. Lesbian health issues: A 10-year review. *Health Education Monograph Series, 19, no. 1* (2002), 40–45.

Freedom to Marry. *The freedom to marry internationally,* 2015. Available: http://www.freedomtomarry.org/landscape/entry/c/international.

Frequently asked questions about same-sex couple households. U.S. Census Bureau, 2013. Available: http://www.census.gov/hhes/samesex/files/SScplfactsheet_final.pdf.

Gates, G. J. *LGBT demographics: Comparisons among population-based surveys.* Williams Institute, 2014. Available: http://williamsinstitute.law.ucla.edu/research/census-lgbt-demographics-studies/lgbt-demogs-sep-2014/.

Gay and lesbian rights. *Gallup.com*, 2015. Available: http://www.gallup.com/poll/1651/gay-lesbian-rights.aspx.

Goodnough, A., & Schwartz, J. Judge topples U.S. rejection of gay unions. *The New York Times* (July 8, 2010). Available: http://www.nytimes.com/2010/07/09/us/09marriage.html.

Goodstein, L. Largest Presbyterian denomination gives final approval for same-sex marriage. *New York Times*, March 17, 2015. Available: http://www.nytimes.com/2015/03/18/us/presbyterians-give-final-approval-for-same-sex-marriage.html?_r=0.

Goodstein, L. Presbyterians approve ordination of gay people. *The New York Times* (May 10, 2011). Available: http://www.nytimes.com/2011/05/11/us/11presbyterian.html.

Hasenbush, A., Flores, A. R., Kastanis, A., Sears, B., & Gates, G. J. The LGBT divide: A data portrait of LGBT people in the Midwestern, Mountain, and Southern states. Williams Institute, 2014. Available: http://williamsinstitute.law.ucla.edu/research/lgbt-divide-dec-2014/.

Herdt, G. H., & Kertzner, R. I do, but I can't: The impact of marriage denial on the mental health and sexual citizenship of lesbians and gay men in the United States. *Sexuality Research & Social Policy, 3, no. 1* (March 2006), 33–44.

Hillard, P., Love, L., Franks, H. M., Laris, B. A., & Coyle, K. K. "They were only joking": Efforts to decrease LGBTQ bullying and harassment in Seattle public schools. *Journal of School Health, 84, 1* (2014), 1–9.

Hoffman, R. M. Conceptualizing heterosexual identity development: Issues and challenges. *Journal of Counseling and Development, 82* (2004), 375–380.

Horvath, K. J., Beadnell, B., & Bowen, A. M. Sensation seeking as a moderator of Internet use on sexual risk taking among men who have sex with men. *Sexual Research and Social Policy, 3, 4* (2006), 77–90.

Individuals with intersex conditions. American Psychological Association, 2015. Available: http://www.apa.org/topics/lgbt/intersex.pdf.

Intersex Society of North America. How Can You Assign A Gender (Boy or Girl) Without Surgery?, 2008. Available: www.isna.org/faq/gender_assignment.

Jacobson, J. Rice U. football coach chastised for comments on gay athletes. *Chronicle of Higher Education, 49, no. 11* (November 18, 2002b), A32.

Kastanis, A., & Wilson, B. D. M. *Race/ethnicity, gender and socioeconomic wellbeing of individuals in same-sex couples.* Williams Institute, 2014. Available: http://williamsinstitute.law.ucla.edu/wp-content/uploads/Census-Compare-Feb-2014.pdf.

Kosciw, J. G., Palmer, N. A., & Boesen, M. J. *The 2013 National School Climate Survey: The experiences of lesbian, gay, bisexual and transgender youth in our nation's schools.* New York: GLSEN, 2014.

Laumann, E. O., Gagnon, J. H., Michael, R. T., & Michaels, S. *The social organization of sexuality: Sexual practices in the United States.* Chicago: University of Chicago Press, 1994.

Levay, S. *Gay, straight and the reasons why: The science of sexual orientation.* Oxford, UK: Oxford University Press, 2011. Available: http://www.simonlevay.com/the-science-of-sexual-orientation.

LGBT terms and definitions. International Spectrum, University of Michigan, 2013. Available: http://internationalspectrum.umich.edu/life/definitions.

McCarthy, J. Satisfaction with acceptance of gay people plateaus at 53%. *Gallup.com*, 2015. Available: http://www.gallup.com/poll/181235/satisfaction-acceptance-gay-people-plateaus.aspx.

Ness, C. PBS shies from show. *San Francisco Examiner* (June 6, 1999).

Newport, F. For first time, majority of Americans favor legal gay marriage. Gallup, May 20, 2011. Available: http://www.gallup.com/poll/147662/first-time-majority-americans-favor-legal-gay-marriage.aspx.

Newport, F., & Gates, G. J. San Francisco metro area ranks highest in LGBT percentage. *Gallup.com*, 2015. Available: http://www.gallup.com/poll/182051/san-francisco-metro-area-ranks-highest-lgbt-percentage.aspx.

New report details high rates of violence, discrimination toward bisexual people. Movement Advancement Project, 2014. Available: http://www.lgbtmap.org/news/understanding-issues-facing-bisexual-americans-release.

Ontario Consultants on Religious Tolerance. Brief descriptions of the six belief systems, 2014. Available: http://www.religioustolerance.org/hom6beli1.htm.

An open letter to religious leaders on marriage equality. Religious Institute on Sexual Morality, Justice, and Healing 2015. http://www.religiousinstitute.org/wp-content/uploads/2013/08/OL-Marriage-Equality.pdf.

Palermo, E. Pansexual: A "new" sexual orientation? *Livescience.com*, 2013. Available: http://www.livescience.com/41163-pansexual-sexual-orientation-pansexuality.html.

Payne, E. C., & Smith, M. The reduction of stigma in schools: A new professional development model for empowering educators to support LGBTQ students. *Journal of LGBT Youth, 8* (2011), 174–200.

Payne, E., & Smith, M. Rethinking Safe schools approaches for LGBTQ students: Changing the questions we ask. *Multicultural Perspectives, 14, 4* (2012), 187–193.

Payne, K. K., & Manning, W. D. *Number of children living in same-sex couple households 2013.* National Center for Family & Marriage Research, 2015. Available: http://www.bgsu.edu/ncfmr/resources/data/family-profiles/number-of-children-living-in-same-sex-couple-households--2013.html.

Point Foundation. *The National LGBTQ Scholarship Fund*, 2015. Available: http://www.pointfoundation.org/.

Poteat, V. P., DiGiovanni, C. D., Sinclair, K. O., Koenig, B. W., & Russell, S. T. Gay–straight alliances are associated with student health: A multischool comparison of LGBTQ and heterosexual youth. *Journal of Research on Adolescence, 23, 2* (2012), 319–3300

Prabhat, S. Difference between bi-sexual and pan sexual. *DifferenceBetween.net*, October 9, 2014. Available: http://www.differencebetween.net/science/nature/difference-between-bi-sexual-and-pan-sexual/.

Presgraves, D. 2009 National School Climate Survey: Nearly 9 out of 10 LGBT students experience harassment in school. Gay, Lesbian and Straight Education Network (September 14, 2010). Available: http://www.glsen.org/cgi-bin/iowa/all/news/record/2624.html.

Pruitt, P. Majority of Americans support legalizing same-sex marriage, poll shows. *ABC News* (June 6, 2012). Available: http://abcnews.go.com/Politics/OTUS/majority-americans-support-legalizing-sex-marriage-poll-shows/story?id=16505633#.UCwBDVZlS2X.

Rahman, Q. The neurodevelopment of human sexual orientation. *Neuroscience & Biobehavioral Reviews, 20, 7* (2005) 1057–1066.

Ranji, U., Beamesderfer, A., Kates, J., & Salganicoff, A. *Health and access to care and coverage for lesbian, gay, bisexual, and transgender individuals in the U.S.* Henry J. Kaiser Family Foundation, 2014. Available: http://kff.org/disparities-policy/issue-brief/health-and-access-to-care-and-coverage-for-lesbian-gay-bisexual-and-transgender-individuals-in-the-u-s/.

Regan, H. The U.S. has appointed its first ever special envoy for LGBT rights. *Time.com*, 2015. Available: http://time.com/3719879/us-special-envoy-lgbt-rights-randy-berry/.

Rice, W. R., Friberg, U., & Gavrilets, S. Homosexuality as a consequence of epigenetically canalized sexual development. *Quarterly Review of Biology, 87, 4* (December 2012), 343–368.

Robinson, J. P., & Esplage, D. Inequities in educational and psychological outcomes between LGBTQ and straight students in middle and high school. *Educational Researcher, 40, 7* (2011), 315–330.

Robinson, J. P., & Esplage, D. Peer victimization and sexual risk differences between lesbian, gay, bisexual, transgender, or questioning and heterosexual youth in grades 7–12. *American Journal of Public Health 103* (2013), 1–10.

Ruscombe-King, R. Homophobia, prejudice and attitudes to gay men and lesbians. AVERT (an international AIDS charity), 2009. Available: http://avert.org/homophobia.htm.

Russell, S. T., Ryan, C., Toomey, R. B., Diaz, R. M., & Sanchez, J. Lesbian, gay, bisexual, and transgender adolescent school victimization: Implications for young adult health and adjustment. *Journal of School Health 81, no. 5* (May, 2011), 223–230.

Ryan, C., Huebner, D., Diaz, R. M., & Sanchez, J. Family rejection as a predictor of negative health outcomes in white and Latino lesbian, gay, and bisexual young adults. *Pediatrics, 123, 1* (January 2009), 346–352.

Saewyc, E. M., Homma, Y., Skay, C. L., Bearinger, L. H., Resnick, M. D., & Reis, E. Protective factors in the lives of bisexual adolescents in North America. *American Journal of Public Health, 99, 1* (January 2009), 110–117.

Saewyc, E. M., Taylor, D., Homma, Y., & Ogilvie, G. Trends in sexual health and risk behaviours among adolescents students in British Columbia. *Canadian Journal of Human Sexuality, 17, 1–2* (2008), 1–13.

Savic, I., Berglund, H., & Lindstrom, P. Brain response to putative pheromones in homosexual men. *Proceedings of the National Academy of Sciences, 102, no. 20* (May 17, 2005), 7356–7361.

Sexual orientation and homosexuality. American Psychological Association, 2015. Available: http://www.apa.org/helpcenter/sexual-orientation.aspx.

SIECUS Policy and Advocacy. A portrait of sexuality education and abstinence-only-until-marriage programs in the states (fiscal year 2008 edition), 2008. Available: http://www.siecus.org/index.cfm?fuseaction=Page.ViewPage&PageID=1164.

SIECUS position statements on sexuality issues, 2015. Available: http://www.siecus.org.

Staley, M., Hussey, W., Roe, K., Harcourt, J., & Roe, K. In the shadow of the rainbow: Identifying and addressing health disparities in the lesbian, gay, bisexual, and transgender population—a research and practice challenge. *Health Promotion Practice, 2, no. 3* (July 2001) 207–211.

Statement by Secretary Kathleen Sebelius on LGBT Health Awareness Week 2012. March 26, 2012. Available: http://www.hhs.gov/news/press/2012pres/03/20120326a.html.

Substance Abuse and Mental Health Services Administration (SAMHSA). *A practitioner's resource guide: Helping families to support their LGBT children.* HHS Publication No. PEP14-LGBTKIDS. Rockville, MD: SAMHSA, 2014.

Swarns, R. L. Male couples face pressure to fill cradles. *The New York Times* (August 9, 2012). Available: http://www.nytimes.com/2012/08/10/us/gay-couples-face-pressure-to-have-children.html?pagewanted=all.

Thomas, K. College team teaches a lesson in acceptance. *The New York Times* (May 7, 2010). Available: http://www.nytimes.com/2010/05/09/sports/09oneonta.html.

Trebay, G. The secret power of lesbian style. *The New York Times* (June 27, 2004).

UNAIDS. HIV prevention hampered by homophobia, 2009. Available: http://www.unaids.org/en/KnowledgeCentre/Resources/FeatureStories/archive/2009/20090113_MSMLATAM.asp.

U.S. Census Bureau. *2013 American Community Survey 1-year data file.* United States Housing Unit Records, 2015. Available: http://factfinder.census.gov/faces/tableservices/jsf/pages/productview.xhtml?pid=ACS_pums_sas_2009_2013&prodType=document.

Ward B.W., Dahlhamer, J.M., Galinsky, A.M., & Joesti, S.S. (July 15, 2014). Sexual Orientation and Health Among U.S. Adults: National Health Interview Survey, 2013. *National Health Statistics Reports 77.*

Weinstein, N., Ryan, W. S., DeHaan, C. R., Przybylski, A. K., Legate, N., & Ryan, R. M. Parental autonomy support and discrepancies between implicit and explicit sexual identities: dynamics of self-acceptance and defense. *Journal of Personality and Social Psychology, 102, no. 4* (April 2012), 815–832.

What Do Intersex and the Same Sex Marriage Debate Have to do With Each Other? Intersex Society of North America, 2008. Available: www.isna.org/faq/marriage.

What Does ISNA Recommend for Children With Intersex?, Instersex Society of North America, 2008. Available: www.isna.org/faq/patient-centered.

Winfield, N. (2014). Vatican Alters Draft Report Translation About Gays. Yahoo News. Available: http://news.yahoo.com/vatican-alters-draft-report-translation-gays-132855337.html

Worthington, R. L., Savoy, H. B., Dillon, F. R., & Vernaglia, E. R. Heterosexual identity development: A multidimensional model of individual and social identity. *The Counseling Psychologist, 30,* (2002), 496–531.

Zivony, A., & Lobel, T. (2014). The invisible stereotypes of bisexual men. *Archives of Sexual Behavior 43, 6* (1165–1176).

CHAPTER 13

Sexuality in Childhood and Adolescence

© Gayvoronskaya Yana/Shutterstock

FEATURES

Communication Dimensions
Tips for Discussing Sexual Messages and Scandals on TV with Children

Communication Dimensions
Resources for Becoming Askable

Ethical Dimensions
Is It Ethical to Ignore Your Child's Developing Sexuality?

Ethical Dimensions
Should Parents Have Their Adolescent Children Vaccinated Against HPV?

Gender Dimensions
How Gender Stereotypes Affect Sexuality

Multicultural Dimensions
Racial and Ethnic Differences in Sexual Behaviors

Global Dimensions
Teenagers and Sexuality Around the World

CHAPTER OBJECTIVES

1 Explain why an infant is a sexual being; include the role that touch plays in development.

2 Explain the sexual development of children from preschool through the early elementary years.

3 Describe the differences in puberty for boys and girls.

4 Identify the three developmental stages of adolescence.

5 Compare the findings of various surveys concerning adolescent sexual behaviors and attitudes.

6 Discuss the prevalence of sexual abuse and sexual harassment of children and adolescents.

INTRODUCTION

Shawna is a precocious 5-year-old who already reads. She's been eating lunch at a nice restaurant with her mother after a morning of shopping. In the restroom before heading for home, she notices a vending machine mounted on the wall and asks, "Mama, why are they selling napkins in the bathroom when they already give them to everyone when they're eating?" Mama, visibly flustered, says, "We'll talk about it later, after we get home." Shawna feels as if she has asked something she shouldn't have mentioned and never brings it up again. Neither does her mother.

A few years later, still a precocious child, she reaches menarche just as she enters fifth grade, before she turns 10. Shawna has used the dictionary and the Internet to try to learn all the "facts of life" she can find. She knows what is happening to her body, but is afraid to tell her mother. She privately rejoices at this sign of her physical maturity. Finally, some stained panties in the laundry disclose her secret. Then she and her mother have "the talk" about menstruation. Shawna's mother shares that when she was growing up, she was expected to announce when every period came at the breakfast table. That was very embarrassing to her, and she doesn't want Shawna to feel the same way. So she suggests, "Just let me know if there is anything you need or if something doesn't seem right." Looking back, that assurance was both positive and comforting. Shawna hopes someday she will be able to treat her own daughter with that kind of respect. But she will have "the talk" sooner and will try to answer questions candidly whenever they come up.

Now as a young mother, Shawna is in a public restroom with both her daughters, aged 3 and 5. Her 5-year-old, Samantha, asks, "Mom, how come they sell 'tampads' in here?" Remembering her own early questions, Shawna *decides to respond on the spot in front of both girls and anyone else that happens to be listening. She says, "The pads are for women or older girls who are having a menstrual period. It's a natural and healthy thing that happens every month. A period helps a girl's body to be able to have babies."*

As you read this chapter, you may want to think about your own life and ask yourself, "How did I become who I am today?" "Which experiences helped promote my sexual health?" "What happened to me that I must overcome as I move into sexual adulthood?"

Learning the sexual values of parents and caregivers happens through observation and nonverbal cues, along with the "talks" that may or may not have helped move one over the speed bumps that happen as children grow up. Reflect on past experience; think about how situations might have been handled differently. Perhaps questions could have been answered more honestly. Puzzling dilemmas might have been discussed more openly.

Today, honest answers, balanced discussion, and decision-making options are more available than ever before. Reliable websites, well-informed educators, and parental resources abound. (See suggestions in Communication Dimensions: Resources for Becoming Askable.) Yet, this open discussion leads to more emphasis on sexuality in the media. Parents are understandably confused about how to answer their children's questions about the most recent scandal related to sexuality.

How much should they tell their children? Should they answer their children's questions directly? Should they try to shield their children from the news?

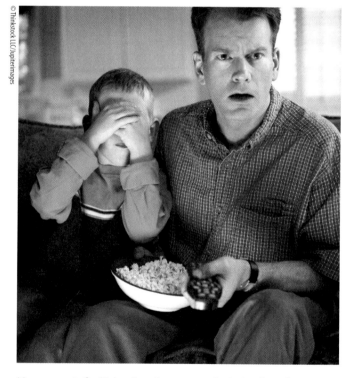

Sexual Development of Infants and Toddlers

Sexuality education begins in the delivery room. Of course, we are not talking about giving newborn babies facts about reproduction or sexual behaviors. But think for a minute: What is the first or second question parents ask after the birth of a child? They ask, "Is it a boy or a girl?" And sexuality education about sex roles begins.

Newborn babies develop sexually. In some ways, the first 18 months of life is one of the most important times for learning about love and touch and developing a sense of trust in the world. It is during their infancy that babies learn they are loved

Many parents find it hard to discuss sexual relationships that are sensationalized in the media. However, it is important to realize that parents teach their children about sexuality with what they say—as well as by what they do not say. By *not* saying anything about the latest incidents in the news, parents may be inadvertently telling their children not to ask questions about sexuality.

Communication
DIMENSIONS

Tips for Discussing Sexual Messages and Scandals on TV with Children

If a sexuality scandal of a high public official or a popular entertainer makes headlines, most likely any child in school will hear about it. Many parents wonder whether they need to discuss these scandals at all. The question parents need to ask is, Who do I want to tell my children about this sad situation? Another child on the playground? An acquaintance on the school bus?

Here are some tips for discussing scandals with your children:

1. Think about values as they relate to the current situation. What are your family values about sexual behavior outside marriage, fidelity, telling the truth?

2. Find out what the children already know. Do not wait for them to ask questions. That may never happen. You can start by saying, "Tell me what you've heard about …." You may be surprised how much they know.

3. Ask them to tell you what certain words mean to them. For example, a child may say that a celebrity had "oral sex" and think that means kissing.

4. Clarify the facts. Give short, age-appropriate answers. A short answer on "oral sex" for a child below the age of 10 years is, "Adults kiss, hug, or touch each other in special ways to show caring and share sexual pleasure. Oral sex is one way." Ask preteens or teenagers for their definition. Then correct any misinformation.

5. Help your children understand the larger issues surrounding sexuality scandals. These issues will affect the families of those involved, careers, and possibly the welfare of the nation.

6. You do not have to answer questions about your personal life. The answer to "Do you and Daddy do that?" is "Daddy's and my sex life is personal. When you are an adult, you will decide what sexual behaviors are comfortable for you."

Television and the Internet have become a primary part of most children's sexuality education. Rather than viewing media as an adversary in efforts to educate, it can become an ally. Suit the conversation to the developmental level of the child.

Age 3–6: Focus on varied family configurations and non-normative sex roles to help little ones learn about different grown-up possibilities.

Age 7–10: Identify concerns about racial and ethnic differences, body image, clothing, and hairstyles, especially unwarranted stereotyping and advertising.

Age 11–13: Programs featuring hidden feelings and deceptions make good lessons as emotions and hormones escalate. Discuss how feelings are expressed and directed.

Age 14–17: Major adolescent concerns involve sexual behaviors and their consequences. Use viewing to discuss issues; muse aloud.

Source: Data from Garrity, J. *Tuning in to TV sex: Using television for dialogue with your children.* Malibu, CA. Center for Media Literacy, 2002. Retrieved Jan 8, 2015, from http://www.medialit.org/reading-room/tuning-tv-sex-how-use-media-dialogue-your-children.

---

and learn how to love when parents kiss them, hug them, and talk to them. Babies also learn whether care providers will meet their needs or whether they will have to tough it out. They learn quickly whether they can count on their care providers to respond to their basic needs.

Actually, biological sexual development begins during pregnancy. Prenatal ultrasound technology has verified that the sexual response system begins to develop in males during the middle stages of gestation. Erectile response begins to appear at around 16 weeks; respiratory function does not begin until almost 12 weeks later. And, although sexual response in female fetuses is not readily observable, it is assumed that the capacity for lubrication begins at this time as well.

During the first few months of life, **infants**, babies from birth to 1 year, begin to discover their bodies. By 7 or 8 months, they discover their hands and toes. About the same time, boys discover their penis. Girls, on average, seem to discover their vulva about 2 months later. Infants love to put their fingers and toes into their mouths, and they love to touch their genitals. Baby boys have erections regularly throughout the day and during sleep, as many as three or more times a night. Infant boys may become erect simply by crying, coughing, stretching, or urinating. Baby girls' vaginas are believed to lubricate about

infants Babies from birth to 1 year old.

just as often, although this is not easily observable, and studies on this topic have not been done.

Psychosexual Development

Cuddling and stroking babies help them learn that their bodies feel good when they are touched and also help cement the parent–child bond. In fact, research shows that parents should hold their babies as much as possible. Touch is one of the first ways that a baby learns he or she is loved. Some psychologists theorize that a loving touch helps set the stage for adult intimacy. Touching and holding infants teach them how parents feel about them. When I am crying, will I be picked up? Can I count on you to show me that you love me? Responding to infants' needs teaches them that the world is a predictable, safe place. It boosts their self-confidence and their ability to believe that when they need help and support, they will get it. When parents and caregivers convey love and delight when they hold their infants, the infants learn they are loved.

Bonding, based on this love, begins at birth when mother and newborn are brought together. It continues during feeding, diapering, smiling, talking, and acknowledging the infant. As active and comfortable participants in parenting, both parents bond with the infant through touch. This fosters trust that all needs will be fulfilled and the infant is **thriving**. Developing a sense of trust in the world is an important foundation for adult mental health, including sexual health. The developmental psychologist Erik H. Erikson wrote that the first psychosocial crisis in life is to resolve "basic trust versus basic mistrust." According to Erikson, between birth and 18 months of age, children learn whether their needs will be met and whether they can trust the people and the world around them. If their needs are met, they develop the ability for intimacy and a sense of hope. Erikson wrote that feeding is the primary way that an infant resolves these issues (Erikson, 1950).

In the early 1960s, two researchers did an important experiment with rhesus monkeys. They separated some monkeys from their mothers at birth and offered them surrogate wire mothers to hold. Some of the surrogates were only wire frames; others were covered with soft fabric. The monkeys would cling to a dummy covered with soft fabric but rejected one made up just of wire, even when it had a bottle of

milk attached. In other words, the baby monkeys preferred a soft touch to being fed. The baby monkeys denied touch grew up to be troubled adult monkeys. They were more likely to bite and scratch; the males did not approach females sexually; and the females were mostly infertile (Bullough & Bullough, 1994). Some psychologists believe that such studies show that a lack of touch in infancy can affect future adult sexual and intimate relationships.

Teaching Body Parts

Bath time and diaper changes are wonderful times to start teaching a child about body parts—*all* the parts of his or her body. Many parents play this game to teach body parts with their 5- or 6-month-old children: "Here is your nose, here's your tummy, here are your knees, here are your toes." In addition to teaching the names of these body parts, these parents may be inadvertently conveying an early message about their willingness to address sexual issues. These parents may be communicating to their child that many (one-third) of the body's parts have no names and that they are different from all the other parts of the body. How much more sex-positive it would be if parents could learn to say, calmly and without flinching, "Here's your nose, here's your tummy, here's your penis (or vulva), here are your knees, here are your toes." Thus all the parts of the body that the baby is exploring have names, and parents can speak about all of them.

Parents should treat all body parts equally. When parents use euphemisms only for the genitals, they give their child a message that these parts of the body are shameful or different. They may, without meaning to or realizing it, even introduce a sense of guilt about certain parts of the body. These feelings sometimes persist into adulthood, making it difficult for grown men and women to be comfortable with their bodies and sexual feelings. They may also affect a child's ability to tell about sexually abusive incidents accurately.

Infant Genital Touching

Babies begin to explore their genitals during diaper changes. This usually happens at about 7 to 10 months, a little after they discover that they have fingers and toes. And they experience for themselves that it feels good to touch all the parts of their bodies.

Many parents are uncomfortable when they see their babies touch their genitals. They wonder what, if anything, they should do. They wonder whether their child is masturbating or is becoming obsessed with this behavior. This type of genital exploration is not the same as masturbation; it is generally not purposeful and not directed at orgasm. It is about exploring and learning more about the body.

psychosexual development The blending of sexual aspects of one's development with other psychological factors.

bonding A process of developing a close physical and psychological relationship with one's caregiver.

thriving Normal physical and psychological pattern of weight gain, neuromuscular development, and other developmental attributes of infants.

Communication
DIMENSIONS

Resources for Becoming Askable

Here are some guidelines for becoming askable—10 healthy hints—as well as examples of questions and answers.

1. Start early, using body language and nonverbal behaviors to convey messages of approachability.
2. Giving "too much" information should not be a concern. Observe reactions to gauge how much is needed.
3. Communicate openly, even acknowledging discomfort.
4. Admit ignorance and offer to find out—together if possible.
5. Concise, simple answers are better than long lectures.
6. Too much technical information won't hurt; it allows children to sort it out and honors their ability to understand.
7. Mistakes will happen; admit them, correct them if possible, and handle them as you would other mistakes.
8. Share your values about sexual matters; children want to know what you believe.
9. Encourage laughing and learning by using a sense of humor.
10. Use books as a springboard for discussion; they are lasting and can be referred to over and over.

Having resources at hand is helpful when talking to children about sexuality issues in the home. See the suggested reading list at the end of the chapter to begin a resource library at home.

Sexuality education often begins with a child's curiosity about his or her body. Let the child set the pace with his or her questions.

If your child points to a body part, simply tell him or her what it is. This is also a good time to talk about which parts of the body are private.

Expect self-stimulation. Teach your child that masturbation is a normal—but private—activity. If it happens in public, try distraction. If that fails, take your child aside for a reminder about the importance of privacy.

Curiosity about others—examining another child's sex organs—is usually normal exploration and far removed from adult sexual activity. It's harmless when only young children are involved, but as a family matter, you may want to set limits on such exploration.

Take advantage of everyday opportunities. Consider these examples:

- **How do babies get inside mommy?** You might say, "A mom and a dad make a baby by holding each other in a special way."
- **How are babies born?** It might be enough to say, "Doctors and nurses help babies who are ready to be born." If your child wants more details, you might say, "Usually a mom pushes the baby out of her vagina."
- **Why doesn't everyone have a penis?** Try a simple explanation such as, "Boys' and girls' bodies are made differently."
- **Why do you have hair down there?** Simplicity often works here, too. You might say, "Our bodies change as we get older." If your child wants more details, add, "Boys grow hair near their penises, and girls grow hair near their vaginas."

Answer specific questions using correct terminology. Even if you're uncomfortable, forge ahead. Remember—you're setting the stage for open, honest discussions in the years to come.

Source: Reproduced from Mayo Clinic Sexual Health (2014). Retrieved Jan 8, 2015, from www.mayoclinic.com/health/sex-education/HQ00547.

Self-exploration lays the foundation for development of a broad range of sexual feelings and behaviors. Parental reaction also impacts development. Consider the effect of punishment—yelling, pushing the hand away, and admonishing the behavior as dirty. Conveying a strong negative message about behavior that is pleasurable creates confusion—ultimately leading to feelings of shame and fear about sexuality.

Some responses that encourage healthy sexual development include viewing exploratory behavior as normal learning, socializing for privacy rather than forbidding, using natural opportunities to provide basic information, and becoming more "askable."

Gender During the Early Years

Many experts believe that there are some innate differences between boy babies and girl babies. In general, boy babies seem to be more active than girl babies. Girl babies may develop faster. This is often shown by girls sitting up, reaching for objects, and talking earlier than boys. However, there can be a

The affection displayed by parents sets an example for their children. Parents who are violent or abusive to each other around a child also set an example for the child to follow.

wide variation of timing in both boys and girls, so we cannot say that all boy babies or all girl babies follow exact timing.

The expectations of parents for their babies can also influence gender development. For example, today many people going through a pregnancy know the sex of their baby well before the baby is born. Some experts believe that these parents start talking differently to their unborn babies and act differently towards them once they know the sex of the baby. This same behavior often occurs after the baby is born. Many parents speak differently to boy infants and girl infants. They may touch and hold them differently as well. They may even react differently to the needs of the baby depending upon its sex.

During the first 18 months of life, children are beginning to learn the differences between males and females (that is, **gender identity**). As they approach 3 years old, most boys and girls can identify dolls and photographs as male or female. They can also tell an adult whether they are a girl or a boy.

In their early years, children encounter many **gender stereotypes**. They identify certain behaviors as male or female. They might think male things and female things are supposed to be different colors. Children learn from the world around them. In their homes they might see (or be told) that males do certain things and females do other things. They might learn that opportunities and behaviors are

supposed to be very different for males and females. Children are also influenced by what they see in the media related to gender stereotypes. Perhaps most important, what adults say and do around children can have a big impact on what these children believe about gender and the amount of gender stereotypes they believe in their own lives.

■ Sexual Development During Preschool and Early Elementary Years

During the years from age 3 years to age 5 years, children begin to develop a strong sense of gender and what that means to them and the people around them. They are finishing with toilet training, and if they are in school or a day care center, they have probably observed other children and learned for themselves that boys and girls have different body parts. At this time the child realizes that he or she will not usually change over the life span. This concept is known as **gender constancy**. Children of this age are very curious about their own and other people's bodies. This is the age when a child is first likely to ask, "Where did I come from?"

Preschool Genital Touching

Three- and 4-year-olds delight in their own bodies. And just as they learn it feels good when they run, jump, and cuddle, they are also discovering that it feels good when they touch their own genitals. Most professionals believe that preschool children touch their genitals as a natural part of child development. In a study of mothers of 2- to 5-year-olds, mothers reported that 25% of their sons and 15% of their daughters touched their genitals in public. Sixteen percent of both preschool boys and girls had been observed masturbating with their hands (Delamater & Friedrich, 2002).

Toddlers and preschoolers touch their genitals in a much less purposeful way than older children and adolescents, and many do so without embarrassment or anxiety. In fact, it is not unusual in a preschool to have several of the boys touching their penis unconsciously throughout the day. Little girls find it pleasurable to touch their vulva and clitoris as well.

Many children appear not even to be aware that they are touching their genitals in this way. Some children do discover that this activity helps them calm down. Many children touch their genitals right before naps or bedtimes to help them fall asleep. (Just as for adults, some children never touch their genitals at all. It is normal for a preschooler to touch the genitals and it is normal for him or her not to.)

gender identity Having an internal sense of self as male or female; part of one's self-image.

gender stereotypes Beliefs about how each sex should behave, which may be overgeneralized or rigidly held.

gender constancy Recognition by a child that he or she will remain the same sex throughout life.

Not only do parents treat boys and girls differently, but children themselves learn sex differences in voices, levels of aggression, and even the colors of toys.

Attraction to Parents

Sigmund Freud felt that 3- to 5-year-old boys develop fantasies of possessing their mother sexually and become jealous of their father. He named it the **Oedipus complex** after the Greek tragedy in which Oedipus unknowingly kills his father and then marries his mother. According to Freud's theory, this period is accompanied by castration anxiety; boys fear that their father will retaliate against their interest in their mother by cutting off their penis. Freud also theorized that girls develop an **Electra complex**; they develop "penis envy" and want to take their father away from their mother. Girls, he said, reject their mother because they blame her for their lack of a penis. Freud named this "complex" the Electra complex after the Greek tragedy in which a princess helps kill her mother.

Most modern psychologists debunk these ideas. Feminist psychologists critique Freud's views as extremely sexist, and anthropologists point out that these "complexes" are not found in all cultures. Still, it is not uncommon for preschool children to prefer the parent of the other sex at this time.

Preschool children love their parents intensely and may be confused about whether all love is expressed romantically. Many children try to kiss their parents romantically. Some even try to imitate adults they have seen in person, on TV, on the Internet, or in the movies by putting their tongue into their parents' mouths. Preschool children sometimes may even seem jealous when their parents show affection to each other.

Preschoolers and Sex Play

Many adults remember playing "doctor" or "house" with other children. Playing doctor, including undressing each other and examining each other's genitals, is quite common. Most child development experts see this type of sex play as expected and natural childhood sexual curiosity. If the children are of the same age and stage of development, experts do not believe that it is harmful. And studies of adults show that engaging in childhood sexual play does not seem to have any effect, either positive or negative, on adult sexuality.

Besides concern about childhood sex play among peers, exposure to nudity or parental sexual intercourse has been studied. The researchers concluded

---

Oedipus complex   Libidinal feelings of a child toward the parent of the other sex and hostile or jealous feelings toward the parent of the same sex.

Electra complex   Freud's theory that 3- to 5-year-old girls want to take their father away from their mother.

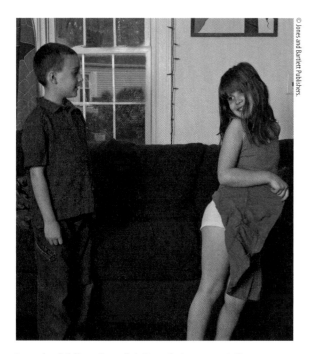

In early childhood, availability of playmates influences interaction. Games that provide opportunities for sex play and exploration such as "doctor" or "nurse" are responses to natural curiosity. According to Erickson's developmental stages (Erikson, 1950), these children need to accomplish autonomy and initiative rather than shame, doubt, or guilt.

that such exposure is not detrimental to the mental health of children. Characterizing exposure as harmful or even a subtle form of abuse might better be conceptualized as myth. Another concern, that of erections among young boys as evidence of romantic interest, is also a myth. Erections come and go, rise and fall, among babies and young boys, even sleeping and waking adults, with odd timing. One study examined the impact of noncoercive sexual contact with similarly aged individuals. Researchers found that adult adjustment problems were no different from those who had no sexual contact experience. Among those who had been abused, problems escalated

according to the amount of coercion reported (Friedrich, Whiteside, & Talley, 2004).

That said, there is a big difference between normally harmless child sexual play and play that is exploitative or abusive. Children do not normally engage in painful sexual behavior, oral–genital contact, or simulated or real intercourse or penetration with fingers or objects with another child, and they do not engage in normal sexual play with children more than a few years older than they are. These behaviors may indicate a child who *may* have been sexually abused. (They could also indicate exposure to inappropriate TV, Internet, or videos.) Table 13.1 provides some guidelines on distinguishing between harmless play and exploitative, inappropriate behaviors.

Questions About Reproduction

Some time between the ages of 2½ and 5 years, children ask, "Where did I come from?" Children at this age are often very curious about pregnancy and birth. According to psychologists, at around the age of 4 years, children understand that babies do not just spontaneously appear and that something must have happened for this process to begin.

The emphasis really is on the *where*: They want to know *where* the baby comes from and *where* it was before it was born. Preschoolers can be offered a very simple answer: "You grew in a special place inside Mom called a uterus. You began from a tiny egg (the size of a pencil dot) from Mom and an even tinier sperm from Dad." This will satisfy most preschoolers. If they ask, "But how did I get into the uterus?" they can be given a very simple definition of sexual intercourse:

> When two grown-ups love each other, they like to kiss and hug and touch each other in ways that feel good. Sometimes, the man and woman place the man's penis into the woman's vagina. The man's penis releases sperm into the woman and sometimes a baby begins.

TABLE 13.1

A Quick Way to Assess Whether Childhood Sex Play Is Likely to Be Harmless or Whether Parents Should Be Concerned

	Expected	Problematic
Age of children	Similar	More than 3 years apart
Children seem	Giggly, curious, happy	Aggressive, angry, fearful, withdrawn
Activities	Undressing, playing doctor ("You show me yours I'll show you mine")	Oral, anal, or vaginal intercourse; penetration with fingers, objects
After parental Intervention	Behavior stops	Behavior continues

Elementary School Years

The early elementary school years (kindergarten to grade 3) are years of tremendous growth and change. Naps and playtime give way to homework and tests. Preschool teacher hugs may be replaced by neutral hellos. The class of 12 now has 20 children, and individual attention is no longer the rule. Children begin to learn about sexuality issues from other children on the bus or the playground.

Freud wrote that the period from 5 to 11 years of age was the **latency period**. Although some blame Freud for mistakenly characterizing this as a period of sexual *dis*interest, Bullough describes it differently. He credits Freud with breaking the taboo on full discussions of sexuality, recognizing it as a prime factor in human development. Rather than *dis*interest, Freud expected active sexual exploration and information seeking, the prepubescent hormone surge and accompanying growth of internal and external sexual organs (Bullough, 2004).

Five- to 8-year-olds continue to be very interested in sexual issues; it is just that their interest is no longer as apparent to the adults in their lives as it used to be. They continue to develop as sexual persons, and they are very curious about pregnancy and birth. They develop strong friendships, and most boys and girls show a strong preference for playing with children of the same sex. They become even more aware of socially defined sex roles. They may continue to engage in sex play with children of both sexes. And in private, their exploration of their genitals may become more purposeful.

Developing Empathy

Some sexologists believe that the period from age 5 years to age 8 years is critical in sexual development. They believe that the elementary school years are the most important time for people to develop as moral thinkers, and that development is important to adult sexual health. While they are preschoolers, children believe that their way of thinking is the only way possible. But in early elementary school, children begin to understand that there may be other points of view and ways to consider a situation. They can begin to understand the "golden rule": Treat others with the same respect you would want for yourself.

Developing an ability to empathize and make good decisions is part of the foundation for adult sexual health. A sexually healthy adult is able, for example, to make decisions about his or her sexuality that are consistent with his or her own values.

The Media as Sexuality Educator of Children

The media—television, movies, the Internet, magazines, even the news—are among many children's most prominent sexuality educators. On average, children ages 2 to 5 years spend 32 hours a week in front of a TV—watching television, DVDs, and DVR, and using a game console. Children ages 6 to 11 years spend about 28 hours a week in front of the TV. TV can be entertaining and help children learn about different cultures and gain exposure to ideas they may never encounter in their own community. However, children can also learn things from TV that may affect their health, behavior, and family life in negative ways. For example, children may learn to accept the stereotypes presented on TV. Research indicates that what children see on TV does affect how they see male and female roles in society. In addition, children can get lots of information about sexuality from TV. Sexual content is a real presence on TV. The number of sex scenes on TV has nearly doubled since 1998. Some researchers are concerned that watching sexual content on TV will influence children to make poor decisions about their own sexual activity (Television and children, 2011).

In addition to television, movies, music videos, video games, print, and the Internet are pervasive forms of media in today's world. According to the *Surgeon General's Call to Action to Promote Sexual Health and Responsible Sexual Behavior* (Satcher, 2001), sexual talk and behavior are increasingly explicit and frequent. Much of the content in videos and films portrays sexual eroticism, and more than half of television programming has sexual content. Thus the media do have potential for providing sexuality

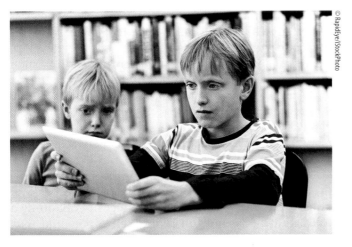

© RapidEye/iStockPhoto

Children are naturally curious about sexuality.

latency period Outdated Freudian theory that children aged 6–12 years old have no sexual feelings or interest.

Young people can learn about people and their roles in many ways. Even TV programs where animals are used to portray human characteristics can be helpful.

information and education. In a national survey, more than half the students said they learned about topics such as birth control, contraception, and preventing pregnancy from television and magazines. Yet the impact of media on actual behavior is controversial and research is indecisive (Weinstein & Rosen, 2006).

Focusing on media literacy rather than potential harm may be a way of enhancing the benefits of media as a source of useful information. More and more schools are embracing the notion that learning how information is assembled and edited will help students read, hear, and view media more critically (Goldstein, 2005). An analytical perspective can help young people entering puberty as they view media norms that present a narrow cultural definition of

physical perfection. The goal is to foster an internal **locus of control** in which one's sense of identity is personally defined and not dependent on the scripts of others. An example of such an educational approach for girls in grades 4–8 is called *Full of Ourselves: A Wellness Program to Advance Girl Power, Health, and Leadership* (Steiner-Adair & Sjostrom, 2006). It is a primary prevention program aimed at helping girls decrease their vulnerability to body preoccupation and eating disorders. One of the units focuses on media literacy, particularly advertising strategies. Both parents and schools are encouraged to create a supportive environment for students entering puberty.

Sexual Development During Puberty

Puberty, teenager, and *adolescence* are not interchangeable words. *Puberty* is the stage of maturation when a human being becomes capable of sexual reproduction. *Teenager* is defined chronologically: A teenager is a young person between the ages of 13 and 19 years. *Adolescence* is actually a relatively new concept: It is the period of development that extends from puberty (or the end of childhood) through the attainment of full adult status. Before 1900, and still today in many developing societies, children marry shortly after puberty and begin their adult responsibilities. Today, as more American young people stretch their college and graduate school education through their 20s and even 30s—and then return to live in their parents' homes—some have wondered when contemporary U.S. adolescence ends: At 30 years? When you buy your own home? Have your own children? Before your midlife crisis?

Preparing for Puberty

Young people, at some time between the ages of 8 and 16 years, go through a predictable process of biological development called *puberty*. Normal pubertal changes, indicated by the development of **secondary sexual characteristics** such as breast buds and pubic hair, may begin as early as age 8 years for girls and as early as age 9 years for boys, but some teens may not begin these changes until they are 15 or 16 years old. The median age for puberty to begin for boys is between 11 and 12 years; for girls, it is between 10 and 11 years. Still, *average* means that half of young people begin this process earlier, and half begin it later. The process of puberty from the first physical changes to obtaining a fully adult body and full reproductive potential may last 4 or 5 years. On average, boys begin and end puberty about 1 year to 2 years later than girls do.

locus of control Refers to an individual's perception of the main causes of events in life. More simply, is life's destiny controlled by the self (*internal locus*) or by external forces such as fate or other people (*external locus*)?

secondary sexual characteristics Changes occurring during adolescence—such as growth of pubic hair, breast development, and testes and penile development.

Many young women in college human sexuality classes say they were not prepared adequately for pubertal changes. Some received little or no education in school. Many who did have some education report that it was poorly done and contained little helpful information. Fortunately, there are some who report good educational programs related to puberty, but they seem to be in a relatively small minority. Other college women report that they received only scant information from their mother or father or older siblings or friends.

Puberty for Girls

The first noticeable sign of puberty in girls is generally the development of **breast buds**; the breast begins to elevate as a small mound. Later, the breast and the nipple get bigger. Light, sparse pubic and underarm hair begins to appear about 6 months later. Girls begin to experience a growth spurt, often growing as much as several inches in a year. Their genital and underarm areas begin to produce sweat glands, and body odor may result. Most girls begin menstrual periods about 2 years after breast budding begins, but some girls have completed breast development before their first period, and some girls' breasts continue to develop for many years after.

Girls today are experiencing first menstruation at earlier ages than girls growing up three or four decades ago. The average age for first menstruation, **menarche** (pronounced "men-ar-key"), in the United States is now 12½ years. That means that many girls have their first period before the end of seventh grade, and many begin as early as fourth or fifth grade. It also means that many girls will at least be in the eighth grade before their first period, and some may be seniors in high school before they get a period. All of these situations are normal.

Many pediatricians use a measurement called a **Tanner scale** to rate physical sexual development in both boys and girls (see Table 13.2).

Puberty for Boys

Puberty in boys begins on average during the sixth or seventh grade, but in some boys it begins at 9 years, and in others puberty does not begin until they are almost 14 years old. Boys experience many of the same changes as girls do. The first physical sign is usually an increase in the size of the testes; unlike breast budding in girls, this is unlikely to be observed by parents. During puberty, they too develop light, sparse pubic and underarm hair, and their sweat glands become activated. Between the ages of 12 and 14 years, their penis and scrotum begin to enlarge. At first, the testes become larger, and the skin on

TABLE 13.2

Tanner Scale for Girls

Tanner Stage	Pubic Hair	Breasts
1	None	None
2	Sparse	Small breast buds
3	Darker, begins to curl	Breasts and nipples enlarged
4	Coarse, less curly than adult	Continued breast development
5	Adult triangle	Mature; nipple projects

Source: Data from Marshall, W. A., & Tanner, J. M. (June 1969). Variations in pattern of pubertal changes in girls. *Archives of Disease in Childhood, 44*, no. 235, 291–303.

the scrotum reddens and coarsens. As boys mature, their penis starts to grow longer. Pubic hair slowly becomes darker, and it starts to curl. During puberty, the penis doubles in size.

By Tanner stage 3 (see Table 13.3), ejaculation has usually occurred, and there may be some production of sperm. In fact, some sexologists call this **semenarche**, to correspond to the first period of girls (menarche). Most often, a boy experiences this as nocturnal emissions, or wet dreams. By Tanner stage 4, males are fertile and able to cause a pregnancy. The average length of time for a boy to go through puberty is 3 years, but it can vary from 2 to 5 years.

Significant numbers of boys are troubled by a condition called **gynecomastia**. During puberty, they begin to develop an increase in the glandular tissue around their breasts; in fact, these boys sometimes are very worried and fearful that they are growing breasts or turning into a girl. Nearly one in five 10-year-olds will have this kind of tissue development. In rare cases, gynecomastia may be the result of diseases that are rare in young people: liver disease, **hypogonadism**, **hyperthyroidism**, or

breast budding First stage of breast development in females, whereby breast tissue elevates as a small mound.

menarche First menstruation for girls.

Tanner scale Scale developed by Dr. John Tanner for measuring pubertal development in boys and girls.

semenarche First ejaculation of semen for boys.

gynecomastia Glandular tissue development in the breasts of males.

hypogonadism Decreased activity of the gonads that may result in retardation of growth and sexual development.

hyperthyroidism Excessive functional activity of the thyroid gland.

TABLE 13.3

Tanner Scale for Boys

Tanner Stage	Pubic Hair	Penis/Scrotum
1	None	Childlike
2	Sparse	Scrotum: reddened, thinner, larger Penis childlike
3	Darker, begins to curl	Penis length increases Scrotum continues to enlarge and darken
4	Coarse, less curly than adult	Penis increases in length and circumference
5	Adult	Adult

Source: Data from Marshall, W. A., & Tanner, J. M. (February 1970). Variations in the pattern of pubertal changes in boys. *Archives of Disease in Childhood, 45,* no. 239, 13–23.

hypothyroidism. It could also be a sign of drug use. However, most of the time it is just a variation of male pubertal development, and it usually resolves itself within 1 year to 1½ years. It continues longer than 2 years in fewer than 1 in 10 boys.

Early and Late Developers

Although the majority of young people finish puberty a few years after the start of their teen years, some begin puberty much earlier and some go through it much later. Both early and late developers face special challenges.

Early-developing girls have special problems. Because they look more mature, adults often expect them to act more mature. A third- or fourth-grade girl with developing breasts may feel awkward and want to hide her body. She may be relentlessly teased by her male and female classmates. She may indeed feel that she is not normal. Conversely, late development in boys may be more of a problem than early development. A 15- or 16-year-old boy who is still short, has no facial hair, and has a high voice may be relentlessly teased.

Some children begin puberty much earlier than age 9 or 10 years. Some children even enter what is

called **precocious puberty** in the first year of life. Interestingly, this seems to be largely the result of genetic coding in girls, and most often there is no underlying disease. Conversely, precocious puberty in boys is much more likely to be an indication that something is wrong. If parents observe pubertal changes in a boy younger than 7 years old, they should see a health practitioner for a medical evaluation and possible interventions.

What Is Normal?

Early, late, and average developers *all* share a common concern: *Am I normal?* Rapid body changes can be very confusing. Nine- to 12-year-olds can become obsessed with their appearance. In fact, psychologists say preteens have an **imaginary audience**: They think that everyone is looking at them. Getting dressed and preparing their hair and faces can take hours. They need adult reassurance that they are attractive, and they need to understand that it is not true that everyone is looking at them.

They are concerned about their height and breast size or penis size, and they wonder whether they are too developed or too underdeveloped. They wonder whether their feelings, which sometimes fluctuate immensely, are normal. It is important to reassure preadolescents that they are developing according to their own personal genetically predetermined clock. When they ask questions like "How come I don't have my period yet?" or "Why am I the shortest boy in the class?" the question behind the question is almost always "Am I normal?"

The reality is that during preadolescence and the years following it, conflicts with parents peak. Yet, it is important to know that only about one in six teenagers and parents experience a severe disruption in their parent–child relationship (Grunbaum et al., 2004). Preadolescents are just beginning to separate from their parents, but they are also still looking to their parents for guidance and support.

Children learn about many aspects of sexuality and relationships from their parents—much of it by astute observation rather than through discussion. Yet, the value of parental involvement and maintaining open lines of communication is well documented as a deterrent to a variety of risky behaviors. Parents can enhance their children's sense of self-worth with assurances of affection and acceptance in spite of the many changes adolescence brings.

Emotional Changes in Preadolescence

The rapid physical changes of puberty we have described initiate many psychosocial changes. Preadolescents are beginning to move toward independence and are often very self-conscious of their

hypothyroidism A deficiency of thyroid activity.

precocious puberty Pubertal development before the age of 7 years.

imaginary audience Belief in early adolescence that other people are looking at you as if you are onstage.

Development of body hair in both boys and girls and facial hair in boys results in shaving, viewed by some as a rite of passage indicating sexual maturity.

bodies. They may even be embarrassed by parents. Children at this age also need to test parental authority and sometimes the authority of teachers and other adult figures in their lives. This may include trying out values that are different from their parents'. The research literature demonstrates that most teenagers go through a period of seeming to reject their parents' values; yet, by the time they reach adulthood, almost all of them adopt values similar to their parents'.

Friends become very important during the preadolescent years. Being popular is of utmost importance. The good news is that needing to be just like friends, known by psychologists as **conformity with peers**, peaks in early adolescence and then starts to decline. The bad news for parents is that peer pressure can be intense during this period and usually dictates the type of clothes that are acceptable. It also can lead to experimentation with cigarettes, alcohol, and sexual activity.

Cliques often emerge during this period. Preadolescents may for the first time feel pressure to engage in certain activities to be part of a group, and, for some young people, that means experimenting with smoking, shoplifting, or cheating on tests.

Preadolescents are also beginning to develop a sense of identity. Their ability to think abstractly has just begun. They frequently daydream and turn inward and imagine acting out different roles. Daydreaming

is normal and actually quite healthy. Giving a child a diary or journal and then respecting his or her right to keep it private can be an effective way to encourage a new adolescent to think about and explore his or her feelings. Children at this age can seem very dramatic. They often feel that they are continuously onstage. They may become convinced that their problems are unique and no one understands them.

Masturbation

During puberty, many boys and girls begin to masturbate for sexual pleasure. In addition to providing relief from sexual tension, masturbation has several physical and mental health benefits (Yudt, 2004). These include relief from migraine headaches and menstrual cramps, and self-knowledge about sexual functioning that can be shared with a partner. In spite of these positive aspects, along with its relative safety—no chance of pregnancy or infection—masturbation creates anxiety. Again, questions arise about what is normal because masturbation is one of the most widely practiced forms of sexual behavior but the least discussed. Data indicate that a majority of boys begin masturbating between the ages of 13 and 15, whereas the onset among girls is more gradual (Bancroft, Herbenick, & Reynolds, 2003). Frequency is also a concern, but is highly individual. Some adults masturbate every day; some, once a year. Some people never masturbate. In fact, teenagers

conformity with peers   Desire to be like everyone else.

need to know that although many preteens, teens, and adults masturbate, some never do.

Sexuality in Adolescence

There is public and professional consensus about what is sexually unhealthy for teenagers. Professionals, politicians, and parents across the political spectrum share a deep concern about unplanned adolescent pregnancy; out-of-wedlock childbearing; STIs, including AIDS; sexual abuse; date rape; and the potential negative emotional consequences of premature sexual behaviors.

However, there is little public, professional, or political consensus about what is sexually healthy for teenagers. The public debate about adolescent sexuality has often focused on which sexual behaviors are appropriate for adolescents and ignored the complex dimensions of sexuality.

Some groups support the "Just say no" approach to adolescent sexuality. They believe that the only healthy adolescent sexuality is abstinence from all sexual behaviors until marriage and that adults should work to eliminate teen sexual experimentation. Another approach could be described as "Just say not now." This philosophy encourages young people to abstain until they are more mature but, given the high rates of teenage sexual involvement in intercourse, recommends that it is important to provide young people with access to contraception and condoms regardless of whether adults approve of their behavior. This approach might also be labeled "If you can't say no, protect yourself!" Other adults adopt a "Don't ask; don't tell" posture and simply pretend that adolescent sexuality and sexual behavior do not exist (Grunbaum et al., 2004).

Sexuality Education

It is important for parents and educators to approach sexuality education in a positive way and handle topics as positively as possible. Sources of sexual information can exert strong influence on adolescents' sexual behavior. Rosengard et al., (2012) reported that many 15- to 18-year-olds identified the family as sexual health information sources. Their primary messages recalled were risks of sexual behavior, protection, and relationship advice. Many portrayed their learning experiences as negative, cautionary, lacking detail, and not always balanced with positive messages. The authors concluded that sexual health messages should be tailored to adolescents' needs for practical and sex-positive guidance regarding mechanics of sex and formation of healthy relationships, and balanced with cautions regarding negative consequences.

Myth vs Fact

Myth: People become sexual at puberty.
Fact: People are sexual from birth to death. Although people sexually mature at puberty and become capable of reproduction, infants and children experience sensual feelings and identify themselves as boys and girls.

Myth: Dressing boys in blue and girls in pink teaches them about their gender.
Fact: By the time they are 3 years old, almost all boys and girls identify themselves by gender. They know that they will have that gender throughout their lifetime (the concept known as gender constancy). Clothes' colors do not make a difference.

Myth: Children in elementary school go through a latency period about sexual issues.
Fact: Elementary school children remain very interested in sexuality-related issues, and many continue to be involved in sex play with friends or genital self-pleasuring. They have just learned to hide this behavior from adults.

Myth: The average age of first intercourse has plummeted in the past 5 years.
Fact: The biggest change in adolescent sexual behavior occurred in the 1970s. The average age of first intercourse has decreased by 1 year since 1971.

Myth: Most teenagers have had sexual intercourse.
Fact: Only about half of teenagers aged 15–19 years have had sexual intercourse.

Myth: Masturbating more than once a week is harmful.
Fact: There is no "standard" for frequency of masturbation. Once is too often if you do not like it. Frequency is highly individual, and it is not harmful as long as it does not interfere with school, work, or relationships.

The Sexuality Information and Education Council of the United States (SIECUS) publishes the *Guidelines for Comprehensive Sexuality Education: Kindergarten–12th Grade*, third edition, compiled by the National Guidelines Task Force. The following sections are adapted with permission. "The primary goal of sexuality education is to promote adult sexual health. It should assist young people in developing a positive view of sexuality, provide them with information they need to take care of their sexual health, and help them acquire skills to make decisions now and in the future. Life behaviors of a sexually healthy adult are essentially outcomes of instruction. The following lists reflect the actions students will be able to take after having applied the information and skills.

Human Development Life Behaviors:
Having applied the human development subconcepts at the appropriate age, the learner will be able to:

• Appreciate one's own body.

• Seek further information about reproduction as needed.

Many adults become concerned when their adolescent children begin to explore their emerging sexuality. But honest communication between an adult and a child can help him or her develop into a sexually healthy adult.

- Affirm that human development includes sexual development, which may or may not include reproduction or sexual experience.

- Interact with all genders in respectful and appropriate ways.

- Affirm one's own sexual orientation and respect the sexual orientations of others.

- Affirm one's own gender identities and respect the gender identities of others.

Relationship Life Behaviors:
Having applied the relationships subconcepts at the appropriate age, the learner will be able to:

- Express love and intimacy in appropriate ways.
- Develop and maintain meaningful relationships.
- Avoid exploitative or manipulative relationships.
- Make informed choices about family options and relationships.
- Exhibit skills that enhance personal relationships.

Personal Skills Life Behaviors:
Having applied the personal skills subconcepts at the appropriate age, the learner will be able to:

- Identify and live according to one's own values.
- Take responsibility for one's own behavior.
- Practice effective decision making.
- Develop critical-thinking skills.
- Communicate effectively with family, peers, and romantic partners.

Sexual Behavior Life Behaviors:
Having applied the sexual behavior subconcepts at the appropriate age, the learner will be able to:

- Enjoy and express one's sexuality throughout life.
- Express one's sexuality in ways that are congruent with one's values.
- Enjoy sexual feelings without necessarily acting on them.
- Discriminate between life-enhancing sexual behaviors and those that are harmful to self and/or others.
- Express one's sexuality while respecting the rights of others.
- Seek new information to enhance one's sexuality.
- Engage in sexual relationships that are consensual, nonexploitative, honest, pleasurable, and protected.

Sexual Health Life Behaviors:
Having applied the sexual health subconcepts at the appropriate age, the learner will be able to:

- Practice health-promoting behaviors, such as regular check-ups, breast and testicular self-exam, and early identification of potential problems.
- Use contraception effectively to avoid unintended pregnancy.
- Avoid contracting or transmitting an STI, including HIV.
- Act consistently with one's own values when dealing with an unintended pregnancy.
- Seek early prenatal care.
- Help prevent sexual abuse.

Society and Culture Life Behaviors:
Having applied the society and culture subconcepts at the appropriate age, the learner will be able to:

- Demonstrate respect for people with different sexual values.
- Exercise democratic responsibility to influence legislation dealing with sexual issues.
- Assess the impact of family, cultural, media, and societal messages on one's thoughts, feelings, values, and behaviors related to sexuality.
- Critically examine the world around them for biases based on gender, sexual orientation, culture, ethnicity, and race.

Ethical DIMENSIONS

Is It Ethical to Ignore Your Child's Developing Sexuality?

One of us once attended a presentation with a group of Swedish sexuality educators who were talking about the difference in sexual mores between Sweden and the United States. One of the Swedish women told us a story about her first sexual experience. She was 17 years old and very much in love. She and her boyfriend told her parents that they were ready to have sexual intercourse, and they asked to make love in her bedroom at home. The next morning, her parents served them breakfast in bed to celebrate this passage! The American educators were stunned.

Whether parents in America would openly accommodate their teens' first experience of sexual intercourse at home or not, it *is* happening. Almost half (46%) of all high school students reported in 2010 they have had sexual intercourse, and sexual activity increased with grade level, while condom use decreased (Eaton et al., 2010). When asked the location, 68% of 16- to 18-year-olds reported their first sexual intercourse occurred in their family home (22%), their partner's family home (34%), or a friend's house (12%).

The boundaries between parents and their teen children about sexuality are often difficult to negotiate and raise many moral and ethical issues. Is it ethical to ignore a teen's developing sexuality? Is it ethical to withhold information about contraception and condoms? Does talking about condoms and contraception encourage teens to experiment with sexual behaviors? Should parents help a teen obtain contraception, or is a teen who is old enough to be having intercourse old enough to go to a clinic or a drug store unassisted? And if you know your teen child is having intercourse, should you allow him or her to do so in your home? While you are out? Overnight? And what is your responsibility to the other child's parent?

How did your parents handle these issues? How do you think you will handle them when you are a parent? Which issues do you need to think about in answering these questions?

- Promote the rights of all people to accurate sexuality information.

- Avoid behaviors that exhibit prejudice and bigotry.

- Reject stereotypes about the sexuality of different populations.

- Educate others about sexuality.

The following four areas contribute to an educational experience that will encourage achievement of the life behaviors listed above.

Information: Sexuality education seeks to provide accurate information about human sexuality, including growth and development, human reproduction, anatomy, physiology, masturbation, family life, pregnancy, childbirth, parenthood, sexual response, sexual orientation, gender identity, contraception, abortion, sexual abuse, HIV/AIDS, and other STIs.

Attitudes, Values, and Insights: Sexuality education seeks to provide an opportunity for young people to question, explore, and assess their own and their community's attitudes about society, gender, and sexuality. This can help young people understand their family's values, develop their own values, improve critical thinking skills, increase self-esteem and self-efficacy, and develop insights concerning relationships with family members, individuals of all genders, sexual partners, and society at large. Sexuality education can help young people understand their obligations and responsibilities to their families and society.

Relationships and Interpersonal Skills: Sexuality education seeks to help young people develop interpersonal skills, including communication, decision making, assertiveness, and peer refusal skills, as well as the ability to create reciprocal and satisfying relationships. Sexuality education programs should prepare students to understand sexuality effectively and creatively in adult roles. This includes helping young people develop the capacity for caring, supportive, noncoercive, and mutually pleasurable intimate and sexual relationships.

Responsibility: Sexuality education seeks to help young people exercise responsibility regarding sexual relationships by addressing such issues as abstinence, how to resist pressures to become involved in unwanted early sexual intercourse, and the use of contraception and other sexual health measures" (National Guidelines Task Force, 2004).

Linking Research and Programs

While the content and goals of a comprehensive sexuality education program are presented as the

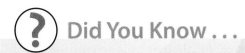

A number of interesting comparisons can be made between comprehensive sexuality education programs and abstinence-only-until-marriage programs. They include:

Comprehensive Sexuality Education Programs	Abstinence-Only-Until-Marriage Programs
Teaches that sexuality is a natural, normal, healthy part of life.	Teaches that sexual activity outside of marriage will have harmful social, psychological, and physical consequences.
Provides values-based education and offers students the opportunity to explore and define their individual values as well as the values of their families and communities.	Teaches one set of values as morally correct for all students.
Includes accurate, factual information about abortion, masturbation, and sexual orientation.	Either omits or contains biased information about topics such as abortion, masturbation, and sexual orientation.
Teaches that consistent use of contraception can greatly reduce a couple's risk of unintended pregnancy.	Discusses contraception only in terms of failure rates; often exaggerates contraceptive failure rates.
Teaches that religious values can play an important role in an individual's decisions about sexual behavior; offers students the opportunity to explore their own and their family's religious values.	Often promotes specific religious beliefs.

Source: Modified from Comparing comprehensive sexuality education with abstinence-only-until-marriage programs. SIECUS Community Action Kit, 2008. Available: http://www.communityactionkit.org/.

ideal, the research literature identifies antecedents of risky sexual behavior and pregnancy that provide implications for program delivery. Five sets of associated factors need to be considered: race and ethnicity; socioeconomic status; social influences; attitudes toward contraception, condoms, and pregnancy; and safer sex behavioral skills. The following is a list of eight programmatic implications designed to reduce high-risk behaviors among adolescents.

- Programs should begin earlier and target younger adolescents.

- New program models for minority teens need to be developed.

- Risk reduction programs need to be systematically linked to other youth programs that directly address socioeconomic disadvantage.

- Professionals need to understand that many youth lack the skills to practice safer sexual activity. A variety of behavioral skills are necessary for condom use; these include communication, negotiation and refusal skills, and technical condom use skills.

- Programs need to effectively address the influence of peer groups, social norms, and pressures to have sexual activity.

- Professionals working with adolescents should not assume that sexual behavior is always freely chosen.

- Professionals should not assume that sexual activity among teens is limited to vaginal sexual activity.

- Professionals cannot assume that teens are unambivalent about preventing pregnancy.

There are also impediments to program success with adolescents. These include learning disabilities and cognitive immaturity, insufficient male involvement, very early sexual activity of males (as yet largely unexplored by research), and single program opportunities due to one-time clinic visits (Kalmus et al., 2003). Another researcher, Dr. Douglas Kirby, has investigated a range of school-based sexuality and HIV education programs over many years to determine program outcomes (Kirby, 2007, 2008). He reported that the evidence that comprehensive programs work has only become stronger over time. The vast majority of these programs have a significant positive impact on behavior. Many program participants either delay or reduce sexual activity or increase condom or other contraceptive use. Kirby reviewed 56 studies that assessed the impact of sexuality education programs. He found that most abstinence programs did not delay initiation of sexual activity and that only three of nine had any significant positive effects on any sexual behavior. In contrast, nearly two-thirds of the comprehensive programs had strong evidence that they positively affect young people's sexual behavior, including both delaying initiation of sexual activity and increasing condom and other contraceptive use. Kirby concluded that abstinence programs have little evidence to warrant their widespread replication; conversely, strong evidence suggests that some comprehensive programs should be disseminated widely.

Risk and Protective Factors
Kirby has contributed to a summary of risk and protective factors affecting teen sexual behavior, pregnancy, childbearing, and STI. More than 400 research studies were analyzed to determine which factors influence adolescents' decisions about sexual behavior and which of these factors can be altered. The likelihood that a teen will have sexual activity, become pregnant or cause a pregnancy, or contract an STI increases as the number of risk factors in a teen's life increases and/or the number of protective factors decreases. These risk and protective factors are as follows: (1) individual biological factors such as age, physical maturity, and gender; (2) disadvantage, disorganization, and dysfunction in the lives of teens, including violence, substance abuse, divorce, and low levels of education; (3) sexual values, attitudes, and modeled behaviors as expressed by teens themselves and by parents, peers, and romantic partners; and (4) connection to adults and organizations that discourage sexual activity, unprotected sex, or early childbearing, such as parents and adults in schools and places of worship (Kirby, Lepore, & Ryan, 2005).

Although more research is certainly warranted, most professionals agree that age-appropriate and targeted sexuality education is one of the best preventive means available for reducing risks and enhancing sexual health. Parents can guide, schools can inform, and other community support can be provided so that adolescents will have the knowledge and self-confidence to make informed decisions regarding their own sexual outcomes.

The Three Stages of Adolescence

Developmental psychologists and health professionals have categorized adolescence into three developmental stages: early adolescence, middle adolescence, and late adolescence. These stages are key to understanding adolescents' behavioral decisions and adolescent sexuality. Table 13.4 summarizes these stages.

While reading this section, it is important to remember that there is no such thing as an "average adolescent." Individual adolescents vary widely in

---

TABLE 13.4

Highlights of Adolescent Developmental Stages

Early Adolescence
Females ages 9–13; males ages 11–15
- Puberty as hallmark
- Adjusting to pubertal changes such as secondary sexual characteristics
- Concern with body image
- Beginning of separation from family, increased parent–child conflict
- Presence of social group cliques
- Identification in reputation-based groups
- Concentration on relationships with peers
- Concrete thinking but beginning of exploration of new ability to think abstractly

Middle Adolescence
Females ages 13–16; males ages 14–17
- Increased independence from family
- Increased importance of peer group
- Experimentation with relationships and sexual behaviors
- Increased abstract thinking ability

Late Adolescence
Females ages 16 and older; males ages 17 and older
- Autonomy nearly secured
- Body image and gender-role definition nearly secured
- Empathetic relationships
- Attainment of abstract thinking
- Defining of adult roles
- Transition to adult roles
- Greater intimacy skills
- Sexual orientation nearly secured

Source: Reprinted with permission from Haffner, D. *Facing facts: Sexual health for America's adolescents.* New York: SIECUS, 1995.

---

the pace of their development. Adolescent sexuality emerges from cultural identities mediated by ethnicity, gender, sexual orientation, class, and physical and emotional capacity. Adolescent development is affected by parents, other family members, and other adults, as well as schools and the peer group.

Early Adolescence
The **early adolescent** (females aged 9–13 years, males aged 11–15 years) experiences body changes more

---

early adolescence First stage of adolescence, defined by pubertal changes—usually ages 9–13 years for females and ages 11–15 years for males.

rapidly than at any time since infancy—secondary sexual characteristics begin to appear; growth accelerates; and physical changes require psychological and social adjustments of the adolescent, family, and other adults. These young people are often concrete thinkers and therefore have difficulty projecting themselves into the future. This phenomenon creates problems when young people are asked to modify their behaviors and delay gratification to achieve a distant future goal. The young adolescent is beginning to separate from the family but usually values parental guidance on important issues. Peer norms, especially identification with a particular group or set of groups, assume increasing importance.

Experimenting with some sexual behaviors is common, but sexual intercourse of any kind is usually limited. Males may initiate intercourse during this stage but most often delay regular sexual activity until middle or late adolescence. Adolescent girls are much less likely to begin having sexual intercourse at this age. Of those who do, many are in relationships with much older males.

Young adolescents seek to develop a sense of identity, connection, power, and joy. For many adolescents in communities that do not support the development of personal identity in other ways, drugs and sexual experimentation may provide a way to achieve it. Early sexual involvement is one way that disadvantaged youth may meet developmental needs for power, identity, connection, and pleasure. Involvement in sexual behaviors may not be motivated by sexual pleasure but rather may reflect peer norms, boredom, conflicts with adults, low self-esteem, and poor ability to control impulsivity.

Middle Adolescence
Middle adolescence (females aged 13–16 years, males aged 14–17 years) is the stage that most typifies the stereotype of "teenager." The transitions in this stage are so dramatic that they seem to occur overnight. The secondary sexual characteristics become fully established, and, for girls, the growth rate decelerates. Abstract thought patterns begin to develop in significant proportions of middle adolescents.

Middle adolescents are sometimes described as feeling omniscient, omnipotent, and invincible. These feelings provide young people with the support to develop increased autonomy but may also put them at risk. In a study of ninth graders, their early sexual decision-making processes highlighted active consideration of health and social risks and benefits, as well as generating options, setting boundaries and limits, and evaluating sexual experiences (Michels et al., 2005).

As adolescents continue the process of separation from the family, they cling more tightly to the peer group that they defined for themselves in early adolescence. The peer group begins to define the rules of behavior. Parents generally place more value on long-term issues such as the importance of education and career preparation than peers do. The desire to be accepted by the peer group often influences experimentation with drugs or sex. By its acceptance or rejection, the peer group influences the adolescent's self-image.

Middle adolescents often focus on themselves and assume others will, too. Many middle adolescents choose to show off their new bodies with revealing clothes. Although adults may define these styles as sexually provocative, that may not be the intent of the middle adolescent.

Middle adolescents often fall in love for the first time. Again, because they are self-centered, their love object may serve as a mirror and reflect characteristics that they admire; that is, they may not love an individual for himself or herself. Sexual experimentation is common, and many adolescents first have intercourse in middle adolescence.

Late Adolescence
Teenagers in **late adolescence** (females aged 16 years and older; males aged 17 years and older) are explicitly moving toward adult roles and responsibilities. Some are beginning full-time jobs; others are beginning families. Many are preparing for these adult roles. The late adolescent completes the process of physical maturation. Many young people at this stage achieve the ability to understand abstract concepts, and they become more aware of what their limitations are and how their past will affect their future. They understand the consequences of their actions and behaviors, and they grapple with the complexities of identity, values, and ethical principles. Within the family, they move to a more adult relationship with their parents. The peer group recedes in importance as a determinant of behavior, and sexuality may become closely tied to commitment and planning for the future.

Adolescent Developmental Tasks

Developmental psychologists have identified six key developmental tasks for adolescents. Becoming a sexually healthy adult depends on the completion

middle adolescence The typical "teenage years," usually ages 13–16 years for females and ages 14–17 years for males.

late adolescence Period of transition to adulthood, beginning usually at age 16 years for females and age 17 years for males.

Ethical DIMENSIONS

Should Parents Have Their Adolescent Children Vaccinated Against HPV?

You will see more information about HPV later, in the chapter on sexually transmitted infections, but at this point we want to raise an interesting dilemma that has developed in the United States since 2008, when an effective vaccine against human papillomavirus (HPV) was approved by the Food and Drug Administration (FDA). This was the first time an effective vaccination against any STI became available. The Centers for Disease Control and Prevention (CDC) recommends that all girls and boys get the HPV vaccination at ages 11 and 12 because it is most effective if done at that time.

As of 2015, however, only 37% of girls and 14% of boys ages 13 to 17 had received the vaccine. Sometimes the fault lies with the physician: Doctors failed to recommend the vaccine to one-third of girls and more than 50% of boys. In other instances, parents have perhaps not been well informed about the vaccine or fear that if they have their child vaccinated against an STI this might be seen as endorsing sexual behavior by the child. There is no evidence that the sexual behavior of those youths who are vaccinated is any different from those not vaccinated.

What do you think? Is it ethical for parents to have their children vaccinated against HPV? Is it more ethical for them not to have their children vaccinated against HPV? Why?

of these key developmental tasks (Grunbaum et al., 2004). The six key tasks are as follows:

1. *Physical and sexual maturation:* Adolescents mature biologically into adults, a process that occurs at an earlier chronological age than it did in the past.

2. *Independence:* Adolescents develop autonomy within the structure that gave them nurture and support during their childhood. This is usually the family but may include some similar surrogate structure. The parent–child relationship is transformed during adolescence, as the young person obtains the skills to maintain satisfying relationships.

3. *Conceptual identity:* Adolescents establish and place themselves within the religious, cultural, ethnic, moral, and political constructs of their environments.

4. *Functional identity:* Adolescents begin to prepare themselves for adult roles in society. By identifying their competencies, they

discover how they will support themselves and contribute to their own families and society.

5. *Cognitive development:* Children and young adolescents are concrete thinkers and focus on real objects, present actions, and immediate benefits. During adolescence they develop a greater ability to think abstractly, plan for their future, and understand the effect of their current actions on their future lives and other people.

6. *Sexual self-concept:* During adolescence, young people tend to experience their first adultlike erotic feelings, experiment with sexual behaviors, and develop a strong sense of their own gender identity and sexual orientation.

The pursuit of these developmental tasks answers three psychosocial questions that adolescents ask themselves: Am I normal? Am I competent? Am I lovable and loving? Many adolescent behaviors can be attributed to the search for affirmative answers to these questions.

Physical and Sexual Maturation

As noted in the section on puberty, sexual maturation differs significantly among young men and young women. On average, young girls begin pubertal events 1 to 2 years before boys. The adolescent

conceptual identity Who am I in my world?

functional identity What adult roles will I play in the world?

cognitive development Explains the ability to think concretely or abstractly.

sexual self-concept Who am I as a sexual being?

female completes the process of puberty in 3 to 5 years, whereas for males, the process lasts 4 to 6 years. Adjusting to the biological changes of puberty is a major task of early adolescence, and society does not adequately prepare or support young people during these changes.

Sexual cognitions of girls appear to change prior to sexual experiences such as breast fondling and genital contact. Because most research focuses on intercourse as a key marker or pivotal event, the importance of attitudes, perceptions, and sexual self-esteem may have been overlooked as an important aspect of sexual development (O'Sullivan & Brooks-Gunn, 2005). The discrepancy between maturation among young women and young men is one factor that may contribute to some young women's seeking partners older than they are. This difference in age places young women at considerable risk for sexual exploitation.

Adolescents express sexual cognitions, social cognitions, peer affiliations, and various aspects of gender identity such as gender role expression, behavior, and conformity as they participate in proms, graduation events, and other social activities that mark passages throughout the teen years.

Cognitive Development

During adolescence, young people develop a range of intellectual characteristics that increase the probability that they will be able to become sexually healthy adults. Ideally, this includes developing the ability to reason abstractly, to foresee consequences of actions, and to understand the social context of behaviors. Adolescents develop an increased ability to control impulsivity, to identify the future implications of their actions, and to obtain control of their future plans.

Although the study of child development from 0 to 3 years of age has recognized the importance of brain development, study of adolescents has tended to focus more on psychological and social factors rather than on physiological ones. Recent imaging advances have allowed neuroscience—the scientific study of the biology of the brain—to demonstrate brain growth patterns. These studies in teens reveal remarkable changes during the second decade of life (Weinberger, Elvevåg, & Giedd, 2005). Of particular interest is the frontal cortex area, which governs impulse control, judgment, and decision making; that portion does not fully mature until around the age of 25. That means that teenagers, though very capable of huge intellectual and creative endeavors, are limited in

strategies, organizing, and recognizing potential consequences. Conversely, the teen brain is adept at learning by example. Thus, modeling behavior to be emulated could be a good tactic for both parents and teachers (Giedd, 2005).

Developmental age and general level of cognitive and emotional development may influence adolescent sexual decisions, contraceptive use, and safer sex practices. An adolescent's degree of cognitive maturity may place limits on his or her ability to plan for sexual relationships, clearly articulate personal values, negotiate with a partner, and obtain contraception and condoms. Further, the adolescent's ability to form empathetic relationships is dependent on **social cognition**: the capacity to see a situation from another person's perspective. Social cognition is one aspect of cognitive development. Understanding one's feelings and the feelings of others is central to emotional growth.

Sexual Self-Concept

Sexual self-concept, an individual's evaluation of his or her sexual feelings and actions, develops during adolescence. Young people develop an increasing sense of gender identity as men and women. An understanding of one's sexual orientation also

sexual cognitions Attitudes, expectations, beliefs, and values framing one's sexual experiences

social cognition Ability to see a situation from another person's point of view.

Gender DIMENSIONS

How Sex-Role Stereotypes Affect Sexuality

Sex-role stereotypes impede both young men and young women in attaining sexual health. Young women may learn that "It is better to be cute and popular than smart," "Girls have few sexual feelings," and "Girls who carry condoms are bad." Boys may learn that "Real men are always ready for sex" and that "Guys should never act like girls." In an online article for teens written by a 17-year-old male staff writer for Sex, Etc., women clearly are short-changed. He says, guys get to enjoy sex but girls are told by society they can't. Females faking orgasm is a laughing matter. Another problem is that many people, especially teens, are focused on sexual intercourse (where the "goal" is for the male to have an orgasm). Other ways of experiencing pleasure are less valued or ignored. Or, as one concerned male suggests, men are afraid they don't know how to please their partner, so they're reluctant to try. Regarding masturbation, there is silence and disdain for women but with men, it's common conversation. The suggested solution is T-A-L-K. When discussing safer sex, pleasure should be included, too. Since communication is the key to better relationships, maybe the real payoff *and* the best pleasure of all is an enhanced sexual connection (Dalal, 2005).

Although patterns of sexual involvement are increasingly similar for boys and girls, persistent sex stereotypes mean that expectations regarding sexual pleasure for young women are still quite different from those for young men.

Why do these different standards continue to exist? Will they ever change?

develops during adolescence: Young people become more aware of their sexual attractions and love interests, and adultlike erotic feelings emerge. Sexual experimentation is common among all groups of adolescents.

Gender Identity

During adolescence, young people solidify their gender identification by observing the gender roles of their parents and other adults. Gender identification includes understanding that one is male or female, as well as understanding the roles, values, duties, and responsibilities of being a man or a woman. Most young people have a firm sense of their maleness or femaleness before adolescence, but in adolescence, clear identification with adult masculine and feminine models emerges. The markers of masculinity and femininity vary by culture and are adopted to a greater or lesser extent by adolescents. *Gender-role behavior, expression,* and *conformity* are all current terms used to describe sex-typed attributes. Differences that have been studied include peer affiliation preference, aggression, and activity level (Zucker & Bradley, 2005).

Sexual Orientation

One's erotic attraction to others is discovered as one matures sexually. Sexual orientation, whatever it may be, does not seem to be something one chooses. Gay, lesbian, and bisexual people are not seduced, recruited, or taught to become LGBTQ people. Rather, one's sexual orientation often emerges in adolescence.

In retrospective studies, many gay and lesbian adults identify adolescence as a period of confusion about their sexual orientation. Although a majority of adult gay men recall feeling different as children, most did not self-identify as gay until their late teenage years.

Adolescent Sexual Behavior

Regardless of one's sexual orientation, almost all American adolescents engage in some type of sexual behavior (Table 13.5). Although policy debates have tended to focus on sexual intercourse and its negative consequences, young people explore dating, relationships, and intimacy from a much wider framework. Sexual behavior is almost universal among American adolescents.

The majority of adolescents move from kissing to other more intimate sexual behaviors during their teenage years.

- Overall, 49% of boys and 48% of girls ages 15 to 19 have engaged in oral sexual activity. Among the younger teens in one survey (ages 15 to 17), these percentages dropped to 38% for boys and 33% for girls. Rates of oral sexual activity have been decreasing

TABLE 13.5

Trends in the Prevalence of Sexual Behaviors and HIV Testing National YRBS: 1991–2013

The national Youth Risk Behavior Survey (YRBS) monitors priority health risk behaviors that contribute to the leading causes of death, disability, and social problems among youth and adults in the United States. The national YRBS is conducted every two years during the spring semester and provides data representative of 9th- through 12th-grade students in public and private schools throughout the United States.

	1991	1993	1995	1997	1999	2001	2003	2005	2007	2009	2011	2013	Long-term Change[1]	Change from 2011–2013[2]
									Percentages					
Ever had sexual intercourse														
	54.1	53.0	53.1	48.4	49.9	45.6	46.7	46.8	47.8	46.0	47.4	46.8	Decreased 1991–2013 Decreased 1991–2001 No change 2001–2013	No change
Had sexual intercourse before age 13 years (for the first time)														
	10.2	9.2	8.9	7.2	8.3	6.6	7.4	6.2	7.1	5.9	6.2	5.6	Decreased 1991–2013 Decreased 1991–1997 Decreased 1997–2013	No change
Had sexual intercourse with four or more persons (during their life)														
	18.7	18.7	17.8	16.0	16.2	14.2	14.4	14.3	14.9	13.8	15.3	15.0	Decreased 1991–2013 Decreased 1991–2003 No change 2003–2013	No change
Were currently sexually active (sexual intercourse with at least one person during the 3 months before the survey)														
	37.5	37.5	37.9	34.8	36.3	33.4	34.3	33.9	35.0	34.2	33.7	34.0	Decreased 1991–2013	No change
Used a condom (during last sexual intercourse among students who were currently sexually active)														
	46.2	52.8	54.4	56.8	58.0	57.9	63.0	62.8	61.5	61.1	60.2	59.1	Increased 1991–2013 Increased 1991–2003 Decreased 2003–2013	No change

Continues

TABLE 13.5

Trends in the Prevalence of Sexual Behaviors and HIV Testing National YRBS: 1991–2013 (Continued)

	Percentages												Long-term Change[1]	Change from 2011–2013[2]
1991	1993	1995	1997	1999	2001	2003	2005	2007	2009	2011	2013		
Used birth control pills (before last sexual intercourse to prevent pregnancy among students who were currently sexually active)														
20.8	18.4	17.4	16.6	16.2	18.2	17.0	17.6	16.0	19.8	18.0	19.0	Decreased 1991–1995 Increased 1995–2013	No change
Did not use any method to prevent pregnancy (during last sexual intercourse among students who were currently sexually active)														
16.5	15.3	15.8	15.2	14.9	13.3	11.3	12.7	12.2	11.9	12.9	13.7	Decreased 1991–2013 Decreased 1991–2007 No change 2007–2013	No change
Drank alcohol or used drugs before last sexual intercourse (among students who were currently sexually active)														
21.6	21.3	24.8	24.7	24.8	25.6	25.4	23.3	22.5	21.6	22.1	22.4	Increased 1991–1999 Decreased 1999–2013	No change
Were ever taught in school about AIDS or HIV infection														
83.3	86.1	86.3	91.5	90.6	89.0	87.9	87.9	89.5	87.0	84.0	85.3	Increased 1991–1997 Decreased 1997–2013	No change
Were ever tested for HIV (not including tests done when donating blood)														
—[3]	—	—	—	—	—	—	11.9	12.9	12.7	12.9	12.9	No change 2003–2013	No change

[1] Based on linear and quadratic trend analyses using logistic regression models controlling for sex, race/ethnicity, and grade, $p < 0.05$. Significant linear trends (if present) across all available years are described first followed by linear changes in each segment of significant quadratic trends (if present).

[2] Based on t-test analysis, $p < 0.05$.

[3] Not available.

Source: Reproduced from Centers for Disease Control and Prevention. *Trends in the prevalence of selected risk behaviors and HIV testing. National YRBS: 1991–2013.* Youth Risk Behavior Survey. Available: http://www.cdc.gov/healthyyouth/yrbs/pdf/trends/us_sexual_trend_yrbs.pdf.

since 2002, when 55% of 15- to 19-year-olds reported having engaged in oral sexual activity. By 2010, that percentage had declined to 48% for boys and 46% for girls (Copen et al., 2012).

- Copen et al. (2012) reported on the first time young people were surveyed about the timing of oral sex relative to intercourse. It was about equally likely for oral sex to happen before intercourse as after. Among females aged 15 to 24, 26% had first oral sex before first intercourse, and 27% after first intercourse. Among males aged 15 to 24, 24% had first oral sex before first intercourse and 24% had first oral sex after first intercourse.

- Teens in the United States and Europe have similar levels of sexual activity. However, European teens are more likely than U.S. teens to use contraceptives generally and to use the most effective methods; as a consequence, they have substantially lower pregnancy rates (*American teens' sexual and reproductive health*, 2014).

- Twelve percent of females ages 18 to 19 report same-sex sexual behaviors (any sexual experience, including oral sexual activity), compared with 4% of males in the same age-group (includes any oral or anal sexual activity) (*American teens' sexual and reproductive health*, 2014).

When data are collected about teen sexual behavior, the focus becomes *what, when,* and *how often,* but rarely *with what emotional intent.* Thus it is difficult to pin down aspects of sexual experience that are nuanced. Much has been written recently about changes in relationship patterns, particularly the phenomenon of "friends with benefits" and hooking up (a euphemism for a sexual encounter, particularly oral sex, without emotional involvement). Much of the discussion is anecdotal and involves use of the Internet to post personal profiles, chat online, and arrange meetings. Whether such interaction is viewed as healthy or harmful may depend on one's age and experience. Many people feel that females may have less to gain than males and the ultimate risk may be increased chance of STIs. The role of commitment and dating seems to be changing, perhaps due to the expectation that marriage and romantic relationships won't happen until later in life.

Clearly, research is needed to measure more than numbers. Detailed studies might discover whether friends with benefits are truly a widespread and long-term change in relationship patterns or a minor blip in reaction to new technology that will be reversed

when another trend appears. Some experts suggest that the progression from kissing to noncoital behaviors to intercourse differs among different groups of adolescents. Many teenagers move through a progression of intimate behaviors; lower-income teenagers may be less likely to follow this progression, moving more rapidly from kissing directly to sexual intercourse.

Sexting and Sexual Behavior

Temple et al. (2012) found that adolescents who engaged in sexting behaviors were more likely to have begun dating and to have had sexual intercourse than those who did not sext. For girls, sexting was also associated with risky sexual behaviors.

Dake et al. (2012) found statistically significant correlations between sexting and sexual behaviors. Of those who had anal sex, 71% had sexted; of those who had 4 or more sexual partners, 65% had sexted; of those who did not use contraceptives at last intercourse, 65% had sexted; of those who had oral sex, 54% had sexted; and of those who had ever had sexual intercourse, 47% had sexted.

In another survey, 15% of adolescents with cell phone access reported sexting, and 54% reported knowing someone who had sent a sext. Adolescents whose peers sexted were more likely to sext themselves. Adolescents who sexted were more likely to report being sexually active. Nonheterosexual students were more likely to report sexting, sexual activity, or unprotected sexual activity at last sexual encounter (Rice et al., 2012). In addition, 13% of 14- to 24-year-olds reported having shared a naked photo or video of themselves via digital communication such as the Internet or text messaging (*Sexual health of adolescents and young adults in the United States,* 2014).

Teenagers Who Have Intercourse

Substantial changes in adolescent sexual behavior have occurred in the past six decades. From the late 1960s until 1988 the proportion of teens who had had sexual intercourse increased. Then the trend reversed, and from 1991 to 2001 the proportion of teens reporting having had sexual intercourse dropped from 54.1% to 45.6%. However, since 2001 the proportion of students who had ever had sexual intercourse has stayed about the same (Eaton et al., 2010) (see Table 13.5).

Contraceptive use among teens has also undergone remarkable change. In the 1970s, the most commonly used method was the birth control pill, followed by condom use and withdrawal. In the 1980s, condom use increased and the use of birth control pills declined. This trend continued into the 1990s, and now condom use among high school students has stabilized at 63% with no significant change from 2003 to 2013 (see Table 13.5).

Rates of teen pregnancy, including births and abortions, have changed dramatically. A record high (96 births per 1,000 teen girls aged 15–19) was reached in 1957, followed by a steady decline to the mid-1980s. Then the birth rate increased again by 24% by 1991. Then there was a decrease of more than 33% in the birth rate, to a low of 41 births per 1,000 teen girls in 2004. After 14 years of decline, the birth rate for teens *increased* by 3% in 2006 and by 1% in 2007. However, it declined 36% from 2007 through 2013, reaching 26.6 births per 1,000 women aged 15 to 19. Rates fell significantly for teenagers in all age groups and for all racial and ethnic groups (Ventura, Hamilton, & Mathews, 2014). The abortion rate for teens rose in the 1970s, was mostly stable in the 1980s, and declined 66% from its 1988 peak and 2010 (from 43.5 abortions per 1,000 teens to 14.7 abortions per 1,000 teens, respectively) (Wind, 2014).

While it is difficult to pinpoint the exact causes, it seems that both delayed initiation of sexual intercourse and improved contraceptive practice contributed equally to the declines in these rates. There was an increase in condom use, a decrease in the use of withdrawal, and decline in use of no contraceptive method. In spite of these trends, the U.S. teen birth rate remains much higher than the rates in other developed countries.

Early Sexual Activity

- Sexual activity is and has long been rare among girls 12 and younger; most of such encounters are nonconsensual.

- Most older teen girls (ages 17 to 19) are sexually active.

- Approximately 30% of girls ages 15 to 16 have had sexual intercourse.

- Contraceptive use among girls as young as 15 is similar to the use among their older counterparts.

- Girls who start having sexual intercourse at age 14 or younger are less likely to have used contraception at first intercourse and take longer to begin using contraception.

- Pregnancy rates range from 0.14 per 1,000 girls at age 12, to 5 per 1,000 girls at age 14, to 36 per 1,000 teens at age 16, to 95 per 1,000 teens at age 18.

- Among sexually active girls, the pregnancy rates range from 12 per 1,000 girls at age 12, to 58 per 1,000 girls at age 14, to 110 per

1,000 girls at age 16, to 157 per 1,000 girls at age 18.

- The abortion rate for teenage girls ranges from 0.07 per 1,000 girls at age 12, to 2 per 1,000 girls at age 14, to 11 per 1,000 girls at age 16, to 25 per 1,000 girls at age 18.

- The birth rate for teenage girls ranges from 0.05 per 1,000 girls at age 12, to 2.3 per 1,000 girls at age 14, to 19 per 1,000 girls at age 16, to 56 per 1,000 girls at age 18 (Finer & Philbin, 2013).

Interestingly, economic status influences rates of teen sexual activity. In households earning $200,000 or more per year, 32% of teens have had sexual intercourse by age 16; in households earning $100,000 to $199,000, 41% have had intercourse by age 16; in households earning $60,000 to $99,000, 46% have had intercourse by age 16; in households earning $30,000 to $59,000, 54% have had intercourse by age 16; and in households earning less than $29,000, 61% have had intercourse by age 16 (Barone, 2014).

Figure 13.1 shows birth rate data from 1940 to 2013. The U.S. teen birth rate remains higher than the rates in most other developed countries. More than one-third of young women become pregnant before they reach the age of 20, and the vast majority of these pregnancies are unintended. A major change has been the significant increase in the proportion of teen births to unmarried teenagers. In a recent year, 89% of births to teens were nonmarital, up from 48% in 1980 and 15% in 1960 (Ventura et al., 2014).

Teen birth rates continue to vary widely by race and Hispanic ethnicity. They range from 9.7 per 1,000 Asian or Pacific Islander (API) girls aged 15 to 19, to 46.3 per 1,000 Hispanic teens. Rates for other groups are 20.5 per 1,000 non-Hispanic white teenagers, 34.9 per 1,000 American Indian or Alaska Native teenagers, and 43.9 per 1,000 non-Hispanic black teenagers. The general downward trend in teen birth rates is apparent for each group. The steepest declines were noted for non-Hispanic and API teens, down 63% and 64% respectively. Rates for other groups fell 53% to 59%. As a result of these trends, differences in birth rates for most racial and Hispanic ethnicity groups have narrowed for teens aged 15 to 19 (Ventura et al., 2014).

Various researchers have added interesting information to the statistics already presented. For example, by state, teen births are lowest in the Northeast and highest in the South. New Hampshire had the lowest rate at 13.8 births per 1,000 teens, and New Mexico had the highest at 47.5 per 1,000. Relatedly, over a recent 5-year period, Colorado saw the highest percentage drop in birth rates among U.S. teens ages 15 to 19. The state's family planning policies

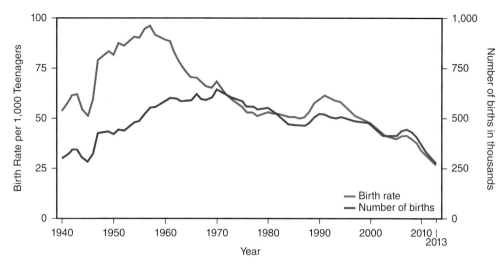

FIGURE 13.1 Teen Birth Rates in the United States, 1940–2013
From 1940 to 1957, the U.S. teen birth rate increased to a record high. This rate dropped fairly steadily from the end of the 1950s through the mid-1980s, but then increased between 1986 and 1991. Between 1991 and 2013, the teen birth rate decreased to a record low of 26.6 births per 1,000 teens in 2013. The teen birth rate in 2013 was one-third lower than the historic high in 1957. This chart reflects births per 1.000 teen girls aged 15 to 19 in the United States and presents the most recent national data available.

Note: Data for 2013 are preliminary.

Source: Ventura, S. J., Hamilton, B. E., & Mathews, T. J. National and state patterns of teen births in the United States, 1940–2013. *National Vital Statistics Report;* vol. 63, no. 4. Hyattsville, MD: National Center for Health Statistics, 2014.

improved teens' access to long-acting reversible contraceptives, which in turn helped to lower its rates. Over the same period, abortion rates fell 35% (*CDC: U.S. teen birth rates down significantly since 1950s,* 2014).

Many experts believe there is a need for better sexuality education as well as use of more effective contraceptives. One report found that approximately 91% of girls ages 15 to 17 reported having taken a formal sexuality education class that discussed contraceptive methods or ways to say no to having sexual activity, while 61% said they had learned about both birth control and abstinence. Further, 76% of these girls said they had discussed contraception, abstinence, or both with their parents. Yet 83% of female teens who reported having had sexual intercourse said they did not receive any sexuality education before the first time they had sexual intercourse (*CDC report: Need for better sex ed, contraceptive use despite record-low teen births,* 2014).

In addition, few pediatricians seem to offer routine sexual health services for teens. Vaccination rates for HPV continue to fall short of the CDC recommendation that all teens receive the shots. Time constraints and a lack of training on how to handle issues related to adolescent sexuality are among the reasons that physicians often fail to discuss this topic, and many pediatricians simply are not comfortable talking about sexuality (*Few pediatricians offer routine sexual health services for teens,* 2014).

Although some people might find their discovery intuitive, Hensel and Sorge (2014) confirmed that sexual intercourse among 14- to 17-year-olds was more frequent (13.5% versus 5.4%) and condom use was less frequent (13.8% versus 33.1%) on weekdays when school was skipped as compared to weekdays when school was attended. From an emotional standpoint, young women reported significantly higher levels of negative mood, sexual interest, and feeling in love, and lower levels of positive mood on weekdays when they skipped school or failed a test.

The self-assessment exercise at the end of this chapter raises many of the questions that a young person—indeed, an adult—needs to consider to determine his or her readiness for a sexual relationship.

Sexual Abuse of Children and Adolescents

Sexual abuse occurs in all types of homes. It happens hundreds of times a day in the United States. The real prevalence of child and adolescent sexual abuse is not known because so many victims do not disclose or report their abuse. There also can

sexual abuse The psychological exploitation or infliction of unwanted sexual contact on one person.

be differences in how child sexual abuse is defined in various studies as well as the time periods over which studies are conducted. Thus, estimates range from 1.2 victims per 1,000 and 1.9 victims per 1,000 in studies focusing on occurrences in 1 year. At the upper end, between 90 and 280 per 1,000 victims have been found in a survey of adults who experienced some sexual abuse or assault in their childhood. It seems that females are more at risk than males. Also, children from low-income families are more at-risk as are children who have been victims of other forms of crime, violence, and abuse. With regard to the perpetrators, men perpetrate most sexual abuse and sex crimes. Sex offenders against children tend to be juveniles or young adults younger than age 30. Most sexual abuse is committed by people who know the victims, followed by family members (Sexual abuse, 2011).

The definition of child sexual abuse is broader than most people think. It can include any sexual act between an adult and a minor, or between two minors, when one exerts power over the other. It also includes forcing, coercing, or persuading a child to engage in any type of sexual act. In addition, it encompasses noncontact acts such as exhibitionism, exposure to pornography, voyeurism, and communicating in a sexual manner by phone or Internet (*The issue of child sexual abuse*, 2015).

Sexual Abuse of Children

Most parents teach their children not to talk to strangers, accept candy from people they do not know, or ever get into a car with a stranger. Many preschools and kindergartens offer "stranger danger" programs. However, the reality is that, in 90% of the cases, the assailant is someone in the child's family or someone close to the family.

It is also possible for children to be sexually abused by other children. This is different from the sex play described earlier in this chapter. In sex play, children are usually of the same age, they are engaging in light-hearted exploration, and they appear to be enjoying themselves—at least until they realize they have been "discovered" by an adult. And, in general, once they are told by an adult that they should stop, they do.

Some children, however, engage in inappropriate behaviors and become sexually abusive to other, usually younger, children. This may include engaging in oral or genital sex with other children, with or without their consent. Many of these children have been sexually abused themselves, and many of them have inappropriately been exposed to sexually explicit materials or adult erotic behavior. Most of the males and females who sexually abuse children have earlier been molested themselves.

Myth (vs) Fact

Kiss and Tell: What Teens Say About Love, Trust, and Other Relationship Stuff

It's a relationship world. Seven in 10 teens say their friends are in romantic relationships.

Relationships

The good news is that most teens (68%) say that their friends are in "healthy" romantic relationships. The proportion saying this is almost identical for teen boys and teen girls.

The not-so-good news is that one in five teens (19%) aged 15–17 say that most of their friends are in *unhealthy* relationships—those without love, trust, mutual respect, and honesty.

Trust and Honesty Rule. When it comes to relationships, teens say it's all about trust—40% of guys and 48% of gals say that *trust* is the most important part of a healthy relationship. Teens say that *honesty* is the second most important factor. Surprisingly, 10% of teen boys say that *compatibility* is most important; yet only 3% of teen girls agree. Fewer than 3% of teens say *looks* or *popularity* matters most.

Pressure

More good news is that most teens (84% of guys and 85% of gals) say they have never felt pressure to be in a romantic relationship before they were ready.

Fast Fact. Teens who are in relationships with someone who is 3 years older are far more likely to say that sex was unwanted.

Role Models

Teens in focus groups indicated that they can learn a lot about what to avoid from seeing unhealthy relationships.

Almost one in five (17%) teens say they don't know *anyone* who serves as an example of a healthy relationship.

Fast Fact. Most teens aged 15–17 say they enjoy spending time with their mother (79%) and father (76%).

Source: Data from Kiss and tell: What teens say about love, trust, and other relationship stuff survey results. National Campaign to Prevent Teen and Unplanned Pregnancy. 2007. Retrieved June 5, 2012, from www.thenationalcampaign.org /resources/pdf/pubs/kiss_tell.pdf.

Family and Acquaintance Sexual Abuse Using the Internet

The Internet and related technologies have transformed many aspects of communication. It is realistic to assume it will have an effect on child mistreatment as well. So far, concern has focused on online meeting crimes in which adult strangers have used the Internet to meet and develop abusive relationships with vulnerable youth. However, just as most face-to-face sexual abuse involves family members and acquaintances of the victim, so it is realistic to assume that Internet sexual abuse would also involve nonstranger sex offenders.

Internet technology provides a number of ways for this to happen. Digital photography has made online production and distribution of child pornography a more frequent component of abuse. Availability and ease of online communication may

Multicultural DIMENSIONS

Racial and Ethnic Differences in Sexual Behaviors

The likelihood of having several sexual partners varies by race and ethnicity, as does condom use. The percentages of high school students who have had four or more sexual partners by race/ethnicity as well as high school students who used condoms (either they or their partner) during their last sexual intercourse are shown here.

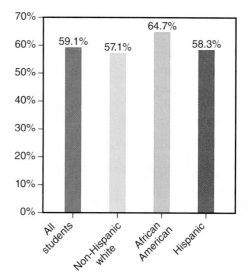

Source: Data from Youth risk behavior surveillance—United States, 2013. *Morbidity and Mortality Weekly Report, 63, no. 4* (June 13, 2014). A-168.

allow acquaintance and family member offenders a means of bypassing parents and other caregivers so as to develop abusive relationships with potential victims. The Internet may provide opportunities for family and acquaintance offenders to seduce children and adolescents by bringing up sexual topics and exposing potential victims to sexual images and materials.

Child sexual abuse researcher David Finkelhor and his colleagues periodically report interesting statistics. For example, they looked at the sexual victimization of more than 4,500 children and youth. Their data revealed that 2.9% of the males and 12.9% of the females had received unwanted Internet sex talk in the past year. Moreover, 4.2% of the males and 21.4% of the females had received unwanted Internet sex talk at some time during their lifetime. In addition, 4.4% of the 10- to 13-year-olds had experienced some form of sexual victimization in the past year. The same was true for 16.4% of the 14- to 17-year-olds. Among the 14- to 17-year-olds, 10.3% of the males and 22.8% of the females had been sexually victimized in the past year. In addition, 20.2% of the males and 34.9% of the females had been subjected to some form of sexual victimization during their lifetime (Finkelhor et al., 2013).

Sexual Harassment

Sexual harassment is a fact of life in most middle and high schools. *Sexual harassment in school* is defined as "unwanted and unwelcome sexual behavior that interferes with the student's life." Sexual harassment includes unwanted sexual comments, jokes, and gestures; receiving from another student sexual pictures, photographs, and notes; sexual graffiti about a specific student in the bathroom or locker room; spreading of sexual rumors; flashing or mooning; touching, grabbing, or pinching in a sexual way; brushing against another student in a sexual way; pulling clothes off; blocking another student in a sexual way; and forcing kissing and other sexual behaviors.

Statistics about sexual harassment in schools vary among studies. A national study of almost 2,000 students conducted by the American Association of University Women found that sexual harassment is part of everyday life in middle and high schools. Nearly half (48%) of the students experienced some form of sexual harassment. Verbal harassment (unwelcome

sexual harassment Unwanted sexual behavior that interferes with the student's life.

Global

DIMENSIONS

Teenagers and Sexuality Around the World

There is no one best way to improve adolescent sexual health, but leaders in the United States can learn from efforts in some other countries. These efforts are often designed to promote the idea that sexuality is a normal and healthy part of being human and being an adolescent. Some examples of the efforts in other countries include the following:

- In France, Germany, and the Netherlands, adults respect adolescents and expect them to act responsibly. Sexuality education for youth is strongly supported by governments.
- Public health policies to reduce unintended pregnancies, abortions, and STIs, including HIV, are based on research and not the whims of political and religious interest groups.
- Easy access to condoms and other contraceptive methods, consistent and effective sexuality education, and widespread public education campaigns support the desire to improve adolescent sexual health.
- Long-term government-supported public education campaigns are provided through the Internet, television, films, radio, billboards, discos,

pharmacies, and healthcare providers. Campaigns are direct and humorous and focus on both safety and pleasure.

- Youth have convenient access to free or low-cost contraception through national health insurance.
- Sexuality education is usually integrated across school subjects and at all grade levels. It is based on accurate and complete information in response to students' questions.
- Families support educators and healthcare providers' efforts to make sexual health information and services available to teens. Families also have open and honest discussions with adolescents about sexuality.
- Sexual relationships are viewed as normal and natural for older adolescents, a positive component of emotionally healthy maturation. Also, young people believe it is "stupid and irresponsible" to have sexual activity without protection.
- The values of responsibility, respect, tolerance, and equity are included in ethical views of sexual behavior.

Source: Adapted from Alford, S., & Hauser, D. Adolescent Sexual Health in Europe and the United States. Advocates for Youth, 2011. Available: www.advocatesforyouth.org/publications/419?task=view.

Sexual harassment in schools is common. What type of program could be instituted to help stop such harassment?

© Richard Hutchings/Science Source

sexual comments, jokes, or gestures) made up the bulk of the incidents, but physical harassment was also common. Sexual harassment by text, email, Facebook, or other electronic means affected nearly one-third (30%) of students. Many of the students who were sexually harassed through cyberspace were also sexually harassed in person. Girls were more likely than boys to be sexually harassed (56% versus 40%). Girls were more likely than boys to be sexually harassed both in person (52% versus 35%) and via text, email, Facebook, or other electronic means (36% versus 24%). Being called gay or lesbian in a negative way was a form of sexual harassment that girls and boys reported in equal numbers (18% of students).

The prevalence of sexual harassment in grades 7 to 12 surprises many people, in part because it is rarely reported. Half of the students who reported being sexually harassed in the American Association of University Women study said they did nothing afterward in response to the harassment. A vicious cycle was noted in which most students who admitted to sexually harassing another person were sexually harassed themselves. Many of the sexually harassed students reported trouble sleeping, not wanting to go to school, and wanting to change the route they took to or from school. These negative emotional effects can take a toll on students, resulting in decreased productivity and increased absenteeism from school. Under Title IX (federal law), schools are required to eliminate sexual harassment and sexual violence, prevent their recurrence, and address their impacts (*Crossing the line: Sexual harassment at school*, 2011; *Sexual harassment and sexual violence in school*, 2015).

Most sexual harassment in schools occurs openly in classrooms and hallways, rather than in secluded areas. Students are usually harassed by other students, but occasionally they are harassed by adult employees.

Schools are supposed to protect students against sexual harassment. Schools need to have sexual harassment policies, with clear penalties for perpetrators, which should be communicated to students and parents. A clear procedure for handling complaints of sexual harassment should be established.

Recognizing a Sexually Healthy Relationship

Although sexual abuse and harassment are critical concepts to define and avoid, the components of a **sexually healthy relationship** are less often discussed. This is unfortunate because development of self-identity, particularly in personal and intimate relationships, is a key developmental task of young adults. Being skilled at recognizing a positive relationship provides protection from being exploited, misled, or victimized. Here the focus is on health rather than harm. To distinguish between potentially healthy and harmful sexual relationships, the following list provides a tool for assessing relationships by applying the defining characteristics to one's own personal relationships or those of others.

Who is your partner? What is your relationship with this person? Sexual activity often involves many feelings and emotions that can be confusing. How will you and your partner handle these feelings if they come up? How will sex change your relationship with this person?

Do you feel safe? Consider your partner, the situation, the location … Do you feel safe and taken care of? Do you feel respected by your partner? Do you respect your partner? Can you talk and listen to him or her? Are you worried that someone might walk in?

Is it consensual? No one has the right to be sexual with another person without that person's explicit permission. Have you talked about which behaviors you give permission for and have permission to start? Have you talked about where you will stop? Do you feel like your partner respects your decisions? Do you respect your partner's decisions?

What is your motivation? Why are you thinking of doing this? People can have many reasons for having sex, like to become closer, to feel loved, to express love, to feel good, to satisfy curiosity, to gain popularity, to get someone to like them, to fit in, or to rebel. Let's face it, some of these aren't very good reasons for getting sexually involved with someone else. Be honest with yourself, what are your reasons?

Is it non-exploitative? Exploitation is when one person uses someone else for selfish reasons. Exploitation should not be part of sexual relationships. Partners should be interested in each other's well-being as well as their own. Are you and your partner looking out for each other?

Are you being honest? Have you talked to your partner about your feelings, what you want to do, and what you don't want to do? Were you truthful in these conversations? Being honest with yourself and your partner can help you have a better relationship.

Is it pleasurable? One reason that many people participate in various sexual activities is because these behaviors provide physical, emotional, and psychological pleasure. Does the sexual activity you are considering or engaging in feel good?

Is it protected? Most sexual behaviors carry some risk of STIs or pregnancy. It's important to protect yourself from these risks—either by avoiding behaviors and eliminating the risk or by using effective protection and reducing the risk. Do you understand the risk involved in each behavior you are considering? Do you understand the benefits of abstaining from some or all risky behaviors? Do you understand how condoms or birth control can reduce your risk? Do you know how to use condoms or birth control correctly?

What does your gut instinct say? A lot of people talk about listening to their inner voice or gut to let them know whether they are making the right decision. Whatever the decision is—if it feels wrong, it is wrong for you. And remember, you can always change your mind. You and your partner always have the right, the ability, and the responsibility to stop if either one of you changes your mind (Kemper & Rodriguez, 2005).

Questions courtesy of SIECUS, www.siecus.org.

---

sexually healthy relationship   Consensual, non-exploitative, honest, mutually pleasurable, safe and protected from unwanted pregnancy, STIs, and other harm (National Guidelines Task Force, 2004).

Exploring the Dimensions of Human Sexuality

Sexual maturation is a time of constant physical and psychological changes. At the same time, deeply rooted sociocultural influences, once able to provide a sense of comfort, now may cause confusion.

Many adolescents feel they have almost no control over physiological changes and the accompanying mood swings. In an attempt to preserve the child's body they once had, some girls attempt to control their food intake. But a girl with a bad self-image may develop an obsession with food intake that leads to an eating disorder.

Boys also feel out of control, experiencing erections and hormonal surges at almost any stimulus.

A cultural double standard does not help. Boys who do not want to be permissive feel out of place, as do girls who want to experience sexual behaviors. Such confusion can lead to sexual experimentation—usually in the form of unsafe sexual practices.

Biological Factors
- Puberty changes boys and girls into men and women.
- Genetic coding affects the onset of puberty and general overall appearance.
- Reproduction becomes possible after menarche and semenarche.
- Sexual arousal and response become important issues in an adolescent's life.
- Physical appearance changes dramatically during puberty, affecting body image.
- Growth and development, in terms of physical and mental maturity, greatly affect a person's self-concept.

Sociocultural Factors
- Socioeconomic status affects sexual behaviors. Lower-economic status youths have sexual intercourse earlier than teens who are more well off, and they experience a higher rate of STIs and births.
- Religion and ethnic heritage affect beliefs about sexuality and permissiveness.
- Many cultures' double standard expects boys to be sexually aggressive and girls to remain sexually passive.
- Media and ad information often convey information to adolescents about sexuality and sexual behavior.
- Friends often convey false information about sexual behaviors to adolescents.
- Use of the Internet can provide access to reliable sexuality information but can also lead to sexually abusive situations.

Psychological Factors
- Emotions are dramatically affected by hormones, which cause dramatic mood swings for adolescents.
- Early or late developers may have issues with securing their body image.
- Sexual experience used to be gained slowly, starting with kissing games, moving to petting, then intercourse. Today's teens often move directly from kissing to intercourse.
- Self-concept is influenced by social status and peers.
- Learned attitudes and behaviors are put to the test as the body goes through constant physical changes.

Summary

- Biological sexual development begins during pregnancy. Infants develop a sense of trust based on loving touch and reliable need fulfillment.

- Healthy sexual development of infants and toddlers is fostered by teaching correct names of all body parts and responding non-punitively to self-stimulation and curiosity about genitals.

- Sex is assigned at birth, usually based on genital appearance. By age 3, a child recognizes gender differences; by age 5, a child has an internal sense of being male or female (gender identity) and knows his or her gender will not change (gender constancy).

- Preschoolers develop autonomy and initiative rather than shame or guilt when curiosity-based sex play is expected as normal behavior and questions about reproduction are answered truthfully.

- Parents can use the media as an effective teaching tool, encouraging elementary-school-age children to develop empathy and to critically examine what they see and hear for sexism, sex-role stereotypes, and other prejudices.

- Puberty—the predictable process of biological sexual development—usually occurs between the ages of 8 and 17; the median age is 10–11 years for girls and 11–12 years for boys. Physical changes during puberty include emergence of secondary sexual characteristics such as body and facial hair, glandular changes, growth spurt in height and weight, and reproductive maturity indicated by menarche (first menstrual period for girls) and semenarche (first ejaculation for boys).

- The goal of comprehensive sexuality education is to promote adult sexual health. Key concepts include human development, relationships, personal skills, sexual behavior, sexual health, and sexual aspects of society and culture. These concepts are learned through obtaining accurate information, exploring attitudes and values, developing interpersonal skills including communication, and exercising responsibility.

- Adolescence—the period of development from puberty to adulthood—consists of three stages during which thinking, emotions, relationship skills, autonomy, body image, sex-role definition, and sexual self-concept become mature.

- Teen sexual behavior is often examined through the lens of risk behaviors, STIs, and teen birthrates. After 14 years of birthrate decline, attributed to decreased sexual intercourse and increased use of condoms, the birthrate among U.S. teens increased 4% from 2005 to 2007. However, it decreased again and reached a record low in 2013. It remains the highest in the Western industrialized world.

- Sexual abuse and harassment can occur online via the Internet—that is, electronically as well as directly.

- A sexually healthy relationship can be recognized as one that is safe, consensual, non-exploitative, honest, pleasurable, and protected.

Discussion Questions

1. Discuss how touch, including genital touching, differs for infants and toddlers versus adolescents.

2. Describe the roles that parents, peers, and the media play in teaching preschoolers and early elementary students about sexuality.

3. Compare and contrast puberty in boys and girls, both physiologically and emotionally.

4. Identify and describe the three stages of adolescence, including the development of sexual self-concept.

5. Describe how trends in sexual behaviors, attitudes, and birthrates have changed since the first YRBS was administered in 1991.

6. Distinguish between expected childhood sex play and behaviors that could be abusive.

Application Questions

Reread the chapter-opening story and answer the following questions.

1. Some people believe that a young child should be told that boys are special on the outside and girls are special on the inside. Is there any reason to tell a young child more than that?

2. Some parents choose to teach their young children about sexual intercourse and reproduction; many other parents do not want their children learning such information. Given that children repeat what they know, is it

important to respect the rights of those who—for religious or cultural reasons—want such information withheld from their children?

3. Given that children do hear explicit sexual references on the national news at some point, how should the mass media handle this content with adequate discretion? If you were a reporter *and* a parent, how would you balance the responsibility to report the news but protect young children?

Critical Thinking Questions

1. You are the parent of a 4-year-old and have just received a phone call from a parent who has a child the same age. It seems the two children were in the garage "examining" each other. The other parent is furious, accusing your child of initiating the "perversities." What do you say to the parent? What do you say to your child?

    You have 10 minutes before your child arrives home, time enough to check out the SIECUS website. Which information will help you talk to your child?

2. Some pressures of adolescence are the result of society's double standard—that it is OK for men but wrong for women to be interested in engaging in sexual behaviors. Given what the chapter says about normal sexual feelings, what pressures does a double standard place on women? On men?

    Is it possible for society to eliminate the double standard and emphasize equality? If so, would society choose that both men and women have an equal right to say yes or no to sexual experiences? Explain your answer.

3. Refer to the Multicultural Dimensions feature when answering these questions. What is the influence of race and ethnicity on condom use? What might account for these differences? What is the influence of race and ethnicity on the number of sexual partners? Why might these differences exist? How might cultural differences influence partner impregnation? How can young people who choose to engage in sexual intercourse be encouraged to use condoms consistently?

Critical Thinking Case

Adolescents have a hard enough time coming to grips with their sexuality even if they receive proper information and support. But few do. In addition, some school-based sexuality education programs have a "fear-based" component. The aim of many fear-based programs is abstinence outside marriage. There is nothing wrong with teaching abstinence; however, many fear-based programs tend to distort information and use incorrect information to make their point.

The SIECUS website features a large section on fear-based programs, with general information and critiques of seven fear-based programs.

Choose one fear-based program and prepare a critique. What are the strong points and weak points of the program? How could it be improved? Would the fear techniques used in the program have prevented you from engaging in sexual activity?

Exploring Personal Dimensions

Readiness for a Sexual Relationship

Teenagers and young adults often wonder, "How do I know if I am ready for sex?" The following checklist may help them assess their readiness for mature sexual relationships.

This checklist may help adolescents *and* adults evaluate whether they are ready for a mature sexual relationship with a partner. Ideally, these criteria would be met *before* a young person or an adult engaged in intimate sexual behaviors, including any type of intercourse. Think about your own decisions or the decisions of people you know. Do they meet these criteria?

Are you and your partner

_____ Physically mature?
_____ Patient and understanding?
_____ Knowledgeable about sexuality and sexual response?
_____ Empathetic and able to be vulnerable?
_____ Committed to preventing unintended pregnancies?
_____ Able to handle responsibility for positive consequences?
_____ Able to handle responsibility for potential negative consequences?
_____ Honestly approving of your behavior?

Is your relationship

_____ Committed, mutually kind, and understanding?
_____ Do you trust and admire each other?
_____ Have you experimented with and found pleasure in nonpenetrative behaviors?
_____ Have you talked about sexual behaviors before they occur?
_____ Is your motivation for a sexual relationship pleasure and intimacy?
_____ Do you have a place for the sexual relationship that is safe and comfortable?

Suggested Readings

Albert, B. *With one voice 2014: America's adults and teens sound off about teen pregnancy.* Washington, DC: The National Campaign to Prevent Teen and Unplanned Pregnancy, 2014. Available: www.thenationalcampaign.org /resources/one-voice–2014.

Boonstra, H. D. What is behind the declines in teen pregnancy rates? *Guttmacher Policy Review, 17, 3* (2014), 15–20. An analysis of what has been behind the decrease in teen pregnancy rates in the United States.

Goldman, L. *Coming out, coming in: Nurturing the well-being and inclusion of gay youth in mainstream society.* New York: Routledge Press, 2007.

Haffner, D. W. *Beyond the big talk: A parent's guide to raising sexually healthy teens, revised and updated edition.* New York: Newmarket Press, 2008.

Haffner, D. W. *From diapers to dating: A parent's guide to raising sexually healthy children,* revised 2nd Ed. New York: Newmarket Press, 2008.

Harris, R. H., & Emberley, M. *A family library: It's not the stork! A book about girls, boys, babies, bodies, families and friends.* Cambridge, MA: Candlewick Press, 2006.

It's perfectly normal. Cambridge, MA: Candlewick Press, 2009.

It's so amazing! A book about eggs, sperm, birth, babies, and families. Cambridge, MA: Candlewick Press, 2009.

Key statistics from the National Survey of Family Growth. Centers for Disease Control and Prevention, 2015. Available: http://www.cdc.gov /nchs/nsfg/key_statistics/s.htm. Data from the National Survey of Family Growth.

Web Resources

Answer/Sex, Etc.
www.sexetc.org

Sex, Etc. is part of the Teen-to-Teen Sexuality Education Project developed by Answer. Answer—part of the Center for Applied Psychology at Rutgers University—is a national organization dedicated to providing and promoting comprehensive sexuality education to young people and the adults who teach them.

Sexuality Information and Education Council of the United States
www.siecus.org

SIECUS has been a national voice for sexuality education, sexual health, and sexual rights for more than 40 years. It provides information, education, public policy, and media outreach to educators, healthcare providers, parents, journalists, policy makers, religious leaders, community members, and young people.

National Campaign to Prevent Teen and Unplanned Pregnancy
www.thenationalcampaign.org

Founded in 1996, this nonprofit, nonpartisan initiative is supported almost entirely by private donations. Its mission is to improve the well-being of children, youth, and families by reducing the nation's teen and unplanned pregnancy rates. It offers a host of research-based resources for teens, parents, faith leaders, researchers, and professionals.

Planned Parenthood Federation of America
www.plannedparenthood.org/teen-talk

Teen-Talk is the official teen outreach website of Planned Parenthood. It provides honest and nonjudgmental information about sexuality in language teens can understand. The goal of this site is for teens to use this knowledge to reduce their risk of unintended pregnancy and sexually transmitted infections.

References

American teens' sexual and reproductive health. Guttmacher Institute, May 2014. Available: http://www.guttmacher.org /pubs/FB-ATSRH.html.

Bancroft, J., Herbenick, D., & Reynolds, M. Masturbation as a marker of sexual development, in *Sexual Development in Childhood,* J. Bancroft, ed. Bloomington, IN: Indiana University Press (2003), 438.

Barone, E. Who we are. *Time, 184, 9–10* (2014), 53–58.

Berk, L. *Exploring lifespan development.* Boston: Allyn & Bacon, 2011.

Bullough, V. L. Children and adolescents as sexual beings: A historical overview. *Child and Adolescent Psychiatric Clinics of North America, 13, no. 3* (2004), 447–459.

Bullough, V. L., & Bullough, B. *Human sexuality: An encyclopedia.* New York: Garland Press, 1994.

CDC: U.S. teen birth rates down significantly since 1950s. National Partnership for Women & Families, 2014. Available: http://go.nationalpartnership.org/site/News2?abbr =daily2_&page=NewsArticle&id=45398.

CDC report: Need for better sexed, contraceptive use despite record-low teen births. National Partnership for Women and Families, 2014. Available: http://go.nationalpartnership.org /site/News2?abbr=daily2_&id=44133&security=1201.

Centers for Disease Control and Prevention. *HIV and AIDS in the United States: A picture of today's epidemic.* Atlanta, GA: Author, 2009. Available: http://www.cdc.gov/hiv/topics /surveillance/united_states.htm.

Copen, C. E., Chandra, A., & Martinez, G. Prevalence and timing of oral sex with opposite-sex partners among females and males aged 15–24 years: United States, 2007-2010. *National Health Statistics Reports, no. 56,* (August 16, 2012), 1–14.

Crossing the line: Sexual harassment at school. American Association of University Women, 2011. Available: http:// www.aauw.org/research/crossing-the-line/.

Dake, J. A., Price, J. H., & Ward, B. Prevalence and correlates of sexting behavior in adolescents. *American Journal of Sexuality Education, 7, no. 1,* (January–March 2012), 1–15.

Dalal, A. Sexual stereotypes stop females from feeling pleasure. *Sex, Etc.* (2005).

Erickson, E. H. *Childhood and society.* New York: Norton, 1950.

Few pediatricians offer routine sexual health services for teens. National Partnership for Women and Families, 2014. Available: http://go.nationalpartnership.org/site/News2?abbr =daily4_&id=45595&security=1521.

Finer, L. B., & Philbin, J. M. Sexual initiation, contraceptive use, and pregnancy among young adolescents. *Pediatrics, 131,* 5 (2013), 886–891.

Finkelhor, D., Turner, H. A., Shattuck, A., & Hamby, S. L. Violence, crime, and abuse exposure in a national sample of children and youth. *JAMA Pediatrics, 167,* 7 (2013), 614–621.

Friedrich, W. N., Fisher, J., Broughton, D., Houston, M., & Shafran, C. R. Normative sexual behavior in children: A contemporary sample. *Pediatrics, 101, no. r* (April 1998), e9.

Giedd, J. Teen brains: Still under construction. Parents play important role. *NIH News in Health* (September 2005). Available: http://newsinhealth.nih.gov.

Goldstein, H. Making movies, mastering the media. *Teenwire .com,* (November 18, 2005).

Grunbaum, J., et. al. Youth Risk Behavior Surveillance—United States, 2003. *Surveillance Summaries, Morbidity and Mortality Weekly Report, 53.SS-2* (May 21, 2004), 1–95. Available: http://www.cdc.gov/nccdphp/dash/yrbs/.

Guttmacher Institute. Can more progress be made? Teenage sexual and reproductive health behaviors in developed countries. In *Executive summary.* New York: Author, 2001, 1–6.

Hensel, D. J., & Sorge, B. H. Adolescent women's daily academic behaviors, sexual behaviors, and sexually related emotions. *Journal of Adolescent Health, 55, 6* (2014), 845–847.

Kalmus, D., Davidson, A., Cohall, A., Laraque, D., & Cassell, C. Preventing sexual risk behaviors and pregnancy among teenagers: Linking research and programs. *Perspectives*

on Sexual and Reproductive Health, 35, no. 2 (March/April 2003).

Kemper, M., & Rodriguez, M. Talk about sex. SIECUS, 2005. Available: http://www.siecus.org/_data/global/images /TalkAboutSex.pdf.

Kirby, D. B. *Emerging answers 2007: Research findings on programs to reduce teen pregnancy and sexually transmitted disease.* Washington, DC: National Campaign to Prevent Teen and Unplanned Pregnancy, 2007.

Kirby, D. B. The impact of abstinence and comprehensive sex and STD/HIV education programs on adolescent behavior. *Sexuality Research and Social Policy, 5, no. 3* (2008), 18–27.

Kirby, D. *Do abstinence-only programs delay the initiation of sex among young people and reduce teen pregnancy?* Washington, DC: National Campaign to Prevent Teen Pregnancy, 2002a.

Kirby, D. Effective approaches to reducing adolescent unprotected sex, pregnancy, and childbearing. *Journal of Sex Research, 39, no. 7* (2002b), 51–58.

Kirby, D., Lepore, G., & Ryan, J. Executive summary: Sexual risk and protective factors, in *Putting what works to work,* ETR Associates (September 2005).

Michels, T. M., Kropp, R. Y., Eyre, S. L., & Halpern-Felsher, B. L. Initiating sexual experiences: How do young adolescents make decisions regarding early sexual activity? *Journal of Research on Adolescence, 15* (2005), 583–607.

Mitchell, K. J., Finkelhor, D., & Wolak, J. The Internet and family and acquaintance sexual abuse. *Child Maltreatment, 10, no. 1* (February 2005), 49–60.

National Guidelines Task Force. *Guidelines for comprehensive sexuality education: Kindergarten–12th grade,* 3rd ed. New York: Sexuality Information and Education Council of the United States, 2004.

Nowhere to hide. Center for Research on Women, University of Memphis, 2009. Available: http://www.memphis.edu/crow /sexualharassment.php.

O'Sullivan, L. F., & Brooks-Gunn, J. The timing of changes in girls' sexual cognitions and behaviors in early adolescence: A prospective, cohort study. *Journal of Adolescent Health, 37, no. 3* (2005), 211–219.

Rice, E., Rhoades, H., Winetrobe, H., Sanchez, M., Montoya, J., Plant, A., & Kordic, T. Sexually explicit cell phone messaging associated with sexual risk among adolescents. *Pediatrics,* 2012. doi: 10.1542/peds.2012-0021.

Rosengard, C., Tannis, C., Dove, D. C., van den Berg, J. J., Lopez, R., Stein, L. A. R., & Morrow, K. M. Family sources of sexual health information, primary messages, and sexual behavior of at-risk, urban adolescents. *American Journal of Health Education, 43, no. 2* (March/April 2012), 83–87.

Satcher, D. *Surgeon General's call to action to promote sexual health and responsible sexual behavior.* United States Department of Health and Human Services, July 9, 2001.

Sexual abuse. Crimes Against Children Research Center, 2011. Available: http://www.unh.edu/ccrc/sexual-abuse/.

Sexual behavior of young adolescents. *Science Says, 3* (Sep. 2003).

Sexual harassment and sexual violence in school. American Association of University Women, 2015. Available: http://www.auw.org.

Sexual health of adolescents and young adults in the United States. Henry J. Kaiser Foundation, 2014. Available: http://kff.org/womens-health-policy/fact-sheet/sexual-health-of-adolescents-and-young-adults-in-the-united-states/.

Steiner-Adair, C., & Sjostrom, L. *Full of ourselves: A wellness program to advance girl power, health, and leadership.* New York: Teachers College Press, 2006.

Teens and oral sex. *Science Says, 17* (September 2005).

Television and children. University of Michigan Health System, 2011. Available: http://www.med.umich.edu/yourchild/topics/tv.htm.

Temple, J. R., Paul, J. A., van den Berg, P., Le, V. D., McElhany, A., & Temple, B. W. Teen sexting and its association with sexual behaviors. *Archives of Pediatrics & Adolescent Medicine,* (2012), 1–6. doi: 10,1001/archpediatrics.2012.835.

The issue of child sexual abuse. Darkness to Light, 2015. Available: http://www.d2l.org/site/c.4dICIJOkGcISE/b.6143427/k.38C5/Child_Sexual_Abuse_Statistics.htm.

Ventura, S. J., & Hamilton, B. E. U.S. teenage birth rate resumes decline. *NCHS Data Brief, no. 58.* Huntsville, MD: National Center for Health Statistics, 2011.

Ventura, S. J., Hamilton, B. E., & Mathews, T. J. National and state patterns of teen births in the United States, 1940–2013. *National Vital Statistics Report;* vol. 63, no. 4. Hyattsville, MD: National Center for Health Statistics, 2014.

Weinberger, D. R., Elvevåg, B., & Giedd, J. N. *The adolescent brain: A work in progress.* National Campaign to Prevent Teen Pregnancy, June 2005. Available: http://www.teenpregnancy.org/resources/reading/pdf/BRAIN.pdf.

Wind, R. *U.S. Teen birth and abortion rates reach historic lows.* Guttmacher Institute, 2014. Available: https://guttmacher.org/media/nr/2014/05/05/index.html.

Yudt, S. Masturbation myths. *Teenwire.com.* Planned Parenthood Federation of America (November 9, 2004).

Zucker, K. J., & Bradley, S. J. Gender identity and psychosexual disorders. *American Psychiatric Association Focus, 3* (2005), 598–617.

CHAPTER 14

Sexuality in Adulthood

© Gayvoronskaya Yana/Shutterstock

CHAPTER OBJECTIVES

1 Discuss the major theories of love and sexuality.

2 Describe the typical college relationship, including sexual activities.

3 Cite the factors that have led to the increase in the number of single people and the postponement of marriage.

4 Evaluate the advantages and disadvantages of cohabitation.

5 Describe the characteristics of a happy marriage.

6 Discuss the reasons for the high number of divorces.

7 Describe changes that occur during the aging process.

8 Discuss the sexuality challenges for the disabled and ill, as well as how to overcome them.

INTRODUCTION

*L*ynn and Chris first met in a small town's only junior high when they were 12 years old. By high school, they had become friends and had their first date at the homecoming dance their sophomore year. After a couple of years of dating, they lost their virginity together at age 16 years. Throughout high school, they stayed together and began planning for college and a life together.

They applied to the same colleges and entered the college where they were both accepted. The struggles of college produced many changes, but they made a conscious effort to change together. As they grew up together, they did things they perceived to be more grown-up: traveling, saving up for an apartment, and the like. During their junior year, they got an off-campus apartment in the heart of the local city.

Although they had been together for more than 5 years and were engaged, they were surprised at their parents' reactions—shock and dismay—to their living together. However, both families had had other relatives who had lived together. Lynn and Chris saw living together as a "next step" toward marriage. Why, they thought, was society so backward?

Surviving college made them more determined to pursue their dream of life together, with children and good jobs. At age 24 years, they married. Four years later, a first child was born; 3 years later, a second child. With each change, they managed to adapt. But slowly—almost imperceptibly—they realized that they were not always changing in the same ways.

As they hit full stride in their careers in their mid-30s, and their children reached school age, decisions had to be made. Holding a high-level management position that requires long hours and travel also requires support at home—with children and housework. The old saying

"Behind every great man, there's a great woman" today would be phrased as "A successful person has family support."

Lynn supported the family by working from a home office and taking care of the children—schools, homework, sick days, vacation days, doctor and dentist appointments, play dates, sports, and extracurricular activities. Chris rarely returned home from work before 7:30 P.M., worked many weekends, and traveled around the world. Conflicts developed over what was important in their lives, and, because Chris made more money than Lynn, issues concerning how to spend also arose. Chris's lack of time at home increased tensions. Eventually, Lynn discovered that Chris was having an affair with a business associate.

After considering the possibility of divorce for several years, Lynn and Chris finally proceeded—after 14 years of marriage and almost 25 years together. The children stayed with Lynn, and Chris was ordered to pay child support and alimony. Both Lynn and Chris expressed a feeling of relief after the divorce was finalized.

Lynn and Chris had a great deal of positive support from friends, many of whom had been divorced themselves. It seemed that society had begun to accept divorce. But once again, they were surprised by the reaction of their parents, who felt that they should stay together and try to work out their problems. Some things never change!

In this chapter we explore how people fall in love, then we follow the life cycle from singlehood, through cohabitation, marriage, and divorce. Finally, we take a look at sexuality and the elderly.

Love and Sexuality

What is love? How do you know when and whether you are in love, whether you are loved, or whether you love another person? These questions have been asked through the ages by young people just beginning to long for and seek intimacy outside their parental families. And through the ages love has never grown any easier to define. There are many types of love—love of one's parents, of a friend, of a pet. Perhaps the most difficult sort of love to describe is love of a person with whom one could potentially share a sexual relationship.

Theories About Love

Love may take a variety of forms, as Greek philosophers long ago demonstrated: *eros*, passionate and/or erotic love; *agape*, a selfless, giving love; *storge*, affectionate love, usually of the type parents have for their children; *ludus*, playful love (partners keep the relationship at a distance by keeping love at a game level); and *mania*, a love consumed by emotional extremes such as misery, possessiveness, and jealousy.

Erich Fromm presented his ideas about love in *The Art of Loving* (1956). He distinguishes brotherly love, motherly love, erotic love, and self-love.

Passionate love is characterized by almost total absorption in another person.

He believes that loving is an art—something that must be learned and practiced. Fromm indicated that immature love is characterized by a dependent relationship between two people, and mature love is characterized by care, responsibility, respect, and knowledge of the loved person. He defines erotic love as a craving for total union with another person that is exclusive and enduring.

Abraham Maslow distinguished between B-love and D-love (1968). Those who experience B-love (short for *Being* love) are unselfish in their love for another; those who experience D-love (short for *Deficiency* love) are selfish and have a strong need for love.

Rempel and Burris (2005) suggested that love is a motive based on the valuing of the other person, and is associated with the goal of preserving or promoting the other's well-being. They said that intense, powerful emotions may serve as eliciting experiences for different types of love. Benefitting the other person can be an ultimate goal for the various forms of love.

Types of Love

Love takes many forms and can be distinguished as romantic love or conscious love. Romantic love, also known as passionate love, is characterized by almost total absorption in another, with strong feelings of elation, sexual desire, anxiety, and arousal. This form of love is often accompanied by physiological reactions—perspiration, stomach churning, blushing, and increased pulse rate.

Intense, passionate love is most likely to occur early in a relationship. At this point people often overlook faults, avoid conflicts, and ignore logic and reasoned consideration. Conscious love, in contrast, is a more realistic view of another person. We see both the strengths and weaknesses of the loved one and do not depend completely on him or her to fulfill our needs and give us what we ourselves lack. The sexual activity in conscious love may be more rewarding than in romantic love because the sexual behavior communicates and expresses loving feelings. People who have an honest view of each other can enjoy giving as well as receiving. People who feel romantic (passionate) love are often intent on receiving pleasure and fulfilling their desires, rather than on giving and taking equally.

In addition to being romantic or conscious, love can take various forms—erotic, friendship, devotional, parental, or altruistic. In erotic love there is a type of biological "chemistry" that binds lovers together and leads them to form a binding relationship. Individuals experiencing erotic love are preoccupied with their love and constantly think about their partner. Erotic love becomes less intense as time goes on, but even at a lower level it can be a positive part of a relationship.

Friendship involves deep and intimate feelings, but these are not physical. The Greek term for this type of friendship or liking is *philia*. Although there are many similar attitudes and feelings among lovers as well as friends, lovers tend to differ from friends in sexual intimacy, exclusiveness, and fascination. Men and women can be friends without becoming sexually involved.

Devotional love does not involve physical contact and is a very specific kind of love. This type of love is most likely to be directed to a god, a country, an ethnic group, or other significant groups or institutions.

Parental love can be intense, but the feelings are different from other forms of love. Infants and children learn this type of love through holding and touching—even very early in life. For some people, parental love represents the most intense form of love they will ever feel.

Altruistic love is a generous giving of the self. Some say this is a special form of parental love; it is seen in people who spend great amounts of time doing church work, volunteering in hospitals, and

FIGURE **14.1** Sternberg's triangular theory of love.

Source: Reproduced from Sternberg, Robert J. (1986). A triangular theory of love. *Psychological Review, 93, no. 2,* 119–135. American Psychiatric Association. Reprinted with permission.

assisting others in a variety of ways. Some people who work in helping professions—for example, as therapists or teachers—might find they have a great capacity for altruistic love.

Sternberg (1986) proposed a triangular theory of love suggesting that there are three components of love: intimacy, passion, and decision/commitment. These components can be visualized as points on a triangle (Figure 14.1); the triangle metaphor is used to show how a couple can be matched or mismatched in the love they have for each other. The top of the triangle is intimacy, which is the emotional component of love, according to Sternberg. Here are feelings of mutual understanding, bondedness, willingness to share, giving of emotional support, and valuing of the other person as part of your life. Passion is the motivational drive of love that includes physical attraction, sexual relations, and romance. Passion can usually differentiate romantic love from love in a friendship or of a family member. This component is usually first in a relationship but is also the first to fade. Passion and intimacy are interwoven and one may precede the other, depending on how the relationship begins.

Decision/commitment is the cognitive component of the triangle, as one makes the decision to love the other person and then makes the long-term commitment to maintain the relationship.

Perfectly matched involvements of partners exist when the vertexes of the triangles are equally matched and are at the same level. Closely matched couples may be slightly off on one of the components, and this is usually not a perilous situation. Moderately mismatched partners exhibit mismatching at one or two of the vertexes and the partners are at different levels within those components. For example, they may be equally matched on the passion vertex, but one partner is slightly more committed and has greater feelings of intimacy than the other. A severely mismatched couple is one whose partners may be equally committed but are very disparate in the passion and intimacy components.

This theory of love may help partners determine whether they are on the right track in their relationship and may help diagnose any problems.

Sternberg (1988) has outlined eight types, or phases, of love based on his triangular model. They are listed in Table 14.1.

Characteristics of Romantic Love

Because we are focusing on human relationships and sexuality in this text, it is appropriate to consider briefly the characteristics of romantic love—companionship, intimacy, caring, commitment, sexual activity, and romance. Companionship involves sharing experiences and receiving emotional support from each other. At first this characteristic

---

TABLE 14.1

Sternberg's Types (Phases) of Love

1. **Nonlove:** All three components of love are absent. Most personal relationships are of this type.

2. **Liking:** Intimacy is present, but passion and commitment are not.

3. **Infatuation:** There are passionate desires, but intimacy and commitment are not present. This is a kind of "love at first sight."

4. **Empty love:** Commitment exists, but passion and intimacy are missing. Relationships that once had passion and intimacy can become stagnant.

5. **Romantic love:** There is no commitment, but there is passion and intimacy.

6. **Companionate love:** A combination of intimacy and commitment exists, but passionate attraction has died down. The relationship becomes a kind of committed friendship.

7. **Fatuous love:** Passion and commitment are present, but intimacy is not. This type is associated with whirlwind romances and "quickie marriages."

8. **Consummate love:** This is the complete measure of love involving passion, intimacy, and commitment. It can be very hard to achieve this type of love, and even harder to maintain it.

Source: Data from Sternberg, Robert J. (1986). A triangular theory of love. *Psychological Review, 93, no. 2,* 119–135.

Intimacy means sharing thoughts and feelings with someone we consider very special.

might not seem as exciting as some of the others, but over time it can be enduring and very necessary.

Intimacy involves sharing thoughts and feelings with a person who is considered very special. Whereas traditionally women and not men revealed their innermost thoughts, in recent years there is a tendency for both sexes to disclose highly personal feelings within a relationship.

Caring is the desire to do things for another person without expecting anything in return. As in most other aspects of a relationship, balance is important. For example, it is possible to think of situations in which there is so much caring that the relationship is completely one-sided.

Commitment means pressing on with a relationship even during difficult times. When conflict or problems exist, commitment is needed to give other aspects of love a chance to grow.

Sexual activity sometimes seems to be the major part of romantic love; however, there are many couples who love each other but have a minimal amount of sexual activity. Sexual activity alone, even when highly pleasurable, is not enough to maintain a poor relationship. There does seem to be a connection between sexual activity and positive relationships, but a good relationship probably has a positive influence on sexual activity, rather than the converse.

The decision to participate in sexual activity can be very simple for some people, and very complicated for others. Sexual activity can have different meanings for different people. It can be a validation of deep intimacy in a relationship, it can be a way to help get to know another person, it can be done to promote reproduction, it can reduce sexual tension, it can produce excitement and risk, and for some it can be a form of recreation.

For many college students it is helpful to base decisions about sexual activity on their values. Some students may have clear guidelines based upon what they have learned from their family, their religion, or their peers; others may not have such guidelines. In either case it may be wise to consider personal values in life and relationships before getting sexually involved. This can mean thinking about the role of relationships and sexual activity in life at that time, which norms are most highly valued and why, and what should be done for protection against unwanted pregnancy and sexually transmitted infections (STIs) if a decision is made to participate in intimate sexual activity. Communication about these decisions with a potential partner is especially important.

The nature of love typically changes as a relationship develops. For example, the passionate or romantic love of an early stage might evolve into a companionship type of love. This does not mean that passion and romance have evaporated, nor does it mean that the relationship is not as good as before. It simply means that there are common stages of relationships, and they can all be of high quality. Relationships can be thought of as having different phases of growth. At any stage there are ways to promote better relationships.

Aron et al. (2005) reported interesting research about romantic love and related changes as relationships develop. They used MRI brain scans and studied 17 college students who were intensely "in love" from 1 to 17 months. Participants alternately viewed a photograph of their beloved and a photograph of a familiar individual. The MRI detected increases or decreases of blood flow to the brain, which reflected changes in neural activity. Based on brain activity, they found that romantic love is a biological urge distinct from sexual arousal. It is close to the neural profile of drives like hunger and drug craving. In its early stages, love can be very intoxicating and the drive for romantic love can be stronger than the will to live. With time, however, the intoxication mellows and brain scans show different findings. The scans show that different parts of the brain are stimulated later in a relationship as compared to the earlier stages. The researchers indicated that, among other processes, new love involves psychologically internalizing a lover, absorbing elements of the other person's opinions, hobbies, expressions, and character, as well as sharing one's own. The expansion of the self happens very rapidly, and it is one of the most exhilarating experiences there is.

Many have traditionally believed that romantic love fades over time and evolves into warm feelings. However, Acevedo and Aron (2009) found that long-term relationships do not necessarily kill the romance. Their research indicates long-term romantic love (with intensity, sexual interest, and engagement, but without the obsessive element common in new relationships) appears to be real and is associated with marital satisfaction, mental health, and overall well-being.

The relationship between love styles and lifetime number of sexual partners has also been explored among college students. Hans (2008) found that the number of sexual partners was positively correlated with age, romantic lovers, and game-playing lovers (who typically value fun and self-indulgence over commitment and emotional involvement), and was negatively correlated with religiosity.

Hormonal and Chemical Aspects of Love

The characteristics and types of love presented so far have been mainly based upon emotional, psychological, and spiritual kinds of feelings. Some experts argue that hormonal and chemical factors are also involved in love. One reason may be related to brain chemistry. Another relates to pheromones, which are chemical substances secreted by some animals that supposedly affect the reproductive behavior of another same-species animal.

Related to brain chemistry, during the intense passion of a developing love relationship some people report a natural high, almost as though they were on drugs. This "high" results from surging levels of three brain chemicals that allow brain cells to communicate with each other. They are similar to amphetamine drugs and cause effects such as giddiness, euphoria, and elation. As with use of amphetamines, the "high" typically does not last—perhaps because the body develops a tolerance for the chemicals just as it does for amphetamines, or perhaps because the intensity of the relationship decreases.

There are also brain chemicals that help explain why some relationships develop into long-term loving relationships. These substances, called endorphins, are morphine-like chemicals that help cause a sense of security, tranquility, and peace. These chemicals help explain why abandoned lovers may feel such a loss: They are not getting their doses of feel-good chemicals.

The topic of pheromones has received greater attention in recent years. For more than a hundred years scientists have documented the effects of pheromones on mating behavior in insects and animals. The big question has been, Do pheromones have the same effects on humans?

In 1986 Dr. Winnifred Cutler began to document the effects of human pheromones (Link & Copeland, 2001). Those who believe in human pheromones claim they send signals that are picked up by organs inside the nose. We cannot smell them, but they supposedly can have a major impact on sex drive, increase in fertility, and regulation of women's menstrual cycles. Behaviors that are reported to increase as a result of pheromones include making conversation, expressing an interest in another person, being responsive to another person, paying unsolicited compliments, overtly flirting, brushing up against another person, and becoming sexually excited.

On the basis of the concept that there are natural human pheromones, entrepreneurs developed numerous products designed to mimic the alleged effects of pheromones. These include towelettes with pheromones as well as creams and oils that are supposed to help with sexual attraction. It is too early to tell whether such products are effective—and even the basic effects of pheromones are not agreed upon by experts.

The overall biology of love is still a mystery. However, many people report that biological factors and changes seem to influence their strong feelings for another person. Obvious things like increased heart rate, slight sweating, and hormonal changes do seem to occur. For example, levels of glucocorticoids and norephinephrine can increase in the bloodstream very quickly when seeing a very attractive person. These reactions, along with the potential influence of pheromones, result in biological impacts on potential love relationships (Gonzales, 2005).

Researchers have indicated that parts of the brain respond strongly when people are around those they love romantically, brain cells make chemicals and send them to different brain regions, and love works chemically in the brain like a drug addiction.

Love Problems

With all its positive aspects, love can also create problems. Perhaps the most obvious ones are rejection, jealousy, and falling out of love. Being turned down by another person (rejection) can be difficult to experience. This can happen at various stages of a relationship, and fear of rejection is natural. Of course, as with so many other aspects of life, obtaining the many positive benefits of a relationship always entails a gamble (such as the possibility of rejection). Dealing with rejection can be difficult for some, but often it simply involves trying again. If a strong relationship already exists, it might be wise to use good communication skills and talk about the rejection with the other person. Couples counseling can help single and married couples. At any rate, rejection can also be used as a learning experience to help in future relationships.

Some jealous feelings are probably natural, but jealousy is also a bothersome feeling that can get in the way of good love relationships. It can be helpful to understand why jealous feelings occur, to use good communication skills to talk about jealousy within a relationship, and to avoid doing things that might contribute to a partner's jealous feelings. For some, effective means of coping with jealousy are thinking about one's positive qualities, selectively ignoring some activities that might be upsetting, and simply containing feelings of jealousy. It might be wise to recognize jealous feelings and accept and deal with them as part of an overall relationship.

Related to love problems, Amber Vennum studied couples in cyclical relationships—the term used for a couple who breaks up and then gets back together. She said that with college-age people, about 40% are currently in a relationship where they have broken up and gotten back together. Generally, the results of getting back together were less than desirable. Couples in a cyclical relationship tended to be more impulsive about major relationship transitions—like moving in together, buying a pet together or having a child together. As a result, they tended to be less satisfied with their partner, had worse communication, made more decisions that negatively affected the relationship, had lower self-esteem, and had a higher uncertainty about their future together. Couples often said they had gotten back together because they believed their partner had changed for the better or that communication had improved, but the results indicated otherwise. She said many studies show that when our relationships are poor, we don't function well. In most cases it does not make sense to get back together (Why Couples Who Have Broken Up Should Not Get Back Together: Relationships Expert, 2012).

What Causes Attraction?

Many factors contribute to attraction and falling in love. Unlike in the fairy tale in which the prince marries the commoner, in real life we are usually attracted to someone we consider attainable. This attraction differs from adolescent crushes on movie stars, sports stars, politicians, or teachers. In adulthood, we seek intimate relationships with someone who can love us in return.

Most North Americans marry someone who has the same sociocultural dimensions, someone whose race and ethnicity, religion, age, and social class are similar to their own. Why do we like people who are like us? One explanation is that doing so provides us with validation for our personality characteristics and beliefs. Similarity is a very powerful determinant of attraction.

It may be hard to deal with feelings if you are attracted to someone who is in a relationship with another person.

Gender also plays a role in mate selection. Researchers interviewed more than 9,000 young adults (males and females), all in their 20s, who lived in 33 countries. Subjects were given a list of 18 traits and asked to rank them in terms of most (1) to least (18) desirable in a potential mate (Buss et al., 1990). The results are listed in Table 14.2.

TABLE 14.2

Ranking of Desirable Traits in a Partner (Male and Female Combined)

1. Mutual attraction (love)
2. Dependable character
3. Emotional stability and maturity
4. Pleasing disposition
5. Good health
6. Education and intelligence
7. Sociability
8. Desire for home and children
9. Refinement, neatness
10. Good looks (ranked higher by males)
11. Ambitious and industrious
12. Good cook and housekeeper
13. Good financial prospects (ranked higher by females)
14. Similar education
15. Favorable social status or rating
16. Chastity (ranked higher by males)
17. Similar religious background
18. Similar political background

Buss and associates found a gender difference as well: Males in all cultures in the study placed an emphasis on youthfulness and attractiveness. Data showed that at the time of marriage, the average male was 2 to 5 years older than his partner. Women, however, placed an emphasis on mates who were somewhat older, had better prospects for financial security, and were industrious. Buss explains the difference in terms of evolutionary needs: Males select younger, physically attractive women because such characteristics are viewed as good indicators of reproductive success. Women select older, more established males because such characteristics are viewed as good indicators of security for their offspring (Buss, 1994).

Attraction, then, can be caused by many characteristics. Features such as height, eye color and size, size of body parts, skin characteristics, musculature, and body symmetry can all play a role for some people. Related to all of this is the waist-to-hip ratio. It is determined by dividing your waist measurement by your hip measurement. For example, a ratio of 0.7 might be considered desirable for a female, while a ratio of 0.9 might be desirable for a male. The hips are measured at the widest part of the buttocks, and the waist is measured at the smaller circumference of the natural waist, usually just above the belly button. Research indicates that people with "apple-shaped" bodies (with more weight around the waist) face more health risks than those with "pear-shaped" bodies who carry more weight around the hips. It has also been found that in most cultures waist-to-hip ratio is viewed as a measure of attractiveness and health for men and women (Singh, 2002).

Whatever causes attraction, it is interesting that many of us have a "love-is-blind bias" (a tendency to perceive romantic partners as more attractive than the self). For example, Swami (2009) found that both gay men and lesbians rated their partners as significantly more attractive than themselves. The author called this a "robust positive illusion in self–partner perceptions."

Sexuality During the College Years

Before the late 1960s, there were strict rules on campuses about men's and women's socializing. Older readers may remember the "one foot on the floor" rule: Women were allowed to have men in their college dorm room only with the door open and only with each person's having one foot on the floor. Curfews were common. Coed dorms were nonexistent. Today, most campuses have long given up these types of rules.

Since 2000, the American College Health Association (2014) has conducted the National College Health Assessment every fall and spring term. Some of the questions relate to sexual behavior, and more than 30,000 college students respond each term. Here are highlights from the most recent findings:

- 22.9% of respondents had ever been tested for HIV infection.
- 16.2% of sexually active women had used emergency contraception within the last 12 months.
- 1.4% of females and 1.5% of males who had vaginal intercourse within the 12 months had become pregnant unintentionally or had gotten someone else pregnant unintentionally.
- 45.5% of students had oral sexual activity in the past 30 days.
- 49.2% of students had vaginal intercourse in the past 30 days.
- 5.2% had anal intercourse in the past 30 days.
- 29.6% had no sexual partner, 44% had one sexual partner, 10.1% had two sexual partners, 6.2% had three sexual partners, and 10.1% had four or more sexual partners in the past 12 months.
- Using a condom within the last 30 days (mostly or always) was reported by 50.7% of those who had vaginal intercourse and 27.2% of those who had anal intercourse.
- The most common forms of birth control used by students or their partners the last time they had vaginal intercourse were male condoms (61.8%), birth control pills, (62.4%), and withdrawal (29.3%).

It is interesting that in general respondents thought that their college peers were participating in much more sexual activity than they actually were. This reminds us that perceptions of other people's sexual behavior are often not accurate.

Seventeen Magazine and the National Campaign to Prevent Teen and Unplanned Pregnancy partnered to conduct a survey of 1,200 15- to 22-year-old males (*What teen guys really think about sex*, 2015). The survey asked the participants how they think and feel when it comes to sexual activity and hooking up. The results were surprising to some people. Notably, teen boys are not all sex-crazed players—most said they were looking for love and relationships instead of casual hookups. Sixty-six percent said they could be happy in a sex-free relationship, and 54% would rather give up sexual activity for a month than give up the Internet for a month. Seventy-five percent would choose to wait to lose their virginity to someone they love than to lose their virginity as soon as possible.

The guys in this survey also said they were confused about sexual activity—both physically and emotionally. There is a huge need for accurate information and more communication. Seventy percent were confused about what a girl expected from them after sexual activity, and 63% were confused about what was pleasurable for a girl. Forty-two percent did not know that a girl can get pregnant during her period, and 34% did not know that using two condoms at the same time is not more effective than just wearing one. Finally, guys felt under tremendous pressure to have sexual activity. They walked a line between what they wanted and what they felt was expected of them. For example, 78% said there is far too much pressure from society to have sexual activity, and 21% had been pressured by a girl to go further sexually than they desired. Sixty percent admitted they had lied about something related to sexual activity, such as how far they had gone in an encounter or how many sexual partners they had (often to appear cooler or more experienced).

Although there can be many motivations to participate in sexual activity, Oswalt (2010) surveyed 422 college students to determine their main motivations. She found that physical gratification was the most constant reason for them to engage in sexual activity.

Something that might relate to relationships and sexual activity is who pays for dates (*Who pays for dates*, 2014). Survey data from more than 17,000 participants were collected to examine this age-old question. Conventional ideas have dictated that on a "date" the man pays, whereas egalitarian ideals suggest sex should not determine who pays. Most men (84%) and women (58%) reported that men pay for most expenses even after dating for a while. More than half (57%) of women claimed they offer to help pay, but many (39%) confessed they hope men will reject their offers to pay. Nearly 44% of women were bothered when men expected women to help pay. Nearly two-thirds of men said that women should contribute to dating expenses, and many felt strongly about that. Nearly half of men (44%) said they would stop dating a woman who never pays. A large majority (76%), however, reported feeling guilty accepting women's money. In terms of actual behavior, 40% of the men and women agreed that dating expenses were at least partly shared within the first month after they began a dating relationship, and 74% of men and 83% of women reported sharing expenses by 6 months into the relationship.

Types of Relationships

The Institute for American Values (Mulhauser, 2001) interviewed 1,000 college women and reported that dating among college students was all but dead. Apparently, college students either participate in random hookups or are in a very serious relationship. For many, there is nothing in between. Hooking up does not have to mean having sexual intercourse. In fact, 39% of the respondents were virgins. Dating, however, was not reported to be very common. One-third of the women said they had been asked on two or fewer dates. Of the seniors interviewed, only 50% said they had been asked on six or more dates since college started. Because few people are asking for dates, what is left is an informal hookup.

The attitudes of high school seniors about marriage and family life can help us understand which thoughts might be influencing the sexual behavior of college students. In one study, 80% of girls and 72% of boys said having a good marriage and family life is "extremely important. This proportion has been relatively stable since the mid-1970s. In addition, 62% of girls and 56% of boys said it is very likely they will stay married to the same person for life. At the same time, there is widespread acceptance by high school seniors of nonmarital lifestyles. Only 30% of girls and 39% of boys agreed that most people will have fuller and happier lives if they choose legal marriage rather than staying single or just living with someone—a belief that runs contrary to the empirical evidence, which consistently indicates the personal and social benefits of being married compared to staying single or just living with someone. Finally, 56% of the total group agreed that having a child without being married is experimenting with a worthwhile lifestyle or

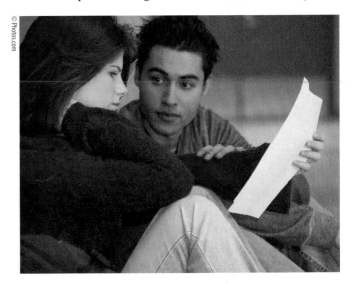

Some researchers indicate that dating among college students is almost dead. Many seem to participate in random hookups or very serious relationships instead.

not affecting anyone else. It seems that overall, high school seniors believe marriage and family life are very important, but they are increasingly accepting of nonmarital lifestyles that seem to counter those goals (Social indicators of marital health and well-being, 2012).

Overall there has been an increase in "casual" sexual relationships among high school and college students (Surveys show change in attitudes toward sex among high school and college students, 2003). Thirteen hundred Ohio seventh- to eleventh-grade students were interviewed about dating, relationships, and sexual activity. About 55% had engaged in intercourse and one-third of those had engaged in intercourse with "someone whose attachment went no further than friendship." The study also reported a significant shift in attitudes toward oral sexual activity, noting that respondents consider it "an acceptable alternative" to intercourse and different from sexual intercourse. The proportion of young adults who have engaged in oral sexual activity has risen; one-third of 15- to 17-year-olds and two-thirds of 18- to 24-year-olds have engaged in oral sexual activity.

Some people have wondered whether relationships that begin as "hookups," "friends with benefits," or casual dating are less satisfying and rewarding than serious sexual involvements. Paik (2010) found that couples who start a relationship based on physical interaction may be less satisfied in the long run than those who delay sexual activity. However, he also pointed out there are people who are mainly interested in sexual activity and people who are mainly interested in long-term relationships. Perhaps this is the reason that the people who delay sexual activity also have more relationship satisfaction. In other words, it might have been the type of people selecting certain relationships and not the timing of the sexual activity that made a difference in relationship satisfaction.

The term "hooking up" can be very vague. In your authors' human sexuality classes we often ask students in the class to define the term. There is never much agreement about what the term means. Some have said it can be anything from kissing on the dance floor to going to someone's room and having various sexual activities and spending the night. It is interesting that the term is used so commonly with little consensus about its meaning. It is also interesting that studies of young adults in the United States have indicated a rise in casual relationships based on sexual activities, but at the same time other studies have shown an increase in the number of young adults who say they are virgins (Studies show shifting paradigm of sexual relationships among young adults, 2011).

It is difficult to know for sure how the "hookup culture" compares to the behaviors of college students in earlier cultures. Interestingly, Monto and Carey (2014) found that college students from the current era did not report more sexual partners since age 18, more frequent sexual activity, or more partners during the past year than respondents from an earlier era (1988–1996). Indeed, these researchers found no evidence of substantial changes in sexual behavior that indicated a new or pervasive pattern of nonrelational sexual activity among contemporary college students.

There are also differing opinions about the effect of sexual activity in such "hookup" relationships. Bersamin et al. (2014) looked at a sample of more than 3,900 college students. A greater percentage of men (18.6%) compared to women (7.4%) reported having casual sexual activity in the month prior to the assessment. The researchers found that casual sexual activity was negatively associated with well-being and positively associated with psychological distress. They concluded that engaging in casual sexual activity may elevate the risk for negative psychological outcomes.

 Did You Know ...

Some people suggest that there is intense pressure on college students to practice unhealthy behavior. They also believe that some of this pressure may stem from environmental factors on campus. For example, many campuses are characterized by mixed-sex dorms, high-risk health behaviors, and insufficient monitoring of sexual behavior by parents and college personnel. In addition, it is common to see ads for sex-toy sales, "fetish" fairs, and other sexually oriented activities on campus.

Others are concerned that "hanging out" and having "friends with benefits" can be problematic. They point out that it would be healthier to return to more traditional dating instead of engaging in these more casual behaviors.

How do you feel about this issue? Does the college campus environment contribute to sexual behavior problems? Is there anything you would change about the environment related to sexuality?

Relatedly, Furman and Collibee (2014) found that for all types of nonromantic partners, more frequent sexual activity was associated with more substance abuse and risky sexual behavior. Women's sexual activity frequency with a nonromantic partner was more commonly associated with poorer psychosocial adjustment than such activity by men. In addition, Willoughby et al. (2014) found that waiting to initiate sexual intimacy in unmarried relationships was generally associated with positive outcomes. Individuals who reported early sexual initiation reported increasingly poorer outcomes.

College students, and others as well, can now explore dating via the communication device they carry and check numerous times during the day. Traditional dating sites like eHarmony and Match.com were designed to narrow down an endless stream of potential matches to that one right fit. Many of the newer apps aimed at a younger audience, however, revel in the wide stream. Their creators developed interfaces designed to keep their user base constantly stimulated, engaged, and plugged in. In these apps, romance is boiled down to the basics. Users specify what they want and are shown corresponding photographs of nearby potential mates along with basic information imported from Facebook. They swipe right for "like" or left for "nope." When two people swipe right for each other and produce a match, they get the option to "send message" or "keep playing." There are a number of these dating apps based on a system of snap judgments that function somewhat like a game (Stampler, 2014).

Some relationships develop over the Internet. The Internet can be a useful technology for meeting potential partners and even carrying out cyber-relationships. It can even be a unique site for sexual experimentation. However, these relationships may make it difficult to be safe when pursuing personal contact with those met via the Internet. Safety strategies include seeking reliability of a person's responses by repeated questioning, conducting Google searches on the person, setting boundaries and limits on sexual activity before the in-person meeting, and relying on intuition and gut feelings. Strategies for achieving safety during in-person encounters include meeting a person by day and in public, making safe calls during the date, using personal transportation, having a friend in the area, and carrying a cell phone. Despite all these precautions, one study showed that one-third of Internet daters had sexual activity on the first personal encounter, and nearly 80% did not use a condom or question the new partner about STIs. Perhaps this was because of "accelerated intimacy" as a result of developing the relationships via the Internet (Ross, 2007).

Global DIMENSIONS

Young People, Unprotected Sexual Activity, and Trustworthy Information

As you might expect, there are a number of differences in various countries related to both obtaining sexual information and participating in sexual activity. Here are some examples:

1. It is not possible to know the quality of the education received, but it seems that about 55% of young people in Europe receive sexuality education in school. In the United States the number is 74% as compared to 78% of young people in Latin America and 76% in Asia Pacific.

2. About 20% of the respondents said that their school does not provide an environment that is comfortable for questions and discussions about sexuality and intimacy.

3. Forty-two percent of respondents in Asia Pacific and 28% in Europe said they could not get contraception when they needed it because they were too embarrassed to ask a healthcare professional.

4. In recent years the number of people having sexual intercourse without contraception with a new partner has increased by 111% in France (from 19% to 40%), 39% in the United States (from 38% to 53%), and 19% in Great Britain (from 36% to 43%).

5. In Egypt a little more than one-third of men and women think that bathing or showering after sexual intercourse is an effective form of contraception.

6. More than a quarter of people in Thailand and India think that having sexual intercourse during menstruation is an effective way to prevent a pregnancy.

Source: Data from The "Clueless or Clued Up: Your Rights to be Informed About Contraception" Survey, 2011. Bayer Healthcare Pharmaceuticals. Available: http://multivu.prnewswire.com/mnr/prne/bayergroup/52124/.

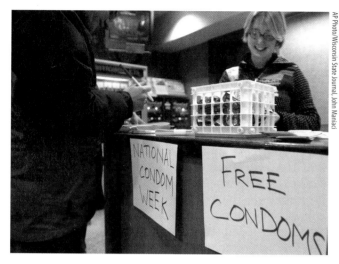

College students need to know about contraception and prevention of HIV and AIDS.

Safer Sexual Activities and College Students

Most studies of condom use among college students date from the early 1990s; the results then indicated that condom use was relatively rare. Studies found that between 15% and 41% of students reported that they always used condoms, and the more partners a person had, the lower the rate of condom use (Lewis et al., 1997). A 1998 telephone survey of college students was much more encouraging; 54% reported that they always or almost always use condoms, and 24% said that they sometimes did. Still, one in five respondents reported that he or she almost never used condoms (Survey USA, 1998). As a result, one in five males and nearly one in three college-age females were infected with an STI (Reinisch et al., 1995).

In 2004 it was found that 84% of adults between the ages of 18 and 35 said they take "necessary" steps to protect themselves against STIs, but their actions did not support their claims. Although 63% of respondents said they were "well informed" about the risks associated with sexual activity, 82% said they never use protection against STIs during oral sexual activity, 64% did not use protection during anal sexual activity, and 47% did not use protection during vaginal sexual activity. In addition, although 93% said they believed their current sexual partners did not have STIs, 33% said they had never discussed the issue with their partners. About 53% said their partners had undergone screening for STIs (Survey finds gaps between safe-sex claims, behavior among U.S. adults, 2004). Sixty-eight percent of respondents said that STI tests should be part of a routine health exam, but only 51% had ever spoken to a healthcare provider about STIs. Also, 68% did not feel concerned about contracting an STI.

Communication is the key to an honest and protected sexual relationship. Yet, most studies indicate that college students do not talk before they have sexual activity.

Planned Parenthood (2009) indicates that these are the most important ways to practice safer sexual activities:

- Understand and be honest about the risks you take.

- Keep your blood, pre-cum, semen, or vaginal fluids out of each other's bodies.

- Always use latex male or female condoms for anal or vaginal intercourse.

- Don't have sex play when you have a sore caused by an STI.

- Find ways to make safer sex as pleasurable as possible.

In addition, be aware of your body and your partner's body. Cuts, sores, or bleeding gums may all increase the risk of spreading STIs. Lubricants can increase sexual stimulation, and they also reduce the chance that condoms or other barriers will break. Of course, abstinence is totally safe. Sexual activity with just one partner is also safe as long as neither of you is infected and neither of you ever has sexual activity or shared needles with anyone else (Safer sex guidelines, 2009).

While there has been little change in the typical age when women have sexual intercourse for the first time over the past several decades, today's college students wait much longer until their first marriage and first birth compared with their counterparts born about 40 years earlier. This gap has increased from about 3 years in the past to 10 years or more today. In turn, today's college females who do not wish to become pregnant must use reliable means of preventing pregnancies for much longer periods of time prior to marriage than did women in past years (Finer & Philbin, 2014).

■ Singlehood

For most heterosexual young adults—male and female—singlehood is a temporary status. The vast majority of people eventually marry, but they are delaying marriage longer than in the past. In 1970, the median age for first marriage was 20.6 years for women and 22.5 years for men (Renzetti & Curran, 1998); by 1997, it had reached 25 years for women and 26.8 years for men (Schmid, 1998). According to the U.S. Census Bureau, it is now about 26.1 years for women and 28.2 years for men.

The Internet is one of the places to meet singles. On singles bulletin boards, singles can read extended personal ads, complete with photos. In chat rooms, singles have the opportunity to "meet" and "talk" to prospective dates in a safe environment. But be wary—experts warn that a first encounter with someone met on the Internet should be in a public place, perhaps among other friends.

While there can be variation from person to person, singles seem to delay or avoid marriage for a number of common reasons. These can include improved social attitudes toward being single, increased caution because of perceived high divorce rates, increased availability of better contraceptives, an enjoyment of freedom from unnecessary commitments, opportunities to meet new people and develop new relationships, and the desire to have a varied sex life free of guilt. Economic constraints probably also contribute to longer periods of singlehood. For example, housing prices have increased significantly at the same time that good jobs are harder to find. In addition, many who have graduated from college might have large debts as a result of college expenses.

This group has been labeled the "twixters." They aren't kids anymore, but they're not adults either. They are a new breed of young people who won't or can't settle down. The percentage of 26-year-olds living with their parents nearly doubled from 1970 to today, from 11% to 20% (Grossman, 2005). While many writers speculate that there are now many more twixters than there were in 2005 (with some estimates suggesting that as many as 50% of 26-year-olds are twixters), we do not know for sure how large this population is—we simply know it seems to have grown significantly. Instead of moving from adolescence to adulthood, some experts feel there is a new, intermediate phase of development for the twixters. They are called this because they are betwixt and between. Some who study this new life phase see it as a good thing—a chance for young people to savor the pleasures of irresponsibility and search their souls for new life paths. Others

are worried that twixters aren't growing up because they can't. They feel that the cultural machinery that used to turn kids into grown-ups has broken down. They fear that society no longer provides young people with the moral backbone and the financial means to take their rightful places in the adult world. They point out that growing up may be harder than it used to be.

The number of people who never marry has increased since 1970. This is true for both males and females and for every age group. In the United States, approximately 30% of females and 36.3% of males 15 years and older have never married. In addition, 52.1% of the population 15 years and older is not currently married. This includes 50.4% of males and 53.8% of females. There are also about 15.2 million families with a female head of household with no husband present and about 5.6 million families with a male head of household with no wife present. In terms of the unmarried-partner households, approximately 0.4% of these partnerships are same-sex couples and 5.7% are other-sex couples (*American Fact Finder*, 2015).

Some people feel that living alone is the new norm. In 1950 people living alone made up only 9% of households. But, in 2011 that number was 28%. People living alone were tied with childless couples as the most prominent residential type, more common than the nuclear family. Some people feel that living alone helps us pursue sacred modern values—individual freedom, personal control, and self-realization. It may mean that living alone is exactly what we need to reconnect (Klinenberg, 2012).

Of course, some people who are single would like to get married. "The majority of people still want to get married, but they see it sort of as dessert now, something that's desirable rather than necessary," said the executive director of the Albany, New York–based Alternatives to Marriage Project, which aims to fight discrimination based on marital status and to seek equality and fairness for unmarried people. He feels that people want to be sure that they don't make a marriage mistake. Also, societal pressures to marry before having children have decreased. About 41% of births are to unmarried women (Births to unmarried women, 2015).

Online dating, once viewed as a refuge for the socially inept and as a faintly disrespectable way to meet other people, has quickly become a fixture of single life for adults of all ages, backgrounds, and interests. Some people feel that the traditional means for getting people together are not working as well as they did previously, and that there is a need for something new. As more people choose to marry later in life, few social institutions have arisen to replace the role that local communities, families, and schools once played. The Internet is filling that need. For many, there is a disconnect between who people say they are online and what they really are like. However, many people have found success through Internet dating and feel that online dating may be making it more acceptable to openly signal what they want.

A Match.com study (2010) found that more than twice as many couples who married in a recent year met through online dating services than in bars, at clubs, and other social events combined. Seventeen percent of those who married in a recent 3-year period met online, making it the third most frequent method of introduction, behind meeting through a mutual acquaintance or at work or school. In addition, 1 out of 5 single people have dated someone they met on an online dating site.

Matchmaking has become a serious and fast-growing business. Today's matchmaking service often offers much more than just dating services; it may also act as a pal, coach, mom, and concierge. Various formats can be used to help participants get to know as many other potential dating partners as possible. Clients may pay a fee, perhaps around $1,000 to $1,500, to join for a year. They are probably guaranteed a minimum number of dates in return for the fee. If a spark is ignited, they can probably put their memberships on hold for a while. Some clients indicate that a short date with no commitment set up by someone else builds self-confidence because it minimizes the fear of rejection.

At least one company provides its clients with calling cards to give to alluring strangers they see every day. Those who get the cards can use an ID code to log in and send a message to their admirer. Some card users indicate that the cards allow them to approach people who otherwise might have been missed connections. This practice also reverses the online dating process—observe someone in person first, then send a message. Other companies are helping singles connect in different ways. For example, a cell phone's global positioning system (GPS) can be used to help users find like-minded people within a reasonable walking distance. Those who sign up for the application create basic profiles with photos and then use an instant message feature to communicate when they are within range of each other.

DatingAdvice.com had its experts thoroughly test every major dating site, and rated each based on safety, date quality, success rate, and more. The top sites were determined to be Match.com, eHarmony, Zoosk, BlackPeopleMeet.com, SeniorPeopleMeet .com, and Chemistry.com. Dating sites for seniors,

Christians, blacks, gays, and lesbians were also rated (10 best dating sites, 2015).

■ Cohabitation

Cohabitation is the situation in which people who live together and share a sexual relationship are not married. Just a generation or two ago people who lived together were said to be "living in sin"— a remark meant as religious scorn, not humor. Today cohabitation is not regarded as negatively as it used to be.

One reason for the increased acceptance of cohabitation is the vast increase in the number who cohabitate—from 439,000 in 1960 to more than 6.66 million in 2010. About a quarter of unmarried women age 25–39 were currently living with a partner of the other sex, and an additional quarter lived with a partner of the other sex in the past. More than 60% of first marriages are preceded by living together, as compared with virtually none 50 years ago. For many, cohabitation is a prelude to marriage. For others, it is simply better than living alone. For a small but growing number it is considered an alternative to marriage (Wilcox & Marquardt, 2010).

In a study conducted by Copen et al. (2013), 48% of women interviewed in 2006–2010 cohabited with a partner as a first union, compared with 34% of women in 1995. During that time, the percentage of women who cohabited as a first union increased for all Hispanic-origin and race groups except for Asian women. Seventy-percent of women with less than a high school diploma, 62% with a high school diploma or GED, 59% with some college, and 47% with a bachelor's degree or higher cohabited as a first union. First premarital cohabitations were longest for foreign-born Hispanic women (33 months) and shortest for white women (19 months). Forty percent of first premarital cohabitations among women transitioned to marriage by 3 years, 32% remained intact, and 27% dissolved. Nearly 20% of women experienced a pregnancy in the first year of their first premarital cohabitation.

Manning and Stykes (2015) examined the profile of women who had ever cohabited since 1987. The percentage of women who had ever cohabited almost doubled since 1987—from one-third of women to two-thirds of women aged 19–44. All age groups experienced an increase in the proportion of women who ever cohabited. The age group experiencing the highest level of cohabitation was women aged 30–34, of whom three-fourths had ever cohabited. The greatest increase (214%) occurred in women aged 40–44, and the smallest increase (45%) occurred to women aged 19–24. The most recent data showed that 65%

cohabitation Situation in which people who live together and share a sexual relationship are not married.

of all women had ever cohabited, including 42% of those aged 19–24, 73% of those aged 25–29, 75% of those aged 30–34, 68% of those aged 35–39, and 69% of those aged 40–44. In addition, 28% of those in current unions were cohabiting, including 65% of those aged 19–24, 37% of those aged 25–29, 23% of those aged 30–34, 15% of those aged 35–39, and 14% of those aged 40–44.

Experts disagree about the effect of cohabitation on divorce. Some believe cohabitation is a good way to avoid a bad marriage and eventual divorce. According to this perspective, cohabiting is not tied to an increased risk of divorce. Others, however, suggest that those who live together before marriage are more likely to break up after marriage.

Manning et al. (2014) pointed out that as the median age at first marriage rose from the mid-1980s to the late 2000s, the median age at first cohabitation slightly decreased, from 22.8% to 21.8% for women, and from 23.9% to 23.5% for men. In other words, even though men and women are delaying marriage until their later 20s, they are not delaying cohabitation.

Vespa (2014) found that cohabitation is becoming increasingly detached from marriage. For example, younger women are more likely to begin cohabiting with intentions to marry than are older women. For an increasing number of couples, it seems that cohabitation is no longer necessarily a "stepping stone into marriage," but rather a decision "motivated by convenience or a desire to spend time together." Vespa also observed that even if a cohabiting person may not have intentions to marry his or her particular partner, cohabitation could be part of a larger strategy to avoid divorce.

Nearly two-thirds of adults who have ever cohabited thought about it as a step toward marriage. Also, public acceptance of cohabiting couples has been increasing through the years. Most Americans now say the rise in unmarried couples living together either makes no difference to society (46%) or is good for society (9%) (Cohn, 2011).

Reasons for Cohabitation

Some people feel that cohabitation has become more acceptable because of the increasing numbers who cohabitate. Another reason for increased acceptance is that some major companies have extended "domestic partner benefits" to both LGBTQ and heterosexual cohabitors. A further reason is the availability of effective contraceptives that reduce the fear of pregnancy for those who want to live together but not start families.

Traditionally, many reasons have been given for living together. They include finding out more about the habits and character of a partner, wanting to test compatibility, avoiding the risks of being trapped in an unhappy marriage, working on personal issues before deciding to marry, and saving money.

Popenoe (2008) pointed out additional reasons why people cohabitate. He suggests that the "sexual revolution" of the 1960s gave premarital sexual activity more of a stamp of approval. Traditional norms were challenged, and relatively reliable birth control for women became available. Some men pulled back from marriage and from having children and simply lived with their sexual partners in cohabitation. Women had gained more equality in many ways and got married many years later, on average. Childbearing was also delayed, and cohabitation was a natural outcome. Also, as the number of divorces increased, people became worried about marriages going wrong. Cohabitation—rather than marriage—became increasingly popular.

Some argue that there are economic benefits to cohabitation. But it seems to play a different role in the lives of adults with or without college degrees. For the most educated, living as an unmarried couple usually is an economically positive way to combine two incomes and is a step towards marriage and having children. But for adults without college degrees, cohabitation is more likely to be a parallel household arrangement to marriage—complete with children—but at a lower economic level than married adults enjoy (Fry & Cohn, 2011).

Disadvantages to Cohabitation

Unmarried couples may experience discrimination in housing, insurance, taxes, child custody, and other areas. They may also face pressure to marry from parents and friends—who may have social and religious backgrounds different from the cohabitors'.

Some people, especially divorced people, become cohabitors because they do not want the legal and economic "entanglements" of another marriage should the relationship end. In reality, though, the legal "entanglements" of marriage can also prove to be legal "entitlements." When cohabitors break up, one partner may lose financially because of inability to prove that assets were jointly purchased. Also, if one partner dies without a will, property would pass to surviving family members—not to the intended surviving partner. For example, in Massachusetts, the property would go half to parents, half to siblings, and none to the partner. Further, if a partner is disabled or hospitalized, the cohabitor has no rights to make medical decisions and can even be legally barred from hospital visits.

After dissolution of a cohabiting relationship, formerly cohabiting men's economic standing declines moderately. However, formerly cohabiting women's economic standing declines a great deal, leaving a substantial proportion of women in poverty. This is particularly true for African American and Hispanic women (Avellar, 2005).

Are Cohabitations Successful?

Do cohabiting couples have a higher rate of success if they marry later than do married couples who did not live together first? A critical look at the body of research fails to prove whether prior cohabitors have better marriages.

In some ways, cohabitation is replacing dating. There also seems to be an increase in "serial cohabitation," or living with one partner for a time and then another. It is interesting that women seem to perceive cohabitation as a step before marriage to that partner, whereas men tend to see cohabitation as something to do before you make a commitment. Men who live with women they eventually marry don't seem to be as committed to the union as those who didn't live with their mates before getting married (Smock et al., 2005).

There is also a growing number of older Americans living together. The reasons vary, but for many it is a combination of bad experiences in previous marriages, the desire to keep their finances separate, and for some, loss of benefits if they remarry. According to U.S. Census Bureau figures, cohabitation numbers for people 65 and older tripled from 193,000 in 2000 to 575,000 in 2010.

Cohabitation seems to differ for older and younger adults. Older cohabitors report significantly higher levels of relationship quality and stability than younger cohabitors, although they are less likely to have plans to marry their partners. Reasons for cohabitation are similar, but assessing compatibility is a more important reason for younger cohabitors. Older cohabitors are more likely to view their relationship as an alternative to marriage, whereas younger cohabitors are more likely to view their relationship as a prelude to it (King, 2005).

A comparison of gay and lesbian cohabiting couples with heterosexual married couples showed that

There is contradictory research about the effects of cohabitation.

in many respects they do not differ. However, it seems that gay or lesbian partners function better in their relationships than heterosexual partners (Kurdek, 2004). According to the U.S. Census Bureau, there are almost 515,000 same-sex unmarried-partner households in the United States (Census Bureau releases estimates of same-sex married couples, 2011).

So, is cohabitation a positive or a negative thing? There are different opinions among different people. For example, some reports indicate that marriages of people who have cohabited and later marry are significantly more likely to end in divorce. Some people feel this is partly because people who choose to live together tend to be younger, to be less religious, or to have other qualities that put them at risk for divorce. Others argue that marriage is too great a commitment and prefer cohabitation.

 Did You Know . . .

The countries with the highest cohabitation rates among persons ages 20 and older are France (14.4%), Luxembourg (14%), Finland and Estonia (11.8%), Denmark (11.5%), and Norway (10.7%). Those with the lowest cohabitation rates are Turkey (0.2%), Cyprus (0.9%), Poland (1.3%), Slovak Republic (1.4%), and Greece (1.7%). The U.S. rate is 5.5%, the Canadian rate is 8.9%, and the U.K. rate is 8.7%.

Source: Partnership and prevalence of cohabitation, recent years. Organization for Economic Cooperation and Development, 2013. Available: http://www.oecd.org/els/soc/SF3_3_Cohabitation_rate _and_prevalence_of_other_forms_of_partnership_Jan2013.pdf.

They feel that the emphasis should be on the commitment between two people and that the quality of the relationship is the most important consideration. They indicate that society discriminates against people who wish to commit themselves to another person and remain unmarried.

Interestingly, cohabitation has emerged as an important precursor or alternative to marriage in many countries for a variety of reasons. Adults may look for more flexibility or freedom in their relationships, or feel they do not have sufficient financial or emotional resources to marry, or perceive marriage as a risky undertaking. On an international scale, cohabitation is rare in Asia and the Middle East. Moderate to high levels of cohabitation occur in North America and Australia, where between 8% (Mexico/United States) and 19% (Canada) of adults aged 18–49 are in cohabiting relationships. Cohabitation levels in sub-Saharan Africa vary considerably, with comparatively high levels in South Africa (13%) and low levels in Ethiopia (4%), Nigeria (2%), and Kenya (4%). High levels of cohabitation are observed in much of Europe: For example, approximately 25% of Swedish and French adults aged 18–49 years are in a cohabiting relationship. Cohabitation is most common among South Americans, where between 12% (Chile) and 39% (Colombia) of adults aged 18–49 live in cohabiting unions. Columbia has the highest level of cohabitation of any country (World Family Map, 2013).

Questions are sometimes asked about the quality of the relationships when comparing cohabiting and married couples. Brown et al. (2014) found directly married couples reported the highest relationship quality, and cohabitors without marriage plans reported the lowest marital quality. In the middle were the two largest groups: marrieds who premaritally cohabited and cohabitors with plans to marry.

Marriage

Marriage has changed over the years, but in many respects it has remained the same. June is still the most popular time to marry, more adults marry than never marry, and marriage is still a legal entity. It involves a fee to the county, a marriage license, and a marriage ceremony—either civil or religious. Although there is no legal requirement that a wife take the husband's last name, she usually does. Most Americans spend most of their lives within a marital relationship.

Although most people marry, the U.S. marriage rate—defined as the number of women's marriages per 1,000 unmarried women 15 years and older—has fluctuated. It was the highest in 1920, at 92.3. It was 76.5 in 1970, but has since declined by almost 60% to the present 31.1 rate. The proportion of women

Marriage customs vary in different cultures.

married was highest in 1950, at approximately 65%. Today, fewer than half (47%) of women 15 years and older are married. The proportion of women married has declined among racial/ethnic groups since the 1950s. This decrease has been most dramatic among Hispanic and black women, who experienced 33% and 60% declines, respectively. Presently, the racial/ethnic group with the lowest proportion married is black women (26%), and the group with the highest proportion married is Asian women (56%). Approximately 43% of Hispanic women and 51% of white women are currently married. Women with at least a bachelor's degree demonstrate the highest proportion of currently married women (60%). The group with the lowest proportion is women with less than a high school diploma (28%) (Cruz, 2013).

The trend toward older age at first marriage has been well documented. Some sources suggest that this increase in age is detrimental to marriage as an institution. They also suggest it might have negative effects such as increased exposure to the hazards of nonmarital sexual activity and childbearing, sexual exploitation, loneliness, and lack of social integration. In contrast, others argue that older age at first marriage has a very positive effect, as it seems to be an important factor in leveling off divorce rates.

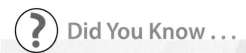

Did You Know...

The Pros and Cons of Cohabitation

Whether cohabitation is a good idea for you can depend on many factors. Some of the most commonly perceived pros and cons are listed here.

The Pros

1. You will know what you're getting into. The realities of living together will be made known.

2. You get accustomed to your partner's habits. Cohabitation allows each of you to become familiar with the other's lifestyle and foibles.

3. You develop a routine and personal space. The adjustment period during the early months of marriage should be less difficult as a result.

4. You solve a lot of practical problems. For example, you can share some of the costs.

The Cons

1. You lose the whole excitement of "being married." If you live together before being married, you will not appreciate the feeling of being married anymore once you are married.

2. You might suffer criticisms of immorality. Given that some people consider it a sin to live together before marriage, you might hear negative feedback.

3. You might just be "playing house." Some couples cohabit for convenience and then break up when they get tired of the relationship.

4. Cohabitation may put off the wedding indefinitely. Some people ask, "Why get married when everything is in place already?" Only one out of every two cohabiting couples ever gets married.

Source: Cohabitation before marriage: The pros vs the cons. *RelationshipPsychology.com*, 2015. Available: http://www.relationshippsychology.com/marriage/cohabitation-before-marriage.

The ages at which men and women marry are at historic highs—27 years for women and 29 years for men—and they seem to still be climbing. The age at which women first have children is also increasing, albeit not as quickly as the age at first marriage. The trend of delayed marriage has elevated the socioeconomic status of women, especially more privileged women and their partners, allowed women to reach other life goals, and reduced the odds of divorce. Even though women have been postponing marriage until their late 20s and beyond, they have not put off childbearing to the same extent. The median age at first birth (25.7 years) now falls below the median age at first marriage (26.5 years). Overall, 48% of first births occur to unmarried women, most of them in their 20s. This pattern is of concern because children born outside of marriage are more likely to experience family instability, school failure, and emotional problems. Most of the first births to unmarried women involve women with lower levels of education, such as high school only or some college. By contrast, college-educated women typically have their first child more than 2 years after marrying.

Overall, 35% of single men and cohabiting men report they are "highly satisfied" with their life, compared to 52% of married men. Likewise, 33% of single women and 29% of cohabiting women are "highly satisfied," compared to 47% of married women (Hymowitz et al., 2013). The question of the optimal age at which to marry, then, remains open. It seems best to wait until the early 20s at least, but how much beyond that is wise cannot be stated definitely.

There are many statistics available about marriage, and many articles are written about it. For example, we already mentioned that age at first marriage has been steadily increasing. Interestingly, the age at remarriage after a divorce has also been increasing. In addition, the number of interracial marriages has increased. Because it is clear that a majority of people choose to be married, it is appropriate to consider the attraction of marriage and marriage partners.

The Attraction of Marriage

The attraction to marriage is the result of several factors:

1. *Marriage provides companionship.* It is nice to have someone committed to spending time with you and sharing important occasions in your life.

2. *Marriage provides for emotional security.* The intimate nature of the marital relationship can help alleviate the anxieties, fears, and insecurities you experience in today's society.

3. *Marriage provides for a sexual outlet.* The knowledge that your sexual needs will be satisfied in a loving, caring relationship can be quite appealing.

4. *Marriage can improve your self-esteem.* Just knowing that you are worthy enough for someone else to marry can make you believe you are an attractive, appealing, valuable person.

5. *Marriage can provide financial security.* The addition of another wage earner, or someone who can earn money while you contribute to the partnership by doing chores that would cost money to pay someone else to do, can make you more financially able to live the life you desire.

6. *Marriage can legitimize reproduction.* If you want children and believe they will do best in a socially sanctioned family—a marriage—you may want to be married.

The benefits include legal and financial benefits ranging from family leave, health care, and parenthood to those involving taxes, property rights, and inheritance. Marriage seems to also provide a wealth-generation bonus. Married people are more likely to save money and become more economically productive. Marriage can also provide couples with an economy of scale (two can live as cheaply as one), and act as a small insurance pool against life's uncertainties such as illness or job loss. In addition, research indicates that married people are not only wealthier but happier, healthier, and having better sex lives. Married people also take fewer risks, have better health habits, and enjoy a wider social support network.

Related to the association between marriage and well-being, Musick and Bumpass (2012) examined the persistence of changes in well-being as marriages and cohabitations progress (and sometimes dissolve) over time. The effects of marriage and cohabitation were found to be similar across a range of measures looking at psychological well-being, health, and social ties. They found that while married couples experienced health gains—likely linked to the formal benefits of marriage such as shared healthcare plans—cohabiting couples experienced greater gains in happiness and self-esteem.

Obviously, marriage has numerous attractions that have made it the predominant family lifestyle. However, not all these attractions are present in all marriages, and, depending on the expectations before the marriage and on other important considerations—such as the personality traits of the partners and their love for each other—the resultant disappointments either are overlooked or are deemed important enough to cause divorce.

Choosing a Life Partner

Interestingly, when and if you choose another person with whom to form a lifelong commitment, that person will most likely be similar to you in many ways. Most people choose others of similar religion, age, social class, race, and education. When two people join together after 20 or 30 or more years of living independently of each other, they have all the problems of adjustment you can imagine. They may have to learn to eat the same foods, wake and go to sleep at the same times, and put up with each other's myriad idiosyncrasies. In other words, they have enough problems without adding still others that occur when they have different religions, social classes, educational backgrounds, and so on. It would be unfair, however, to overlook the relationships that work in spite of the partners' dissimilarities. That elusive concept, love, can do wonders with problems. However, the odds against partners of dissimilar backgrounds are greater than those for similar partners.

Although similar characteristics are important to many people when choosing a life partner, marriages between whites and blacks in the United States have increased. Thirty-five years ago just 5% of black men were married to a white woman, but that figure has risen almost threefold to 14%. The proportion of black women marrying white partners has increased from 1% to 6% during the same time (Qian & Lichter, 2011).

Over the last several decades, the American public has grown increasingly accepting of interracial dating and marriage. About 85% of millennials (those age 18–29 years) say they would be fine with a family member's marriage to a person from another racial group. The amount of support drops to about 73% among those 30–49 years, 55% among those 50–64

Married people can enjoy a wide variety of activities together throughout their marriage.

Communication
DIMENSIONS

How to Make Someone Fall in Love with You

When researchers asked people to tell the stories of how they fell in love, they most commonly cited the 11 factors listed here. Note how many of them relate to the various types of communication discussed in this book.

1. Similarity in attitudes, background, and personality traits
2. Geographic proximity
3. Desirable characteristics of personality and appearance
4. Reciprocal affection, the fact that the other likes us
5. Satisfying needs
6. Physical and emotional arousal
7. Social influences, norms, and the approval of people in our circle
8. Specific cues in the beloved's voice, eyes, posture, or way of moving
9. Readiness for a romantic relationship
10. Opportunities to be alone together
11. Mystery, in the situation or the person

Source: Barker, E. How to make someone fall in love with you. *Time.com*, June 25, 2014. Available: http://time.com/2918758/how-to-make-someone-fall-in-love-with-you/.

years, and 39% among those ages 65 and older (Almost all millennials accept interracial dating and marriage, 2010).

There has been a large increase in the approval of black–white marriages in the past five to six decades (Newport, 2013). A Gallup poll showed that 87% of Americans now approve of black–white marriage, as compared to only 4% in 1958. This is one of the largest shifts or public opinion in Gallup history. Ninety-six percent of blacks and 84% of whites approve of such marriages. Approval of black–white marriage is higher among younger Americans and lowest among those age 65 and older. Americans living in the South are slightly below average in their approval, while approval is above average in the West. Census data, however, indicate that black–white marriages remain fairly rare—such unions account for only about 1% of all married couples.

Many factors come into play when choosing a person for a relationship. For example, research has found that women who believed the men liked them a lot were more attracted to the men than women who thought the men liked them only an average amount. However, women who found the men most attractive were the ones who were not sure whether those men were into them or not. Perhaps keeping people in the dark about now much we like them will increase how much they think about us and will pique their interest (Whitchurch et al., 2011).

Stritof (2015) brought together a variety of widely used premarital inventories (http://marriage.about.com/od/premaritaltests/a/premaritaltest.htm). The purpose of such an inventory is to provide two people with an objective assessment of the potential problems and issues in their relationship. Such inventories are not designed to indicate whether the couple should get married, but rather to help them realize and deal with differences in expectations, family backgrounds, and personality traits. Ignoring potential issues could result in serious marital problems.

As noted by Rhoades and Stanley (2014), the typical relationship sequence today is radically different than it was for much of American history. In the past, especially for women, the typical sequence was courtship, which then led to marriage, which then led to sexual activity, cohabitation, and children. Today, marriage comes near the end of the line, with approximately 90% of couples having sexual intercourse before marriage and nearly 40% of babies being born to unmarried parents. Given that many partners live together before being married, couples build a lot of history, both together and with prior partners, before deciding to spend their lives together. Rhoades and Stanley wondered if the change in relationship sequence would influence the ability to have a successful marriage. To find out, they analyzed data from the Relationship Development Study (a national study to investigate romantic relationships over several years to learn how they develop and change over time). These authors looked closely at 418 new marriages and analyzed the history of the spouses' relationship. They came to three major conclusions:

1. Men and women who had sexual intercourse only with their future spouse prior to marriage reported higher marital quality than those who had sexual partners other than their future spouse. Rhodes and Stanley pointed out that this finding does not mean that sexual intercourse before marriage will doom a marriage, but rather indicates that having many partners may be risky if you are looking for a high-quality marriage.

2. How couples handle choices prior to marriage seems to matter. Rather than consciously deciding how and when to transition to the next stage of a relationship, some couples seem to slide through milestones without prior planning. Couples who ignore their relationship transitions have poorer marital quality than those who make intentional decisions about major milestones.

3. Having more guests at the wedding is associated with higher marital quality. This pattern held even when Rhodes and Stanley controlled for factors such as income and education. It may be that having community support both while dating and through the marriage is important for marriage quality.

It is wise to learn a lot about a potential marriage partner before getting married.

Promoting a Happy Lifelong Commitment

Many sources give you advice about how to be happy in a relationship. For example, here are "nine psychological tasks for a good marriage" from the American Psychological Association (2015):

1. To separate emotionally from the family of one's childhood so as to invest fully in the relationship.

2. To build togetherness based on mutual identification, shared intimacy, and an expanded conscience that includes both partners and protects each partner's autonomy.

3. To establish a rich and pleasurable sexual relationship.

4. For couples with children, while protecting their own privacy, to embrace the roles of parenthood and to absorb the effect of a baby's entrance into the marriage.

5. To confront and master the inevitable crises of life.

6. To maintain the strength of the relationship in the face of adversity. It should be a safe haven in which partners are able to express their differences, anger, and conflict.

7. To use humor and laughter to keep things in perspective.

8. To nurture and comfort each other, satisfying each partner's needs for dependency and offering continuing encouragement and support.

9. To keep alive the early romantic, idealized images of falling in love while facing the sober realities of the changes wrought by time.

Many other factors can relate to the quality of marriage. For example, Kiecolt-Glaser (2009) reported that couples whose disagreements were nastier or hostile showed large increases in stress hormones during and after an argument. Among other potential problems, it was found that women who were unhappy in their marriages had higher risks of heart and circulatory problems. This gives medical support for the need to follow the advice given previously for promoting a happy lifelong commitment.

Also, the increase in "boomerangers" can be stressful on marriages. These are people who are young adults or even in their 30s or 40s who move back in with their parents. This practice commonly occurs for economic reasons, and it can cause tensions for both the older and younger generations. Suggestions for dealing with this situation include talking about expectations, building in privacy for all concerned, sharing household expenses, realizing that the house is the property of the parents (grandparents?), and being realistic about expectations (Koss-Feder, 2009).

Fortunately, there seems to be increased attention given to promoting healthy marriages and relationships. One example was explained in "Facilitating Forever" (Hawkins & VanDenBerghe, 2014). This report documented federal and state policy experiments designed to help couples form and sustain healthy relationships and enduring marriages. A strategic set of relationship education activities was advocated, including the following measures:

• Relationship literacy education for youth and young adults to help them avoid the dangerous detours that make it difficult to form healthy marriages

- Relationship development education for cohabiting couples and unmarried parents with aspirations for marriage to help them assess and improve the prospects for successful relationships

- Marriage preparation education for engaged couples to help them strengthen the foundation for an enduring marriage

- Marriage maintenance education for married couples to counter the forces of marital disorder

DiBenedetto (2014) suggested 10 rules to make a relationship last. Here are some of them:

- Start the day with a small kindness. Think: *What can I do to make his or her day just a little happier?*

- Remember that being close does not mean you are the same. Everyone has his or her own ideas about the world. The other person is still another person.

- Nurture the friendship. Many things will challenge relationships, but an abiding friendship is at the basis of a solid marriage.

- Surround yourself with happy couples. Success imitates success.

- Repeat back to each other. Disagreements often happen because we do not understand where the other person is coming from.

- Divvy up chores based on your strengths. Sharing is necessary.

- Take breaks. If conflict occurs, there is a Chinese saying, "Take a step back, and you can see the whole sky."

- Know that there is always more to learn. A relationship is a process. You never get there; you are always in process. Maintaining a relationship is often a lot of work.

Types of Marriage

In some states couples who have lived together for a specified period and who have represented themselves as married are recognized as legally married. These associations are called **common-law marriages**.

common-law marriage The recognition by some states that couples who have lived together for a specified period and have represented themselves as married are in fact legally married.

nuclear family A father and mother and their children.

peer marriage Relationship in which partners have equal status.

A **nuclear family** is usually defined as a father and mother and their children. According to the U.S. Census Bureau, there were 1.3 million fewer nuclear families in the United States in 2010 than in 2000. Not all parts of the country changed in the same ways. Two-thirds of the decline came in only eight states, seven of which are in the Northeast and Midwest. Nuclear families account for about one-fifth of all households (Francese, 2011).

Peer marriages are relationships in which couples have worked out at least a 60–40 split on child rearing, housework, and control of discretionary funds and consider themselves equal. Most partners in peer marriages work outside the home. Partners in peer marriages require lots of honesty, a dedication to fair play, flexibility, generosity, and maturity.

Related to peer marriages, the past 40 years have seen the emergence of the working mom, the supermom, the soccer mom, and—because full-time motherhood is often considered a choice rather than a given—the stay-at-home mom. The title of "dad" has rarely been linked to a modifier. However, the majority of men today are vastly more involved in the rearing of children and maintenance of households than their fathers ever were. In straining to manage responsibilities at work and at home, many men say they don't feel an adequate sense of control in either realm. As with women of a generation ago, men are experiencing the notion of a second shift, and they are doing so in a shaky economy. They must contend with buyouts, layoffs, mergers, and a need to keep up with changing job skills. There is sometimes also uncertainty in men's roles at home.

According to the American Time Use Survey done by the Bureau of Labor Statistics, on an average day in all types of marriages combined 83% of women and 65% of men spent some time doing household activities such as housework, cooking, lawn care, or

Wavebreak/iStock

Some couples like to do online inventories and questions about relationships to learn more about themselves and each other.

financial and other household management. On the days they did household activities, women spent an average of 2.6 hours on such activities and men spent 2.1 hours. On an average day, 19% of men did housework, such as cleaning or doing laundry, compared with 49% of women. Forty-two percent of men did food preparation or cleanup, compared with 68% of women. However, married men and women with full-time jobs have almost equal total workloads, with or without children younger than age 18 (American Time Use Survey, 2014).

About 20% of American women end their childbearing years without having a child, compared with about 10% in the 1970s. Childlessness has risen for all racial and ethnic groups and most education levels. It has fallen for women with advanced degrees. Various reasons have been given for an increase in childlessness. They include decreased social pressure to bear children and more recognition of the decision to have children as an individual choice. Also, improved job opportunities for women and improved contraceptive methods have created alternatives for women who choose not to have children (Livingston & Cohn, 2010).

Sandler (2013) pointed out interesting information about childless couples. About 1 in 5 American women ends her childbearing years maternity free, compared with 1 in 10 in the 1970s. The proportion of women ages 40 to 44 who have never given birth grew by 80% over the same period, from 10% to 18%. Of these women, 49% are voluntarily childless. Women who choose not to become mothers are finding they can lead a fulfilling, childless life. They have invented a new female archetype, one for whom having it all does not mean having a baby. American women expecting to remain childless include 1 in 8 with high incomes, 1 in 14 with middle incomes, and 1 in 20 with low incomes.

An increasing number of children live in a **stepfamily**. Stepfamilies can be more complex than the families of first marriages, but, contrary to myth, stepfamilies have a high rate of success in raising healthy children. Stepkids seem to be very resilient. Their major source of problems is parental conflict left over from a first marriage. Stepfamilies experience most of their troubles in the first 2 years; after 5 years, stepfamilies are more stable than first-marriage families, because second marriages are generally happier than first marriages. Stepfamilies are not just make-do households limping along after loss. All members experience real gains, notably the opportunity to thrive in a happier relationship.

Some people choose a **same-sex marriage**. Because of differences in laws and opinions related to same-sex marriage, it is difficult to get accurate information about such relationships. However, the U.S. Census Bureau indicated that there are almost 132,000 same-sex married couple households and about 515,000 same-sex unmarried partner households in the United States (Census Bureau releases estimates of same-sex married couples,

stepfamily A family with children that is formed as a result of remarriage.

same-sex marriage A marriage between two people who perceive themselves to be of the same sex.

2011). In 1996, when Gallup first asked Americans if they supported same-sex marriages, 68% were opposed, with 27% supporting it (McCarthy, 2014). Since then, support has steadily grown, reaching 42% by 2004. In 2001, support for same-sex marriage topped the 50% mark for the first time, and it reached 54% in 2014. Nevertheless, there are some dramatic divisions in opinion between age groups. For example, adults between 18 and 29 years of age are nearly twice as likely to support marriage equality as adults aged 65 or older. In 2014, same-sex marriage was supported by 78% of those 18 to 29 years old, 54% of those 30 to 49 years old, 46% of those 50 to 64 years old, and 41% of those 65 and older.

With many new marriages in the United States destined to end in divorce, an increasing number of couples are turning to prenuptial agreements to protect their assets in the event of a marital breakup. Most such agreements simply state how assets will be divided in case of divorce or death. Some people argue that prenuptial agreements contribute to marital happiness; others believe they contribute to distrust and overemphasize personal assets.

In some states, it is legal to back up marriage laws with tougher, individually designed and legally mandated divorce standards. This is called a *covenant marriage*. In this marriage style, the option of walking out is eliminated. For example, Louisiana's covenant marriage requires premarital counseling and, for divorce, 2 years of living apart plus mandated marital counseling. The goal is to make marriage more committed.

So, how does the American public feel about the changes in the structure of the family and marriage relationships that have occurred over the past 50 years? The Pew Research Center surveyed a nationally representative sample of almost 2,700 adults to answer this question. Respondents were asked whether they considered the following seven trends to be good, bad, or of no consequence to society: more unmarried couples raising children, more gay and lesbian couples raising children, more single women having children without a male partner to help raise them, more people living together without getting married, more mothers of young children working outside the home, more people of different races marrying each other, and more women not ever having children. Although views can vary on different trends, overall about a third (31%) of the subjects were "accepters," indicating that these trends make no difference to society. A similar share of the public (32%) rejected virtually every trend that the acceptors endorsed. The third group, the "skeptics" (37%) generally shared most of the tolerant views of the accepters, but expressed concern about the potential impact of the trends on society (Morin, 2011).

Building a good relationship obviously takes a lot of effort. There are sources of help for couples desiring to use them. For example, the Association for Couples in Marriage Enrichment is an organization designed to preserve and strengthen relationships.

Many experts say that the American family is in the midst of unprecedented change (Jensen, 2014). When baby boomers were children in the 1950s, 60% of U.S. families consisted of two married parents: a breadwinner and a homemaker. Today, only 20% of American children live in such a family. Instead, many couples divorce—or never marry in the first place—and form new households, raising their children as a mixture of step-siblings and half-siblings. Although the divorce rate is declining among younger couples, among older couples it has increased 50% in the last 20 years. There are definitely shifting family configurations. For example, the percentage of households consisting of a married couple and their children has decreased from 40% in 1970 to about 19% today. The percentage of adults who are married has decreased from 72% in 1960 to 51%. Births to unmarried women have increased from 5% of all births in 1960 to 42%, and the share of Americans living in multi-generational households has increased from 12% in 1980 to 17%. Fifty-one percent of men aged 18–24 lived with their parents in 2010, compared to 47% of women. Twenty-one percent of same-sex households include children, and 8.4% of all married people in the United States have a spouse of a different race.

Blended families come in many sizes and can look very different from each other.

Sexual Behavior in Marriage

Nonmarital sexual behavior has received more attention than marital sexual behavior from researchers for many decades. It still does today. While the information about marital sexual behavior is comparatively limited, it is still appropriate to consider what is known.

Today's married couples have sexual intercourse more often, experience more sexual pleasure, and engage in a greater variety of sexual activities and techniques than the people surveyed in the 1950s. There is now more precoital activity and it tends to last longer than in earlier years. Oral stimulation of the breasts and manual stimulation of the genitals have increased, as has oral–genital contact.

We can ascribe these changes to a loosening up of society in general and to the fact that even heterosexual sexual activity has come out of the closet. It is now permissible to talk about sexual behavior freely with one's partner and with others. Thus, communication between partners has become more open and honest and certainly has had an effect on their lovemaking. Women have become more aware of their capacity for and their right to sexual satisfaction through orgasm. As a result they have been assuming an active role in lovemaking and in communicating what turns them on. When their partners have responded positively, one result has been that partners spend more time exploring each other sexually, attending to each other's bodies, and experimenting with various coital positions that may better satisfy women's needs.

Many married people also masturbate. The reasons married people cite for masturbating vary. Some people masturbate when they are separated from their partner. Some do so as a variation on their sexual experience. Also some couples like to watch each other masturbate as part of their mutual sexual activity. Others masturbate because they do not achieve satisfaction with their partner and are unwilling to forgo it altogether.

The frequency of sexual interactions is a factor of age, relationship duration, and marital status. In general, married couples engage in sexual activities more frequently than singles; cohabiting couples engage in sexual activities more often than married couples (Laumann et al., 1994). Nearly 40% of married couples engage in sexual activities twice a week, compared with 25% of singles (Elmer-Dewitt, 1994).

Some people wonder whether their sex life is "normal." Statistics on sexual behavior can be misleading. For example, if a couple heard that the average married couple had sexual intercourse three times a week, they may not realize that the average includes a wide range. The frequency of intercourse might range from zero for some to 15 to 20 times a week for others. So, even if their frequency of intercourse is more or less than three times a week, their behavior is within the range of normal human

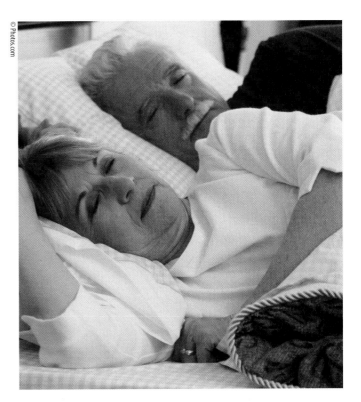

Today's married couples experience much more sexual pleasure than those of past decades.

experience. The most important consideration isn't whether their frequency and pattern of sexual activity matches some numerical average, but whether each partner is satisfied and comfortable with the sexual relationship. There should be a feeling of overall satisfaction, relaxation, and enjoyment following sexual activity.

As with other research, the data about frequency of marital sexual activity will vary in different research studies. However, it is generally agreed that the frequency of sexual intercourse in marriage tends to decrease the longer a couple is married. For example, for newly married couples the average rate of sexual intercourse is about three times per week. In early middle age, the average rate is about one-and-a-half to two times a week. After age 50 years the rate is about once a week or less. This does not mean that sexual activity is not important or that the marriage is no longer satisfactory. The decrease may be the result of biological aging, fatigue, and a decrease in sex drive. Higher levels of sexual satisfaction and pleasure seem to be found in marriage than in extramarital relationships or in singlehood.

The decline of marital sexual activity is explained by several factors. First, the "honeymoon effect" leads to the highest rates among the recently married, and those recently married tend to be younger. Second, biological aging reduces hormonal output, and poor health in general and sexual arousal

Myth (vs) Fact

Myth: Single adults have more sexual activity than married adults.
Fact: Research indicates that married adults have more sexual activity than single adults.

Myth: Liberals enjoy sex more than conservatives.
Fact: Married couples, regardless of religious or political background or past sexual history, have roughly the same amount of sexual activity. And conservative women report more frequent orgasm than liberal women.

Myth: Almost all married couples have affairs.
Fact: Only 25% of men and 15% of women report that they have had an extramarital affair.

Myth: People lose interest in sexual activity as they get older, and, by their 60s, few people are having sexual relationships.
Fact: People can have a satisfying sexual life as they age. Sexual relationships may change as a couple ages, but many couples in their 60s, 70s, and 80s report pleasurable, exciting sexual relationships.

problems increase with age. As a result, even among couples who consider their marriages to be very happy and say they are still in love, frequency of intercourse goes down with age. Third, some research indicates that the quality of sexual activity declines with marital duration and that might reduce frequency. Among married people, intercourse is more frequent among those who have happier marriages.

Related to the above, data from the National Survey of Sexual Health and Behavior (2010) also indicated that the frequency of heterosexual intercourse for married men and women tends to decline with age. For example, for 18- to 24-year-olds 83% of men and 73% of women reported vaginal intercourse at least a few times per month. However, comparable numbers for older married couples were 89% for males and 85% for females age 25–29, 80% for males and 77% for females age 30–39, 75% for males and 70% for females age 40–49, 54% for both males and females age 50–59, 45% for males and 42% for females age 60–69, and 22% for males and 21% for females age 70 and older.

Stritof and Stritof (2010) reported that 44% of married couples are fully satisfied with their sex lives. They also reported twice as many men (64%) as women regularly have orgasms and that those older than age 65 are still having sexual intercourse more than once a week. Mutual respect plays a vital role in a satisfying sex life, with 82% of those who are sexually satisfied saying they feel respected by their partner.

Also, Baron (2010) indicated that midlifers seem to be the ones most dissatisfied with their sex lives. Nearly half of 44- to 55-year-old men reported dissatisfaction with their sex lives. Just 28% of adult men

younger than age 45 felt that way, as did 17% of the 66-plus seniors. Perhaps age, expectations, and quality of the relationship can all influence satisfaction with one's sex life.

It seems that both married men and married women tend to believe that sexual activity is integral to a good marriage, and that men may be more interested in sexual activity than women. Sometimes husbands and wives experience conflict related to sexual activity and need to work emotionally to manage their own and their spouse's feelings about sexual activity (Elliott & Umberson, 2008).

One factor that can contribute to problems in marital sexual activities is timing—particularly in the years when couples are both raising children and working hard at their jobs. Married people often have sexual activities late in the evening after a long day and just before sleep. The presence of children in the family can make it hard for parents to find time to be alone. Because many people feel that a quiet and private time is necessary for sexual activities, there may be pressure to "work sex in" during the short evening.

Emotional and social issues can influence sexual activity. For example, tension and emotional distance in a relationship can be detrimental to a couple's sex life. A preoccupation with one's own appearance or that of a partner can prevent some people from initiating or responding to sexual advances. Stress and fatigue are major libido sappers. Also, with so many demands on time and attention, a couple may neglect to nurture their relationship. Chronic illnesses, commonly used medications, and emotional issues can influence sexual capacities. Even so, there are various medical treatments, counseling, and self-help techniques to address the most common types of sexual problems (*Sexuality in midlife and beyond*, 2013).

Extramarital Relationships

Despite all the media hype over the past few years about extramarital sexual activity by government officials and others, the reality is that most people are faithful to their spouses. There are probably more scientifically worthless "facts" on extramarital relations than on any other facet of human behavior. Experts point out that extramarital relations are less prevalent than pop and pseudo-scientific accounts contend. The best estimates are that 3% to 4% of currently married people have a sexual partner other than their spouse in a given year. About 15% to 18% of people have had a sexual partner other than their spouse while married. It does not seem that levels have changed much in the past 30 years. The rates of extramarital relations are about twice as high among husbands as among wives. They are also more common among African Americans, those with lower incomes, those who attend church less frequently, those who have been separated or divorced, and those who are unhappy with their marriage.

Wilcox and Marquardt (2010) indicated that marital infidelity is more common among the lower educated than among the highly educated. For example, 21% of the least educated, 19% of the moderately educated, and 13% of the highly educated had sexual intercourse with someone other than their spouse while married during the 2000s.

Because husbands are involved in extramarital sexual relations more often than wives are, presumably without their spouses' knowledge, more women may be at risk of STIs than has been thought. Research is not available on what proportion of husbands have same-sex relationships outside their marriage. However, married men and women who perceive themselves to be at no (or low) risk of STIs and HIV may, in fact, be at risk because of their partner's extramarital sexual activities.

Extramarital sexual activity can take place in two different contexts: one in which the partners have no agreement (nonconsensual context) and one in which the partners agree to have sexual relations with someone else (consensual context).

Nonconsensual Extramarital Sexual Activity
Married people engage in **nonconsensual**—and therefore usually secret—extramarital relationships for many and complex reasons. On a practical level, one's spouse may be unable to have sexual intercourse because of illness, or a couple may be separated for a long period. Thus the person deciding on an extramarital relationship does so to have sexual relations at all. But in other situations an individual might search for someone outside the marriage simply to add excitement or variety to life. Another might feel dissatisfied sexually with his or her partner and look for a more satisfactory emotional and physical relationship while maintaining the marriage. Or a person might feel drawn to someone outside the marriage by sexual attraction alone and choose to act on that attraction.

A number of forces tend to restrain or increase extramarital sexual activity:

1. Because religiously devout people tend to have lower rates of extramarital sexual activity, rising rates can be predicted from the decline in traditional religious activity.

2. Those who participate in nonmarital sexual intercourse are more likely to participate in extramarital activity, too.

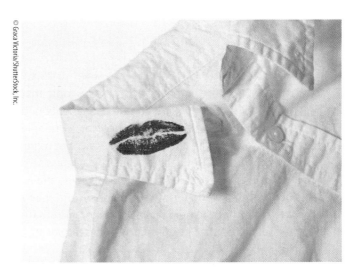

Extramarital affairs are less common than the media might lead us to believe.

3. Because women are more aware of their right to sexual satisfaction than in years past, some females are more likely to now seek sexual pleasures outside marriage.

4. The more money a person has, the greater is the opportunity for extramarital sexual activity.

5. The changing role of women in the labor force is also a factor; women who work outside the home have a greater opportunity for extramarital activity than women who do not.

Although there are cultures in which it is expected that married people will have affairs, most people in the United States say they believe in monogamy and want it in their marriage. However, two of three married couples experience an affair during their marriage, and 17% of divorces are caused by infidelity. Traditionally, more men than women take part in affairs, but women are catching up. Affairs are a sign that the wandering spouse is dissatisfied in the marriage. They can be a way of expressing pain and confusion that the person cannot verbally articulate. However, an affair does not necessarily mean that he or she wants to end the marriage. An affair can be a way of expressing that there are problems that need to be resolved (Stanton, 2001).

What are the effects of extramarital sexual relationships on a marriage? Initially, many people who learn their spouse has been having affairs feel both betrayed and emotionally devastated, especially if

nonconsensual In this context, a married person's engaging in sexual intercourse without the consent of the spouse.

Tempted by Digital Dalliances

Internet infidelity is a topic that would not have been mentioned many years ago. Not all people see Internet infidelity as a real act of betrayal, but many see this as not only real infidelity but as also having as serious an impact on the couple as a traditional offline affair.

The Internet's anonymity, convenience, and ready access to potential partners make it easy to participate in cyber-sex with other people. Cyber-infidelity occurs when a partner in a committed relationship uses a computer to violate agreements of sexual exclusivity. Internet affairs often go through progressive steps: non-sexually explicit flirting, sexual innuendo and explicit repartee, scheduling sex-laced chats, discussing sexual preferences and fantasies, simultaneous masturbation online, and planning or (in fewer cases) conducting face-to-face meetings and physical contact. Women are as likely to engage in cyber-affairs as men. For therapists, treating Internet affairs is no different than treating other affairs.

they believe their spouse to be honest, loyal, and loving. When they learn of the affair, there is a chance that the marriage will fall apart quickly. However, if the couple can talk about the situation, taking the opportunity to improve their communication and assess their own relationship, the marriage does not necessarily dissolve.

Sometimes the type of extramarital relationship has a great effect on the eventual outcome. When a spouse has engaged in a one-night stand, the other spouse might be likely to forgive and forget. If the extramarital affair was intimate, was long-lasting, and involved a strong emotional commitment, however, the other spouse may find it difficult to get over the unfaithfulness.

Consensual Extramarital Sexual Activity

There are many types of **consensual** activities; we discuss the two major ones—open marriage and swinging. **Open marriage** became publicized with the appearance of George and Nena O'Neill's book, *Open Marriage*, in 1972. The O'Neills believed that traditional marriage was too confining and limiting for the partners and that one partner could not fulfill all the intimate needs and expectations of the other. They described an open marriage as one in which the partners allow each other to have intimate and emotional relationships—sexual or nonsexual—with others. For instance, the married couple might decide that each partner is entitled to one night a week alone to engage in another intimate relationship. The idea is that this arrangement allows the married couple to grow and contribute more to the marriage. Another aspect of the open marriage is the renewable contract. The partners formally agree that extramarital relationships are permitted in the marriage and might even foster support, loyalty, and trust between partners but that the partners may change their contract regarding extramarital activity as they continue to grow. The idea here is that the agreement is flexible and renewable so that neither partner is forced to stand by a commitment that he or she no longer feels.

Swinging is the exchange of partners among married couples. (This practice used to be called *wife-swapping*, but the term lost favor with the rise of the women's movement because of its suggestion that wives were property and that men made the decisions.) All those involved participate willingly, and both partners in a marriage usually engage in it simultaneously.

Swingers object to calling this type of activity extramarital, because they view it as part of the marriage relationship. Most swingers do not want emotional involvements outside the marriage. Most often swingers find one another by advertising in tabloids or in special magazines devoted to swinging. People who engage in swinging are apparently very ordinary outside their sexual life.

Like other aspects of society, some for-profit ventures have developed related to extramarital sexual activity. For example, in 2002 the Ashley Madison Agency launched its website to the public. It is designed to promote social networking. As it says on the website, the agency deals with "risqué business." Its purpose is to cater to people who are already in relationships, but still want to date. In its first

consensual In this context, a married person's engaging in extramarital sexual activity with the knowledge and permission of the spouse.

open marriage A marriage in which partners allow each other to have intimate and emotional relationships with others.

swinging Swapping of mates for sexual activities.

3 years the agency signed up more than 500,000 members, with about 8.5 men signing up for every 1.5 women. In July 2011 Ashley Madison hit 10 million members, ensuring that it is the most popular and successful website for heterosexual married dating services. Ashley Madison Down Low has also had enormous success in breaking into the same-sex market for bisexual married men who want to have an affair with another man (Ashley Madison News, 2011).

In 2013, the website Ashley Madison, whose tagline is "Life is short—have an affair," polled its members to see where unfaithful spouses are most likely to live. The results showed that the highest number of cheaters lived in Washington, D.C.; Houston, Texas; Miami, Florida; Pittsburgh, Pennsylvania; and Los Angeles, California. Fifty-four percent of Americans say they know someone who has an unfaithful spouse. Ninety-one percent say men and women having affairs is morally wrong. If their spouse were having an affair, 61% would not forgive the partner—only 37% would forgive the cheating spouse. Fifty-five percent of currently married adults would get a divorce in the face of such infidelity, and 37% would not (Here's where all the cheating spouses in America live, 2013).

In 2014, Ashley Madison sought to discover the link between religion and infidelity by polling 105,000 of its members—60,000 in the United States. About one in four who responded described themselves as "born-again evangelist Christians" (25.1%). Catholics were the next largest group at 22.75%, followed by Protestants at 22.7% (You may be surprised at how many born-again Christians use Ashley Madison, 2014.) As of 2015, Ashley Madison had more than 15 million members.

Divorce

There are many reasons that marriages break up. Among these are greater economic independence of women, greater ease of getting a divorce, decreased stigma attached to divorce, unrealistic expectations for marriage, communication difficulties, infidelity, and feelings of incompatibility.

The current U.S. divorce rate is much higher than in 1960, but much lower than the peak rate during the 1980s. Two probable reasons for the decline in the divorce rate are an increase in the age at which people marry for the first time and the higher educational level of those marrying, both of which are associated with greater marital stability.

There are various ways that divorce statistics are given. For example, the U.S. Census Bureau indicated that in the overall U.S. population, 9.7% of males and 12.3% of females 15 years and older were divorced as

Communication difficulties are one of the major reasons for divorce.

of 2013. Those numbers had been relatively stable for several years (U.S. Census Bureau, 2013).

Another way to look at divorce statistics is the number of divorces per 1,000 population. Using this approach, in 2013 the United States had 3.4 divorces per 1,000 population. This was the sixth highest rate in the world, with Russia (5 per 1,000), Belarus (3.8 per 1,000), and Ukraine (3.6 per 1,000) being the top three. The bottom three were Australia (2.2 per 1,000), Japan (2.0 per 1,000), and Mongolia (0.7 per 1,000) (Divorce rate, 2015).

In contrast to the seeming stabilization in divorce rates for the general population over recent years, the "gray divorce rate" has increased. Married individuals aged 50 and older, including college-educated persons, are twice as likely to experience a divorce today as they were in 1990. For married individuals aged 65 and older, the risk of divorce has more than doubled since 1990. It is interesting that for younger couples (aged 25–49), the divorce rate for those with a college degree is about 50% lower than the rate for those with a high school diploma. Possible reasons for the higher gray rate include higher standards for marriage than in the past, much greater opportunities for older people to meet new partners, the reality that Americans are living longer and healthier lives, and the rise in female labor force participation, which offers women a way out of marriage that was not available in the past (Brown & Lin, 2014).

Trail and Karney (2012) wanted to separate myth from reality related to divorces among various groups. They found that people with lower incomes value the institution of marriage just as much as those with higher incomes and have similar romantic standards for marriage. However, low-income respondents were more likely than more affluent couples to say that their romantic relationships were negatively affected by economic and social issues such as money problems, drinking, and drug use. They concluded that initiatives to strengthen marriage among low-income populations should move beyond promoting the value of marriage and instead focus on the actual problems that low-income couples face.

The significant effect of divorce on family life cannot be exaggerated. The spouse who maintains custody of the children has to supervise their care, earn enough money to meet their needs, and provide, often without help, the love and affection all children crave. In addition, the divorced parent must reestablish a social life at the same time the emotional scars from the failed marriage are healing. The children may blame themselves for the divorce and must manage without the constant contact with one parent. Many experts feel that the most important factor in how divorce affects a child's life is how the parents treat each other and their children during and after the divorce.

The question of whether divorce creates long-term negative effects for children has long been debated. Some studies indicate that about twice as many children of divorced parents have emotional problems. In addition, they have greater challenges negotiating relationships once they are older, have a greater chance of choosing the "wrong" partner, and are much more likely to divorce. Critics of this research question these findings. They point out that most of the studies do not involve interviews with the children, but instead are colored by caregivers' views of how a divorce affects children. Some researchers indicate that children of divorce often have a greater sense of responsibility, independence, and maturity than their counterparts whose parents have remained together. In addition, if there has been great discord and constant fighting in the household, a divorce can provide relief to the children who have been living in that highly stressful setting.

Interestingly, children of wealthy families that come apart seem to have a bigger spike in behavior problems than children of poor families who experience the same disruption. However, wealthier children seem to benefit more from being incorporated into stepfamilies than poorer children do. The children's age when their parents separate plays a key role, with the most vulnerable age being from 3 to 5 years old. It is not known for sure why children of high-income parents have more problems after separation than children from low-income parents. It may be that fathers, who are often breadwinners,

move out of the home, leading to a dip in household income. It could also be that the children may move to a new neighborhood/school/friend group, with the ensuing instability taking a toll. Another possible explanation is that parental separation is more common among lower-income families, so perhaps they do not take the instability so hard. In such families, parents and children may perceive family changes as more normative, more predictable, and therefore less stressful (Luscombe, 2014).

Problems with the economy can also contribute to divorce. Money issues can drive a wedge between couples. They can lead couples to either withdraw from each other or attack each other about things that don't have anything to do with financial matters. Financial anxiety can lead spouses to alcohol or substance abuse, gambling, or extramarital affairs. At the same time, however, many couples may be motivated to make their marriages work. People are realizing it is more expensive to break up a family than it is to stay together.

With the share of married adults at an all-time low in the United States, some researchers have found that one of the main reasons why couples do not get married is that they fear divorce (Miller et al., 2011). Among cohabiting couples, more than two-thirds had concerns about dealing with the social, legal, emotional, and economic consequences of possible divorce. Middle-class subjects spoke more favorably about marriage and viewed cohabitation as a natural stepping stone to marriage compared to their working-class counterparts. Lower-income women, in particular, disproportionately expressed doubts about the "trap" of marriage, fearing it could be hard to exit if things go wrong or it would lead to additional domestic responsibilities but few benefits. Working-class cohabiting couples were more apt to view marriage as "just a piece of paper," nearly identical to their existing relationship.

When everything is considered, your chances of divorce may be much lower than you think. While it has been said that the national divorce rate is close to 50%, for many people the actual chances of divorce are much less. If you are a reasonably well-educated person with a decent income, come from an intact family, are religious, and marry after age 25 without having a baby first, your chances of divorce are very low indeed (Wilcox & Marquardt, 2010).

Single-Parent Families

Families with a single parent (**single-parent families**) are becoming increasingly prevalent. According to the U.S. Census Bureau, the number of single-parent families has increased greatly. In 1980, for example,

single-parent family For whatever reason, only one parent who is living with a child or children.

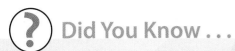

Did You Know . . .

Chances of Divorce

Most people have heard that the national divorce rate is almost 50%. While this is true for the married population as a whole, for many people the actual risk is far smaller.

The background characteristics of people entering marriage have major implications for their risk of divorce. Some percentage-point decreases in the risk of divorce or separation during the first 10 years of marriage are noted below.

Factor	Percentage-Point Decrease in Risk of Divorce
Annual income more than $50,000 (versus less than $25,000)	–30
Having a baby 7 months or more after marriage (versus before marriage)	–24
Marrying after age 25 (versus before age 18)	–24
Family of origin intact (versus divorced parents)	–14
Religious affiliation (versus none)	–14
College education (versus high school dropout)	–25

Thus, if you are a reasonably well-educated person with a decent income, come from an intact family, are religious, and marry after age 25 without having a baby first, your chances of having a divorce are very low indeed.

Source: Your chances of divorce may be much lower than you think. National Marriage Project, 2011. Available: http://www.stateofourunions.org.

Single-parent families are becoming more common.

19.5% of all households with children were single-parent households. In 1990 it was 24%, in 2000 it was 27%, in 2010 it was 34%, and in 2012 it was 35%. This meant that 24,725,000 children were living in single-parent households in 2012 (*Kids count data book*, 2014).

Reasons for the increase in the number of children living with single parents include a larger proportion of births occurring to unmarried women; the delay of marriage, which means that adults were single for more years; and the growth in divorce among couples with children (Fields, 2004). More than half of births to American women under 30 occur outside of marriage (two-thirds of U.S. children are born to mothers under 30). The fastest growth of this number has occurred in white women in their 20s who have some college education but no four-year degree. In the mid 1990s a third of Americans were born outside marriage. In 2012 the figure was 41% (DeParle and Tavernise 2012). Usually when we think of single-parent families, we think of them as being headed by women. However, the number of households headed by single fathers has been growing significantly.

Father-headed single-parent families often place the father in a new role. We say "often" because nowadays men in two-parent families more and more are

Global DIMENSIONS

Single-Parent Households in Various Countries

Although the reasons for these differences are not known, it is interesting to look at the percent of single-parent households in other countries. In declining order, they are:

1. United Kingdom   25.0%
2. Canada   24.6%

3. Ireland   22.6%
4. Denmark   21.7%
5. Germany   21.7%
6. France   19.8%
7. Sweden   18.7%
8. Netherlands   16.0%
9. Japan   10.2%

Source: Data from Section 30—International Statistics, Statistical Abstract of the United States. U.S. Census Bureau, 2012.

helping with what were heretofore considered to be the wife's household chores and responsibilities. For these husbands the adjustment to heading a single-parent family will be less difficult because they are accustomed to cooking, cleaning, nurturing, and changing diapers. For the more traditional husband, the adoption of these necessary chores and responsibilities, added to the financial and emotional burdens of divorce, means that a more significant adjustment is required.

Life in a single-parent family can be stressful for both the adult and the children. Members may unrealistically expect that the family can function as a two-parent family does and may feel that something is wrong if it cannot. The single parent may feel overwhelmed by the responsibility of caring for the children, maintaining a job, and keeping up with the bills and household chores. Typically, the family's finances and resources are drastically reduced by the parents' breakup.

Single-parent families deal with pressures and potential problem areas that the nuclear family does not have to face, such as the following:

- Visitation and custody problems

- The negative effects of continuing conflict between the parents

- Fewer opportunities for parents and children to spend time together

- Negative effects of the breakup on children's school performance and peer relations

- Disruptions of extended family relationships

- Problems caused by parents' dating and entering new relationships

The demand for social services to meet the special needs of single-parent families is growing. Because single-parent families often have financial,

psychological, custodial, and other needs that are more acute than those of conventional two-parent families, they need counseling and/or support groups. Many single parents have the added responsibility of providing role models for their other-sex children. Day care, a virtual necessity (as it also is for many two-parent households), solves some problems, yet it may also be a source of anxiety, or at least concern, for financial, educational, psychological, or other reasons.

As Zill (2015) pointed out, many studies have found that young people raised in single-parent families demonstrate greater achievement and behavior problems than those who grow up with two parents. These developmental problems are often attributed to the meager financial resources of single parents

© Ami Beyer/ShutterStock, Inc.

Children in single-parent families can be just as successful as other children.

and the less adequate supervision they may be able to exercise over their children. Childhood disturbances are often linked to conflict between parents, especially when the conflict is intense or prolonged. Children of divorced and never-married parents are more likely to have been exposed to domestic violence than children in married two-parent families.

Although some of these research findings might seem discouraging—or they might seem wrong to readers who come from single-parent families—it is important to remember that these findings refer to trends in groups and have no bearing on particular individuals. Children in single-parent families are often very successful. Our intention here is to suggest that single parenthood does require special care and consideration. Perhaps most of all, the special needs of single-parent families should be understood both by family members themselves and by teachers, employers, and others with whom they interact. To meet this need for understanding, a group called Parents without Partners serves as a sounding board and a source of counsel for single parents.

The need for good parenting skills remains constant regardless of the parent's marital status. However, the situation can be more demanding for both the parents and the children in single-parent households. The following are some suggested guidelines.

1. Be honest with your children about the situation that caused you to become a single parent.

2. In case of a separation or divorce, assure children that they are not responsible for the breakup of the relationship.

3. Try to maintain as much of the same routine as possible.

4. Do not try to be both mother and father to the children. Establish a family atmosphere of teamwork.

5. In the case of divorce, acknowledge that the relationship between you and your former partner is over, and do not encourage your children to hope for reconciliation.

6. Reassure children that they will continue to be loved and cared for (by both parents, if true).

7. Do not use children to gain bargaining power with a separated or divorced spouse.

8. Encourage relatives to help children maintain a sense of belonging to a continuing family.

Wilcox & Marquardt (2010) have provided helpful information to summarize this section. For example, they indicate that the percentage of children who grow up in fragile—typically fatherless—families has grown enormously over the past five decades. This is mainly due to increases in divorce, out-of-wedlock births, and unmarried cohabitation. Children in such families have negative outcomes at two to three times the rate of children in married two-parent families. In earlier times, most single mothers were divorced or widowed. Today the number of never-married single mothers is higher than that of divorced mothers. A major reason for the increase in number of never-married single mothers is that single motherhood has become a permanent status for many women.

Sexuality and Aging

There was a time when it was believed that sexual desire and functioning became unimportant with age. Although a gradual decline in sexual activity occurs around age 50 years and accelerates after age 70 years, sexuality remains an important part of life into old age.

Understanding the sexuality of elders is important because of the rapidly increasing elderly population. The population of U.S. citizens aged 65 years and older grew from 25.5 million in 1980 to 35 million in 2000. It was more than 40.4 million in 2010.

As people get older they can continue to have excellent relationships that include sexual activity.

Between 2012 and 2050, the United States will experience considerable growth in its older population. In 2050, the population aged 65 and older is projected to total 83.7 million persons, almost double the estimated 43.1 million elderly people living in the country in 2012 (Ortman et al., 2014). As people live longer, it is important to understand how sexuality is affected in later years.

Many studies have confirmed that people remain sexually active into their 70s and 80s. Griebling (2011) provided data related to sexual behaviors of Americans older than age 50. Regarding men aged 50–80, within the past year 25.8% had masturbated a few times per year, 20% a few times per month, 13.2% two or three times per week, and 4.5% four or more times per week. Within the past year, 37.1% had given oral sex and 39.3% had received oral sex. Within the past year, 17.8% had penile–vaginal intercourse a few times during the year, 24.6% a few times per month, 10.2% two or three times per week, and 0.9% four or more times per week. Regarding women aged 50–80, within the past year 34.3% had masturbated a few times per year, 10.7% a few times per month, 1.3% two or three times per week, and 0.5% four or more times per week. Within the past year, 25.8% had given oral sex and 25.6% had received oral sex. Within the past year, 13.5% had penile–vaginal intercourse a few times per year, 20.3% a few times per month, 6.8% two or three times per week, and 1.4% four or more times per week.

As Stein (2014) indicates, there is no age limit on sexuality and sexual activity. If one stays interested, stays healthy, stays off medications, and has a good mate, one can have good sexual activity all the way to the end of life. Among a 45- to 59-year-old sample with sexual partners, 56% of respondents said they had sexual intercourse once a week or more. Among 60- to 70-year-olds with partners, 46% of men and 38% of women had sexual intercourse at least once a week, as did 34% of those 70 and older.

Lee et al. (2015) surveyed more than 6,200 people in England aged 50–90 about their sexual activity. Slightly more than 31% of the 80- to 90-year-old men had sexual intercourse or masturbated in the last year, compared with 59% of those in the 70–79 age group. Among women in the same age brackets, the figures were 14% and 34%, respectively, though more than 41% of 80- to 90-year-old women who lived with a partner reported some sexual activity in the previous year. Problems most frequently reported by sexually active women related to becoming sexually aroused (32%) and achieving orgasm (27%), while for men the major problem was erectile difficulties (39%).

A study of sexually active older women (mean age of 67; 63% were postmenopausal) found that sexual satisfaction increased with age and that those

The Abkhasian people of Georgia (a republic of the former Soviet Union) often live to be more than 100 years old. One reason they believe they live so long is their sexual customs. The Abkhasian people believe that sexual energy should be conserved. They do not marry until about age 30 years and do not believe in premarital sexual activity. It is essential that a bride be a virgin. In marriage, sexual activity is considered a pleasure to enjoy, but for the sake of one's health it should not be overdone.

not engaging in sexual activity were satisfied with their sex lives. Half of the respondents who reported having a sexual partner had been sexually active in the last 4 weeks. The majority of the sexually active women (67%) achieved orgasm most of the time or always. The youngest and oldest women in the study reported the highest frequency of orgasm satisfaction. Regardless of partner status or sexual activity, 61% of all women in this study were satisfied with their overall sex life (Trompeter et al., 2012).

Many people of all ages believe that sexual behavior is a lifelong need, that it has beneficial effects for older people, that it is a critical part of a good relationship, and that it is important to their overall quality of life. Some use sexual performance-enhancing medications to ensure that they can continue to enjoy such activities.

Prevalent in our society is the performance ethic, which is concerned with the frequency of intercourse and orgasm. As we mature (age, if you will), it becomes apparent that other types of sexual activity become important. These include caressing, hugging, petting, kissing, and sharing of intimacies. People who experience a satisfying sexual life in their early years will most likely continue this pursuit. However, those people who are today 65 years and older lived under very different mores. Your grandparents and possibly your parents led more restricted sexual lives, especially the women. Women were not taught about masturbation, nor were they taught to ask that they be sexually satisfied.

Communication DIMENSIONS

20 Ways to Fall in Love All Over Again

There are many advantages to a long-term relationship, including better health and overall well-being. A loving partner can offer companionship, comfort, and physical and emotional support when needed. While the following tips are designed specifically for older couples, most of them can be helpful for couples of all ages:

1. Be more touchy-feely. When we touch—especially skin-to-skin—we get a little rush of the brain chemicals that help trigger those loving feelings.
2. Sleep closer together. Sleeping skin-to-skin, even if it is just touching small parts of the body, can have relationship benefits. Even snuggling for a few minutes can be helpful.
3. Limit technology. Smartphones and other devices may interfere with communication and love lives. Cutting out their use at certain times can be beneficial.
4. Take a vacation. Getting away may help you focus on each other. It is a good idea to discuss expectations before going.
5. Say "thank you." It is easy to take for granted the nice things a partner does, but gratitude is important and showing it in even small ways can be helpful.
6. Pucker up. Locking lips can play an important role in the quality of a long-term relationship. A hug and a kiss give warm, fuzzy, safe bonding feelings.
7. Compliment each other. Try to focus more on the good things. Letting your partner know what you love about him or her—whether physical, intellectual, or emotional—can help you see the partner in a more positive light.
8. Incorporate surprise. Incorporate novelty, excitement, and surprise into the relationship. Planning secret activities, having a date night with something new, or going to a new place can all be enjoyable and helpful to the relationship.
9. Cultivate your own interests. Make sure your life contains something you feel passionate about. This may also ensure a better relationship with your partner.
10. Observe your partner's passions. Find a way to witness your loved one in a passionate state—in a business, with children, at a hobby the partner loves.
11. Create something together. When you work on things you both care about (e.g., children, home remodeling, volunteer work), you can see your partner in a different light.
12. Go on double dates. Watching your other half interact with friends can help you remember what you love about him or her.
13. Flirt with each other. Excitement, novelty, and mystery can result from flirting with each other as if you have just met.
14. Work out together. Breaking a sweat together may increase your physical attraction as well as your emotional bond.
15. Engage in pillow talk. Spend a few extra minutes after sexual activity chatting and snuggling. Disclose positive feelings to each other during this time.
16. Scheduling regular time to be by yourselves as a couple, away from work and home, can help you stay connected and remember what you love about each other.
17. Be there for each other. Having your partner's back and knowing that your partner has yours can increase feelings of security and promote higher self-esteem.
18. Adjust your expectations. No relationship will be perfect. All long-term unions have their ups and downs, and love can be felt and expressed in many different ways.

Older people can not only be sexually satisfied by having relationships with others, but can also experience active sexual behaviors by themselves. Masturbation is a viable activity for older people, especially women. If the male loses the capacity to maintain erections, women can masturbate; or men can masturbate to orgasm even after they can no longer become erect. Mutual masturbation becomes popular, once again, as it may have been when they were younger.

Physiological changes are often attributed to changes in sexuality associated with aging. However,

A phenomena in Hollywood, both on-and-off screen, is that of a romantic involvement between a younger man and an older woman. The term "cougar" is used to refer to older women who have relationships with younger men.

onset of menopause for women and declining levels of testosterone for men represent only one factor in sexuality changes. Psychological and sociocultural changes occur as well.

Some sexual dysfunction associated with aging, such as erectile disorder, can now be overcome with pharmacology. Drugs such as Viagra and Cialis can restore the physical ability to have an erection; however, it does not rekindle the psychological or social aspects that make for a loving relationship. These drugs pose special problems to a relationship: A woman may wonder whether the erection is caused by the drug or by attraction to her.

Psychological changes also occur across the aging process, such as changes in mood. For women, causes may include stress, health problems, menopause, hormone replacement therapy, and other lifestyle changes. For men, they may include a shift in focus from career to increased focus on family, challenge to the traditional male role as leader and protector of the family, increased need for affirmation and acceptance, or irritation and anger with aging (especially the physical changes).

Social factors affecting psychological changes include the fact that socialization of people in their 70s, 80s, or 90s in regard to sexuality is substantially different from that of those in their 30s or 40s. For example, images of sexual attractiveness tend to be youth oriented and may affect the self-esteem of aging women. Ironically, men are sometimes viewed as more attractive as they age. And Hollywood movies often capitalize on this double standard by pairing an older, experienced male actor with a young actress.

The term "cougar" is used to refer to older women who have relationships with younger men. Easton et al. (2011) reported that older women have evolved a reproduction-expediting physiological adaptation designed to capitalize on their remaining fertility. These women experience increased sexual motivation and sexual behaviors compared to women not facing a similar fertility decline. Easton's research showed that women with declining fertility think more about sexual activity, have more frequent and intense sexual fantasies, are more willing to engage in sexual intercourse, and report engaging in sexual intercourse more frequently than women in other age groups.

Interestingly, some long-married couples experience more sexual satisfaction during their older years. Once their offspring are out of the house and they are retired from working, they can devote more time to each other and have more fulfilling and rewarding lovemaking.

On a related, but different, note, an increasing number of older men and women are deciding to have children. Many older moms and dads are happy to devote what might have been leisure-filled years to the frenzy of child care and related responsibilities. People might have to be creative to achieve this goal—for example, using techniques such as frozen embryos, fertility treatments and drugs, and adoption. Many older parents feel they do a better job of parenting than they would have done while they were younger.

In recent years, more attention has been paid to the needs of the lesbian, gay, bisexual, and transgender (LGBT) people as they get older. Many issues are the same as those for older heterosexuals, but there are also some that are unique to LGBT people. For example, there may be limited access to LGBT-friendly health care. They might experience homophobia, deal with stigmas, and be socially isolated. Denial of hospital and nursing home visitation rights for their partners may also be a problem. In addition, ageism may exist within the gay and lesbian community.

The National Institute on Aging suggests the following ways for women to stay healthy after menopause (Menopause, 2010):

- Don't smoke.

- Eat a healthy diet, low in fat, high in fiber, with plenty of fruits, vegetables, and whole-grain foods, as well as all the important vitamins and minerals.

- Make sure you get enough calcium and vitamin D—either in your diet or with vitamin/mineral supplements.

- Learn what your healthy weight is, and try to stay there.

- Do weight-bearing exercise, such as walking, jogging, or dancing, at least 3 days each week for healthy bones. Also try to be physically active in other ways for your general health.

Menopause

Usually between the ages of 40 and 55 years, women produce progressively less estrogen and progesterone, as an effect of aging on the ovaries. Whereas the pituitary continues to produce follicle-stimulating hormone (FSH) and luteinizing hormone (LH), the ovaries can no longer respond to these pituitary hormones as they once could. This decrease in estrogen and progesterone occurs over approximately a 5- to 10-year period and results in a cessation of menstruation. The period when these changes take place is called the **perimenopause**, or the **climacteric**; when menstruation has not occurred for a year, we call that **menopause**.

Symptoms of Perimenopause and Menopause

Most perimenopausal women report mild symptoms or no symptoms at all; only about 20% report symptoms severe enough to cause them to seek medical attention. The symptoms that perimenopausal and menopausal women experience can vary from headaches, dizziness, palpitations, insomnia, anxiety, depression, and weight gain to hot flashes and vaginal dryness. **Hot flashes** (sometimes referred to as *hot flushes*) are sudden waves of heat felt throughout the body, often accompanied by reddening and sweating (Menopause, 2010). Some women experience hot flashes infrequently, whereas others may have them every few hours or so. They may last a few seconds or, in severe cases, a full 30 minutes. And some women never have hot flashes. Because hot flashes tend to occur more frequently at night, they often disturb sleep, causing the woman to awaken in a sweat. In particularly bothersome cases, they may contribute to insomnia. Hot flashes appear to be caused by hormonal fluctuations that affect the nerves governing the dilatation or constriction of the blood vessels. When the blood vessels rapidly dilate in response to hormonal secretions, a sense of warmth may result. Generally, hot flashes cease after 2 years, but in some cases they may last longer.

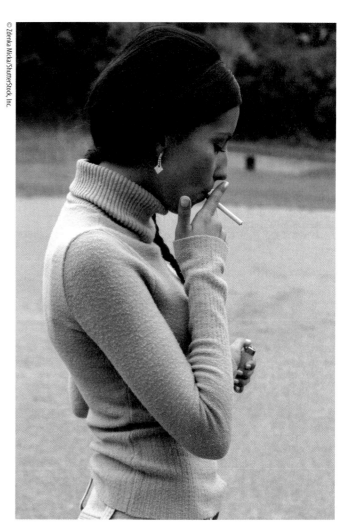

Increased risk factors for osteoporosis include smoking, consumption of alcohol, physical inactivity, being underweight, and having a diet low in calcium.

Vaginal dryness results from the lowered amount of estrogen in the vaginal walls, which causes shrinking and thinning and causes the vaginal mucosa to become thinner. The net result is that both the length and the width of the vagina become smaller and the vagina cannot expand during penile insertion as it once could. In addition, there is diminished vaginal lubrication during perimenopause and menopause. These changes can mean painful intercourse as well as an increased risk of vaginal infection (Menopause, 2010). Over-the-counter lubricants can be helpful in these cases.

perimenopause (climacteric) The period just before menopause when the production of estrogen and progesterone is decreasing, usually a 5- to 10-year period.

menopause The time when a woman's menstrual cycle ceases, usually between 40 and 55 years of age.

hot flashes Intermittent sensations of heat reported by menopausal women, possibly caused by decreased estrogen production.

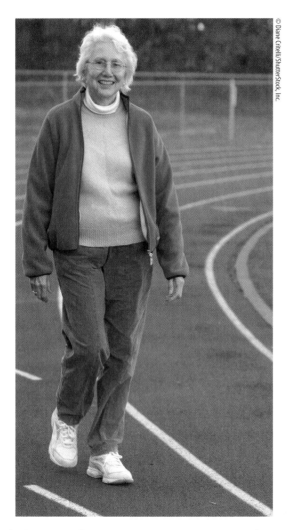

Exercise is one way for women to prevent osteoporosis, the weakening of their bones. Thus exercise, along with proper nutrition, not smoking, and refraining from drinking alcoholic beverages, is helpful in preventing bone fractures.

A significant symptom caused by the decrease in estrogen production is the decalcification of the bones. **Osteoporosis** is the disease that results when enough calcium is lost in the bones to make the person susceptible to bone fractures and bending (for example, curvature of the back—sometimes called "dowager's hump" because it is common among older women). Women older than 50 years of age lose about 10% of their bone mass every 10 years; the result is an increased risk of bone fractures. Women

osteoporosis A condition of weakened bones resulting from decalcification (loss of calcium) of bone that increases in the absence of estrogen and is of particular concern in postmenopausal women.

menopausal hormone therapy (MHT) Replacement of hormones that a woman's ovaries stop making at the time of menopause, easing some of the symptoms of menopause.

older than 60 years of age suffer many more bone fractures than do men (Osteoporosis handout on health, 2011). It seems that osteoporosis occurs more frequently in white women who are fair skinned (especially blonds and redheads), who smoke cigarettes, who drink alcohol, who are physically inactive, who are underweight, and whose diet is low in calcium. Osteoporosis can develop in men, too.

Treatment for Menopause
As we have mentioned, only a minority of women have menopausal symptoms severe enough to make them seek medical attention. To help relieve these symptoms, some women use hormones. This is called **menopausal hormone therapy (MHT)**. It used to be called *hormone replacement therapy* (HRT). MHT is a more current umbrella term that describes different hormone combinations available in a variety of forms and doses. The form of MHT a doctor suggests may depend on the woman's symptoms. For example, an estrogen patch or pill can relieve hot flashes, night sweats, and vaginal dryness. Other forms—vaginal creams, tablets, or rings—are used mostly for vaginal dryness. The vaginal ring insert might also help some urinary tract symptoms. The dose can also vary, as can the timing of these doses. Some women might even take estrogen or progesterone continuously—every day of the month (Hormones and menopause, 2009).

The use of MHT can be controversial. It is important for a woman to discuss the pros and cons of MHT with her physician and see if the potential benefits are worth the potential risks. For example, research indicates that for some women the use of MHT poses some serious risks, such as increasing the risk for breast cancer, heart disease, stroke, and pulmonary embolism (blood clot in the lung). Women

As if smoking weren't enough of a risk of cancer, it has been found that women who replace estrogen after menopause are at an increased risk of contracting breast cancer and ovarian cancer, not to mention the increased risk of stroke and heart disease.

who choose to use MHT should use the lowest dose that helps for the shortest time needed (Womenshealth.gov, 2011).

Other treatments for menopause disorders specific to preventing osteoporosis include sufficient physical exercise to strengthen the bones, a diet rich in calcium to slow bone decalcification, refraining from smoking of cigarettes and drinking of alcohol, and avoidance of carbonated soft drinks that contain high levels of phosphorus, which may contribute to a phosphorus–calcium imbalance associated with osteoporosis. Foods such as milk, sardines and salmon canned with bones, oysters, and dark green vegetables are recommended because they are all high in calcium.

Some physicians may also prescribe tranquilizers for women who have difficulty with the psychological aspects of menopause. It is unclear whether the depression some women report during menopause is a cause of that condition or is caused by other changes that usually occur during that stage of life (for example, children leaving home, aged parents needing more attention, or a woman's life taking a new direction).

Treatment for vaginal dryness can include the use of lubricated creams, vegetable oils, or water-soluble jellies (such as K-Y or Lubifax) and suppositories. In addition, it appears that regular masturbation or participation in sexual intercourse helps reduce vaginal soreness.

It would be unfortunate to close this section without citing the benefits and positive aspects of menopause. Because women can no longer conceive, the fear of pregnancy is removed, and lovemaking is often more enjoyable as a result. However, a woman who has ceased to menstruate has not necessarily ceased to ovulate. So-called **change-of-life babies** have been known to surprise women just entering menopause who thought they could no longer conceive. Especially during perimenopause—when the menses occurs, however infrequently—caution is advised.

The anthropologist Margaret Mead talked of "postmenopausal zest" to describe the excitement, stimulation, and enjoyment that can result from menopause. If viewed in this way, the postmenopausal years can be rich with new opportunities and experiences. If its negative aspects become the focus, menopausal symptoms will probably increase, and psychological discomfort will result. It is up to a woman's friends, relatives, and colleagues at work to help her focus on the positive aspects of menopause rather than its less desirable components. In addition, many women now turn to support groups (for example, The Red Hot Mamas) or online forums to share strategies on ways to manage menopausal symptoms.

Male Climacteric

Do men have an experience analogous to menopause (termed the **male climacteric**)? The answer to this question is not clear. There is evidence that at approximately the same age at which women experience menopause, some men experience what is called a **midlife crisis**. Men wonder about the meaning of their lives thus far and worry about what the future holds for them. They may become more people oriented and less job-and-task oriented. They may grow concerned about a diminishing interest in sexual activity and a reduction of sexual potency. Some men, to reassure themselves about their sexual capabilities, begin to date younger women or initiate extramarital affairs.

The hormonal evidence usually cited for this male climacteric is a decrease in testosterone production at about age 40 to 50 years. However, the decrease in the testosterone level is believed by many experts to be minimal, too insignificant to influence male behavior. Furthermore, middle-aged women face many of the same concerns and fears about the past and the future and put themselves through similarly agonizing self-examinations. In trying to decide what accounts for the midlife crisis, researchers' difficulties in distinguishing the psychological and sociological influences from clearly identifiable physiological and hormonal changes are practically insurmountable. In women, decreased estrogen production and increased FSH production, as well as a lack of menstrual flow, serve as irrefutable evidence of menopause. No similar evidence exists for a male climacteric. Still, most observers admit that males often go through a change of life—whether hormonally, psychologically, or culturally based—that deserves recognition and attention.

Hormone Therapy

Hormone therapy is sometimes administered to men. For instance, testosterone supplements are sometimes administered to treat erectile dysfunction in older men (although testosterone levels are not low in all men who have trouble maintaining erection). Sometimes this treatment for erectile dysfunction is

change-of-life baby A baby born to a menopausal woman who, in spite of not menstruating regularly, ovulated.

male climacteric Sometimes termed "male menopause," which occurs at about the same age that women experience menopause, when men experience slightly decreased testosterone production and begin to question the directions in which their lives are headed.

midlife crisis A time of life, usually between 40 and 50 years of age, during which men question the path their lives have taken and make plans for changing their goals.

effective; other times it is not. The reason for this inconsistency is unclear; however, it is safe to say that the complex nature of sexuality makes it only partially responsive to hormone treatment. Testosterone supplements may not have much effect when personality, past experiences, the sexual partner, effectiveness in communication, setting, and so on, continue to have negative effects.

Other Aging-Related Physiological Changes

Direct physical changes do occur in men as they age: The testes become smaller, the scrotal skin becomes thinner and less elastic, seminal fluid may become thinner and be produced in lower quantities, and sperm become less lively. Erections occur more slowly and the plateau phase lasts longer. Another important occurrence is that older men do not feel imminent ejaculation—it is less forceful. It is common for the refractory period to become longer as men age. One possible advantage of slower response is the likelihood that middle-aged and older men can prolong sexual activity and actually be better sexual partners. It should be remembered, however, that even elderly men continue to produce sperm and can become fathers if appropriate precautions are not taken.

The capacity to enjoy sexual experiences is not lost in older men, as it is not lost in older women. Masters and Johnson (1966) maintain the importance of continued and frequent sexual experiences for aging males:

> If elevated levels of sexual activity are maintained from earlier years and neither acute nor chronic physical incapacity intervenes, aging males usually are able to continue some form of active sexual expression into the 70- and even 80-year age groups.

Masters and Johnson further indicate that women who do not regularly participate in sexual activity tend to have difficulty accommodating a penis when they do attempt sexual intercourse. Those who can accommodate a penis and have adequate lubrication are likely to have maintained regular sexual response (once or twice a week).

If an older woman has not been sexually active for a long time, it may take a little time and patience to be able to resume sexual activity. For example, it may take longer for the vagina to swell and lubricate. Longer foreplay can be helpful, as can the use of a lubricant, such as K-Y Jelly. For some women, vaginal treatment with estrogen works well. It may also take time to stretch out the vagina so it can accommodate a penis if the woman has not had sexual intercourse for a long time. Touching, cuddling, and good communication between partners help to promote sexual satisfaction (Sexuality in later life, 2010).

Influences on Sexual Activity in Later Years

Many older adults say their sex lives improve as they age. Improvements probably require more communication with partners and possible small changes both people can make. Here are a few examples (Intimacy and aging: Tips for sexual health and happiness, 2003):

- *Expand your definition of sex.* It is more than intercourse. Other options for sexual activity might be more comfortable and more fulfilling. Touching, holding, sensual massage, masturbation, and oral sexual activity are all possibilities.

- *Communicate with your partner.* Discuss changes and possible accommodations. Try different positions and activities. Ask your partner about his or her interests and needs and how you can be helpful. Communication itself can be arousing.

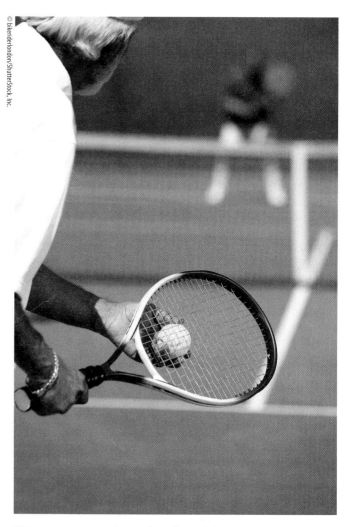

With age, men experience physiological changes that slow their sexual response.

- *Make changes to your routine*. Change the time of day to a time when you have the most energy. Take more time to set the stage, such as a romantic dinner or an evening of dancing. Try new sexual activities.

- *Manage your expectations*. Be realistic. For example, if you didn't have much sexual activity when you were younger, you probably won't when you are older.

- *Take care of yourself*. Healthy living habits can help improve sexual activity at any age.

Although health problems can interfere with sexual activity for older people, they need not end all sexual activity. For example, arthritis or lower back pain might require understanding and a variety of sexual positions. Diabetes can result in diminished sexual response, but sexual pleasuring can still provide satisfaction. Stroke victims might lose some control of speech or movements but still be capable of sexual response under appropriate conditions.

Heart attacks are sometimes of particular concern in relation to sexual activity. Some people think that sexual activity may bring about a heart attack, and although in reality this is not a common problem, heart attack victims often hesitate to return to sexual activity. In general, those who have been sexually active before the heart attack will have little, if any, problem being sexually active again. Of course it makes sense to improve personal health as much as possible after a heart attack. Those who have a proper diet, exercise appropriately, and control stress responses are most likely to have satisfactory sexual activity as well.

The availability of partners for the older divorced or widowed person can present severe restrictions on intimacy. How can one have a successful relationship if there are no possible mates? Older women outnumber older men; they tend to live 7 years longer and they generally marry men a few years older than they are. Hence the older woman, who is supposed to have sexual relationships only with her spouse, is alone.

Another problem that exists for older men and women is that their sphere of friendships may be couples—that is, pairs. If one of only a few single people, the person may be omitted from social activities or may appear to be a fifth wheel, and so he or she is not very comfortable with other couples. This indeed limits sexual activity; even more importantly, it may limit intimacy and friendships in later life.

For older people living in nursing homes, there might be additional problems. For example, nursing home personnel sometimes resist sexuality programs. People may be segregated to discourage sexual activities. Medications may be prescribed without

Ethical DIMENSIONS

Should Donor Eggs Be Used to Let Women Older Than 50 Years Produce Viable Babies?

Women older than 50 years are just as likely to conceive and deliver a baby with donor eggs as younger women are. Many people argue that there is no medical reason why healthy women in their 50s should not have babies with donor eggs. They say that people in their 60s and 70s are much more active than in past years, so they have enough stamina to raise a child. Also, knowing that they can reproduce after age 50 will take the pressure off some women to reproduce when they are younger. They can concentrate more on their marriage and their careers and not worry about child rearing until later in life.

Others feel that it is wrong for a woman older than 50 years to reproduce. They feel that there is a much higher possibility of their offspring's being orphaned at a young age. Even if people are healthy and active, statistics show that many people die in their 60s and 70s. If that happens, relatively young children will be without parents for more of their lives. Also, for healthy people, raising a child takes a lot of energy and it is more likely younger parents will have that energy. Women older than age 50 who get pregnant using donor eggs do not appear to face greater risks of complications than younger women using the same technologies. Births to women 50 and older are increasing through the availability of in vitro fertilization with eggs donated from younger women. Nevertheless, some clinics remain reluctant to accept older women.

Do you think donor eggs should be used to let women older than 50 years reproduce? At what ages should women be allowed to reproduce?

Source: Egg donation news. *Pollenrtree.com*, 2015. Available: http://www.pollenrtree.com/egg-donation/news/egg-donation-news/older-mothers-using-donor-eggs.

considering their effects on sexual functioning; for example, some high blood pressure or arthritis medications can lessen sexual response. Fortunately, attitudes of the staff in nursing homes as well as the families of those in the homes are changing. This is an excellent example of the need to accept people of all ages as sexual beings.

It should be noted that there are times when couples may want to sleep apart, because medication may cause a person to snore loudly, shake violently, or talk loudly, making it uncomfortable for the other partner. As well as elderly adults, some younger couples choose to sleep in separate bedrooms for similar reasons. It should be remembered that sexual activity can occur in either bedroom and at any time during the day or evening.

Aging and Safer Sexual Activity

STIs and HIV are generally thought of as diseases that the young must worry about. But the number of older Americans with various STIs and HIV is steadily rising. Some of this is related to the fact that more older people are sexually active. However, older adults can also be more vulnerable to HIV infection because the linings of the vagina and anus become more fragile and more susceptible to tears during sexual activity, providing a direct path into the bloodstream for the virus. The immune system also tends to grow weaker with advancing age. To make matters worse, older people are much less likely than younger people to be tested for STIs or HIV. As a result, diseases are typically not diagnosed until a late stage. It is important that older adults take the same precautions to promote safer sexual activity as younger people are encouraged to do.

One problem is that many people may not think to use a condom—after all, pregnancy is not possible among older women. But condom use and safer sexual practices are still needed throughout life to prevent transmission of STIs and HIV, and because an elderly man can impregnate a woman late into his life, safer sexual practices must include contraception.

Because of concern for the overall health of older people, the American Association for Retired People (AARP) surveyed over 2,000 older adults on their sexual attitudes and practices (Fisher, 2010). Results showed that a sort of "sexual revolution" continues in the older population. For example, opposition to sexual activity among those who are not married was down by half over a 10-year period. Also, the belief that there is too much emphasis on sexuality in our culture was also down. However, both the frequency of self-stimulation and sexual thoughts and fantasies did not change. The researchers pointed out that an economic environment that adds to stress

and financial anxiety has previously been shown to decrease sexual satisfaction. Men continue to think about sexual activity more than women, see it as more important to their quality of life, engage in sexual activities more often, are less satisfied if without a partner, and are twice as likely as women (21% versus 11%) to admit to sexual activity outside of their relationship.

Lesbian and Gay People Among the Aging

Like all sexual beings, lesbian and gay people eventually become old and need to deal with problems caused by aging. The loss of partners and friends may be compounded for older gay men, who saw many of their friends die of AIDS during the 1980s and 1990s. For them, AIDS meant that the good-byes that would have been said as they approached old age were made not only to lifelong friends but also to younger and younger men.

Because they grew up in such a sharply homophobic society, many gays are still cautious about coming out. Many elderly lesbians are still careful about coming out in today's somewhat more accepting society because they have become accustomed to hiding their identity. When older gay men or lesbians do not disclose their sexual identity, they prevent themselves and others from sharing in a comprehensive understanding of their lives.

Many gays may decide to keep their sexual identities secret because of fears of receiving biased or inferior services from doctors, attendants, or nursing homes. Help is available from Senior Action in a Gay Environment (SAGE), an organization concerned with gay, lesbian, bisexual, and transgender elders. It provides social services, individual and group therapy, and home visits for the homebound. It also acts as advocates on behalf of older lesbians and gays.

As people and society in general have become more open and accepting about lesbian and gay people, changes have slowly occurred related to lesbian and gay people and aging as well. One germane example is the opening of retirement communities especially for lesbian and gay people. However, retirement communities for gays and lesbians have experienced some of the same problems as other community developments in recent years. For example, RainbowVision opened its doors in 2006 as one of the first retirement communities in the country to proudly serve gays and lesbians. Its problems were similar to other gay retirement communities, and other new communities in general—a weakened housing market and a deflated economy. These factors make it difficult for anyone to sell a home and move to a new community or perhaps even to have enough money to think about making such a change. A number of communities planned for gay and lesbian retirees never opened because of a lack of finances and a decline in real estate values. As a result, housing options tailored to the estimated 1.5 million elderly people in the United States who are gay are still rather limited. Many are growing older without the support of children or extended family members. Gay and lesbian seniors are twice as likely to live alone (Frosch, 2011).

Sexuality for the Physically and Mentally Challenged

In July 2005, the U.S. Surgeon General released a report related to disabilities. More than 54 million Americans, or one in five people, were living with at least one disability. Most Americans will experience a disability some time during the course of their lives. The Surgeon General's report emphasized that people with disabilities can learn, get married, have a family, worship, vote, work, and live long, productive lives. There is a need to treat them as active members of society. In this spirit, the four goals of the Surgeon General's Call to Action to Improve the Health and Wellness of Persons with Disabilities were (U.S. Surgeon General issues first call to action on disability, 2005):

- Increase understanding nationwide that people with disabilities can lead long, healthy, and productive lives.

- Increase knowledge among healthcare professionals and provide them with tools to screen, diagnose, and treat the person with a disability with dignity.

- Increase awareness among people with disabilities regarding the steps they can take to develop and maintain a healthy lifestyle.

- Increase accessible health care and support services to promote independence for people with disabilities.

There are implications related to sexuality for each of the four goals. For example, a healthy lifestyle is important related to sexual interest and activity. It is also important for healthcare professionals to understand the whole person—including his or her sexuality.

Although we think of physical or mental challenges and illness as physical (biological) dimensions of sexuality, psychological and sociocultural dimensions also come into play. Mild depression is common among not only those with a chronic illness but

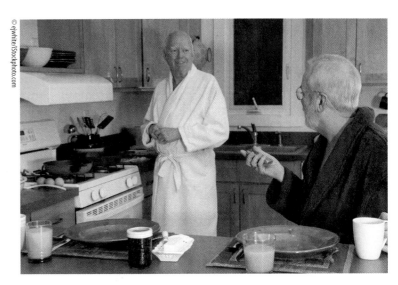

Some older gay and lesbian partners recall sanctions applied to them when they were younger and choose to remain "closeted," whereas others are adamant about expressing their sexuality openly in a more tolerant society.

also their caregivers and spouses, and it affects the couple's sexual activities. Further, an illness or disability may force a person to withdraw from normal social activities, thereby removing himself or herself from social support. Those who suffer from a disability also may suffer from body-image or gender-identity problems.

As with any sexual problem, it is not just the ill or disabled spouse who suffers. Both partners have to come to terms with changes in sexuality. Communication becomes a critical tool for acceptance of these changes and the best ways to adjust to them.

Physical Challenges

Physical challenge can result in any number of specific problems—for example, low energy levels, blindness or limited vision, movement problems, sensory loss, and the need to manage bags or tubes. Nevertheless, the challenged can generally find, or be helped to find, creative ways of overcoming such impediments to physical intimacy. For example, although most of us tend to focus on stimulating the genital area, in fact, the whole body can be stimulated and aroused. We can achieve sexual satisfaction—and possibly orgasm—without an erect penis or a well-lubricated vagina. With conscious intention and learning, anyone can use any part of the body in an infinite number of ways to achieve sexual satisfaction. For the challenged—as well as for the able-bodied—such learning can lead to a rich sexual life.

Even though sensory challenges, such as blindness and deafness, do not directly influence overall sexual responsiveness, they may affect sexuality. For

Disabilities do not have to prevent individuals from experiencing all the dimensions of human sexuality.

example, people who have been blind for most or all of their life may have difficulty in understanding a partner's anatomy. Fortunately, educational programs, including learning about sexual anatomy and intercourse positions through the use of models, can be very helpful.

People who are deaf may also have special challenges related to sexuality. For example, some of the usual communication routes may be blocked. People who are deaf may miss words in lipreading or may be misunderstood when using sign language if others are not familiar with it. As people without such challenges do, those with sensory challenges may feel afraid or embarrassed when attempting to communicate about sexuality. Educational programs are needed for the sensory challenged just as they are needed for people without such challenges.

Cerebral palsy usually does not preclude interest in sexual activity, fertility, or ability to experience orgasm. Depending upon the nature and extent of problems with muscle control, those with cerebral palsy may have difficulty with certain sexual activities or positions. In addition, social rejection or feelings of inadequacy may become problems. Fortunately, education and counseling to help those with cerebral palsy understand their sexuality and learn appropriate social skills can help improve body image and ability to have intimate relationships.

Sometimes challenged people have to adapt their behavior to meet new conditions. For example, a woman with severe arthritis of the hip joints may find she cannot spread her legs wide enough for intercourse in the standard frontal position or that the weight of a partner's body may produce pain. She can employ rear entry or side-by-side coital positions that reduce or eliminate discomfort.

It is important to recognize certain aspects of sexual functioning in paralyzed individuals. Even though the following statements were made many years ago, they are still pertinent today (Woods, 1979):

1. Some components of the human sexual response cycle (such as erection) are mediated by spinal cord reflexes. Therefore, it is not necessary to have pathways from the brain to the sex organs. For example, stimuli resulting from pressure or tension in the pelvic organs or from touch excite impulses that can cause erection.

2. The level of the spinal cord lesion and the degree of interruption of nerve impulses influence the nature of sexual functioning. For example, the local reflexes important in female orgasm are thought to be integrated into the lumbar and sacral regions of the cord.

3. Gratification can be obtained from sexual responses other than those from the sex organs during sexual stimulation. Many physically challenged people develop other areas of stimulation to high levels.

It is important to consider the sexuality of ill people just as we consider the sexuality of all other people.

Gender
DIMENSIONS

Coming to Terms: Masculinity and Physical Challenges

Men with physical challenges may be marginalized and stigmatized in American society. The image and reality of men with challenges undermine cultural beliefs about men's bodies and physicality. The body is a central foundation of how men define themselves and how they are defined by others. Men consider their bodies as vehicles for determining value, which in turn translates into status and prestige. Men's bodies allow them to demonstrate the socially valuable characteristics of toughness, competitiveness, and ability .... Thus, one's

body and relationship to it provide a way to comprehend the world and one's place in it. The bodies of men with challenges serve as a continual reminder that they are at odds with cultural expectations.

Men with physical challenges may have conflicting expectations placed on them as men and as people with disabilities. Contemporary masculinity often expects men to be strong, courageous, aggressive, independent, and self-reliant, while people with disabilities may be seen as weak, passive, and dependent. Because of this for men with physical disabilities, being recognized as masculine by others may be difficult.

4. Adaptation of previous sexual practices may be needed after spinal cord injury. Sexual activity may need to take place in different positions, and sexual aids may be helpful.

5. Fertility and the ability to bear children are usually not lost by women with spinal cord injuries.

Sexuality and Illness

The ill are another group whose sexuality has mainly been ignored. In the past both patients and medical personnel avoided any mention of sexual topics, no doubt because both were too embarrassed to discuss them. Now questions about sexual history are often asked in addition to standard questions about medical history. And physicians, patients, and partners are encouraged to discuss, when relevant, the effects of illness or other medical problems on sexual functioning.

Diabetes, neurological disorders, gynecological disorders, inflammation of the male's prostate gland, castration, rectal surgery, and heart attacks usually have a direct (or assumed) effect on sexual functioning. But people with other nonrelated physical medical problems often experience sexual problems caused by psychological factors. Some of us, for example, feel guilty when we get sick and try to determine where the fault lies. Because the topic of sexuality is a leading producer of guilt, we may consciously or unconsciously avoid sexual activity. We may even allow illness to restrict our sexual life, not because restriction is necessary but because we failed to ask medical personnel whether restriction was actually required.

To reduce sexual problems associated with illness, we need to feel that sexuality is appropriate to discuss, and we need to be aware of guilty feelings. And, in all cases of illness, we need to take responsibility for finding out the earliest and safest time to resume normal sexual activity to prevent other detrimental effects on interpersonal relationships, as well as on self-concept.

After a heart attack, it is important to talk with one's doctor about guidelines for sexual activity. In general, having heart disease, a heart attack, or undergoing heart surgery does not mean an end to a satisfying sex life. Sexual activity is not generally risky for the heart. If a person does not get short of breath, have chest pain, or get tired when climbing two flights of stairs, the heart can meet the demands needed for sexual activity.

A person is usually able to resume sexual activity 3 to 4 weeks after a heart attack and 2 to 3 weeks after heart surgery. A decrease in sexual desire after a heart attack or surgery can be expected—this is normal and should be only temporary.

When people who have heart disease engage in sexual activities, they should choose a time when they are rested and relaxed, and free of stressful feelings. They should wait 1 to 3 hours after eating a full meal so that digestion can take place. It makes sense to select a familiar, peaceful setting that is free from interruptions. Medicine should be taken before sexual relations if prescribed by a physician.

Alzheimer's disease also affects sexuality. Some Alzheimer's sufferers develop a loss of libido, whereas others develop hypersexuality—a constant desire to engage in sexual activities. However, an affected spouse may demand sexual activity but not even recognize his or her own spouse. Caregivers

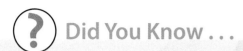

? Did You Know . . .

Persons with physical, cognitive, or emotional challenges have a right to sexuality education, sexual health care, and opportunities for socializing and for sexual expression. Family, healthcare workers, and other caregivers should receive training in understanding and supporting sexual development and behavior, comprehensive sexuality education, and related health care for individuals who have these challenges. The policies and procedures of social agencies and healthcare delivery systems should ensure that services and benefits are provided to all persons without discrimination and their caregivers have information and education about ways to minimize the risk of sexual abuse and exploitation.

Source: Modified from Position statement of Sexuality Information and Education Council of the United States, 2015. Available at http://www.siecus.org/index.cfm?fuseaction=Page.viewPage&pageId=494&parentID=472

---

say that the sexual encounter may be emotionless, mechanical, or marred by inappropriate behavior, such as giggling.

We also need to realize that sexual problems can be expressed through physical symptoms; a person who asks for an examination of the genital area because of a supposed concern about cancer may actually be seeking an acceptable way to talk about a sexual difficulty. The relationship between illness and sexuality needs to be understood to help reduce the incidence of problems in medical settings and to increase our acceptance of both ourselves and others when illness is present—either in or out of the hospital.

Emotional Challenges

Throughout this text we have emphasized a comprehensive concept of human sexuality. One excellent example of this concept is the influence of emotional states upon sexual responsiveness. Many life problems, such as stress, problems at work, death of a friend or relative, or work overload, may interfere with sexual interest or response. Apprehension about intimacy, fear of pregnancy, or possibly fear of contracting an STI may influence relationships with others. Depression or poor self-esteem can also create problems related to intimate relationships.

Whatever the reason, emotional well-being has a strong influence on overall sexuality and on sexual response. It can be helpful to understand that, at times, lack of interest in sexual activity or even inability to respond can be natural and common. Fortunately, these situations are usually temporary and can be effectively handled through personal understanding or professional counseling if needed.

Sexuality of the Mentally Challenged

For many years, the sexuality of the mentally challenged was dealt with by restricting or preventing sexual behavior; indeed, the mentally challenged were sterilized to prevent any chance of pregnancy. The societal fear was that the mentally challenged would have mentally challenged children and that they would not be able to care for their children properly—thus costly medical care would be needed. A turning point in the rights of the mentally challenged occurred with the election of President John F. Kennedy in 1960. His mentally challenged sister, Rosemary, had a profound effect on him and was a major factor in his proposing of legislation to educate and help the mentally challenged.

© Mark Richards/PhotoEdit

Despite many factors that must be considered, including safe sex and the ability to make proper decisions regarding sexuality, the mentally challenged are certainly capable of participating in sexual relationships. With the support of education and counseling, mentally challenged individuals can often greatly benefit from the affection and intimacy encountered through a sexual relationship.

The American Association on Intellectual and Developmental Disabilities has a position statement (Sexuality and Intellectual Disability, 2012) related to human sexuality. Among other points it says:

1. People with intellectual disabilities have sexuality, regardless of their degree of disability.

2. A person's ability to participate depends upon his or her functional social understanding.

3. Many adults with intellectual disability can develop meaningful, mutual relationships that may include a range of sexual activity and/or marriage.

4. People with intellectual disabilities have the right to be sexually active and the right and responsibility to be educated about sexuality, just like everyone else.

5. Some individuals who exhibit inappropriate sexual behavior do so as the result of limited communication and social skills.

6. Culturally acceptable, personally enjoyable social behaviors are the best safeguards from abuse for people with intellectual disabilities.

Mentally challenged people who are allowed to have sexual relationships can and do build feelings of affection and tenderness that appear to contribute to their happiness and tranquility. In 1970, the United Nations passed a resolution supporting the right of mentally challenged individuals to sexuality education, cohabitation, and marriage. Although the rights of the mentally challenged are indisputable, their ability to make proper decisions regarding sexuality is often disputed.

Just as everyone else, mentally challenged people can benefit from sexuality education and counseling. Because being challenged is just one more dimension of human sexuality, it should be factored into the decision-making process. For example, a long-term contraceptive might be selected instead of oral contraceptive pills so that contraceptive effectiveness would not depend on remembering to take a pill every day. Through factual knowledge, role playing, and personal experience, mentally challenged people are able to have fulfilling sexual lives.

Personal and Social Support

Society in general continues to deny the sexuality of the ill and the challenged. If this situation is to change, we need to remember that these people are sexual beings in the same way as everyone else. We also need to prevent public service personnel from denying the sexuality of their clientele. Attention must be paid to policy decisions influencing human services; to approaches used to serve the ill and the challenged; and to attitudes of those working with these people, as well as of society in general. Organizations that provide services to the ill and challenged need to teach classes in sexuality, not only for their patients but also for their patients' relatives and those who work with them.

© Gayvoronskaya Yana/Shutterstock

Case Study

The life cycle of sexuality, from high school graduation through aging, offers many opportunities to see the interaction of the dimensions of human sexuality.

Consider the aging process: Biological changes, especially in levels of hormones, can bring about psychological changes, such as in mood. In addition, a psychological shift occurs in men as they shift their attention from career to family. Cultural expectations affect elderly adults' perceptions and expectations of their sexuality.

New advances in pharmacology such as the introduction of Viagra and Cialis may solve a biological problem, but the couple must then solve the psychological and social problems related to reintegrating the ability to have an erection in the relationship. Although medication can solve most erectile disorder issues, an erection is also a function of psychosocial sexual attraction—something that cannot yet be purchased.

Biological Factors

When a sperm with a Y chromosome meets an egg, a male will develop. Biological factors continue to influence development throughout life.

- Genetic coding affects physical appearance, including height; coloration of skin, hair, and eyes; muscularity; and many aspects of health.
- Physiological changes result at puberty from the hormone testosterone, which in turn affects muscle development and body size. Testosterone also increases aggression and leads to increased rates of heart attacks.
- Toward middle age, testosterone levels begin to drop, resulting in decreased muscle mass, increased fat, and a reduced sex drive.

Sociocultural Factors

Sociocultural factors interact with biological factors to influence health.

- Laws affect what health insurers must cover. The Affordable Care Act contains requirements that will influence this.
- Religion may affect the decision as to whether to circumcise the penis.
- The cultural bias allowing men to be sexually permissive can compromise a man's sexual health and wellness.
- Ethnic heritage influences health; for example, African American males tend to have higher levels of stress and heart disease than white men do.
- Media and ads portray the ideal man with extreme muscularity which is achievable only with tremendous work and, in many cases, illegal steroids.
- Family, neighbors, and friends often reinforce gender stereotypes.
- Behavior proscribed by society as illegal can influence health; for instance, a man can compromise his health by taking anabolic steroids.

Psychological Factors

Biological and sociocultural factors combine to influence psychological factors.

- Body image and self-concept is enhanced for many men through exercise and competitive sports.
- Men often suppress their emotions, which can result in increased levels of stress.
- Learned attitudes and behaviors about sex roles can lead to unhealthy lifestyles for men.

Summary

- There are many theories about the types of love.

- It is important to understand sexual development during the college years. Many experiences and relationships with others will lay the foundation for future happiness.

- Although most people eventually marry, many are delaying marriage longer than in the past. Some people decide to remain single throughout life. In the United States, approximately 30% of women and 36.3% of men have never married.

- Cohabitation has drastically increased through the years. There are a number of advantages and disadvantages related to cohabitation.

- Marriage is attractive to people for many reasons. A little less than half of males and females older than age 15 are married in the United States.

- There are many types of marriage—including the nuclear family, peer marriages, and stepfamilies.

- Extramarital relationships may be consensual or nonconsensual. Many worthless facts exist about extramarital relationships.

- The divorce rate has declined in the last two decades largely because of people getting married later and being better educated.

- Most older people remain interested in sexual activity and participate in various forms of sexual activity. Some health difficulties associated with aging may impede sexual activities.

- Today there is increased recognition of the sexuality of physically and mentally challenged people.

Discussion Questions

1. Compare and contrast the different theories about love. Which do you agree with? Explain why.

2. Summarize the studies about college relationships and sexual activities.

3. Discuss why increased numbers of people are remaining single.

4. Compare the advantages and disadvantages of cohabitation versus marriage.

5. Discuss why marriage is popular.

6. Discuss the reasons for divorce. What can be done to help protect children?

7. Discuss how and why the aging process affects sexuality.

Application Questions

Reread the chapter-opening story and answer the following questions.

1. The names Lynn and Chris were deliberately used as pseudonyms because they are names used by both sexes. When you read the story, who did you think was the male? The female? Explain your answer. Then switch the sexes of Lynn and Chris and reread the story. Does it strike you differently now? Why?

2. What advice from the chapter might have helped Lynn and Chris have a better marriage?

Critical Thinking Questions

1. Should mildly mentally challenged people be allowed to have children? Would they be any better or worse than typical parents (who have to learn from the start as well)? If mentally challenged parents are denied reproduction rights, what about those who have diagnosed psychiatric illness (such as depression)?

2. An increasing percentage of the population is remaining permanently single. Discuss whether this trend appears to be long term or just temporary. What are its implications for population growth? The future of Social Security?

3. Because of all the problems that divorce causes, should it be outlawed? What effects would such a law have on families?

4. Write a prenuptial agreement, indicating your expectations and responsibilities in marriage. Be sure to include how financial decisions, household tasks, child-rearing responsibilities, and so on, will be handled. Would such a document help or hinder a marriage?

Critical Thinking Case

Although dual-income families have become very common, equal sharing of work around the house is not as common. It is common for women to be responsible for things like shopping, cooking, and cleaning. It is common for men to more often be responsible for maintenance and repairs around the house.

The responsibility of women for more of the housework has been referred to as the "second shift." The first shift is the paid job outside the home, and the second shift is all the work at home. Putting the two shifts together, women put in much more work time than men.

In addition, many of women's tasks with children involve maintenance activities such as feeding, bathing, taking them to the doctor, and helping with homework. In contrast, men often help out with the more fun activities like going to the movies or playing in the park.

Consider which dimensions of human sexuality influence the continuation of this phenomenon. What could be done to break out of the stereotyped roles and create a more equal home environment? Should there be a more equal home environment?

Exploring Personal Dimensions

Are You Ready for Marriage?

The following quiz can help you decide whether marriage is right for you at this point in your life. Respond as honestly as you can to the following statements. Indicate which of the two choices more closely reflects your personal opinions and priorities by placing a check before line "a" or "b." (If you have a mate, you might each fill out the quiz separately, and then compare your answers.)

1. _____ a I wouldn't feel alive unless I were married.

   _____ b Give me liberty or give me death.

2. _____ a My "favorite things to do" are typical of married people.

   _____ b My hobbies and interests are those of a single person.

3. _____ a Being married can give me more of the security I want.

   _____ b Being single can probably give me more of the career opportunities I want.

4. _____ a I'd love to vacation alone somewhere with my spouse.

   _____ b I'd love to vacation with different people at different times.

5. _____ a Married means being sexually content.

   _____ b Single means being sexually content.

6. _____ a I prefer the stability and security of married life.

   _____ b I prefer the self-reliance and adventure of single life.

7. _____ a I want sex and affection from one reliable person.

   _____ b I want a variety of lovers.

8. _____ a Marriage is underrated.

   _____ b Marriage is overrated.

9. _____ a I'm willing to work to make my spouse happy.

   _____ b I don't want to be responsible for my mate's happiness.

10. _____ a It's morally more correct to live a married life.

    _____ b I'd like to do things when I want, without family constraints.

11. _____ a I'm ready to share my life and my credit cards.

    _____ b I'm ready to share good times, but let's not get too serious.

12. _____ a I believe that people should be married.

    _____ b I think people are happier if they are single.

13. _____ a Sex is best with one's spouse.

    _____ b Sex is too delicious to limit it to one person.

14. _____ a My career plans can tolerate or maybe even benefit from my being married.

    _____ b My career plans benefit from my being single.

15. _____ a I prefer the majority of my friends to be married.

    _____ b I prefer the majority of my friends to be single.

16. _____ a Marriage can be a beautiful experience.

    _____ b Marriage can be a trap.

17. _____ a I'd like to know whom I'll be sleeping with for the rest of my life.

    _____ b I don't want to know whom I'll be sleeping with for the rest of my life.

18. _____ a Today's smart people are getting married.

    _____ b Today's smart people are single and enjoying it.

19. _____ a The pleasures of marriage are wonderful.

_____ b The risk of a bad marriage more than offsets any pleasure.

20. _____ a "Love" and "marriage" go together.

_____ b "Love" and "independence" go together.

21. _____ a I don't mind sharing bank accounts and expenses.

_____ b I'm too independent to enjoy sharing my money with a spouse.

22. _____ a I want to pour all my love into a permanent relationship.

_____ b I'm not happy with an exclusive love relationship.

23. _____ a The economic advantages of being married are important to me.

_____ b I like the idea of being single so I can spend my money as I wish.

24. _____ a Being married is important from a moral/religious standpoint.

_____ b Morality and religion have little to do with marital status.

25. _____ a Lovemaking with one's spouse is certainly best.

_____ b The many sexual opportunities of being single are a great advantage.

26. _____ a My greatest chance for personal growth is through marriage.

_____ b My greatest chance for personal growth is through independence.

27. _____ a I'd prefer to share the risks of life with a spouse.

_____ b My privacy is too important for me to enjoy being married.

28. _____ a I want a reliable lifetime relationship in marriage.

_____ b I'd rather live free and easy and singly.

29. _____ a I'd be willing to make major changes, such as moving to another state, to help a spouse.

_____ b I'm not ready to move, or make other major changes, to help a spouse.

30. _____ a Marriages are made in heaven.

_____ b Marriages are too often made in hell.

31. _____ a My recreational interests are family oriented.

_____ b My recreational interests are for singles.

32. _____ a I'd enjoy the security involved in being married.

_____ b I prefer the freedom of being single.

33. _____ a I would love to have children.

_____ b I don't want the responsibility of a family.

34. _____ a Being married offers joint tax returns and other financial benefits.

_____ b I prefer to spend my money the way I want to.

35. _____ a I prefer sex and affection with my spouse for life.

_____ b I prefer love affairs with many people.

36. _____ a I prefer the steady companionship of being married.

_____ b I prefer the excitement of companionship with many lovers.

37. _____ a I'd enjoy spending leisure time with my spouse.

_____ b I like spending my leisure time as I please.

38. _____ a If I have to choose between career advancement and marriage, I choose marriage.

_____ b If I have to choose between career advancement and marriage, I'll take career.

39. _____ a Married people can count on sexual satisfaction from a trusted partner.

_____ b Single people can find lovers from an endless pool of possibilities.

40. _____ a Marriage requires major compromises, and I'm willing to make them.

_____ b Marriage requires major compromises, and I'm not yet ready to make them.

Scoring the Quiz

1. Count the number of your "a" responses and write the total here: _____
2. Compare your number of "a" responses with the following scale to determine your level.

   0–20 = Low readiness

   21–30 = Medium readiness

   31–40 = High readiness

Interpreting Your Score

Low marriage readiness: If you scored here, your values are heavily weighted toward a single lifestyle. Even if you've found a partner who shares your interests and values, the importance you attach to marriage at this time isn't enough to ensure success. Don't marry on the assumption that your values will change. They may not. And you shouldn't marry on the basis of other people's expectations or views about being married. *Yours* are the only ones that really count when it comes to marriage.

Though you may not value married life now, marriage readiness can develop rapidly. You may grow tired of the freedom and lifestyle that characterize being single, or come to appreciate more those elements associated with being married. Continue to review your marriage readiness from time to time, but do NOT marry until your values will support it.

Medium marriage readiness: Your values blend support for both single and married lifestyles, which means there's a certain level of risk if you choose to get married at this time. Probably the most important issue for you to consider is your potential mate's marriage readiness. Someone with a high readiness level can add stability to the relationship, increasing the likelihood of its success. Conversely, someone without it would dramatically reduce your already uncertain potential for a good marriage.

If he/she is less ready for marriage than you, be wary of demands for concessions. For example, he/she may say, in effect, "Do what I want or I'm getting out. I don't really want to be married as much as you do anyway." This is a destructive gambit; don't be pushed into a decision you're not ready to make.

A second major issue for you is the parity "fit" between you and your potential mate—your approximate equality in terms of personality, status, and appearance. Medium marriage readiness provides little cushion against the costs of an unequal match. High parity may lead to a successful marriage even if one or both partners possess only medium marriage readiness. But as the parity levels decrease, the greater the need for both partners to have a strong commitment to their marriage.

High marriage readiness: Your values strongly support married life, and your only challenge will be to find the right match. Be on guard, however, against projecting your own high level of marriage readiness onto a potential mate. The key for you is to realize that although you may be ready, you still need to choose your partner wisely.

Suggested Readings

AgePage: Sexuality in later life. National Institute on Aging, 2015. Available: http://www.nia.nih.gov /health/publication/sexuality-later-life.

Kim, H. S. Consequences of parental divorce for child development. *American Sociological Review, 77, no. 30* (2011), 487–511.

Marquardt, E., Blankenhorn, D., Lerman, R. I., Malone-Colon, L., & Wilcox, W. B. State of our unions: The president's agenda for the forgotten sixty percent. *The state of our unions.* National Marriage Project and Institute for American Values, 2012. Available: http://nationalmarriageproject.org/reports/.

Menopausal symptoms and complementary health approaches. National Center for Complementary and Integrative Health, 2015. Available: https://nccih.nih.gov/health /menopause/menopausesymptoms.

Parker-Pope, T. *For Better: The science of good marriage.* New York: Dutton, 2010.

Sexual difficulties: Healthy aging. Office of Women's Health, U.S. Department of Health and Human Services, 2015. Available: http://www .womenshealth.gov/aging/sexual-health/sexual -difficulties.html.

Singles in America 2015. *Match.com.* Available: http://www.singlesinamerica.com/.

Web Resources

Child Trends Data Bank
www.childtrends/databank.org

Information about the well-being of children, family structure, and family trends.

The National Marriage Project
www.nationalmarriageproject.org

Information about marriage, divorce, cohabitation, and some international comparisons.

Hawkins, A. J., & VanDenBerge, B. *Facilitating forever.* National Marriage Project, 2014. Available: http://nationalmarriageproject.org/wp-content /uploads/2014/03/FacilitatingForeverFINAL_Web 031114.pdf.

Documents federal and state policy experiments designed to help couples form and sustain health relationships and enduring marriages.

U.S. Census Bureau
www.census.gov

Statistics on marriages, divorces, and various types of families and living arrangements.

Mayo Clinic.com
www.mayoclinic.com

Information on sexual health of various groups of people.

References

10 best dating sites. *DatingAdvice.com*, 2015. Available: http://datingadvice.com/rankings.

Acevedo, B. P., & Aron, A. Does a long-term relationship kill romantic love? *Review of General Psychology, 13, 1* (2009), 59–65.

Almost all millennials accept interracial dating and marriage. Pew Research Publications, 2010. Available: http://pewresearch.org/pubs/1480/millennials-accept-iinterracial-dating-marriage-friends-different-race-generations.

American College Health Association. American College Health Association—National College Health Assessment II: 2014.

American Fact Finder. U.S. Bureau of the Census, 2015. Available: http://factfinder.census.gov/faces/nav/jsf/pages/guided_search.xhtml.

American Time Use Survey. U. S. Bureau of Labor Statistics, June 18, 2017. Available: http://www.bls.gov/news.release/pdf/atus.pdf.

Aron, A., Fisher, H. A., Mashek, D. J., Strong, G., Li, H., & Brown, L. L. Reward, motivation and emotion systems associated with early-stage intense romantic love. *Journal of Neurophysiology, 94* (May 31, 2005), 327–337.

Ashley Madison News, 2011. Available: http://www.ashleymadison.com/cheating/news.html.

Avellar, S. The economic consequences of the dissolution of cohabiting unions. *Journal of Marriage and Family 67, no. 2* (May 2005), 315–327.

Baron, K. New poll reveals that we are not happy with our sex lives. Associated Press LifGoesStrong.com poll, 2010. Available: http://www.lifegoesstrong.com/sex-poll.

Bersamin, M. M., Zamboanga, B. L., Schwartz, S. J., Donnellan, M. B., Hudson, M., Weisskirch, R. S., et al. Risky business: Is there an association between casual sex and mental health in emerging adults? *Journal of Sex Research, 51, 1* (2014), 43–51.

Births to unmarried women. Child Trends Data Bank, 2015. Available: http://www.childtrends.org/?indicators=births-to-unmarried-women.

The boomer sandwich. *Modern Maturity, 44, no. 5* (September/October 2001), 94.

Brown, S. L., & Lin, I. F. *Gray divorce: A growing risk regardless of class or education.* Council on Contemporary Families, 2014. Available: https://contemporaryfamilies.org/growing-risk-brief-report/.

Brown, S. L., Manning, W. D., & Payne, K. K. *Relationship quality among cohabiting versus married couples.* National Center for Family and Marriage Research, 2014. Available: http://www.bgsu.edu/content/dam/BGSU/college-of-arts-and-sciences/NCFMR/documents/WP/WP-14-03.pdf.

Buss, D. *The evolution of desire: Strategies of human mating.* New York: Basic Books, 1994.

Buss, D., et al. International preferences in selecting mates. *Journal of Cross-Cultural Psychology, 21* (1990), 5–47.

Census Bureau releases estimates of same-sex married couples. U.S. Census Bureau, 2011. Available: http://2010.census.gov/news/releases/operations/cb11-cn181.html.

Cohn, D. New Facts About Families. Pew Research Center Publications, 2011.

Copen, C. E., Daniels, K., & Mosher, W. D. First premarital cohabitation in the U.S.: 2006–2010 National Survey of Family Growth. *National Health Statistics Reports, 64* (April 4, 2013).

Cruz, J. *Marriage: More than a century of change.* National Center for Family and Marriage Research, 2013. Available: https://www.bgsu.edu/content/dam/BGSU/college-of-arts-and-sciences/NCFMR/documents/FP/FP-13-13.pdf.

DeBeauvoir, S. *The coming of age.* New York: Warner Books, 1973.

DiBenedetto, C. *10 rules to make your relationship last,* 2014. Available: http://news.health.com/2015/01/13/marriage-rules-make-your-relationship-last//

DeParle, J., & Tavernise, S. For women under 30, most births occur outside marriage. *The New York Times,* February 17, 2012. Available: http://www.nytimes.com/2012/02/18/us/for-women-under-30-most-births-occur-outside-marriage.html?pagewanted=all.

Divorce rate. *Divorcepad.com*, 2015. Available: http://www.divorcepad.com/rate/.

Easton, J. A., Confer, J. C., Goetz, C. D., & Buss, D. M. Reproduction expediting: Sexual motivations, fantasies, and the ticking biological clock. *Personality and Individual Differences, 49* (2010), 516–520.

Elliott, S., & Umberson, D. The performance of desire: Gender and sexual negotiation in long-term marriages. *Journal of Marriage and Family, 70, 2* (April 2008), 391–406.

Finer, L. B., & Philbin, J. M. Trends in ages at key reproductive transitions in the United States, 1951–2010. *Women's Health Issues, 24, 3* (2014), e1–e9.

Francese, P. Stat of the day: Census finds 1.3 million fewer nuclear families. ADAGESTAT, June 8, 2011. Available: http://adage.com/article/adagestat/census-finds-1-3-million-fewer-nuclear-families/228057/.

Fromm, E. *The art of loving.* New York: Harper and Row, 1956.

Frosch, D. Hard times for gay retirement havens. *The New York Times,* October 28, 2011. Available: http://www.nytimes.com/2011/10/29/us/gay-retirement-communities-struggling-in-the-recession.html?pagewanted=all.

Fry, R., & Cohn, D. Living together: The economics of Cohabitation. Pew Research Center Publications, 2011.

Furman, W., & Collibee, C. Sexual activity with romantic and nonromantic partners and psychosocial adjustment in young adults. *Archives of Sexual Behavior, 43, 7* (2014), 1327–1341.

Gonzales, L. The biology of attraction. *Men's Health, 20, no. 6* (September 2005), 186–193.

Griebling, T. L. Sexual behaviors, condom use, and sexual health of Americans over 50: Implications for sexual health promotion for older adults. *Journal of Urology, 185, 6* (2011), 2275–2276.

Hans, J. D. Do love styles predict lifetime number of sex partners? *American Journal of Sexuality Education, 3, 2* (2008), 149–159.

Hawkins, A. J., & VanDenBerghe, B. *Facilitating forever.* National Marriage Project, 2014. Available: http://nationalmarriageproject.org/resources/facilitatingforever/.

Here's where all the cheating spouses in American live. *Huffington Post*, 2013. Available: http://www.huffingtonpost.com/2013/12/16/where-people-cheat_n_4425534.html.

Hymowitz, K., Carroll, J. S., Wilcox, J. B., & Kaye, K. *Knot yet: The benefits and costs of delayed marriage in America.* National Campaign to Prevent Teen and Unplanned Pregnancy, 2013. Available: http://nationalmarriageproject.org/wp-content/uploads/2013/03/KnotYet-FinalForWeb.pdf.

Intimacy and aging: Tips for sexual health and happiness. *MayoClinic.com* (November 18, 2003). Available: http://www.mayoclinic.com/invoke.cfm?id=HA00035.

Jensen, B. The new American family. *AARP The Magazine* (June–July 2014), 30–36.

Kids count data book. Annie E. Casey Foundation, 2014. Available: http://www.aecf.org/2014db.

Kaplan, H. S. *The new sex therapy: Active treatment of sexual dysfunction.* New York: Brunner/Mazel, 1974.

Kids Count Data Center, 2011. Children in Single-Parent Families (Number)-2010; Children in Single-Parent Families (Percent)-2010. Available: http://datacenter.kidscount.org/data/acrossstates/Rankings.aspx?.

Kiecolt-Glaser, J. The risks of marital discord. *U.S. News & World Report* (January 28 2009). Available: http://researchnews.osu.edu/archive/fighting.htm.

King, V. A Comparison of cohabiting relationships among older and younger adults. *Journal of Marriage & Family, 67, no. 2* (January 2005), 271–285.

Klinenberg, E. Living alone is the new norm. *Time, 197, no. 10* (March 12, 2012), 60–62.

Koss-Feder, L. Bunking in with mom and dad. *Time, 173, 8* (March 2, 2009), 537.

Kurdek, L. A. Are gay and lesbian cohabiting couples really different from heterosexual married couples? *Journal of Marriage & Family, 66, no. 4* (November 2004), 880–900.

Lewis, J. E., Malow, R. M., & Ireland, S. J. HIV/AIDS risk in heterosexual college students: A review of a decade of literature. *Journal of American College Health, 45, no. 4* (1997), 147–158.

LGBT older adults in long-term care facilities: Stories from the field. National Senior Citizens Law Center, 2011. Available: http://lgbtlongtermcare.org/.

Lindau, S. T., Schumm, L. P., Laumannm, E. O., Levinson, W., O'Muircheartaigh, C. A., & Waite, L. J. A study of sexuality and health among older adults in the United States. *New England Journal of Medicine, 357, 8* (August 23, 2007), 762–774.

Link, A., & Copeland, P. Sexual magnetism: Pheromones—the scent of sex. *Urban Male Magazine* (Winter 2001), 38–39.

Livingston, G., & Cohn, D. More women without children. Pew Research Center, June 25, 2010. Available: http://pewresearch.org/pubs/1642/more-women-without-children.

Luscombe, B. Wealthy kids are more affected by divorce than poor kids. *Time.com*, 2014. Available: http://time.com/3311733/divorce-wealthy-families-georgetown/.

Manning, W. D., Brown, S. L., & Payne, K. K. Two decades of stability and change in age at first union formation. *Journal of Marriage and Family, 76, 2* (2014), 247–260.

Manning, W. D., & Styles, B. *Twenty-five years of change in cohabitation in the U.S., 1987–2013.* National Center for Family and Marriage Research, 2015. Available: http://www.bgsu.edu/content/dam/BGSU/college-of-arts-and-sciences/NCFMR/documents/FP/FP-15-01-twenty-five-yrs-cohab-us.pdf.

Marriage Project, Rutgers, the State University of New Jersey, 2005. Available: http://marriage.rutgers.edu.

Maslow, A. H. *Toward a psychology of being*, 2nd ed. Princeton, NJ: Van Nostrand, 1968.

Masters, W. H., & Johnson, V. E. *Human sexual response.* Boston: Little, Brown, 1966.

Match.com and Chadwick Martin Bailey 2009–2010 studies: Recent trends: Online dating, 2010. Available: http://cp.match.com/cppp/media/CMB_Study.pdf.

McCarthy, J. Same-sex marriage support reaches new high at 55%. *Gallup.com*, 2014. Available: http://www.gallup.com/poll/169640/sex-marriage-support-reaches-new-high.aspx?version=print.

Menopause. National Institute on Aging, 2010. Available: http://www.nia.nih.gov/health/publication/menopause.

Menopause. National Institute on Aging, 2010. Available: http://www.nia.nih.gov/HealthInformation/Publications/menopause.htm.

Miller, A. J., Sassler, S., & Kusi-Appouh, D. The specter of divorce: Views from working-class and middle class cohabitors. *Family Relations, 60* (2011), 602–616.

Monto, M. A., & Carey, A. G. A new standard of sexual behavior? Are claims associated with the "hookup culture" supported by general social survey data? *Journal of Sex Research, 51, 6* (2014), 605–615.

Morin, R. The public renders a split verdict on changes in family structure. Pew Research Center, February 6, 2011. Available: http://pewsocialtrends.org/files/2011/02/Pew-Social-Trends-Changes-In-Family-Structure.pdf.

Mulhauser, D. Dating among college students is all but dead, survey finds. *Chronicle of Higher Education, 47, no. 48* (August 10, 2001), A51.

Musick, K., & Bumpass, L. Reexamining the case for marriage: union formation and changes in well-being. *Journal of Marriage and Family, 74, no. 1* (February 2012), 1–18.

National Marriage Project. Available: http://nationalmarriageproject.org/wp-content/uploads/2014/08/NMP-BeforeIDoReport-Final.pdf.

National Survey of Sexual Health and Behavior. Indiana University Center for Sexual Health Promotion, 2010. Available: http://www.nationalsexstudy.indiana.edu/.

Newport, F. In U.S., 87% approve of black–white marriage, vs 4% in 1958. *Gallup.com*, 2013. Available: http://www.gallup.com/poll/163697/approve-marriage-blacks-whites.aspx.

Nine psychological tasks for a good marriage. American Psychological Association, 2015. Available: http://www.apa.org/helpcenter/marriage.aspx.

Ortman, J. M., Velkoff, V. A., & Hogan, H. An aging nation: The older population in the United States. U.S. Census Bureau, 2014. Available: http://www.census.gov/prod/2014pubs/p25-1140.pdf.

Osteoporosis Handout on Health. National Institute of Health Osteoporosis and Related Bone Diseases National Resource Center, 2011. Available: http://www.niams.nih.gov/Health_Info/Bone/Osteoporosis/osteoporosis_hoh.asp.

Oswalt, S. B. Beyond risk: Examining college students' sexual decision making. *American Journal of Sexuality Education 5, no. 3* (July–September, 2010), 217–239.

Paik, A. "Hookups," dating, and relationship quality: Does the type of sexual involvement matter? *Social Science Research 39, no. 5* (September, 2010), 739–753.

Planned Parenthood Federation. *Thinking about adoption*, 2009. Available: http://www.plannedparenthood.org/health-topics/pregnancy/adoption-21520.htm.

Popenoe, D. Cohabitation, marriage and child wellbeing. National Marriage Project, 2008. Available: http://marriage.rutgers.edu/Publications/2008cohabreport.html.

Popenoe, D., & Whitehead, B. D. The state of our unions 2005. The National Population 65 years and older in the United States, 2011. U.S. Census Bureau, American Fact Finder. Available: http://factfinder2.census.gov/faces/tableservices/jsf/pages/productview.xhtml?pid=ACS_10_1YR_S0103&prodType=table.

Qian, Z., & Lichter, D. T. Changing patterns of interracial marriage in a multicultural society. *Journal of Marriage and Family, 73, no. 5* (October, 2011), 1065–1084.

Reinisch, J. M., Hill, C. A., Sanders, S. A., & Zembia-Davis, M. High-risk sexual behavior at a Midwestern university—a confirmation survey. *Family Planning Perspectives, 27, no. 2* (March/April 1995), 79–82.

Rempel, J. K., & Burris, C. T. Let me count the ways: An integrative theory of love and hate. *Personal Relationships, 12, no. 2* (June 2005), 297–313.

Renzetti, C. M., & Curren, D. J. *Living sociology*. Needham Heights, MA: Allyn & Bacon, 1998.

Rhoades, G. K., & Stanley, S. M. Before "I do": What do premarital experiences have to do with marital quality among today's young adults? 2014.

Ross, M. W. Situating sexuality electronically: The Internet and sexual expression. *Sexuality Research & Public Policy, 4, 2* (June 2007), 1–4.

Safer sex guidelines. Information. Education. Action (2009). Available: http://www.aids.org/factSheets/151-Safer-Sex-Guidelines.html.

Sandler, L. None is enough. *Time, 182, 7* (2013), 40–45.

Schmid, R. E. Unmarried couples top 4 million. *AP/AOL* (July 27, 1998).

Sexuality and Intellectual Disability. American Association on Intellectual and Developmental Disabilities, 2012. Available: http://www.aamr.org/content_198.cfm.

Sexuality in midlife and beyond. Cambridge, MA: Harvard Health Publications, 2013.

Singh, D. Female mate value at a glance: Relationship of waist-to-hip ratio to health, fecundity, and attractiveness. *Human Ethology & Evolutionary Psychology, 23* (December 2002), 81–91.

Smock, P. J., Bergstrom, C., Huang, P., & Manning, W. Why shack up? Motivations to cohabit among young adults in the U.S. Presented at 37th World Congress of the International Institute of Sociology, Stockholm, Sweden, July 5–9, 2005.

Social indicators of marital health and well-being. *The state of our unions.* National Marriage Project, 2012. Available: http://www.stateofourunions.org/2012/social_indicators.php#teens.

Stampler, L. The new dating game. *Time, 183, 6* (2014), 41–45.

Stanton, A. Affairs, part 2: Understanding what went wrong. Health and age. Novartis Foundation for Gerontology, 2001. Available: http://www.healthandage.com/Home/gid2=1258.

Stein, L. Sex and seniors: The 70-year itch. *HealthDay*, 2014. Available: http://consumer.healthday.com/encyclopedia/aging-1/misc-aging-news-10/sex-and-seniors-the-70-year-itch-647575.html.

Sternberg, R. A triangular theory of love. *Psychological Review, 93* (1986), 119–135.

Sternberg, R. *The triangle of love: Intimacy, passion, commitment.* New York: Basic Books, 1988.

Stritof, S. *Most widely used premarital inventories,* 2015. Available: http://marriage.about.com/od/premaritaltests/a/premaritaltest.htm.

Stritof, S., & Stritof, B. Marital sex statistics. About.com. Marriage, 2010. Available: http://marriage.about.com/cs/sexualstatistics/a/sexstatistics.htm.

Studies show shifting paradigm of sexual relationships among young adults. National Partnership for Women and Health, April 4, 2011. Available: http://www.nationalpartnership.org/site/News2?abbr=daily2_&page=NewsArticle&id=28190.

Survey finds gaps between safe-sex claims, behavior among U.S. adults. *Kaiser Daily Reproductive Health Report*, (April 7, 2004). Available: http://www.kaisernetwork.org.

Survey USA public opinion poll (1998). Available: http://www.surveyusa.com.

Surveys show change in attitudes toward sex among high school and college students, higher incidences of "casual" and oral sex. *Kaiser Daily Reproductive Health Report* (January 21, 2003). Available: http://www.kaisernetwork.org.

Swami, V. An examination of the love-is-blind bias among gay men and lesbians. *Body Image* (February 3, 2009).

That's what he said. Seventeen Magazine and the National Campaign to Prevent Teen and Unplanned Pregnancy, 2010. Available: http://www.thenationalcampaign.org.

Trail, T. E., & Karney, B. R. What's (not) wrong with low-income marriages. *Journal of Marriage and Family, 74, no. 3* (June 2012), 413–427.

Trompeter, S. E., Bettencourt, R., & Barnett-Connor, E. Sexual activity and satisfaction in health community-dwelling older women. *American Journal of Medicine 125, no. 1* (January 2012), 37–43.

U.S. Bureau of Labor Statistics. Single-parent households by country, September 30, 2011. Updated and Revised from Families and Work in Transition in 12 Countries, 1980–2001, *Monthly Labor Review* (September 2003), with national sources, some of which may be unpublished.

U.S. Census Bureau. *2011–2013 3-year American Community Survey,* 2013. Available: http://factfinder.census.gov/faces/tableservices/jsf/pages/productview.xhtml?pid=ACS_13_3YR_DP02&prodType=table.

U.S. Surgeon General issues first call to action on disability. United States Department of Health and Human Services, July 26, 2005. Available: http://www.surgeongeneral.gov.

Vespa, J. Historical trends in the marital intentions of one-time and serial cohabitors. *Journal of Marriage and Family, 77, 1* (2014), 207–217.

What guys really think about sex. Seventeen & National Campaign to Prevent Teen and Unplanned Pregnancy, 2015. Available: http://www.seventeen.com/health/tips/boys-and-sex.

Whitchurch, E. R., Wilson, T. D., & Gilbert, D. T. "He loves me, ne loves me not ...", uncertainty can increase romantic attraction. *Psychological Science, 22, no. 2* (February 2011), 172–175.

Who pays for dates? Schmid College of Science and Technology, 2014. Available: http://blogs.chapman.edu/scst/2014/02/13/who-pays-for-dates/.

Why couples who have broken up should not get back together: Relationships expert. Health, Medical, and Science Updates. Stone Hearth News, February 20, 2012. Available: http://www.stonehearthnewsletters.com/why-couples-who-have-broken-up-should-not-get-back-together-relationships-expert/relationships/.

Willoughby, B. J., Carroll, J. S., & Busby, D. M. Differing relationship outcomes when sex happens before, on, or after first dates. *Journal of Sex Research, 51, 1* (2014), 52–61.

Womenshealth.gov. Menopausal Hormone Therapy (MHT), 2011. Available: http://womenshealth.gov/glossary/index.cfm#M.

Woods, N. F. *Human sexuality in health and illness*. St. Louis: Mosby, 1979.

World Family Map. *Mapping family change and child well-being outcomes*, 2013. Available: http://worldfamilymap.org/2013/articles/world-family-indicators/family-structure.

You may be surprised how many born-again Christians use Ashley Madison. *Huffington Post*, 2014. Available: http://www.huffingtonpost.com/2014/06/04/infidelity-and-religion_n_5447526.html.

Zill, N. *Kids of single parents more likely to witness domestic violence*, 2015. Available: http://family-studies.org/children-in-single-parent-families-are-more-likely-to-witness-domestic-violence/.

CHAPTER 15

Sexual Techniques and Behavior

© Gayvoronskaya Yana/Shutterstock

FEATURES

Global Dimensions
Global Religious Views on Sexuality

Gender Dimensions
Differences Between Male and Female Sexual Fantasies

Ethical Dimensions
Should People Who Do Not Feel Comfortable with Oral or Anal Sexual Activity Learn to Enjoy These Activities?

Multicultural Dimensions
Does Level of Education Influence Sexuality?

Global Dimensions
Gay and Lesbian Rights Around the World

Communication Dimensions
The use of Sexual words and the Resulting Confusion

CHAPTER OBJECTIVES

1 Identify the historical basis for present-day societal, religious, and/or cultural attitudes toward masturbation.

2 Cite the prevalence of sexual fantasy, describe its content and function, and note differences in male and female sexual fantasies.

3 Describe the role of touch, sight, smell, sound, and taste in sexual foreplay. Then list and describe various positions of sexual intercourse, including their advantages and disadvantages.

INTRODUCTION

*O*ne often hears that the 20th century's sexual revolution has led to more promiscuity and sexual freedom. The following excerpt, written before a different sort of revolution—the American Revolution—shows that many sexual techniques have not changed in a long time:

> As I kept hesitating and disconcerted under this soft distraction, Charles, with a fond impatience, took the pains to undress me; and all I can remember amidst the flutter and discomposure of my senses was some flattering exclamations of joy and admiration, more specially at the feel of my breasts now set at liberty from my stays, and which panting and rising in tumultuous throbs, swell'd upon his dear touch, and gave it the welcome pleasure of finding them well form'd, and unfail'd in firmness.

> I was soon laid in bed, and scarce languish'd an instant for the darling partner of it, before he was undress'd and got between the sheets, with his arms clasp'd round me, giving and taking, with gust inexpressible, a kiss of welcome, that my heart rising to my lips stamp'd with its warmest impression, concurring to my bliss, with that delicate and voluptuous emotion which Charles alone had the secret to excite, and which constitutes the very life, the essence of pleasure....

> But as action was now a necessity to desires so much on edge as ours, Charles, after a very short prelusive dalliance, lifting up my linen and his own, laid the broad treasures of his manly chest close to my bosom, both beating with the tenderest alarms: when now, the sense of his glowing body, in naked touch with mine, took all power over my thoughts out of my own disposal, and deliver'd up every faculty of the soul to the sensiblest of joys, that affecting me infinitely more with my distinction of the person than of the sex, now brought my conscious heart deliciously into play: my heart, which eternally constant to Charles, had never taken any part in my occasional sacrifices to the calls of constitution, complaisance, or interest.

The preceding excerpt, from John Cleland's 1749 novel Fanny Hill, or Letters of a Woman of Pleasure, *shows that erotic literature has detailed sexual liaisons for centuries.*

Relatively few people actually set out to learn effective sexual arousal techniques. What learning takes place often occurs through trial and error *(with plenty of both). The results may be total pleasure, or they may be shame and embarrassment, confusion, and perhaps sexual dysfunction. Furthermore, such naivete and ignorance too often result in unwanted pregnancies. We believe that a strong foundation of sexual knowledge includes not only anatomical and physiological facts but also specific information about what people find sexually stimulating. Therefore, this chapter covers nonphysical means of arousal, as well as techniques in beginning play (foreplay), sexual intercourse, and oral–genital sexual activity.*

■ Autoerotic Sexual Behaviors

The two solitary sexual behaviors we discuss in this section are masturbation and fantasy. We should note, however, that although these are usually solitary behaviors, they can also be engaged in with a partner in the form of mutual masturbation or shared sexual fantasizing.

Masturbation

One need not have a partner to be sexually stimulated. **Masturbation** is the stimulation of one's own genitals for sexual pleasure. As Woody Allen said in the movie *Annie Hall*, masturbation is sex with the person you love most.

Negative Attitudes: A Matter of History
Many of our attitudes regarding sexual activity are part of our cultural past. Masturbation is a good example of this. Ancient Hebrews believed they were partners of God in replenishing the Earth. In addition, they needed male offspring to maintain the patriarchal system and to supply needed labor. Consequently, laws were enacted to discourage nonprocreative sexual behavior. Any sexual activity that did not potentially lead to conception was devalued.

Many believe this attitude is best represented by the story of Onan in Genesis in the Old Testament. Onan was the brother of Er, whom God slayed because he was "wicked." However, Er had not yet conceived any children with his wife, Tamar. It was Judaic law that the next of kin of the husband must impregnate the widow so that the dead man had an heir. God, therefore, ordered Onan to impregnate Tamar, but Onan, not wanting to sire a child who would not be his, "wasted his seed" on the ground by withdrawing his penis just before ejaculation. The Lord killed Onan for this indiscretion, and, erroneously,

masturbation came to be nicknamed *onanism*. Christian mores were influenced greatly by Jewish codes of behavior, and, consequently, masturbation was condemned by Christian law as well.

To this day our attitudes toward masturbation are colored by these ancient proscriptions. For example, although Freud believed masturbation to be a normal childhood practice, he feared that if carried into adulthood it would interfere with the formation of healthy sexual relationships. As recently as 1976 the Vatican stated in a Declaration on Sexual Ethics that masturbation was an "intrinsically and seriously disordered act."

The Danger
No physiological harm can be attributed to masturbation. It will not cause insanity, sterility, sexual dysfunction, or any other physical affliction. Nor is there evidence that masturbation leads to an inability to establish meaningful sexual relationships. The primary danger associated with masturbation is within the individual's own mind—the guilt or shame he or she may feel about masturbating. Masturbation is so common that human sexuality experts now consider it a normal sexual act. It is normal to masturbate, and it is normal not to. As all sexual behaviors are, masturbation is a matter of personal choice. Awareness of this current thinking should go a long way toward alleviating a good deal of the guilt and shame people feel about engaging in this behavior.

Prevalence
Sexual research is fraught with limitations. Consequently we can only present data from several different studies and present a composite view about the prevalence of masturbatory behavior. The majority of studies have found that approximately 90% of adult males and slightly more than 60% of adult females report having masturbated (Arafat & Cotton, 1974; Downey, 1980; Hunt, 1974; Kinsey, Pomeroy, & Martin, 1948, 1953). These figures have remained

---

masturbation Self-stimulation of the genitals.

Global DIMENSIONS

Global Religious Views on Sexuality

Different religions confront sexual behaviors and sexual mores differently. For example, in Judaism, a *mikva* (ritual bath) is prescribed for women who have just finished menstruating to cleanse them physically and spiritually. Muslims and Jews perform circumcisions as part of their religious rituals, although they perform them at different times and for different reasons. Muslim circumcision of men is a rite of passage into manhood and of women is a means to prevent them from being easily sexually aroused and, therefore, potentially unfaithful to their husbands.

In Jewish practice, circumcision is performed only on young male infants 8 days old and represents a covenant with God. In Catholicism, abortion is a sin, because the religion teaches that life begins when fertilization occurs; the mother has no more status than does the unborn. In several other religions, abortion is allowed to remain a decision between the pregnant woman and her physician.

If you have a religion, what does it teach about sexuality? Perhaps you will want to interview a member of the clergy to understand better the rules, regulations, rituals, and rationale behind these teachings.

remarkably consistent through the years (Clement, 1990). In fact, studies in the 1990s found that 60% of American men and 40% of American women had masturbated in the past year. Among couples living together, 85% of the men and 45% of the women had masturbated within the past year (Laumann et al., 1994; Michael et al., 1995). More recently, the Center for Sexual Health Promotion at Indiana University reported results from the National Survey of Sexual Health and Behavior (Herbenick et al., 2010). It found that 92% of men ages 20 to 24 and 94% of men ages 25 to 29 had ever masturbated. For women, 77% ages 20 to 24 and 85% ages 25 to 29 had ever masturbated.

A number of sociodemographic and behavioral factors are associated with their masturbation. Among both men and women, masturbation increased with higher levels of education and social class, and was more common among those reporting sexual function problems. For women, masturbation was more likely among those who had more frequent vaginal sex, who had a greater repertoire of sexual activity (such as oral and anal sex), and who had more sexual partners in the past year. In contrast, the prevalence of masturbation was lower among men reporting more frequent vaginal sex. Furthermore, both men and women reporting same-gender partners were more likely to masturbate than heterosexual partners.

Techniques

Males masturbate by stroking the shaft of the penis, often stimulated by erotic literature, films, or the Internet. Some men use gadgets to assist them. Artificial vaginas, furlike clothes, inflatable dolls, and other devices have been reported as masturbatory aids.

Women masturbate by rubbing the vulva—in particular, the clitoris—or inserting an object (a finger, a dildo, a banana, or a similarly shaped object) into the vagina. There are, of course, many variations on this theme, and the use of a vibrator to stimulate the vulva, cream to decrease friction on the area rubbed, pillows or other soft objects to rub the genitals against, and squeezing together of the thighs are all common adjuncts to the standard masturbatory techniques (see Figure 15.1).

Masturbation is a pleasurable, common, and varied sexual behavior; it is devoid of physical harm; it is more prevalent in men than women; and it continues even after marriage. The appropriateness of this and other sexual behaviors, however, relates to one's acceptance of them without guilt or shame and one's religious and moral points of view. As with other sexual behaviors, whether to masturbate is a personal choice.

The G Spot

Some women report experiencing heightened sexual arousal when an area of the interior wall of the vagina is stimulated. This area's sensitivity was first noted by the gynecologist Ernst Grafenberg; hence it is called the G spot. To stimulate the G spot, two fingers should be inserted into the vagina. The fingers should be pressed deeply into the tissue of the anterior wall of the vagina between the posterior side of the pubic bone and the cervix. Initially a woman may report a slight feeling of discomfort, a pleasurable feeling, or a sensation of needing to urinate. This latter reaction is probably due to pressure on the bladder. After a short period the tissue may swell, and unpleasant sensations may be replaced with erotic sensations. Women who experience orgasms from stimulation of the G spot often report them to be

FIGURE **15.1** Masturbatory techniques.

intense. Perry and Whipple (1981) describe this orgasm as resulting in a more intense uterine contraction than orgasm from stimulation of either clitoris or the vagina. Other researchers do not agree that a "uterine orgasm" distinct from other orgasms exists (Pastor, 2010).

Recently evidence has been found that might verify the existence of what appears to be a G spot in some women (Geddes, 2008; Henderson, 2008). Using vaginal ultrasound, researchers compared women who reported experiencing a vaginal orgasm with women who did not (Gravina et al., 2008). They found the tissue in the area thought to contain the G spot to be thicker in women who experienced vaginal orgasm. Still, some experts suggest this might really be a result of the size of the clitoris rather than a distinct G spot. Others wonder if the thicker vaginal wall is a result of women learning to orgasm vaginally, thereby altering their anatomy, much like exercising a muscle makes it grow. Even more recently, researchers reviewed past studies of the existence of the G spot and highlighted the controversy surrounding its existence (Kilchevsky et al., 2012). The researchers concluded that "objective measures have failed to provide strong and consistent evidence for the existence of an anatomical site that could be related to the famed G-spot." They did temper their conclusion by pointing out that

reports and anecdotal testimonials raise the question of whether research studies and the methods used by researchers have been adequate to definitively identify the existence or nonexistence of the G spot. With subsequent research, perhaps the existence of the G spot will be either validated or refuted. In the meantime, the controversy continues.

Fantasy

Fantasies are thoughts and images, daydreams, and scenarios. In a sexual context, we call these **sexual fantasies**.

Prevalence of Sexual Fantasies

Sexual fantasies are quite commonplace (Halderman, Zelhart, & Jackson, 1984). One researcher surveyed middle-class women and found that only 7% had never experienced sexual daydreams or fantasies (Hariton, 1973). Earlier, Kinsey had found that 84% of men and 67% of women had sexual fantasies. Other researchers have also found sexual fantasies prevalent; for example, when studying college students, Sue (1979) found that 60% of men and women fantasized during sexual intercourse; Crepault and associates (1977) reported that 94% of their sample of women engaged in sexual fantasies; Zimmer and colleagues (1983) found that 71% of men and 72% of women fantasized about sex to become more sexually aroused; and Masters, Johnson, and Kolodny (1985) reported

sexual fantasies Thoughts, images, and daydreams of a sexual nature.

Gender DIMENSIONS

Differences Between Male and Female Sexual Fantasies

In one of the author's college classes, students are asked to write their most erotic fantasy on one side of a sheet of paper. They are then instructed to write the letter M or F on the back to indicate male or female. Of course, students can opt out of this exercise regarding what males and females find erotic, but they seldom do. The papers are collected and placed face up on a long table. Students read the fantasies, one at a time, and try to determine whether a male or a female wrote each. When all the fantasies are read, the males meet in one room and the females in another and generalize about what the opposite sex seems to find erotic. The following are typical observations:

1. In both male and female fantasies, the males were active and the females passive. In other words, males were doing "it" (whatever "it" happened to be) to the females.

2. The female fantasies involved more of a relationship between the sexual partners than did the male fantasies. For example, many females described sexual activity after a walk on the beach, dinner, or long conversation. Many female fantasies involved people with whom the writer actually had had a long-term relationship, whereas the male fantasies included more quick sex. For instance, some male fantasies involved picking up a hitchhiker and doing "it" in the back seat of the car. Others described encounters with strangers in elevators, shopping malls, or locker rooms.

3. The male fantasies were more likely to include more than one opposite-sex partner; for example, "I walked into my apartment and there were the Dallas Cowboy Cheerleaders. Boy did we get it on!" The female fantasies seldom included more than one sexual partner, but when they did, they were more likely to include both opposite-sex and same-sex partners.

4. Female fantasies included a more detailed description of the setting than did male fantasies. Females described the colors in the room, the music in the background, the candles flickering, or the bright sun-filled, leafy knoll of grass. If males described anything, it was the sexy clothing the objects of their fantasies were in the process of shedding.

The findings from our sexuality class are similar to those reported by other sexuality experts. For example, Hicks and Leitenberg (2001) studied university students and found a larger proportion of males have sexual fantasies involving someone other than their current partner than do females. They cite other studies that found "women's sexual fantasies are more likely to involve an emotional connection with a particular partner, whereas men's fantasies are more focused on explicit sexual imagery, often without romantic or emotional context" (Leitenberg & Henning, 1995, 48). Plesa (2013) reports that men's top fantasies are watching others having sex, sex with a stranger, sex with a virgin, a threesome with another woman, role playing (for example, patient–nurse, cop–bad girl, teacher–student), no-strings sex, sex with a woman who is off limits (a boss, neighbor, or best friend), erotic locations, getting caught in the act, and being controlled/dominated by a woman. Dubberley (2014) describes women's sexual fantasies as falling into one of five categories: submissive fantasies (such as in the book *Fifty Shades of Grey*), dominant fantasies (being in control), exhibitionist and voyeuristic fantasies (watching and being watched in the act of having sex), group-sex fantasies, and partner fantasies (sex with just one particular partner, often one's own actual partner). Obviously, there are many exceptions to these findings. Some men include romantic elements in their fantasies and some women do not. Some women include explicit, active sexual behavior by them and some men do not. However, as a generalization, it appears the findings of our students are valid.

that 86% of the women they studied fantasized abut sex. More recently, in a study of university students and employees, 98% of men and 80% of women reported having sexual fantasies about someone other than their current partners during the past 2 months (Hicks & Leitenberg, 2001). Studies have consistently shown males have more frequent sexual fantasies than females (Leitenberg & Henning, 1995; Hicks & Leitenberg, 2001; Ellis & Symons, 1990). Fantasies also come in many varieties. A recent study, for example, evaluated the rape fantasies of female undergraduates and found 62% of women have had a rape fantasy, which is somewhat higher than previous estimates (Bivona & Critelli, 2008).

A more recent study of more than 1,500 adults, average age of 30, found sexual fantasies to be prevalent among both men and women (Joyal, Cossette, & Lapierre, 2014). Five sexual fantasies were experienced by more than 84% of participants: feeling romantic emotions during a sexual relationship, fantasies in which atmosphere and location were important, fantasies involving a romantic location, receiving oral sex, and having sexual intercourse with two women (typical for men). A relatively large number of women acknowledged submissive fantasies: being sexually dominated (65%), being tied up for sexual pleasure (52%), being spanked or whipped (36%), and being forced to have sex (29%). Interestingly, these same sexual fantasies were reported by significant proportions of men (54%, 46%, 29%, and 31%, respectively).

However, significant differences were found between genders for specific fantasies. For instance, feeling romantic and pleasurable emotions during a sexual relationship, fantasies in which atmosphere and location were important, and fantasies involving a romantic location were more prevalent among women than among men. For men, receiving oral sex and having sex with someone other than their current partners were rated higher than for women. There was also a gender difference regarding anal sex: 64% of men fantasized about anal sex, compared with only one-third of women. Furthermore, more than half of women reported have fantasized about having sex with two men, and 29% of them reported having fantasized about having sex with more than three men.

Surprisingly, the percentages of women and men fantasizing about homosexual activities were greater than the percentages who stated they were bisexual or homosexual. For instance, 36% of women fantasized about giving cunnilingus, 37% about having sex with another woman, and 42% about watching two other women having sex, despite only 19% considering themselves either bisexual (13%) or homosexual (6%). Likewise, 27% of men fantasized about giving fellatio and a 21% fantasized about having sex with another man, although 90% considered themselves heterosexual.

In a study of gay and straight men, both groups' most arousing sexual fantasies involved oral sex (Keating & Over, 1990). Heterosexual men next found the following to be most arousing (presented in order of arousal): vaginal intercourse, undressing a woman, woman manually caressing penis, and being undressed by a woman. After oral sex, homosexual men found the following to be most arousing (presented in order of arousal): man manually caresses penis, anal intercourse, and kissing a man on the lips.

Most people realize that it is permissible to have sexual fantasies. A *New York Times* poll (The way we live now, 2000) found that 55% of people younger than 30 years of age think it is okay to fantasize about having sex with someone other than their partners. Even many older people believed that—27% of those older than 70 thought it okay to fantasize about sex with someone other than their partners. One of the benefits of these fantasies is being able to imagine whatever one wishes unencumbered by "social convention, practical and legal barriers, or by fears of embarrassment, criticism, or rejection" (Wilson, 1997, 43). Research has demonstrated that sexual fantasizing can be healthy for both men and women (Strassberg & Lockerd, 1998; Chick & Gold, 1987–1988; Davidson, 1985; Knafo & Jaffe, 1984).

Sexual fantasies may be triggered externally, such as by a movie or by photographs. Or, they may be triggered by internal stimuli, such as thoughts of another person or a sexual situation. Alternatively, fantasies may be generated by a combination of external and internal triggers (Jones & Barlow, 1990). In addition, sexual experience appears related to sexual fantasies. For example, in two studies, women with more coital experience reported more sexual fantasies than women who were virgins or had less sexual experience (Hicks & Leitenberg, 2001; Knafo & Jaffe, 1984).

Another source of fantasy images is the Internet. Although fraught with limitations (Are students being truthful?), several studies have explored the prevalence of college students' use of the Internet to view sexually explicit material. In one study of 506 college students, 44% reported accessing sexually explicit material online (Goodson, McCormick, & Evans, 2001). In another study of 985 university students, 38% reported they used the Internet to view sexually explicit images (Rumbough, 2001). Others have reported that 64% of male and 18% of female college students spend some time viewing Internet porn (Leahy, 2009). More specifically, 51% percent of male students and 16% of female students spend less than 5 hours per week viewing Internet porn, whereas 11% of male students and 1% of female students spend 5 to 20 hours per week at online porn sites.

Content of Sexual Fantasies

The content of sexual fantasies is both similar and dissimilar when gender is the variable. Interestingly, when males and females are by themselves they tend to fantasize about engaging in sexual activities with their usual partners; however, when they are engaged in sex with their usual partners, they fantasize about sex with someone else (for example, a movie star or a model) (Leitenberg & Henning, 1995). Although quite

TABLE 15.1

Men's Favorite Sexual Fantasies

- Seeing woman nude
- Having sex with a new partner
- Having sex with multiple partners at the same time
- Having the power to drive women "wild"

Source: Reproduced from Leitenberg, H., & Henning, K. Sexual fantasy. *Psychological Bulletin, 117* (1995), 469–496.

a diversity in the content of sexual fantasies exists, other prevalent fantasies are having oral–genital sex, being found sexually irresistible by others, and having sex forced upon oneself. The most prevalent female sexual fantasies include having sex in a secluded setting, engaging in sexual activity in a different place than usual (such as a hotel), and having thoughts about an imaginary lover (Strassberg & Lockerd, 1998). Table 15.1 presents favorite male sexual fantasies. Table 15.2 lists favorite sexual fantasies of gays and lesbians. Sexual fantasies may also include group sex, sex with celebrities, voyeuristic activities (peeping or watching others engaged in sex), sadomasochism, or experimentation with other partners or other activities. In a 1995 study that reviewed more than

TABLE 15.2

Gays' and Lesbians' Favorite Sexual Fantasies

Gays' Fantasies

- Unspecified sexual activity with another man
- Performing oral sex
- Having partner perform oral sex
- Participating in anal sexual intercourse
- Sex with another man not previously involved with

Lesbians' Fantasies

- Unspecified sexual activity with another woman
- Having partner perform oral sex
- Performing oral sex
- Anticipating sexual activity with a partner
- Being held and touched

Source: Reproduced from Price, J. H., & Miller, P. A. Sexual fantasies of black and white college students. *Psychological Reports, 54* (1984), 1007–1014. © *Psychological Reports* 1984.

200 other studies of sexual fantasies, the researchers concluded that women's fantasies tended to include sex with a new male partner, sex with a celebrity, seduction of a younger man or boy, and sex with an older man. Men's favorite fantasies included seeing women nude and having sex with a new female partner, multiple sex partners, and the power to drive women wild (Leitenberg & Henning, 1995).

Functions of Sexual Fantasies

Sexual fantasies serve several purposes. They are a source of pleasure, and, as such, they enhance sexual arousal. Furthermore, sexual fantasies allow people to test and rehearse various sexual activities if they are concerned about being judged by their partners. In this way the activity is tested in a nonthreatening setting and no one knows whether it works out. And sexual fantasies allow people to acknowledge sexual feelings without acting on them.

There is also research to indicate that sexual fantasies may be helpful in overcoming sexual anxiety (Coen, 1978; Leitenberg & Henning, 1995; Hicks & Leitenberg, 2001). Consequently, many sexual therapists encourage fantasies in counseling clients with sexual dysfunctions. In fact, low sexual desire in women has been found to be associated with a lack of sexual fantasizing (Nutter & Condron, 1983).

In addition, sexual fantasies allow us to be "better" than we really are—that is, better lovers, more confident, more experienced, more risky, and more desirable. They also provide us with a safe means of engaging in sexual activities in which we may never wish to participate. For example, though some women fantasize about being forced to have sex, few would actually want that fantasy to come true. It is hypothesized that the frequency with which a woman reports this forced-sex fantasy is a function of her desire to be risqué in her sexual behavior but not accountable for it, because our society generally frowns on sexually adventurous women. Another interpretation of this forced-sex fantasy is that women seek greater power rather than less, so they fantasize that they are so desirable that the man cannot resist (Hawley & Hensley, 2009; Critelli & Bivona, 2008). Although Hunt (1974) found twice as many women had this fantasy as men, he did find 10% of men also had submission fantasies.

Sexual fantasies also provide us with a means of fulfilling our every desire while not hurting ourselves or those we love. It is a private and safe way of doing anything we want. It is a means of acting out our wildest dreams while never acting improperly. For example, we may wonder what sex with an animal would be like, or what the experience of sex with our lover's friend would feel like. By fantasizing about these situations we do not harm ourselves, our lovers, or our pets, yet we can experience the situation vicariously. Fantasies of this kind are safe as long as they do not become obsessive. If they do, therapy may be indicated.

There are those who argue that sexual fantasies are unhealthy. For example, Apfelbaum (1980) believes fantasizing during sex with a partner can decrease the degree of trust and intimacy in the relationship. Others have taken a similar point of view (Hollender, 1970; Shainess & Greenwald, 1971).

Maltz and Boss (2001) provide a list of nine questions to ask to determine whether, and to what extent, a sexual fantasy may be causing problems:

- Does the fantasy lead to risky or dangerous behavior?

- Does the fantasy feel out of control or compulsive?

- Is the content of the fantasy disturbing or repulsive?

- Does the fantasy hinder recovery or personal growth?

- Does the fantasy lower my self-esteem or block self-acceptance?

- Does the fantasy distance me from my real-life partner?

- Does the fantasy harm my intimate partner or anyone else?

- Does the fantasy cause sexual problems?

- Does the fantasy really belong to someone else?

The predominant view is that sexual fantasizing can enhance sexual relationships as long as it does not become obsessive and as long as there is no compulsion to act out the fantasy. Some fantasies may be acted out with the consent of the sexual partner, but if one person feels uncomfortable, problems may arise. Guilt or shame may lead to other psychological and/or sexual problems. With the willing consent of both partners, however, acting out sexual fantasies can actually enhance sexual satisfaction and improve the relationship. It appears, though, that most sexual fantasizers do not intend to act out their fantasies, and, if they do, they may be disappointed. Nancy Friday (1975) reports that most individuals who have acted out their sexual fantasies were disappointed. It seems that reality seldom matches fantasy.

Sexual Behavior with Others

Foreplay is the physical contact that usually precedes coitus or oral–genital sexual activity. Generally foreplay includes touching, kissing, biting, and genital fondling. The word *foreplay* is really a misnomer, because this behavior can be enjoyed for itself and need not be a prelude (*fore-*) to anything. All such activity is meant to express love, sensuousness, desire, or all these feelings. We might more appropriately term this activity *pleasuring each other*. However, foreplay does also serve to prepare the participants, both psychologically and physically, for coitus.

The importance of foreplay to sexual enjoyment has been widely acknowledged. Data in the 1970s (Hunt, 1974) showed that unmarried people younger than 25 years of age spent an average of 15 minutes in foreplay and another 15 minutes in intercourse. More recently, researchers found that heterosexual couples averaged approximately 12 minutes of foreplay and 7 minutes of intercourse during their sexual encounters (Miller & Byers, 2004). Still other researchers found respondents spent an average of 15 minutes of foreplay and 16 minutes of sexual intercourse

Myth vs Fact

Myth: Sexual fantasies mean a person is fixating on sex and needs either to get professional help or to work hard to stop fantasizing.
Fact: Sexual fantasizing is prevalent and is not indicative of a sexual problem. Many males and females fantasize both before and during sexual intercourse, even if engaged in sexual intercourse with their usual partner.

Myth: Women who fantasize about being raped are "sick" and, if raped, get what they deserve.
Fact: First of all, no one "deserves" to be forced to engage in any sexual activity against his or her will. Second, having a fantasy does not indicate that someone actually wants the fantasy to come true. Rape fantasies may even indicate a woman's wish to be so desirable that men cannot resist her rather than a desire to give up control to a male.

Myth: Masturbation is normal for young people but can interfere

with the healthy sexual relationship of older people, especially if they are married.
Fact: There is no evidence that masturbation is harmful either physically or psychologically. In fact, there are some times when a sexual partner is unavailable and masturbation can serve as a healthy sexual outlet. Furthermore, many married people with regular sexual intercourse still enjoy masturbating.

Myth: People with disabilities cannot have a meaningful sex life because of the restrictions placed on them by their disabilities.
Fact: Certainly some disabilities place restrictions on sexual positions or sexual stamina. Still, there are many accommodations that can be made so that people who have heart disease, who are physically disabled, or who are ill can achieve and maintain meaningful sexual lives.

---

foreplay Physical contact preceding sexual intercourse.

(Weiss & Brody, 2009). Interestingly, one study (Weiss & Brody, 2009) found that the amount of time spent by heterosexual couples on foreplay had no relationship to the likelihood of female orgasm. Instead, the duration of penile–vaginal intercourse did. For same-sex couples, both male and female, the use of vibrators to enhance sexual pleasure is prevalent (Reece et al., 2010; Schick et al., 2011). Interestingly, some men are fearful of foreplay. They worry about losing their erection or ejaculating before intercourse (Elder, 2009). This is unfortunate because foreplay is the perfect time for communicating with your partner to find out what he or she likes (Srovney, 2009). To rush through it is to lose this opportunity.

Whereas Kinsey's 1948 data showed that a majority of males reached orgasm just 2 minutes after penile insertion. Michael and colleagues (1994) found that for 69% of men and 71% of women, intercourse took from 15 minutes to 1 hour. Because women need more time to be vaginally lubricated sufficiently for intercourse than men do to achieve erection and be ready perhaps this acknowledgment represents an increased understanding of women's needs to be sexually stimulated for a longer period than men before coitus. Nevertheless, a recent study of the time Americans spend during sexual intercourse found a range between a high of 7.01 minutes and a low of 1.21 minutes (Hakala, 2014). The researchers compiled their data by state, finding that residents of New Mexico spent the most time during coitus and residents of Alaska the least. Table 15.3 presents these data. Where did your state rank in this listing, and why do you think that is so?

The Importance of the Senses

Sexual stimulation in foreplay, intercourse, or any other activity involves the imagination and all of the senses: touch, sight, smell, hearing, and taste.

Touch

Sensual touching is central to sexual stimulation. Although the skin is not a sexual organ as such, stroking the skin on any part of the body can contribute to and even initiate sexual arousal. The gentle stroking of a partner's face, ear, or neck can be both exciting and effective at communicating affection. Furthermore, each manner and intensity of body contact carries its own kind of stimulation. Gentle touching, where the fingers barely make contact with the skin and perhaps focus on one part of the body, can be tantalizing. Caressing—gentle stroking or rubbing—is firmer than gentle touching and communicates affection or appreciation. Firmer touches, too, can be sexually arousing. Hugs, embraces, and squeezes are all expressions of caring. Some might

TABLE 15.3

Time Spent (in Minutes) During Sexual Intercourse: State by State

1. New Mexico (7:01)	27. Iowa (2:50)
2. West Virginia (5:38)	28. Illinois (2:49)
3. Idaho (5:11)	29. North Carolina (2:47)
4. South Carolina (4:48)	30. Tennessee (2:46)
5. Missouri (4:22)	31. Kansas (2:38)
6. Michigan (4:14)	32. California (2:38)
7. Utah (3:55)	33. Massachusetts (2:31)
8. Oregon (3:51)	34. Florida (2:29)
9. Nebraska (3:47)	35. New Jersey (2:28)
10. Alabama (3:38)	36. Indiana (2:26)
11. Delaware (3:33)	37. Virginia (2:23)
12. Hawaii (3:28)	38. Oklahoma (2:21)
13. Wisconsin (3:22)	39. Colorado (2:21)
14. North Dakota (3:18)	40. Minnesota (2:19)
15. Arizona (3:17)	41. Ohio (2:18)
16. Maryland (3:15)	42. Louisiana (2:17)
17. Mississippi (3:10)	43. Kentucky (2:14)
18. Rhode Island (3:09)	44. Arkansas (2:08)
19. Connecticut (3:07)	45. District of Columbia (2:08)
20. Texas (3:06)	46. Nevada (2:07)
21. New Hampshire (3:04)	47. Georgia (2:07)
22. Wyoming (3:03)	48. Montana (2:03)
23. New York (3:01)	49. Vermont (1:48)
24. Pennsylvania (2:58)	50. South Dakota (1:30)
25. Maine (2:58)	51. Alaska (1:21)
26. Washington (2:51)	

Source: Hakala, K. A study of sex duration in America, Nerve, February 19, 2014. Available: http://www.nerve.com/love-sex/which-states-have-the-longest-and-shortest-sex.

consider a full-body massage the ultimate expression of the sensual touch.

So sensual touching is not necessarily focused on the genitals. But once the body and emotions are primed for sexual activity, touching in and around specific areas of the body is intensely stimulating. The breast (especially the nipple), the inner thighs, the clitoris, the penis, the neck, the ears, and the navel are particularly receptive to sensual touching because of an abundance of nerve endings. However, touching of some of the sensitive genital areas (for example, the vulva or the glans) can result in irritation unless some kind of lubricant is used. Of course, the best lubricant is that produced vaginally by the woman herself. However, any lotion, such as hydroxyethyl cellulose (K-Y) jelly, that does not contain alcohol is also safe and useful for this purpose (unless you are using a condom, in which case Vaseline should not be used). Touching on all parts of the body can be of a teasing nature: moving here, then there, but not there (though almost), then back here. Genital touching should be done in a gentle manner, because rough handling (for example, of a testicle) could result in injury.

We should not overlook the use of touching for sexual self-stimulation. Masturbation is often the method by which people learn which body areas and which types of touching are most stimulating for them. Vibrators have become popular both for masturbating and for sexually stimulating partners. Many couples masturbate each other to orgasm and find this form of sexual activity very exciting and a safe alternative to intercourse.

As with other sexual behaviors, good communication is important for guiding partners in touching each other effectively. Such phrases as "I like that," "That hurts," and "Keep doing that, but just a little more gently (or more firmly)" will help your partner use touching on the specific areas and in the particular ways most stimulating to you. If you are the toucher and do not get this feedback, ask for it.

Sight

The power of visual images is clear everywhere in modern society—for example, in advertising, in films, and in television. These images sometimes work on us without our notice, but it is possible to use sexual imagery consciously for sexual stimulation. Sexual partners sometimes use sexual imagery in books, magazines, videos, and photographs to become aroused together. Clothing can also serve this purpose. Men and women often dress in a manner termed sexy, not only to attract others but to add to their partners' or their own sexual excitement. Some people are excited by the sight of hair, eyes, legs, or other body parts. Partners can learn to make use of each other's particular visual stimulants to initiate or enhance sexual arousal.

Smell

The popularity of perfumes and colognes is probably attributable to their potential for arousing sexual interest. It is no small wonder that the old-time

Smell can be sexually stimulating. Research with both animals and humans demonstrates the sexually arousing nature of certain smells. Perfume manufacturers have long recognized this fact.

bordello is associated with highly perfumed and painted women (even though these ladies might have been a far sight raunchier than their counterparts in the modern media). Animal studies have identified smell as being more important in many species than sight or sound in attracting a mate (Bhutta, 2007). Substances called **pheromones** are secreted by some female animals to attract male sexual partners. Conversely, unpleasant smells such as bad breath can interfere with sexual arousal. Attention to normal body hygiene can prevent these problems.

Although it has long been suspected that humans produce pheromones, it was only in the late 1980s that scientists verified this. Human pheromones do not actually serve as sexual attractants, but they do alter the timing of women's menstrual cycles. The Monell Chemical Studies Center and the University of Pennsylvania Medical School (Cutler et al., 1986) studied this issue for several years and found that women who experience coitus weekly are more likely to have normal menstrual cycles, fewer infertility problems, and milder menopauses than women who either are celibate or have sexual intercourse only sporadically (Rensberger, 1986). It seems that male aromatic chemicals secreted from sweat glands in the armpits, nipples, and genitalia are transmitted to their sexual partners by smell and skin absorption. Once transmitted, these chemicals affect the woman's reproductive system (Mostafa, Elkhooly, & Hassan, 2012).

Women also produce a pheromone that affects other women's menstrual cycles. For years anecdotal reports indicated that women who live together or who work together seem to have synchronous

---

pheromones Substances that when secreted have a specific scent found to be sexually arousing.

menstrual cycles. These reports now have evidence both to support and to explain them (Preti et al., 1986; Preti et al., 2003).

The manner in which human pheromones work is not fully understood. The suspicion is that molecules of the substances reach receptors of the nervous and endocrine systems and act on them to stimulate signals transmitted in the brain (Keverne, 2004). These brain signals influence the endocrine system's secretion of hormones, and these hormones influence the woman's reproductive system (Lanuza et al., 2008; Spors & Sobel, 2007).

There are several potential practical applications of this knowledge regarding human pheromones. For example, nasal sprays might be developed to alleviate certain kinds of infertility problems, to regulate the menstrual cycle (for instance, to make the rhythm method of birth control more effective), or to effect the onset of menopause or minimize its effects.

Hearing

Have you ever heard the expression "Whisper sweet nothings in my ear"? Well, those murmurings are not just nothings! Words and sounds before and during coitus can be sexually stimulating, as can music that contributes to an erotic atmosphere. Sexual talk can take many forms. Some people are aroused by "dirty words," and others are completely turned off by them. Similarly, some people find moaning during sexual activity to be exciting, whereas others are unimpressed with such guttural goings-on. Furthermore, some people report that saying or hearing "I love you" after orgasm can be one of the most exciting and romantic experiences in the world (Haffner & Schwartz, 1998). Once again, communication between sexual partners is the key.

Taste

The use of the mouth can be quite sexually arousing. Kissing, when both partners attend to it, can be intensely stimulating, whatever the variation: open mouth, closed mouth, a nibble here, a nibble there, a tongue darting from spot to spot, and lips or teeth closing gently on a sensitive body part. Kissing with tongues touching (soul kissing, French kissing, deep kissing) can also take various forms. More on the use of the mouth, tongue, and teeth is discussed in the section on oral–genital sexual behavior. As with the other senses, taste can also be a turnoff. Obviously French kissing someone who has bad breath or licking a smelly body can be anything but arousing. Proper body hygiene and communication on such simple matters between sexual partners can go a long way toward improving sexual relations.

© Gerjan Hooijer/ShutterStock, Inc.

Kissing can be a very erotic, sensual activity in and of itself.

In the following sections, we discuss specific sexual behaviors and provide guidance for enhancing sexual satisfaction through the use of these activities.

Oral–Genital Sexual Behavior

Oral–genital sexual behavior involves contact between the mouth, lips, and tongue of one partner and the genitals of another. When a female's genitals are orally stimulated, the act is called **cunnilingus** (meaning in Latin "one who licks the vulva"). When the penis is taken into the partner's mouth, the act is called **fellatio** (from the Latin *fellare*, meaning "to suck"). As with most sexual acts, some find oral–genital sexual contact sexually arousing; others are indifferent to it or find it repulsive. It is generally agreed, however, that oral–genital activity is quite common. Hunt's (1974) study, for example, indicated that 90% of married couples younger than age 25 years had experienced oral–genital sexual stimulation. Another large-scale study of oral sex was conducted by Michael and associates (1994), found that 77% of men and 68% of women reported having given oral sex *to* a partner, and 79% of men and 73% of women had received oral sex *from* a partner.

More recently, a study by the National Center for Health Statistics (Copen, Chandra, & Martinez, 2012) reported that approximately two-thirds of females and males ages 15 to 24 years had participated in oral

cunnilingus Stimulation of the female genitalia by the mouth, lips, and/or tongue of the sexual partner.

fellatio Oral contact with a male's penis.

FIGURE 15.2 Simultaneous oral–genital stimulation.

sex. The National Survey of Family Growth (2011) found even higher rates for older adults (ages 25 to 44): 89% of women and 90% of men had experienced oral sex with an opposite-sex partner. Even teenagers reported experiencing oral sex: 7% of females and 9% of males have had oral sex with an opposite-sex partner. Furthermore, 5% of males ages 15 to 44 reported having experienced oral sex with another male (Chandra, Copen, & Mosher, 2013).

Many of the techniques described as foreplay are applicable to oral–genital sexual activity. Thus a teasing approach, gentle in nature and varied in form, involving the mouth, lips, and tongue is particularly stimulating. Some women report especially enjoying the licking or sucking of the clitoris and labia minora or a thrusting of the tongue into the vagina. Men are often aroused when their partners lick the underside of the penile shaft and the glans or lick or lightly hold a testicle in the mouth. Again, the testicles and clitoris are very sensitive and should be treated gently. And, of course, attention to personal hygiene is important to maximal—and even minimal—pleasure.

Sexual partners need to discuss whether ejaculation should occur in the mouth during fellatio. Contrary to rumor, the ejaculate is not fattening when swallowed; however, it does have a unique taste. Some like or are indifferent to the taste; others dislike it. One word of caution here, though: Because the ejaculate can contain HIV if the male is infected, unless the relationship has been monogamous for some time and both partners are known to be HIV-free,

the ejaculate should not be swallowed. In any case, whether the ejaculate is swallowed does not need to diminish the pleasure of either partner.

When couples orally stimulate one another simultaneously, the act is referred to as **69** (because their bodies in position resemble the numbers 6 and 9 (Figure 15.2). Couples can perform 69 side by side or with one partner on top of the other, depending on which position they consider more comfortable and stimulating. Some couples prefer to stimulate one another simultaneously, whereas others find they cannot concentrate on their own pleasurable sensations while concentrating on pleasuring someone else.

Partners also need to discuss the need for a male to wear a condom and a female to wear a dental dam during oral–genital contact. These behaviors decrease, although they do not eliminate, the possibility of contracting HIV, as well as other STIs. That is why they are called "safer sex" behaviors. To be "safer," partners should consider agreeing to engage in these behaviors.

Anal Stimulation

Some people enjoy becoming sexually aroused anally, because there are numerous nerve endings in that area. Partners can stimulate each other by inserting a finger into the anus, stroking the anal opening, or licking the area. However, licking the anus, termed **analingus**—also commonly referred to as "rimming"—is risky to one's health. Intestinal infections, such as *Escherichia coli*, can be spread through analingus, as can hepatitis and STIs. This threat exists even though the anus may be carefully washed. In addition, minute tears that occur in the anus during **anal intercourse** provide easy entry into the body for organisms that cause STIs. This is especially likely if a

69 Two partners' simultaneous stimulation of each other's genitalia orally. The numerals 6 and 9 visually describe the body positions.

analingus Licking of the anus.

anal intercourse Insertion of the penis into the anus.

**Should People
Who Do Not Feel
Comfortable
with Oral or Anal
Sexual Activity
Learn to Enjoy
These Activities?**

Some people believe that the more sexual acts one experiences, the more sexually satisfied one will be, and that to enhance our sexual lives, we need a variety of sexual expressions and sexual excitation. They feel that those who are not comfortable with oral–genital sexual activity or anal intercourse ought to be instructed in how to engage in these activities and given counseling to relieve any shame, guilt, or anxiety associated with them. People with this viewpoint argue that to ignore this discomfort is to forever accept a less satisfying sexual life than is possible; and when sexual partners have different desires related to

oral and anal sexual activity, there is a threat to the relationship itself.

Others believe that sexual expression can occur in many forms and that no one person need accept all forms for himself or herself. If some sexual activities are uncomfortable, these people argue, choose other activities to include in your sexual repertoire. People should not be coerced into behaviors that they find repulsive; that is not fair. Furthermore, if one partner desires oral or anal sexual activity and the other does not, a good relationship will result if the one who does want these activities understands and accepts the other's feelings. Anything short of that and the relationship is probably not worthwhile anyhow.

What do you believe a couple who disagrees on this issue should do?

condom is not used. Penile penetration of the anus is also possible, for both heterosexual and homosexual couples. **Dildos** (fake penises) can also be used for anal insertion. Because of the nature of the anus, one should take care not to tear the surrounding tissue (a lubricant should be used), and to prevent infection the penis should be thoroughly cleansed immediately after anal insertion. Because anal intercourse is one of the risk behaviors for HIV, a condom should be used whenever this sexual activity is performed.

Sexual Intercourse

Variety may truly be the spice of life, at least relative to coital (penile–vaginal intercourse) positions. Although most authorities recognize four basic positions of sexual intercourse, the variations on these themes are infinite. A leg thrown over here, an arm positioned there, a hand fondling this, lips doing that can all slightly alter the sexual experience so that it differs from past experiences. Consequently this section can serve only as a guide, not the last word, on coital positions.

In addition to the desire for variety, other situations—such as pregnancy, obesity, or poor health—may dictate certain modifications. For example, it is more comfortable for a pregnant or obese woman to be on top rather than have her partner press down on her abdomen. Similarly, a man with arthritic knees may not be comfortable with his knees bent in the on-top position. In addition, some coital positions

may influence the effectiveness of a condom—male or female. As an example, when the man lies on his back with the woman on top, there may be some seepage of semen from the condom, especially if it is not placed on the penis correctly. When the man is on top, this is not as likely.

1. *Man on top.* The man-on-top position (Figure 15.3) is sometimes called the "missionary position" or the male superior position. The position has a lot going for it: It allows full frontal body contact, which is usually pleasurable; because the couple is lying down, their hands are free to roam; and because they are facing each other, partners can kiss, talk, and watch each other's expressions. This position is also considered the most effective for increasing the chances of pregnancy, but whether you call that an advantage depends on your circumstances. On the negative side, sexuality therapists do not recommend this position for men who have difficulty controlling ejaculation.

2. *Woman on top.* In the woman-on-top position, also called the female superior position (Figure 15.4), the woman can be either prone or on her knees. In either case this position permits more clitoral stimulation by either

dildos Artificial penises.

FIGURE **15.3** Man-on-top position.

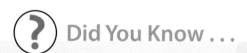

Did You Know . . .

Sex can be enjoyable at any age. Studies have found that the elderly engage in sex well into their 70s and 80s. For example, Lindau (2007) found that many older adults are sexually active, but that about half of the men and women surveyed reported at least one sexual problem and about a third reported at least two problems. Specifically:

1. *In general, older adults are sexually active.* A large portion of respondents said they were sexually active in the preceding 12 months, but the percentage declined with age—from 73% of those age 57–64 to 53% of those age 65–74, to 26% of those age 75–85. Older women, however, were significantly less likely to report sexual activity than older men and less likely to be in intimate relationships, due in part to women's status as widows and the earlier mortality, on average, of men.

2. *Healthier people are more likely to report being sexually active.* Eighty-one percent of men and 51% of women reporting excellent or very good health said they had been sexually active in the past 12 months. Of those in fair or poor health, a considerably lower percentage (47% of men and 26% of women) reported activity in the previous year. Diabetes and hypertension were strongly associated with some sexual concerns.

3. *About half of sexually active older adults report at least one "bothersome" sexual problem.* Thirty-seven percent of sexually active men said they had erectile difficulties. Women most often reported low desire (43%), difficulty with vaginal lubrication (39%), and inability to climax (34%).

partner than the man-on-top position. Thus a woman who does not receive sufficient clitoral stimulation to achieve orgasm through coitus alone can reach orgasm through manual stimulation in this position while her partner's penis is inside her vagina. In this way she can experience the pleasure of orgasm around an erect penis while the man has the pleasure of feeling her orgasmic contractions on his penis. In addition, the woman is free to move rather than being pinned under her partner. This is a good

position for men who are attempting to control their orgasms; the squeeze technique is easy to use because the penis is relatively accessible. Another advantage is that both partners' hands are free, allowing them to caress each other. The one disadvantage of this position is that the effort by the man necessary for thrusting his penis can be tiring because the woman's weight is bearing down on his pelvis. Consequently women might do more of the movement in this position than in some others.

FIGURE **15.4** Woman-on-top position.

3. *Side-by-side.* In the side-by-side position
   (Figure 15.5), neither person is bearing
   the weight of the other. This is a relaxing
   position, because pelvic thrusts do not meet
   as much resistance as with the woman or
   man on top. However, because arms and
   legs may be pinned under other arms and
   legs, blood circulation can be temporarily
   cut off, making periodic switching or
   adjustment necessary for comfort. The side-
   by-side position also allows for kissing and
   face watching, and it too frees the hands
   for stroking and caressing. However, it is
   sometimes difficult to keep the penis in the

vagina in this position, and even vigorous
thrusting can result in little or no clitoral
contact. Still, hands work well here too, as in
the woman-on-top position.

4. *Rear entry.* The rear-entry position (Figure 15.6)
   can be performed in two ways: with both
   people lying down, either side-by-side or with
   the woman atop the man, or with the partners
   kneeling (called the "dog position" for reasons
   clear to anyone who has seen dogs copulating).
   In either case the male's hands are free to fondle
   his partner's breasts and stimulate her clitoris.
   The disadvantages of this position include the

FIGURE **15.5** The side-by-side position. Note the subtle variations that are possible.

Multicultural DIMENSIONS

Does Level of Education Influence Sexuality?

Sexual practices vary greatly from person to person and from couple to couple. Yet, these practices seem to be influenced by education. Laumann and colleagues (1994) found that sex and education were related in the following ways.

1. Whereas 72% of men with any college education reported their last sexual encounter took between 15 minutes and 1 hour, only 61% of men with less than a high school education reported it took that long. With women, the results were comparable. Seventy-four percent of women with any college education reported their last sexual encounter took between 15 minutes and 1 hour, whereas only 60% of women with less than a high school education reported it took that long.

2. Although 81% of men and 78% of women with some college education reported having ever performed oral sex on a partner, only 59% of men and 41% of women with less than a high school education reported having ever performed oral sex on a partner. And although 84% of men and 82% of women with some college education reported ever having oral sex performed on them, only 61% of men and 50% of women with less than a high school education reported ever having oral sex performed on them.

3. In terms of anal intercourse, 28% of college educated men and 24% of college-educated women reported ever having that experience, whereas only 21% of men and 13% of women with less than a high school education reported experiencing anal intercourse.

It appears that being educated results in being less conservative sexually. Why do you think that is the case?

FIGURE 15.6 The rear-entry position.

Global DIMENSIONS

Gay and Lesbian Rights around the World

Being lesbian, gay, bisexual, or transgender is illegal in almost 80 countries around the world. More than 2.7 billion people live in countries where being gay is a crime. In fact, five countries—Iran, Mauritania, Saudi Arabia, Sudan, and Yemen—have statutes specifying the death penalty for gay and lesbian sexual activity.

However, some progress in overturning laws discriminating against LGBT people has occurred in recent years. For example, in 2014 more than 1.3 billion people lived in countries with some form of legal protection from discrimination against LGBT people, while 780 million lived in countries that permitted same-sex marriage or civil unions. Furthermore, more than 1 billion people live in countries that ban workplace discrimination against LGBT people.

The map below shows the status of legal rights of LGBT people around the world.

(Continues)

Global DIMENSIONS

Gay and Lesbian Rights around the World (Continued)

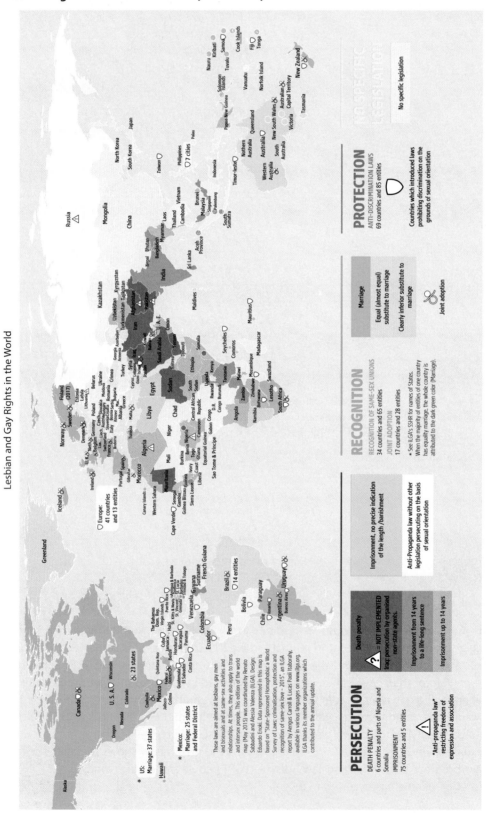

Lesbian and Gay Rights in the World

These laws are aimed at lesbians, gay men and bisexuals and at same-sex activities and relationships. At times, they also apply to trans and intersex people. This edition of the world map (May 2015) was coordinated by Renato Sabbadini and Aleesia Valenza (ILGA). Design: Eduardo Enoki. Data represented in this map is based on "State-Sponsored Homophobia: A World Survey of Laws: criminalisation, protection and recognition of same-sex love – 2015", an ILGA report by Aengus Carroll & Lucas Paoli Itaborahy, available in various languages on www.ilga.org. ILGA thanks its member organizations which contributed to the annual update.

* US:
Marriage: 37 states

* Mexico:
Marriage: 25 states
and Federal District

* Europe:
41 countries
and 13 entities

PERSECUTION

DEATH PENALTY
6 countries and parts of Nigeria and Somalia

IMPRISONMENT
75 countries and 5 entities

⚠ "Anti-propaganda law"
restricting freedom of
expression and association

	Death penalty
⚠	= NOT IMPLEMENTED Iraq: persecution by organised non-state agents.
	Imprisonment from 14 years to a life-long sentence
	Imprisonment up to 14 years

	Imprisonment, no precise indication of the length /banishment
	Anti-Propaganda law without other legislation persecuting on the basis of sexual orientation

RECOGNITION

RECOGNITION OF SAME-SEX UNIONS
34 countries and 65 entities

JOINT ADOPTION
17 countries and 28 entities

* See ILGA's SSHR for names of States.
When the majority of entities of one country has equality marriage, the whole country is attributed to the dark green color (Marriage).

	Marriage
	Equal (almost equal) substitute to marriage
	Clearly inferior substitute to marriage

✂	Joint adoption

PROTECTION

ANTI-DISCRIMINATION LAWS
69 countries and 85 entities

	Countries which introduced laws prohibiting discrimination on the grounds of sexual orientation

NO SPECIFIC LEGISLATION

	No specific legislation

Source: International Lesbian, Gay, Bisexual, Transsexual and Intersex Association. *Lesbian and gay rights in the world*, 2014. Available: http://old.ilga.org/Statehomophobia/ILGA_Map_2014_ENG.pdf.

lack of face-to-face contact and the feeling of some people that they are being animal-like (others find this position sexually stimulating for this very reason). People who try the rear-entry position for the first time may be surprised by the sound effects: Air may enter the vagina and produce noises when it leaves (some sexologists have termed this sound a "vart").

Once again we should say that the variety of coital positions is limited only by your imagination. Coitus, or any other sexual activity, can be pleasurable and exciting when the technique is pleasurable and exciting and when partners follow their inclinations. However, sexual techniques alone may not always be satisfying. The bond between sex makers that sometimes turns them into lovemakers can be as important as technique. A loving relationship of responsible people can add much to the pleasure obtained from sexual activity. Still, the very nature of sexual expression is pleasing, and it is obvious that sexual behavior can be enjoyed by people who are not in love but still care for each other. Whether such sexual behavior is moral or legal, however, is another issue, which depends on your ethics and society's.

Sexual Behavior of Gays and Lesbians

Although study findings vary, approximately 12.5% of U.S. females have engaged in sex with same-gender partners, as have 5.2% of males. Over 9% of females and 5% of males have engaged in oral sex with a same-gender partner, and 2.9% of males have engaged in anal sex with a same-gender partner (Chandra et al., 2011). With regard to the sexual activity of gays and lesbians, they enjoy most of the same activities as heterosexuals (Figures 15.7 and 15.8). One difference that has been noted, however (Tripp, 1976), is that intimacy and closeness seem to be more important than what is specifically done by the partners. For example, a study of gay men (Rosenberger et al., 2011) found that the most commonly reported behavior was kissing a partner on the mouth (75%), followed by oral sex (73%), and partnered masturbation (68%). Anal intercourse occurred among fewer than half of participants (37%) and was most common among men 18 to 24 years of age (43%). The number of behaviors engaged in during last sexual event varied, with most (63%) including five to nine different sexual behaviors. Findings from this study suggest that gay and bisexual men have a diverse sexual repertoire and that partnered sexual behaviors are not limited solely to acts of penile insertion.

Yet, more recently it has been reported that more gay men who have been living with a partner for 2 to 10 years have sex with someone other than their partner (79%) than do heterosexual males living with a partner 2 to 10 years (11%). In addition, gays tend to have more sexual partners than do lesbians (Peplau & Cochran, 1990; Blumstein & Schwartz, 1990). People seem to have stereotyped ideas of specific sexual acts in which homosexuals participate (Spalding & Peplau, 1997). In contrast to these myths, both male

FIGURE 15.7 Gay men engage in varied sexual activities.

FIGURE 15.8 Oral and manual stimulation, and touching, are some of the sexual activities enjoyed by lesbians.

and female homosexuals appear to take their time and make sexual activity last longer. They seem to prolong the pleasure rather than rush to orgasm (Masters & Johnson, 1979). Perhaps this is due to the fact that a person stimulating another person of the same sex can better understand what that person enjoys. Contrary to popular belief, male homosexuals do not generally have a preference to receive or insert the penis (Rathus, Nevid, & Fichner-Rathus, 2008, 300–301). Some people are under the misconception that one man plays the male and the other plays the female. This is not the case.

Masters and Johnson (1979), on the basis of their study of homosexuality, reported a number of findings about the specific sexual behavior of homosexual men and women.

1. There are no major differences between the fantasy patterns of homosexuals and heterosexuals.

2. Homosexuality is learned and is definable only by overt behavior.

3. Homosexuality is a pattern of sexual interaction that a person can move into or out of at any time in life.

4. Physiologically homosexuals respond exactly as heterosexuals do to the same sexual stimuli—no sexual stimulus is unique to homosexuals.

5. Homosexuals are as amenable to treatment (with partners of their own choice) for sexual inadequacy as are heterosexuals.

6. Among established couples, homosexuals get more pleasure from lovemaking, even without intercourse, than do heterosexuals.

From a developmental standpoint, it is common for male and female homosexuals and bisexuals to have a history of sexual activity with the same and opposite genders, and to become sexually active during their early teens. No significant gender differences are found in lifetime prevalence rates or ages at initiating homosexual practices, but females tend to become sexually active at an older age than males and engage in more heterosexual activity. Sexual practices follow an initiation sequence beginning with manual sexual activity during their early teens and leading to further sexual activities during the middle and late teens (Rosaria, 1996).

Lesbian Sexual Activities

In lesbian lovemaking, oral sexual activities are common, as are manual stimulation and tribadism. **Tribadism** is the rubbing of genitals against someone's body or genital area. Touching, caressing, and hugging—the emotional components of lovemaking—play a large role in lesbian lovemaking. Specifically, the following lesbian sexual activities have been reported (Dibble & Robertson, 2010):

- 95% engage in oral sex

- 85% engage in digital–vaginal contact (fingering and fisting)

- 60% insert dildos in the vagina and 25% insert dildos in the anus

- 25% engage in anal sex

- 35% engage in rimming (oral–anal contact)

- 95% engage in tribadism

Generally, lesbians tend to do more overall genital stimulation, rather than direct clitoral stimulation, as is often the case in heterosexual relationships (Masters & Johnson, 1979).

Gay Sexual Activities

Homosexual men engage in foreplay activities similar to those of heterosexuals, such as hugging, kissing, petting, and nipple stimulation. Anal intercourse is actually the least frequent male homosexual activity. More often, gay men participate in mutual masturbation or fellatio (oral sex). Laboratory studies by Masters and Johnson (1979) showed that gay men were likely to pay more attention to the area of the penis on the lower side than heterosexual couples.

Keeping It Going

College-age students sometimes wonder how long-term partners can maintain monogamous sexual relationships over many years. Doesn't it get stale after a while? Certainly, for some couples, it does. For many others, sex remains exciting and fulfilling. This must be the case if so many older people are still sexually active. For example, one study found that 60% of women ages 42 to 52 reported having regular sexual intercourse and 24% experienced oral sex on a regular basis (Cain et al., 2003). Another study conducted by the American Association of Retired Persons found that 19% of men 75 years of age or older have sexual intercourse at least once a week (AARP, 1999).

Even more recently (Lindau et al., 2007), a survey of more than 3,000 U.S. adults 57 to 85 years old found that most remained sexually active, with frequent and varied sexual behavior. Approximately 28% of men

tribadism Rubbing genitals against someone's body or genital area.

Communication DIMENSIONS

The Use of Sexual Words and the Resulting Confusion

When President Bill Clinton was accused of having inappropriate sexual interaction with Monica Lewinsky, he insisted, "I did not have sex with that woman!" What did *sex* mean in that context? Likewise, authors often write of *sex*—its frequency, duration, and prevalence. What do they mean by *sex*? The issue becomes even more problematic when researchers refer to sex when reporting results of their studies. Does *sex* mean solely sexual intercourse, which is what President Clinton meant when he denied having sex with Monica Lewinsky, or does *sex* refer to any sexual activity?

Of course, President Clinton was accused of engaging in oral sex, not coitus, with Monica Lewinsky. Even so, what is meant by *oral sex*? In any particular context, does it mean fellatio, or cunnilingus, or analingus? When we read about oral sex, what is being referred to? Is it referring to women performing oral sex? If so, is it fellatio performed on a male, cunnilingus performed on a female, or analingus performed on a male or a female? Or, is it referring to a men performing oral sex? In that case, does it refer to cunnilingus performed on a female, fellatio performed on a male, or analingus performed on a female or a male?

Then there is the issue of *rape*. Does *rape* refer only to a male forcing a female to engage in unwanted sexual intercourse? Or can it include forcing a woman to engage in any sexual activity? Does *rape* also include a female forcing a male to engage in any unwanted sexual behavior? Does this term, in the context in which it is being used, refer to statutory rape (that is, with an underage male or female), date rape, acquaintance rape, or other forms of forcing unwanted sexual activity upon another person?

We might also read about *sexual satisfaction*. For example, it is often reported that communication is related to couples' *sexual satisfaction*. Does that refer to their enjoyment of the sexual behaviors in which they engage? Does it refer to the frequency of their sexual encounters? Does it refer to the variety of sexual activities in which they participate?

The point is that when reading articles, research reports, or other written materials, or when listening to experts or reporters discussing issues related to sexual activities and behaviors, we need to be sure about what is being referenced. That may not be as clearly evident as you suspect, or should desire.

and 14% of women said sex was very important to them, and about three-fourths of those with partners reported still being sexually active, defined as having had mutually voluntary sexual contact with another person within the past 12 months. Although the proportion of those having sex declined with age, 39% of men and 17% of women 75 to 85 years of age were still sexually active. Furthermore, 54% of those who were sexually active reported having sex at least two to three times per month, and 23% reported having sex once a week or more. The most common sexual activity was vaginal intercourse, but a significant proportion of the elderly reported engaging in oral sex, both giving and receiving, as well as masturbation.

Although the frequency of sexual activity may decrease with age due to physical changes, such as taking longer to achieve an erection or vaginal lubrication, accommodations can be made to account for these changes. Foreplay may have to be extended, and the goal may have to be changed from achieving orgasm to intimacy and sexual pleasure.

In addition, as we've stated elsewhere in this text, variety can be vital in maintaining a satisfying sexual relationship over time. Some couples use sexual aids such as vibrators, others make use of pornographic materials to spice up their sex lives, and still others use sexual fantasy or role playing. In addition, long-term partners have learned what is sexually stimulating for each other, and the level of intimacy they develop over time goes a long way toward their still finding sex exciting.

Exploring the Dimensions of Human Sexuality

© Gayvoronskaya Yana/Shutterstock

Case Study

Many factors influence what we find sexually arousing. Biologically, a physical disability may limit some sexual activities; however, it may also lead to other activities that are equally stimulating for a partner.

Psychologically, emotional attachment lends itself to sexual pleasuring. The greater the emotional attachment to someone we feel, often the greater the sexual pleasuring.

Schools play a broad role in developing our sense of what is acceptable or unacceptable. Community standards have an influence on what is taught, and that in turn influences student perceptions. Some fundamentalist religions ask young people to sign a public pledge to abstain from premarital sexual activity.

Communication is an important dimension. You and your partner need to be able to communicate which techniques you find sexually arousing. In addition, you must be able to communicate your love.

Family and friends influence sexual opinions as well. For example, comments by family and friends about Tiger Woods' affair may have influenced your perception of extramarital activity.

Biological Factors

- Sexual stimulation involves all five senses—touching, seeing, hearing, smelling, and tasting.
- Physical characteristics can enhance or inhibit sexual activities. For example, varying positions of intercourse offer varying degrees of comfort, depending on weight, physical stamina, or physical limitations.
- Foreplay allows for vaginal lubrication and erection before penile insertion.
- Physical disabilities may limit some sexual activities.
- Safer sexual activities decrease the risk of STI or HIV transmission.

Sociocultural Factors

- Sexual experience plays a role in what you find arousing.
- Sodomy laws prohibited certain sexual activities; however, these laws have been largely overturned.
- People who have more education tend to be less conservative sexually.
- Many religions prohibit certain sexual activities, such as premarital sex and masturbation.
- School sexuality education programs often reflect community standards about what is perceived to be acceptable sexual behaviors. Parent and peer reactions to sexual information affect your perception of sexual activities.

Psychological Factors

- Emotional involvement with a partner plays a role in sexual pleasuring.
- Sexual fantasies are common among males and females.

Summary

- Two autoerotic, or solitary, sexual behaviors are *masturbation* and *sexual fantasy*. These activities are considered normal with a majority of people engaging in them at one time or another. There are usually no negative physical or psychological effects of either.

- Some women report experiencing heightened sexual arousal when an area of the interior wall of the vagina is stimulated. This area is known as the *G spot*, named after Ernst Grafenberg who first discovered it. Although recent evidence has been found that might verify the presence of the G spot, experts still disagree as to its existence.

- *Foreplay* is usually the name given to the physical contact preceding coitus or oral sex. Foreplay includes touching, kissing, biting, and genital fondling. However, the term foreplay is a misnomer since it may not precede any other sexual activity but might be engaged in just for its own pleasure.

- Sexual stimulation involves all the senses: touch, sight, smell, hearing, and taste. Among these senses, the secretion of *pheromones*—substances that attract sexual partners—has long been recognized to be produced by animals. In the late 1980s, scientists verified the secretion of pheromones in humans as well.

- Oral–genital sexual behavior includes three activities. *Cunnilingus* is the oral stimulation of the female genitalia. *Fellatio* is the oral stimulation of the male genitalia. *Analingus*—commonly referred to as *rimming*—is the oral stimulation of the female or male anus.

- Sexual intercourse can include many different positions. Among the most prevalent of these are the man on top, the woman on top, side-by-side, and the rear entry positions.

- Homosexuals enjoy many of the same sexual activities as heterosexuals. Lesbian sexual activities often involve rubbing the genitals against someone's body or genital area. This is called *tribadism*.

- One of the challenges faced by long-term sexual partners is to remain monogamous over many years. Although the frequency of sexual activity may decrease with age due to physical changes, accommodations can be made to account for these changes. Foreplay may be extended, and a variety of sexual behaviors may be engaged in to spice up the relationship.

Discussion Questions

1. Discuss the many dimensions that shape current attitudes toward masturbation and fantasies. How do male and female fantasies differ?

2. Explore the role of the senses, oral–genital contact, and various intercourse positions and sexual stimulation. Describe how sexual contact with another person can be made safer.

Application Questions

Reread the chapter-opening story and answer the following questions.

1. Many people are surprised to find that such an erotic novel dates back to the mid-18th century. Given that your ancestors reproduced (if they had not, you would not be reading this text), why is it widely believed that sexuality in the 1700s was inferior to today's sexuality?

2. One major change in sexual techniques since the novel was written is the more common prevalence of oral–genital sex. What might have prompted such a change?

3. This novel, as well as *Lady Chatterly's Lover* and many others, was banned in Boston, meaning that the book was not allowed to be sold in the city. The ban was finally rendered legally useless by the mid-20th century. How do current efforts to ban or limit the distribution of sexually explicit materials differ from the efforts of our ancestors?

Critical Thinking Questions

1. If you are in a sexual relationship, is it inappropriate to masturbate? Some people believe to do so is to risk fantasizing about someone else, which is tantamount to infidelity; that it uses sexual energy that is better directed toward one's partner; and that it is an expression of dissatisfaction with one's partner, thereby insulting him or her. Others argue that masturbation has no effect on the sexual relationship; it is merely another means of sexual expression. They also believe that fantasizing about having sex with someone else is perfectly acceptable, as long as one doesn't act on that fantasy. Lastly, fantasizing can lead to uncovering new and exciting sexual activities that can be shared with one's partner. What do you think?

2. Is it better to do what is natural during sexual activity with a partner or to act according to what is learned in books such as this one?

Critical Thinking Case

The author Susan Minot, in her short story "Lust," mentions sexual technique: "I lay back with my eyes closed, luxuriating because he knew all sorts of expert angles, his hands never fumbling, going over my whole body, pressing the hair up and off the back of my head, giving an extra hip shove, as if to say *There*" (p. 15). But Minot continues the description as though the "expert" was very cold and unloving in his sexual activities.

Critics of sexuality education argue that knowing of the existence of the Grafenberg spot, erogenous zones, and the like makes sexual relationships too mechanistic. Each partner is trying so hard to recall what is stimulating and how to stimulate it that the spontaneity that makes sexual relationships so enjoyable is lost. People would be better off just "flying by the seat of their pants." Is that not the way sex has been conducted for eons? Have we not done all right with that system for generation after generation? Why add science to a nonscientific experience? Just lie back and enjoy yourself.

Others agree that sexual relationships have been adequate in the face of little knowledge of sexual arousal and response. However, they argue, adequate is not good enough. With knowledge of how the body is organized—for example, where nerve endings are accumulated—and how to achieve increased sexual excitement, sexual relationships could be enhanced. Further, there is nothing wrong with consciously, even during a highly emotional sexual encounter, thinking of how best to please your partner, because that means that your partner will be thinking of how best to please you. The result will be a more sexually satisfying relationship.

What do you think? Spontaneous sexual experiences or mechanistic ones? Thoughtless sexual experiences or thoughtful ones?

Exploring Personal Dimensions

Assessing Your Sexual Fantasies

Are your sexual fantasies similar or dissimilar to other people's sexual fantasies? In what ways are they similar? In what ways are they dissimilar? To find out, answer the following questions. A discussion follows.

1. Do you fantasize about sex? How often?
2. What do you fantasize about when you fantasize about sex?
3. Do your sexual fantasies when you are with your partner differ from those when you are alone? If so, describe the difference.

4. Do you discuss your sexual fantasies with anyone else? If so, why? If not, why not?

Discussion

In a summary of research on sexual fantasies that reviewed more than 200 studies, the *Washington Post* reported the following information. Compare your responses to the typical responses of other adults.

1. Men average seven sexual fantasies a day, five of these triggered by outside stimuli such as watching a beautiful woman and two by inner thoughts. Women average five sexual fantasies a day, three from outside stimuli and two from their internal selves.
2. Women's favorite sexual fantasies involve a new sexual partner, sex with a celebrity, and sex with either a younger man or boy or an older "gent." Men's sexual fantasies include observing women nude and having sex with a new partner, sex with multiple partners at the same time, and having the sexual prowess to "drive women wild."
3. When men and women are alone, their sexual fantasies tend to be of their usual sexual partner, if they have one. Ironically, though, when they are actually engaged in sexual activity with their usual sexual partner, they tend to fantasize about sex with someone else. Often, this fantasy involves a celebrity.
4. Because many men and women feel guilty about fantasizing about someone else while being engaged in sexual activity with their usual partner they do not discuss their sexual fantasies with their partner. A mere 26% of men and only 32% of women tell their sexual partner about their fantasies.

Well, how do you compare with the average adult female or male? Is there anything about your sexual fantasies that you will work to change?

Source: Tasker, F. X marks the fantasy, *The Washington Post* (July 27, 1995), D5.

Suggested Readings

Bakos, S. C. *The little book of the big orgasm: More techniques and games for amazing orgasms than you could possibly imagine trying.* Beverly, MA: Quiver, 2010.

Bakos, S. C. *The orgasm bible: The latest research and techniques for reaching more powerful climaxes more often.* Beverly, MA: Quiver, 2008.

Bakos, S. C. *The sex bible: the complete guide to sexual love.* Beverly, MA: Quiver, 2008.

Bennett, M. *Fifty shades of pleasure: A bedside companion: Sex secrets that hurt so good.* New York, NY: Skyhorse, 2012.

Blue, V. *Seal it with a kiss: Tips, tricks, and techniques for delivering the knockout kiss.* Berkeley, CA: Viva Editions, 2010.

Borg, S. *Spectacular sex moves he'll never forget: Ingenious positions and techniques that will blow his mind.* Minneapolis, MN: Quiver, 2010.

Chia, M., & Wei, W. U. *Chi kung for women's health and sexual vitality: A handbook of simple exercises and techniques.* Rochester, VT: Destiny Books, 2014.

Davis, P. *The passion parties guide to great sex: Secrets and techniques to keep your relationship red hot.* Bel Air, CA: Broadway, 2007.

Hutchins, D. C., & Sinclair, A. *The sensuous couple's (flip over) guide to seismic oral sex.* Philadelphia, PA: JPS, 2008.

Leman, K. *Sheet music: Uncovering the secrets of sexual intimacy in marriage.* Carol Stream, IL: Tyndale House, 2011.

McCarthy, B., & McCarthy, E. *Sexual awareness: Your guide to healthy couple sexuality.* New York, NY: Routledge, 2012.

Schell, J. *Lesbian sex: 101 lovemaking positions.* Berkeley, CA: Celestial Arts, 2008.

Spurr, P. *Naughty tricks and sexy tips: A couple's guide to uninhibited erotic pleasure.* Berkeley, CA: Amorata Press, 2007.

Winston, S. *Women's anatomy of arousal: Secret maps to buried pleasure.* Kingston, NY: Mango Garden Press, 2011.

Zilbergeld, B. *The new male sexuality: The truth about men, sex, and pleasure.* New York, NY: Bantam, 2013.

Web Resources

Good Vibrations
www.goodvibes.com

A website that provides links related to sexual techniques and behaviors. Included are links to sex toys, sex education, erotic and informative books, adult DVDs, and other sexual-related materials. Products may be purchased at this website.

AllSex Guide
www.allsexguide.com

Offers links on matters pertaining to sex. Information made available in the form of guides on various topics, including couples sex, solo sex, kinky sex, safe sex, how to, and sex toys.

Sex Information Associates: Sex Positions and Techniques
www.sex-techniques-and-positions.com

A guide to a variety of sexual positions and techniques to enhance sexual pleasure. The guide includes photographs of people demonstrating the sexual positions. Also offers videos of sexual positions and sexual techniques.

SexualHealthConnection.com: Sex Tips and Advice
www.healthcentral.com/sexual-health/sextechniques.html

Recommendations for enhancing one's sex life. Among the topics included are speaking up for better sex, salvaging so-so sex, tantric sex, multiple orgasms, 5 steps to a healthy sex life, and 10 sexy gifts to give your partner.

References

AARP. *American Association of Retired Persons/Modern Maturity sexuality study.* Washington, DC: Author, 1999.

Apfelbaum, B. Why we should not accept sexual fantasies, in *Expanding the boundaries of sex therapy.* Berkeley, CA: Berkeley Sex Therapy Group, 1980.

Arafat, I., & Cotton, W. L. Masturbation practices of males and females. *Journal of Sex Research, 10* (1974), 293–307.

Bhutta, M. F. Sex and the nose: Human pheromonal response. *Journal of the Royal Society of Medicine, 100* (2007), 268–274.

Bivona, J., & Critelli, J. The nature of women's rape fantasies: An analysis of prevalence, frequency, and contents. *Journal of Sex Research, 45* (2008), 1–13.

Blumstein, P., & Schwartz, P. *American couples.* New York: William Morrow, 1983.

Blumstein, P., & Schwartz, P. Intimate relationships and the creation of sexuality. In *Homosexuality/heterosexuality: Concepts of sexual orientation,* McWhirter, D. P., Sanders, S. A., & Reinisch, J. M., eds. New York: Oxford Press, 1990, pp. 307–320.

Cain, V. S., Johannes, C. B., Avis, N. E., Mohr, B., Schocken, M., Skurnick, J., & Ory, M. Sexual functioning and practices in a multi-ethnic study of midlife women: Baseline results from SWAN. *Journal of Sex Research, 40* (2003), 266–276.

Copen, C. E., Chandra, A., & Martinez, G. Prevalence and timing of oral sex with opposite-sex partners among females and males aged 15–24 Years: United States, 2007–2010. *National Health Statistics Reports, 56* (August 16, 2012).

Chandra, A., Copen, C. E., & Mosher, W. D. Sexual behavior, sexual attraction, and sexual identity in the United States: Data from the 2006–2010. National Survey of Family Growth. In: Baumle, A. K. (Ed.), *International handbooks of population: International handbook on the demography of sexuality* (Vol. VI, pp. 45–66). Dordrecht, Germany: Springer Science and Business Media, 2013.

Chandra, A., Mosher, W. D., Copen, C., & Sionean, C. Sexual behavior, sexual attraction, and sexual identity in the United States: Data from the 2006–2008 National Survey of Family Growth. *National Health Statistics Reports, 36* (March 3, 2011).

Chick, D., & Gold, S. R. A review of influences on sexual fantasy: Attitudes, experiences, guilt and gender. *Imagination and Cognitive Personality, 7* (1987–1988), 61–76.

Christensen, F. M. *Pornography: The other side*. New York: Praeger, 1990.

Clement, U. Surveys of heterosexual behavior, in *Annual Review of Sex Research, Vol. 1*, Bancroft, J., Davis, C. M., & Weinstein, D., eds. New York: Society for the Scientific Study of Sex Research, 1990, 45–74.

Coen, S. Sexual interviewing, evaluation, and therapy: Psychoanalytic emphasis on the use of sexual fantasy. *Archives of Sexual Behavior, 7* (1978), 229–41.

Crepault, C. C., et al. Erotic imagery in women, in *Progress in sexuality*. Gemme, R., & C. C. Wheeler, ed. New York: Plenum, 1977.

Critelli, J. W., & Bivona, J. M. Women's erotic rape fantasies: An evaluation of theory and research. *Journal of Sex Research, 45* (2008), 57–70.

Cutler, W., Berg, G. P., Krieger, A., Huggins, G. R., Garcia, C. R., & Lawley, H. J. Human axillary secretions influence women's menstrual cycles: The role of donor extract from men. *Hormones and Behavior, 20* (1986), 463–473.

Das, A. Masturbaton in the United States. *Journal of Sex and Marital Therapy, 33* (2007), 301–317.

Davidson, J. K. The utilization of sexual fantasies by sexually experienced university students. *Journal of American College Health, 34* (1985), 24–32.

Dibble, S. L., & Robertson, P. A. *Lesbian health 101: A clinician's guide*. San Francisco, CA: UCSF Nursing Press, 2010.

Downey, L. International change in sex behavior: A belated look at Kinsey's males. *Archives of Sexual Behavior, 9* (1980), 267–317.

Dubberley, E. *Garden of desires: The evolution of women's sexual fantasies*. London: Virgin Books, 2014.

Elder, S. Sexual foreplay: What's in it for men? *WebMD*, 2009. Available: http://men.webmd.com/guide/sexual-foreplay-whats-for-men.

Ellis, B. J., & Symons, D. Sex differences in sexual fantasy: An evolutionary psychological approach. *Journal of Sex Research, 27* (1990), 527–555.

Friday, N. *Forbidden flowers*. New York: Pocket Books, 1975.

Frye, M. Lesbian sex, in *Through the prism of difference: Readings on sex and gender*, Zinn, M. B., Hondagneu-Sotelo, P., & Messner, M. A., eds. Boston: Allyn & Bacon, 1997.

Geddes, L. Ultrasound nails location of the elusive G spot. *Independent* (February 20, 2008). Available: http://www.sensualism.com/sex/g-spot.html.

Gerressu, M., Mercer, C. H., Graham, C. A., Wellings, K., & Johnson, A. M. Prevalence of masturbation and associated factors in a British national probability survey. *Archives of Sexual Behavior, 37* (2008), 266–278.

Goodson, P., McCormick, D., & Evans, A. Searching for sexually explicit materials on the Internet: An exploratory study of college students' behavior and attitudes. *Archives of Sexual Behavior, 30* (2001), 101–118.

Gravina, G. L., Brandetti, F., Martini, P., Carosa, E., Di Stasi, S. M., Morano, S., Lenzi, A., & Jannini, E. A. Measurement of the thickness of the urethrovaginal space in women with or without vaginal orgasm. *Journal of Sexual Medicine, 5* (2008), 610–618.

Haffner, D. W., & Schwartz, P. *What I've learned about sex*. New York: Perigee Books, 1998.

Hakala, K. A study of sex duration in America, *Nerve*, February 19, 2014. Available: http://www.nerve.com/love-sex/which-states-have-the-longest-and-shortest-sex.

Halderman, B. L., Zelhart, P. F., & Jackson, T. T. The study of fantasy: Determinants of fantasy function and content. *Journal of Clinical Psychology, 41* (1984), 325–330.

Hariton, B. E. The sexual fantasies of women. In *Psychology Today* (editors). *The female experience*. Del Mar, CA: Communications/Research/Machines, 1973.

Hawley, P. H., & Hensley, W. A. Social dominance and forceful submission fantasies: Feminine pathology or power? *Journal of Sex Research, 46* (2009), 568–585.

Henderson, M. Scientist may be first man to find the female G-spot. *The Times* (February 21, 2008). Available: http://www.timesonline.co.uk/tol/news/uk/science/article3406113.ece.

Herbenick, D., Reece, M., Schick, V., Sanders, S. A., Dodge, B., & Fortenberry, J. D. Sexual behavior in the United States: Results from a national probability sample of men and women ages 14–94. *Journal of Sexual Medicine, Special Issue: Findings from the National Survey of Sexual Health and Behavior (NSSHB), Center for Sexual Health Promotion, Indiana University, 7* (suppl 5) (2010): 255–265.

Hicks, T., & Leitenberg, H. Sexual fantasies about one's partner versus someone else: Gender differences in incidence and frequency. *Journal of Sex Research, 38* (2001), 43–50.

Hollender, M. H. Women's wish to be held: Sexual and nonsexual aspects. *Medical Aspects of Human Sexuality*, (October 1970), 12–26.

Hunt, M. *Sexual behavior in the 1970's*. Chicago: Playboy Press, 1974.

Jones, J. C., & Barlow, D. H. Self-reported frequency of sexual urges, fantasies, and masturbatory fantasies in heterosexual males and females. *Archives of Sexual Behavior, 19* (1990), 269–279.

Joyal, C. C., Cossette, A., & Lapierre, V. What exactly is an unusual sexual fantasy? *Journal of Sexual Medicine*, October 30, 2014. Available: http://onlinelibrary.wiley.com.proxyum.researchport.umd.edu/doi/10.1111/jsm.12734/full.

Keating, J., & Over, R. Sexual fantasies of heterosexual and homosexual men. *Archives of Sexual Behavior, 19* (1990), 461–475.

Keverne, E. B. Importance of olfactory and vomeronasal systems for male sexual function. *Physiology and Behavior, 83* (2004), 177–187.

Kinsey, A. C., Pomeroy, W. B., & Martin, C. E. *Sexual behavior in the human female*. Philadelphia: Saunders, 1953.

Kinsey, A. C., Pomeroy, W. B., & Martin, C. E. *Sexual behavior in the human male*. Philadelphia: Saunders, 1948.

Knafo, G., & Jaffe, Y. Sexual fantasizing in males and females. *Journal of Research in Personality, 19* (1984), 451–462.

Lanuza, E., Novejarque, A., Martinez-Hernandez, J., Agustin-Pavon, C., & Martinez-Garcia, F. Sexual pheromones and the evolution of the reward system of the brain: The chemosensory function of the amygdala. *Brain Research Bulletin, 75* (2008), 460–466.

Laumann, E. O., Gagnon, J. H., Michael, R. T., & Michaels, S. *The social organization of sexuality: Sexual practices in the United States.* Chicago: University of Chicago Press, 1994.

Leahy, M. *Porn university: What college students are really saying about sex on campus.* Chicago: Northfield Publishers, 2009.

Leitenberg, H., & Henning, K. Sexual fantasy. *Psychological Bulletin, 117* (1995), 469–496.

Lindau, S. T., Schumm, L. P., Laumann, E. O., Levinson, W., O'Muircheartaigh, C. A., & Waite, L. J. A study of sexuality and health among older adults in the United States. *New England Journal of Medicine, 357* (2007), 762–774.

Maltz, W., & Boss, S. *Private thoughts.* Novalo, CA: New World Library, 2001.

Masters, W. H., & Johnson, V. E. *Homosexuality in perspective.* Boston: Little, Brown, 1979.

Masters, W. H., & Johnson, V. E. *Human sexual response.* Boston: Little, Brown, 1966.

Masters, W. H., Johnson, V. E., & Kolodny, R. C. *Human sexuality*, 2nd ed. Boston: Little, Brown, 1985.

Michael, R. T., Gagnon, J. H., Laumann, E. O., & Kolata, G. *Sex in America: A definitive survey.* New York: Warner Books, 1995.

Michael, R., Gagnon, J., Laumann, E., & Kolata, G. *Sex in America.* Boston: Little, Brown, 1994.

Miller, S. A., & Byers, E. S. Actual and desired duration of foreplay and intercourse: Discordance and misperceptions within heterosexual couples. *Journal of Sex Research, 41* (2004), 301–309.

Mostafa, T., El Khouly, G., & Hassan, A. Pheromones in sex and reproduction: Do they have a role in humans? *Journal of Advanced Research, 3* (2012), 1–9.

Nutter, D., & Condron, M. Sexual fantasy and activity patterns of females with inhibited sexual desire versus normal controls. *Journal of Sex and Marital Therapy, 9* (1983), 276–282.

Pastor, Z. [G spot—myths and reality.] *Ceska Gynekologie, 75* (2010), 211–217.

Peplau, L. A., & Cochran, S. D. A relationship perspective on homosexuality, in *Homosexuality/heterosexuality: Concepts of sexual orientation*, McWhirter, D. P., Sanders, S. A., & Reinisch, J. M., eds. New York: Oxford Press, 1990, pp. 321–349.

Perry, J. D., & Whipple, B. Pelvic muscle strength of female ejaculators: Evidence in support of a new theory of orgasm. *Journal of Sex Research, 17* (1981), 22–39.

Plesa, A. Top ten sexual fantasies for men. *Examiner.com*, 2013. Available: http://www.examiner.com/article/top-ten-sexual-fantasies-for-men.

Preti, G., Winnifred, C., Celso, R., Garcia, G. Huggins, R., & Lawley, H. J. Human axillary secretions influence women's menstrual cycles: The role of donor extract of females. *Hormones and Behavior, 20* (1986), 474–482.

Preti, G., Wysocki, C. J., Barnhart, K. T., Sondheimer, S. J., & Leyden, J. J. Male axillary extracts contain pheromones that affect pulsatile secretion of luteinizing hormone and mood in women recipients. *Biological Reproduction, 68* (2003), 2107–2113.

Rathus, S. A., Nevid, J. S., & Fichner-Rathus, L. *Human sexuality in a world of diversity.* Boston, MA: Pearson, 2008.

Reece, M., Rosenberger, J. G., Schick, V., Herbenick, D., Dodge, B., & Novak, D. S. Characteristics of vibrator use by gay and bisexually identified men in the United States. *Journal of Sexual Medicine, 7* (2010), 3467–3476.

Religious tolerance. About Masturbation: Diversity of Beliefs within the Roman Catholic Church, 2008. Available: http://www.religoustolerance.org/masturba10.htm.

Rensberger, R. Pheromones discovered in humans: Substances help regulate female reproductive cycle. *Washington Post* (November 1986) A1, A7.

Rosaria, M. The psychosexual development of urban lesbian, gay, and bisexual youth. *Journal of Sex Research, 33, no. 2* (1996), 113–126.

Rosenberger, J. G., Reece, M., Schick, V., Herbenick, D., Novak, D. S., Van Der Pol, B., & Fortenberry, J. D. Sexual behaviors and situational characteristics of most recent male-partnered sexual event among gay and bisexually identified men in the United States. *Journal of Sexual Medicine, 8* (2011), 3040–3050.

Rumbough, T. B. *Controversial uses of the Internet by college students*, 2001. Available: http://www.eucuase.edu/ir/library/pdf/C5D1618.pdf.

Schick, V., Herbenick, D., Rosenberger, J. G., & Reece, M. Prevalence and characteristics of vibrator use among women who have sex with women. *Journal of Sexual Medicine, 8* (2011), 3306–3315.

Shainess, N., & Greenwald, H. Debate: Are fantasies during sexual relations a sign of difficulty? *Sexual Behavior, 1* (1971), 38–54.

Spalding, L. R., & Peplau, L. A. The unfaithful lover: Heterosexuals' perceptions of bisexuals and their relationships. *Psychology of Women Quarterly, 21* (1997), 611–625.

Spors, H., & Sobel, N. Male behavior by knockout. *Neuron, 55* (2007), 689–693.

Strassberg, D. S., & Lockerd, L. K. Force in women's sexual fantasies. *Journal of Sexual Behavior, 27* (1998), 403–414.

Strovny, D. The importance of foreplay. *AskMen.com*, 2009. Available: http://www.askmen.com/dating/love_tip/sextip18.html.

Sue, D. Erotic fantasies of college students during coitus. *Journal of Sex Research, 15* (1979), 299–305.

Tripp, C. A. *The homosexual matrix.* New York: New American Library, 1976.

The way we live now. *New York Times* (May 7, 2000), p. 18.

Weiss, P., & Brody, S. Women's partnered orgasm consistency is associated with greater duration of penile–vaginal intercourse but not of foreplay. *Journal of Sexual Medicine, 6* (2009), 135–141.

Wilson, G. D. Gender differences in sexual fantasy: An evolutionary analysis. *Personality and Individual Differences, 22* (1997): 27–31.

Zimmer, D. E., Borchardt, E., & Fischle, C. Sexual fantasies of sexually distressed and nondistressed men and women: An empirical comparison. *Journal of Sex and Marital Therapy, 9* (1983), 38–50.

CHAPTER 16

Alternative Sexual Behavior

© Gayvoronskaya Yana/Shutterstock

FEATURES

Communication Dimensions
Communicating Accurately

Multicultural Dimensions
Paraphilias Across Cultures

Gender Dimensions
Paraphilias and Gender Differences

Ethical Dimensions
The Ethics of Chemical Treatment for Paraphilias

CHAPTER OBJECTIVES

1 Discuss how some alternative sexual behaviors exist on a continuum of sexual activity.

2 Describe the most common paraphilias.

3 Name and define paraphilias other than the most common ones.

4 Explain what can be done to treat paraphilias.

5 Summarize what is known about sexual addiction.

© Gayvoronskaya Yana/Shutterstock

INTRODUCTION

*V*arieties of sexual behaviors have been around a long time, as have many opinions about them. Many people were surprised when a well-known sportscaster was indicted on charges of assault and sodomy. His accuser, a 41-year-old female friend whom he had known for 10 years, claimed that he viciously bit her several times on the back during an argument in his hotel room.

The woman claimed that her partner became enraged when she refused to join in a "three-way" with him and another man and that he threw her on the bed and bit her on the back 10 to 15 times. Then, according to court documents, he forced her to perform oral sexual activity. After the woman sought treatment at a local hospital, the police were notified.

To many people, the charges against the sportscaster seemed very much out of character. One of his producers said that on both a professional and a personal level he was a joy to be around. The executive producer of the network sports said he was "in total shock" about the charges.

As the allegations were investigated, additional stories came out about the sportscaster's sexual behavior, including his alleged fondness for wearing women's underwear and participating in threesomes. As a result, he was removed from sportscasting and taken off network shows. About 3 years later, he returned to broadcasting as the radio voice of a pro sports team.

Stories like this cause people to wonder about varieties of sexual behavior and talk more about them. Although many varieties of sexual behavior are relatively uncommon, it can be important to know more about them.

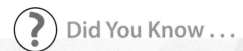

Did You Know . . .

Elsewhere in this chapter, you will read that theories about causes of paraphilias can be grouped into psychoanalytical, behavioral, and sociobiological theories. Related to this, and perhaps including aspects of two or more of the theories, is the concept of erotic target location error (ETLE). This condition entails having a strong sexual interest in features that are somewhere other than on one's sexual partner(s). Examples could include children, real animals, and plush animals. Some aspects of the most common paraphilias are described in this chapter.

Common Versus Atypical Sexual Behaviors

A few points about atypical sexual behavior in general should be noted before we consider specific behaviors. First, in many instances there are gradations of a sexual behavior existing on a continuum. For example, most people enjoy looking at other people. However, if someone spends many hours each day just looking at others, we would probably assume that person has a problem. There would be spots on the continuum between these two extremes that might be hard to judge. Is the behavior common or is it atypical? Is it acceptable or unacceptable? It is up to each individual, and society, to decide where on the continuum of sexual behavior activities become unacceptable. For instance, when is behavior obsessive (that is, the individual does not freely choose the behavior); when is it associated with emotional distress or with the inability to interact satisfactorily with other people; when is it forced on another person; when is it illegal?

Because many behaviors vary in degree, it is not surprising that many of us may recognize some degree of atypical behaviors or feelings in ourselves—perhaps only in private fantasies. In most instances, such behaviors or feelings should be accepted as natural—as long as they do not interfere with our optimal functioning or with the rights of others.

It is also common for us not to know a great deal about atypical sexual behaviors. Because in most cases such behavior is not common, and in most cases it is performed in private, it is difficult to study. Therefore, as we consider atypical sexual behaviors, many questions will be left unanswered.

It is also interesting that atypical sexual behaviors often occur in combination. For example, one well-known celebrity apparently did some cross-dressing along with participating in group sexual activity and violence.

Some people wonder about causes of paraphilias. Not a great deal is known about this topic, but theories can be grouped into psychoanalytical, behavioral, and sociobiological (Brannon & Carroll, 2008). Psychoanalytical theory centers on possible distortion of courtship phases. Some people are unable to adhere to socially acceptable norms and develop deviant or unconventional sexual practices. Behavioral theory attributes the development of certain paraphilias to the process of conditioning. For example, if nonsexual objects are frequently associated with a pleasurable sexual activity, the objects can become sexually arousing. In some cases, the constant threat of discovery may be as arousing as the act itself. Sociobiological theory includes the idea that even atypical sexual behavior relates to survival of the species. For example, different paraphilias may be responsible for enhancing society's level of sexual excitation. In turn, this increases the likelihood of people engaging in sexual acts that would ultimately lead to procreation.

Within this chapter, we briefly discuss some of the most common atypical sexual behaviors.

The Most Common Paraphilias

Unusual or problematic sexual behaviors are scientifically known as paraphilias. **Paraphilia** means love (*philia*) beyond the usual (*para*). There are about 50 different paraphilias, and each exists in fantasy and in reality. It is generally accepted that the prevalence and variety of paraphilias are greater in males than in females, but as indicated previously, in most instances little is known about them.

Paraphilic behaviors are unconventional sexual behaviors that are obsessive and compulsive. They can interfere with love relationships and intimacy. Paraphilias are defined as recurrent, intense sexually arousing fantasies, sexual urges, or behaviors involving (1) nonhuman objects, (2) the suffering or humiliation of oneself or one's partner, or (3) children or other nonconsenting persons. Also, the behavior, urges, or fantasies cause significant stress in social,

---

paraphilia Literally meaning "love (*philia*) beyond the usual (*para*)," this term refers to various sexual behaviors previously referred to as deviant.

occupational, or other important areas of functioning. Some behaviors, such as sadomasochism, when they are consensual and do not impair life functioning, are not considered to be a paraphilia because they do not meet all of the diagnostic criteria.

Paraphilias include sexual behaviors that many people view as distasteful, unusual, or abnormal. In descending order, the most common are pedophilia, exhibitionism, voyeurism, and frotteurism. Far less common are fetishism, sexual masochism, sexual sadism, and transvestism (Paraphilias, 2014).

Exhibitionism

Exhibitionism (commonly called *flashing* or *indecent exposure*) occurs when an individual achieves sexual gratification by exhibiting the genitals to observers. One definition of exhibitionism is that it is characterized by intense, sexually arousing fantasies, urges, or behaviors involving exposure of the individual's genitals to an unsuspecting stranger. The exhibitionist feels a need to surprise, shock, or impress his or her victims. The condition is usually limited to exposure, with no other harmful advances made (Definition of exhibitionism, 2014). Though exhibitionism is a good example of a sexual behavior that is difficult to classify as one that causes problems, we would probably agree that if someone's primary motivation in life is exhibitionism, that person has a problem. At what point does the behavior become abnormal?

Although exhibitionists are often portrayed comically, in real life the phenomenon is quite different. Exhibitionists gain sexual pleasure from eliciting a harsh reaction to their unprovoked actions. It is best to ignore one if you are ever flashed.

There are three key features of true exhibitionism: (1) There is sexual arousal directly related to the shock; (2) the victim is unwilling; and (3) no further sexual contact is desired.

A few facts about exhibitionists might help to put this behavior into perspective. The exhibitionist receives sexual gratification through the victim's (observer's) response. Exhibitionists might achieve orgasm by the very act of exposure, but more likely they will masturbate either while exhibiting or later. Exhibitionists feel inadequate, they are afraid of rejection, they are shy, and commonly they have had unsatisfactory sexual relationships. They may be looking for attention or affirmation of their masculinity (most exhibitionists are male) or attempting to frighten others.

Exhibitionism, though often discussed as a humorous topic, is a very serious behavior that can frighten the victim. The exhibitionist is typically male, and the victim is usually a female (adult or child), and usually an unsuspecting stranger. The unusual behavior may sometimes become the major sexual activity in the exhibitionist's life (Exhibitionism, 2015).

Although people often think exhibitionists are violent and aggressive, they usually are not. It is extremely rare for exhibitionists to do more than display the genitals. They do not want contact with a person. Punishment and imprisonment do not seem to prevent the recurrence of exhibitionism. Although it may be difficult, generally the best response is to ignore an exhibitionist and continue usual activities. In this way the exhibitionistic behavior is not reinforced.

The incidence of exhibitionism in the general population is difficult to estimate because, as with most other paraphilias, persons with this disorder do not usually seek counseling by their own free will. Exhibitionism is one of the three most common sexual offenses in police records. The other two are voyeurism and pedophilia (Exhibitionism, 2011).

Voyeurism

In a very general sense, the term **voyeurism** (or **scopophilia**, "love of viewing") means obtaining sexual pleasure from observing unsuspecting individuals who are naked, in the process of undressing, or engaging in sexual acts. The person being observed is usually a stranger to the observer. The act of

exhibitionism Achievement of sexual gratification by exhibiting the genitals to observers.

voyeurism (scopophilia) Obtaining pleasure from watching people who are undressing or engaging in sexual behavior.

looking is done for the purpose of achieving sexual excitement. The observer generally does not seek to have sexual contact or activity with the person being observed. If orgasm is sought it is generally achieved through masturbation. This may occur during the act of observation or later, relying on the memory of the act that was observed (Voyeurism, 2011). A "peeping Tom" is a voyeur. The voyeur learns from experience where to find people to watch. His erotic excitement lies in the forbidden act of looking at the person.

The fantasies, sexual urges, or behaviors cause clinically significant distress or impairment in social, occupational, or other important areas of functioning. Voyeurs derive sexual gratification from seeing sex organs and sexual acts.

Voyeurs, who are often shy and lonely and lack social skills, commonly fantasize about having sexual relations with the people they are watching and often masturbate while fantasizing. Voyeurs derive satisfaction from the fear of being caught, the anonymity of the person being watched, and the fact that the person does not know he or she is being watched. Generally voyeurs are not violent and, in fact, are fearful of any contact with the people they observe.

Some degree of voyeurism probably exists in everyone. Society even condones some forms of voyeurism; for example, some magazines are designed to satisfy peoples' voyeuristic tendencies, and the popularity of sexually explicit movies and websites is due to voyeurism.

Obscene Communication

The most common and traditional form of obscene communication has been obscene phone calls. Obscene letter writing is also relatively common. However, more recently, there has been a rapid rise in *sexting*—a general term that includes obscene emails and text messages.

Regardless of the form, erotic communication is a form of erotic distancing. As do the exhibitionist and the voyeur, the obscene communicator obtains sexual pleasure from a distance and not from direct contact with another person. Communicators may receive sexual gratification from making obscene remarks over a telephone or sending obscene messages with a computer or phone. They might suggest that the person meet them to have sexual relations, even though they would probably never go through with this act. The recipient of the obscene communication may be a stranger or a consenting message receiver.

It seems that the majority of females receive obscene messages of some type at some time in their life. Historically, the typical communicator has been

Females living in major metropolitan areas are the most likely victims of obscene communication.

an adult male unknown to the victim. While this still happens today, many individuals who send sexts and texts are already known to the person receiving the message.

Obscene communicators have counterparts whose main turn-on is not genital sexual activity with a partner, but rather sending erotic messages of some type. These communicators are often hoping for sexual gratification as well.

According to the U.S. Department of Justice, "Any comment, request, suggestion, proposal, image, or other communication which is obscene or indecent, knowing that the recipient of the communication is under 18 years of age" is illegal. In addition, "any indecent communication for commercial purposes which is available to any person under 18 years of age or to any other person without that person's consent" is illegal. These offenses are punishable by a fine up to $50,000 for each violation or imprisonment of up to 6 months or both (United States Code Annotated Title 47, 2014). Note that this covers any telecommunication device, including computers.

What should someone who receives an obscene communication do? Above all, one should remain calm and not reveal shock or fright: These reactions can reinforce the message sender and increase the likelihood of repeated contact. The recommended response is to not respond at all and end the communication. Most people who send obscene messages are not dangerous, and most do not make repeat contacts with the same person. In the case of obscene phone calls, it might be helpful to get an unlisted phone number, obtain caller ID capabilities, and/or contact the police about threatening or repeated calls.

Communication
DIMENSIONS

Communicating Accurately

With any sexual behavior, the concept of consent is crucial. For example, if a partner wants to be tied up, that might be fine; however, prior communication about the goal is important. A student once confessed (under the influence of alcohol) to a group of people that she wanted to be tied up. Another time, though, she said that her fantasy really involved being tied down with silk ribbons to a luxurious four-poster bed. Still later she said that what she really wanted was a partner who would initiate sexual activity with her. Thus she did not always like being the aggressor, and her fantasy was really about having her lover "take charge." But in respect to her original assertions, that underlying desire would not have been known to a partner, nor would her desire for an initiating partner be fulfilled when she engaged in nonbondage activities. As always, effective communication is a must.

First, it is crucial to explain desires and intentions clearly in such situations. The student in our example was not clear, and this could have led to behavior or attempts at behavior that were not desired. This, in turn, could have caused overall relationship problems. Second, as with any form of sexual behavior, it is important to obtain consent. It is not enough to assume that you know what your partner meant or that consent is implicit because you have a good relationship. Without consent, sexual behavior is forcible. With consent, it can be enjoyable for everyone and contribute to a positive relationship.

Masochism and Sadism

Sexual masochism refers to engaging in or fantasizing about being beaten, bound, or otherwise made to suffer, resulting in sexual satisfaction. Blindfolding, spanking, and humiliation in the form of defecation, urination, or forced imitation of animals are other methods used. Masochists may inflict pain on themselves through shocking, pricking, or choking. Approximately 30% of masochists also participate in sadistic behavior (Sexual masochism, 2015).

Sexual masochism, therefore, is sexual gratification that results from experiencing pain. In addition to the methods mentioned above, this might also include scratching, biting, beating, and the use of various devices. The pain involved must be planned as a part of an overall experience; accidentally hitting a finger with a hammer is not the kind of experience the masochist wants. **Sexual sadism** occurs when an individual gets sexual gratification from inflicting pain on another person—the hallmark of sadism is intentional torture of the victim to sexually arouse the offender. Sadists have persistent fantasies in which sexual excitement results from inflicting psychological or physical suffering (including humiliation and terror) on a sexual partner. At its most extreme, sadism involves illegal activities such as rape, torture, and even murder, in which case the death of the victim produces sexual excitement (Paraphilias, 2009). Sadists obviously make good partners for masochists, but sadomasochistic partner matching is difficult to achieve because it requires that the fantasies of the two people match completely. There are also some times when sexual gratification for a sadist might require that there is an unsuspecting partner or a stranger subjected to sexual abuse. Sadism does not seem to be as common as masochism.

Domination and degradation are important to both the sadist and the masochist. Some psychiatrists feel that sadism is an expression of anger and hostility. Masochism, in contrast, is sometimes thought to result from a belief that sexual activity is dirty and evil; therefore, the activity could be viewed as just punishment for sexual sins. It is difficult to understand the true psychology of these behaviors.

Sadomasochism is a paraphilia that combines both sadistic and masochistic sexual behavior. The main characteristic is the eroticizing of pain. What appears to the outsider to be painful is experienced as somewhat painful but mostly pleasurable and very sexually arousing to the sadomasochist. Sadomasochistic sexual encounters usually occur in the context of scripted scenes that simulate interactions between master and slave, employer and servant, and parent and child. Sadomasochists tend to alternate

sexual masochism Sexual gratification that results from experiencing pain.

sexual sadism Sexual gratification that results from inflicting pain on another person.

between masochistic and sadistic roles. In milder forms, dominance and submissive behaviors may be found in many relationships or may be an element of fantasy life.

There is more information available on masochism and sadism than on most other paraphilias, and a brief chronological review of a few studies will help to shed some light on these two behaviors. Baumeister (1997) pointed out that masochism fosters temporary escape from the stressful awareness of one's ordinary identity. Litman (1997) suggested that sexual masochism is more widespread and can be more dangerous than current literature indicates. Danger can arise from being humiliated, endangered, and enslaved and being physically bound, restrained, and rendered helpless to the degree that life is threatened. He indicates that **bondage perversion** (deriving pleasure from being bound, tied up, or otherwise restricted) can be fatal—a mix of suicide and accident.

Sexual masochism is more common in males, but the incidence in females is on the rise. Masochists often seek partners to tie up, humiliate, blindfold, or hurt. They may enjoy being whipped, beaten, shocked, or cut. Verbal abuse is common. Some masochists require pain or humiliation to function sexually (Masochism, 2001). Some sadists also require the pain or humiliation of a partner to function sexually. As long as it occurs with a consenting partner, sadism is not considered a psychological disorder. It is considered a disorder when it causes the person unhappiness or causes problems with work, social setting, or family. If the other person is not willing, sadism can be a severe and even criminal disorder. Sadism is much more common in males (Sadism, 2001). People who engage in masochism and sadism must be especially careful about diseases transmitted by body fluids, such as hepatitis and HIV.

Masochism can range from mild to extreme versions. Examples of mild versions might include bondage (being tied up for the purpose of sexual arousal), or being spanked or overpowered by physical force. The crucial point is that they are mainly symbolic enactments done under carefully controlled conditions with a trusted partner. At the opposite end of the spectrum are genuinely painful and harmful activities (Discovery Health: Paraphilia, 2005).

Sadism can also be a consensual activity in milder forms. For example, it might involve role-playing with dominant and submissive roles such as master and slave. Like masochism, however, it is important

to have controlled conditions with a trusted partner to avoid unplanned injuries. Sadomasochistic relationships need to be well planned, with partners deciding on a special word the masochist will use to indicate that the sadist should stop. Sadism is commonly found in association with other paraphilias—particularly masochism, fetishism, and transvestism.

Sadism and masochism are good examples of sexual behaviors in which we need to differentiate between fantasy and behavior. For example, many more people have reported sexual fantasies involving masochism and sadism than have actually participated in such behavior. It is possible to enjoy a sexual fantasy without needing to act it out in real life.

Transvestism

Transvestism is sometimes confused with transsexualism and homosexuality. A **transvestite** takes pleasure in wearing clothing of the other sex and is likely to achieve sexual gratification from doing so but has no interest in having a sex-change operation or in relating sexually to members of the same sex. While transvestites may be male or female, they typically are heterosexual married males.

Transvestism is also known as cross-dressing or dressing in drag. Some homosexual men dress in drag for fun. Some people with a gender identity

© Karen Struthers/ShutterStock, Inc.

Transvestites can be of many different sizes and have various appearances.

---

bondage perversion Getting sexual pleasure from being bound, tied up, or otherwise restricted.

transvestite A person who achieves sexual satisfaction from wearing clothes usually worn by the other sex.

disorder dress in clothes of the other sex to try to pass as the other sex or because they simply feel that is their proper sex. Transvestites, however, generally cross-dress for sexual arousal. Most are male and do not wish to be mistaken for women. Transvestism is considered to be a psychological disorder only when the person meets the following conditions (Transvestism, 2005). He:

- Is heterosexual, or straight.
- Has intense sexual fantasies, urges, or behaviors involving dressing in women's clothing.
- Is distressed by these fantasies, urges, or behaviors and they cause problems in his life.

Some transvestites cross-dress only periodically, and the use of female clothes (most transvestites are males) may approximate a fetish. Others may wear female clothing under their male clothes. No one knows for sure why some people are transvestites, and it is interesting to note that most transvestites have quite normal heterosexual relationships.

Most transvestites begin to experiment with cross-dressing when they are children or adolescents. Some feel guilty and uncomfortable about this preference; others do not. Many are happily married to people who understand their behaviors. Others have had relationships ruined by cross-dressing. There are numerous support groups for transvestites and their partners.

It is common for transvestism to be classified as a fetish. It is usually done in private, although undergarments can also be worn in public under regular street clothes. Transvestites will often masturbate while wearing female clothing and/or make-up while fondling specific items. Transvestism, by itself, is usually not associated with criminal behavior, although it could be combined with other fetishes or disorders that result in criminal behavior (Transvestic fetishism, 2005).

Fetishism

Fetishism is a disorder in which there is pathological assignment of sexual fixation, fantasies, or behaviors toward an inanimate object—frequently an item of clothing, such as underclothing or a high-heeled shoe. The fetishist usually holds, rubs, or smells the fetish for sexual gratification or asks the partner to wear the object during sexual activity. Fetishism is more common in males, and the causes are not clearly known (Fetishism, 2015).

The fetishist may masturbate while engaging in fetishistic behavior or may just enjoy stimulation from the objects. In a related paraphilia, **partialism**, people

Various items, articles of clothing, and materials can be fetishistic objects.

are aroused by a particular body part (breasts, muscular chests, feet, and so on). Most fetishes are practiced in private or with a willing partner.

Generally, a person who has fetishism must have the fetish present to become sexually excited. It usually begins in childhood or adolescence and is most common among males. Although many people are aroused by undergarments or other items, this is not considered fetishism except when a person cannot perform sexually unless the partner is wearing the items.

It is difficult to obtain statistical information related to fetishes, but one rather large study found that among those with fetishes, body part fetishes were the most common (33%), followed by objects associated with the body (30%), preferences for other people's behavior (18%), own behavior (7%), and objects unrelated to the body (5%). Feet (and objects associated with feet) were by far the most common fetishes (Griffiths, 2014b).

The fetish may replace sexual activity with a partner or may be integrated into sexual activity with a willing partner. When the fetish becomes the sole object of sexual desire, sexual relationships often are avoided (Paraphilias, 2009). Most fetishes and partialisms are harmless. However, occasionally someone may commit burglary to obtain the fetish object.

Inanimate object fetishes can be categorized into two types: form fetishes and media fetishes. In a form

fetishism Paraphilia in which there is a disorder with pathological assignment of sexual fixation, fantasies, or behaviors toward an inanimate object.

partialism Paraphilia in which sexual arousal is associated with a particular body part.

fetish, it is the object and its shape that are important, such as with high-heeled shoes. In a media fetish, it is the material from which the object is made that is important, such as silk or leather. Although the list of objects that fetishists can use for sexual gratification is inexhaustible, among the more common inanimate objects are panties, bras, slips, stockings or panty hose, negligees, shoes, boots, and gloves. Common media objects include leather, rubber, silk, and fur. In most cases, the person with a fetish is no danger to others and pursues the use of the fetish objects in private, usually through masturbation. The causes of fetishism are not clearly understood. Some experts believe that it develops from early childhood experiences, in which an object was associated with a particularly powerful form of sexual arousal or gratification (Fetishism, 2005).

Other Paraphilias

Bestiality

Bestiality (or **zoophilia**) is sexual contact with animals. In Kinsey's research (1948, 1953), about 8% of males and 4% of females reported having had sexual experiences with animals at some time. The frequency of bestiality was higher (17% for males) for those raised in rural areas. Men most often had sexual contact with farm animals; women most often had sexual contact with household pets.

There are few, if any, more recent statistics related to bestiality. It does not seem to be a topic on which current research is being done. This lack of research interest could stem from many reasons, including the "taboo" nature of the topic, the illegality of the practice in many states, and the difficulty of finding subjects willing to talk about the topic.

Human sexual relationships with animals have been an interesting topic for some people for hundreds of years. Stories of human–animal contact are found throughout ancient folklore. For example, Zeus, in the form of a swan, had sexual intercourse with Leda, the queen of Sparta. Greek and Roman mythology portrayed females having sexual relationships with bears, apes, bulls, goats, horses, wolves, snakes, and crocodiles. Historically, taboos against human–animal contact have been severe. The laws in many states treated bestiality as a felony. In eight states, the maximal penalty was life imprisonment. Many such laws remain on the books.

Sexual experience with animals is usually only a transitory experience for young people who do not have acceptable sexual partners. It most likely occurs during adolescence, and most people move on to more common adult sexual relations with humans. It is generally agreed that a condition is really zoophilia only if someone prefers sexual contact with animals even if other forms of sexual activity are available.

There has been very little research on bestiality. Even though it has been present throughout history, addressing the subject often seems to evoke prejudices and emotional reactions rather than objective reflection. A large part of the information on bestiality stems from criminological reports, and this is a very limited sampling (Beetz, 2004).

Frottage

Frottage is the act of obtaining sexual pleasure from rubbing or pressing against a nonconsenting person.

---

bestiality Sexual contact with animals—also called *zoophilia*.

zoophilia Sexual contact with animals—also called *bestiality*.

frottage Obtaining of sexual pleasure from rubbing or pressing against another person.

The overcrowding of subways in Tokyo and other Japanese cities lends itself to frottage, or deriving sexual pleasure from rubbing up against a nonconsenting person. The situation is exacerbated by the male-dominated Japanese culture, which prevents police from dealing with the problem.

The American Psychiatric Association's official definition (2015) is "over a period of at least six months, recurrent, intense sexually arousing fantasies, sexual urges, or behaviors involving touching and rubbing against a nonconsenting person." It is likely to occur in crowds, on elevators, and in buses and subways. It is even possible that the frotteur will achieve orgasm. Women and girls, the usual recipients, generally find this behavior offensive. Normally no additional contact or other form of behavior follows.

Necrophilia

Necrophilia is a rather rare behavior in which a person receives sexual pleasure from viewing or having sexual relations with a dead person. Sometimes necrophiliacs (almost all of whom are men) pay women to pretend to be dead so as to provide sexual pleasure. This might even include dressing in a certain way, using white powder to look very pale, and lying very still. In this way the participants are simulated corpses.

Necrophiliacs are usually severely emotionally disturbed, sexually and socially inept, and hate and fear women. Although local newspapers do not report instances, law enforcement officers indicate that bodies are sometimes stolen for this purpose.

It is interesting to note that necrophilia was depicted within the range of normal expression in the television program, *Buffy the Vampire Slayer*. The sexual encounter of Buffy with Angel, two characters in the show, was presented as the natural culmination of their love for each other. The fact that Buffy was technically making love to a corpse was

overlooked entirely by the audience. Over the years, a staple of the show was Buffy's relationship with vampire lovers—first Angel and then Spike. The connection between love and death and the acceptance of the undead or necrophilic lover was presented (Spaise, 2005). *Buffy the Vampire Slayer* was on TV from 1997 to 2003, but chances are that some of the readers of this book have seen the show in reruns since then.

Troilism

Troilism is having sexual relations with another person while a third person watches. In one respect, troilism combines elements of exhibitionism and voyeurism. In another respect, it represents an illusion of prostitution, because there are elaborate ruses and pretenses of prostitution. An example might be a husband's inviting another man to have intercourse with his wife. The husband watches and is able to get an erection. He then achieves penetration and orgasm, which are not possible unless his wife plays the role of a prostitute.

Troilism clearly does not qualify as a safe sexual activity. Because multiple partners are involved, this is a high-risk activity.

Asphyxiophilia

Asphyxiophilia is the desire for a state of oxygen deficiency to enhance sexual excitement and orgasm. It has also been called *erotic* or *autoerotic suicide, sexual suicide, autoerotic strangulation, autoerotic asphyxiation, hypoxophilia,* and *autoerotic accident.* Most information about asphyxiophilia is found in reports from police or doctors of forensic medicine who examine people who have died during this behavior.

Self-induced oxygen deficiency is used to produce sexual euphoria, increased excitement, or heightened orgasm during masturbatory activities. Reduced supply of oxygen to the brain results in giddiness, lightheadedness, or exhilaration that is reported to enhance sexual climax.

Oxygen deficiency can be induced in many ways. Because the circumstances and features of autoerotic deaths are not commonly known, they are often misinterpreted as suicides or homicides. And death can easily result, because cutting off the flow of blood to the brain can produce unconsciousness in as little as 5 to 10 seconds. Although the person probably

necrophilia Sexual relations with a dead person.

troilism Having sexual relations with another person while a third person watches.

asphyxiophilia Desire for a state of oxygen deficiency to enhance sexual excitement.

did not intend to die, death results when an escape mechanism fails or the person cannot recover from self-induced oxygen deprivation.

Because of the nature of asphyxiophilia and the fact that it is often covered up, it is difficult to get accurate statistics about it. However, Jenkins (2000) indicated that cases are often reported as intentional suicide; conservative estimates place it at 6.5% of all adolescent suicides and at least 31% of all adolescent hangings. The deceased victims are most often white, middle-class unmarried males. Although it might seem that practitioners of this dangerous behavior suffer mental illness, this is usually not the case. The victims are usually well-adjusted, nondepressed, high achievers.

Asphyxiophilia is really a subcategory of sexual masochism. Although it could be practiced with a partner, it is usually a solitary act. The practice is intended to produce sexual pleasure, but practitioners are well aware of the inherent risk element. Because of that, they use some kind of safety mechanism to prevent accidental death in the event of unconsciousness. There is no evidence that deaths from asphyxiophilia are a form of disguised suicide. Such deaths are usually a complete surprise to family and friends. Nearly all reported deaths have been males, and most under 40 years of age. However, the practice can begin at puberty for some. There are no known signs of predisposition to this behavior or the existence of the paraphilia. In many cases of death from asphyxiophilia, the cause of death has been attributed to suicide even though that is not the case (Hypoxyphilia/auto-erotic asphyxia, 2005).

Hypoxyphilia (near-asphyxiation) is caused by reducing the oxygen level in the brain. An article in *Psychology Today* indicated that this practice results in 1 to 2 accidental deaths per 1 million people per year. To achieve near-asphyxiation, the individual might place a noose around the neck, use chest compression, put airtight bags over the head, or use amyl nitrates ("poppers") (Sexual masochism, 2015).

Klismaphilia

In **klismaphilia** sexual arousal is obtained from enema use. Klismaphiles most often prefer the receiving role, but less commonly erotic arousal may be associated with administering an enema. The background of many individuals who show klismaphilia often indicates that as infants or young children they were frequently given enemas by concerned and loving mothers. This association with loving attention, or

perhaps even sexual pleasure, learned early in life may eroticize the experience for some people, so they show a need to receive an enema for sexual satisfaction as adults. Because klismaphilia involves anal contact, it is not a safe sexual activity unless latex gloves are used and there is great attention to cleanliness.

Klismaphilia is a term that was coined in the reporting of two case studies in the 1970s (*klisma* is a Greek word meaning "enema"). Typically, warm water is used to clean the lower rectum in this practice, although use of other substances has been reported, including coffee, yogurt, air, whisky, wine, beer, cocaine, and epoxy resin. Kinsey's surveys of sexual behavior of males and females in the late 1940s and early 1950s mentioned women using enemas as a masturbatory aid, but no such practice was reported by males. However, it is typically males who are more likely to be klismaphiliacs. Published research on this topic is rare, and it is thought that most klismaphiliacs are very secretive about their engagement in this activity. The little research that has been done suggests that receiving enemas can cause intense stimulation and produce pleasurable sensations (gaining pleasure from a large, water-distended belly or the feeling of internal pressure). Supposedly, drugs administered rectally are absorbed rapidly and have a "mainlining" effect similar to that of intravenous drug injection. Accidental rectal trauma and the lodging of foreign bodies in the gastrointestinal tract have been widely reported in the medical literature (Griffiths, 2014a).

Coprophilia

In **coprophilia**, sexual pleasure is associated with feces. People who show coprophilia reach high levels of sexual excitement by watching someone defecate or by defecating on someone. The connection of feces with sexual arousal may also go back to childhood. Some children seem to enjoy holding back on a bowel movement and then carefully expelling the feces. It could also be that the connection between changing of soiled diapers and sexual stimulation during infancy eroticizes feces. Because it appears that HIV can be present in any body tissue or fluids, coprophilia is not a safe sexual activity.

Some coprophiliacs engage in coprophagia (the eating of feces), which is potentially hazardous activity due to the risks of infection, including development of diseases such as hepatitis. Even consuming one's own feces is potentially harmful because the bowel bacteria are not safe to ingest. Coprophile activities are sometimes referred to by the euphemism "hardsports," supposedly by analogy with the use of the euphemism "watersports" for urophilia. The term "brown showers" refers to the practice of defecating on a person to derive sexual pleasure.

klismaphilia Sexual arousal produced by the use of enemas.

coprophilia Sexual pleasure associated with feces.

Gender DIMENSIONS

Paraphilias and Gender Differences

Because it is hard to find accurate statistics about the incidence of paraphilias, it is also difficult to find a great deal of information about paraphilias and sex differences. We know that the majority of paraphilias occur among men.

How common are paraphilias in general? (How common are paraphilias?, 2011)

a. Most are rare.

b. Most are more common among males than females by about 20 to 1.

c. The reason for the disparity between males and females is not clear.

d. Several paraphilias are associated with aggressive behavior.

e. Most paraphilias are not considered aggressive or harmful.

Coprophilia may be expressed by constantly joking about defecation and feces, hoarding feces or soiled clothing, fecal fantasies, sexual excitement during evacuation, and, less commonly, smearing feces on walls or other objects (Coprophilia, 2014).

Urophilia

In **urophilia**, sexual pleasure is associated with urine. Similarly to coprophilia, the person may want to urinate on someone or be urinated on. As with coprophilia, there may be childhood beginnings for urophilia. For example, stimulation of the urethra during urination may become associated with pleasure, or there may have been stimulation from the changing of wet diapers. Urophilia has been referred to as "golden showers" or "water sports." Urophilia is not a safe sexual activity because HIV and other STIs can be transmitted through urine.

Some urophiliacs may enjoy swallowing urine. In contrast to coprophagia, this practice is generally considered relatively harmless, as the urine of healthy individuals is sterile. A small risk exists if disease or bacterial infection of the urethra is present. There may also be secondary effects, such as skin rashes in individuals sensitive to urine. HIV can also be spread through the urine of an infected person. In the absence of any STIs, however, urine is generally safe to drink in small quantities. The main dangers are the high salt and mineral content. The high salt content usually does not pose a problem if the urine is sufficiently diluted and not consumed in large quantities. The person whose urine will be consumed may want to drink some water (or diet soda) several hours before the act to dilute the urine. Because artificial sweeteners are excreted in urine, consuming artificial sweetener before urine play can lend a sweet taste to the urine. Drinking diet soda or other beverages containing artificial sweeteners before urine play will have

the dual effect of diluting the urine and sweetening it. If you taste sugar in your own or your partner's urine and neither of you has consumed artificial sweetener, this may be a sign of diabetes and you should see a doctor. The participants should use caution or avoid drinking urine if one or both of them are taking vitamins or mineral supplements or medication, as many of these substances are excreted in urine (Urophilia: Symptom, cause and treatment, 2014).

Treatment for Paraphilias

A number of issues surface when one considers treatment for paraphilias. For example, people with paraphilias often do not want treatment. Also, they often feel they cannot control their urges, so they cannot accept personal responsibility for their actions. However, personal responsibility is usually a prerequisite for successful behavior change. In addition, some helping professionals think it is not their responsibility to provide treatment for paraphilias—they believe it is the responsibility of the criminal justice system. In spite of these issues, it is appropriate to consider what might be done to help those with paraphilias. Possible treatments fall into three categories: (1) psychotherapy, (2) behavior therapy, and (3) pharmacological approaches (drug therapy).

Psychotherapy

Not much information is available about successful treatment of paraphilias by psychotherapy. The purpose of psychoanalysis is to discover unconscious conflicts that are believed to originate in childhood. If conflicts can be drawn to the surface and

urophilia Sexual pleasure associated with urine.

Ethical DIMENSIONS

The Ethics of Chemical Treatment for Paraphilias

Is it ethical to force paraphilic sex offenders to take hormones or tranquilizers to reduce their drives for paraphilic behaviors? Although in some cases Depo-Provera reduces the paraphilic sex drive to a level that allows the person to have a more normal sex drive, in others it causes a complete elimination of the sex drive—meaning that the individual has almost no interest in any sexual behavior.

One difficulty is that some paraphilics enjoy their behavior. Therefore, they do not want treatment because they do not view their behavior as a problem.

Some experts would argue that chemical treatment for paraphilic offenders should be required to protect other people from them. Others feel that such treatments should be required only for people who have paraphilias that violate the rights of others or harm them.

When faced with the possibility of arrest or imprisonment, paraphilic sex offenders could waive their right of informed consent and sign up for treatment just to avoid legal action. It can be difficult to balance the right of society to be protected from harm against the right of a person to avoid being given chemicals that may have undesired side effects.

resolved, the hope is that the particular behavior can be changed.

Group therapy involves breaking through the denial so commonly found in people with paraphilias by surrounding them with others who share their condition. Once they begin to admit that they have a sexual divergence, the therapist begins to address individual issues such as past sexual abuse or other problems that may have led to the sexual disorder. When these issues have been identified, individual therapy may be used to help patients get past the guilt and shame that might be associated with their particular paraphilia.

Behavior Therapy

Behavior therapy applies learning principles to help people change their behavior. Many techniques have been used to help change paraphilic behavior. For example, in systematic desensitization the therapist tries to break the link between a sexual stimulus (such as leather for a fetishist) and the inappropriate response (sexual stimulation). The client is taught to relax muscle groups so that relaxation replaces sexual arousal in response to the stimulus.

behavior therapy Applying learning principles to help people change behavior.

aversion therapy Pairing an undesirable sexual behavior with a painful response.

social training Improving a person's social skills.

orgasmic reconditioning Increasing sexual arousal to socially appropriate stimuli.

antiandrogen drugs Chemicals that reduce the sex drive by lowering the testosterone level in the bloodstream.

In **aversion therapy** the undesirable behavior (such as masturbation for a voyeur) is paired repeatedly with a negative stimulus, such as a painful (but harmless) electric shock. The objective is that negative reactions to the paraphilic behavior will develop.

In **social training** the individual is helped to improve his or her social skills. It is hoped that if the person can better relate to people, he or she will be able to develop sexual relationships that would be considered more typical.

In **orgasmic reconditioning** the goal is to increase sexual arousal by socially appropriate stimuli. For example, if the person becomes sexually aroused by masturbating, as he or she approaches orgasm, "socially appropriate imagery" such as pictures of attractive people would be used. The hope is that orgasm will then be connected with these images and not the paraphilic ones.

Drug Therapy

Although no drug can eliminate paraphilic behavior, some chemicals can sometimes be helpful in reducing the intensity of sexual drives and establishing an environment for more successful treatment using one of the other approaches. For example, Prozac, which is commonly used for treating depression, has been used to help some people reduce obsessions and compulsions. Also, **antiandrogen drugs**, chemicals that reduce the sex drive by lowering the testosterone level in the bloodstream, can reduce sexual desire and erections in males. Such a drug is Depo-Provera, which must be injected weekly to be effective. However, even Depo-Provera does not change the nature of sexual stimuli for people; it only reduces the intensity of their reactions.

The International Association for the Treatment of Sexual Offenders (IATSO; http://iatso.org) was founded in 1998 in Caracas, Venezuela. Its goals include the following (Welcome to IATSO, 2015):

- Sponsoring biennial international conferences on the treatment of sexual offenders for the dissemination of new research and treatment methods, and to provide continuing education and networking opportunities

- Promotion of international, regional and local conferences on the treatment of sexual offenders

- Updating the IATSO Standards of Care for the Treatment of Adult Sexual Offenders and the IATSO Standards of Care for the Treatment of Juvenile Sexual Offenders consistent with advances of knowledge of the treatment of sexual offenders

- Advocacy of humane, dignified, comprehensive, ethical, and effective treatment of sexual offenders throughout the world

Sexual Addiction

In 1998 President Clinton's sexual activity stirred up the debate over "sexual addiction." The idea that some people might have very strong, or even insatiable, sexual needs has been around a long time. The term **nymphomania** refers to an excessive, insatiable sexual drive in women. The same condition in men is referred to as **satyriasis**, or **Don Juanism**. Many professionals have argued about the appropriateness of these labels for years. They contend that the labels should not be used at all because judgments about how much sexual behavior is "normal" or "excessive" are subjective.

Some experts believe that sexual addiction is mainly a male abnormality caused by childhood trauma that usually requires intense psychotherapy. Many others say this is nonsense because there is no such thing as too much sexual behavior, unless it is with the wrong partner. They say that some people who have the symptoms do not experience conflict and are not really troubled by it. Still others are concerned that use of the label *sexual addiction* may help people inappropriately excuse their behavior.

Experts are not in agreement with regard to the causes of sexual addiction. Some experts blame biological factors such as mood disorders (such as bipolar disorders) (Kaplan & Krueger, 2010) or brain differences such as frontal lobe dysfunction or temporal lobe abnormalities (Chughtai et al., 2010). Other experts blame psychological factors such as negative early childhood experiences (Birchard, 2011).

Cybersex addiction has become more common in recent years.

Obviously, most people engage in various forms of sexual activity without it becoming disruptive related to other behaviors. Some experts argue that some people become addicts because of changes in the chemistry of the brain. Other experts believe that this view is not correct, and the question of whether addicts experience differences in the way their brains work is still hotly debated (Bodo, 2008).

Dodge et al. (2004) found that college students who are sexually compulsive are more likely to participate in sexual behaviors that are high risk in terms of HIV and STI infections. Bancroft and Vukadinovic (2004) reported that out-of-control sexual behavior seems to result from a variety of mechanisms. They also said that sexual addicts tend to experience increased sexual interest when they are depressed or anxious about something.

A more clinical name for sexual addiction is *hypersexual disorder*. Hypersexual disorder is characterized by recurrent and intense sexual fantasies, sexual urges, or sexual behaviors. The behavior has some of the following characteristics: (1) interferes with other goals and obligations, (2) is used as a distraction from negative moods or stressful life events, (3) is engaged in without regard for physical or emotional safety, and (4) repeated attempts to stop or limit behavior have been unsuccessful (Kafka, 2010). Other popular nonclinical terms for sexual addiction are *out-of-control sexual behavior* and *sexual compulsivity*.

---

nymphomania An excessive, insatiable sexual drive in women.

satyriasis An excessive, insatiable sexual drive in men—also called *Don Juanism*.

Did You Know . . .

Sexual Addiction Recovery Resources

Email Groups

Sex/Porn Addiction: *S-panon@ontos.usa.com*

Addiction research and treatment: *Addict-L@listserv.kent.edu*

Internet addiction support group: *listserv@netcom.com*

Open self-help discussion: *solution@sjuvm.stjohns.edu*

Resource and Recovery Sites

www.kicksexaddiction.com

www.themeadows.org

www.sexualrecovery.com

www.gentlepath.com

National Resources

Sex Addicts Anonymous (SAA)

www.sexaa.org

(713) 869-4902

PO Box 70949

Houston, TX 77270

Sex and Love Addicts Anonymous (SLAA)

www.slaafws.org

(210) 828-7900

1550 NE Loop 410, Suite 118

San Antonio, TX 78209

Sexual Compulsives Anonymous (SCA)

www.sca-recovery.org

(212) 606-3778

1-800-977-HEAL

PO Box 1585, Old Chelsea Station

New York, NY 10011

email: *info@sca-recovery.org*

Source: Data from Sex Addiction Help. Available: www.sexaddicthelp .com/Links/index.htm.

Sexual addiction can involve a wide variety of practices. They can include compulsive masturbation, multiple affairs, multiple or anonymous sexual partners and/or one-night stands, consistent use of pornography, unsafe sexual behaviors, phone or computer sex, prostitution or use of prostitutes, exhibitionism, obsessive dating through personal ads, voyeurism, sexual harassment, and molestation/ rape (Sexual addiction, 2009.) Sometimes an addict has trouble with just one unwanted behavior, sometimes with many. As in other addictions, the sexual addict experiences powerlessness over a compulsive behavior. The addict may wish to stop but repeatedly fails to do so. The consequences can be loss of relationships, difficulties with work, arrests, financial troubles, a loss of interest in matters not sexual, low self-esteem, and despair.

Herkov (2015) describes sexual addiction as a progressive intimacy disorder characterized by compulsive sexual thoughts and acts. Its negative impact on the addict and on family members increases as the disorder progresses. Over time, the addict usually must intensify the addictive behavior to get the same results. For some addicts, behavior does not progress beyond compulsive masturbation or the extensive use of pornography or phone or computer sex services. For others, addiction can involve illegal activities such as exhibitionism, child molestation, and rape. Roughly 55% of convicted sex offenders can be considered sex addicts. Approximately 71% of child molesters are sex addicts. Society has accepted

that sex offenders act not for sexual gratification, but rather out of a disturbed need for power, dominance, control or revenge, or a perverted expression of anger. The National Council on Sexual Addiction and Compulsivity defines sexual addiction as "engaging in persistent and escalating patterns of sexual behavior acted out despite increasing negative consequences to self and others."

The main way to identify any addictive behavior is to consider whether it is causing negative or unwelcome problems and yet the person continues it anyway. Sexual addicts are often unable to make and keep commitments to themselves and others about stopping or changing particular sexual behaviors over the long term, and most have problems with real intimacy.

Sex Addicts Anonymous is a group that operates very much like Alcoholics Anonymous. The group recognizes that sex addicts may act out sexually in many different ways. However, there are common elements that seem to characterize "our addiction" (*Are you a sex addict?*, 2015):

- Powerlessness over addictive sexual behavior

- Resulting unmanageability of the individual's life

- Feelings of shame, pain, and self-loathing

- Failed promises and attempts to stop acting out

- Preoccupation with sex leading to a ritual

- Progressive worsening of negative consequences.

A more recent form of sexual addiction is cybersex addiction. Typical symptoms of cybersex addiction include (1) spending increasing amounts of online time focused on sexual or romantic intrigue or involvement, (2) failed attempts to cut back on frequency of online sexual involvement, (3) online use that interferes with work and personal life, (4) secretiveness or lying about the amount of time spent on online sexual activity, and (5) a primary focus of sexual activity related to computer activity (Cybersex addiction checklist, 2014).

Most addicts live in denial of their addiction. Success in treating addiction depends on the person accepting and admitting that he or she has a problem. In many cases, like with other addictions, it takes a significant event—such as the loss of a job, the breakup of a marriage, or an arrest—to force the addict to admit his or her problem.

Even though there is no agreement about how to deal with compulsive sexual activity—if it can be done at all—organizations have been formed to help people deal with their activities if they feel there is a problem; for example, there is a 12-step program modeled after Alcoholics Anonymous called Sex and Love Addicts Anonymous. Other such groups are called Sex Addicts Anonymous, Sexaholics Anonymous, and Sexual Compulsives Anonymous.

Finally, many issues remain unresolved with regard to sexual addiction. For example, some argue over whether it is a real disease or an excuse for people to cheat and spend hours watching porn and participating in other ways to sexually stimulate themselves. If it is a disease, should insurance companies have to pay for sex addiction treatment?

Exploring the Dimensions of Human Sexuality

Varieties of sexual behaviors have been around a long time—as have opinions about them. Some of them were mentioned in historical documents centuries ago. Some of them are heard about frequently today, whereas others are rarely mentioned. Some students believe there are degrees of behaviors that might be considered "normal," but stages at which that behavior (such as exhibitionism) becomes problematic. For example, is it exhibitionistic if someone gets pleasure out of dressing in certain ways to look attractive? Is it acceptable to reveal many parts of the body, consistent with some clothing styles today? Is it problematic if someone wants to look nice most of the time? At what point might behaviors become exhibitionistic and then become problematic?

In contrast, there is little disagreement among most students that some behaviors—such as necrophilia, coprophilia, and asphyxiophilia—are problematic at almost any degree of behavior. Think about the behaviors discussed in this chapter and decide where you would place them on a "normal" to "not normal" continuum.

Biological Factors

- More men than women seem to participate in many of the alternative sexual behaviors. Are there biological differences that account for this discrepancy?
- Different people will probably respond differently to thinking about and participating in the alternative sexual behaviors discussed in this chapter.
- Not much is known about the relationship between hormones and alternative sexual behaviors.
- Do individuals participate in alternative sexual behaviors because of their biological make-up or because of learned behavior?
- Drugs, alcohol, and some aphrodisiacs may make it more or less likely that some people will participate in alternative sexual behaviors.

Sociocultural Factors

- People from different cultures may view some of the alternative sexual behavior differently.
- How do laws relate to alternative sexual behaviors? Should any of them be changed?
- As long as all participants legally consent, should there be laws against alternative sexual behaviors?
- Is there a "double standard" related to which alternative sexual behaviors would be more acceptable for women or men?
- There is a need for much more research about alternative behaviors.

Psychological Factors

- It is often quite difficult to treat or "cure" people who consistently participate in some of the alternative sexual behaviors.
- Experts continue to argue about whether there is such a thing as "sex addiction."
- Are the various alternative sexual behaviors learned or do some people naturally participate in them?
- What do we learn from other people related to alternative sexual behaviors?
- Our self-concept may influence whether we want to participate in any alternative sexual behaviors, and so will the self-concept of our partner.

Summary

- Because many sexual behaviors vary in degree, it is not surprising that many of us recognize some amount of atypical behaviors or feelings in ourselves.

- There is not a great deal known about atypical sexual behaviors.

- The most common paraphilias are exhibitionism, voyeurism, obscene communication, masochism and sadism, transvestism, and fetishism.

- Other paraphilias include bestiality, frottage, necrophilia, troilism, asphyxiophilia, klismaphilia, coprophilia, and urophilia.

- Possible treatments for paraphilias fall into three categories: psychotherapy, behavior therapy, and drug therapy.

- Some people have very strong, or even insatiable, sexual needs and may be sex addicts. Most treatment programs for sexual addiction resemble treatment programs for people addicted to other behaviors.

Discussion Questions

1. Describe how sexual feelings or behaviors vary from common to atypical along a continuum.

2. What are the most common forms of paraphilia? Describe the type of person who might practice them.

3. What are the less common forms of paraphilia? Discuss why someone would practice them.

4. Describe the major types of treatment programs for paraphilias, including the ways they work and their effectiveness.

5. Is "sexual addiction" a true disorder? Explain your answer.

Application Questions

Reread the chapter-opening story and answer the following questions:

1. In spite of his well-publicized sexual behavior, the sportscaster's fiancée married him. Would you have advised her to go through with the wedding? Explain your answer.

2. Discuss the issues of safer sex surrounding the sexual acts engaged in by the sportscaster.

3. In addition to causing immense embarrassment, the sportscaster's sexual habits cost him his job (and probably some friends as well). What might have caused him to take such risks?

Which therapies are available to help him with his atypical behaviors?

Critical Thinking Questions

1. Look over the American Psychiatric Association's definitions for the varied paraphilias supplied throughout the chapter. What are the common elements? On the basis of that information, how would you define "atypical sexual behavior"?

2. Given that the pornography industry takes in billions of dollars each year, are we a nation of voyeurs? What differentiates a diagnosed voyeur from someone who views porn? Explain your answers.

Critical Thinking Case

Bill and Anne, college juniors, were in a monogamous relationship for about 5 months when Bill said that he wanted to add some "variety" to their sex life. Anne's immediate reaction was to feel that she was not giving Bill enough sexual satisfaction, so she did not respond to his suggestion. As much as she loved Bill, she felt unsure about his request for variety.

After he broached the subject several more times, she finally asked him what he wanted. He said that a former girlfriend had enjoyed having another girl join them from time to time. Anne was initially aghast at the idea of including a third person, especially a girl. But a few months later, Anne and a female friend had a brief sexual encounter after drinking heavily. Anne did not enjoy it. When she told Bill what had happened, he reacted sharply: What was she doing with another sexual partner?

Why did Bill react as he did? What did Bill really want from the encounter—another girl for his girlfriend or a threesome for himself? Why was it important for him to communicate correctly what he wanted?

You want something your partner does not want. How do you approach it? How do you make sure you are comfortable?

Exploring Personal Dimensions

Respond about only your sexual activity. If you do not participate in any sexual activity, skip this assessment. Check the following items that apply to you.

_____ 1. I tell my partner what feels good.

_____ 2. I tell my partner what hurts, if anything.

_____ 3. I avoid frequent sexual encounters because I do not like them.

_____ 4. I let myself just go with my feelings and behave the way I want to act during sexual encounters.

_____ 5. My partner and I have talked about and resolved how often to have sexual activity.

_____ 6. Sexual activity is a problem for me and my partner.

_____ 7. I have told my partner what I want during sexual activity.

_____ 8. My partner and I enjoy holding hands, kissing, and just talking as much as we do having sexual activity.

_____ 9. It is important that each time we express love or go on a date that it culminate in sexual intercourse to be a really meaningful experience.

Scoring

Give yourself the following points for the items you check, and total your score.

1.	2	4.	2	7.	2
2.	2	5.	2	8.	2
3.	–2	6.	–2	9.	–2

Interpretation

This exercise indicates whether you have healthy communication in your sexual relationship. Interpret your score as follows:

6–10	=	Your communication is healthy.
0–5	=	Your communication is moderately healthy.
–1 – –6	=	You need to improve your communication skills.

Source: Bruess, C., & Richardson, G. *Decisions for health.* Madison, WI: Brown & Benchmark, 1995.

Suggested Readings

Cloud, J. The truth about sex addiction. *Time, 177,* no. 8 (February 28, 2011), 42–50.

Kaplan, M. S., & Krueger, R. B. Diagnosis, assessment, and treatment of hypersexuality. *Journal of Sex Research, 47, 2–3* (March 2010), 181–198.

Paraphilias. Encyclopedia of Mental Disorders, 2015. Available: http://www.minddisorders.com /Ob-Ps/Paraphilias.html.

Paraphilias. *MedicineNet.com,* 2015. Available: http:// www.medicinenet.com/paraphilia/article.htm.

Paraphilias. Sexual Conditions Health Center. *WebMD,* 2015. Available: http://www.webmd .com/sexual-conditions/guide/paraphilias -overview.

Sagarin, B. The surprising psychology of BDSM. *Psychology Today,* 2015. Available: https://www .psychologytoday.com/blog/the-wide-wide -world-psychology/201502/the-surprising -psychology-bdsm.

Sexual Addiction and Compulsion: The Journal of Treatment and Prevention. Available: http:// www.tandfonline.com/toc/usac20/current# .VNync_nF9pt.

Web Resources

BDSM Backroom
www.bcwsd.com/backroom

Contains information about bondage, dominance, sadism, and masochism for those who are curious about what BDSM is and want to learn more about it.

Society for the Scientific Study of Sexuality: What Sexual Scientists Know About Compulsive Sexual Behavior
www.sexscience.org/dashboard/articleImages/SSSS-CompulsiveSexualBehavior.pdf

Summarizes scientific information about compulsive sexual behavior.

The Society of Janus
www.soj.org

The Society of Janus is a support and educational group for people interested in learning about BDSM. It emphasizes safe, consensual, and nonexploitative activities.

Discovery Health: Paraphilia
http://health.howstuffworks.com/sexual-health /sexuality/paraphilia-dictionary.htm

Contains information about many forms of atypical sexual behavior.

Medicine.Net.com
http://www.medicinenet.com/paraphilia/article.htm

Gives facts about paraphilias related to causes and risk factors, symptoms, treatment, prognosis, and prevention.

References

American Psychiatric Association. *Diagnostic and statistical manual of mental disorders.* Washington, DC: Author, 2005.

Are you a sex addict? Sex Addicts Anonymous, 2015. Available: http://saa-recovery.org/IsSAAForYou/AreYouASexAddict/.

Bancroft, J., & Vukadinovic, Z. Sexual addiction, sexual compulsivity, sexual impulsivity, or what? Toward a theoretical model. *Journal of Sex Research, 42, 3* (Aug. 2004), 225–234.

Baumeister, R. F. The enigmatic appeal of sexual masochism: Why people desire pain, bondage, and humiliation in sex. *Journal of Social and Clinical Psychology, 16, 2* (1997), 133–150.

Beetz, A. M. Bestiality/zoophilia: A scarcely investigated phenomenon between crime, paraphilia, and love. *Journal of Forensic Psychology Practice, 4, 2* (2004), 1–36.

Birchard, T. Sexual addiction and paraphilias. *Sexual Addiction and Compulsivity: The Journal of Treatment and Prevention, 18, 3* (2011), 157–187.

Bodo, C. Addicted to love. National Sexuality Resource Center, 2008. Available: http://nsrc.sfsu.edu/print/2835.

Chughtai, B., Sciullo, D., Khan, S. A., Rehman, H., Mohan, E., & Rehman, J. Etiology, diagnosis and management of hypersexuality: A review. *Internet Journal of Urology, 6,* no. 2 (2010). Available: http://www.ispub.com/journal/the-internet-journal-of-urology/volume-6-number-2/etiology-diagnosis-amp-management-of-hypersexuality-a-review.html.

Coleman, E. What sexual scientists know …: About compulsive sexual behavior. *Society for the Scientific Study of Sexuality* (2005). Available: http://www.sexscience.org.

Coprophilia. *Depression-guide.com,* 2014. Available: http://www.depression-guide.com/coprophilia.htm.

Cyber sex addiction checklist. Counseling Solutions, 2014. Available: http://www.marriagecounseling.org/cyber-sex-addiction-checklist/.

Definition of exhibitionism. *MedicineNet,* 2014. Available: http://www.medicinenet.com/script/main/art.asp?articlekey=46421.

Discovery Health. Paraphilia 2005. Available: http://health.discovery.com/centers/sex/sexpedia/paraphilia_print.html.

Dodge, B., Reece, M., Cole, S. L., & Sandfort, T. G. Sexual compulsivity among heterosexual college students. *Journal of Sex Research, 41, 4* (November 2004), 343–350.

Exhibitionism. Encyclopedia of Mental Disorders, 2011. Available: http://www.minddisorders.com/Del-Fi/Exhibitionism.html.

Exhibitionism. Psychology Today's Conditions Center (2005). Available: http://cms.psychologytoday.com/conditions/index.php?term=exhibitionism&print=1.

Exhibitionism. *Psychology Today,* 2015. Available: https://www.psychologytoday.com/conditions/exhibitionism.

Fetishism. Discovery Health, 2005. Available: http://health.discovery.com/centers/sex/sexpedia/fetishism_print.html

Fetishism. *Psychology Today,* 2015. Available: https://www.psychologytoday.com/conditions/fetishism.

Griffiths, M. D. Behind enema lines. *Psychology Today,* March 5, 2014a. Available: https://www.psychologytoday.com/blog/in-excess/201403/behind-enema-lines.

Griffiths, M. D. Survival of the fetish: A brief overview of bizarre sexual behaviors. *Psychology Today,* 2014b. Available: https://www.psychologytoday.com/blog/in-excess/201401/survival-the-fetish.

Herkov, M. What is sexual addiction? *PsychCentral,* 2015. Available: http://psychcentral.com/lib/what-is-sexual-addiction/000748.

How common are paraphilias? WebMD, 2011. Available: http://www.webmd.com/sexual-conditions/paraphilias?page=3.

Hypoxyphilia/auto-erotic asphyxia. PsychDirect, 2005. Available: http://www.psychdirect.com/forensic/Criminology/para/aea.htm.

Janus, S., & Janus, C. *The Janus report on sexual behavior.* New York: Wiley, 1993.

Jenkins, A. P. When self-pleasuring becomes self-destruction: Autoerotic asphyxiation paraphilia. *International Electronic Journal of Health Education, 3, 3* (2000), 208–216.

Kafka, M. P. Hypersexual disorder: A proposed diagnosis for DSM-V. *Archives of Sexual Behavior, 39* (2010), 377–400.

Kaplan, M. S., & Krueger, R. B. Diagnosis, assessment, and treatment of hypersexuality. *Journal of Sex Research, 47* (2010), 181–198.

Kinsey, A. C., Pomeroy, W. B., & Martin, C. E. *Sexual behavior in the human female.* Philadelphia: Saunders, 1953.

Kinsey, A. C., Pomeroy, W. B., & Martin, C. E. *Sexual behavior in the human male.* Philadelphia: Saunders, 1948.

Litman, R. E. Bondage and sadomasochism, in *Sexual dynamics of anti-social behavior,* 2nd ed., Schlesinger, L. B. & Revitch, E., eds. Springfield, IL: Charles C. Thomas, 1997.

Masochism. University of Iowa Health Care, 2001. Available: www.uihealthcare.com/topics/mentalemotionalhealth/ment3155.html.

Paraphilias. *MedicineNet.com,* 2009. Available: http://www.medicinenet.com/paraphilia/article.htm.

Paraphilias. *Psychology Today's Conditions Center,* 2014. Available: https://www.psychologytoday.com/conditions/paraphilias.

Person, E. S., Terestman, N., Myers, W. A., & Goldberg, E. L. Gender differences in sexual behaviors and fantasies in a college population. *Journal of Sex and Marital Therapy, 15, 3* (1989), 187–214.

Sadism. University of Iowa Health Care, 2001. Available: http://www.uihealthcare.com/topics/mentalemotionalhealth/ment3168.html.

Sexual masochism. *Psychology Today,* 2015. Available: https://www.psychologytoday.com/conditions/sexual-masochism.

Spaise, T. L. Necrophilia and SM: The deviant side of *Buffy the Vampire Slayer. Journal of Popular Culture, 38, 4* (May 2005), 744–762.

Transvestic fetishism. *PsychDirect,* 2005. Available: http://www.psychdirect.com/forensic/Criminology/para/transfetishism.htm.

Transvestism. University of Iowa Health Care, 2001. Available: http://www.uihealthcare.com/topics/mentalemotionalhealth/ment3174.html.

United States Code Annotated Title 47. U.S. Department of Justice (2014). Available: uscode.house.gov.

Urophilia: Symptom, cause and treatment. *Depression-guide.com,* 2014. Available: http://www.depression-guide.com/urophilia.htm.

Voyeurism. Encyclopedia of Mental Disorders, 2011. Available: http://www.minddisorders.com/Py-Z/Voyeurism.html.

CHAPTER 17

Forcible Sexual Behaviors

© Gayvoronskaya Yana/Shutterstock

FEATURES

Multicultural Dimensions
Sexual Violence

Ethical Dimensions
Should the Media Reveal the Names of Rape Survivors?

Multicultural Dimensions
Sexual Contact in Various Cultures

Global Dimensions
Examples of Child Sexual Abuse Attitudes in Other Countries

Communication Dimensions
Helping Survivors of Rape and Sexual Abuse

Global Dimensions
The Countries That Give the Most Severe Punishments for Rape

Ethical Dimensions
Is It Ethical to Publicly Identify Sexual Offenders?

Multicultural Dimensions
Examples of Sexual Violence in Other Countries

Gender Dimensions
Same-Gender Sexual Harassment

CHAPTER OBJECTIVES

1 Differentiate among rape, statutory rape, stranger rape, and date (acquaintance) rape. Discuss what makes someone rape. Discuss the myths surrounding rape.

2 Discuss pedophilia, including the profile of the pedophiliac, incidence and effects of pedophilia, and prevention.

3 Describe the incidence of incest and the typical effects on incest victims.

4 Summarize important information about violence in marriage, including marital rape and domestic abuse.

5 Discuss sexual harassment in the workplace, in schools, on campus, and in the military, and indicate what can be done to prevent and deal with it.

INTRODUCTION

*A*fter a discussion about forcible sexual behavior in my sexuality class, a female student who was in her late 20s asked to go to my office to talk for a few minutes. When we got there, she said that she had found the information and the discussion on forcible sexual behavior interesting and enlightening. She also said she was feeling personally troubled because it reminded her of something that had happened to her. She then told me about it.

She remembered when she was 15 years old. She said she was a typical middle-class high school girl. Although her parents and her teachers did not say a lot about sexuality, she had heard quite a bit about rape on TV and seen stories about it in magazines, newspapers and on the Internet. Her parents, as had many of her friends, warned her about being careful and about not trusting strangers. She dated Ed, a neighbor who lived just a block away. Ed's parents and her parents sometimes got together socially, and they had been friends for at least 10 years. Ed's parents had always been friendly to her too, and she probably saw them at least two or three times each week.

Ed was 2 years older and a star basketball player. He was an excellent student and considered a leader and one of the most popular boys at school. She remembered that he had always seemed to be one of the best athletes as they were growing up. After a few dates, they had started to become intimate. She enjoyed the closeness with him and found him very attractive. She had some tears in her eyes when she said that on one date, after an exciting basketball game, he had intercourse with her while she was crying and asking him not to do it. Although he was a little forceful, he did not raise his voice and he did not hit her. He just paid no attention to what she was saying.

At the time she said she did not realize it was rape. She asked him why he was doing this to her, but he did not answer. Afterward she did not want to date him anymore, and her parents wondered why. Her friends thought she was crazy not to want to go out with him. She said she had not told anyone about this before, but that she just had to get it out. When we talked about forcible sexual behavior in class, all the memories rushed back to her.

Many readers of this chapter are probably survivors of forcible sexual behavior—whether it was rape, child sexual abuse, sexual harassment, or another form of forcible sexual behavior. Sometimes it can be difficult and painful to think about these topics. However, most people, such as the student in our story, find it helpful to learn more about such topics and to deal more directly with their feelings about them.

Many sexual behaviors exist and various factors contribute to these behaviors. Most often people voluntarily choose a particular behavior, but some sexual behaviors are not voluntary. In this chapter we focus on rape and child sexual abuse because of their seriousness. By no means, however, are these the only forcible sexual behaviors. Other representative forcible sexual behaviors are also considered. A characteristic of all these behaviors is that we know very little about them because of their obvious secretive and private nature. Although knowledge about forcible sexual behavior has rapidly increased, a great need for continued study and research is evident.

■ Sexual Violence

Sexual violence is a serious problem that affects millions of people each year. The victims of sexual violence are at increased risk of being abused again. Sexual violence perpetrators are also at increased risk of perpetrating again. Statistics about sexual violence are given throughout this chapter. It is important to remember, however, that statistics about sexual violence vary due to differences in definition and how data are collected. Such data usually come from police, clinical settings, nongovernmental organizations, and survey research.

For more than 30 years, researchers have noted that sexual violence is a relatively common experience. For example, at least 20% of all females in the United States will be victims of sexual violence during their lives. It is a life-altering experience for many who experience sexual violence. The effects are often experienced long after the event, with many psychological, physical, and behavioral consequences such as STIs,

chronic pain disorders and other physical ailments, as well as anxiety, depression, substance use, sexual problems, and interpersonal difficulties being documented in survivors of sexual violence. Even though much is known, there is a need for continued work related to research, public policy, providing treatment and prevention services, and educating the public about sexual violence. Knowing important facts will help people better understand and deal with sexual violence.

Sexual assault and abuse is any nonconsensual sexual activity, including:

- Inappropriate touching
- Vaginal, anal, or oral penetration
- Sexual intercourse after you say no
- Rape
- Attempted rape
- Child molestation

Sexual assault can be verbal, visual, or anything that forces a person to join in unwanted sexual contact or attention.

Each year the American College Health Association surveys more than 100,000 college students about a variety of behaviors related to their health. In a recent year, 3.3% of males and 8.9% of females were sexually touched against their will. seven-tenths of 1 percent of males and 3.9% of females said sexual penetration (vaginal, oral, or anal) was attempted against their will. Seven-tenths of 1 percent of males and 2.5% of females said they were sexually penetrated (vaginal, oral, or anal) without their consent. Of the males, 6.3% reported an emotionally abusive intimate relationship, as did 10.5% of the females. A sexually abusive intimate relationship was reported by 1.1% of the males and 2.1% of the females (American College Health Association, 2014).

As can be seen from these numbers, both males and females can be victims of sexual violence. It is true that females are victims far more often than males, and males are perpetrators of sexual violence much more often than females. Nevertheless, it is estimated that one in 6 boys and one in 4 girls will experience a sexual assault before the age of 18. One in 5 women and one in 71 men will be raped at some point in their lives. A majority of women (79.6%) who report being raped at some point in their life experienced their first rape before the age of 25, and 42.2 % experienced their first completed rape before the age of 18. More than 25% of male victims in a national sample reported their first rape occurred when they were 10 years of age or younger. Rape is far more extensive than reported in official statistics, and the majority of rapists are never apprehended (*Understanding sexual violence: Tips for parents and caregivers of children*, 2015). As can be seen, adult men are also victims of sexual violence. The experience of sexual assault can be very confusing for men because our society and culture often associate sexual assault only with women.

In 2014, the Centers for Disease Control and Prevention (CDC) provided additional information about sexual violence. About 1 in 5 men (6.7%) reported they were made to penetrate someone else during their lifetime. An estimated 12.5% of women and 5.8% of men reported sexual coercion in their lifetime (i.e., unwanted sexual penetration after being pressured in a nonphysical way). More than one-fourth of women (27.3%) and about 1 in 9 men (10.8%) experienced some form of unwanted sexual contact in their lifetime, and nearly one-third of women (32.1%) and nearly one in 8 men (13.3%) experienced some type of noncontact unwanted sexual experience in their lifetime (Basile et al., 2014).

It has also been found that rape and sexual violence often have negative health-related repercussions,

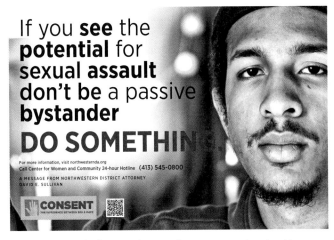

What can people do to make sure they are never involved in forced sexual activity?

such as higher incidences of asthma, irritable bowel syndrome, and diabetes in victims. Victims of sexual violence were also more likely to report symptoms of post-traumatic stress disorder, frequent headaches, chronic pain, and difficulty sleeping.

It is very difficult to obtain truthful and accurate rape statistics, but another source can help illustrate the extent of the problem. The U.S. Bureau of Justice reported in 2014 that, on average, 89,000 rapes are reported in the United States annually. Sixteen percent of women and 3% of men experienced an attempted or completed rape. Since 1993, the rape rate has declined 60%. It is estimated that 60% of rapes and 95% of college rapes are never reported to the authorities. Both survivor and perpetrator had been drinking in 47% of the rapes. Thirty-eight percent of the perpetrators were a friend or acquaintance, 28% were an "intimate," 26% were strangers, and 7% were a relative. Approximately 31% of rapes occurred at the perpetrator's home, and 27% occurred at the survivor's home. The United States has a rape rate of 28.6 per 100,000 population, which places it about sixth in the world. The highest rape rate in the world is 91.6 per 100,000 population in the small South African country of Lesotho, and the lowest rate—0.1 per 100,000 population—is in Egypt (*Rape statistics*, 2014).

Rape

Rape is a forcible act. Legal definitions of rape and law enforcement procedures for handling rape cases are changing, and they differ from state to state. However, a practical definition of **rape** is "forcible sexual

rape Forcible sexual intercourse with a person who does not give consent.

intercourse." This can include forced oral sexual activity, penile–vaginal sexual activity, and anal sexual activity. Penetration may be made by a body part or an object. If a person is forced to do any of these things when he or she does not want to, that is rape. In 2012 the U.S. Attorney General announced changes to the Uniform Crime Report's definition of rape (Siegelbaum, 2012). The Justice Department stated that the new definition would better reflect state criminal codes and focus on the various forms of sexual penetration understood to be rape. It was also felt that these long-overdue updates to the definition of rape would also help ensure justice for those whose lives have been devastated by sexual violence. The Uniform Crime Report's previous definition of rape, first adopted in 1929, was limited only to forcible penetration of a vagina. The new definition of rape is: "The penetration, no matter how slight, of the vagina or anus with any body part or object, or oral penetration by a sex organ of another person, without the consent of the victim." The revised definition includes "any gender of victim or perpetrator, and includes instances in which the victim is incapable of giving consent because of temporary or permanent mental or physical incapacity, including due to the influence of drugs or alcohol or because of age."

The legal definition of penetration has also been clarified. Sexual penetration crimes include the penetration of the vagina, anus, or mouth by the penis or other body part, and also include the penetration of the vagina, anus, or, in rare cases, the mouth by an object. Vaginal penetration occurs, under the law, when the penis, other body part, or object enters the vulva or between the labia majora, which is the outermost part of the female genital organ. Anal penetration occurs, under the law, when the penis, other body part, or object enters the anal opening. Oral penetration occurs when the penis, other body part, or other object enters the lips of a victim's mouth. If penetration is not proved beyond a reasonable doubt, the accused will probably be acquitted or convicted of a less serious offense (Long et al., 2015). Note that these definitions are the same regardless of the sex (male or female) of the individuals involved in the activity.

Rape victims may be forced through threats or physical means. In about 8 out of 10 rapes, no weapon is used other than physical force. Anyone may be a victim of rape: women, men, or children, straight or gay (Was I raped?, 2011).

Sexual assault is unwanted sexual contact that stops short of rape or attempted rape. This includes sexual touching and fondling. This terminology can be confusing because some states use this term interchangeably with rape.

Some people wonder how to determine if what happened was rape. There are three main considerations in judging whether a sexual act is consensual (that is, both people are old enough to consent, have the capacity to consent, and agreed to the sexual contact) or it is a crime. Laws vary from state to state, but here are some examples related to these three considerations (Was I raped?, 2011).

Are the participants old enough to consent? Each state has an "age of consent" that varies from age 14 to 18. Commonly it is 16 or 18. It might also vary according to the age difference between the participants. It is not enough to assume that someone is old enough to legally participate. It is up to both participants to be sure that each is old enough.

Do both people have the capacity to consent? States also define who has the mental and legal capacity to consent. Those with diminished capacity, such as people with disabilities, some elderly people, and those who have been drugged or unconscious, may not have the legal ability to agree to have sexual activity.

Did both participants agree to take part? Using physical force or threats means that it is rape. Also, it does not matter if you think your partner means yes, or if you have already started intimate behavior, "no" means "stop." If you proceed despite your partner's expressed instruction to stop, you have not only violated basic codes of morality and decency, you may have also committed a crime.

Within the category of rape, there are several types. For example, **statutory rape** is intercourse with a person who is younger than the age of consent (ranging from 14 to 18 years from state to state). Even with consent, statutory rape is considered to have occurred if one of the participants is not of legal age. **Stranger rape** is rape of a person by an unknown assailant. If a rape is committed by someone known to the victim, it is **acquaintance rape**, or **date rape**, both of which are discussed later in this chapter.

Rape Myths

In spite of the increased attention given to the topic of rape in recent years, rape myths remain prevalent (see Myth vs. Fact on page 579). It is important for people to know the facts about rape to help reduce some related problems. For example, some of the more prevalent rape myths include that women lead men on and therefore deserve to be raped, people

sexual assault Unwanted sexual contact that stops short of rape or attempted rape.

statutory rape Intercourse with a person younger than the legal age of consent.

stranger rape Rape of a person by an unknown person.

acquaintance rape Rape by a friend, acquaintance, or date; also known as *date rape*.

Did You Know . . .

Rape as a Weapon of War

Organized rape has been an integral aspect of war for a long time. In war rape, a male soldier attacks a civilian woman and does this indirectly with the aim of holding or taking a territory. The main purpose is to inflict trauma and through this to destroy family ties and group solidarity within the enemy camp. Rape is the mark of sovereignty stamped directly on the body. Through war rape, something is introduced within the woman's body (sperm or forced pregnancy), transforming her into someone who is rejected by the family, excluded by the community, and often the object of self-hate, sometimes to the point of suicide. The penetration of the woman's body works as a metaphor for the penetration

of enemy lines. Warring groups have used rape as a weapon because it destroys communities. You punish the men, and you punish the women, doing it in front of the men (*Rape: Weapon of war*, 2015).

Rape has also been used as a weapon of war against men. Some men have been abducted by combatants, held for a long time, and repeatedly raped. Armed combatants have also forced men to have sexual activity with family members, objects, or even the ground. When these men returned to their communities, they faced a wide variety of psychosocial challenges, including stigmatization, as did their families (*Rape as a weapon of war against men*, 2015).

often make false accusations of rape, no person can be raped against his or her will, and most rapists are strangers. *All of these statements are false!* We know that men tend to believe rape myths more than women, that those who believe rape myths are more likely to assign blame to the victim, and that those who believe rape myths are more tolerant of the rapist and less tolerant of the victims (Notice to readers: Sexual Assault Awareness Month, 2005).

Society and Rape

Some people have wondered whether particular characteristics of a given society help promote rape. Even after many years of research, we don't have a definitive answer to this question. The United States has the highest rape rate among Western countries, but the reasons for this are not clear. Some people feel that the reasons may relate to the relative roles of males and females, the presence of pornography that endorses and legitimizes rape, and the fact that rape is a crime of violence in an already violent society. Others feel that these characteristics have nothing to do with the issue.

Rape is one of the most underreported crimes. This makes it difficult to accurately count the number of cases. Some researchers believe that as many as 84% of victims do not report sexual assault to the police. A primary reason given for the underreporting is cultural norms that stigmatize and blame victims for their assaults (Notice to readers: Sexual Assault Awareness Month, 2005).

Victims of rape are generally viewed more sympathetically by females than by males, and by whites more than by African Americans. However, the effect

of race disappears when socioeconomic variables are controlled. Younger people and those with higher education levels are also more likely to view sexual assault victims more sympathetically (Nagel et al., 2005).

Although experts agree that statistics regarding rape and other sexual assault are not totally accurate because many cases are not reported, it is important to consider some statistics to get a clearer view of the overall situation. For example, 15% of sexual assault and rape victims are younger than age 12, 44% are younger than 18, and 80% are younger than 30. One out of every 6 American women has been the victim of an attempted or completed rape, which is a total of 17.7 million women. One out of every 6 American women has been the victim of an attempted rape in her lifetime (14.8% completed rape; 2.8 % attempted rape), and about 3% of men have also experienced an attempted or completed rape. Each year there are about 213,000 victims of sexual assault, which is about one every 2 minutes. Sixty percent are not reported to the police, and 15 of 16 rapists will never spend a day in jail. Fortunately, the incidence of sexual assault has fallen more than 60% in recent years. Victims of sexual assault are 3 times more likely to suffer from depression, 6 times more likely to suffer from post-traumatic stress disorder, 13 times more likely to abuse alcohol, 26 times more likely to abuse drugs, and 4 times more likely to contemplate suicide (Statistics, 2011).

Evidence based on almost 300,000 sexual assaults showed that the modal age of victims was 15 years, regardless of the age of the offender, the gender of the offender, or the gender of the victim. It seems that adolescents have the highest risk of victimization because of their sexual attractiveness, vulnerability, and exposure to motivated offenders. The sexual attractiveness of young people also has implications for the age of offenders. Older men have much higher rates of sexual assault than physical assault. In addition, gay men are at least as likely as heterosexual men to commit sexual assault (Felson & Cundiff, 2014).

Although sexual assault against women has received increasing attention over the past decades, the sexual assault of the elderly has not been well addressed. Print media and the Internet regularly report on these cases and the crises and trauma that follow for the victim and their families. Elderly victims of sexual violence represent a vulnerable and poorly understood population. They may be sexually assaulted in their homes or communities, in an assisted living facility, or in a nursing home environment. Offenders can be strangers, domestic partners, family members, nursing home residents, or caregivers. There is a need for education about sexual abuse of the elderly.

Apparently, steps need to be taken to reduce the cultural acceptance of violence and to restructure male and female sex roles to specify equality, warmth, and supportiveness. In the past, male dominance, toughness, and violence have often been emphasized.

A restructuring of the relationships between sexes might reduce the high incidence of rape in American society. Steps to reduce your personal risk of sexual assault are found in Table 17.1.

The Rapist

The topics of rape and rapists are hot-button issues in American society. Some theorists argue that rape is an act of uncontrolled passion or the result of a lack of sexual partners; others suggest that it is an extreme expression of male power and violence. For others, rape is a biologically driven phenomenon whereby men forcefully try to maximize the number of women with whom they procreate.

Most rapists rape to be aggressive, to wield their power, or to degrade the victim. In most instances their motivations and satisfactions are not sexual. In fact, it is unlikely that they achieve any sexual satisfaction from the act of rape.

Many experts have developed theories about why people commit rape. For example, some believe that rape occurs to enhance the offender's sense of masculinity and power, while others believe that the rapist is angry toward women or men and wants

TABLE 17.1

How Can I Protect Myself from Being Sexually Assaulted?

There are things you can do to reduce your chances of being sexually assaulted. Here are some tips from the National Crime Prevention Council (www.ncpc.org):

- Be aware of your surroundings—who's out there and what's going on.
- Walk with confidence. The more confident you look, the stronger you appear.
- Don't let drugs or alcohol cloud your judgment.
- Be assertive—don't let anyone violate your space.
- Trust your instincts. If you feel uncomfortable in your surroundings, leave.
- Don't prop open self-locking doors.
- Lock your doors and your windows, even if you leave for just a few minutes.
- Watch your keys. Don't lend them. Don't leave them. Don't lose them. And don't put your name and address on the key ring.
- Watch out for unwanted visitors. Know who's on the other side of the door before you open it.
- Be wary of isolated spots, like underground garages, offices after business hours, and apartment laundry rooms.
- Avoid walking or jogging alone, especially at night. Vary your route. Stay in well-traveled, well-lit areas.
- Have your key ready to use before you reach the door—home, car, or work.
- Park in well-lit areas and lock the car, even if you'll be gone only a few minutes.
- Drive on well-traveled streets, with doors and windows locked.
- Never hitchhike or pick up a hitchhiker.
- Keep your car in good shape with plenty of gas in the tank.
- In case of car trouble, call for help on your cellular phone. If you don't have a phone, put the hood up, lock the doors, and put a banner in the rear mirror that says, "Help. Call police."

to hurt, humiliate, or degrade someone. Still others believe that sadistic rapists may be sexually aroused in response to assault and violence, or that, for some rapists, sexual offenses may be only one component of an extensive criminal history.

It is also possible that the reasons for a rape might vary depending on the situation. For example, perhaps with separated couples, the rape might be used to punish the victim. Or, in a dating situation, the rape might occur as part of a feeling of conquest. The reason an individual commits rape can be difficult to determine in each particular instance.

Rapists can be classified into different types (*Types of rapists*, 2015). Sometimes only four classifications are used (the first four listed below), but others are often mentioned (such as the last two listed below).

The power-assertive rapist is the most common type (about 44%). This rapist will claim to have a weapon, but will use it only to ensure the victim's cooperation. The motivation seems to be domination and control of the victim. The anger-retaliation rapist is different because he or she is out to punish someone. Because of his or her hate, this type of rapist will often injure the victim to the point where the victim needs medical treatment. Approximately 30% of rapes fall into this category. Anger might also be expressed as a way to humiliate victims and put them in their place.

The power-reassurance (or opportunity) rapist takes advantage of an opportunity to commit a rape. This is usually done in conjunction with another crime such as robbery or kidnapping. The motivation seems to be reassurance of the rapist's personal status and abilities.

The anger-excitement (or sadistic) rapist is the most dangerous type. These perpetrators want the victim to be hurt. They want to live out personal fantasies on an unwilling victim. The victim is often killed. Fortunately, only 5% of rapists are in this category.

The other two types are juvenile sex offenders and women offenders. Juvenile sex offenders have problems with authority such as school authorities and police. In turn, they seek to take their anger out on or punish victims. This type of crime seems to be on the rise. Women can be both perpetrators and accomplices, luring unsuspecting victims into traps to be raped by others. There is an overlap of characteristics among all six types of rapists, making the picture very complex.

Rapists commonly give excuses for their behavior. Some justify their actions in various ways. Others point out that sexual assault is not their fault because it is beyond their control. Some excuse their behavior because of the presence of alcohol or drugs. Still others feel their behavior was appropriate in the situation. Finally, some feel that their victims "got what they deserved."

There are three categories of stranger rape (*Stranger rape*, 2012). The first is blitz sexual assault, where the perpetrator rapidly and brutally assaults the victim with no prior contact. Blitz assaults usually occur at night in a public place. The second is contact sexual assault, where the suspect contacts the victim and tries to gain her or his trust and confidence before the assault. Contact perpetrators pick their victims in bars, lure them into their cars, or otherwise try to coerce them into a situation of sexual

 Did You Know . . .

What should you do if you've been sexually assaulted? Take these steps right away:

- Get away from the attacker to a safe place as fast as you can. Then call 911 or the police.
- Call a friend or family member you trust. You can also call a crisis center or hotline to talk with a counselor—for example, the National Sexual Assault Hotline at 800-656-HOPE (4673) or the National Domestic Violence Hotline at 800-799-SAFE (7233). It is important to get help from a trusted professional.
- Do not wash, comb, or clean any part of your body. Do not change clothes if possible, so the hospital staff can collect evidence. Do not touch or change anything at the scene of the assault.

- Go to the nearest hospital emergency room as soon as possible. You need to be examined, treated for any injuries, and screened for possible STIs or pregnancy.
- You or the hospital staff can call the police from the emergency room to file a report.
- Ask the hospital staff about possible support groups you can attend right away.

How can you help someone who has been sexually assaulted? Listen and offer comfort. Go with her or him to the police, the hospital, or counseling. Reinforce the message that she or he is not at fault and that it is natural to feel angry and ashamed.

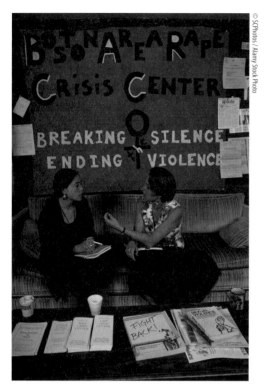

Today most communities have services available to help anyone who has been sexually attacked or abused.

Most rapists rape to demonstrate power and not to obtain sexual satisfaction.

assault. The third is home-invasion assault, where a stranger breaks into the victim's home to commit the assault.

As already indicated, in most cases the rapist isn't a stranger. In addition, more than 50% of rapes and sexual assaults occur in the victim's home or within a mile of their home (The offenders, 2012).

Date Rape

Date rape, or acquaintance rape, is much more common than most people realize, although because of its nature gathering reliable data on this topic is difficult. It is suspected that some incidents of date rape might be a result of poor communication, because many people still have a difficult time talking about sexuality. At any rate, it might help those dating to realize the following: Spending money on a date does not justify expecting sexual favors; a person who participates in other forms of sexual behavior does not necessarily find intercourse acceptable; and if a date uses sexual behavior as a means of proving masculinity or femininity, it might be better to date other people.

Unfortunately, forced sexual contact has always happened between dating partners. Women often blamed themselves for "leading a date on." It was not until the mid-1970s that the term *date rape* was coined and women had legal rights to go after assailants they had dated.

Some statistics related to date rape are included in the periodic Youth Risk Behavior Surveillance (YRBS; Kann et al., 2014). With regard to dating violence, among the 73.9% of grade 9–12 students nationwide who dated or went out with someone during the 12 months before the survey, 10.3% had been hit, slammed into something, or injured with an object or a weapon on purpose by their boyfriend or girlfriend. Rates of physical dating violence were higher among female (13%) than male

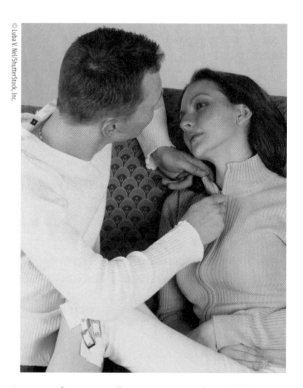

In cases of rape on college campuses, about 80% are committed by an acquaintance.

Myth vs Fact

Myth: Rape is an impulsive act of passion—meaning that men cannot control their sex drive.
Fact: Rapists themselves do not see rape as compulsive sexual behavior. The objective for rape is not usually sexual pleasure; it is to have power and to commit violence. Sexual activity is used to carry out nonsexual needs.

Myth: Women want to be raped—meaning that women have fantasies that reflect their desire to be raped.
Fact: Rape is an act of violent aggression. No healthy individual desires to be dehumanized and violated.

Myth: Women ask to be raped—meaning they tempt the man. "She should have worn a bra," "Hitchhikers get what they deserve," and "She shouldn't have been out so late at night" are examples of this thinking.
Fact: The blame and responsibility for a criminal assault are the assailant's, not the victim's.

Myth: A woman can run faster with her skirt up than a man can with his pants down—meaning a woman cannot be raped against her will.
Fact: Rape is an aggression committed under force or the threat of force on an unconsenting person. A knife, gun, or even verbal threat is often understandably stronger than a person's will.

Myth: You cannot blame a man for trying—meaning the responsibility for stopping a man is the woman's; therefore, it is her fault if matters get out of hand.
Fact: A criminal, not a victim, is responsible for criminal acts. Rape is not an impulsive act of passion. It is done for power and control.

Myth: The rapist is usually of a different race from the victim—meaning rape usually reflects ethnic or racial hatred.
Fact: In most instances the rapist and the victim are of the same race.

Myth vs Fact

Myth: If a person is going to be raped, he or she might as well relax and enjoy it—meaning it is just sexual activity.
Fact: Rape victims experience intense psychological and physical trauma. Rape is a violent, dehumanizing, and intimate invasion of a person's privacy and integrity as a human being. The motive for rape is power; it is not sexual enjoyment. Rape is anything but enjoyable!

Myth: Most rapes are committed by strangers—meaning we are safe with people we know.
Fact: It is common for the rapist and the victim to know each other, to have been acquainted, or at least to have seen each other on the street, in the grocery store, in the student union, and so on.

Myth: It's not sexual assault if it happens after drinking or taking drugs.
Fact: A person under the influence of drugs or alcohol does not cause others to assault him or her. Many state laws say that a person who is impaired due to the influence of drugs or alcohol is not able to consent to sexual activity.

Myth: A person who has really been sexually assaulted will be hysterical.
Fact: Victims of sexual violence can show a wide variety of responses, including calm, hysteria, withdrawal, anger, apathy, denial, and shock. Reactions and the length of time needed to work through the experience vary.

Myth: Only young, attractive people are assaulted.
Fact: Sexual assault is a crime of power and control, and offenders often choose people they view as vulnerable to attack or over whom they believe they can assert power. Victims come from all walks of life and represent all ages—including males, females, and persons with disabilities.

Myth: Men can't be raped.
Fact: About 92,700 men are raped each year in the United States

Myth: I don't know anyone who's ever been raped.
Fact: Rape victims are doctors, lawyers, nurses, military personnel, cooks, accountants, or anyone. Fewer than one-third of sexual assaults are reported to the police.

(7.4%) students. They were also higher among white female (12.9%), black female (12.3%), and Hispanic female (13.6%) students than among white male (6.4%), black male (8.2%), and Hispanic male (7%) students, respectively. Nationwide, 7.3% of students had ever been physically forced to have sexual intercourse when they did not want to participate. The prevalence of such reports was higher among female (10.5%) than male (4.2%) students, and higher among white female (9.1%), black female (11.5%), and Hispanic female (12.2%) students than among white male (3.1%), black male (5.2%), and Hispanic male (5.2%) students, respectively.

While experts do not understand a great deal about date rape, many researchers have studied the topic. Because of the relationship of date rape to overall dating violence, information about the two topics is often put together in research studies. From these studies we know that the vast majority of rapes on college campuses are committed by someone with whom the victim is acquainted. Many are committed on dates, and drinking alcohol and date rape often go together. Many people who are date raped do not

report the assault to authorities because of feelings of self-blame and embarrassment.

Like other forms of sexual assault, acquaintance assault is motivated by a need to control, to humiliate, and to harm. It is important to remember that a prior or current relationship or previous acts of intimacy are insufficient indicators of consent. Also, verbal consent must be obtained both in each instance of sexual intimacy and as the level of sexual intimacy increases (for example, moving from kissing to petting, from petting to oral sexual activity, from oral activity to intercourse or anal activity, etc.) (Acquaintance rape, 2012).

McEwan et al. (2005) studied the relationship between date rape, ego-identity achievement, and locus of control. They found that, compared to women who had not been assaulted, date rape survivors reported lower ego-identity achievement and greater beliefs that the outcomes of their lives were controlled by luck, chance, or powerful others.

Marelich et al. (2008) studied the use of deception in association with sexual encounters. The three components of sexual deception used were blatant lying, self-serving lying, and avoiding confrontation. Those persons who used any of these deceptions reported more sexual partners and one-night stands. Those telling blatant lies to have sexual activity were more likely to report greater needs for sexual activity, while those using self-serving lies or having sexual intercourse to avoid confrontation experienced greater worry about partner loss. Men were more likely to use blatant lies to have sexual activity, while women were more likely to have sexual activity to avoid confrontation.

Collibee and Furman (2014) looked at the effect of sexual coercion on romantic relationship quality and dating experiences. Tracking youth for more than 8 years, they found that negative interactions immediately increased following coercion. Jealousy in romantic relationships also increased. Serious dating decelerated following the coercive incident. Results were consistent across gender and severity of the coercive incident. Overall—perhaps not surprisingly—sexual coercion had a negative impact on romantic experiences.

Ways to Help Prevent Acquaintance Rape

Because of the magnitude of date rape, many steps have been taken to help deal with and reduce the problem. Awareness is the first step, and materials have been developed to help college students understand date rape and how to prevent it. The American College Health Association (2014) has developed a pamphlet titled *Sexual Violence: What Everyone Should Know*, which contains suggestions for both men and women.

For example, the pamphlet indicates that alcohol and other drugs can inhibit clear thinking, make talking and listening more difficult, and make it harder to assess risk. Consenting sexual activity doesn't just happen. It requires sober, verbal communication without intimidation or threats. Many states' laws recognize that someone must be sober to give true consent. Also, being drunk or high is never an excuse for raping someone.

The pamphlet also has a section titled "What You Can Do," which indicates that you can think about how to respond to social pressures and ask yourself:

- How does sex fit into my definition of being a man or a woman?

- What role do I want sex to play in my life?

Alcohol can play a role in acquaintance rape.

- How does alcohol affect my sexual decision-making?

- How do I learn someone's desires and limits?

- How do I express my own desires and limits?

The pamphlet emphasizes the need to communicate effectively. It suggests expressing your limits clearly, listening carefully to what the other person is saying, asking rather than assuming, trusting your instincts, and remembering that effective and assertive communication may not always work. Sometimes people simply don't listen. However, no one ever *deserves* to be raped!

Preventing and Dealing with Sexual Violence on Campus

Much has happened in recent years related to preventing and dealing with sexual violence on campus. A brief chronological review of some of the events should promote a better understanding of the overall situation. For a number of years, many colleges and universities have struggled to develop and implement effective policies related to sexual violence on campus. One example of how this struggle played out is found at Grinnell College in Iowa. In the spring of 2012, the Grinnell College student body voted overwhelmingly to revise the Sexual Harassment and Misconduct policy to incorporate affirmative consent. Table 17.2 lists a few important elements of that 68-page document.

In April 2014, *Not Alone*—the first report of the White House Task Force to Protect Students from Sexual Assault—was published (http://www.whitehouse.gov/sites/default/files/docs/report_0.pdf). The name of the companion website, NotAlone.gov, was chosen to reassure sexual assault survivors that they are not alone. Also, the Task Force wanted institutions

TABLE 17.2

Important Elements of a Campus Sexual Violence Policy

Many terms are defined in the Grinnell College Sexual Harassment and Misconduct Policy; however, it is of basic importance to understand "affirmative consent." Here are some points related to affirmative consent:

1. Consent to engage in sexual activity must be given knowingly, voluntarily, and affirmatively.
2. Consent to engage in sexual activity must exist from the beginning to end of each instance of sexual activity, and for each form of sexual contact.
3. Consent is demonstrated through mutually understandable words and/or clear, unambiguous actions that indicate a willingness to engage freely in sexual activity.
4. Each participant in a sexual encounter is expected to obtain and give consent to each act of sexual activity. Consent to one form of sexual activity does not constitute consent to engage in all forms of sexual activity.
5. Relying on nonverbal communication can lead to misunderstandings. Consent may not be inferred from silence, passivity, lack of resistance, or lack of an active response alone.
6. Consent may be withdrawn by either party at any time. This must also be outwardly demonstrated by mutually understandable words and/or clear, unambiguous actions that indicate a desire to end sexual activity.
7. Individuals with a previous or current intimate relationship do not automatically give initial or continued consent to sexual activity.
8. Consent is not affirmative if it results from the use or threat of physical force, intimidation, coercion, or any other factor that inhibits an individual's free will.
9. Any individual who is physically incapacitated from alcohol and/or other drug consumption, or is unconscious, unaware, or otherwise physically helpless is unable to give consent.
10. Consent can never be given by minors under the legal age of consent.

The entire policy may be seen at http://www.grinnell.edu/sites/default/files/documents/Grinnell%20College%20Sexual%20Harassment%20and%20Misconduct%20Policy_2.pdf .

to live up to their obligation to protect students from sexual violence.

The first action step of the Task Force was providing institutions with a toolkit to conduct campus surveys to identify and help solve the problem of sexual violence on campus. The second action step was to identify a number of promising prevention strategies that institutions could undertake immediately. In addition, an effort was made to engage men as allies in the cause. Most men are not perpetrators, and it was felt that empowering men to step in when someone is in trouble would be an important part of the solution.

The third action step was encouraging institutions to develop plans for effectively responding when a student is sexually assaulted. That should include someone to whom a survivor can talk in confidence, a comprehensive sexual misconduct policy, trauma-informed training for institution officials, better school disciplinary systems, and partnerships with the community (such as rape crisis services or working with local law enforcement) to better meet students' needs.

The fourth action step was to increase transparency and improve enforcement. For example, on the NotAlone.gov website, sexual assault survivors can locate an array of services by typing in their ZIP codes. They can also learn about their legal rights and get understandable definitions of legal terms and concepts.

In September 2014, California became the first state in the nation to define when "yes means yes" and adopt requirements for colleges to follow when investigating sexual assault reports. The text of the bill is available at https://leginfo.legislature.ca.gov/faces/billNavClient.xhtml?bill_id=201320140SB967. The definition of "consent" under California's law requires "an affirmative, conscious and voluntary agreement to engage in sexual activity." In particular, silence or lack of resistance does not constitute consent. Someone who is drunk, drugged, unconscious, or asleep cannot grant consent. Consent can be nonverbal, such as nodding the head or moving in closer to the person. The California law also requires training for faculty reviewing complaints so that victims are not asked inappropriate questions when filing complaints, as well as access to counseling, healthcare services, and other resources for victims.

Also in September 2014, President Barack Obama joined Vice President Joe Biden and Americans across the country in launching the "It's on Us" initiative—a campaign to help put an end to sexual assault on college campuses. The president's message was clear: "It is on all of us to reject the quiet tolerance of sexual assault and to refuse to accept what's unacceptable." That is, it's on us—all of us—to stop sexual assault. The aim of this awareness campaign is to fundamentally shift the way we think about sexual assault, by inspiring everyone to see it as their responsibility to do something, big or small, to prevent such assaults. A long list of "It's on Us" partners was quickly established, including groups such as the NCAA, the American Association of University Women, Viacom (a media company whose TV networks include MTV, VH1, BET, and CMT), Participant Media, Electronic Arts (a leading video gaming company), Mekanism (an advertising company), the Big Ten, the ACC, the Big 12, the PAC 12, Clear Channel, *Newsweek*, National Women's Law Center, National Campus Leadership Council, and many others. More information about this effort is available at http://www.whitehouse.gov /the-press-office/2014/09/19/fact-sheet-launch-it-s-us -public-awareness-campaign-help-prevent-campus-.

On October 20, 2014, the amendments to the Violence Against Women Act (also called the Clery Act) were published in the *Federal Register*. The major provisions included the following:

- Require higher education institutions to maintain statistics about the number of incidents of dating violence, domestic violence, sexual assault, and stalking that meet the definition of these terms

- Revise the definition of "rape" to reflect the Federal Bureau of Investigation's (FBI) updated definition

- Require institutions to provide primary prevention and awareness programs for incoming students and new employees

- Require institutions to provide and describe ongoing prevention and awareness programs for students and employees

- Require institutions to describe each type of disciplinary proceeding used by the institution, the steps' anticipated timelines, and the decision-making process for each type of disciplinary proceeding

- Require institutions to list all of the possible sanctions that the institution may impose following the results of any institutional disciplinary proceedings for an allegation of dating violence, domestic violence, sexual assault, or stalking

- Require institutions to provide for a prompt, fair, and impartial disciplinary proceeding with a number of requirements

Even after all of these developments related to preventing and dealing with sexual violence on campus, a number of questions and issues have arisen in regard to management of such assaults:

- Why should colleges, rather than the local police, handle campus sexual assault cases? In the past, the rationale was that federal gender-equity law compels colleges to investigate and resolve students' reports. Should this system continue to be used?

- How can college lawyers keep up with the evolving array of laws and regulations on campus assault?

- Some people argue that colleges do not have the ability to investigate sexual crimes or the right to properly punish perpetrators. Do college sexual assault trials belong in court, and not on campus?

- How should reports of sexual violence best be handled?

- Should campus officials talk about alcohol when it comes to sexual assault? If this element is emphasized, students who get drunk and are assaulted will be blamed—and may blame themselves. In turn, they may not report the attacks to their colleges and not get the help they need.

- Will efforts to convict the alleged perpetrators go too far, perhaps having a lower burden of proof, and result in innocent students being labeled as rapists?

- When a student confides a rape to a professor, should the professor have to report it?

- The pressure on colleges to prevent and handle sexual assault cases more effectively has grown steadily in recent years. Some institutions have hired a full-time person to handle issues related to campus sexual assault. Is it worth it for colleges to take on this additional expense?

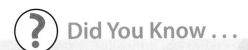

? Did You Know . . .

U.S. Department of Education Guidelines for Colleges' Sexual-Assault Investigations

In 2011 the U.S. Department of Education announced a set of thorough guidelines for how colleges should respond to allegations of sexual assault. One of the key recommendations lowers the burden of proof for finding someone guilty of sexual assault from "clear and convincing" evidence to "more likely than not," which makes it easier for institutions to reprimand the harasser.

There are three key provisions outlined by the guidelines that institutions must follow:

1. Every school must have and distribute a policy against sex discrimination
2. Every school must have a Title IX coordinator
3. Every school must have and make known procedures for students to file complaints of sex discrimination.

Under the new guidelines, the grievance procedures may include voluntary informal methods (e.g., mediation) for resolving some types of sexual harassment complaints. However, the complainant must be notified of the right to end the informal process at any time and begin the formal stage of the complaint process. In cases involving allegations of sexual assault, mediation is not appropriate. In addition, the person who filed the complaint has the right to be notified, in writing, of the outcome. Schools must also disclose to them information about the sanction imposed on the harasser when the sanction directly relates to the harassed student.

If a school knows or reasonably should know about sexual harassment or sexual violence that creates a hostile environment, the school must take immediate action to eliminate the sexual harassment or sexual violence, prevent its recurrence, and address its effects.

In 2014, after working under the guidelines for several years, the U.S Department of Education published *Questions and Answers on Title IX and Sexual Violence* (http://www2.ed.gov/about/offices/list/ocr/docs/qa-201404-title-ix.pdf). The goal was to clarify the legal requirements and give guidance related to the guidelines.

Source: Modified from Know Your Rights: Title IX Prohibits Sexual Harassment and Sexual Violence Where You Go to School. Office for Civil Rights, U.S. Department of Education. (2011).

Many institutions have been trying a variety of approaches to prevent and deal with sexual violence on campus. At some colleges, students can use smartphone apps to ask friends for help if they are in danger. Some colleges have removed students from panels that determine sanctions for campus sexual assault and harassment, replacing them with specially trained employees. Some experts indicate that students are less likely to report sexual misconduct when they know they will be judged by a peer. Other institutions have strengthened their disciplinary policies to require mandatory expulsion for sexual assault perpetrators. Some large universities are using computer-based courses on assault to reach the widest audience with education on this topic. All incoming students might be required to take the courses, and there might also be refresher courses later. More colleges are offering training aimed at teaching students how to intervene in assaults before they happen; such programs target the "bystander" who wants to step in, but does not know how.

Date-Rape Drugs

In the early 1990s the topic of date rape was further complicated by the availability of **date-rape drugs**. These drugs are sometimes used to assist a sexual assault. They are powerful and dangerous. They can be slipped into your drink when you are not looking. The drugs often have no color, smell, or taste, so you can't tell if you are being drugged. They can make you become weak and confused—or even pass out—so that you are unable to refuse sexual activity or defend yourself. If you are drugged, you might not remember what happened while you were drugged. Date-rape drugs are used on both females and males.

One early date-rape drug was flunitrazepam (Rohypnol). It is a prescription drug marketed legally in many countries around the world. It is used as a sedative hypnotic and as a preanesthetic medication in those countries. However, it is not approved for medical use in the United States. Because of its sedative hypnotic action and amnesialike effect, it is ideal for use in date-rape situations. Rohypnol can be administered without consent to produce disinhibition and

date-rape drugs Sedative hypnotic drugs used to incapacitate victims who are then sexually molested or raped.

Date rape drugs have no taste and no odor. They are undetectable when added to a drink.

to obtain sexual activity. It has no taste or odor when mixed with alcohol. People drugged with Rohypnol may remember nothing about what happened or have only a very sketchy memory. They are often unsure that they have been raped, except that they may wake the next morning feeling genital discomfort or finding themselves undressed. Assailants typically claim the victims consented to sexual activity, and there is no way to know for sure. The effects of Rohypnol can be felt within 30 minutes and can last for several hours (Date rape drugs, 2015).

Another date-rape drug is gammahydroxybutyrate (GHB). It can be used by sexual predators to render their victims almost instantly helpless and to leave them with little or no memory of the attack. It is similar to the drug Rohypnol. GHB has no approved medical use, and it can cause depression, seizures, coma, and death. Kits can be purchased to make the drug at home for less than $100. Many argue that GHB should be an illegal substance.

A third drug being used as a date-rape drug is ketamine hydrochloride. It is used medically as an anesthetic for diagnostic and surgical purposes. It produces anesthesia within 40 seconds of intravenous administration and within 8 minutes of intramuscular administration. It is currently widely used by veterinarians. In the United States the popular method of use involves heating of the liquid until it turns into a white powder, which is then smoked or snorted. Full effects of ketamine occur in about 5 to 10 minutes and last up to 1 hour (Date rape drugs, 2008).

Other date rape drugs include gamma-butyrolactone (GBL), benzodiazepines, and Ecstasy (Drug facilitated sexual assault, 2012). GBL, a GHB-like product, is often sold under the guise of a dietary supplement or an industrial cleaner. When the body metabolizes GBL, it becomes twice as potent as GHB. It now comes in flavors and, once ingested, it takes about 30 to 45 minutes to take effect. Benzodiazepines are legal substances commonly prescribed as antianxiety and sleeping medications in the United States. They can be put into an alcoholic drink or soft drink in power or liquid form. They can markedly impair and even abolish functions that normally enable a person to resist, or even want to resist, sexual aggression or assault. Ecstasy is a toxic hallucinogenic and stimulant that has psychedelic effects. It is illegal to sell or produce it in the United States. Ecstasy causes individuals to feel extreme relaxation and positivity towards others and increases sensitivity to touch. Under its influence, individuals are less likely to be able to sense danger, making it difficult to protect themselves from attack.

In 1996 President Clinton signed a bill outlawing Rohypnol and other date-rape drugs and adding 20 years to the sentence of a rapist who uses these drugs on a victim. The law also included increased penalties for illegal manufacturing, distribution,

 Did You Know . . .

Gray Rape

"Gray rape" has been defined as "sexual activity that falls somewhere between consent and denial and is even more confusing than date rape because often both parties are unsure of who wanted what." For example, both parties may have been very drunk during the incident and do not recall what they had said to each other the next morning. Or an accuser may not remember the events of the evening, but insist that he or she was too intoxicated to be able to consciously consent to sexual activity. The person who initiated the sexual encounter, however, may not have been aware that the accuser was drunk.

Some people reject the idea of "gray rape," saying it does not exist. They define rape as forcible sexual relations with a person against their will. The term "gray rape," they say, promotes the communication myth that sexual assault can sometimes be an accident, when in reality it is a deliberate act of violence. Consent must be obtained for sexual activity to be acceptable to all those involved. There is no gray area for consent—either it exists or it doesn't.

What do you think? Should we recognize the existence of "gray rape" or should we believe that there is no such thing? Why?

dispensing, or possession of the drugs. It was the first time that using a drug as a weapon was classified as a crime in the United States.

Alcohol is also a date-rape drug. In fact, it is the drug most commonly used to commit sexual assault. When a person drinks too much alcohol, it is difficult to think clearly, set limits and make good choices, and tell when a situation could be dangerous. It is also more difficult to say "no" to sexual advances and to fight back if a sexual assault occurs. Alcohol can cause a blackout and memory loss as well (Date rape drugs, 2015).

Although the term "date rape" is commonly used, many experts prefer the term "drug-facilitated sexual assault" when referring to these drugs. The drugs can affect a person very quickly, and the length of time that the effect lasts varies, depending on how much is taken and whether it is mixed with other substances such as alcohol. Alcohol can worsen the drug's effects. Here are some ways to protect yourself from being a victim of "drug-facilitated sexual assault" (Date rape drugs, 2015):

- Don't accept drinks from other people.

- Open containers yourself.

- Keep your drink with you at all times, even when you go into the bathroom.

- Don't share drinks.

- Don't drink from punch bowls or other large, common, open containers. They may already have drugs in them.

- Don't drink anything that tastes or smells strange. Sometimes GHB tastes salty.

- Have a nondrinking friend with you to make sure nothing happens.

- If you think you have been drugged and raped:

  - Go to the police station or hospital right away.

  - Get a urine test as soon as possible. The drugs leave your system quickly.

  - Don't urinate before getting help.

  - Don't douche, bathe, or change clothes before getting help. These actions eliminate evidence of the rape.

  - Call the National Domestic Violence Hotline at 800-799-SAFE or 800-787-3224 (TTY).

Are there ways to detect date-rape drugs before ingesting them? The answer to that question varies depending on who you ask. For example, some

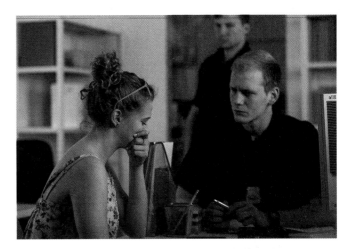

It is important to get help if sexual assault does occur.

people believe that a special nail polish designed to change color if a person stirs a drink containing a date-rape drug is effective. Specially designed cups, coasters, and stirrers have also been promoted as being able to change color or in some other way detect the presence of date-rape drugs. Some sources also claim that the pd.id (personal drink identification device) can quickly and discreetly inform a user if someone has tampered with a drink. This battery-powered device is about the size of a keychain and can be slipped into a drink. If the drink is safe, an LED light flashes green; if it has been spiked, the light goes red. The pd.id sells for about $75 and can be reused about 40 times before the battery needs to be recharged. While some people believe one or more of these devices can be very helpful, others are not yet convinced of their effectiveness.

Consequences of Rape

The survivor of a rape and the survivor's friends, family, and spouse or lover usually respond to the crime's sexual aspects rather than the violent ones. Rape survivors and their loved ones need the same kinds of help to get through this difficult time as survivors of other violent acts. And beyond that, they need assistance with the specific problems that follow such a personally destructive attack.

Traumatic events, such as war, accidents, natural disasters, and sexual violence can result in serious stress and detrimental consequences for survivors and their families. Although most individuals will be able to absorb the trauma over time, many survivors will experience long-lasting problems. About 8% of survivors of traumatic events develop post-traumatic stress disorder (PTSD). PTSD symptoms include nightmares, insomnia, somatic disturbances, difficulty with intimate relationships, fear, anxiety,

Sexual Violence

Sexual violence may be viewed and handled differently in various cultures. For example, sexual violence against Norwegian women is common but rarely reported. Despite being known for its progressive stance on gender equality, Norway has rates of sexual violence on par with much more unequal societies. According to Norway's largest shelter organization, 1 in 10 Norwegian women older than age 15 has been raped. Of these cases, at least 80% are never brought to official attention and only 10% of those that are end in a conviction. Also, Norway is one of 127 countries in the world that do not explicitly criminalize rape within marriage. Every county in Norway has a rape assault center and a medical facility where rape survivors are offered no-cost counseling and medical care and examined for forensic evidence. Yet, most rape survivors do not go to the hospital for forensic exams or press charges. Even when cases are reported to the police, they don't always pick up the evidence that was collected.

Hate crimes can also be viewed as relating to various cultures. By definition, they are victimization of an individual based on that individual's race, religion, national origin, ethnic identification, gender, or sexual orientation. While any group can experience rape and sexual assault as a form of hate crime, two groups are often noted for being victims of this form of hate crime—women and people in the LGBT community.

Many believe that all violence against women, including rape and sexual assault, is a hate crime because it is not simply a violent act, but that it is "an act of misogyny, or hatred of women." Members of the LGBT community are often targets of hate crimes, many of which include rape or sexual assault. In one study of almost 2,000 lesbian and gay individuals, about one-fifth of the women and one-fourth of the men had been victimized at some point during the past 5 years.

Sources: Data from Sexual violence against Norwegian women common but rarely reported. Women's Health Policy Report. National Partnership for Women & Families, October 29, 2011. Available: http://go.nationalpartnership.org/site/News2?page=NewsArticle&id=30763&news_iv_ctrl=0&abbr=daily2_; modified from Hate crimes. Rape, Abuse, & Incest National Network, 2012. Available: www.rainn.org/get-information/types-of-sexual-assault/hate-crimes.

anger, shame, aggression, suicidal behaviors, loss of trust, and isolation (*The effects of trauma do not have to last a lifetime*, 2015).

The **rape trauma syndrome** has two phases. The acute phase can last from days to weeks, and is characterized by general stress responses such as lack of sleep, irritability, and difficulty in thinking clearly. The long-term phase can last several years and the symptoms are similar to those described for PTSD. Some experts believe that the long-term phase of the rape trauma syndrome is actually a subset of PTSD.

In addition to the psychological consequences mentioned previously, physical consequences of rape include the possibility of a pregnancy and/or an STI. Other physical consequences could be chronic pelvic pain, gastrointestinal disorders, migraines and other frequent headaches, back pain, and facial pain. Social consequences include strained family relations, less frequent contact with friends and relatives, and less emotional support from friends and family.

Some rape survivors engage in more sexually risky behaviors after experiencing a sexual assault than they did before the attack, while others significantly reduce their risky behavior, and many abstain from sexual activity after their assault. Sexually risky behavior can include sexual activity with multiple partners, without contraception, and while under the influence of alcohol or other drugs. Rape survivors who had negative interactions with police and medical professionals, and reported experiencing blame for their assault from these sources, tended to fall into the group of women who increased their sexually risky behaviors.

It is clear that individuals who are victims of sexual violence are more likely to experience depression, anxiety, and traumatic symptoms compared to nonvictims. However, the impact of sexual violence is not limited to the act itself. Instead, so-called secondary victimization may result from negative experiences within one's social group or with authorities who may hold negative attitudes toward victims of rape.

rape trauma syndrome A two-phase reaction to rape. An acute phase involves intense emotional responses for several weeks. The long-term phase may last several years and involves reorganization and establishment of control.

Adult rape survivors experience effects on their personal stability and adjustment. Many do not wish to confide in another person and try to hold in their feelings. Some are hesitant to participate in their usual sexual relations. Personal feelings of privacy, dignity, and trust are undermined, and feelings of vulnerability are common. Many feel they live in a world filled with threats. Anger, rage, shame, and fear profoundly influence the recovery of rape survivors. Although some women suffer physical trauma from rape, requiring surgical repair of the perineum, vulva, or urethra, it is emotional scars that take longest to heal.

In summary, victims of sexual assault are 3 times more likely to suffer from depression, 6 times more likely to suffer from PTSD, and 13 times more likely to abuse alcohol. In addition, they are 26 times more likely to abuse drugs, and 4 times more likely to contemplate suicide (Who are the victims?, 2015).

Many survivors of sexual assault do heal and do just fine in their lives. They probably do not forget, but they do move on. There is a great deal of hope today for such survivors.

Rape of Males

Much of the information on rape presented so far has focused on rapes of females. This is appropriate because the vast majority of survivors are females. However, in recent years there has been an increased recognition that males can be sexually assaulted, too. Even the rape laws in many states now recognize the existence of male rape. Generally, male rape falls into one of three categories: male rape in prison, male rape by other males outside prison, and male rape by females.

After decades of research, it is still unknown how much rape and sexually violent activity occur in prisons and jails. What is clear is that, as with rape in free society, prison rape goes largely unreported. It is very difficult to determine the extent of the problem. It is estimated that 4.0% of state and federal inmates and 3.2% of jail inmates experienced one or more incidents of sexual victimization by another inmate or facility staff in the past 12 months. Rates were higher among females than males, higher among whites than blacks, and higher among inmates with a college degree than those who had not completed high school. Among state and federal inmates, about 6.3% of those identified with serious psychological distress reported they were sexually victimized by another inmate. In comparison, among prisoners with no indication of mental illness, 0.7% reported being victimized by another inmate (Beck et al., 2014). Even though research about prison rape is not conclusive, many people believe that the likelihood

A person/entertainer who has recently been involved in child pornography. One that comes to mind is Jared from the Subway commercials.

of being raped in prison is so great that a judge who sentences a young man to prison passes a sentence of male rape on him as surely as the prison sentence. It appears that male prison rape is an act of heterosexuals rather than LGBTQ people. This may sound strange at first, but in a prison situation rape is viewed as validation of masculinity and a violent act of conquest.

As one sign of concern about prison rape, in 2003 Congress passed the Prison Rape Elimination Act. This legislation calls for all correction systems to have a zero-tolerance policy regarding prison rape. It requires standards for detection, prevention, reduction, and punishment of prison rape. It standardizes collection and dissemination of information on the incidence of prison rape, and awards grants to implement the act's provisions (About the Prison Rape Elimination Act of 2003, 2007).

Prison rape is usually the act of heterosexuals rather than LGBT People.

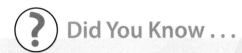

Did You Know . . .

Stalking

The exact definition of stalking varies by state, but generally it refers to a "course of conduct directed at a specific person that involves repeated visual or physical proximity, nonconsensual communication, or verbal, written, or implied threats, or a combination thereof, that would cause a reasonable person fear." Examples of stalking include:

1. Repeated undesired contact (phone calls, emails, letters, showing up unexpectedly, etc.).
2. Following or laying in wait for the individual.
3. Making threats to the individual or her/his family.
4. Any other behavior used to contact, harass, track, or threaten the individual.

Each year about 3.4 million people in the United States are victims of stalking. The majority of victims are 18 to 24 years old. Most victims know their stalker. About 1 in 4 victims experience some form of cyberstalking.

If you are ever stalked, you should consider:

1. Avoiding all contact with the stalker.
2. Informing family, friends, supervisors, and coworkers of what is going on.
3. Reporting the stalking to the local police.
4. Keeping an accurate journal or log of all incidents connected to the stalking.
5. Keeping all evidence received from the stalker, such as letters, packages, taped phone messages, etc.

All 50 states and Washington D.C. have antistalking laws. The impact of stalking can be life altering. Those who are stalked often change many of their behaviors and can have strong emotional responses, including anxiety, fear, depression, nervousness, and isolation. Many resources are available to help people prevent and deal with stalking.

Source: Modified from Stalking. Rape, Abuse, & Incest National Network, 2012. Available: www.rainn.org/newsroom/sexual-assault-issues/stalking.

Even outside prison, it is probable that most rapes of males are committed by heterosexual men. This is perhaps more understandable when we consider that violence and power, rather than sexual satisfaction, are the primary motivations for rape. Statistics on the frequency of male rape are almost impossible to obtain. Perhaps this is because of the lack of research on the subject combined with the hesitation of male victims to report an attack. In addition to the reasons females hesitate to report a rape, males often feel they are supposed to be strong and "macho." To report being raped would not be consistent with this image.

A male being raped by a female is hard for many people to imagine. This is because of traditional feelings about sexuality—particularly the ideas that all males are "at the ready" for sexual activity and that males cannot be forced into submission. Although the first attitude is open to question (often based on incorrect logic), the second relates to physiological functioning. People seem to think that a male could not respond sexually while being threatened because he could not achieve a penile erection. It has been found, however, that such emotions as anger, fright, and pain can cause a sexual response, including all the usual physiological changes. This, of course, can be quite upsetting to the victim because it might be interpreted as indicating willingness. Guilt and other negative feelings can occur as well. Consequently, the responses of male rape survivors are very similar to those of female rape survivors.

Walker et al. (2005) investigated the effects of rape on a sample of 40 men recruited by media advertising. They found that most assaults had been carried out using physical or violent force, in a variety of circumstances. All victims reported some form of psychological disturbance as a result of being raped. Long-term effects included anxiety, depression, increased feelings of anger and vulnerability, loss of self-image, emotional distancing, self-blame, and self-harming behaviors.

Stermac et al. (2004) examined victim and assault characteristics among adult male victims of sexual assaults. They found that male victims presenting to an urban sexual assault care center were young, often single adults with significant vulnerabilities (living on the street or in a shelter, unemployed, and with physical disabilities). These same characteristics were not so common with female victims. Males overall were more likely to be victims of an anal and/or fellatio assault. Male stranger assailant victims were also more likely to be attacked by multiple assailants than were female victims, and more likely to be assaulted outdoors. In contrast, male acquaintance assailant victims were more likely to be assaulted in an institutional setting. Male stranger assault victims were more likely to experience assaults involving weapons. Acquaintance male assaults, however, were more likely to involve victims' alcohol use.

As with rape of females, there are many stereotypes and myths about rape of males. Many of these impact the male survivor's ability to face the sexual assault. Some of these myths are that: (1) men are immune to victimization; (2) men should be able to fight off attacks; (3) men should not express emotion; (4) men enjoy all sexual activity, so they must have enjoyed the assault; and (5) male survivors are more likely to become sexual predators. Of course, all of these statements are false. These stereotypes and myths can lead to certain results for male victims of sexual abuse, including dramatic loss of self-esteem; loss of belief in their masculinity; self-blame; feelings of shame, guilt, and anger; feelings of powerlessness, apprehension, withdrawal, and embarrassment; fears that they will not be able to protect and support their families; sexual difficulties; self-destructive behavior (such as drinking, drug use, and aggression); intimacy issues; and questioning of sexual identity (Male sexual assault, 2011).

Most of what was discussed regarding rape trauma syndrome and post-traumatic stress disorder for female victims of sexual violence also applies to male victims. In addition, a male victim often feels that he has totally lost control over the insides of his own body, resulting in feelings of vulnerability and powerlessness. Men are generally brought up to defend themselves against attack, and may consider total helplessness incompatible with masculinity. They may feel that their gender identity as a male has been compromised or even demolished and reversed.

There is very little information about the prevalence and health impacts of sexual aggression among males who have experienced severe partner violence. However, Hines and Douglas (2014) surveyed 611 men who experienced physical partner violence from their female partners and sought help. Almost half of the men experienced sexual aggression in their relationship, and 28% experienced severe sexual aggression. Increasing levels of severity of sexual aggression were associated with greater prevalence and types of other forms of partner violence. In addition, men with greater levels of sexual aggression had significantly more depression symptoms, post-traumatic stress disorder symptoms, physical health symptoms, and poor health.

Social Responses to Rape

In many communities, sexual assault crisis centers, workshops dealing with prevention of sexual assault, and improved methods of helping survivors have become priorities. Shelters for survivors of assault have been provided so they have a place to receive help. In general, there is a better understanding of the problems in communities and the need for more support.

On many college campuses there are laudable attempts to deal with sexual assault. An effective program (1) defines and demystifies sexual assault,

Myth vs Fact

Myths About Male Rape

Myth: Men can't be sexually assaulted.
Fact: Men are sexually assaulted—regardless of size, strength, appearance, or sexual orientation.

Myth: Only gay men are sexually assaulted.
Fact: Heterosexual and LGBTQ men are equally likely to be sexually assaulted.

Myth: Only gay men sexually assault other men.
Fact: Most men who sexually assault other men are heterosexuals.

Myth: Men can't be sexually assaulted by women.
Fact: Although most perpetrators are men, women can also sexually assault men.

Myth: Erection or ejaculation during sexual assault means you "really wanted it" or consented to it.
Fact: Erection and ejaculation are physiological responses that may result from mere physical contact or even extreme stress. These responses do not imply that you wanted or enjoyed the sexual assault.

Source: Modified from Myths about male rape. South Eastern Centre Against Sexual Assault 2015. Available: www.secasa.com.au.

(2) offers educational programs, (3) empowers women to be assertive, (4) exposes the link between alcohol abuse and unwanted sexual behavior, (5) conducts institutional surveys, and (6) identifies a specific individual on campus to coordinate efforts and clinical services.

It is important for the various aspects of a campus effort to be tied together. Table 17.3 shows how those working with prevention measures can cooperate for the best results.

There is also greater recognition on college campuses of the need for more attention to the problem of sexual assault. Lighting and security on campuses have improved; courses in sexual assault prevention and self-defense are offered; and escort services are available so women need not be alone on campus, particularly after dark.

There have also been major changes in laws related to rape in the past few decades. Many of the newer rape laws (1) establish "degrees" of rape to describe types of sexual assault more accurately; (2) are gender neutral and do not apply only to attacks by men on women; (3) eliminate requirements that victims prove they resisted by "fighting back" and that corroborating evidence be presented; (4) shield victims from inquiries into past sexual experience; and (5) allow a husband to be charged with raping his wife. In fact, in many states the term *forced sex* or *sexual assault* has replaced the word *rape*. The convicted rapist can often be sentenced to life in prison.

TABLE 17.3

A Spectrum of Prevention

Level 1: Strengthening Individual Knowledge and Skills

This level includes workshops for students, faculty, and staff about the definition of sexual assault, its impact, ways to respond to disclosures, campus policies, and local resources.

Level 2: Promoting Community Education

Campus events are usually intended to reach a lot of people at once about sexual violence. These events are more effective when they are a part of a larger conversation.

Level 3: Educating Providers

Campus leaders, including administrators, healthcare providers, discipline officers, security personnel, advocates, resident advisors, student government leaders, and appropriate others, can play a key role in these efforts.

Level 4: Fostering Coalitions and Networks (Individuals and Groups) for Broader Goals and Greater Impact

Collaboration brings more resources. This might include partnerships among campus organizations and coordination with community resources.

Level 5: Changing Organizational Practices

It is important to adopt policies and practices for improving the internal culture and norms around gender, sexual violence, and relationships throughout the campus community.

Source: Adapted from *Overview: Campus sexual violence prevention.* National Sexual Violence Resource Center, 2015. Available: http://www.nsvrc.org/saam.

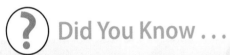 **Did You Know . . .**

Where to Find Help

The following numbers can be helpful if you want to find out more about reporting abuse or if you want more information about abuse:

Child abuse: (800) 4-A-CHILD (422-4453)

Elder abuse: (800) 677-1116

Sexual assault: (800) 656-4673

Domestic violence: (800) 799-7233

Changes have also been made in relation to law enforcement personnel. Training has been designed to help them become more sensitive to the problem of sexual assault. More female officers are used, and there is improved cooperation between law enforcement personnel and medical and support personnel. Guidelines for handling survivors of sexual assault have also been established.

Women who have been assaulted have begun to fight back in civil court as well. For example, a Seattle woman was awarded $300,000 from three men who raped her and a fourth who prevented her escape; a Vermont woman received $450,000 even after a defendant was acquitted of rape charges; and a Minnesota woman received $21,500 from a physician (who had been her lover) for rape.

But even with the increased emphasis on prevention, a great deal must be done. Major priorities include more changes in legislation, law enforcement policies and practices, educational intervention, and media strategies. The codification of women's equality and rights is an important part of a strategy for preventing assault. Skills training, which includes avoidance strategies, appropriate resistance, and self-defense training, is also needed.

■ Pedophilia

The term **pedophilia** denotes feelings of adult sexual attraction to children. Even though physical force may not be used, an adult who performs a sexual act with a child is forcing himself or herself on a helpless minor in the eyes of the law. Pedophiliacs may expose their genitals to a child or fondle and even penetrate a child. There are countless ways a child might be molested; most often the term *child molestation* refers to pedophilia. For all practical purposes the terms are used interchangeably.

The Pedophiliac

A pedophile is a person who has sustained sexual orientation toward children, generally aged 13 or younger. Not all pedophiles are child molesters,

pedophilia   Sexual behavior in which a child is the sexual object.

Ethical
DIMENSIONS

Should the Media Reveal the Names of Rape Survivors?

The names of rape survivors traditionally have been withheld by the news media to "protect" them. Does this special treatment do rape survivors a disservice by separating them from other survivors of violent crimes? Should the privacy of rape survivors be protected more than the privacy of survivors of other violent crimes? This issue has often been debated, and it arose again when two California teenagers were kidnapped. Their names and pictures were widely distributed to help locate them. When, after their rescue, a sheriff said they had been raped during the abduction, "What should be done now?" asked many journalists. Some media representatives stuck to their own rule and did not refer to the teenagers by name. Others called them by name, reasoning that their names had already been released.

Some people believe that the bright lights of publicity may harm the innocent in crimes of rape. They assert that rape survivors are unwillingly thrust into the limelight, their right to choose is once again removed, and their feeling of powerlessness is perpetuated. They argue that publicly identifying rape survivors without their consent compounds the trauma of rape and may discourage future survivors from reporting crimes.

Others point out that in most states it is legal to publish the names of rape survivors, and, in fact, their names should be published just as the names of people who are victims of other violent crimes are. They point out that it is discriminatory to publish the names of alleged assailants, but not the alleged survivors. They also indicate that not naming the survivors contributes to the perception that rape is a different type of crime and helps to perpetuate the notion that there is some blame or disgrace attached. It is also argued that special treatment by the news media inhibits society from treating rape as a violent crime.

Do you think it is ethical, and the best thing to do, for the media to give the names of rape survivors?

and vice versa. Child molesters are defined by their acts, but pedophiles are defined by their desires. Some pedophiles, for example, might refrain from ever approaching children. The American Psychiatric Association has defined pedophilia as "recurrent, intense sexually arousing fantasies, sexual urges, or behaviors that involve children." More recent definitions might refer to a "pedophilic disorder." Such a disorder exists if a person's attraction toward children causes the individual guilt, anxiety, alienation, or difficulty pursuing other goals, or if those urges cause the individual to approach children for gratification in real life (What is pedophilia?, 2015).

There has not been a great deal of research on pedophilia. It is very difficult to treat, and effective treatment needs to be intensive, long term, and comprehensive, possibly with lifetime follow-up.

A man or a woman can be a pedophiliac, but most commonly we hear about males being the offenders. The objects of their desires may be boys, girls, or both. Their preferences with respect to practices vary from exhibition to penetration. Some have fleeting contacts with a series of children, while others look for long-term relationships, which may be sort of caring or manipulative. Many are considerate in their behavior toward children; others use force. Only a few use violent means. There are instances

of consensual sexual activity between adults and children, but this raises the question: Can there ever be sexual consensus between adults and children? Also, there are many cases of nonconsensual sexual contacts between adults and children that are not traumatic for the child, although they do indeed violate the child's right of self-determination. Sexual contacts between adults and children pose a risk of lasting trauma for the latter even when they do not involve violence or the use of force.

Most victims of child sexual abuse do not become pedophiles. However, particular experiences and patterns of childhood behavior are associated with an increased risk of victims becoming abusers in later life. These include neglect, lack of supervision, sexual abuse by a female person, being cruel to animals, and witnessing serious intrafamilial violence.

Although there are many biological and psychological theories, no one really knows how pedophilia develops. The tendency may be established early in life, perhaps genetically or before birth. Hormones may be involved, but consistent hormonal abnormalities are not found in pedophiles. Some experts think that brain function may have something to do with the development of pedophilia, but no one knows for sure. Risk factors for pedophilia—and sexual offenses of all kinds—include childhood emotional

Multicultural
DIMENSIONS

Sexual Contact in Various Cultures

Sexual contact between children and adults may be viewed differently in various cultures. The people following these practices in certain cultures are not pedophiles, but are following cultural or religious tradition.

Historically, in one North African country, men and boys have routinely engaged in anal intercourse. Men are considered peculiar if they do not practice this behavior. In Central Australia, an unmarried man often takes a 10- to 12-year-old boy as his "wife" for several years. In one part of New Guinea, from about age 10, boys would have regular oral sexual activity with older men, swallowing their semen, supposedly to facilitate growth. Practices in some countries have involved young girls as well as young boys.

Publications of the U.S. Army have discussed widespread cultural pedophilia in Afghanistan. For example, one training manual mentioned that some Muslim adult males marry girls as young as 10. Soldiers might pass an older man walking hand-in-hand with a young boy, with the pair's behavior suggesting the man is not the boy's father. For centuries, Afghan men have taken boys, roughly 9 to 15 years old, as lovers. These men often like to boast about it.

Source: U.S. Army admits to widespread cultural pedophilia in Afghanistan. *Examiner.com*, 2012. Available: http://www.examiner.com/article/u-s-army-admits-to-widespread-cultural-s-s-a-pedophilia-afghanistan.

---

abuse, family conflict, childhood behavior problems, substance abuse, and personality disorders—particularly antisocial personality. According to one theory, pedophiles compensate for feelings of powerlessness by engaging in a type of sexual activity that provides them more control than adult relationships permit. Another theory indicates that pedophilia results from a diversion of sexual development that allows immature forms of desire to persist into adulthood. Another common view is that child molestation creates pedophiles. However, as pointed out earlier, most child sex abusers are not pedophiles.

Incidence of Pedophilia

As with other sexual offenses, it is difficult to know for sure how often pedophilia occurs. It is even more complicated because statistics do not differentiate between pedophilia and **child sexual abuse**. However, it is still germane to consider overall statistics regarding adult sexual contact with children.

According to statistics from the Rape, Abuse, and Incest National Network (Who are the victims?, 2015), approximately 44% of sexual assault and rape victims are younger than the age of 18 years. Fifteen percent are younger than age 12. Seven percent of girls in grades 5–8 and 12% of girls in grades 9–12 say they have been sexually abused. Three percent of

boys in grades 5–8 and 5% of boys in grades 9–12 say they have been sexually abused. Ninety-three percent of juvenile sexual assault victims knew their attacker (34% of attackers were family members, 59% were acquaintances, and only 7% were strangers to the victim). About 75% of the sexual abuse victims are girls. Nearly 30% of child victims are between the ages of 4 and 7 years.

Regarding males, about one-sixth of men report having had unwanted sexual contact with an older person by the age of 16. On average, boys first experience sexual abuse at age 10. The age range at which boys are first abused, however, is from infancy to later adolescence. Boys are most often abused by males (between 50% and 75%). However, it is hard to estimate the extent of abuse by females, because abuse by women is often covert. Also, a boy may consider it a "sexual initiation" and deny that it was abusive even though he may suffer significant trauma from the experience. A smaller proportion of sexually abused boys than sexually abused girls reports sexual abuse to authorities. While a majority of perpetrators (about 80%) were themselves abused, the vast majority of sexually abused boys (about 80%) never become adult perpetrators. Boys often feel physical sexual arousal during abuse even if they are repulsed by what is happening (Overcoming sexual victimization of boys and men, 2005).

People often think of child sexual abuse only as having sexual activity with a child. However, it includes a variety of possibilities, including fondling, obscene phone calls, exhibitionism, masturbation, intercourse, oral or anal sexual activity, prostitution, pornography, and any other sexual conduct that is

---

child sexual abuse Any sexual abuse involving fondling, erotic kissing, oral sexual activity, or genital penetration between an adult and a child, including pedophilia and incest.

Examples of Child Sexual Abuse Attitudes in Other Countries

A study carried out in six countries in the eastern Caribbean analyzed the perceptions of women and men aged 18 and older about child sexual abuse. Researchers asked if respondents felt that men's negative attitudes toward women were one of the causes of child sexual abuse. Most respondents either disagreed (60%) or were unsure (27%). However, 77% said that the way a girl dresses draws sexual attention from men.

Most respondents in the eastern Caribbean (85%) considered sexual abuse to be emotionally damaging to children in the long term. However, research showed a range of opinions in other parts of the world. In Norway, for instance, respondents expressed uncertainty about whether sexual contact was damaging to a child. In Nigeria, 61% of parents surveyed believed that abuse could have a serious health impact only when it involved intercourse.

Source: Hidden in plain sight: A statistical analysis of violence against children. UNICEF Division of Data, Research and Policy, September 2014. Available: http://www.unicef.org/publications/index_74865.html.

harmful to a child's mental, emotional, or physical welfare. It may consist of a single incident or many acts over a long period of time. It often escalates over time, especially if the abuser is a family member (Child sexual abuse, 2012).

The absence of force or coercion does not diminish the abusive nature of the conduct, but it may cause the child to feel responsible for what happened. Physical signs of child abuse may include difficulty walking or sitting; bloody, torn, or stained underclothes; bleeding, itching, or burning in the genital area; and frequent urinary or yeast infections. Common reactions of the child being abused can include withdrawal, depression, sleeping or eating disorders, school problems, anxiety, guilt, and possibly other reactions as well (Child sexual abuse, 2012).

In 2011 many people were shocked by the unaddressed child sexual abuse that occurred at Penn State University. Many questions arose, but the major one was: "What is it about the nature of intimate sexual violence that stops so many bystanders from taking action?" One lesson learned from the Penn State situation was that if you hear or witness sexual abuse or harassment it is important to speak up. In cases of abuse, it is never a time to keep silent; abuse should always be reported. It is also important to "abuse-proof" children. For example, the programs children attend should have strong policies on keeping children safe, including screening and background checks for volunteers and employees and ensuring that they are never alone with children. Children need to know that most people would never hurt them, but an older, bigger, or stronger person should never touch a child's genitals. They should know that adults do not ask children to be their "friend" or to keep secrets, and if someone makes them feel bad, funny, or uncomfortable with their touch or their words, they should tell a parent or other trusted adult. Children should realize that their body belongs to them, and they can say no to unwanted touch. If someone does touch them inappropriately, they need to tell the parent or other trusted adult (Haffner, 2011).

Online Pedophilia

As the Internet has developed, so have opportunities for Internet-related crimes such as pedophilia. Children are particularly vulnerable to sexual predators, such as pedophiles, on the Internet. Pedophiles have been known to use the Internet in at least two different ways. One is a trust-based seductive model in which the pedophile tries to build up trust with the child and then attempts to plan a meeting with the child. The other is a direct sexual model in which the pedophile hopes to make contact with the child.

Wolak et al. (2004) reported on a national sample of online sex abuse cases from a national sample of law enforcement agencies. They indicated that most offenders did not deceive victims about the fact that they were adults interested in sexual relationships. The victims, mainly 13 to 15 years of age, met and had sexual relations with the adults on more than one occasion. Half of the victims were described as being in love with or feeling close bonds with the offenders. Few offenders abducted or used force to sexually abuse their victims. Offenders targeted adolescents and not younger children. Ninety-nine percent were 13 to 17 years of age and none were younger than 12 years old. Victims and offenders had typically communicated, both online and by telephone, for more than a month prior to meeting in person.

Wolak et al. (2009) reported additional information related to online predators. There was dramatic growth nationwide in the number of arrests of online predators who solicited law enforcement investigators posing online as juveniles. While online predator arrests were increasing, overall sex offenses against children and adolescents were declining. Arrests of online predators constituted only 1% of all arrests for sex crimes committed against children and youth. These researchers also found that victims were adolescents and not younger children. Most offenders were open about their sexual motives in their online communications with youth. Few crimes (5%) involved violence.

In 2011 police smashed the world's largest online pedophilia ring. They rescued 230 children from abuse and arrested 184 suspects—including teachers and police officers. The 3-year investigation, code named Operation Rescue, uncovered 670 suspects and identified and safeguarded children in more than 30 countries by arresting people accused of abusing them. The ring was centered on an Amsterdam-based online forum called boylover.net. It was intended as a discussion forum where pedophiles could share their sexual interest in young boys (Foundation to Abolish Child Sex Abuse, 2011).

Guidelines for Internet safety related to online pedophilia are similar to more general guidelines for Internet safety. For example, children need to know not to reveal personal information or information about accounts or passwords online. Emails from unknown sources should be deleted, and mean, threatening, or off-color comments made online should be reported to parents. In addition, children need to remember that nothing they write on the Web is completely private. Parents should help their children learn the difference between credible sources of information and those that are not, establish rules for ordering products or participating in Internet discussions, and tell them to end online experiences when they feel uncomfortable (Internet safety, 2011).

Effects of Pedophilia

As with rape survivors, there can be a tendency to blame survivors of pedophilia. This blame can have psychological effects on the young people involved. There has been a great deal of debate about the effects of pedophilia and sexual abuse of children. Some studies connect sexual abuse to many future

Communication DIMENSIONS

Helping Survivors of Rape and Sexual Abuse

Even if you are not a trained counselor, if someone who has been raped or sexually abused talks with you about what has happened, you can be helpful by remembering the following points:

1. Listen in a supportive and nonjudgmental way, showing sympathy and concern. Ask questions and do not argue.
2. Encourage the person to express his or her feelings about the incident(s).
3. Control your own emotions. Do not react strongly and do not question the judgment of the survivor.
4. Indicate that you believe the account of what happened.
5. Let the survivor know that it was not his or her fault and that he or she is not to blame.
6. Give comfort and support.
7. Help the person focus on actions that might be needed, such as seeking medical treatment or reporting to police.
8. Try not to interrupt or ask a lot of questions.
9. Do not tell others what happened without your friend's permission.
10. The survivor must decide what to do; you cannot force him or her or make any decision you've determined.
11. Help the person find professional follow-up services—professional counseling, crisis center or domestic violence center guidance, legal assistance, medical follow-up—and accompany the person if that is appropriate and if the person desires it.
12. Survivors of rape and/or sexual abuse can respond in almost any way. They may be hysterical, amazingly calm, or anything in between. Almost any (or no) reaction is "normal."
13. Let the person know you are available to help or give support in the future.
14. Check as often as necessary to see how the person is progressing toward full recovery.

Source: Adapted from Bruess, C., & Richardson, G. *Decisions for health.* Madison, WI: Brown & Benchmark, 1995; Rape and sexual assault: Information for victims and friends. West Virginia Foundation for Rape Information and Services, 2015. Available: http://www.fris.org /VictimInformationGuide/VictimGuide.html.

DIMENSIONS

The Countries That Give the Most Severe Punishments for Rape

Number 5: Afghanistan. Afghanistan is a Muslim country and its laws are based on Islam. The punishment for committing rape is a bullet to the head within 4 days of the rape.

Number 4: United Arab Emirates. In Dubai, a rapist will be hanged. The rapist will die within 7 days of being found guilty.

Number 3: Egypt. Egypt is another country that hangs rapists. Recently, 10 men gang-raped a woman, and all of them got the death penalty.

Number 2: Iran. Iran offers capital punishment for many crimes, and 10% to 15% of executions in Iran are for rape.

Number 1: Saudi Arabia. The punishment for rape is very brutal. The person who commits rape will be stoned to death. The death is not easy or quick. The criminal has to go through the pain and torture of the stoning and suffer until death finally occurs.

Source: 10 countries which give most severe punishment for rape. *Spot On Lists,* 2015. Available: http://spotonlists.com/crime/10-countries-which-gives-most-severe-punishment-for-rape/.

problems, while others show little or no indication of negative effects of sexual victimization. In fact, a percentage of both men and women reported the experience as positive.

Obviously all children do not react the same way to child abuse. Some research has identified effects of child abuse that include sleeping and eating disturbances, anger, withdrawal, and guilt. Or there might be sexual preoccupation (excessive masturbation and an unusual interest in sexual organs and nudity) and a host of physical complaints such as rashes, vomiting, and headaches without medical explanation. Other common symptoms include shame, poor body image, self-destructive behavior, nightmares, relational and/or sexual dysfunction, and compulsive behaviors like drug addiction, gambling, or overeating. Other related effects could include depression, phobias, psychosomatic symptoms (such as stomachaches or headaches), school problems, poor hygiene or excessive bathing, anxiety, and regressive behaviors (thumb-sucking, etc.) (Child sexual abuse, 2012).

Although not a lot of information is available on the topic, the effects among LGBT people and heterosexuals seem to be very similar. For example, Arreola et al. (2008) studied the effects of forced, consensual, and no childhood sexual experiences on health outcomes among a sample of adult men who have sexual activity with men. They found that the forced-sex group had the highest levels of psychological distress, substance use, and HIV risk.

Often, sexual assault experiences are less traumatic for the child than for the parents. It is important that adults understand children's feelings and reactions, because a child often suffers no lasting trauma if parents can control their reactions.

Prevention

Preventing child sexual abuse demands attention. Fortunately, in recent years programs have been designed to educate children and adults to distinguish between appropriate and inappropriate touch, to say no to unwanted or uncomfortable touch, to tell a trusted adult if inappropriate touch occurs, and to identify their family and community support systems. In addition, adolescents have been encouraged to consider the risks related to certain behaviors, the selection of a mate who will not abuse their children, and ways in which they will protect children from sexual abuse.

Developing children's competence is essential, with the objective of helping children to recognize abusive situations and disclose victimization. In addition, parents can help children learn about sexual abuse in appropriate ways. They can also help children know some basic ways to help prevent sexual abuse such as (Pedophilia: Who are the men who "love" children in intolerable ways?, 2005):

- Never disclose personal information, such as your address, to strangers online.

- Never meet privately in person with anyone you have met online.

- Never get close to a car if a stranger stops and asks for directions.

- Never accept a ride from, or go anywhere alone with, an adult you don't know.

- No adult should touch you or ask you to touch him or her in any way that is confusing or frightening. If this happens, refuse and tell your parent immediately.

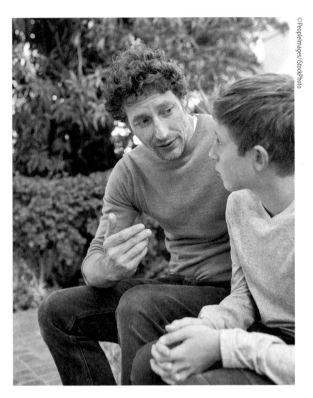

It is important to communicate about sexual abuse and how to prevent it.

- No adult should ever ask you to keep a touch or a kiss secret. If this happens, tell your parent immediately.

- If any of these things happen, you will not be punished even if you have broken a rule.

A major challenge for prevention is the population of young teens who are willing to enter into voluntary sexual relationships with adults whom they meet online. People are often reluctant to confront these situations, but effective prevention requires public and private recognition of what actually happens in these cases. Teens may benefit from being told directly about why such relationships are a bad idea and made to understand that adults who care about their well-being would not propose sexual relationships or involve them in risky encounters. Efforts should be focused on the most vulnerable teens, such as those who have poor relationships with their parents, those who are lonely or depressed, or gay teens or those who are questioning their sexual orientation and turn to others on the Internet for support or information. Training is also needed for law enforcement personnel because teens may not initially see themselves as victims and may require sensitive interviewing to cooperate with investigators.

Educators, parents, and other adults need to learn to recognize physical and behavioral signs of sexual abuse and pay attention to indirectly related comments made by a child. Physical signs may include irritation, pain, or injury in the genital area. Behavioral signs may include nervous, aggressive, hostile, or disruptive behavior toward adults, especially parents. It is wise to remember that one sign alone may not be a positive indication, but if a number of signs are present, the possibility of sexual abuse should be considered. One should believe the child, remain calm, avoid blaming the child, avoid leading questions such as "You did that a lot?" and know where to seek help for counseling services. Adults also need to help children learn that they do not have to agree to demands for physical closeness; that touching can be good, bad, or confusing; that some secrets should not be kept; that at times adults make mistakes and do things they should not; and that there are times to ask for help and to give help when asked for help by a friend.

Another way to help prevent sexual abuse is to carefully screen professionals who work with children. For example, in many states it is necessary for teachers and other school personnel to have a background check before they can assume their responsibilities. This is usually done by requiring fingerprinting of such professionals before they are hired.

A vivid example of the need to screen individuals working with children carefully was seen when a Boston church scandal started a chain reaction.

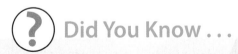

? Did You Know . . .

Law enforcement personnel are recognizing the need for special training to handle child sexual abuse cases. Without proper training, innocent people can be falsely charged, valid cases may have to be dismissed, and children and others involved may not be treated as well as possible.

Training includes the dynamics of child sexual abuse, the science of interviewing children, and approaches to verifying and corroborating allegations. Understanding the psychological needs of the victim, recognizing the sometimes vague symptoms of abuse, and knowing how to elicit sensitive information about sexual behavior from children are essential skills for law enforcement personnel.

In January 2002, Boston's Cardinal Bernard Law acknowledged that he had moved a priest from parish to parish despite evidence that he had molested children. Soon afterward, church files revealed that another priest had abused children and advocated sexual activities between men and boys but still received the archdiocese's support. Before the year was over, thousands of adults filed lawsuits over abuse they said occurred when they were boys and girls—some as long as 50 years earlier. Five U.S. bishops, including Cardinal Law, resigned for reasons related to sexual abuse of children. Although he was not personally accused of abuse, Law resigned because of his failure to deal effectively with abusers who were priests. Interestingly, Law then abruptly moved to Rome and took up a series of positions in the Vatican. He was appointed archpriest of the Basilica di Santa Maria Maggiore, and also took full part in a conclave that selected the successor to Pope John Paul II (Hitchens, 2008). This certainly sent mixed signals regarding the Vatican's feelings about Law's actions.

As a result of this scandal, Roman Catholic bishops adopted a new policy for handling priests accused of sexual abuse. If a priest is found guilty by a board composed mostly of lay Catholics and at least one priest, he cannot wear a collar or give Communion, and he may be stripped of his status. In addition, most priests indicated they will tell the police about sexual abuse allegations in the future. A set of guidelines called the Charter for the Protection of Children and Young People was also developed and adopted by the nation's Roman Catholic Bishops in 2002. In 2011 they voted overwhelmingly to maintain those church policies on the sexual abuse of children. This was a controversial move, because many victims' advocates felt the policies are weak and unenforceable and have not stopped child sexual abuse by Catholic church leaders (Burke, 2011).

In recent years, all 50 states have passed laws requiring sex offenders to alert the community to their presence. Many states run Internet sites listing such criminals. In some states judges have ordered offenders to post signs outside their homes, mandated bumper stickers, and even required temporary placards for traveling in someone else's car. Some people argue these laws are appropriate to help protect society from sex offenders; others consider it inappropriate to brand people and even punish their families.

In many states there is a law requiring rapists and child molesters to register each year for inclusion in a database of sex offenders. Failure to register is usually a felony and can result in more jail time. Even so, the state of California lost track of more than 33,000 sex offenders, or 44% of the total number of registered offenders. They simply vanished after registering. Nationally, 52% of rapists are arrested for new crimes within 3 years of leaving prison, according to the U.S. Justice Department (Curtis, 2003).

In 2006, the Adam Walsh Child Protection and Safety Act was passed by the U.S. Congress. It requires all states to adopt strict standards for registering sex offenders and is meant to prevent offenders from eluding authorities, especially when they move out of state. The act made it a federal crime (a felony) to fail to reregister as a sex offender, after moving to another state and requires states to toughen their penalties for failing to register at all; currently, many states treat such failure as a misdemeanor. An estimated 100,000 sex offenders are not living where they are registered. A number of controversial points have been raised in relation to the act. State officials complain about the law's cost, may believe they have more effective laws than the federal one, and say the federal requirements violate the states' right to set their own policies. In addition, some sex offenders and civil liberties groups have argued that juvenile sex offenders should not have to be on public registries for life and note that the law does not take into account the individual circumstances of each sex offender.

College officials have to decide how to best deal with the Campus Sex Crimes Prevention Act, a federal law that requires sex offenders, when they register with the state, to indicate whether and where they are enrolled, employed, or volunteering on a college campus. College officials must tell students, faculty, and administrators where information on registered sex offenders can be obtained. Most have chosen to make the registry available for perusal in the campus police department and made its existence known either through the college's website or by mailing of pamphlets that direct students and others to its location.

In many states treatment for those convicted of sexual abuse of children is required by law. It is hoped that such treatment will help prevent future sexual abuse, but much remains to be learned about effective treatment. Many treatment methods have been tried. For example, aversion therapy is used to associate a pedophilic fantasy or desire with an unpleasant sensation such as nausea or an electric shock. Behavior therapy is also used to help offenders exercise self-control by changing their beliefs and attitudes as well as their behavior. Many other psychological techniques have been tried, such as externalization where the offender learns how his or her actions look and feel to the child. A number of medications have also been tried with the hope of diminishing sexual desire. It is difficult to tell for sure just how effective various treatments have been. Research results about treatments have not been conclusive.

Ethical DIMENSIONS

Is It Ethical to Publicly Identify Sexual Offenders?

Named after Megan Kanka, a 7-year-old New Jersey child who was raped and murdered by a convicted sex offender who lived across the street from her, "Megan's Law" requires that authorities and the community be notified when a convicted sex offender is released or moves into their neighborhood. Variations of Megan's Law are found in a number of states. For example, Alabama's Megan's Law also forbids a convicted offender to live near a school, day care center, or past victim.

Some people want a law requiring that the identity of convicted child molesters be made known to community members. This means that if a convicted child molester moved into your community, you and all your neighbors would be informed that he or she was there and that he or she had been a child molester. Many people support such a law because they feel they have a right to protect their children.

Other people think it is a violation of individual rights and personal privacy if a convicted child molester's identity is made public. They believe that the molester, as

has any other person convicted of a crime, has paid for the crime through a prison sentence and in other possible ways, and it is not ethical to reveal his or her identity to the public. The person has a right to live privately and to start a new life if he or she desires. On the basis of these arguments, there have been legal challenges to Megan's Law in New Jersey, and similar laws have been found unconstitutional in other states.

In Virginia, state police developed a website that lists the names of violent sex offenders. They guessed that 5,000 people would log on on the first day. In fact, in the first 12 hours, it was visited more than 45,000 times. By the second day, the site was so jammed that many people could not get through because the site can handle only six "hits" per second. Some people express the point of view that we should not be concerned about former sex offenders being harassed, because "If they don't want their names in the paper, they shouldn't commit the crime." Others question the ethics of this website and feel it treats sex offenders unfairly.

Do you think it is ethical to require that identities of sexual offenders be made public?

Incest

Incest is sexual behavior between relatives who are too closely related to be legally married. Much of what has been said about child sexual abuse also applies to incest. However, it is helpful to consider incest separately because it is rapidly changing from a private subject to a public one.

Most contemporary research studies related to incest seem to focus on the offenders, family relationships, and possible treatments. There is not much new information about incest statistics. Because of that, there are very few reliable statistics about how often incest occurs.

The most commonly reported form of incest is father–daughter, but in practice brother–sister incest probably happens more often. Mother–child incest has traditionally been thought to be virtually nonexistent, but today many experts feel that the amount of sexual abuse of children by women has been underestimated.

It is hard to know how many people are affected by incest because many incest situations never get reported. The victim might not report the abuse for a variety of reasons. For example:

1. The victim has been told that what is happening is normal and doesn't realize that it is a form of abuse.

2. The victim may not know that help is available or who he or she can talk to.

3. The victim may be afraid of what will happen if he or she tells someone. (The abuser may have threatened the victim, the victim may be afraid of what will happen, or the victim may care about the abuser and be afraid of what might happen to the abuser.)

4. The victim may be concerned about how people might react when they hear about the abuse. (Maybe no one will believe him or her, maybe someone will tell the abuser, maybe people will say that she or he did something wrong) (Incest, 2012).

incest Sexual behavior between relatives who are too closely related to be married.

Incest victims look and act like anyone else. However, they may suffer from long-term psychological consequences.

Guilt and shame also play a big part in a child's decision not to ask for help after incest has occurred. This is especially true if the child was raised in a home where sexual behavior is considered dirty or sinful. Also, the child may be uncertain what to think about the experience. With this uncertainty, he/she may decide it is safer not to say anything.

Those who commit incest usually appear to be very nice people. The vast majority of offenders (often estimated at 95%) are probably male, and there is often a patriarchal family structure. Contrary to what many think, stepfathers do not seem to be involved in incest any more often than biological fathers. When confronted, most offenders are truly sorry for their actions, but the vast majority do not believe they have done anything particularly wrong. Many believe they have a right to educate their children about sexual behavior and to use their children to meet their own sexual needs. Many refuse to believe that they really hurt their children.

The incest taboo seems universal in human culture. Anthropologists often consider it to be the foundation of all kinship structures and even the basis of human social order. Nevertheless, incest occurs in all social classes, in all geographic areas, and among all ethnic and racial groups.

Many of the reactions to and effects from incest are similar to those related to sexual abuse of children in general. However, incest can be especially damaging because it disrupts the child's primary support system, the family. When the abuser is someone in the family, the family may not be able to provide support or a sense of security. Because children often have limited resources outside the family, it can be hard for them to recover from incest. Incest can damage a child's ability to trust, because the people who were supposed to protect and care for them abused them. It can also be very damaging for a child if a nonabusing parent is aware of the abuse and chooses—for whatever reason—not to take action to stop it. This might happen because the nonabusing parent feels dependent on the abuser for financial support, is afraid of losing the partner, thinks incest is normal in families, or feels that the child was "asking for it" or blames the child for some other reason (Incest, 2012).

The possible behavioral signs of incest are also similar to those of sexual abuse in general. They can include eating disorders or loss of appetite, extreme changes in behavioral patterns, lack of self-confidence, unexplained fear of a particular person, unusual knowledge of sexual matters, regressing to infantile behavior, poor interpersonal relationships, or attempts to run away. Obviously, some of the symptoms of incest can also be normal adolescent problems, but parents and teachers need to at least be aware of the possibility that incest has occurred.

Sexual abuse experts say some victims of incest use overeating to escape inner turmoil and downplay their femininity. They might gain weight so their bodies do not look so good. They might also avoid unwanted attention to their bodies by wearing baggy clothes along with gaining too much weight (McGee, 2007).

Various community organizations offer help for incest survivors and their families—for example, child-protection agencies, rape crisis centers, women's centers, and organizations that offer help for parents who are under extreme stress or are frightened about their feelings toward their children. The best strategy for preventing incest is to provide information to children as well as to parents. This means providing sexuality education at the elementary school level and above, including specific information about incest. For example, children should be taught that Uncle Charlie or Aunt Mary does not automatically have the right to touch them all over. In addition, information about pedophilia and other sexual practices should be provided at the appropriate level of understanding.

The initial focus of crisis intervention should be on stopping the sexual abuse and establishing a safe environment in the family. Once the incest is reported, it is controversial whether the child should be temporarily removed from the home. This might be destructive to children because they may feel that they have done something wrong, that they are being punished, or that both parents are against them. It is also difficult to find an appropriate place to put the child; however, removal from the home may be the only way to ensure the child's safety.

There is also a nationwide group called Survivors of Incest Anonymous that works very much like Alcoholics Anonymous. It is a self-help group of women and men, 18 years and older, who are guided by a set of 12 Suggested Steps and 12 Traditions. The only requirement for membership is that you are a victim of child sexual abuse, and that you are not abusing any child. More information about Survivors of Incest Anonymous can be found at www.siawso.org.

■ Relationship Abuse

According to the Center for Relationship Abuse Awareness, relationship abuse is a pattern of abusive and coercive behaviors used to maintain power and control over a former or current intimate partner. Many types of abuse are possible, including emotional, financial, sexual, and physical. Relationship abuse can include threats, isolation, and intimidation. Abuse tends to escalate over time. When someone levies this kind of abuse against a partner, it is part of a larger pattern of control. The majority of relationship abuse is committed by men against women in heterosexual relationships, but it happens at the same rate in LGBTQ relationships. For the most part, what is said about relationship abuse applies to both males and females and to both heterosexual and LGBTQ relationships (*What is relationship abuse?*, 2014).

Worldwide, including in the United States, one partner commits relationship abuse or sexual assault against the other partner in at least one-third of relationships. Nevertheless, this kind of abuse probably does not show up in statistics as often as it actually occurs. Relationship abuse occurs in all socioeconomic groups, to people of all ages. To stem this tide of abuse, abusers must be held accountable to send a message to others that abuse of any kind will not be tolerated in the community.

Many types of abuse have been documented, as the following examples illustrate (*What is relationship abuse?*, 2014):

- Technology abuse: using an online identity to post false information, using GPS devices to monitor a partner's location, sending repeated messages, or monitoring a partner's email

- Physical abuse: withholding foods, medications, or medical treatment; locking a partner out of the house; slapping, beating, or threatening physical harm to a partner

- Academic abuse: making fun of a partner for studying too much, preventing a partner from working on papers or tests, taking all the same classes as a partner, blaming a partner for poor grades

- Economic abuse: preventing a partner from having or keeping a job, harassing a partner at work, refusing to work, not involving a partner in financial decisions, making the partner ask for money, demanding an account of everything a partner buys

Regardless of the type of relationship or its stage, there are important signs of relationship abuse. When these appear, it is wise to take steps to deal with them effectively or get out of the relationship. They are (1) isolation, (2) jealousy, (3) possessiveness, (4) double standards, (5) name-calling, (6) controlling behavior, (7) threats of self-harm, (8) playing rough, (9) nonconsensual sexual activity, and (10) violence (Ten signs of relationship abuse, 2008).

Marital Rape

Until the late 1970s, most states did not consider spousal rape to be a crime. In most cases, spouses were exempted from the sexual assault laws. For example, until 1993 North Carolina law stated that "a person may not be prosecuted under this article if the victim is the person's legal spouse at the time of the commission of the alleged rape or sexual offense unless the parties are living separate and apart." These laws date all the way back to the seventeenth century, when it was said that "for by their mutual matrimonial consent and contract the wife hath given up herself in this kind unto the husband which she cannot retract." In the late 1970s, feminists began efforts to change these laws. Currently, rape of a spouse is a crime in all 50 states and the District of Columbia (Spousal rape laws: 20 years later, 2004).

Although it is probably the most underreported rape, marital rape is prevalent. Of all reported rapes in the United States, 25% are marital rapes. It is estimated that between 10% and 14% of married women are raped by their husbands. Many of these women have also been battered by their husbands (How commonplace is marital rape?, 2015).

It was not until 1993 that it became illegal in every state to rape one's spouse. States took three different approaches to criminalizing marital rape. Some states just abolished the marital rape exception by striking it from the books. With this approach, which most states followed, marital rape is treated the same as other forms of rape. A second approach was to explicitly eliminate marriage as a defense to the charge of rape. A third approach was to leave the marital rape exemption in the code and create a separate offense of marital rape (sometimes with lesser penalties than for other forms of rape).

Special issues faced by marital rape victims, as distinguished from other rape victims, include the following (*Marital rape*, 2015):

- Longer recovery from trauma. This is probably because of lack of recognition and ability to share the pain, and the strong sense of betrayal of trust.

- Higher likelihood of repeated assaults. Marital rape victims are more likely to experience repeated assaults than other rape victims.

- Tendency of married perpetrators to use anal and oral rape to humiliate, punish, and take "full" ownership of their partners.

- Pressure to stay with the perpetrator. There may be financial dependence on the spouse and/or pressure from friends or family members to stay with the perpetrator.

- Negative effects on children in the household. Such children may witness the violence or otherwise be affected by it.

- Difficulty identifying what happened as a crime. Victims may find it hard, for cultural reasons, to define a spouse's conduct as rape or to identify someone they married as a "rapist."

Marital rape remains a controversial issue, if only because some people still believe myths and misinformation about spousal rape. Some people believe that spousal rape is contractually impossible because they believe that spouses give up their right to not give consent when they marry their partner. Others believe in the concept of marital unity and insist that the spouses are one person under the law, which means that the legal existence of the other person is suspended. Some people also voice concerns that the potential for marriage reconciliation might be negated by rape laws. In addition, in some countries a wife is still considered property of the husband, so a husband cannot be convicted of hurting his own property. There are also people who do not believe that marital rape is as physically and emotionally damaging as stranger rape. Some people suggest that, out of revenge or for their own personal gain, one spouse might destroy the other's life by making false allegations of marital rape. Finally, some worry that the legal system, in trying to deal with marital rape, might become bogged down by cases that are impossible to prove (Stritof, 2015).

It seems that women raped by a spouse are more likely to experience long-term effects than are women raped by an acquaintance or a stranger. Possible long-term effects include (1) negative feelings toward men; (2) low self-esteem; (3) fear; (4) anxiety; (5) guilt; (6) embarrassment; (7) outrage; (8) changes in behaviors, including an increase in drinking and refusal to consider remarriage; and (9) depression.

Domestic violence is a pattern of behavior used to establish power and control over another person through fear and intimidation, often including the threat or use of violence. Other terms used to describe this behavior include intimate-partner violence, battering, spousal abuse, and family violence. Domestic violence can happen to anyone, regardless of gender, race, ethnicity, sexual orientation, income, or other factors. Women and men can be both victims or perpetrators of domestic violence. Men are victims of nearly 3 million domestic physical assaults in the United States, and 1 in 4 women will experience domestic violence during her lifetime. More than 60% of domestic violence incidents happen in the home. Domestic violence is the third leading cause of homelessness among families, and women ages 20 to 24 are at greatest risk of becoming victims of domestic violence. One in 3 homicide victims is murdered by a current or former partner every year. More than 3 million children witness domestic violence in their homes every year. Children who grow up in homes where there is domestic violence are more likely to suffer domestic violence as adults, have health problems including becoming sick more often, have frequent headaches or stomachaches, and be more tired and lethargic. Domestic violence victims face high rates of depression, sleep disturbances, anxiety, flashbacks, and other emotional distress. In the United States, domestic violence costs more than $37 billion per year in law enforcement involvement, legal work, medical and mental health treatment, and lost productivity at companies (*Domestic violence: Statistics and facts*, 2015).

Domestic violence often follows a repeating cycle within each relationship. Not all abusive relationships follow this pattern, but many survivors describe their relationships this way. First, there is a *tension building phase* in which victims may feel they are "walking on eggshells" around the abuser. This phase can last for a few hours or for months, or anything in between. The victim cannot be sure exactly what will be "the straw that breaks the camel's back." The *abusive incident* usually occurs when the tension finally breaks and the abuser lashes out at the victim. The abuser may hit, rape, or try to rape the victim; he or she may also use psychological tactics

In the movie *Gone with the Wind*, the husband, Rhett Butler (played by Clark Gable), carries his wife, Scarlett O'Hara (Vivien Leigh), kicking and screaming up a staircase, implying sexual activity is to follow. Portrayed as sensual more than 75 years ago, could it be considered spousal rape by today's standards?

such as denying the victim basic necessities (e.g., by changing locks on the doors or cutting off access to a shared checking account), calling the victim humiliating names, or making threats of violence. Next, a *honeymoon phase* may occur, in which the abuser may apologize, buy gifts, or be extra-affectionate to "make up" for the abuse. Many abusers promise to change and stop abusing, or swear that the abuse will never happen again. This reassurance is intended to persuade the survivor to stay in the relationship. Not all abusive relationships have a honeymoon phase, however. In some cases, the abusive incident is soon followed by mounting tension that leads to the next incident. In most cases, the abuser will not really change, and the only way to end the abuse is for the victim to end the relationship. Unfortunately, the most dangerous time can be when the victim tries to leave. Victims of relationship abuse are encouraged to access the National Domestic Violence hotline (1-800-799-SAFE [7233]), which can be called at any time of day or night, seven days a week, to speak to someone trained to help (Focht, 2013).

Children may also become involved in intimate-partner violence. Many adults who abuse their intimate partners frequently abuse their children as well. Many victims of relationship violence live in homes with children younger than age 12. Even if they are not objects of violence themselves, many children witness some form of domestic violence.

Experts suggest that domestic violence against men is understudied and often hidden. Indeed, there are some commonly held misconceptions about domestic violence against men. For example, one myth is that few men experience domestic violence. When 400 randomly selected men were interviewed by phone, it was found that 5% experienced domestic violence in the previous year, 10% in the past 5 years, and 29% at some point during their lifetime. Even if the abuse was not physical in nature, the men who were abused suffered serious, long-term mental health effects. Depression symptoms were nearly 3 times as common in older men who had experienced abuse. Most men in abusive relationships stayed in the relationships, through multiple episodes, for years. Although some people believe that domestic violence affects only the poor, the survey revealed that men from all walks of life were affected by this issue. Many men were ashamed to speak out about their abuse because of society's expectations that men should be strong and in control. Older men, for example, were less likely to speak out than younger men (Schimelpfening, 2013).

There are several types of marital rape. *Battering rape* is when beating and rape are combined. Some may experience physical abuse during the sexual assault. Others may experience sexual assault after a physical assault as an attempt to "make up." *Force-only rape* is motivated by a need to demonstrate power and maintain control. Therefore, the perpetrator asserts his or her feelings or entitlement over the partner in the form of forced sexual contact. *Obsessive/sadistic rape* involves torture and perverse sexual acts. It is characteristically violent and often leads to physical injury. Survivors of partner rape are more likely to be raped multiple times when compared to stranger and acquaintance rape survivors. Therefore, partner rape survivors are more likely to suffer severe and long-lasting physical and psychological injuries (Partner rape, 2012).

Intimate-Partner Violence

Domestic violence is a significant health and social problem in the United States and many other industrialized societies. In some industrialized societies, however, it is considered to be almost nonexistent. The reasons for the variability from culture to culture have not been established. Intimate-partner violence occurs for many reasons. It can be an indication of manhood, a means of personal control, a reflection of personal animosity, and an expression of social jealousy. Many who are victims of violence are often unable or afraid to seek health care, and violence also has serious consequences for maternal mortality and child survival.

It is difficult to estimate rates of intimate-partner violence. Many factors inhibit people from reporting these crimes. The private nature of the event,

NO MORE is a unifying symbol and movement to raise public awareness and engage bystanders around ending domestic violence and sexual assault. Many advertising groups, celebrities, and public figures are part of this Public Service Announcement campaign.

the perceived stigma, and the belief that no purpose would be served by reporting the crime prevent an unknown percentage of survivors from talking about the event. Therefore, available statistics are at best estimates.

Those who are battered may stay with a batterer for a number of reasons, including financial dependence, lack of social support (the batterer may have controlled the victim's contact with other people), fear of severe physical attack, self-blame (believing the abuse is a result of the victim's real or imagined offenses), or belief that the violence is temporary or caused by unusual circumstances. Many battered women believe the abuse will stop when "things return to normal" (Dating and domestic violence, 2009).

We have been slow to recognize the problem of intimate-partner violence. In the past, laws and common practice encouraged husbands to discipline their wives by force if they saw fit. But conditions have changed. Family violence research has made it clear that the problem of battering is too widespread to ignore or to explain away by blaming the victim. Many new resources are available. Battered women's shelters are particularly helpful in providing services for battered women and their children and in continuing efforts to educate people about intimate- partner violence.

Most of the research discussed so far has been about heterosexual couples. However, existing studies show that the prevalence as well as the types of abuse and the dynamics of abuse are very similar between heterosexual and LGBT couples.

There are ways we can combat intimate-partner violence. Here are some possibilities (101 ways to combat domestic violence, 2003):

1. Make violence unacceptable in your life.

2. Contact your local school board and ask its members to address dating violence.

3. Contact your local media representatives and remind them that October is Domestic Violence Awareness Month. Ask them what they plan to do. Tell them about the National Domestic Violence Hotline (800-799-SAFE), and ask them to publicize it.

4. Contact community businesses and agencies, and ask them to display the number of the National Domestic Violence Hotline in prominent places.

5. Contact local schools and colleges and let students know about resources available on the Internet concerning intimate-partner violence.

6. Ask the local police department to be sure officers are trained in handling intimate-partner violence.

7. Ask your priest, pastor, rabbi, or other religious leader to have a special service devoted to intimate-partner violence.

8. Do not let jokes about violent behavior go unchallenged.

9. Work with day care centers to make information about intimate-partner violence available to their customers.

10. Learn more about policies and facilities related to intimate-partner violence in your community.

Services for survivors of intimate-partner violence have been improved through the years, but more and better services are still needed. In 1994, the Violence Against Women Act was passed by Congress; it was extended in 2000. Its purpose was to broaden the range of services and counseling available to women victims of abuse. In 2005, the act was reauthorized, and it increased funding for new rape crisis centers and increased grant money to organizations working on intimate-partner violence issues. In 2014, the act was reauthorized again. Much of the revised provisions focused on college campuses. For example, institutions were required to maintain statistics about domestic violence and sexual assaults, provide prevention and awareness programs to incoming

Multicultural DIMENSIONS

Examples of Sexual Violence in Other Countries

Many South African girls have enduring experiences of sexual violence both in and out of school. There is often a general fear of boys and men in schools, in the neighborhood, and even in the home. Male sexual violence seems to be one of the gender norms in this country. The freedom of girls is compromised as a result, so this pattern is often viewed as a human rights issue (Bhana, 2012).

In much of China, violence among adolescent dating partners remains a largely ignored and invisible phenomenon. Data collected from a probability sample of 976 adolescents from Taiwan, Hong Kong, and Shanghai revealed a high prevalence of dating violence (including physical violence, sexual violence, and controlling behavior), with a victimization rate of 39%. Adolescents who endorse traditional gender-role beliefs are more likely to view dating violence as acceptable behavior (Shen et al., 2013).

Among Ethiopian higher education students, affirmative action policies benefit women at the entry point into the educational system. However, prejudice against women and sexual violence are key expressions of qualitative gender inequalities in higher education. The institutions seem to be male dominated, hierarchical, and hostile to women. Furthermore, taken-for-granted gender assumptions and beliefs at institutional and individual levels operate to make women conform to structures of disadvantage and in effect sustain the repressive gender relations (Molla & Cuthbert, 2014).

 ## Did You Know . . .

Violence by women received little attention until the mid-1970s. Now we know that women in relationships engage in violent acts as often as men. In about half of violent relationships, the violence is mutual. When there is a sole perpetrator, it is just as likely to be a female as a male. However, female use of violence, even when intended to cause harm, is mainly self-defensive.

Men tend to inflict more severe damage on women than the converse. Reasons given for this are that women tend to cease violent behaviors before causing serious injury and that men are usually physically larger and stronger than women.

The needs of battered men are somewhat different from those of battered women. Abused women have varied needs, including safety for themselves and often for their children; abused men's needs are more limited. Because they usually have the necessary resources to leave the relationship, their primary needs are legal assistance and psychological counseling.

students and new employees, provide descriptions of any disciplinary proceedings, and develop more sophisticated procedures for record-keeping and reporting among other requirements (*Federal Register*, 2014).

Also, the Office for Victims of Crime of the U.S. Department of Justice provided funding in 1997 to develop Sexual Assault Nurse Examiner (SANE) programs designed to improve the community response to sexual assault victims. There are now hundreds of these programs around the country, and new ones are started every month. The goal is to see that every victim receives fundamental justice and needed services.

One excellent example is the Summit County SANE program in Colorado. The specialized nurses who participate in SANE provide comprehensive medical care and evidence collection in the local hospital's emergency department. The nurses are also trained and available to provide expert witness testimony in court. The SANE program provides a valuable community service that should help increase victim reporting rates and the prosecution of perpetrators (Sexual Assault Nurse Examiner [SANE] Program, 2015).

■ Sexual Harassment

Since the mid-1970s, courts, popular and professional periodicals, newspapers, and books have focused on **sexual harassment**. Hundreds of articles have appeared in print, increasing the national attention

sexual harassment Unwelcome verbal, physical, or sexual conduct that has the effect of creating an intimidating, hostile, or offensive environment paid to the subject. It is not easy to define sexual harassment. Sometimes it is hard to draw the line between harassment and other behaviors, but it can include touching, verbal abuse, demanding of sexual favors, or use of threatening tones.

The U.S. Equal Employment Opportunity Commission (EEOC) says that sexual harassment is a form of sex discrimination that violates Title VII of the Civil Rights Act of 1964. It defines sexual harassment as unwelcome sexual advances, requests for sexual favors, and other verbal or physical conduct of a sexual nature when this conduct explicitly or implicitly affects an individual's employment, unreasonably interferes with an individual's work performance, or creates an intimidating, hostile, or offensive work environment (Facts about sexual harassment, 2015). The EEOC also says that sexual harassment can occur in a variety of circumstances, including but not limited to the following:

- The victim as well as the harasser may be a woman or a man. The victim does not have to be of the other sex.

- The harasser can be the victim's supervisor, an agent of the employer, a supervisor in another area, a coworker, or a non-employee.

- The victim does not have to be the person harassed but could be anyone affected by the offensive conduct.

- Unlawful sexual harassment may occur without economic injury to or discharge of the victim.

- The harasser's conduct must be unwelcome.

The Commission further says that it is helpful for the victim to inform the harasser directly that the conduct is unwelcome and must stop. The victim should use any employer complaint mechanism or grievance system available.

Sexual harassment may include verbal abuse; sexist remarks regarding a person's clothing or body; patting, pinching, or brushing up against a person's body; leering or ogling; demand for sexual favors in return for hiring, promotion, or tenure; physical assault; and rape. Two categories of sexual harassment have been described. In the first, something is to be exchanged. Perhaps a boss offers a person a job opportunity in exchange for sexual favors or threatens loss of a job opportunity if the person does not comply. In the second, there is no promise or threat; however, there are sexual remarks, touching/stroking, or lewd looks.

Legally speaking, then, there are two kinds of sexual harassment. The first is quid pro quo (Latin for "something for something"): Something is to be exchanged. For example, a perpetrator might make conditions of employment contingent on the victim

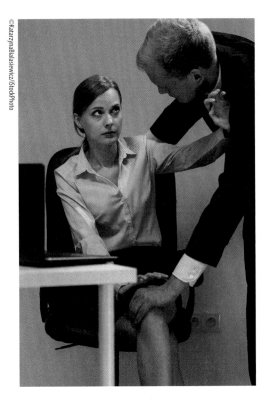

Workplace sexual harassment can include various behaviors. Coworkers need to indicate when behavior is inappropriate and unwanted.

providing sexual favors. The second is a hostile environment. This is when unwelcome severe and persistent sexual conduct by the perpetrator creates an uncomfortable and hostile environment (for example, jokes, lewd postures, leering, inappropriate touching, etc.). This type of harassment constitutes up to 95% of all sexual harassment cases (Sexual harassment, 2012).

In 1991 Anita Hill's testimony at confirmation hearings for Supreme Court Justice Clarence Thomas brought into the open the problem of sexual harassment. Previously, it had been an issue that millions of victims privately recognized but rarely discussed before Hill told her story. Since that time, many employers started training programs to deter sexual harassment, but it is thought that even today only a small proportion of sexual harassment victims risk stigma and potential job losses to pursue claims.

The EEOC has kept statistics related to sexual harassment since 1997. The number of charges filed with the EEOC each year has remained relatively consistent, but has decreased somewhat over the years. For example, there were almost 16,000 charges in 1997, almost 14,000 in 2008, and about 11,300 in 2011. The percentage of charges filed by males increased from 11.6% in 1997 to 16.3% in 2011 (Sexual harassment charges, 2015).

In 2009, the U.S. Supreme Court ruled that workers who cooperate with an internal investigation and

In recent years, more attention has been paid to sexual harassment in schools. All too often, reports cite a teacher sexually harassing his or her students. If you were a parent, what would you recommend that your child do if he or she believes sexual harassment is occurring?

report uncouth behavior by a supervisor are protected from retaliation under civil rights laws (Sexual harassment, 2009). This ruling further strengthened laws against sexual harassment in the workplace.

Efforts to end sexual harassment that rely mainly on target reporting are unlikely to be successful because most targets do not report their experiences. They tend to deny the harassment, avoid the harasser, or treat the harassment as a joke rather than confronting the harasser or reporting the behavior. It seems that the targets don't report the offenses because they want to avoid reprisal by the harasser and maintain their reputation and status in the workgroup. For this reason, some experts feel that one way for progress to be made against sexual harassment is for those who observe the harassment to be the ones who report it.

In addition to being upsetting and distracting, workplace sexual harassment can even be hazardous to health. For example, common emotional and physical reactions include poor concentration at work, staff turnover, increased absenteeism, lower staff productivity, poor staff morale, less teamwork, fear/anxiety, and stress on personal relationships (*Sexual harassment*, 2015). Harassment may be hazardous not only to targets' health, but also to the bottom line of the organization in the form of costly worker's compensation claims.

Online Sexual Harassment

As use of the Internet has grown, so has sexual harassment on the Internet. While it is impossible to know the extent of sexual harassment on the Internet, it seems that most victims are women. The three general types of offline sexual harassment also exist online:

(1) gender harassment—unwelcome comments that insult individuals because of their gender or that use stimuli intended to provoke negative emotions; (2) unwanted sexual attention—uninvited behaviors that communicate sexual desires or intentions toward another individual; and (3) sexual coercion—putting pressure on a person to elicit sexual cooperation.

Online sexual coercion can become actual coercion if a perpetrator uses technical knowledge to break into a person's computer and cause damage or threaten to do so. Technology—such as digital photos, videos, apps, and social media—can be used to engage in harassing, unsolicited, or nonconsensual sexual interactions. Such attacks can leave the recipient feeling manipulated, unsafe, and exposed—for example, when someone forwards a text, photo, or "sext" intended only for the original recipient. Digital technology can be used to hurt others by distributing sexual images of someone without their consent, sending unwanted or unsolicited sexually explicit photos or messages (sexting), harrassment through an online gaming platform, and posting embarrassing or inappropriate information on social media or other public sites (*Using technology to hurt others*, 2015).

Stalking is defined as a pattern of repeated and unwanted attention, harassment, contact, or any other course of conduct directed at a specific person that would cause a reasonable person to feel fear. One of the ways perpetrators may stalk victims is through technology—a practice called cyberstalking. Cyberstalking may include using someone's computer or spyware to track that person's computer activity, posting personal information about someone on public Internet forums, installing video cameras that give the stalker access to someone's personal life, or persistently sending unwanted communication through the Internet. Each year in the United States, approximately 33 million people ages 18 and older are victims of stalking. Most are young (between 18 and 24 years old) and know their stalker. People being stalked are right to be concerned. Possible things to do when faced with a stalker include avoiding the person stalking you; making it clear that you wish to stop contact (and not responding to further communication); keeping evidence received from the stalker; informing family, friends, and coworkers about the situation; and reporting the stalking to local law enforcement (*Stalking*, 2015).

What are ways to try to stay safe online? Here are some suggestions (*RAINN's top five ways to stay safe online*, 2015):

- *Protect your identity.* Avoid sharing personal information through social networks and online forums.

- *Report inappropriate images.* If inappropriate or sexual images are received via text message or online, report it to police or to www.cybertipline.com.

- *Use a secure Internet connection.* Make sure you are using a secure and reputable website.

- *Be mindful of privacy settings.* Check privacy settings, such as location services and contact information, when using social media.

- *If you have children, talk with them about Internet safety issues.* Be familiar with online privacy settings and help children set up social media accounts.

Sexual Harassment in Schools

Initial concerns about sexual harassment focused on the workplace; however, more attention has also been given to schools and colleges. Verbal and physical sexual harassment often begin in elementary school. Many girls, and almost as many boys, experience some form of sexual harassment.

Using a nationally representative survey of 1,965 students in grades 7–12, the American Association of University Women reported on student experiences with sexual harassment during the past school year (Crossing the line: Sexual harassment at school, 2011). Nearly half (48%) of the students experienced some form of sexual harassment, and 87% of them said it had a negative effect on them. Verbal harassment made up the bulk of the incidents, but physical harassment was also common. Sexual harassment by text, email, Facebook, or other electronic means affected nearly one-third of students. Many students who were sexually harassed through cyberspace were also sexually harassed in person. Girls were more likely than boys to be sexually harassed (56% versus 40%). This was true both in person (52% versus 35%) and electronically (36% versus 24%). The girls' experiences tended to be more physical and intrusive than the boys' experiences. Being called gay or lesbian in a negative way was reported equally (18%) by both sexes. Witnessing sexual harassment at school was also common (33% of girls and 24% of boys), and 56% of these students witnessed sexual harassment more than once during the school year. Among those who were sexually harassed, 12% of girls and 5% of boys reported the incident to an adult at school. About one-quarter said they talked about it with parents or family members, and 23% spoke with friends. Boys were more likely than girls to say they sexually harassed other students (18% versus 14%). Almost one-third of students who experienced sexual harassment also identified themselves as harassers. Many who admitted to sexually harassing others did not think of it as a big deal, and many were trying to be funny.

Mitchell et al. (2014) examined variations in rates of experiencing sexual harassment among students of different sexual orientation and gender identity. These researchers conducted an online survey of almost 6,000 students ages 13 to 18. Past-year sexual harassment was reported by 23% to 72% of youth, depending on their sexual orientation. The highest rates were reported by lesbian/queer girls (72%), bisexual girls (66%), and gay/queer boys (66%). When the data were examined by gender identity, transgender youth reported the highest rates of sexual harassment (81%). Overall, the most common modes for sexual harassment were in-person harassment followed by online harassment. Distress in the form of interference with school, family, and/or friends; creating a hostile environment; or being very/extremely upset was reported by about half of the sexually harassed bisexual girls and lesbian/queer girls, 65% of the gender-nonconforming/other-gender youth, and 63% of the transgender youth. Youth with high levels of social support and self-esteem were less likely to report sexual harassment. These findings point to the importance of sexual harassment prevention for all adolescents, with particular emphasis on the unique needs and experiences of youth of different sexual orientations and gender identities.

The question of whether schools should be held liable when students sexually harass their peers is extremely sensitive. Some people argue that schools should be responsible only for taking reasonable action rather than for ensuring that the behavior ends—although it can be hard to determine the definition of "reasonable." Others feel school personnel have a responsibility to take strong actions to prevent behaviors often associated with typical child growth and development—such as sexual comments, touching, and jeering. It is a real challenge to design appropriate policies and procedures related to students' sexually harassing their peers.

It is important to talk about sexual harassment with children in appropriate ways and at the appropriate level. For example, elementary school children should know that sexual harassment is unwanted and uninvited sexual attention such as teasing, touching, or taunting; sexual harassment is against the law; and they should be taught their school's sexual harassment policy. In addition, students aged 12 to 15 should know that sexual harassment can occur in a variety of settings including schools, the workplace, and extracurricular programs. They should also know where they can call for information about sexual harassment. Students aged 15 to 18 should also know that whether to report sexual harassment is a personal decision that can be hard to make, and

Gender DIMENSIONS

Same-Gender Sexual Harassment

Sexual harassment is obviously a problem for women in the workplace—and sometimes for men. Most often, the instances we hear about involve other-sex situations. However, more and more same-sex harassment cases have been filed, and lower courts have been inconsistent in their findings. One judge allowed a case to proceed only because the supervisor, accused of harassing, was admittedly gay.

The Equal Employment Opportunity Commission has for years taken the position that Title VII of the Civil Rights Act does not care which sexes are involved. In one case the Supreme Court allowed a case to proceed in which a man working on an oil rig charged two male co

workers with making taunting comments and threatening rape.

Men and women often deal with sexual harassment differently. Whereas a woman may be more inclined to report harassing conduct, the traditional inclination of many men is just to "deal with it." This attitude has possibly led to less frequent reporting of male same-sex harassment.

Same-sex harassment cases will probably receive heavy media coverage. Treatment in the press will likely have a strong influence on whether men (or women in same-sex harassment situations) will keep harassment complaints to themselves or report them in the future.

---

that people who experience sexual harassment may need help and support to deal with the situation (Keeping kids sexually safe, 2004).

Sexual harassment in schools can take many forms. Its milder forms include looks, jokes, graffiti on bathroom walls, and comments about body parts. More severe forms include physical intrusion into personal space, grabbing, and brushing up against someone in a sexual way. Students can have a variety of reactions to sexual harassment in schools; however, common ones are feeling less confident, being more self-conscious, feeling ashamed, feeling embarrassed, and consequently getting lower grades (*Sexual harassment in the schools*, 2015).

Sexual Harassment on Campus

Sexual harassment exists on all types of university campuses. In many cases it is unreported—and is often ignored altogether. In general, women are more likely to define behaviors as harassing and men are more likely to believe victims have contributed to their own problem. There are costs to individuals and to the institution. Victims tend to sacrifice self-confidence, academic and work opportunities, letters of recommendation, and grades. The student's professional development is hindered, and the university acquires a negative image.

Nearly two-thirds of college students experience some type of sexual harassment. Yet, less than 10% tell a college or university employee about it, and an even smaller fraction officially report the harasser to a Title IX officer. These, and other interesting facts, are part of a major report from the American Association

Bullying, teasing, and sexual harassment can be common in schools.

of University Women (Sexual harassment on campus: Drawing the line, 2005). Key research findings in the report are highlighted here:

- Sexual harassment is common on college campuses. More than one-third of college students encounter sexual harassment during their first year on campus.

- Men and women are equally likely to be harassed, but in different ways and with different responses. Females are more likely to be the target of sexual jokes, comments, gestures, or looks. Males are more likely to be called gay or a homophobic name. Females are more likely to be upset and to feel embarrassed, angry, less confident, afraid, confused, and disappointed in their college experience.

- Lesbian, gay, bisexual, and transgender students are more likely to be harassed.

- Different racial and ethnic groups experience sexual harassment in similar, but not identical ways. Generally, white, African American, and Hispanic students perceive and react to sexual harassment in similar ways.

- Men are more likely than women to harass. Both males and females are more likely to be harassed by a male.

- More than half of harassers think their actions are funny.

- Most victims don't report sexual harassment.

Some university officials feel there should be a general statement of the university's position on sexual harassment because it is not possible to cover specific situations adequately. Others feel that the specifics should be clearly spelled out to prevent potential confusion. Some officials feel policies should prohibit even consensual sexual relationships between students and faculty members. They argue that although such relationships may appear to be consensual, they are not because of the faculty member's position of authority. Others feel that consensual relationships are not the business of the university.

As part of the emphasis on sexual harassment on campuses, many colleges and universities have developed various types of educational programs for students and faculty. It is important to understand and protect the rights of both complainants and accusers and to avoid either sensationalizing or minimizing allegations. It is also crucial for all concerned to understand the institution's policies against harassment and its procedures for handling complaints.

Sexual Harassment/Assault and the Military

It is important to understand the difference between sexual harassment and sexual assault. These terms are defined as part of current SHARP (Sexual Harassment/Assault Response and Prevention) training at all U.S. military installations. The Department of Defense (2003) defines sexual harassment as a form of sex discrimination involving unwelcomed verbal, nonverbal and/or physical behaviors of a sexual nature. It defines sexual assault as "intentional sexual contact characterized by use of force, threats, intimidation, or abuse of authority or when the victim

does not or cannot consent" (Department of Defense, 2015). It is also critical to understand that these are two related issues, as, according to SHARP training statistics, approximately one-third of all reported sexual assaults within the Army have been preceded by sexual harassment (U.S. Military Academy, 2011).

In 2003 the National Organization for Women (NOW) reported instances of rape and sexual harassment at the U.S. Air Force Academy. It also indicated that a 1994 Congressional report found that 78% of the 90 female cadets in attendance at the Academy at that time reported either sexual assaults or unwanted sexual advances (NOW staff, 2003).

At about the same time, Sadler et al. (2003) reported that 79% of 558 female military veterans reported experiencing sexual harassment during their military service. Thirty percent of the women reported an attempted or completed rape. The report indicated findings consistent with research in civilian populations showing that younger women entering male-dominated work groups at lower levels of authority are those most likely to be harassed. Findings also indicated that military women working with superiors who made sexually demeaning comments or allowed such behavior were found to have a nearly fourfold risk of rape.

Cohen (2005) reported that women in the Israeli Defense Force reported hundreds of incidents of sexual harassment and rape, yet harassers often went unpunished. Some felt that the hierarchal structure encouraged males to misuse their power. Under Israeli law, those found guilty of harassment can be sentenced for up to 3 years of imprisonment. In reality, senior military officers accused of sexual harassment are rarely sent to jail.

Tyson (2005) wrote about a Department of Veterans Affairs report indicating that 60% of women and 27% of men in the military reserves and the National Guard suffered sexual assault or harassment during their service. Eleven percent of women experienced rape or attempted rape, compared with 1.2% of males. More than half of the incidents took place at a military worksite during duty hours, and in most cases military personnel were the offenders. Fewer than 19% said that they received any help for the trauma.

Sexual harassment has been consistently correlated with negative consequences for working women, including changes in job attitudes (e.g., lower satisfaction) and behaviors (e.g., increased work withdrawal). Sims et al. (2005) surveyed more than 11,500 military servicewomen and found that experiences of harassment led to increased turnover. These findings have important implications not only for individual women, but also for organizations.

Kimerling et al. (2010) examined military-related sexual trauma among deployed Operation Enduring

Did You Know . . .

Addressing Sexual Harassment in the Military

A climate that negatively affects teamwork within a military unit impacts mission effectiveness. Consequently, the Department of Defense has specific policies and programs that support a zero-tolerance philosophy toward sexual harassment in the armed forces. Because a diverse and talented workforce is essential to mission accomplishment, this is an issue that is addressed at every level of every military unit.

As gender-related incidents are investigated, they have been accompanied by a concerted effort on the part of the Department of Defense to prevent future recurrences. This has been demonstrated by the development and continual reevaluation of programs designed to educate service members as to what constitutes sexual harassment, how to deal with it, and how to report incidents without fear of reprisal.

In an appearance before the Senate Armed Services Committee in 1997, Edwin Dorn, the Undersecretary of Defense for Personnel and Readiness, underscored the importance of military units' functioning as a team. He mentioned trust, loyalty, and self-sacrifice, issues not often found in large organizations. According to Dorn, a climate of discrimination and harassment will erode these elements that are essential for unit effectiveness.

Nevertheless, a policy can only be as strong as the program it supports. According to Sheila Widnall, former Secretary of the Air Force, an Equal Opportunity program to support a zero-tolerance policy on harassment needs to be based on the following five principles:

1. A commander's personal commitment
2. The establishment of goals, principles, and standards of performance
3. Clear, concise written policies
4. Continual training throughout a military member's career
5. Complaint systems that are prompt, thorough, fair, and allow for resolution, support, reprisal prevention, and sanctions.

The military leadership has taken the initiative for monitoring the climate within the services. Programs have been developed to improve the climate through training, prevention, and resolution. These programs have been evaluated using instruments such as command climate surveys, sensing sessions, and other internal review processes. They have also been examined by the media, congressional inquiry, and watchdog organizations. In 2000, an assessment of four key Department of Defense human relations programs that had been fielded or modified since 1997—the Command Climate Survey, The Army

Values Program, the Consideration of Others Program, and Equal Opportunity Training Programs—was conducted. The purpose of this reassessment was to see if the establishment or revision of these programs had improved human relations in the Army. A total of 24,000 Army leaders and soldiers were surveyed and interviewed. Among the findings were indications that although the Army provides a generally effective human relations environment, many service members did not yet consider human relations an important component of combat readiness.

Since the 2000 survey, focus has shifted to the issue of sexual assault in the military. A total of 26,505 active duty members responded to a survey entitled "2010 Workplace and Gender Relations Survey of Active Duty Members, Overview Report on Sexual Assault." A summary of the results indicated that despite efforts to educate service members annually concerning prevention and response to sexual harassment and assault, these incidents still occur. Additional findings indicated that not all service members are aware of resources available, many incidents remain unreported, and incidents of sexual harassment or stalking occurred either before or after an assault incident.

In January 2012, Defense Secretary Leon Panetta said that although 3,200 sexual assaults were reported across all active duty services in 2011, he felt that the number was realistically closer to 19,000, knowing that most crimes go unreported. Commenting on a report on sexual harassment and violence across all U.S. service academies, he reinforced the fact that this was a leadership issue and that further initiatives will be prepared to eliminate such behavior.

Commanders are constantly working toward achieving zero tolerance for sexual harassment; there is still much work to do. The process for reporting incidents has been improved, thus increasing the prospect of investigation and resolution. This sends a clear message that members of the various armed services must be willing to report and be vigilant, and that these behaviors are not tolerated.

Susan M. Tendy, EdD, Professor, Retired, Department of Physical Education, United States Military Academy

Sources: Data from Dorn, E. DoD committed to zero tolerance of sexual harassment. *Defense Issues*, 12, *no.* 9 (1997), 1–4; Widnall, S., Dorn, E. To stop harassment, leaders must lead. *Defense Issues. 10, no.* 64 (1995), 1–5; Johnson, E., Harris, B. Special report 46: Human relations update 2000 executive summary (March 2001); Rock, L., Lipari, R., Cook, P., Hale, A. *2010 Workplace and Gender Relations Survey of Active Duty Members, Overview Report on Sexual Assault.* Arlington, VA: Defense Manpower Data Center; March 2011; 2010–2025; Elliott, D. No simple explanation in AF academy sex crime data. *Denver Post* (January 22, 2012). Available: www.denverpost.com/dontmiss/ci_19795071.

Freedom and Operation Iraqi Freedom veterans. Among almost 126,000 veterans, 15.1% of the women and 0.7% of the men reported military sexual trauma. This trauma was associated with increased chance of a mental disorder diagnosis, including post-traumatic stress disorder, other anxiety disorders, depression, and substance abuse disorders.

With these studies as a backdrop, the National Lawyers Guild launched a Women's Military Rights Project to challenge the long-term problem of sexual harassment and abuse within the military system through a combined program of education, legal assistance and litigation, and support for political action (Boghosian, 2005). This was a result of many events through the years—particularly the Navy Tailhook Association convention in 1991, the court martial of the most senior enlisted man in the U.S. Army for sexual harassment in 1997, the accusation of the Army's most senior enlisted man in Europe of sexual harassment in 1999, the substantiated accusation of an Army Major General of sexual harassment by the highest-ranking woman in Army history in 2000, and the Air Force Academy scandal in 2003, which erupted when 142 cadets made sexual assault charges that resulted in zero convictions. In addition, as part of her congressional testimony in June 2006, Christine Hansen, Executive Director of the Miles Foundation, reported that she had previously testified before the Senate Armed Services Committee and presented written testimony to the House Armed Services Military Personnel Subcommittee in February 2004. During her testimony two and a half years later, Hansen reported that in 2005 alone, 2,374 acknowledged reports of sexual assault were investigated by military criminal units, 518 of which occurred in the Central Command Area of Responsibility (CENTCOM AOR)—the Middle East (Hansen, 2006). She also noted that there was no "centralized database available that would accurately reflect" the total number of reports registered throughout all of the Armed Forces.

As a result of these continued incidents, new educational training and awareness programs have been developed to help military personnel recognize potential harassment and assault behaviors, apply intervention techniques, provide victim assistance and counseling, and hold offenders accountable (Department of the Army, 2011a). For example, the Army has instituted the "I. A.M. STRONG" campaign, the purpose of which is to educate all soldiers that assault prevention is a total team effort. The Army (Department of the Army, 2011b) has developed a four-phase strategy for this program, consisting of the following:

Phase I: A committed Army leadership that aggressively condemns sexual harassment/assault.

Phase II: Army-wide ownership of sexual assault prevention strategies to stop them before they occur.

Phase III: Change the culture, whereby Army values are inculcated, and assaults are eliminated within the ranks.

Phase IV: Sustain, refine and share best practices, as well as lessons learned.

In 2012 the Navy adopted new strategies for addressing sexual assault among sailors, including a skit-based program that urges troops to help protect each other. The program teaches troops not to stand by if another person is attacked by a sexual predator. According to Navy data, 2,485 sailors and 1,453 Marines were sexually assaulted in 2011. Internal surveys suggested that sexual assaults among sailors and Marines declined after the program was implemented (Navy Expands Training to Address Sexual Assaults Among Sailors, 2012).

Notwithstanding this campaign, the Women's Rights Project and the Service Woman's Action Network have joined forces in challenging the alleged lack of oversight of sexual abuse and harassment on the part of the U.S. military by continuing to seek detailed and consolidated records from the Departments of Defense and Veterans Affairs regarding the disposition of sexual assault, sexual harassment, and domestic violence incidents in the military. These follow-up records are being sought to further investigate the annual release by the Department of Defense of separate statistics on the prevalence of sexual assault within each branch (Park & Natelson, 2012).

In 2012 Defense Secretary Leon Panetta announced new policies with regard to sexual assault in the military. The plan's initiatives mandate sexual assault cases to be handled by high-level senior officers within the chain of command. The plan also created new special victims' units to handle sexual assault cases, required all new service members be briefed on sexual assault policies within 2 weeks of reporting for duty, required that records be kept on all disciplinary actions related to sexual assault cases, and allowed National Guard and reserve troops to remain on active duty to obtain proper treatment and support while their cases are investigated (Defense Sec. Panetta Announces Initiative to Address Sexual Assault in the Military, 2012).

In preparation for the announcement of these initiatives, an open letter to Secretary Panetta was coauthored by Protect Our Defenders and the Service Women's Action Network, outlining their concerns that allowing the military chain of command to control the direction of these cases, and affording them the power to use command discretion to proceed or dismiss, was a central flaw in his proposal, and does not account for potential conflicts of interest (Parrish & Jacob, 2011).

The debate continues concerning how the military investigates and prosecutes sexual assault cases. After interviewing countless military personnel who were victims of sexual assault, Senator Kirsten Gillibrand of New York introduced the Military Justice Improvement Act in March 2014. This bill addressed the conflict of interest concerns by seeking to remove prosecution of sexual assault crimes from the typical military chain of command and place these cases with specially trained legal military prosecutors. It was met with strong resistance from the military and its supporters, and was narrowly defeated in the Senate. A follow-up bill with a more moderate tone was immediately introduced by Senator Claire McCaskill of Missouri, called the 2014 Victim's Protection Act. This legislation, which was passed unanimously by the Senate and was awaiting House approval in 2015, recommends the establishment of a review process that stays within the prosecutorial authority of the military chain of command, and assumes that recent Congressional oversight will hasten the reform process long sought by victims of sexual assault (Draper, 2014). However, according to Caslen et al. (2015, p. 2), "Congress and the American people are 'fed up' with the ongoing issues, and the military must continue to take its obligation seriously."

Five principles based on lessons learned at the U.S. Military Academy at West Point have been offered as a framework to eliminate sexual harassment and assault not only at the military academies and within the military, but also on college campuses and in the workplace environment:

1. *Leaders identify and break negative chains of circumstance.* This principle points out the importance of commander involvement as well as bystander involvement to prevent a critical incident before it occurs. This not only includes looking out for one's "battle buddy" in social situations, but also suggests the monitoring and elimination of sexist and gendered terms that differentiate females from the rest of the population as "others." For example, using the term "female soldiers" versus "soldiers," or "coeds" versus "students," connotes a bias that should be treated similarly to a racial slur.

2. *Education is preferable to litigation.* Proper training should include the empowerment of soldiers to make immediate, on-the-spot corrections when improper behavior is observed.

3. *What is electronic is public.* Postings to websites and anonymous web applications are the same as bullying and assault. Such postings also

signal the culture of the unit, and commanders should be aware of these activities.

4. *Do not ignore pornography.* The authors documented research that has shown that the display of pornography in the workplace and in barracks has a negative effect on behavior (Caslen et al., 2015, p. 18). Living areas such as barracks and dorm rooms should be considered work spaces, and applicable standards should apply.

5. *Unit climate is the commander's responsibility.* This principle further defines the obvious: Commanders must be well trained and actively engaged in SHARP training, they must be held accountable for unit activities both on and off a military installation where the military culture extends, and proper bearing and expectations should be made clear.

Reactions to Sexual Harassment

Reactions to sexual harassment are influenced by individual characteristics and the severity of the harassing behavior. Gender, attitudes toward both women and men, religiosity, and confidence all influence the way people might react to sexual harassment. Responses can range from avoidance or defusion to negotiation or confrontation. Avoidance (ignoring the harassment or doing nothing) is quite common. Defusion (which includes responses such as going along, stalling, or making a joke of it) is a more active way to minimize the impact of conflict. Negotiation is a more assertive response and involves a direct request to the harasser to stop. This shifts the focus of the interaction to the victim's needs and priorities in the relationship. Confrontation, the most assertive response on this continuum, has two components: aggressive personal responses (such as telling the harasser to stop rather than simply asking) and use of the organizational power structure (such as making a formal complaint through channels).

A person being harassed usually has several options—personal action, grievance to an employer (if applicable), union grievance (if applicable), and legal action. Each situation influences the best way to handle the harassment. There are two objectives for personal action: Attempt to stop the harassment and, if that fails, document it. If this fails and there is a grievance procedure, a complaint can be filed through prescribed channels. If none of these routes works, it may be necessary to pursue legal action.

Sexual harassment is against the law, and each institution is obliged to create a safe environment for its students. Here are some steps you can take if you experience sexual harassment on campus (*Sexual*

The sexual harasser is often a person who has authority or power over others.

harassment on campus: What are students' rights?, 2015):

- *Tell the harasser to stop.* Promptly let the person know that his or her behavior makes you uncomfortable. Do not mince words—use precise language indicating that you want the harassment to stop immediately.

- *Document the abuse.* Write down what happened, when it occurred, who witnessed the harassment, and how it affected you. If harrassment occurs on separate occasions, record every instance as quickly as possible while details are fresh in your mind.

- *Consider confronting the harasser via a letter.* In this letter, include a factual summary of what happened, describe how you felt, and make a straightforward request that the behavior never occur again. Keep a copy for your records; it can be a powerful piece of evidence if you ultimately involve authorities.

- *Report the harassment.* Check your school's policies and procedures for reporting sexual harassment. School officials are legally required to follow up on your report. You might also wish to make a police report.

- *Tell someone.* It is important to tell at least one other person about the harassment. It can help to talk about the incident with a trusted friend, family member, or faculty member. If you find it difficult to get past the abuse, look into counseling services at your school's counseling center.

- *Do not blame yourself.* You did nothing wrong, and you are not to blame for the incident. The law is designed to protect you from harassment. Anything less than full protection is not acceptable. As you pursue your options, stay firm in your conviction that you and other students at your school deserve to be safe and feel comfortable on campus.

Case Study

Many positive social changes have occurred over the past few decades to help the victims of forcible sexual behaviors. Although child sexual abuse has long occurred—Freud wrote about it almost 100 years ago—it was a hushed, taboo topic. Many victims thought that they were the "only one," or that they had done something wrong. Not anymore.

The media have been a positive force for change by giving coverage to forcible sexual behavior cases. The surrounding coverage about battered women—gave many victims the courage to step forward. Many TV shows inform children about what to do in case someone touches them in a way that makes them feel "uncomfortable."

The legal system has made huge strides in recent years, creating and enforcing laws and helping victims of forced sexual behaviors. Police have been trained to take intimate-partner violence calls seriously, and not to let the perpetrator of violence off the hook.

Laws have been passed to help victims of sexual harassment at work or school. And, whereas in 1976 no man could be legally accused of raping his spouse, now marital rape laws have been passed in all 50 states.

Biological Factors

- Alcohol is a factor in 50% of rapes.
- Date-rape drugs produce disinhibition and an amnesia-like effect, so that victims do not remember what happened.
- Younger people commit violent acts more often than older people do.
- Although men and women attack each other at about the same rate (12%), as a result of the usually greater strength of men, women are hurt more often and live in fear of further attacks.

Sociocultural Factors

- Socioeconomic status plays a role in forcible sexual behaviors, as higher levels of aggression are found among lower-income populations. Pedophiles and the children they abuse are members of all socioeconomic and educational groups.
- People who believe in rape myths assign less blame to the perpetrator and more blame to the victim.
- Laws regarding sexual activity of teens vary among countries.
- Deliberate interracial rape is uncommon; 88% of victims are the same race as the perpetrator.
- A cultural belief in patriarchy, whereby males have a dominant role over women, can promote abusive behavior.

Psychological Factors

- Sexual abuse in childhood contributes significantly to the risk of development of mental disorders later in life. Adolescent rape survivors have more behavioral problems compared to older survivors. Women with low self-esteem tend not to end an abusive relationship.

Summary

- Millions of people are affected by sexual violence each year. Sexual assault and abuse include inappropriate touching; vaginal, anal, or oral penetration; sexual intercourse after a person says no; rape; attempted rape; and child molestation.

- Rape is one of the most underreported crimes. There are many myths about rape.

- Date rape, also known as acquaintance rape, is much more common than most people realize. There are many ways to help prevent acquaintance rape.

- Pedophilia entails feelings of adult sexual attraction to children. Children are particularly vulnerable to sexual predators, such as pedophiles, on the Internet.

- Preventing sexual abuse demands attention. There is a need to help children and adults distinguish between appropriate and inappropriate touch, say no to unwanted or uncomfortable touch, tell a trusted adult if inappropriate touch occurs, and identify family and community support systems.

- Incest is sexual behavior between relatives who are too closely related to be legally married. The most commonly reported form is father–daughter.

- Intimate-partner abuse is a significant health and social problem in the United States. In addition to physical abuse, it can include sexual abuse, emotional abuse, or property/economic abuse.

- Sexual harassment is unwelcome verbal, physical, or sexual conduct that has the effect of creating an intimidating, hostile, or offensive environment. It is a problem in schools, colleges, and the workplace.

Discussion Questions

1. What are the different categories of rape? Who are the rapists in these categories? What are the effects on the victims?

2. What effects does child abuse have on its survivors?

3. Describe the type of person who commits incest. What drives a seemingly "normal" individual to commit incest?

4. Explain why someone in an abusive marriage stays in the relationship. Can one be absolutely sure when a spouse should leave? Or is every situation different?

5. In what ways is sexual harassment the same and different in the workplace, in schools, in colleges, and in the military? Is the intent of harassment the same in each situation?

Application Questions

Reread the chapter-opening story and answer the following questions.

1. Is date rape a form of miscommunication or a form of sexual violence? Put another way, did Ed simply misinterpret the woman's resistance, assuming that "she wanted to be convinced to have sex"? Even if that were the case, did he have the right to continue sexual activity before she consented?

2. Assume for a moment that you are the woman who has just been date raped. Which actions can and should you take? What might the consequences of those actions be for both you and the rapist?

Critical Thinking Questions

1. A Florida federal judge ruled that pictures of naked and scantily clad women displayed in a workplace qualified as sexual harassment under Title VII of the 1964 Civil Rights Act. In his written opinion, the judge said that such a "boys' club" atmosphere is "no less destructive to workplace equality than a sign declaring 'Men Only.'" At the same time, the Florida branch of the American Civil Liberties Union denounced the decision as a possible violation of free speech. Under the federal court ruling, the company involved had to institute an antiharassment policy and take down the photos. In your opinion, what was the right decision in this situation?

2. Several women in an office complained to their human resources department that a male colleague had a photo of a woman in a bikini on his desk and that the photo created a "hostile working environment." When the man was confronted by his supervisor, he stated that the photo was of his wife, and he refused to remove it. What rights does the man have to display a photo of his wife? What rights do the women in the department have to object to the photo?

3. The goal of this question/activity is to increase your awareness of relationship abuse while enabling you to reflect on your own values about what would constitute an abusive romantic or sexual relationship. Read each statement, consider how you feel about it, and discuss your feelings with others in your class to explore the various opinions that might exist in your class.

Is it abuse if ...

1. a man and a woman are arguing when she begins to cry hysterically, and he gives her a light slap to calm her down?

2. a husband takes his wife to work every morning, meets her for lunch every day, and picks her up at the end of each afternoon?

3. a wife tells her husband that he would look better if he lost a few pounds?

4. every time a lesbian couple argues, one of the partners threatens to "out" the other to her family?

5. an 18-year-old has a sexual relationship with a 14-year-old?

6. a woman who wears tight clothing and short skirts walks down the street and men whistle and make sexual comments to her?

7. a man says he wants to have sexual intercourse, his girlfriend says she's not ready, but after talking about it, she gives in and has sexual intercourse with him, even though she doesn't really want to?

Source: Adapted from Schroeder, E. Is it abuse if ...? *American Journal of Sexuality Education, 1, 1* (2005), 141–149.

Critical Thinking Cases

A deputy in the sheriff's department in Olympia, Washington, suddenly found himself accused of child abuse. His two daughters, aged 18 and 22 years, had just returned from a spiritual retreat when they suddenly recalled that their father had sexually abused them when they were children. During the retreat, a charismatic preacher had said that someone in the audience had been molested as a child—a plausible assumption in any audience given prevalence rates. The more the daughters remembered, the more their stories kept changing. The father was stunned, claiming he remembered no sexual abuse toward his daughters. But he also believed his daughters would never lie. Eventually,

he confessed to abusing his daughters. In fact, the more he remembered, the clearer his memories of the events became. A psychologist tried an experiment, in which false information about abusing his children was told to him. Within days, he claimed to "remember" these made-up events. When told that these events had never taken place, he tried to retract his other statements from the legal process. Unfortunately, he was too late. He was convicted and sentenced to jail for his initial recalled memories.

Given this true case study of recovered memories, is it ethical to use them for treatment of a sexual abuse survivor? Is it ethical to use them to charge someone else with sexual assault or sexual abuse many years later?

Explain your answer.

Exploring Personal Dimensions

Date Rape
This exercise is for those who are single and dating. Mark all that apply to you.

_____ 1. When dating, most of the excitement is to see what degree of intimacy I will be able to reach with this person (that is, how far we will go).

_____ 2. I test how far I will go (physical intimacy) with someone by progressive fondling (holding hands, putting arm around waist, rubbing back, chest, or breast and genitals) to see at what point the person will stop me.

_____ 3. When dating, I generally go with others or go somewhere public until I know someone.

_____ 4. I ask around about someone before I go out with her or him.

_____ 5. I make it very clear what my values are about physical intimacy when dating before difficult situations arise.

_____ 6. I have tried to coerce or talk someone into having sexual activity with me.

Scoring
Give yourself the following points for the items you checked, and total your score.
1. 3
2. 3
3. -2
4. -3
5. -3
6. 5

Interpretation

3–11	You are potentially infringing on someone else's right to live within her or his value system and legal rights. You may be "date raping" or attempting date rape.
0–2	You have tendencies to infringe on someone else's right to live within her or his value system.
(–1)–(–3)	You are practicing moderately healthy dating precautions to avoid date rape.
(–4)–(–8)	You are practicing healthy dating precautions to avoid date rape.

Suggested Readings

Acquaintance rape. Rape, Abuse, and Incest National Network, 2015. Available: http://www.rainn.orglget-information/types-of-sexual-assauIt/acquaintance-rape.

Child sexual abuse. Rape, Abuse, and Incest National Network, 2015. Available: http://www.rainn.org/get-information/types-of-sexual-assault/child-sexual-abuse.

Dating and domestic violence. Rape, Abuse, and Incest National Network, 2015. Available: http://www.rainn.org/get-information/types-of-sexual-assault/dating-and-domestic-violence.

Humphreys, T. P., & Brousseau, M. M. The sexual consent scale-revised: Development, reliability, and preliminary validity. *Journal of Sex Research, 47,* 5 (September 2010), 420–428.

Preventing sexual violence on college campuses: Lessons from research and practice. White House Task Force to Protect Students from Sexual Assault, April, 2014. Available: https://www.notalone.gov/assets/preventing-sexual-violence-on-college-campuses-lessons-from-research-and-practice.pdf.

Sexual exploitation by helping professionals. Rape, Abuse, and Incest National Network, 2015. Available: http://www.rainn.org/get-information/types-of-sexual-assault/sexual-exploitation-by-helpingprofessional.

Types of sexual violence. Rape, Abuse, and Incest National Network, 2015. Available: http://www.rainn.org/get-information/types-of-sexual-assault.

What is healthy sexuality and consent? National Sexual Violence Resource Center, 2015. Available: http://www.nsvrc.org/sites/default/files/saam_2015_what-is-healthy-sexuality-and-consent.pdf.

Web Resources

MaleSurvivor
www.malesurvivor.org

Provides extensive information about sexual victimization of boys and men designed to help them overcome their sexual victimization experiences.

Men Can Stop Rape
www.mencanstoprape.org

This organization works with male youth to help them be allies with women in preventing rape and other forms of men's violence. Gender equity is promoted along with men's capacity to be strong without being violent.

National Coalition Against Domestic Violence
www.ncadv.org

The mission of the National Coalition Against Domestic Violence (NCADV) is to organize for collective power to end the violence in our lives. NCADV believes violence against women and children results from the use of force or threat to achieve and maintain control over others in intimate relationships. NCADV works for major societal changes necessary to eliminate both personal and societal violence against all women and children.

Violence Against Women—Office of Women's Health
www.womenshealth.gov/blog/category/violence-against-women.html

The Office of Women's Health coordinates the efforts of all of the federal Health and Human Services agencies and offices involved in women's health. Its purpose is to improve the health and well-being of women and girls in the United States through education, programs, and motivating behavior change.

U.S. Department of Justice: Office on Violence Against Women
www.justice.gov/ovw

The mission of the Office on Violence Against Women (OVW), a component of the U.S. Department of Justice, is to provide federal leadership in developing the national capacity to reduce violence against women and administer justice for and strengthen services to victims of domestic violence, dating violence, sexual assault, and stalking.

Rape, Abuse, and Incest National Network
www.rainn.org

The Rape, Abuse, and Incest National Network is the nation's largest anti-sexual assault organization. RAINN operates the National Sexual Assault Hotline and carries out programs to prevent sexual assault, help victims, and ensure that rapists are brought to justice.

REFERENCES

101 ways to combat domestic violence. Feminists Against Violence Network, 2003. Available: http://www.geocities.com/ Heartland/Meadows/7905/101.htm.

About SSSS: Mission statement: A special note about Sexual Harassment. Society for the Scientific Study of Sexuality (June 3, 2005). Available: http://www.sexscience.org.

About the Prison Rape Elimination Act of 2003. National Institute of Justice, 2007. Available: http://www.ojp.usdoj.gov/nij/topics/corrections/prison-rape/prea.htm.

Acquaintance rape. Rape, Abuse, & Incest National Network, 2012. Available: http://www.rainn.org/get-information/types-of-sexual-assault/acquaintance-rape.

American College Health Association. American College Health Association-National College Health Assessment II: Reference Group Executive Summary Spring 2014. Hanover, MD: American College Health Association, 2014.

American College Health Association. National College Health Assessment. *Journal of American College Health, 56, 5* (March/April 2008), 469–479.

American Psychiatric Association. Statement: Diagnostic criteria for pedophilia (June 17, 2003).

Arreola, S., Neilands, T., Pollack, L., Paul, J., & Datania, J. Childhood sexual experiences and adult health sequelae among gay and bisexual men: Defining childhood sexual abuse. *Journal of Sex Research, 45, 3* (July 2008), 246–252.

Basile, K. C., Smith, S. G., Breiding, M. J., Black, M. C, & Mahendra, R. *Sexual violence surveillance: Uniform definitions and recommended data elements.* Centers for Disease Control and Prevention, 2014. Available: http://www.cdc.gov/violenceprevention/pdf/sv_surveillance_definitionsl-2009-a.pdf.

Beck, A., Berzofsky, M., Caspar, R., & Krebs, C. *Sexual victimization in prisons and jails reported by inmates, 2011–2012 update.* Bureau of Justice Statistics, 2014. Available: http://www.bjs.gov/index.cfm?ty=pbdetail&iid=4654.

Bhana, D. "Girls are not free"—in and out of the South African school. *International Journal of Educational Development, 32, 2* (2012), 352–358.

Black, M. C., Basile, K. C., Breiding, M. J., Smith, S. G., Walters, M. L., Merrick, M. T., Chen, J., & Stevens, M. R. The National Intimate Partner Sexual Violence Survey (NISVS): 2010 summary report. Atlanta, GA: National Center for Injury Prevention and Control, Centers for Disease Control and Prevention, November 2011.

Boghosian, H. Gauntlet of change. *National Lawyers Guild Foundation: Guild Notes, 30, 2* (Summer 2005), 1–14.

Burke, D. Bishops leave sex abuse policies largely intact. Pew Forum on Religion and Public Life, June 16, 2011. Available: http://pewforum,org/Religion-NewsLRNS-Bishops-leave-abuse-policies-Iargely-intact.aspx.

Caslen, R. L., Jebb, C. R., Gade, D., & Landsem, H. C. *Getting to the left of SHARP: Lessons learned from West Point's efforts to combat sexual harassment and assault.* Carlisle Barracks, PA: Strategic Studies Institute and U.S. Army War College Press, January 2015. Monograph no. 1244. Available: http://strategicstudiesinstitute.army.mil/pubs/display.cfm?pubID=1244.

Child sexual abuse. Rape, Abuse, & Incest National Network, 2012. Available: http://www.rainn.org/get-information/types-of-sexual-assault/child-sexual-abuse.

Cohen, A. Harassment complaints ignored. *Horizons, 19, 1* (Summer 2005), 11–12.

Collibee, C., & Furman, W. Impact of sexual coercion on romantic experiences of adolescents and young adults. *Archives of Sexual Behavior, 43, 7* (2014), 1431–1441.

Craig, M. E. Coercive sexuality in dating relationships: A situational model. *Clinical Psychology Review, 10* (1990), 395–423.

Crossing the line: Sexual harassment at school. Washington, DC: American Association of University Women, 2011.

Curtis, K. California loses track of 33,000 sex offenders. *The Birmingham News* (January 8, 2003), 8A.

Date rape drugs. *Medicine Net.com*, 2015. Available: http://www.medicinenet.com/date_rape_drugs/article.htm.

Date rape drugs. U.S. Department of Health and Human Services, Office on Women's Health, 2008. Available: http://www.womenshealth.gov/faq/date-rape-drugs.cfm.

Date rape drugs fact sheet. Office on Women's Health, U.S. Department of Health and Human Services, 2015. Available: http://womenshealth.gov/publications/our-publications/fact-sheet/date-rape-drugs.html.

Dating and domestic violence. Rape, Abuse & Incest National Network, 2005. Available: http://www.rainn.org/get-information/types-of-sexual-assault/dating-and-domestic-violence.

Defense Sec. Panetta announces initiative to address sexual assault in the military. Women's Health Policy Report, April 18, 2012. Available: http://go.nationalpartnership.org/site/News2?abbr=daily2_&page=NewsArticle&id=33119.

Department of Defense. Military equal opportunity (MEO) program. In Directive Number 1350.2 (p. 18), 2003. Available: http://www.dtic.mil/whs/directives/corres/pdf/135002p.pdf.

Department of Defense. Sexual assault prevention and response program procedures. In Directive NUMBER 6495.01 (p. 21), 2015. Available: http://www.dtic.mil/whs/directives/corres/pdf/649501p.pdf.

Department of the Army. Sexual assault prevention and response program. In AR 600-20, Army Command Policy. Rapid Action Revision (RAR), (pp. 66–77), 2011a. Available: http://www.apd.army.mil/pdffiles/r600_20.pdf.

Department of the Army. Sexual assault prevention strategy goals. In I. A.M. STRONG: Unit commander's guide, sexual harassment/assault response & prevention (SHARP), (p. 5). Washington, DC: Military OneSource, 2011b.

Domestic homicides. Domestic violence is a serious, widespread social problem in America: The facts 2005. Family Violence Prevention Fund. Available: http://endabuse.org.

Domestic violence: Statistics and facts. Safehorizon, 2015. Available: http://www.safehorizon.org/page/domestic -violence-statistics--facts-52.html.

Draper, R. The military's rough justice on sexual assault. *New York Times Magazine* (November 26, 2014). Available: http://www.nytimes.com/2014/11/30/magazine/the-militarys -rough-justice-on-sexual-assault.html.

The effects of trauma do not have to last a lifetime. American Psychological Association, 2015. Available: http://www.apa .org/research/action/ptsd.aspx.

Fact sheet. National Center for Injury Prevention and Control, U.S. Centers for Disease Control, 2005. Available: http:// www.cdc.gov/ncipc/factsheets/svfacts.htm.

Facts about sexual harassment. U.S. Equal Employment Opportunity Commission, 2015. Available: http://www .eeoc.gov/eeoc/publications/fs-sex.cfm.

Federal Register, June 20, 2014. Available: https://www .federalregister.gov/articles/2014/10/20/2014-24284 /violence-against-women-act#table_of_contents.

Felson, R. B., & Cundiff, P. R. Sexual assault as a crime against young people. *Archives of Sexual Behavior, 43, 2* (2014), 273–284.

Focht, J. *The cycle of domestic violence.* National Center for Health Research, 2013. Available: http://center4research .org/violence-risky-behavior/violence-and-threats-in-the- home/cycle-of-domestic-violence/.

Foundation to Abolish Child Sex Abuse. Police smash "world's largest" online pedophilia ring. March 16, 2011. Available: http://www.abolishsexabuse.org/index.php70ption-com content&view-article&id-904:policesmash-gworlds-largestg -online-pedophilia-ring&catid-54:latest-news&ltemid-179.

Haffner, D. From the executive director. News from the Religious Institute, The Religious Institute. Westport, CT, November 15, 2011.

Hansen, C. Statement to the House, Subcommittee on National Security, Emerging Threats and International Relations of the Committee on Government Reform. *Sexual assault and violence against women in the military and at the academies*, Hearing, June 27, 2006 (Serial 109-220). Available: http://www.gpo.gov/fdsys/pkg/CHRG-109hhrg 33682/html/CHRG-109hhrg33682.htm.

Hines, D., & Douglas, E. M. Sexual aggression experiences among male victims of physical partner violence: Prevalence, severity, and health correlates for male victims and their children. *Archives of Sexual Behavior* (December 12, 2014). DOI: 10.1007/s10508-014-0393-0.

Hitchens, C. Cardinal's law: Two questions for the pope, *Slate*, April 14, 2008. Available: http://www.slate.com/id/2188971.

How commonplace is marital rape? About dating and relationships. *About.com*, 2015. Available: http://marriage .about.com/cs/maritalrape/f/maritalrape9.htm.

Humphreys, T. Perceptions of sexual consent: The impact of relationship history and gender. *Journal of Sex Research, 44, 4* (October 2007), 307–315.

Incest. Rape, Abuse, & Incest National Network, 2012. Available: http://www.rainn.org/get-information/types-of-sexual -assault/incest.

Internet safety. Counter Pedophilia Investigative Unit, 2011. Available: http://www.cpiu.us/internet-safety.

Kann, L., Kinchen, S., Shanklin, S. L., et al. Youth Risk Behavior Surveillance—United States, 2013. *Morbidity and Mortality Weekly Report, 63, 4* (June 13, 2014), 1–168.

Keeping kids sexually safe. *Families Are Talking 3, 3* (2004), 1–4.

Kimerling, R., Street, A. E., Pavao, J., Smith, M. W., Cronkite, R. C., Holmes, T. J., & Frayne, S. M. Military related sexual trauma among Veterans Health Administration patients returning from Afghanistan and Iraq. *American Journal of Public Health, 97, 8* (June 2010), 1409–1412.

LaFraniere, S. Entrenched epidemic: Wife-beatings in Africa. *The New York Times* (August 11, 2005).

Lee, J., Pomeroy, E. C., Yoo, S. K., & Rheinboldt, K. T. Attitudes toward rape—a comparison between Asian and Caucasian college students. *Violence Against Women, 11, 2* (February 2005), 177–196.

Long J. G., Kristiansson, V., & Whitman-Barr, C. Establishing penetration in sexual assault cases. *Strategies in Brief, 24* (January 2015). Available: http://www.aequitasresource.org /Establishing-Penetration-in-Sexual-Assault-Cases-SIB24.pdf.

Male sexual assault. Rape, Abuse, and Incest National Network, 2011. Available: http://www.rainn.org/get-information/types -of-sexual-assualt/male-sexualassault.

Marelich, W. D., Lundquist, J., Painter, K., & Mechanic, M. B. Sexual deception as a social exchange process: Development of a behavior-based deception scale. *Journal of Sex Research, 45, 1* (January 2008), 27–35.

Marital rape. Rape Abuse & Incest National Network, 2015. Available: https://www.rainn.org/public-policy/sexual -assault-issues/marital-rape.

McEwan, S. L., DeMan, A. F., & Simpson-Housley, P. Acquaintance rape, ego-identity achievement, and locus of control. *Social Behavior and Personality, 33, 6* (2005), 587–592.

McGee, R. Don't look at me. National Sexuality Resource Center, April 17, 2007. Available: http://nsrc.sfsu.edu/print/2641.

Mitchell, K. J., Ybarra, M. L., & Korchmaros, J. D. Sexual harassment among adolescents of different sexual orientations and gender orientations. *Child Abuse & Neglect, 38, 2* (February 2014), 280–295.

Molla, T., & Cuthbert, D. Qualitative inequality: Experiences of women in Ethiopian higher education. *Gender and Education 26, 7* (2014).

Navy expands training to address sexual assault among sailors. Women's Health Policy Report, August 17, 2012. Available: http://www.nationalpartnership.org/site/News2?news_iv _ctrl=-1&abbr=daily2_&page=NewsArticle&id=34957.

Notice to readers: Sexual Assault Awareness Month—April 2005. U.S. Centers for Disease Control. Available: http://www.cdc .gov/mmwr/preview/mmwrhtml/mm5412a8.htm.

NOW Staff. Military "don't tell" policy hushes up rape and sexual assault. National Organization for Women, 2003. Available: http://www.now.org/issues/military/031103airforce.html.

The offenders. Rape, Abuse, & Incest National Network, 2012. Available: http://www.rainn.orgiget-information/statistics /sexual-assault-offenders.

Pakistan lifts travel ban on raped women. *The Birmingham News* (June 16, 2005), A4.

Park, S., & Natelson, R. Exposing the ugly details of the military sexual violence epidemic. American Civil Liberties Union, 2012. Available: http://www.aclu.org/blog/womens-rights /exposing-ugly-details-military-sexual-violence-epidemic.

Partner rape. Rape, Abuse, & Incest National Network, 2012. Available: http://www.rainn.org/get-information/types-of -sexual-assault/partner-rape.

Parrish, N., & Jacob, G. *A call for fundamental change: An open letter to the Honorable Leon Panetta, Secretary of Defense, on the need to fix how rape and sexual assault is handled in the military.* Protect Our Defenders & Service Women's Action Network, December 29, 2011. Available: http://www .protectourdefenders.com/open-letter-to-secretary-panetta/.

RAINN's top five ways to stay safe online. Rape, Abuse & Incest National Network, 2015. Available: https://rainn.org/news -room/rainns-top-five-ways-to-stay-safe-online.

Rape statistics. Statistic Brain, 2014. Available: http://www .statisticbrain.com/rape-statistics/.

Rape: Weapon of war. United Nations Human Rights, 2015. Available: http://www.ohchr.org/en/newsevents/pages /rapeweaponwar.aspx.

Rape as a weapon of war against men. IRIN Humanitarian News and Analysis, 2015. Available: http://www.irinnews.org /report/93960/health-rape-as-a-weapon-of-war-against-men.

Rempala, D. M., & Bernien, F. J. The consideration of rape: The effect of target information disparity on judgments of guilt. *Journal of Applied Social Psychology, 35, 3* (March 2005), 536–550.

Rodriguez, A. Kidnapped, forced to wed. *The Chicago Tribune* (July 24, 2005).

Sadler, A., Booth, B., Cook, B., & Doebbeling, B. Factors associated with women's risk of rape in the military environment. *American Journal of Industrial Medicine, 43* (2003), 262–273.

Schimelpfening, N. Battered men: The hidden side of domestic violence. *About.com*, 2013. Available: http://depression .about.com/b/2013/08/31/battered-men-the-hidden-side-of -domestic-violence-2.htm.

Sexual Assault Nurse Examiner (SANE) Program, 2015. Available: http://www.summitmedicalcenter.org/smc /specialties/sexual-assault-nurse-examiner-sane-program/.

Sexual harassment. Rape, Abuse & Incest National Network, 2015. Available: https://rainn.org/get-information/types-of -sexual-assault/sexual-harassment.

Sexual Harassment Charges. U.S. Equal Employment Opportunity Commission, 2011. Available: http://eeoc.gov /eeoc/statistics/enforcement/sexual_harassment.cfm.

Sexual harassment in the schools. Rape, Abuse & Incest National Network, 2015. Available: https://www.rainn.org/get -information/types-of-sexual-assault/sexual-harassment.

Sexual harassment on campus: Drawing the line. American Association of University Women Educational Foundation, 2005. Available: http://www.aauw.org/research/dtl.cfm.

Sexual harassment on campus: What are students' rights? Education-portal.com, 2015. Available: http://education -portal.com/articles/How_to_Address_Sexual_Harassment _on_Campus.html.

Sexual harassment. Rape, Abuse, & Incest National Network, 2012. Available: http://www.rainn.org!get-information /types-of-sexual-assault/sexual-harassment.

Sexual harassment. U.S. Equal Employment Opportunity Commission, 2009. Available: http://www.eeoc.gov/types /sexual_harassment.html.

Shen, A. C., Chiu, M. Y., & Gao, J. Predictors of dating violence among Chinese adolescents. *Journal of Interpersonal Violence, 27, 6* (2013), 1066–1089.

Siegelbaum, D. Justice expands definition of rape. The Hill, January 6, 2012. Available: http://thehill.com/homenews /administration/202757-department-of-justice-expands -definition-of-rape-to-increase-reporting.

Sims, C. S., Drasgow, F., & Fitzgerald, L. F. The effects of sexual harassment on turnover in the military: time-dependent modeling. *Journal of Applied Psychology 90, 6* (November 2005), 1141–1152.

Snyder, M., & Ickes, W. Personality and social behavior, in *The handbook of social psychology,* Lindzey, G., & Aronsen, E., eds. New York: Random House, 1985, 883–937.

South African anti-rape condom could reduce risk of pregnancy, HIV, STDs. *Kaiser Daily HIV/AIDS Report* (September 02, 2005). Available: http://www.kaisernetwork.org.

Spousal rape laws: 20 years later. National Center for Victims of Crime, 2004. Available: http://www.ncvc.org/ncvc/main.aspx?dbName=DocumentViewer&DocumentID=32701.

Stalking. Rape, Abuse & Incest National Network, 2015. Available: https://rainn.org/news-room/sexual-assault-issues/stalking.

Statistics. Rape, Abuse, & Incest National Network, 2012. Available: http://www.rainn.org/statistics.

Stermac, L., Del Bove, G., & Addison, M. Stranger and acquaintance sexual assault of adult males. *Journal of Interpersonal Violence, 19, 8* (Aug. 2004), 901–915.

Stranger rape. Rape, Abuse, & Incest National Network, 2012. Available: http://www.rainn.org!get-information!tvpes-of-sexual-assauIt/stranger-rape.

Stritof, S. Why is marital rape a controversial issue? *About.com,* 2015. Available: http://marriage.about.com/cs/maritalrape/f/maritalrape3.htm.

Ten signs of relationship abuse. Human Relations Media. Mount Kisco, NY, 2008.

Types of rapists. Hope for Healing, 2015. Available: http://www.hopeforhealing.org/types.html.

Tyson, A. Sexual abuse is called rife in Guard and Reserves. *Washington Post* (September 30, 2005), p. A2.

Understanding sexual violence: Tips for parents and caregivers of children. National Sexual Violence Resource Center, 2015. Available: http://www.nsvrc.org/saam.

U.S. Military Academy. *SHARP annual training program: Leading the charge against sexual harassment and assault.* West Point, NY: Simon Center for the Professional Military Ethic, 2011.

Using technology to hurt others. Rape, Abuse & Incest National Network, 2015. Available: https://rainn.org/get-information/types-of-sexual-assault/using-technology-to-hurt-others.

Walker, J., Archer, J., & Davies, M. Effects of rape on men: A descriptive analysis. *Archives of Sexual Behavior 34, 1* (February 2005), 69–80.

Was I raped? Rape, abuse, & Incest National Network, 2012. Available: http://www.rainn.orglget-information/types-of-sexual-assault/was-it-rape.

Whatley, M. A. The effect of participant sex, victim dress, and traditional attitudes on causal judgments for marital rape victims. *Journal of Family Violence 20, 3* (June 2005), 191–200.

What is pedophilia? Mental Health Center. *WebMD,* 2015. Available: http://www.webmd.com/mental-health/features/explaining-pedophilia.

What is relationship abuse? Center for Relationship Abuse Awareness, 2014. Available: http://stoprelationshipabuse.org/educated/what-is-relationship-abuse/.

Who are the victims? Rape, Abuse & Incest National Network, 2005. Available: http://www.rainn.org/get-information/statistics/sexual-assault-victims.

Wolak, J., Finkelhor, D., & Mitchell, K. *Trends in arrests of "online predators."* Durham, NH. Crimes Against Children Research Center, March 31, 2009.

CHAPTER 18

Sexually Transmitted Infections

FEATURES

Global Dimensions
STIs Around
the World

Communication Dimensions
Talking with a Partner
About STI Prevention

Multicultural Dimensions
STIs and Minorities

Ethical Dimensions
Notifying Partners
About STIs

CHAPTER OBJECTIVES

1 Define sexually transmitted infections (STIs) and sexually related diseases (SRDs), describe how are they transmitted, and discuss the reasons for their prevalence.

2 Discuss the bacterially based STIs, including incidence, transmission, symptoms and complications, and diagnosis and treatment.

3 Discuss the virally based STIs, including incidence, transmission, symptoms and complications, and diagnosis and treatment.

4 Discuss the ectoparasitic infestations, including transmission, symptoms and complications, and diagnosis and treatment.

5 Describe ways that STIs and SRDs can be prevented.

INTRODUCTION

*J*essica was enrolled in one of our human sexuality classes. One day after class, she asked whether she could stop in during office hours to discuss something "private." Over the years, we have learned that "private" can mean many things: a student just found out she is pregnant, is being abused by a romantic partner, or is concerned about a sexual disorder. In Jessica's case, though, it was a concern that she might have an STI.

Jessica went on to describe a sexual encounter with Rodney that culminated in vaginal sex. Shortly afterward, Jessica noticed a rash on her inner thighs and became alarmed. As soon as she described her concern about having contracted an STI, I knew I would have to refer Jessica to the campus health center for testing and diagnosis. I am an educator, not a medical doctor, I know my limitations. Still, I could not refer her immediately for fear that she would think I was uninterested and be disinclined to discuss with me other concerns she might have in the future. Consequently, we discussed the reasons for her concern—the rash appeared, Rodney had not used a condom, they had not employed any other method of birth control, she met Rodney only the week before at a party and she did not really know him well—and we explored other symptoms she described. Although I did not feel qualified to discuss whether Jessica had an STI, I did take advantage of our private time together to talk about the benefits of using condoms and other methods of birth control and explored with her the decision to engage in sex with someone she had only recently met.

It turned out that all Jessica had was a rash caused by nylon underpants she wore while exercising. The relief on her face said it all, and I doubt that Jessica forgot that scare the next time she was faced with a *decision regarding whether to engage in sex. That is not to say that she will refrain or become abstinent, although those are certainly possibilities and decisions others have made, but rather that she will understand better that any choice to engage in sexual activity is accompanied by both potentially pleasurable and potentially disturbing consequences. Contracting an STI— one of those disturbing consequences—is always a possibility.*

Although Jessica did not have an STI, we have encountered other students who did. Fortunately, most of those students were diagnosed early enough and treated successfully. This chapter describes the more common STIs, ways they can be prevented, and ways they are treated when they are not prevented.

What Are Sexually Transmitted Infections?

The term **sexually transmitted infections (STIs)** describes infections that can be contracted through sexual intimacy. Sexual intimacy includes oral, vaginal, and anal sex as well as genital-to-genital contact that is not penetrative. At least 20 STIs have been identified. There are also diseases of the sexual organs referred to as **sexually related diseases (SRDs)**, which are disorders of the reproductive tract that occur in both sexually active and sexually abstinent individuals. These can be caused by organisms that live in the healthy body but under certain conditions, such as stress, diabetes, drug use, and other health-related problems, affect the delicate chemical balance of the body and cause disease conditions of the sexual organs. Some cancers are also considered to be SRDs. A sexually related infection can sometimes be transmitted to a sexual partner, and the conditions under which this occurs are discussed in this chapter.

Whatever the sexual disease, whether contracted during sexual activity or occurring in an abstinent individual, it affects the individual's feelings about his or her sexuality. Some people believe that anyone with a disease of the sexual organs is unclean, evil, and immoral; that a sexual disease is a punishment for sexual intimacy; and that only those of low socioeconomic and low educational status contract these diseases.

There is no truth to any of these beliefs. Organisms live in our bodies and can multiply when our resistance is low or, as mentioned earlier, when other conditions exist. Pathogenic organisms can sometimes adjust to their habitat, proliferate, and change in ways that cause symptoms of disease. Not only can they affect the body of an infected individual, but they can also be transferred to another individual through sexual activity.

Prevalence of Sexually Transmitted Infections

STIs have become quite common, even though the rates of some STIs have declined in recent years. There are many reasons for the high prevalence of STIs. For example, whereas most states now require physicians to report HIV and AIDS, chlamydia, gonorrhea, and syphilis cases to their state health departments, this was not always the case. Therefore, to compare current STI rates with periods in which reporting was not required would certainly make it appear as if there are more cases today; in fact, there may not be. In addition, since the 1960s, there has been a change in attitudes toward sexual behavior. The trends toward more frequent sexual encounters and sexual activity at earlier ages have meant an increase in the number of people subjected to STIs. Other variables include the following:

1. There is considerable social pressure for social and sexual contact, along with widespread ignorance about sexual health and disease transmission.

2. The traditional restraints on sexual behavior are weakening as families and society in

---

sexually transmitted infections (STIs) Infections that are primarily contracted through sexual contact.

sexually related diseases (SRDs) Diseases of the reproductive system that can occur in either sexually active or sexually inactive individuals.

general become more loosely knit. Families are more mobile; relocation can threaten the stability of family members as they move away from the support system offered by the extended family and community. Adolescents and young adults are now reared in an atmosphere favoring more personal freedom and less adult supervision. More and more families have two parents in the workforce, adolescent and young adult family members are frequently employed while attending school, and many more adolescents today than in the past are unattended during certain times of the day.

3. Adolescence is a time of physical, psychological, and biochemical change and development. The pace of adolescent development varies widely. In particular, physiological maturing occurs at a faster rate than do intellectual, social, and emotional maturing. This places young people in a position of biological readiness for activities that have physical and emotional consequences for which they are not always prepared. Often they face sexual decisions that affect their interests and are not able to judge the best course of action.

4. Current social values have led to widespread expectations of instant gratification. Learning, growing, and achieving goals require persistence—yet young people tend to have a strong sense of urgency to act now, accompanied by a need for immediate satisfaction.

5. An "everybody does it" attitude undermines convictions about individual responsibility. Thus adolescents who feel stifled by external controls and are eager for independence often take action, frequently sexual in nature, for which they are unprepared.

6. Contraceptive methods have not eliminated unwanted pregnancy, but they have essentially eliminated the fear of it. In the past, this fear effectively inhibited sexual activity among many people of childbearing age.

One result of the combination of these factors has been an increase in sexual activity in general—not just the young. This increase, in turn, has led to higher incidence of STIs. There is no doubt the risk of exposure is greater in people who are sexually active, especially with more than one person, because the chance of contracting an STI increases with the number of sexual contacts.

Global DIMENSIONS

STIs Around the World

There are wide variations in the numbers and types of STI cases encountered around the world. Some countries have a high incidence; others have a lower one. The reasons for these differences might at first appear obvious, but on further inspection prove extremely complex.

For example, it is assumed that lack of education is related to STIs, and, in fact, in some countries this is true. Better-educated people have access to more information about STIs, their transmission, and their prevention. Furthermore, better-educated people are more likely to have better-paying jobs, allowing them to act on their STI knowledge (purchase condoms, for example). Yet, this is not always the case. For example, in the early years of the HIV/AIDS epidemic in sub-Saharan Africa, most HIV infections occurred among more educated people. Speculated causes for this difference included ideas that individuals with more education

were wealthier, were more mobile, and had broader networks of sexual partners. However, once educational campaigns were implemented in the region, the HIV rates started to shift, with educated individuals being among the first to adopt protective behaviors. This change could in part reflect the fact that HIV campaigns were often incorporated into schools, so those who stayed in school longer might have been exposed to more health education messages (Hargreaves & Glynn, 2002). Today, education plays a large role in HIV prevention in Africa, with several studies demonstrating that cognitive ability and increased time in school are correlated with lower risk levels for HIV (Baker et al., 2009; Peters et al., 2010).

The reason people contract STIs varies from country to country and even within subpopulations in any one country. The key to preventing STIs at a policy level is understanding these differences and responding to them systematically.

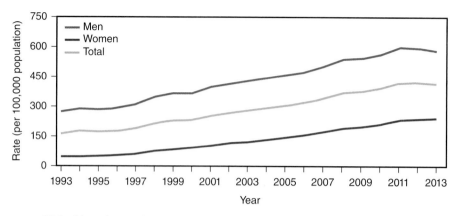

FIGURE **18.1** Chlamydia: rates by sex, United States, 1993–2013.

Source: Reproduced from Centers for Disease Control and Prevention. *Sexually transmitted diseases surveillance, 2013.* Atlanta, GA: U.S. Department of Health and Human Services, 2014. Available: http://www.cdc.gov/std/stats13/figures/1.htm.

In spite of these social factors, and because of several other variables such as the fear of HIV infection, the rates of several STIs have decreased in recent decades. However, accompanying this decrease in rates for some STIs is an increase in rates for others. The rates, signs, symptoms, potential complications, and means of diagnosing and treating the more prevalent STIs are presented in the following sections.

▧ Bacterial Infections

Some STIs are caused by bacteria. Among these are chlamydia, gonorrhea, nongonococcal urethritis, and syphilis. It is not uncommon for these bacterial infections to be transmitted from one partner to the other, so treatment often requires refraining from sexual activity until the bacteria have been eliminated.

Chlamydia

Incidence
Chlamydial infections, caused by the intracellular parasite **Chlamydia trachomatis**, are the most commonly reported STIs in the United States today. According to the Centers for Disease Control and Prevention (CDC, 2014c), because case reporting remains incomplete, estimating the total number of **chlamydia** cases is extremely difficult. However, in 2013 there

were more than 1.4 million chlamydial infections reported—a rate of 446.6 cases per 100,000 population. There are three times more chlamydia cases than gonorrhea cases. From 1993 through 2011, reported cases of chlamydia increased from 178.0 cases per 100,000 population to 453.4 cases per 100,000 population (Figure 18.1). This increase reflects increased screening, recognition of the nature of asymptomatic infection (especially in women), and more consistent reporting as well as actual increases in the infection. The recent small decline may be related to decreases in incidence or decreases in screening.

Reported cases of chlamydia in women far exceed reported cases in men (623.1 cases per 100,000 versus 262.6 per 100,000, respectively). Rates for women are highest in the 15- to 19-year-old (3,043.3 per 100,000 persons) and 20- to 24-year-old age groups (3,621.1 per 100,000) (Figure 18.2) (CDC, 2014c).

Chlamydial infection is an umbrella term that encompasses four major diseases caused by *C. trachomatis*: (1) a genitourinary tract infection in adults, (2) inclusion conjunctivitis (an acute eye infection) in newborns and chlamydial pneumonia in infants, (3) trachoma (a chronic eye infection), and (4) lymphogranuloma venereum. The two diseases of most concern in the United States are adult genitourinary tract infection and infant conjunctivitis and pneumonia.

Symptoms and Complications
Genitourinary tract chlamydial infection has been called "the silent STI." Early symptoms of this infection are often mild and, therefore, unrecognized. Most infected people are asymptomatic. Symptoms, in those who exhibit them, occur 1 to 3 weeks after exposure. In men, the most common symptoms include pain or burning on urination and a white, watery discharge from the penis. Women may note

Chlamydia trachomatis An intracellular parasite that causes chlamydial infections.

chlamydia A term that encompasses several major diseases caused by *Chlamydia trachomatis*, including genitourinary tract infection, a type of conjunctivitis in newborns, a type of pneumonia in infants, lymphogranuloma venereum, and trachoma.

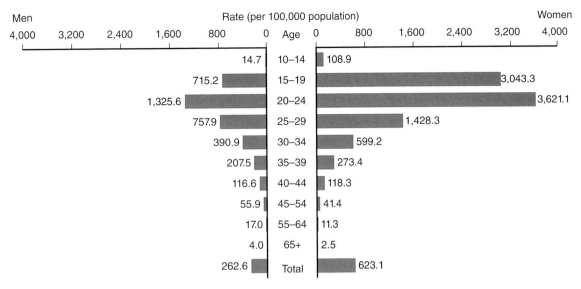

FIGURE 18.2 Chlamydia: rates by age and sex, United States, 2013.

Source: Reproduced from Centers for Disease Control and Prevention. *Sexually transmitted diseases surveillance, 2013.* Atlanta, GA: U.S. Department of Health and Human Services, 2014. Available: http://www.cdc.gov/std/stats13/figures/5.htm.

painful urination, a vaginal discharge, and abdominal pain. Individuals who engage in receptive anal sex can become infected with chlamydia in the anus. Symptoms can include rectal pain, discharge, or bleeding. For those performing oral sex on an infected partner, chlamydia can also be transmitted to the throat.

Diagnosis

To diagnose chlamydia, a layer of cells is scraped from the infected area or a urine sample is tested. The type of laboratory test used depends on the collection method. Nucleic acid amplification tests are the most sensitive tests for endocervical specimens and urethral swab and they are also FDA approved for use with urine. Because of the increased sensitivity, it is less likely that a false-negative result will be obtained with this testing method.

Although most samples are collected by a healthcare practitioner, self-service and self-collected samples are becoming more common. For example, the Los Angeles County Department of Public Health successfully launched an at-home testing campaign in which women requested kits through the phone or online. More than half of the women returned the kits and 8.5% tested positive for chlamydia or gonorrhea (Rotblatt et al., 2013). A similar program on a university campus was not successful, however—fewer than 5% of the women who received kits returned them for analysis (Jenkins et al., 2012). However, another study that used self-collected vaginal swabs to test for multiple STIs (chlamydia, gonorrhea, and trichomoniasis) with collection occurring at a university health center was well received; the swabs were easy to use and considered a favorable testing method by first-year female students (Fielder et al., 2013).

Infants born to women with genitourinary chlamydial infections are at risk of acquiring either inclusion conjunctivitis (pinkeye) or chlamydial pneumonia during delivery (American Sexual Health Association [ASHA], 2014). In the United States, an estimated 100,000 pregnant women have a chlamydia infection. Because of the magnitude of this health threat, the CDC (2010b) recommends that all pregnant women be screened for chlamydia at their first prenatal visit, whether or not they exhibit symptoms of infection. Additionally, high-risk women should be screened again in their third trimester to prevent complications at birth.

Treatment

Chlamydial infections are easily treated in their early stages with antibiotics. The treatment of choice is a single 1-g dose of azithromycin administered orally or 100 mg of doxycycline administered orally twice a day for 7 days. Alternatively, either erythromycin or ofloxacin may be used. Pregnant women should not use doxycycline; erythromycin can be substituted in such individuals.

To minimize the risk of reinfection, patients are asked to refer their sexual partners for evaluation, testing, and treatment and to refrain from sexual intercourse with any partners who have not been treated. Prevention of reinfection is critically important. Many health organizations, including the American Medical Association, the American College of Obstetrics and Gynecologists, the Society for Adolescent Health and Medicine, and the American

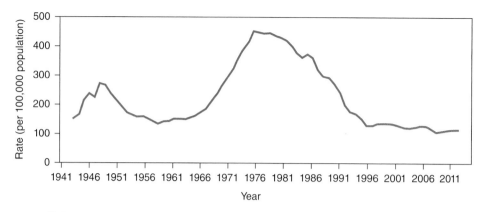

FIGURE 18.3 Gonorrhea: rates, United States, 1941–2013.

Source: Reproduced from Centers for Disease Control and Prevention. *Sexually transmitted diseases surveillance, 2013.* Atlanta, GA: U.S. Department of Health and Human Services, 2014. Available: http://www.cdc.gov/std/stats13/figures/11.htm.

Academy of Pediatrics, recommend the use of expedited partner therapy (EPT) for chlamydia and gonorrhea in states where the practice is legal. EPT entails treating sex partners of patients diagnosed with chlamydia or gonorrhea by providing prescriptions or medications to the patient to take to his or her partner without the healthcare provider first examining the partner. As of June 2015, EPT is permitted in 38 states and the District of Columbia and potentially allowable in an additional 8 states and Puerto Rico. The 4 remaining states have statutes that prohibit EPT (CDC, 2015a). In states where the legality of EPT is not clear, the American College of Obstetrics and Gynecologists (2011) encourages clinicians to advocate for its legality because evidence indicates that this practice can decrease the risk of reinfection.

Unfortunately, because of the asymptomatic nature of the infection and the similarity of symptoms of chlamydia and gonorrhea, many cases of chlamydia are either improperly treated or untreated. Untreated chlamydia can lead to pelvic inflammatory disease (PID) in women and to epididymitis in men. In both genders, the possibility of sterility exists. Because of the high prevalence of chlamydia infections, annual screening for this STI is recommended for all sexually active women 25 years of age and younger (CDC, 2010b).

Gonorrhea

Incidence
Gonorrhea ranks high on the list of reportable communicable diseases. Only chlamydia is more prevalent. The incidence of gonorrhea declined 74% from

1975 to 1997 after implementation of a national gonorrhea control program, with the lowest rate being reached in 2009—98.1 cases per 100,000 individuals. In 2013, the rate increased slightly to 106.1 cases per 100,000 individuals, with 333,004 cases reported in the United States (CDC, 2014c) (Figure 18.3).

Rates of gonorrhea are not equal between the sexes and racial/ethnic groups. Rates are slightly higher among men (109.5 cases per 100,000) than among women (102.4 cases per 100,000), although this is a recent change (Figure 18.4). Regarding ethnicity, the 2013 gonorrhea rates remained highest among blacks at 426.6 cases per 100,000, which is more than 12 times the rate among whites (34.5 per 100,000). Rates among other ethnicities were also higher than those among whites: The rates for American Indians/ Alaska Natives were 4 times those of whites (137.4 per 100,000), the rates for Native Hawaiians/other Pacific Islanders were 2.7 times those of whites (94.0 cases per 100,000), and the rates for Hispanics were almost 2 times those of whites (65.8 per 100,000). While the gonorrhea rate among black individuals is the highest, there was a 9.1% decrease in the rate among blacks from 2009 to 2013; rates for all other ethnicities increased during the same time period (CDC, 2014c).

While a person's sexual behavior certainly affects his or her risk of acquiring gonorrhea, public health studies increasingly indicate that social determinants of health have a critical influence on susceptibility. Social determinants of health are the circumstances in which people are born and live (World Health Organization [WHO], 2015); these physical and social factors of people's lives can affect unhealthy or risky behavior through behavioral influences as well as limited preventive and healthcare access. Notably, living in a neighborhood with a high population density, high female proportion, high percentage of single mothers, high proportion of unmarried family

gonorrhea An STI that commonly starts with inflammation of the mucous membrane lining of the openings of the body (e.g., mouth, vagina).

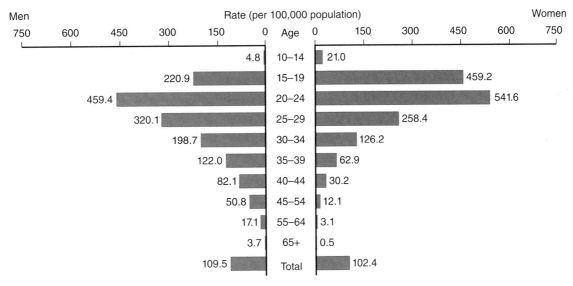

FIGURE 18.4 Gonorrhea: rates by age and sex, United States, 2013.

Source: Reproduced from Centers for Disease Control and Prevention. *Sexually transmitted diseases surveillance, 2013.* Atlanta, GA: U.S. Department of Health and Human Services, 2014. Available: http://www.cdc.gov/std/stats13/figures/16.htm.

units, high proportion of vacant housing units, high proportion of black or other racial minorities, and low socioeconomic status may influence gonorrhea risk (Moonesinghe et al., 2012; Stenger et al., 2014; Sullivan et al., 2011).

Transmission

Gonorrhea is caused by a bacterium known as ***Neisseria gonorrhoeae***, also called *gonococcus*. This bacterium grows in the mucous membranes, the moist protective coat that lines all orifices (openings) of the body. The mucous membranes lining the mouth, throat, vagina, cervix, urethra, and anal canal are all very receptive to gonococcus. When contact occurs between the site of gonococcus in one person and the moist membrane of another—as in all forms of sexual activity—bacteria may be transferred. Thus oral–vaginal, oral–anal, penile–anal, oral–penile, oral–oral, and genital–genital contact can result in the transmission of the bacterium from an infected person to the other partner. Outside the body, however, the gonococcus dies in a few seconds, making it almost impossible to transmit via toilet seats, cups, towels, or other articles used by an infected person.

Interestingly enough, although bacteria may travel from the mucous membranes of the infected partner to the mucous membranes of the uninfected partner, they sometimes die during transfer. Thus exposure does not always result in infection.

The risk of transmission from an infected female to a male through vaginal sex is about 20%. This risk increases to 60% to 80% if there are four or more exposures via vaginal sex. However, for a woman, the risk per episode of vaginal sex for transmission from

an infected partner is in the range of 50% to 70% (CDC, 2013c). This difference occurs because the mucous membrane lining of the vagina, which has a large surface area, is particularly receptive to the bacteria. Any small irritation in this lining can allow the organism rapid entry into the woman's system. Rates of transmission through anal sex have not been quantified, but this route appears to be an efficient mode of transmission; pharyngeal gonorrhea (gonorrhea of the throat) is easily acquired when performing oral sex on a male but transmission to someone performing oral sex on a female is less likely (CDC, 2013c).

Symptoms and Complications

Males are more likely than females to exhibit symptoms of gonorrhea, and most males will experience symptoms severe enough to seek treatment. It is estimated that 90% to 95% of men infected with gonorrhea have symptoms. The males who exhibit symptoms do so within 1 to 14 days after contact; 2 to 5 days is the most likely interval (CDC, 2013c). The primary infection sites in males are the urethra and the rectum.

Symptoms include the sudden onset of frequent, painful urination (dysuria) and a discharge of pus from the urethra. Some males have tenderness in the groin area and noticeable swelling of lymph nodes. In anal gonorrhea, symptoms include membrane irritation, discharge, and painful defecation.

Neisseria gonorrhoeae The bacterium that causes gonorrhea; also known as *gonococcus*. Street names include "clap" and "drip."

Most males with gonorrhea experience some symptoms, but most females are asymptomatic. For males, the gonorrhea "drip" is a common symptom.

Gonorrhea lesions on the tongue.

Neisseria gonorrhoeae is the cause of gonorrhea.

Complications in the male are seen within 2 to 3 weeks without treatment. Infection spreads up the *genitourinary tract*, the posterior urethra, the prostate, the seminal vesicles, and the epididymis. Sometimes acute inflammation of the prostate occurs, accompanied by pelvic tenderness and pain, fever, and urinary retention. Inflammation of the epididymis may

pelvic inflammatory disease (PID) Infection of the reproductive organs, particularly the uterus and fallopian tubes, and the pelvic cavity.

occur; it can be recognized by a feeling of heaviness in the affected testicle, inflammation of the scrotal skin, and sometimes swelling in the lower part of the testicles. If the gonococcal infection spreads to the other testicle, infertility is a possible complication.

Approximately 50% of all females who contract gonorrhea have no symptoms (CDC, 2013c). The cervix is the primary infection site in females; although it may be inflamed, symptoms may not be evident. Inflammation of the Bartholin's glands is possible but not common. A yellowish discharge may be present but may remain undetected. In fact, most females do not realize they have a gonorrheal infection until the infected partner tells them or they have a smear and culture done in a routine gynecologic examination. This point alone should encourage sexually active women to ask for a gonorrhea test as part of their regular checkups.

A potential complication of gonorrhea in women is **pelvic inflammatory disease (PID)**. In PID cases, the most common cause is gonorrhea. If the gonorrhea goes untreated in a woman, within 2 months the gonococcal organisms may cause an ascending infection into the internal reproductive organs and pelvic cavity. During menstruation and immediately after, the organisms travel rapidly. Symptoms include dyspareunia (painful intercourse), occasional nonmenstrual uterine bleeding, inflammation of the fallopian tubes with subsequent tubal infection, vaginal discharge, general abdominal pain, and fever up to 102°F. PID is a common complication in women. As the body defenses try to wall off the infection, scarring of the fallopian tubes can occur and infertility can result.

Disseminated gonococcal infections are systemic infections that occur elsewhere in the body; these are rare, with the incidence ranging from 0.5% to 3% (CDC, 2013c). Examples include *gonococcal arthritis* and *gonococcal dermatitis*. Gonococcal arthritis affects the hands, wrists, ankles, knees, and elbows. Gonorrhea is the primary cause of arthritis in pregnant women and the most common cause of infectious arthritis in the United States. Gonococcal dermatitis, a rash, is most frequently seen on the hands and lower extremities. White blisters appear and eventually darken, leaving the body without scars. *Gonococcal endocarditis*, inflammation of the heart valves, is a serious but rare gonorrheal complication. Finally, *gonococcal ophthalmic infection* can occur in the newborn; that complication has been reduced by treating the eyes of all babies with silver nitrate tetracycline, or penicillin, at birth.

Diagnosis and Treatment
Diagnosis of gonorrhea is usually made through analysis of a urine sample. In some cases, discharge

from body sites will be examined. Throat and rectal cultures are taken if the patient's sexual activity with an infected person involves these body areas. Otherwise, discharge from the urethra in a male and the cervix of a female will be examined. When gonococci are present, approximately 96% of the organisms are isolated in these areas.

For many years, the treatment of choice for gonorrhea was penicillin. In 1976, however, a strain of gonococcus resistant to penicillin appeared. This first antibiotic-resistant strain produced a substance that inactivates penicillin. Since then, other antibiotic-resistant strains of gonorrhea have appeared, including those demonstrating resistance to tetracycline and ciprofloxacin. Consequently, only one class of antimicrobials, the cephalosporins, is recommended and available for the treatment of gonorrhea in the United States. Unfortunately, in Japan in 2011 a strain of gonorrhea was found to be resistant to all forms of antibiotics—including all cephalosporin-class drugs (Ohnishi et al., 2011). There are concerns that this gonorrhea strain could spread worldwide in a few decades, especially as the bacteria's susceptibility to cephalosporins has been decreasing rapidly in the United States as well (Bolan et al., 2012). It is estimated that 20% to 30% of gonococci in the United States are resistant to one or more antimicrobial agents (CDC, 2013c). Because of this concern, the current treatment of choice for uncomplicated gonorrhea infections of the cervix, urethra, and rectum consists of dual therapy of ceftriaxone and either azithromycin or doxycycline (CDC, 2014c). As with all drug regimens, special populations, such as pregnant women, require special precautions and alterations.

Nongonococcal Urethritis

Incidence
Nongonococcal urethritis (NGU) and its potential companion, *nongonococcal cervicitis* (in females), are STIs characterized by inflammation of the urethra and cervix, respectively. The signs and symptoms of NGU are similar to those of gonorrhea. If there are indications of urethritis and a laboratory test rules out gonorrhea, NGU is diagnosed.

Before the 1990s, this condition was called *nonspecific urethritis* because its causes were unknown. Today, researchers have identified that most cases of NGU are caused by *Chlamydia trachomatis*. In most cases of nonchlamydial NGU, no pathogen can be detected, although some research shows that *M. genitalium* may account for 15% to 25% of NGU cases (CDC, 2010b). Other potential causes of NGU include *Ureaplasma urealyticum*, adenovirus, *Haemophilus vaginalis*, *Trichomonas vaginalis* (rare), and herpes simplex virus (rare) (ASHA, 2015d).

Symptoms
NGU symptoms in males include discharge from the penis, itching, irritation and tenderness, and a burning sensation during urination. Nevertheless, 10% of infected men may be asymptomatic. Women who have a NGU-related infection sometimes report a mild vaginal irritation, burning, or discharge. At least 70% of infected women, however, are believed to be asymptomatic. If a woman experiences abdominal pain or abnormal vaginal bleeding, it may indicate that the infection has advanced to pelvic inflammatory disease.

NGU is not a reportable communicable disease, so there is no official count of cases in the United States. It is estimated that cases of NGU equal or surpass those of gonorrhea.

Treatment
Treatment of NGU consists of either 100 mg of doxycycline taken twice a day for 7 days or a single dose of 1 g of azithromycin; both of these medications are administered orally. Alternatively, erythromycin, levofloxacin, or ofloxacin may be used (CDC, 2010b).

Syphilis

Incidence
After falling to an all-time low in 2000, the **syphilis** rate in the United States has risen and is currently at the highest level since 1996 (CDC, 2014c). In 2013, a total of 56,471 syphilis cases (primary and secondary, early latent, late, late latent, and congenital) were reported. In terms of primary and secondary syphilis cases only, 17,375 cases were reported, giving a rate of 5.5 cases per 100,000 people (Figure 18.5).

Outbreaks of syphilis among men who have sex with men (MSM) are largely responsible for the increasing syphilis rate. High-risk sexual behaviors and HIV coinfection contribute to the rate among MSM. In 2013, 75% of primary and secondary syphilis cases in the 49 states and the District of Columbia that provided information about the sex of sex partners occurred among MSM (CDC, 2014c).

Wide disparities exist in the rate of syphilis among racial and ethnic groups. While the rate among blacks has decreased in recent years to 16.8 cases per 100,000, this rate is 5.6 times higher than the rate for whites (3 cases per 100,000). Rates among

nongonococcal urethritis (NGU) Inflammation of the urethra caused by *Chlamydia trachomatis*, *Ureaplasma urealyticum*, *Mycoplasma hominis*, *Trichomonas vaginalis*, herpes simplex virus, and unknown organisms.

syphilis An STI caused by the spirochete *Treponema pallidum*.

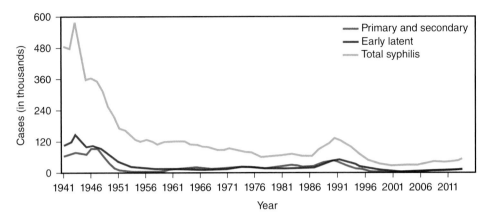

FIGURE **18.5** Syphilis: reported cases by stage of infection, United States, 1941–2013.

Source: Centers for Disease Control and Prevention. *Sexually transmitted diseases surveillance, 2013.* Atlanta, GA: U.S. Department of Health and Human Services, 2014. Available: http://www.cdc.gov/std/stats13 /figures/30.htm.

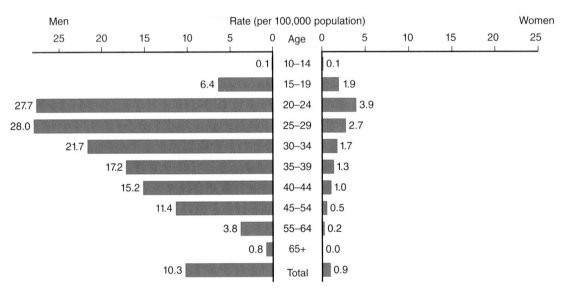

FIGURE **18.6** Primary and secondary syphilis: rates by age and sex, United States, 2013.

Source: Centers for Disease Control and Prevention. *Sexually transmitted diseases surveillance, 2013.* Atlanta, GA: U.S. Department of Health and Human Services, 2014. Available: http://www.cdc.gov/std/stats13/figures/36.htm.

Hispanics have also been increasing, to reach a rate 2 times that of whites (6.3 cases per 100,000). In terms of distribution based on sex, males contract syphilis at a rate 10 times higher than females (CDC, 2014c) (Figure 18.6).

Congenital syphilis—that is, babies born with syphilis—is still a concern in the United States. As with other forms of syphilis, rates of congenital syphilis declined in the 1990s and early 2000s but have increased relatively steadily since then. In 2013, there were 8.7 cases of congenital syphilis per 100,000 live births (CDC, 2014c).

Transmission

The cause of syphilis is *Treponema pallidum*, a spirochete organism that requires a warm, moist area to survive. The **spirochete** is thin and corkscrew shaped; it is transmitted from the open lesions of the infected person to the mucous membranes or cuts in the skin of the other person. The organism can be transmitted by vaginal, anal, or oral sex; however, it can also be spread via genital-to-genital contact without penetration if the individual comes in contact with the open lesion (chancre). Only a few hours after the time of contact, the spirochete reaches the bloodstream of the newly infected person.

T. pallidum can also be transmitted by an infected pregnant woman through the placenta to the unborn child. Syphilis bacteria cannot cross the placenta to

spirochete A spiral-shaped bacterium, one of which—*Treponema pallidum*—causes syphilis.

? Did You Know . . .

In 1932, the U.S. Public Health Service began a study to determine if syphilis developed differently in African Americans than in whites. The study was conducted in Alabama under the guidance of the Tuskegee Institute, one of the foremost black universities in the United States; it became known as the Tuskegee Study. The Tuskegee Study followed 399 black subjects, all with syphilis—and 201 control subjects who had not contracted the disease—for 40 years.

In 1951, when penicillin became available to treat syphilis, the researchers withheld treatment from the study's subjects because of concern it would interfere with their results. Even in 1966, when the morality of withholding treatment to subjects of the Tuskegee Study was raised with the director of the U.S. Public Health Service's Division of Venereal Disease, a committee specifically organized to decide this issue voted to continue the study and continue to withhold treatment from the subjects. Not until a concerned

researcher went public in 1972, and another committee chaired by Senator Edward Kennedy in 1973 was formed to study the issue, was a directive ordered to stop the study and treat the remaining subjects. Guidelines were subsequently developed to prevent researchers conducting studies under the aegis of the federal government to ever again behave in such an immoral manner. The remaining subjects of the Tuskegee Study sued the government and eventually settled for $10 million.

Unfortunately, a similar study conducted by U.S. researchers in Guatemala in the 1940s was revealed in 2011 in a review of historical documents. In this case, 1,300 Guatemalan patients were intentionally infected with syphilis, gonorrhea, or chancroid (Presidential Commission for the Study of Bioethical Issues, 2011). Because of such incidents, suspicion of researchers, especially among underserved populations, is often widespread.

infect the fetus until after the fourth month of pregnancy because of protection provided by a membrane known as Langhan's layer. Therefore, if the mother is treated before the fourth month of pregnancy, the baby will be free of the disease. Women should be tested early in pregnancy, and if they suspect exposure at any time during pregnancy, they must be retested. Additionally, high-risk women should be retested in the third trimester (CDC, 2010b).

Symptoms and Complications

Syphilis proceeds through three stages of development: primary, secondary, and late (tertiary). There is also a latent stage after the secondary stage that lacks any clinical symptoms; it can be subdivided into early latent and late latent stages. Latent syphilis acquired within the last year is referred to as early latent syphilis. Syphilis is infectious during the primary, secondary, and early latent stages. In the late latent and late periods, blood tests of untreated persons yield positive findings for the spirochete, although the disease is not infectious at this stage (except to a fetus).

Primary syphilis manifests itself by the appearance of a painless lesion, called a **chancre**. The chancre can appear from 10 to 90 days after exposure; on average, it appears in 21 days. Usually one lesion forms, generally on the glans penis in the male and the cervix in the female; however, the walls of the vagina and the tissues of the labia can also be sites of chancres. Because the lesions occur most frequently

Courtesy of CDC

Chancres of primary syphilis on penis.

on hidden genital areas, they often remain undetected. Lesions can also appear on the nipples, anus, scrotum, or mouth.

The chancre disappears with or without treatment within 3 to 6 weeks, so a person who suspects that he or she has been exposed to syphilis should have a blood test and not assume that the disappearance of the lesion means absence of an infection. During the primary stage, however, a blood test result may be negative; thus the test should be repeated. If possible, material exuding from a lesion suspected of being syphilitic should be examined under a microscope in

primary syphilis The first stage of syphilis most generally manifested by the appearance of a painless lesion called a *chancre*.

chancre A painless lesion that is symptomatic of the primary stage of syphilis and appears at the site of contact.

A chancre is symptomatic of the primary stage of syphilis. Often, though, the chancre can appear on hidden parts of the female genital areas, making the disease asymptomatic by appearance. A woman who suspects that her partner has syphilis should request a medical exam or test.

In the secondary stage of syphilis, a generalized rash can appear on the body 6 weeks to several months after initial exposure. Although the rash disappears within a few weeks, medical treatment should be sought to eradicate the underlying syphilis bacteria, *Treponema pallidum*.

what is called the *darkfield technique*. Sometimes this procedure, too, is repeated.

Secondary syphilis is usually characterized by a generalized rash that appears on the body 6 weeks to several months after initial exposure. The rash does not itch, and it too subsides without treatment. Sometimes in this stage mucous patches are found in the mouth. Other symptoms during secondary syphilis may include fever, swollen lymph glands, sore throat, patchy hair loss, headaches, weight loss, muscle aches, and fatigue (CDC, 2014d). `

Latent syphilis has no visible symptoms, and this stage may last for years. The early latent period begins when the secondary symptoms disappear and ends 1 to 4 years later. Approximately 30% of all individuals infected in the latent stage progress to **late syphilis** (also called tertiary syphilis) within 1 to 20 years of infection; the rate is relatively low because of widespread use of antibiotics. In the late stage, symptoms may involve the nervous system or cardio-vascular system. The infection can cause blindness, paralysis, crippling, dementia, and possibly death.

Diagnosis and Treatment
As noted, early diagnosis of syphilis is made through a darkfield microscope examination of the material

exuding from the chancre or rash, if possible, and through blood testing. Penicillin G is the current method of choice for all stages of syphilis. The preparation used, the dosage, and the length of treatment all depend on the stage and clinical manifestations of the disease (CDC, 2010b).

■ Viral Infections

Some STIs are caused by viruses. Among these are genital warts, genital herpes, and hepatitis B. The human immunodeficiency virus (HIV) causes acquired immunodeficiency syndrome (AIDS); both HIV and AIDS are discussed elsewhere in this text.

secondary syphilis The second stage of syphilis, often characterized by a rash.

latent syphilis A stage of syphilis that may last for years. Early latent syphilis typically lasts 1 to 4 years and individuals can still be infectious. Late latent syphilis also lasts multiple years, but individuals are not infectious to others except for transmission in utero to the fetus.

late (tertiary) syphilis The final stage of syphilis, which is characterized by systemic complications including damage to the nervous and circulatory systems, and possibly death. This stage is rare because of widespread use of antibiotics to treat syphilis.

HPV is the most common STI in the United States. Some strains of HPV cause genital warts. Although the symptoms and conditions associated with HPV are treatable, HPV infection cannot be cured.

Viral STIs are among the most difficult to eradicate because the viruses that cause them remain in the body even after symptoms subside. However, as we discuss, there are effective treatments for viral STIs.

Human Papillomavirus

The most common sexually transmitted infection in the United States is caused by **human papillomavirus (HPV)**. The estimated overall prevalence rate for all types of HPV is 42.5%. Ninety percent of these infections are asymptomatic and resolve themselves within 2 years; however, persistent infection with the virus is associated with the development of cervical cancer and/or genital warts, depending on the type of HPV. While more than 40 distinct types of HPV can infect the genitals, only a few have a widespread impact; HPV-6 and HPV-11 account for 90% of all genital warts, and HPV-16 and HPV-18 are responsible for 70% of all cervical cancers worldwide (CDC, 2014c). Since 2006, an HPV vaccine has been available in the United States.

Transmission

HPV is different than some STIs as it is transmitted via contact with the infected area; contact with vaginal fluid, semen, or blood is not required for transmission. As a result, oral, vaginal, and anal sex can transmit the virus, but genital-to-genital contact can also be a risky behavior. Similarly, because condoms do not cover the entire genital area, they can reduce but not eliminate risk.

Genital Warts

Genital warts can occur in most areas of the genitals and anus. In females, the warts appear on the labia, in the lower area of the vagina, on the cervix, or around the anus. In males, they appear on the glans, foreskin, and shaft of the penis; on the scrotum; and in the anal area. Genital warts are growths or bumps that vary in appearance; they may be raised or flat, single or multiple, small or large. Usually, they are flesh colored or whitish in appearance. Typically, warts do not cause itching, burning, or pain.

Warts may appear within several weeks after sex with someone infected with a strain of HPV that causes warts, or it may take several months or years to appear. This extended incubation period makes determining the infection date difficult. It is also possible to transmit the virus to sexual partners when no warts are present; however, it is believed that HPV is more likely transmitted when warts are present.

There is some evidence that the incidence of genital warts may be decreasing based on a variety of measures that examine clinical reports of genital warts (see Figure 18.7 for example). However, more years of data collection are needed to determine whether this minor decrease indicates a sustained pattern and how the introduction of the HPV vaccines might be affecting these rates (CDC, 2014c).

human papillomavirus (HPV) A persistent STI caused by any of a group of viruses associated with the development of cervical cancer and/or genital warts.

Communication
DIMENSIONS

Talking with a Partner About STI Prevention

Many of our students react incredulously when we suggest they speak with a potential partner about STIs before engaging in sex. "It would ruin the moment," they argue. In frustration, we sometimes respond, "Contract an STI and then let us know about ruining the moment!" If that were all we offer our students, they would be right to be angry. Instead, we also provide them with suggestions about ways to communicate with a potential sexual partner about preventing STIs:

- Begin the conversation before matters are "hot and heavy." Once people are sexually excited, it is more difficult for them to make sensible decisions or to participate in meaningful conversation.
- While many STIs are asymptomatic, examining your partner's genitals can be part of familiarizing yourself with what is normal for your partner. Laughing, soft touch, and expressions of admiration can make the moment enjoyable rather than clinical. Offering to be "examined" first can help reduce your partner's anxiety about the process.

- Discuss your prior sexual history, as it relates to STI risk, with your partner before asking your partner to share his or her history. Engage in this discussion by disclosing as much detail as you feel comfortable discussing. If expressed in an erotic manner, this discussion can be sexually stimulating as it concurrently accomplishes the purpose of preventing exposure to disease-causing organisms.
- Suggest a "testing" date where you and your partner visit a clinic and get tested together. This can help reduce the pressure or anxiety that you or your partner may feel.
- Demonstrate effective communication skills. Lean forward, nod your head, and look your partner in the eyes to communicate interest. Periodically paraphrase what your partner has said and what you guess he or she is feeling to demonstrate you have been listening. Do not interrupt, raise your voice, or frown in a way that interferes with your partner's communication.

There are ways to make communicating about STIs less embarrassing, less confrontational, and more effective. Discussing STIs with sexual partners is important. Your health—and maybe even your life—may depend on it!

Some clinical data indicate individuals presenting with genital warts differ based on sex of partner (male or female) and geographic location.

Diagnosis and Treatment of Genital Warts

Genital warts are typically diagnosed through visual exam, although in some cases the warts may be too small to see with the naked eye. A clinician may use acetic acid (vinegar) to "highlight" the warts, because the solution turns warts white. However, because this is not a specific test for HPV, it is not a recommended practice (CDC, 2010b).

Treatment of genital warts can vary depending on the size, location, and number of warts; changes

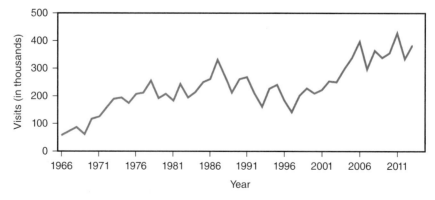

FIGURE **18.7** Genital warts: initial visits to physicians' offices, United States, 1966–2013.

Source: Data from Centers for Disease Control and Prevention. *Sexually transmitted diseases surveillance, 2013.* Atlanta, GA: U.S. Department of Health and Human Services, 2014. Available: http://www.cdc.gov/std/stats13/figures/49.htm.

in the warts; patient preference; treatment cost; convenience; adverse effects; and a clinician's experience with the treatments. Some methods are applied in a clinician's office; others are administered at home by the patient.

A number of in-office procedures are available. With cryotherapy, the wart is frozen with liquid nitrogen. The tissue then dies and is replaced with healthy normal tissue. Trichloracetic acid is another chemical applied to the surface of the wart by a doctor or a nurse. The warts can also be cut off, which has the advantage of getting rid of warts in a single office visit. With electrocautery, the warts are burned off with an electrical current. Laser therapy uses an intense light to destroy warts. This type of therapy usually is reserved for cases with larger wart clusters, especially those that have not responded well to other treatments.

Two prescription creams can also be used at home by the patient to treat warts. Podofilox cream or gel may be less expensive than treatment done in a clinic and is easy to use, but its use must be continued for about 4 weeks. The other cream, imiquimod cream, is also effective and easy to use. Because this cream boosts the immune system's ability to fight HPV, it may reduce the frequency of recurrences (ASHA, 2015a).

HPV, Cervical Changes, and Cancer

HPV can cause normal cells on infected skin to become abnormal. As previously discussed, some strains of HPV can cause visible changes in the form of genital warts. Other strains may cause cell changes that could represent precancerous changes in the cervix or other areas related to HPV infection: vulva, vagina, penis, anus, and oropharynx (back of the throat including the base of the tongue and the tonsils).

Recent media attention around oral cancers and HPV may have some students wondering about their level of risk. Studies have shown that oral HPV is found in less than 7% of the population, and only 1% of cases involve the type that causes oropharyngeal cancer. Rates have been determined to be higher in men, current cigarette smokers, heavy users of alcohol, and current and former users of marijuana (Gillison et al., 2012). The transmission route for oral HPV is not clear; some studies suggest that oral sex and "French" (wet) kissing can transmit the virus (CDC, 2013b), but other studies show that partners of individuals with oral cancers have oral HPV rates equal to the general population (D'Souza et al., 2014). More research is needed to better understand the transmissibility of this virus and to quantify the risk related to oral HPV.

When HPV infection leads to precancerous changes in the cervix, in many cases the immune system is able to fight off HPV naturally, and the infected cells return to normal. In other cases, the body is not able to fight the virus and persistent infection, and possible complications result. For men who have sex with men, there is an increased risk of anal cancer due to HPV infection.

Risk of any type of HPV infection increases for people who have unprotected sex, especially at a young age, and who have many sex partners (although people with just one sexual partner can also contract HPV). Because most people can clear the infection, other factors may contribute to the increased risk of developing cervical cancer, including smoking, a weakened immune system, a large number of childbirths, and long-term use of oral contraceptives (American Cancer Society, 2015).

Diagnosis and Treatment of Cervical Changes

HPV is usually diagnosed as part of a woman's health or gynecologic exam. The Pap test looks for abnormal cells in a woman's cervix that may be caused by HPV, but it is not a diagnostic test for HPV. Tests are available for women older than 30 years that look for viral DNA or RNA or capsid proteins related to specific HPV strains. These tests are not recommended for women younger than 20 years of age, for men, or as a general test for STIs. In women younger than 21 years of age, the rate of spontaneous clearance of HPV is high; in turn, limiting HPV screening reduces the possibility of unnecessary treatment. Unfortunately for men, there is no way to diagnose HPV strains related to these cancers before symptoms develop.

For women who are diagnosed with HPV strains related to cancer, the treatment will vary depending on the woman's age and pregnancy status, the location of the abnormality, and the severity of the cell changes. Because the immune system may be able to combat HPV, in some cases monitoring the cervix and retesting in a few months may be the recommended strategy. In other cases, treatment to remove the affected area may be suggested; this can be done through cryotherapy (freezing the cells with liquid nitrogen), loop electrosurgical excision procedure (LEEP), or a cone biopsy (sometimes called conization) (ASHA, 2015c).

Prevention of HPV

Three vaccines have been approved for use in the United States to prevent infection with HPV. Cervarix protects against the two strains of HPV most associated with cervical cancer and has been approved for use in girls and women. Gardasil protects against the four different strains of HPV that are associated with 70% of cervical cancers, 80% of anal cancers (HPV types 16 and 18), and 90% of genital wart infections (HPV types 6 and 11). Some research has shown that Gardasil may provide some protection against anal cancer caused by HPV in MSM (Palefsky et al., 2011).

In December 2014, the FDA approved Gardasil 9; this new version of the vaccine covers nine HPV types: HPV types 6 and 11, the two strains responsible for most genital wart infections, and the seven types that can cause cell changes leading to cervical and other cancers (types 16, 18, 31, 33, 45, 52, and 58). Both versions of Gardasil are approved for use in males and females. Because the vaccine will be most effective if received before becoming sexually active, it is recommended that girls and boys between 11 and 12 years old receive the vaccine (although it can be administered as early as 9 years of age).

All three vaccines consist of a series of three shots given over a 6-month period, with the second dose being given 1 to 2 months after the first and the third dose being given 6 months after the first dose. The three doses of the HPV vaccine cost $130 per injection ($390 for the entire series). As a result of the Affordable Care Act mandates, all private insurance must cover the cost of the HPV vaccine. For those individuals without private insurance, the Vaccines for Children (VFC) program provides federal funds to cover the cost of vaccines in children ages 18 and younger who are either Medicaid eligible, uninsured, American Indian, Alaska Native, or underinsured. Other support options may be available for those children who do not qualify for VFC coverage (Kaiser Family Foundation, 2015).

Whereas health advocates welcome and support the recommendation that all preteens be inoculated, this support is not universal. Some people believe that the vaccine encourages sexual behavior, and some parents question the value of vaccinating young children for a STI. Currently no federal law requires this vaccination, and state laws vary regarding requirements for the HPV vaccine prior to school entry. In spite of widespread media coverage and financial support, in 2013 only two-thirds (37.6%) of girls and 14% of boys between 13 and 17 received all three doses of an HPV vaccine. There are many reasons for the slow uptake of the vaccine, including parents' lack of knowledge about the vaccine, concerns about safety, and belief that their child is not sexually active. While you may hear "horror stories" about the side effects of the vaccine, few adverse events have actually been reported and the frequency of these incidents is similar to that for other vaccinations (Kaiser Family Foundation, 2015). Research has also shown that sexual activity of young adults is not impacted by receiving the vaccine (Jena et al., 2015).

genital herpes An STI characterized by tiny fluid-filled blisters that appear on the genitals and in the genital tract.

herpes simplex virus (HSV) The virus that causes oral and genital herpes infections.

Genital Herpes

Incidence

The cause of **genital herpes** is a virus called **herpes simplex virus (HSV)**, which belongs to a family of more than 70 herpes viruses. Humans play host to four herpes viruses:

- Herpes simplex virus: the agent that causes fever blisters and genital herpes

- Cytomegalovirus: a virus that can cause death or retardation if acquired by a fetus

- Varicella-zoster virus: the agent that causes chickenpox and shingles

- Epstein-Barr virus: the agent that causes Burkitt's lymphoma in humans

In 1961, it was found that two types of HSV exist: type 1 (HSV-1) and type II (HSV-2). Previously, HSV-1 was more commonly found in the mouth and HSV-2 was more commonly observed in the genital and anal areas. However, HSV-1 is becoming increasingly common in the genital area, and some research indicates that it may be more common than HSV-2, especially among young women and MSM (Bernstein et al., 2013; Ryder et al., 2009). Rates of HSV-1 are also higher among white women, whereas rates of HSV-2 are higher among black and Hispanic women (Bernstein et al., 2013). Possible reasons for the increase in HSV-1 prevalence include differences in sex practices between young and older individuals, with younger persons being more likely to practice oral sex (Bernstein et al., 2013). In addition, as acquisition of HSV-1 through nonsexual means as a child decreases, it leaves individuals without the protective antibodies when they are exposed to HSV-1 as adolescents during their initial sexual activities (Bradley et al., 2014).

Most patients who experience a first episode of HSV-2 infection experience recurrent episodes of genital lesions. However, clinical recurrences are much less frequent for HSV-1 infection than for HSV-2 infection. Therefore, identifying the causative agent has implications for treatment and counseling.

Overall rates of genital herpes in the United States appear to be consistent, with about 1 in 6 individuals having genital herpes (CDC, 2014a). Over the past decade, this rate has remained relatively stable, although increases in initial clinic visits (Figure 18.8) may indicate that more people are recognizing and identifying the infection. This change would be a positive one, as 87.4% of individuals who are infected with genital HSV do not know it (CDC, 2014a).

Women are more likely than men to be infected; in opposite-sex sexual experiences, transmission from a male partner to a female partner is more likely than

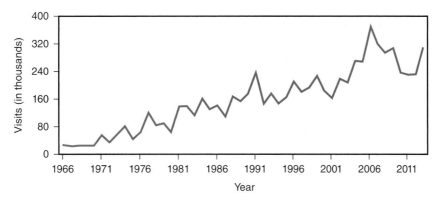

FIGURE **18.8** Genital herpes: initial visits to physicians' offices, United States, 1966–2013.

Source: Data from Centers for Disease Control and Prevention. *Sexually transmitted diseases surveillance, 2013.* Atlanta, GA: U.S. Department of Health and Human Services, 2014. Available: http://www.cdc.gov/std/stats13/figures/53.htm.

from a female partner to a male partner. There are also racial/ethnic group differences, with black individuals disproportionately at risk for herpes; black Americans have a 41.8% prevalence rate compared to a rate of 11.3% for whites. This disparity persists even after controlling for sexual experience; for example, among individuals with 2 to 4 lifetime sexual partners, HSV-2 infection is still more prevalent among blacks (34.3%) compared to whites (9.1%) or Hispanics (13%) (CDC, 2014a). As with gonorrhea, the social determinants of health are a factor in herpes rates.

Transmission
Herpes is similar to HPV in that it is transmitted via contact with the infected area. While oral, vaginal, and anal sex can transmit the virus, so can genital-to-genital contact. Infected individuals also need to be aware of potential self-transmission. For example, if individuals with oral herpes touch their mouth and then genitals, they can spread the herpes infection to their genitals. Additionally, because condoms do not cover the entire genital area, condoms reduce but do not eliminate risk.

Symptoms and Complications
Primary genital herpes corresponds to the time of actual infection by the herpes virus and the formation of antibodies. A primary (first occurrence) herpes infection can be very painful but can also be completely symptom free. Almost 90% of individuals who test positive for HSV-2 infection are asymptomatic or have symptoms that were unrecognized as herpes (CDC, 2014a). Many of these infected individuals are carriers of HSV who are unaware of their infection and as a result pose a potential risk to sexual partners.

The first outbreak usually occurs approximately 4 days after the initial infection (though the range is 2 to 12 days), and the sores typically heal within 2 to 4 weeks (CDC, 2014a). During this initial outbreak, symptoms may include painful lesions, a sluggish feeling, and fever, along with possible lymph-node enlargement. Tiny blisters form; these are filled with a clear fluid in which the virus thrives. The area may become reddened and infected. When blisters appear, the site is in its most infectious state. The open lesions crust over as healing begins. In addition to the internal and external genitals and the anus, blisters can sometimes appear on the thighs and buttocks. Some people experience itching, tingling, or burning sensations on the legs, hips, and buttocks occurring hours to days before a lesion will appear, known as the **prodrome**.

Courtesy of CDC/Dr. Hermann.

Herpes simplex type 1 can manifest itself as a cold sore.

primary genital herpes The first stage of a genital herpes infection; it begins with infection by the herpes virus and the formation of antibodies. Common symptoms include painful lesions in or around the genital area, a sluggish feeling, fever, and possibly swollen lymph nodes.

prodrome Itching, tingling, or burning sensations that occur where a herpes lesion will appear.

Symptoms of primary genital herpes include painful lesions, a sluggish feeling, and fever, along with lymph-node enlargement.

Once antibodies are formed, the virus enters the **latent genital herpes** stage. Antibodies do not protect against reinfection, but they do tend to make any recurrent outbreaks less severe. During the latent stage HSV travels up the afferent nerve to the sacral ganglion, where it remains inactive (Figure 18.9). At this point in the infection there are no signs and symptoms.

The virus can become reactivated in the sacral ganglion without producing clinical signs, a process termed **viral shedding**. During this stage, the virus is excreted from the body even though the infected individual is experiencing no symptoms. HSV is readily transmitted when blisters or ulcers are present. However, the infection can occur through asymptomatic viral shedding.

Recurrent genital herpes is characterized by reactivation of the virus with clinical manifestations. During this stage the virus travels down the nerve root to the skin, often causing new herpes blisters to erupt. Approximately half of individuals experience prodrome symptoms before a recurrence. Recurrent infections are usually shorter and have milder symptoms than a primary herpes infection. They are common during the first year, but their frequency can vary. Those persons with HSV-1 infection average fewer than 1 outbreak per year, while those with HSV-2 infection average 4 to 5 outbreaks per year. While recurrence is individualized, some common triggers have been identified: poor diet, emotional or physical stress, friction in the genitals, surgical trauma, illness, and some steroid medications such as those used for asthma. Initial infections and recurrences are not always apparent, as blisters may appear inside the genital tract where they cannot be seen, symptoms may be so mild they go unnoticed, or symptoms are confused with other conditions. Sometimes the infection may look like a red spot, a pimple, an ingrown hair, razor burn, hemorrhoids, or an insect bite (ASHA, 2015e).

Diagnosis and Treatment

Traditionally, HSV was diagnosed visually based on symptoms, with a culture taken of fluid from the blisters to confirm the diagnosis. While this method is still preferred if genital ulcers are present for less than 48 hours, the sensitivity of this method decreases for recurrent lesions and as lesions begin to heal. If a clinician is able to get a culture from a new lesion, then it can also be typed as HSV-1 or HSV-2. Unfortunately, because of the decreased efficacy for recurrent infections and healing lesions, there is a high risk of a false-negative result (meaning that the results appear to be negative, but the person actually has herpes).

Blood tests are available for individuals without symptoms or those past the 48-hour window of initial symptoms. Two different tests are used to measure antibodies: immunoglobulin M (IgM) and immunoglobulin G (IgG). The IgG test offers greater accuracy in detecting HSV type and is the only one

latent genital herpes   The stage of genital herpes characterized by inactivity of the herpes virus, during which an infected individual is asymptomatic.

viral shedding   HSV is excreted from the body even though an infected individual experiences no signs or symptoms.

recurrent genital herpes   The stage of a genital herpes infection that is characterized by a reactivation of the virus and the appearance of blisters on the skin. Not all people with herpes have recurrences.

Herpes simplex on penis.

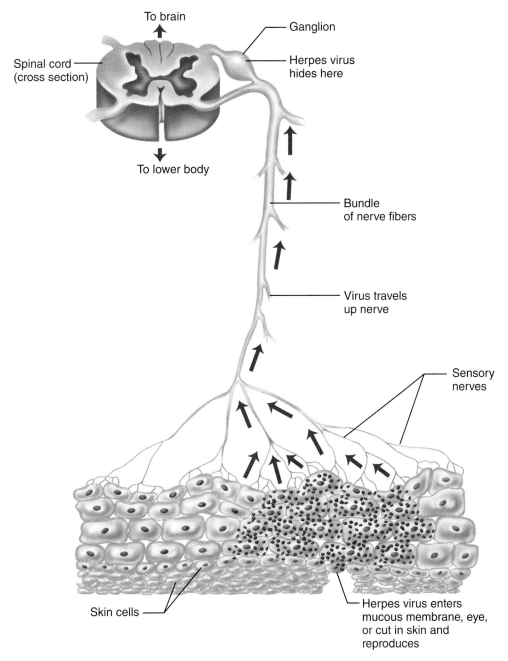

To brain

Ganglion

Spinal cord
(cross section)

Herpes virus
hides here

To lower body

Bundle
of nerve fibers

Virus travels
up nerve

Sensory
nerves

Skin cells

Herpes virus enters
mucous membrane, eye,
or cut in skin and
reproduces

FIGURE **18.9** An initial herpes infection takes place when the virus (dots) enters cells of the mucous membranes, eyes, or skin. It reproduces and travels up (arrows) the sensory nerves until it reaches a ganglion (cluster of nerve cell bodies). There it hides, protected from attack by the body's immune system, which overcomes the infection at the place of entry. Although the entry wound soon heals, when conditions allow, the virus may later travel back down the nerve pathway to reinfect skin cells.

recommended by the American Sexual Health Association (2015b).

One limitation of blood tests is that they do not indicate the location of infection. Because almost all HSV-2 infections are sexually transmitted, the presence of HSV-2 antibodies implies a genital infection. However, if test results show only HSV-1 antibodies, it is more difficult to interpret. Many people with HSV-1 antibodies have an oral HSV infection acquired during childhood, which might be asymptomatic. However, genital HSV-1 infection appears to be increasing, and genital HSV-1 also can be asymptomatic. In the absence of clinical symptoms, a genital HSV-1 infection may be more difficult to confirm (CDC, 2010b).

Treatment for HSV does not remove the virus from the body, but it can help to alleviate symptoms, including outbreaks and viral shedding. Antiviral medication can be used in two primary ways: episodic treatment and suppressive treatment. Episodic treatment is administered during the prodrome or within 1 day of a lesion developing; the goal is to diminish symptom severity and shorten the duration of lesions. Suppressive treatment is usually the treatment option for those persons with frequent lesion recurrences; it requires a daily dosage of antiviral medication. Studies have shown that suppressive therapy reduces the frequency of genital herpes recurrences by 70% to 80% in patients who have frequent recurrences, and some individuals have reported no symptomatic outbreaks while being on the therapy (CDC, 2010b). Suppression therapy with one type of antiviral (valacyclovir) has also been shown to reduce transmission among serodiscordant heterosexual couples (when one individual has HSV and the other does not). Suppression therapy also reduces the risk of viral shedding (Corey et al., 2004), although even high doses of antiviral medication do not eliminate viral shedding (Johnston et al., 2012).

Because many people are not aware they have genital herpes, prevention can be difficult. Using condoms, regardless of whether a person knows his or her infection status, will reduce—but not eliminate—risk. Persons with genital herpes should refrain from sexual activity when lesions or symptoms (prodrome) are present and inform their sexual partners that they have herpes. Pregnant women with herpes infection need to inform their healthcare providers of their status, as there is a risk of transmitting herpes to a fetus neonatally. Individuals with herpes should consider whether episodic or suppression medications are options for them. Individuals can also track recurrences to identify their individual triggers, such as stress or illness, to better reduce the risk that they might transmit their infection to other people. To help prevent infections in other areas, persons with genital herpes should thoroughly wash their hands after touching their genitals.

One rare but serious risk associated with genital herpes is potentially fatal infections in babies. It is important that women avoid contracting herpes during pregnancy because a newly acquired infection during late pregnancy poses a greater risk of transmission to the baby (CDC, 2010b). As already noted, the contagious virus is contained within the lesions. If vaginal lesions leak fluid during childbirth, the virus may be transmitted to the infant and can result in encephalitis, brain damage, or both. Although less common, HSV can also be transmitted to a fetus through the placenta, thereby causing infection before birth.

At this time it is not considered practical or feasible to test all women for herpes during their pregnancies, but women with a history of herpes definitely should be examined weekly from 32 weeks gestation until delivery to see whether lesions recur. Any primary genital herpes lesions are likely to be detected in the frequent routine prenatal visits. If genital herpes is present at the time of delivery, the infant should be delivered by cesarean section. If examinations for active herpes virus yield negative findings at delivery, the infant can be delivered vaginally with little risk of infection.

Hepatitis

There are five hepatitis viruses: A, B, C, D, and E. In the United States, hepatitis D and E are rare. The other three types (A, B, and C) can cause similar symptoms but have different modes of transmission and can affect the liver differently. Hepatitis A is usually associated with oral–fecal contamination of water and food, but transmission through oral–anal contact has been increasingly documented, especially among MSM. Hepatitis B is transmitted in a variety of ways, including sexual contact. Transmission of hepatitis C usually occurs via blood-to-blood contact through needles or other drug paraphernalia. Hepatitis C can also be spread through sexual contact, although it is unclear how frequently this type of transmission occurs. Having an STI or HIV, sex with multiple partners, or rough sex appears to increase a person's risk for contracting hepatitis C.

In addition to transmission differences, manifestations of the viruses differ. Hepatitis A appears only as an acute (self-limited) infection and does not become chronic; people infected with hepatitis A usually improve without treatment. Hepatitis B and hepatitis C can also begin as acute infections, but in some people the virus remains in the body, resulting in chronic disease and long-term liver problems. Vaccines are available to prevent hepatitis A and B, but there is not a vaccine for hepatitis C. Because transmission of the hepatitis B virus (HBV) is often sexual, specifically through blood or blood products, semen, vaginal secretions, and saliva, the discussion here will focus on that virus.

Hepatitis B Incidence

The incidence of acute hepatitis B has been declining since 1990, mainly due to effective vaccination strategies. Nevertheless, chronic HBV infection remains widespread, affecting an estimated 700,000 to 1.4 million people in the United States. In 2012, 2,895 cases of acute hepatitis B in the United States were reported to CDC. Many cases are not reported, however, so the estimated number of acute cases is actually 18,760 (CDC, 2015b).

Primary risk factors for HBV infection include unprotected sex with an infected partner, birth from an

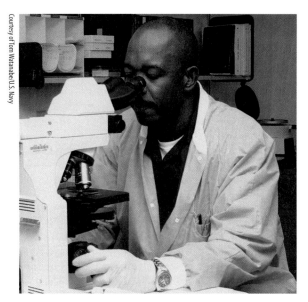

Hepatitis B is diagnosed by a blood test that looks for antibodies or antigens that are present when a person has been exposed to the hepatitis B virus.

? Did You Know . . .

Individuals infected with an STI are at a higher risk for becoming infected with HIV, the virus that causes AIDS. The genital lesions characteristic of STIs—such as the blisters associated with herpes infection—provide HIV with an easy entry point into the body. Thus individuals who engage in unsafe sexual practices while an open lesion exists on the genitals lose an important line of defense against infection—unbroken skin.

Photomicrograph of cells infected with the herpes simplex virus.

infected mother, unprotected sex with more than one partner, MSM, history of other STIs, and illegal injection drug use (CDC, 2012). About half of all chronic HBV infections are found among persons born in Asia and Asian Americans who were born to HBV-infected mothers in the United States (CDC, 2015b).

Hepatitis B Symptoms and Complications

Only about half of adults who contract HBV are symptomatic, with fewer than 1% of reported cases resulting in rapid onset of liver failure and death. If symptoms are present, they can include fatigue, loss of appetite, nausea, vomiting, abdominal pain, dark urine, and jaundice (yellowing of the skin and eyes). Risk of chronic infection decreases with age; 90% of infants and 30% of children younger than 5 years are likely to become chronically affected, compared to 2% to 6% of adults (CDC, 2012). Persons with chronic HBV infection might be asymptomatic, or they may experience more severe conditions such as cirrhosis and liver cancer. In the United States, chronic HBV infection results in approximately 2,000 deaths per year (CDC, 2015b).

Hepatitis B Diagnosis, Treatment, and Prevention

Diagnosis of acute or chronic HBV infection requires blood tests for HBV antibodies. Specific antibodies may be present with an acute infection, so clinicians can determine if it is an acute or chronic infection based on the results of the blood tests (CDC, 2010b).

No specific therapy is available for persons with acute hepatitis B; treatment is supportive in that it can address any nausea, aches, or other pain. For individuals with chronic HBV, several antiviral drugs are available. A medical evaluation and regular monitoring should be undertaken to determine whether the disease is progressing and to identify any damage to the liver.

The prime method of HBV prevention is widespread vaccination. Most traditional-age college students have been vaccinated because of school requirements. If vaccination has not been undertaken, individuals should consider vaccination, and in the meantime take steps to reduce their risk. HBV is a highly stable virus that can survive outside the body for at least 7 days and still be infectious (CDC, 2014b). Likewise, HBV is easily transmitted during sexual activity, so using a condom to reduce risk is essential. Not handling blood or blood products, semen, and vaginal secretions and not sharing items that might contain blood (such as razors or toothbrushes) are other critical strategies to reduce risk.

▪ Vaginal Infections

One category of infection, vaginitis or vaginal infections, occurs in response to changes in an individual's own body, and therefore has been referred to as a *sexually related disease*. Two types of vaginitis,

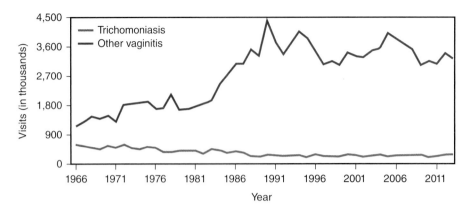

FIGURE **18.10** Trichomoniasis and other vaginal infections: women, initial visits to physicians' offices, United States, 1966–2013.

Source: Data from Centers for Disease Control and Prevention. *Sexually transmitted diseases surveillance, 2013.* Atlanta, GA: U.S. Department of Health and Human Services, 2014. Available: http://www.cdc.gov/std/stats13/figures/55.htm.

trichomoniasis and candidiasis, can also be transmitted from partner to partner and are considered relatively common in women.

Trichomoniasis

Trichomonas vaginalis is a one-celled organism that burrows under the vaginal mucosa to cause **trichomoniasis**, or **trich**. The prevalence rate for this infection, estimated based on the number of clinician visits, is 3.1%, although the rate among black women is much higher—13.1% (CDC, 2014c) (Figure 18.10). The most common mode of transmission is through sexual contact with an infected partner; vaginal sex, sharing sex toys, and mutual masturbation can all transmit the one-celled protozoan if fluids from one partner are passed to the genitals of the other.

For those women who exhibit symptoms, the main ones are an odorous, foamy, white or yellow-green discharge that irritates the vagina and vulva. Frequent and some painful urination can also occur. Men rarely have symptoms, but if they do occur it is usually a discharge from the urethra or frequent and sometimes painful urination.

Trichomoniasis can be passed back and forth between partners; therefore it is important that all sexual partners of an infected individual receive treatment, especially because of the high rates of asymptomatic infections. Metronidazole (Flagyl) is the drug

Micrograph of a vaginal discharge revealing the presence of *Trichomonas vaginalis*, a common infection.

of choice, although tinidazole has also been used as a treatment. Those individuals undergoing treatment should refrain from alcohol use because of undesirable side effects.

Trichomoniasis in pregnant women has been associated with premature rupture of membranes, preterm delivery, and low birth weight. Previous studies identified concerns with treatment during pregnancy, but guidelines today indicate treatment with metronidazole during any stage of pregnancy is acceptable (CDC, 2010b). Some studies have shown that infection with trichomoniasis causes an increased risk of HIV infection (McClelland et al., 2007; Van Der Pol et al., 2008).

Candidiasis

The second most common form of vaginitis, **candidiasis**, also called *moniliasis, Monilia,* or *yeast infection,* is caused by the fungus *Candida albicans.* This

trichomoniasis (trich) A type of vaginitis that can be an STI or an SRD. Symptoms include a foul-smelling, foamy white or yellow-green discharge that irritates the vagina and vulva. Urethritis may also be present.

candidiasis A common form of vaginitis, sometimes called a yeast infection, which is caused by the fungus *Candida albicans.*

fungus normally lives and grows in the vagina. It is also known to be present in the mouth and intestine of many men and women.

On occasion, when the **lactobacilli**, or *Doderlein bacilli*, that are necessary for a healthy vaginal condition become reduced in number, the *C. albicans* yeast may multiply rapidly, with its growth outpacing that of other vaginal organisms. Women normally have these lactobacilli in the vagina, where they are necessary to maintain a healthy environment. They protect against a variety of infections, particularly those caused by bacteria in the urinary tract and the colon. The protective lactobacilli can be reduced by general poor health or lowered resistance, by douching, and by use of antibiotics (which can kill the lactobacilli as well as the bacteria causing the disease for which the antibiotic is prescribed). When the normally acid environment is changed, the excessive growth of the yeast results in a white and curdy discharge. Examination reveals a whitish plaque around the vagina and on its walls. Itching, frequently associated with a rash or redness of the vulva, is common. In advanced cases, intercourse is painful, and burning and discomfort occur during urination.

The second most common form of vaginitis is candidiasis, or yeast infection. It can result in white and curdy discharge, as shown here.

Women with compromised immune systems, with glucose intolerance, or who are receiving antibiotics may be at increased risk for yeast infections. Prolonged exposure to wet, synthetic material, such as bathing suits, also prevents air from circulating around the vulva and keeps normal discharge in contact with vaginal tissues, contributing to yeast growth. It is important to keep the area around the vulva as dry as possible. Letting towels dry before reuse and not sharing towels can also help. Avoiding panty hose, tight-fitting clothing, and noncotton underwear are other strategies to decrease risk. In addition, if material from the anus is carried to the vagina, the person becomes more susceptible to moniliasis, because the anus harbors the *Candida* fungus.

A variety of over-the-counter and prescription intravaginal creams and suppositories are available for treatment of yeast infections. A woman should visit a clinician if she has never been diagnosed with a yeast infection before using any over-the-counter treatment. In addition, the creams and suppositories available are oil based, so pregnancy prevention methods should be considered because they may weaken latex condoms and diaphragms. Because yeast infections in women are not typically transmitted sexually, no data support the need for partner testing or treatment.

Ectoparasitic Infestations

There are two common STIs that are not diseases as such, but rather infestations of parasites—namely, pubic lice and scabies. Parasites are found among all socioeconomic classes and are spread by close physical contact.

Pubic Lice

Pubic lice, commonly referred to as crabs, are parasites. Actually there are three different kinds of lice, known as **pediculosis lice**, and each seems to prefer its own habitat. *Pediculus corporis* is a body louse, *Pediculus capitus* is a head louse, and *Pediculus pubis* is the louse of the pubic area. Pubic lice are usually transmitted from person to person by sexual contact. Infection from infected bedding, clothing,

lactobacilli Bacteria in the vagina that aid in keeping it healthy; also called *Doderlein bacilli*.

pubic lice A parasite, commonly referred to as crabs; a louse that grips the pubic hair and feeds on tiny blood vessels of the skin.

pediculosis lice A parasite of three common types: *Pediculus corporis*, a body louse; *Pediculus capitis*, a head louse; and *Pediculus pubis*, a pubic louse.

Multicultural DIMENSIONS

STIs and Minorities Surveillance data show high rates of STIs for some minority racial or ethnic groups compared with rates for whites. Race and ethnicity in the United States are risk markers that correlate with other more fundamental determinants of health status such as poverty, access to high-quality health care, healthcare-seeking behavior, illicit drug use, and residence in communities with high prevalence of STIs.

- In 2013, the chlamydia rate for blacks was more than 6 times that for whites. The chlamydia rate for African American women was almost 6 times higher than the rate for white women. The chlamydia rate for African American men was almost 8 times higher than the rate for white men.
- Overall, in 2013, the chlamydia rate for Hispanics was more than 2 times higher than the rate for whites. The chlamydia rate for American Indians/Alaska Natives was almost 4 times higher than the rate for whites.
- In 2013, almost 59% of the total number of reported cases of gonorrhea occurred among blacks. Overall, the rate of gonorrhea among blacks in the United States was more than 12 times greater than that among whites, with similar rates being noted for black men (12.7 times greater) and black women (12.0 times greater). Among those persons aged 20 to 24 years, the gonorrhea rate for blacks was more than 11 times greater than that for whites (1,842.6 versus 161.6 cases per 100,000).
- In 2013, the gonorrhea rate for American Indians/Alaska Natives was 137.4 cases per 100,000

individuals, which was 4.0 times higher than the rate for whites; the rate for Hispanics was almost 2 times that for whites. The gonorrhea rate for Asians was half that for whites.

- In 2013, more than one-third (37.3%) of all cases of primary and secondary syphilis occurred in blacks. Compared to whites, the overall 2013 rate of primary and secondary syphilis for blacks was 5.6 times higher, with black women having a rate 15 times that for white women.
- Compared to whites, the 2013 primary and secondary syphilis rate among American Indians/Alaska Natives was 1.5 times higher, and the rate among Hispanics was 2.1 times higher.

Reducing the prevalence of many of these STIs in minority populations will require a combination of strategies. Of course, education about prevention is important. Even so, education will not have a significant effect in minority populations if social determinants of health are not addressed at the same time. Strategies need to include poverty reduction, increased job opportunities, increased general education, instillation of a positive sense of future among youth, increased access to good-quality health care, and creation of comprehensive sexuality education programs that start in schools at early ages and continue through community agencies into the adult years.

Source: Data from Centers for Disease Control and Prevention. *Sexually transmitted diseases surveillance, 2013.* Atlanta, GA: U.S. Department of Health and Human Services, 2014. Available: http://www.cdc.gov/std/stats13/surv2013-print.pdf.

upholstered furniture, and toilet seats is rare. The organism grips the pubic hair and feeds on tiny blood vessels of the skin.

Female crabs live 1 to 2 months and lay up to 10 eggs per day. As they feed on the human skin

Pubic lice, commonly called "crabs," are usually transmitted from person to person by sexual contact. Direct treatment, plus cleaning of clothes and bedding, eliminate the lice.

and blood, they irritate the skin, causing itching and occasionally swelling of glands in the groin. The nits, or eggs, stick to the pubic hair with a thick substance. Aided by body warmth, the eggs hatch. The new lice then perpetuate the cycle of feeding on the human before dropping off. They can live for 1 to 2 days off the body and are visible to the naked eye on clothing and bed sheets.

Treatment usually involves a cream rinse applied to the affected area. Reports of resistance to typical treatment methods have been increasing and are widespread. An alternative method is available, though not preferred, because of its strong odor and the longer required application time. Clothing and bed linen used before treatment should be washed but fumigation of living areas is not considered necessary.

Scabies

Scabies is caused by a tiny mite that can barely be seen. This organism generally lives for up to 2 months. The female burrows under the skin at night, probably seeking the warmth of the human host, and the results are intense itching and the formation of pus. There is a characteristic distribution pattern of scabies. It is seen most commonly on the wrists, in the spaces between the fingers, under the breasts, and on the buttocks. Nodular scabies (raised lesions) can last up to 1 year. The mites lay two to three eggs per day, and in 2 or 3 weeks a new cycle begins. Because the incubation period is 4 to 6 weeks for those who have never been infected, one individual can transmit scabies to another before being aware of its existence. Close contact that is usually (but not exclusively) sexual can transmit the mites. Scabies can spread rapidly under crowded conditions where close body and skin contact is frequent. Institutions such as nursing homes, extended-care facilities, and prisons are often sites of scabies outbreaks. Child care facilities also are a common site of scabies infestations.

A severe form of scabies, called crusted scabies or Norwegian scabies, can occur in persons who are immunocompromised, malnourished, or debilitated. These individuals will have thick crusts of skin that contain large numbers of scabies mites and eggs;

Scabies lesions can last for up to a year. The organism that causes scabies may be transmitted before a person is even aware of its presence.

they may not show the typical signs and symptoms of scabies and should be considered very contagious.

Diagnosis is usually based on the customary appearance and distribution of the rash and the presence of burrows. However, if possible, the diagnosis should be confirmed by identifying the mite, mite eggs, or mite fecal matter by removing a mite from the end of its burrow using the tip of a needle or by obtaining a skin scraping to examine under a microscope for mites, eggs, or mite fecal matter (CDC, 2010a). Typical treatment is application of permethrin cream to all areas of the body (except the head), with the cream then being washed off after 8 to 14 hours. Lindane (Kwell) is no longer recommended as a primary treatment because of its toxicity; however, if other treatments fail, it can be used under strict guidelines (CDC, 2010b). Sexual contacts and those with close personal or household contact within the last month should be examined and treated.

■ Prevention

On the one hand, STIs are often like other conditions in that, for many, there are effective treatments that result in elimination of the infection. On the other hand, for some STIs, even though there are effective treatments, there are no cures (for example, genital herpes). Still other STIs have only recently had effective treatments developed to treat them, and before that, they inevitably led to incapacity and death (for example, syphilis). Even when cured, people who have contracted some STIs can be affected for their entire lives—for example, when the disease results in infertility. STIs, therefore, are serious conditions that we would be best advised to prevent. Fortunately, there are actions we can take to prevent contracting an STI or at least minimize the likelihood of contracting one.

Abstinence

The most certain way to avoid contracting an STI is to abstain from sexual activity. Because STIs can be contracted through oral sex, vaginal sex, anal sex, and skin-to-skin contact, refraining from all penetrative behaviors and contact with the genitals is needed to completely eliminate the risk.

Some may choose abstinence until they are married or until they are in a committed relationship. Others may practice abstinence at different points in

scabies Skin irritation caused by a tiny mite that is transferred from one person to another by close contact, sexual or otherwise.

Ethical DIMENSIONS

Notifying Partners About STIs

There are many reasons why people with STIs choose not to notify their sexual partner(s) about their infection. They may be embarrassed to do so, they may be in a relationship and have contracted the STI from another partner, or they may not want anyone to know about their infection for fear they will not be able to get dates or other sexual partners.

Similarly, there are many reasons people with STIs choose to notify their sexual partners. They may believe that all sexual partners, past and present, should be notified of a sexual partner's STI status. In this way, they can get tested and retested if they are infected. Also, they can prevent the spread of the infection by refraining from sex with other people until they are disease free.

On the one hand, some people argue that absent any signs or symptoms, notifying a sexual partner might do more harm than good. For example, if the infection was contracted during an extramarital affair, notification might result in divorce. Notification might unduly frighten the unsuspecting partner, causing potentially unhealthy consequences associated with stress.

On the other hand, some people argue that to disclose an STI is consistent with the ethical principles of honesty and nonmaleficence (do no harm). Even if the result of the sexual behavior is accompanied by sanctions (such as divorce), they believe it further compounds the violation of trust to withhold information that a loved one can use to protect his or her health.

What do you think is the ethical thing to do? Does the fact that many STIs are asymptomatic affect your decision?

their lives, such as after a recent divorce. The option of refraining from sexual activity is available to everyone at all times. However, for many people, abstinence is not acceptable for a variety of reasons. Perhaps they have an interest in sex and find it so pleasurable that they are not willing to forgo it. They may have no moral or ethical objections to premarital sex or they may have no intention of marrying in the future. For those not willing to remain abstinent, other strategies to reduce the risk of contracting an STI are available.

Monogamy

If a sexual partner is STI free, and he or she is the only person with whom you engage in sexual activity, then you will not contract an STI. Monogamy with an uninfected partner, though, can be problematic. How can you make sure your partner is uninfected?

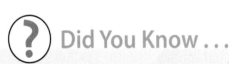

Did You Know . . .

The Centers for Disease Control and Prevention estimates 20 million new sexually transmitted infections occur in the United States each year. The direct cost of medical care of these new infections is estimated to be $16 billion (Owusu-Edusei et al., 2013). This cost does not include existing conditions, which bring the total prevalence to 110 million infections in the United States (Satterwhite et al., 2013).

How can you make sure that your partner is also monogamous? Without seeing the STI testing results and following your partner everywhere (which is usually not recommended), you can never really be sure that your partner is STI free and monogamous. Moreover, in some cases, as with the lack of a test for HPV in men or with herpes infections that can go unnoticed and be "discovered" years after the initial infection, even testing and stalking may not prove adequate. For all of these reasons, relying on

If sexually active, the best way to prevent contracting an STI is by maintaining a monogamous relationship in which both partners are STI free.

Myth vs Fact

Myth: If you get syphilis, you will know it because a rash will break out.

Fact: A rash may not appear until secondary syphilis has developed. Furthermore, although a chancre (a sore) may develop early in the course of the infection, it may not be visible or may be dismissed as inconsequential. Also, in women, the early signs of syphilis may not be readily visible on the genitals.

Myth: Gonorrhea is no more serious than the common cold and can be cured easily.

Fact: Gonorrhea can cause infertility, arthritis, or endocarditis (inflammation of the heart valves). In addition, certain antibiotic-resistant strains of gonorrhea raise concern about the ability to continue to treat this STI with current medications.

Myth: If you get an STI once, you acquire an immunity to it and cannot contract it a second time.

Fact: You do not have immunity to STIs and can contract them anew each time you have contact with the disease-causing organisms.

Myth: STIs occur only in or on the genital organs.

Fact: You can acquire an STI through oral–genital contact, in which case the signs of the infection would occur in the mouth and on the face. Or, you can have contact with an STI-causing organism by touching an infected area with your fingers, in which case the signs of the infection could appear on other body areas (like eyes and mouth) if you touch those areas.

monogamy with an uninfected partner as protection against contracting an STI can be risky.

Reduce the Number of Sexual Partners

If a person is unwilling or unable to maintain a monogamous relationship, decreasing the number of sexual partners lessens his or her odds of contracting an STI. The greater number of sexual partners, the greater the likelihood that one of them will be infected.

Refrain from the Use of Alcohol and Other Drugs

Decisions regarding important aspects of your life deserve thoughtful consideration. What more important decision is there than that concerning whether you will engage in an activity that has the potential of causing serious illness? Alcohol and other drugs can interfere with decision-making by decreasing inhibitions and affecting judgment. Therefore, protection against STIs should include abstention from the use of mind-altering drugs.

Discuss STI Concerns with Potential Sexual Partners

Any new sexual partners should discuss concern about STIs before engaging in sexual activity. Whether they know they are infected, they should share information about the high-risk behaviors they have engaged in and the results of any medical screenings they have had. This kind of a conversation can lead to concern about a potential sexual partner and a decision to refrain from sex altogether—or at least until a new medical screening can be obtained.

Be Observant

We used to recommend an examination of your own genitals and your partners' genitals for any obvious signs of an STI. However, this is no longer recommended because so many STIs are asymptomatic and the "exam" can give individuals a false sense of security that they are infection free.

At the same time, becoming familiar with your own body and examining your genitals for any lesions, blisters, or infected sores can help you recognize when something abnormal develops. If so, it is important to refrain from sexual activity until you know the cause. If you experience any unusual growth or sore or a foul-smelling odor, you need to see a healthcare provider for an exam and possible testing.

You also want to be observant of your partners' genitals. If you see something that may be a sign of an STI, ask questions and do not continue to engage in any sexual activity until you are certain there is no risk to you. One of us had a student who saw a blister on his partner's vulva, asked her about it, and was informed that it was "a pimple." When he later contracted genital herpes, he was devastated and wished he had trusted his instinct that it could be a symptom of an STI.

Use Condoms and Other Barriers

Male condom use is something that is often discussed as a prevention strategy for STIs. For all methods that are intended to reduce the risk of STI transmission, accurately estimating the effectiveness is challenging from a research perspective. Measuring consistent and correct use of the method, determining whether the infection identified is new or preexisting, and determining whether the individuals have had exposure to the STI of interest during the study all pose challenges.

The research on male latex condoms demonstrates that they protect well against STIs that are transmitted through genital fluids (e.g., pre-ejaculate, semen, vaginal secretions). These STIs include HIV, hepatitis B, gonorrhea, chlamydia, and trichomoniasis. The numerous studies on HIV transmission are the most methodologically strong, but epidemiological evidence also supports condoms' ability to prevent transmission of the other fluid-carried STIs. In all cases, male latex condoms provide a barrier to particles the size of STI pathogens; no "holes" exist in which HIV, another virus, or bacteria could penetrate (CDC, 2013a).

For infections that are transmitted by skin-to-skin contact (syphilis, HPV and herpes), studies have not shown the same level of protection by male condoms. Consistent and correct male condom use can reduce the risk of genital herpes and syphilis only for the covered area. Other studies have shown that condom use may reduce the risk of HPV infection; condom use has also been associated with higher rates of clearance of HPV infection in women and with regression of HPV lesions on the penis in men. In addition, a few prospective studies have shown condoms as having a protective effect on the acquisition of genital HPV (CDC, 2013a).

Research is very limited on polyisoprene male condoms, female condoms, latex dams (used during oral sex on a female or oral–anal contact), gloves, or other latex-protective barriers and the extent to which these items protect against STIs. In general, female condoms (Gallo et al., 2012), polyisoprene male condoms, and latex dams are believed to provide protection from fluid-transmitted STIs and from skin-to-skin STIs on the portion of the body covered.

Avoid High-Risk Behaviors

Because organisms that cause STIs are present in semen and vaginal secretions, the goal is to prevent them from being transmitted from an infected person to a person not infected. Penile–vaginal sex without the use of a condom can result in the depositing of semen that includes infection-causing organisms within a partner's body. So can fellatio (oral-penile sex) without a condom and cunnilingus (oral-vulva sex) without a dental dam. Anal sex is a particularly high-risk behavior because the friction creates fissures (tears in the lining) in the anus, allowing easy entrance of infection-causing organisms into the bloodstream. Furthermore, because some organisms that cause STIs reside in the blood, using needles or other products that may contain drops of blood from another person puts an individual at high risk for infection. Sharing needles is one of the more common ways of contracting HIV in the United States.

Other Protective Measures

Still other behaviors can lessen the likelihood of contracting an STI or increase the likelihood of detecting one at an early stage:

- Wash the genitals before and after sex.

- Obtain regular medical checkups.

- Inspect your genitals regularly.

- Do not share razors, hypodermic needles, or scissors.

- Do not handle towels, wet bedding, or undergarments immediately after these have been in contact with another person.

If you suspect you have been exposed to an STI, see a clinician or visit a health clinic in your community or on your campus. It is unwise to try to diagnose and treat the condition yourself. It is also extremely important to comply with the treatment regimen, which includes taking all the medication prescribed at the appropriate times and returning for any follow-up visits. Also, if you have an STI, notify your partner(s). Failing to tell a partner of the possibility of infection could result in the spread of the infection, not just to a single individual but possibly to many individuals (Figure 18.11).

Sexuality Education and STIs

Alarmed at what it called the "hidden epidemic," the Institute of Medicine (IOM) convened a 15-member expert panel in 1994 to strategize ways to address the STI problem. The IOM concluded that society's unwillingness to confront sexual issues is the main barrier to responding to STIs (Eng & Butler, 1996). The IOM report went on to explain that this attitude hinders the dissemination of accurate, straightforward information about STIs in educational

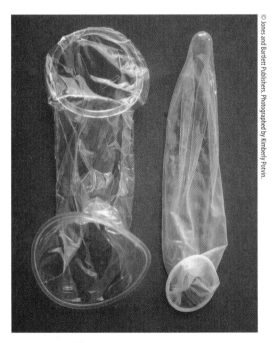

The male and female condoms prevent STIs by establishing a barrier between the infection-causing organism and the body. This barrier prevents the organism from finding a pathway into the body.

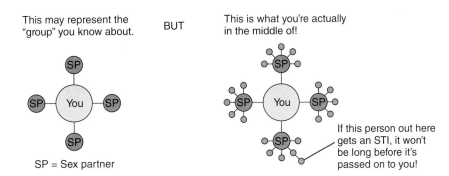

This may represent the "group" you know about. BUT This is what you're actually in the middle of!

SP = Sex partner

If this person out here gets an STI, it won't be long before it's passed on to you!

FIGURE 18.11 STIs: a fact of life for the sexually active. By "sexually active," we do not mean having a lot of sex. Instead, we mean having sex with different people. In general, the fact of life is that, sooner or later, sexually active people will either be exposed to an STI or contract one.

programs for adolescents and interferes with communication between parents and their children and between sexual partners. Furthermore, this attitude compromises healthcare professionals' ability to counsel patients, impedes research on sexual behavior, and leads to unbalanced messages being sent via the media. The members of the expert panel noted several studies that found that almost two-thirds of respondents knew little or nothing about STIs other than HIV and AIDS and that most people seriously underestimate their risk of acquiring an STI, as well as its consequences. Not much has changed in the intervening years.

The need for education about STIs is evident, has long been overlooked, and requires the involvement of many different segments of our society, working together to prevent their occurrence and to develop more effective treatments if and when they do occur.

Case Study

Sexually transmitted infections are quite prevalent, especially among young people. Some STIs and SRDs are curable; some are treatable but chronic. Because many cases are asymptomatic or early symptoms are ignored, treatment does not always occur. The STI can then be transmitted further.

Having a curable STI is, at a minimum, embarrassing. Yet having a chronic STI such as genital herpes or genital warts can have a profound psychological impact on a person's life. The STI will affect the individual's sexual activities for an entire lifetime. The fear of rejection after informing a potential sexual partner might cause the individual to say nothing. Self-esteem can diminish.

Socially, race and ethnicity correlate with fundamental determinants of health status such as poverty, access to health care, healthcare-seeking behavior, and residence in areas with a high prevalence of STIs. Thus a higher prevalence of gonorrhea or syphilis among African Americans has social—not biological—underpinnings.

STI risk can be reduced in a number of ways, including abstinence, monogamy, reduction in the number of sexual partners, refraining from alcohol or other drugs, communication with partners, use of latex condoms and other barrier methods, and avoidance of high-risk behaviors. However, if we belong to a community that has high rates of infection, our risk will still be greater unless we practice abstinence from oral, vaginal, and anal sex and genital contact. Simply engaging in sex with members of our community should not be an increased factor, and society as a whole needs to consider how to address these underlying influences as well as general STI awareness, education, and prevention practices.

Biological Factors

- STIs are contracted primarily through sexual contact.
- SRDs are diseases of the reproductive system that can occur in either sexually active or sexually inactive individuals.
- Individuals with an STI have a higher risk of becoming infected with HIV, possibly because the genital lesions characteristic of some STIs give HIV access to the body.
- STIs can be passed to a baby both before and during birth.

Sociocultural Factors

- Society's unwillingness to confront sexual issues is a major barrier in responding to STIs.
- Some ethnic groups have higher rates of STIs than others. Southern states have higher rates of syphilis than the national average.
- Economically, the direct medical cost of treating new STIs is $16 billion per year.
- Social determinants of health play a critical role in some groups increased risk for STIs.

Psychological Factors

- Biological and sociocultural factors combine to influence psychological factors.
- Having an STI affects an individual's feelings about his or her sexuality.
- Learning later in life that you became sterile due to an undiagnosed STI can have a devastating psychological effect.
- Psychological stress increases for individuals with genital herpes because they are constantly concerned that symptoms will reappear. They must decide whether to tell new partners of their condition, which can lead to rejection.

Summary

- Sexually transmitted infections (STIs) are infections contracted through sexual activities. There are also diseases of the sexual organs referred to as sexually related diseases (SRDs), which can occur in both sexually active and sexually abstinent individuals.

- Chlamydia is the most frequently reported STI in the United States. More than 1.4 million cases were reported in 2013, more than 4 times the number of gonorrhea cases reported. Symptoms are often asymptomatic, although men may notice pain or burning during urination and women may notice a vaginal discharge and abdominal pain.

- Gonorrhea is the second most reported STI. In 2013, more than 333,000 cases were reported in the United States. Males are more likely to experience symptoms from gonorrhea infection than females. Males may experience frequent and painful urination and a discharge of pus from the urethra. Females are usually asymptomatic, although some may notice a yellowish discharge.

- Total syphilis rates are now the highest reported since 1996. Initial symptoms include the development of a lesion (chancre), which disappears in 2 to 4 weeks. Soon afterward, a rash, fever, and some hair loss can occur. If syphilis goes untreated, blindness, paralysis, brain damage, and death are possible.

- Human papillomavirus (HPV), which is associated with the development of genital warts and cervical cancer, is a viral infection and the most common STI in the US. Vaccines are available, and Gardasil and Gardasil 9 can prevent as much as 70% of cervical cancers, 80% of anal cancers, and 90% of genital warts caused by HPV.

- Other viral causes of STIs include herpes simplex virus (HSV), which is associated with the development of genital herpes, and hepatitis B virus (HBV), which is associated with the development of hepatitis B.

- Sexually related diseases include vaginal infections (such as trichomoniasis and candidiasis) and ectoparasitic infections (such as pubic lice and scabies).

- Ways to prevent or minimize the risk of contracting an STI include practicing sexual abstinence, maintaining a monogamous sexual relationship, reducing the number of sexual partners, refraining from the use of alcohol or other drugs, and using latex or polyisoprene male condoms or female condoms.

Discussion Questions

1. What are STIs, how are they transmitted, and what are the reasons for their increasing prevalence?

2. What are the bacterially based STIs? Include their incidence, transmission, symptoms and complications, and diagnosis and treatment in your answer.

3. What are the virally based STIs? Include their incidence, transmission, symptoms and complications, and diagnosis and treatment in your answer.

4. What are the ectoparasitic infestations? Include their incidence, transmission, symptoms and complications, and diagnosis and treatment in your answer.

5. List the key ways to prevent STIs, evaluating the theoretical and user effectiveness of each in the real world.

Application Questions

Reread the chapter-opening story and answer the following questions.

1. Jessica chose to ask her human sexuality professor about her potential STI. Why didn't she go to the student health clinic or her primary care clinician?

2. The author describes several of the "private" conversations students wish to have with human sexuality professors concerning pregnancy, abuse, sexual disorders, and STIs. Where on your campus (or in your community) could you go for help for each of these problems? Be specific, creating a list with phone numbers.

3. Should professors discuss personal sexuality issues with students? Explain why or why not.

Critical Thinking Questions

1. Until July 2012, applications for marriage licenses in Mississippi required a blood test for syphilis but not for the other STIs. Because many STIs are asymptomatic, should marriage tests require testing for all the major STIs? Identify potential difficulties to implement such a program? (*Hint:* Consider how each infection is diagnosed.)

2. How can undetected STIs affect fetuses and newborns?

3. Criminal laws generally provide that someone who deliberately inflicts harm on another person should be punished. Civil laws allow the victim to seek compensation for harm done. Should people who know they are infected with STIs but who have unprotected sex with others and infect them be prosecuted? Should the people they infect be able to sue for physical and psychological damages?

Critical Thinking Case

Most of us believe that STIs afflict young people. In reality, STIs strike people of all ages—including senior citizens. People who are widowed or divorced do not become asexual; rather, they usually begin dating new people. In fact, 90% of postmenopausal women remain sexually active.

Dr. Peter Leone, medical director of the Wake County, North Carolina, STI Clinic, says: "Women who are past menopause often think they can't get an STI. People link pregnancy and STI risk. But methods to prevent pregnancy aren't the best ones for preventing STIs. Some post-menopausal women may think, 'Why should I use a condom? I can't get pregnant.' "

The STI incidence rates per 100,000 people have remained low for older individuals compared to younger groups; however, there is evidence that these rates are increasing. At the same time, the risk is not equivalent across groups. For example, compared with their heterosexual peers, older MSM are at higher risk for developing STIs and HIV infection. In addition to the growing number of elderly people with new infections, owing to improvements in longevity, the number of older individuals with an existing infection is also expected to increase (Poynten et al., 2013).

Consider your parents or your parents' friends who are divorced or widowed. How could you, as a student in this class, give them information about taking responsibility for their sexual behavior?

In an odd twist, it seems that senior citizens share the attitude of young people regarding sexual behavior: It cannot happen to me. Explain this attitude. Do young people and seniors have different reasons for their beliefs?

Exploring Personal Dimensions

Can You Be Assertive When You Need to Be?

To take the necessary actions to prevent contracting an STI, you will have to be assertive—that is, you will need to resist pressure to engage in sexual activity if you choose not to, and you will need to insist on the use of a condom and other safer sex precautions if you decide to engage in sex. Do you have assertiveness skills? To find out, write an assertive response to each of the situations described.

1. You are on a date and your partner insists on engaging in a sexual activity that you decide is not for you at that time. You say:

   _____

   _____

   _____

2. Your partner argues that condoms or latex barriers diminish the sensation. You respond by saying:

   _____

   _____

   _____

3. Your partner states that she or he has been tested for STIs and the test result was negative. Therefore, there are no reasons for using safer sex techniques. You respond by saying:

   _____

   _____

   _____

To be assertive, you need to:

1. Specify the behavior or situation to which the statement refers.

2. Relate your feelings about that situation.

3. Suggest a remedy or what your preference is.

4. Identify the consequences of the change: what will happen if it occurs and what will happen if it does not occur.

   Now check your responses and revise them to be consistent with these assertiveness principles.

Suggested Readings

Grimes, J. A., Smith, L. A., & Fagerberg, K., eds. *Sexually transmitted disease: An encyclopedia of diseases, prevention, treatment, and issues.* Santa Barbara, CA: Greenwood, 2013.

Joannides, P. Condoms: For the ride of your life (pp. 323–332) and Gnarly sex germs (pp. 683–716), in *Guide to getting it on! A book about the wonders of sex* (7th ed.). Waldport, OR: Goofy Foot Press, 2013.

Lowy, I. *A woman's disease: The history of cervical cancer.* New York: Oxford University Press, 2011.

Nack, A. *Damaged goods? Women living with incurable sexually transmitted diseases.* Philadelphia, PA: Temple University Press, 2008.

Schwartz, P., & Kempner, M. STIs and protection: The risks of romance (pp. 167–189), in *50 great myths of human sexuality.* West Sussex, UK: Wiley, 2015.

Web Resources

For links to the websites below, visit *go.jblearning.com/dimensions6e* and click on Resource Links.

Centers for Disease Control and Prevention: Sexually Transmitted Diseases
www.cdc.gov/std

This site provides statistics and reports pertaining to STIs. In addition, there are fact sheets and basic descriptive information for all common bacterial and viral STIs. While some material is directed toward healthcare providers, much of the information is written in basic terminology for individuals of all knowledge levels.

American Sexual Health Association
www.ashastd.org

The American Sexual Health Association develops and delivers accurate, medically reliable information about sexual health including STIs. ASHA publishes educational pamphlets and books for clients and students. It helps community-based organizations communicate about risk, transmission, prevention, testing, and treatment of STIs. Links to statistics, prevention tips, and information about particular STIs are included on this website.

STD Wizard
www.stdwizard.org/#/home

This interactive tool has visitors provide personal information about their sexual health and then creates recommendations for testing and relevant vaccination based on the details provided. While not a substitute for a visit to a healthcare provider, the results can help identify needs and familiarize someone with the questions a healthcare provider will ask to assess risk and needed medical attention.

References

American Cancer Society. *Cancer facts & figures 2015.* Atlanta, GA: American Cancer Society; 2015. Available: http://www.cancer.org/acs/groups/content/@editorial/documents/document/acspc-044552.pdf.

American College of Obstetrics and Gynecologists, Committee on Adolescent Health Care and Committee on Gynecologic Practice. Committee Opinion No. 506: Expedited partner therapy in the management of gonorrhea and chlamydia by obstetrician-gynecologists. *Obstetrics & Gynecology, 118,* 3 (2011), 761–766.

American Sexual Health Association (ASHA). *Chlamydia,* 2014. Available: http://www.ashasexualhealth.org/stdsstis/chlamydia/.

American Sexual Health Association (ASHA). *Genital warts,* 2015a. Available: http://www.ashasexualhealth.org/stdsstis/hpv/genital-warts/.

American Sexual Health Association (ASHA). *Herpes testing,* 2015b. Available: http://www.ashasexualhealth.org/stdsstis/herpes/herpes-testing/.

American Sexual Health Association (ASHA). *HPV and cervical cancer,* 2015c. Available: http://www.ashasexualhealth.org/stdsstis/hpv/hpv-cervical-cancer/.

American Sexual Health Association (ASHA). *NGU,* 2015d. Available: http://www.ashasexualhealth.org/stdsstis/ngu/.

American Sexual Health Association (ASHA). *Signs & symptoms,* 2015e. Available: http://www.ashasexualhealth.org/stdsstis/herpes/signs-symptoms/.

Baker, D., Collins, J., & Leon, J. Risk factor or social vaccine? The historical progression of the role of education in HIV/AIDS infection in sub-Saharan Africa. *Prospects: Quarterly Review of Comparative Education, 38,* 4 (2009), 467–486.

Bernstein, D. I., Bellamy, A. R., Hook, E. W., Levin, M. J., Wald, A., Ewell, M. G., et al. Epidemiology, clinical presentation, and antibody response to primary infection with herpes simplex virus type 1 and type 2 in young women. *Clinical Infectious Diseases, 56* (2013), 344–351.

Bolan, G. A., Sparling, P. F., & Wasserheit, J. N. The emerging threat of untreatable gonococcal infection. *New England Journal of Medicine, 366* (2012), 485–487.

Bradley, H., Markowitz, L. E., Gibson, T., & McQuillan, G. M. (2013). Seroprevalence of herpes simplex virus types 1 and 2—United States, 1999–2010. *Journal of Infectious Diseases, 209* (2014), 325–33. doi: 10.1093/infdis/jit458.

Centers for Disease Control and Prevention (CDC). *Scabies frequently asked questions*, 2010a. Available: http://www.cdc.gov/parasites/scabies/gen_info/faqs.html.

Centers for Disease Control and Prevention (CDC). *Sexually transmitted diseases treatment guidelines 2010*, 2010b. Available: http://www.cdc.gov/std/stats10/surv2010.pdf.

Centers for Disease Control and Prevention (CDC). *Hepatitis B information for health professionals*, 2012. Available: http://www.cdc.gov/hepatitis/HBV/index.htm.

Centers for Disease Control and Prevention (CDC). *Condom effectiveness: Fact sheet for public health personnel*, 2013a. Available: http://www.cdc.gov/condomeffectiveness/latex.html.

Centers for Disease Control and Prevention (CDC). *Human papillomavirus (HPV) and oropharyngeal cancer: Fact sheet*, 2013b. Available: http://www.cdc.gov/std/HPV/STDFact-HPVandoralcancer.htm.

Centers for Disease Control and Prevention (CDC). *Ready-to-use STD curriculum for clinical educators: Gonorrhea module (notes)*, 2013c. Available: http://www2a.cdc.gov/stdtraining/ready-to-use/Manuals/Gonorrhea/gonorrhea-notes-April-2013.pdf.

Centers for Disease Control and Prevention (CDC). *Genital herpes: CDC fact sheet*, 2014a. Available: http://www.cdc.gov/std/herpes/stdfact-herpes-detailed.htm.

Centers for Disease Control and Prevention (CDC). *Hepatitis B FAQs for health professionals*, 2014b. Available: http://www.cdc.gov/hepatitis/HBV/HBVfaq.htm#.

Centers for Disease Control and Prevention (CDC). *Sexually transmitted diseases surveillance, 2013*, 2014c. Available: http://www.cdc.gov/std/stats13/surv2013-print.pdf.

Centers for Disease Control and Prevention (CDC). *Syphilis: CDC fact sheet*, 2014d. Available: http://www.cdc.gov/std/syphilis/stdfact-syphilis.htm.

Centers for Disease Control and Prevention (CDC). *Legal status of expedited partner therapy (EPT)*, 2015a. Available: http://www.cdc.gov/std/ept/legal/default.htm.

Centers for Disease Control and Prevention (CDC). *Surveillance for viral hepatitis—United States, 2012*, 2015b. Available: http://www.cdc.gov/hepatitis/Statistics/2012Surveillance/Commentary.htm#hepB.

Corey, L., Wald, A., & Patel, R., et al. Once-daily valacyclovir to reduce the risk of transmission of genital herpes. *New England Journal of Medicine, 350* (2004), 11–20.

D'Souza, G., Gross, N. D., Pai, S. I., Haddad, R., Anderson, K. S., Rajan, S., et al. Oral human papillomavirus (HPV) infection in HPV-positive patients with oropharyngeal cancer and their partners. *Journal of Clinical Oncology, 32* (2014), 2408–2415. doi: 10.1200/JCO.2014.55.1341.

Eng, T. R., & Butler, W. T., eds. *The hidden epidemic: Confronting sexually transmitted diseases*. Washington, DC: Institute of Medicine, 1996.

Fielder, R. L., Carey, K. B., & Carey, M. P. Acceptability of STI testing using self-collected vaginal swabs among college women. *Journal of American College Health, 61*(2013), 46–53. doi: 10.1080/07448481.2012.750610.

Gallo, M. F., Kilbourne-Brook, M., & Coffey, P. S. (2012). A review of the effectiveness and acceptability of the female condom for dual protection. *Sexual Health, 9* (2012), 18–26.

Gillison, M. L., Broutian, T., Pickard, R. K., Tong, Z. Y., Xiao, W., Kahle, L., et al. Prevalence of oral HPV infection in the United States, 2009–2010. *Journal of the American Medical Association, 307* (2012), 693–703.

Hargreaves, J. R., & Glynn, J. R. Educational attainment and HIV-1 infection in developing countries: A systematic review. *Tropical Medicine and International Health, 7, 6* (2002), 489–498.

Jena, A. B., Goldman, D. P., & Seabury, S. A. incidence of sexually transmitted infections after human papillomavirus vaccination among adolescent females. *Journal of the American Medical Association: Internal Medicine* (2015). [Epub ahead of print]. doi: 10.1001/jamainternmed.2014.7886.

Jenkins, W. D., Weis, R., Campbell, P., Barnes, M., Barnes, P., & Gaydos, C. Comparative effectiveness of two self-collected sample kit distribution systems for chlamydia screening on a university campus. *Sexually Transmitted Infections, 88* (2012), 363–367. doi: 10.1136/sextrans-2011-050379.

Johnston, C., Saracino, M., Kuntz, S., Magaret, A., Selke, S., Huang, M. L., et al. Standard-dose and high-dose daily antiviral therapy for short episodes of genital HSV-2 reactivation: Three randomised, open-label, cross-over trials. *Lancet, 379* (2012), 641–647.

Kaiser Family Foundation. *The HPV vaccine: Access and use in the U.S.*, 2015. Available: http://files.kff.org/attachment/the-hpv-vaccine-access-and-use-in-the-u-s-fact-sheet.

McClelland, R. S., Sangare, L., & Hassan, W. M., et al. Infection with *Trichomonas vaginalis* increases the risk of HIV-1 acquisition. *Journal of Infectious Disease, 195* (2007), 698–702.

Moonesinghe, R., Fleming, E., Truman, B. I., & Dean, H. D. Linear and non-linear associations of gonorrhea diagnosis rates with social determinants of health. *International Journal of Environmental Research and Public Health, 9* (2012), 3149–3165.

Ohnishi, M., Golparian, D., Shimuta, K., Saika, T., Hoshina, S., Iwasaku, K., et al. Is *Neisseria gonorrhoeae* initiating a future era of untreatable gonorrhea? Detailed characterization of the first strain with high-level resistance to ceftriaxone. *Antimicrobial Agents and Chemotherapy, 55, 7* (2011), 3538–3545.

Owusu-Edusei, K. Jr, Chesson, H. W., Gift, T. L., Tao, G., Mahajan, R., Ocfemia, M. C. B., & Kent, C. K. The estimated direct medical cost of selected sexually transmitted infections in the United States, 2008. *Sexually Transmitted Diseases, 40* (2013), 197–201.

Palefsky, J. M., Giuliano, A. R., Goldstone, S., Moreira Jr, E. D., Aranda, C., Jessen, H., et al. HPV vaccine against anal HPV infection and anal intraepithelial neoplasia. *New England Journal of Medicine, 365* (2011), 1576–1585.

Peters, E., Baker, D., Deickmann, N., Leon, J., & Collins, J. Explaining the education effect on health: A field-study from Ghana. *Psychological Science, 21, 10* (2010), 1369–1376.

Poynten, I. M., Grulich, A. E., & Templeton, D. J. Sexually transmitted infections in older populations. *Current Opinion in Infectious Diseases, 26* (2013), 80–85.

Presidential Commission for the Study of Bioethical Issues. *"Ethically impossible": STD research in Guatemala from 1946 to 1948*, 2011. Available: http://bioethics.gov/cms/sites/default/files/Ethically-Impossible_PCSBI.pdf.

Rotblatt, H., Montoya, J. A., Plant, A., Guerry, S., & Kerndt, P. R. There's no place like home: First-year use of the "I know" home testing program for chlamydia and gonorrhea. *American Journal of Public Health, 103* (2013), 1376–1380.

Ryder, N., Jin, F., & McNulty, A. M., et al. Increasing role of herpes simplex virus type 1 in first-episode anogenital herpes in heterosexual women and younger men who have sex with men, 1992–2006. *Sexually Transmitted Infections, 85* (2009), 416–419.

Satterwhite, C. L., Torrone, E., Meites, E., Dunne, E. F., Mahajan, R., Ocfemia, M. C. B., et al. Sexually transmitted infections among US women and men: Prevalence and incidence estimates, 2008. *Sexually Transmitted Diseases, 40* (2013), 187–193.

Stenger, M. R., Samuel, M. C., Anschuetz, G. L., Pugsley, R., Eaglin, M., Klingler, E., et al. Neighborhoods at risk: Estimating risk of higher *Neisseria gonorrhoeae* incidence among women at the census tract level. *Sexually Transmitted Diseases, 41, 11* (2014), 649–655.

Sullivan, A. B., Gesink, D. C., Brown, P., Zhou, L., Kaufman, J. S., Fitch, M., et al. Are neighborhood sociocultural factors influencing the spatial pattern of gonorrhea in North Carolina? *Annals of Epidemiology, 21, 4* (2011), 245–252.

Van Der Pol, B., Kwok, C., Pierre-Louis, B., Rinaldi, A., Salata, R. A., Chen, P. L. et al. *Trichomonas vaginalis* infection and human immunodeficiency virus acquisition in African women. *Journal of Infectious Disease, 197* (2008), 548–454.

World Health Organization (WHO). *Social determinants of health*, 2015. Available: http://www.who.int/social_determinants/thecommission/finalreport/key_concepts/en/.

CHAPTER
19

HIV and AIDS

© Gayvoronskaya Yana/Shutterstock

CHAPTER OBJECTIVES

1 Describe the way in which the human immunodeficiency virus (HIV) invades the body and causes acquired immunodeficiency syndrome (AIDS) and the opportunistic infections associated with AIDS.

2 Discuss different treatments for HIV infection and AIDS, including how the mortality rate has declined as a result of these treatments.

3 Review prevention strategies for HIV infection.

4 Identify specific risk factors for young adults.

INTRODUCTION

*J*uan was a third-year student in our department and had taken several classes with me. During class, he was a vocal contributor to discussions, offering examples from both the readings and his own personal stories. He also regularly attended office hours to clarify concepts, so I got to know him fairly well both in and out of the classroom. He was, quite honestly, an ideal student in that he was engaged with the content and a pleasure to interact with even when challenging me or the ideas presented in a course.

During his fourth year, Juan had registered to take another course with me, but before the semester started, he withdrew from the class. Because the course was required and offered only once each year, I knew not taking it would delay his graduation, so I reached out to Juan via email. After several weeks with no response, I emailed him again. When he did respond a few weeks later, he said that he needed to take some time off and hoped to be back in school soon. I was concerned. Although I felt we had a good relationship, I did not feel comfortable as his instructor in pressing him for details. A few weeks after that, Juan got back in touch with me and asked if he could make an appointment.

When Juan arrived at my office, I knew something was seriously wrong. He looked pale, had lost weight and had large black circles under his eyes. When I asked what was going on, Juan was nervous and did not respond immediately. Finally, with a great sigh, he said that he had tested positive for HIV and was having a hard time dealing with it; he had not been sleeping or eating regularly for several months. From our class discussions, I knew Juan was gay, and I also knew that his family did not know about his sexual orientation. He was hesitant to seek medical care because he did not want his parents to find out and *he was still covered by their health insurance, but he knew the importance of early treatment. During our meeting, I contacted a colleague at a local clinic to discuss options for Juan that would allow him access to medical care while addressing his parental issues and made an appointment for him later that week. After that, Juan and I kept in regular contact about his health and his disclosure to his parents about his sexual orientation and HIV status. While his parents were initially shocked and upset by the information, they eventually supported Juan both emotionally and financially in obtaining medical care.*

Today, Juan is regularly taking his antiviral medications, while living a healthy lifestyle of eating right, exercising, sleeping, and limiting alcohol use. He is also in graduate school pursuing his PhD in biostatistics. Thanks to the currently available medications for HIV, it is likely that Juan will lead a long and healthy life.

While Juan's story has a happy ending, many others are not so fortunate. All too frequently, homonegativity and stigma attached to HIV infection continue to prevail in some regions, social groups, and families in the United States. We hope that this chapter, by presenting information about HIV and AIDS, will help us all become more understanding of those who are wrestling with not only the physical and psychological effects of HIV infection, but also the social consequences.

Human Immunodeficiency Virus and Acquired Immune Deficiency Syndrome

For students in their 20s, **human immunodeficiency virus (HIV)**, the virus that causes **acquired immune deficiency syndrome (AIDS)**, may be perceived as just another infection that has always existed. In reality, HIV and AIDS have been known to the medical community for less than 40 years.

In the early 1980s, the cause of AIDS was unknown. The disease was named acquired immune deficiency syndrome because of its attack on and

slow destruction of the body's immune system. At that time, physicians noted the unusual occurrence of five cases of *Pneumocystis carinii* pneumonia among previously healthy gay men in Los Angeles. Soon after, reports surfaced of a rare form of cancer, Kaposi's sarcoma, also among young gay men in New York and California. These observations led to the recognition of AIDS, a disease characterized by **opportunistic infections** in immunocompromised individuals. Illnesses such as *P. carinii* pneumonia and Kaposi's sarcoma are labeled "opportunistic" because they rarely occur in young healthy individuals, instead capitalizing on the vulnerability presented by a depressed immune system. Because it is characterized by a range of opportunistic infections, rather than one particular disease, AIDS is considered a syndrome (Table 19.1).

Research conducted by Robert Gallo at the National Institutes of Health and by Luc Montagnier and colleagues at the Pasteur Institute in Paris eventually led to the discovery of a new virus believed to cause AIDS. Gallo named the virus human T-lymphotropic virus type III (HTLV-III); Montagnier identified it by

human immunodeficiency virus (HIV) A retrovirus that causes AIDS.

acquired immune deficiency syndrome (AIDS) A syndrome caused by the human immunodeficiency virus (HIV), characterized by a depressed immune system and the presence of one or more opportunistic infections.

opportunistic infections A major manifestation of AIDS; conditions that occur in the presence of a suppressed immune system.

TABLE 19.1

AIDS-Defining Conditions*

Cancers
- Invasive cervical cancer
- Kaposi's sarcoma
- Lymphoma, multiple forms

Fungal Infections
- Candidiasis of bronchi, trachea, esophagus, or lungs
- Cryptococcosis
- Histoplasmosis
- *Pneumocystis carinii* pneumonia

Protozoan, Spore, and Parasite Infections
- Cryptosporidiosis, chronic intestinal (greater than 1 month's duration)
- Coccidioidomycosis
- Isosporiasis, chronic intestinal (greater than 1 month's duration)
- Toxoplasmosis of brain

Viral Infections
- Cytomegalovirus disease (particularly CMV retinitis)
- Herpes simplex: chronic ulcer(s) (greater than 1 month's duration); or bronchitis, pneumonitis, or esophagitis
- Progressive multifocal leukoencephalopathy

Bacterial Infections
- *Mycobacterium avium* complex
- Tuberculosis
- *Salmonella* septicemia, recurrent

Other conditions
- Encephalopathy, HIV-related
- Pneumonia, recurrent
- Wasting syndrome due to HIV

* If someone has HIV and one or more of these opportunistic infections, the person will be diagnosed with AIDS regardless of CD4 count.

Source: Data from Department of Health and Human Services. *Opportunistic infections*, 2010. Available: http://www.aids.gov/hiv-aids-basics/staying-healthy-with-hiv-aids/potential-related-health-problems/opportunistic-infections/.

Today we know that HIV belongs to a special class of viruses called **retroviruses**. Retroviruses consist of a protein shell surrounding the genetic material ribonucleic acid (RNA) (Figure 19.1). For HIV to attack a human cell, it must first attach itself to a special receptor on the cell's surface. In humans, HIV attaches to CD4 lymphocytes, a type of white blood cell that plays an important role in the immune response to disease. Once attached to the CD4 (also called T4) cell, HIV enters the cell and releases its RNA. The RNA is then converted into DNA by an enzyme (reverse transcriptase) also carried by HIV. This HIV DNA combines with the cell's DNA, causing the cell to reproduce HIV (Figure 19.2). In essence, HIV converts the cells it attacks into factories producing HIV, which then goes on to infect other CD4 cells. As this process progresses, CD4 cells are destroyed and the body becomes unable to defend itself against organisms that would normally pose no threat to health. Thus the opportunistic infections that characterize AIDS are able to more readily infect the individual.

Incidence of HIV and AIDS

As noted in Table 19.2, through December 2013, more than 1.1 million adults and adolescents had acquired AIDS in the United States (Centers for Disease Control and Prevention [CDC], 2015d). HIV infection disproportionately affects African Americans. In 2013, the rate for black/African Americans was 55.9 per 100,000 people, compared to 18.7 per 100,000 for Hispanics/Latinos, 16.8 per 100,000 for persons of multiple races, 12.7 per 100,000 for Native Hawaiians/other Pacific Islanders, 9.4 per 100,000 for American Indians/Alaska Natives, 6.6 per 100,000 for whites, and 6.0 per 100,000 for Asians. Unless there are changes in the patterns of HIV in the United States, an estimated 1 in 16 black men and 1 in 32 black women will be diagnosed with HIV infection at some point in their life (CDC, 2014c). Most black women with HIV acquired it through heterosexual sex (Figure 19.3) (CDC, 2014c).

In the United States, HIV affects different age groups at different rates. In 2013, the rate of HIV infection was highest among persons aged 25–29 years (36.3 per 100,000 individuals), followed by the rate among those aged 20–24 years (35.3 per 100,000 individuals) (CDC, 2015d). Because HIV treatment strategies are becoming increasingly effective, more people are living longer after infection with HIV and even

the name lymphadenopathy-associated virus (LAV). In May 1986, the International Committee on Taxonomy of Viruses announced its recommendation that the virus be consistently identified by the name *human immunodeficiency virus* (AIDS virus gets new name amid feuding, 1986).

retroviruses A group of viruses consisting of ribonucleic acid (RNA) surrounded by a protein coat that can convert their RNA into deoxyribonucleic acid (DNA) once they have invaded a living cell, allowing them to take over the cell and reproduce themselves.

FIGURE **19.1** HIV consists of an outer shell, or protein envelope, that surrounds a protein core that protects the ribonucleic acid (RNA) and the enzyme reverse transcriptase.

Source: Reproduced from *FDA Consumer* (October 1987), 10.

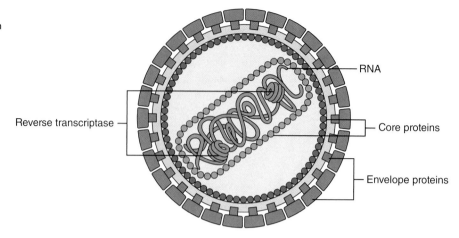

FIGURE **19.2** HIV infection and replication in a human cell. The virus enters the cell and releases RNA, its genetic material. Using the enzyme reverse transcriptase (RT), the virus converts its RNA into deoxyribonucleic acid (DNA), which enters the cell nucleus and combines with the cell DNA. The cell's altered genetic material then produces messenger RNA (mRNA), which codes for new virus.

Source: Reproduced from *FDA Consumer* (October 1987), 10.

TABLE 19.2

Estimated AIDS Cases by Transmission Category and Sex, 2013 & Cumulative, United States

Adult or Adolescent Transmission Category	2013—Males		2013—Females		Cumulative (Both Males and Females)	
	Number	%	Number	%	Number	%
Male-to-Male sexual contact	14,611	72.13	—	—	577,403	50.01
Male-to-male sexual contact & injection drug use	1,026	5.07	—	—	83,828	7.26
Injection drug use	1,610	7.95	1,143	17.79	277,008	23.99
Heterosexual Contact*	2,865	14.14	5,109	79.53	228,986	19.83
Other**	144	0.71	172	2.677	17,413	1.51
Total	20,256		6,424		1,154,618	

*Heterosexual contact with a person known to have, or to be at high risk for, HIV infection.

**Includes hemophilia, blood transfusion, perinatal exposure, and risk factors not reported or not identified.

Source: Data from Centers for Disease Control and Prevention. Diagnoses of HIV Infection in the United States and Dependent Areas, 2013. *HIV Surveillance Report,* 2015; vol 25. Available: http://www.cdc.gov/hiv/pdf/g-l/hiv_surveillance_report_vol_25.pdf#Page=17.

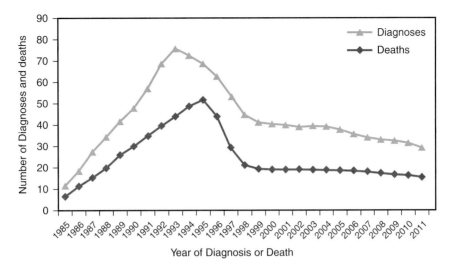

FIGURE **19.3** Classifications and deaths of persons with HIV infection ever classified as AIDS, among adults and adolescents, 1985–2011, United States and six dependent areas.

Note: All displayed data have been statistically adjusted to account for reporting delays, but not for incomplete reporting. Deaths of persons with an AIDS diagnosis may be due to any cause.

Source: Reproduced from Centers for Disease Control and Prevention. *Epidemiology of HIV infection through 2012*, Slide 24, 2014. Available: http://www.cdc.gov/hiv/pdf/statistics_surveillance_epi-hiv-infection.pdf.

after a diagnosis of AIDS; the highest rates of people living with AIDS are among persons aged 45–49 years (17.8 per 100,000), followed by the rate for persons aged 40–44 years (16.8 per 100,000). Death rates are decreasing or remaining stable for all age groups except those 60 years and older (CDC, 2015d); Figure 19.4 presents overall rates of diagnoses of AIDS and death among those with AIDS.

Similar to the situation within the United States, the global issue of HIV has stabilized in recent

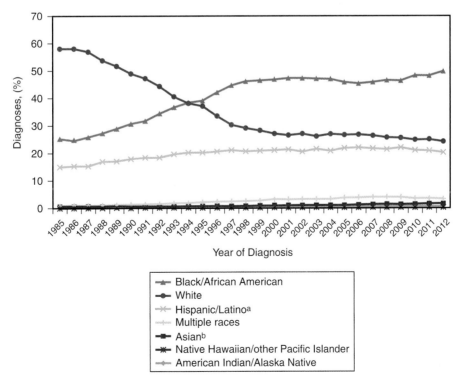

FIGURE **19.4** Percentages of AIDS classifications among adults and adolescents with HIV infection, by race/ethnicity and year of diagnosis, 1985–2012, United States and six dependent areas.

Source: Reproduced from Centers for Disease Control and Prevention. *Epidemiology of HIV infection through 2012*, Slide 26, 2014. Available: http://www.cdc.gov/hiv/pdf/statistics_surveillance_epi-hiv-infection.pdf.

Multicultural DIMENSIONS

HIV in American Indians and Alaskan Natives

Because the total number of individuals affected is small and the proportional rate is equivalent to the population rate, little attention is focused on HIV in American Indians and Alaskan Natives. However, these groups warrant special focus because of the unique challenges affecting HIV in their communities—specifically, the higher rate of transmission through injectable drug use. In 2013 in the United States, both male and female American Indians and Alaskan Natives (AI/AN) had the highest percentage of estimated diagnoses of HIV infection attributed to injection drug use among all races/ethnicities. Among AI/AN men, 13.0% of new HIV diagnoses were attributed to injection drug use and 5.9% were attributed to both male-to-male sex and injection drug use; this compares to the rates of 5.6% and 2.1%, respectively, for black men, who have the next highest percentages of these transmission categories. Among AI/AN women, 28.6% of the estimated new HIV diagnoses were attributed to injection drug use, compared to 24.9% for white women (CDC, 2015d). In addition to the direct risk through injection drug use, general substance use among AI/AN individuals is a risk factor for HIV infection. Compared with other racial/ethnic groups, AI/AN individuals tend to use alcohol and drugs at a younger age, use them more often and in higher

quantities, and experience more negative consequences from their use (CDC, 2015b).

Other issues also influence HIV risk within AI/AN communities, such as the vast diversity within these groups: There are more than 560 federally recognized AI/AN tribes, whose members speak more than 170 languages. Because each tribe has its own culture, beliefs, and practices and can be subdivided into language groups, it can be challenging to create culturally appropriate prevention programs for each group (CDC, 2015b).

Poverty both directly and indirectly increases the risk for HIV infection and affects the health of people living with and at risk for HIV infection. Compared with other racial/ethnic groups, members of AI/AN communities have higher poverty rates, have completed fewer years of education, are younger, are less likely to be employed, and have lower rates of health insurance coverage (CDC, 2015b).

AI/AN individuals are entitled to use the federally funded Indian Health Service (IHS), which encompasses services delivered directly, tribally operated healthcare programs, and urban Indian healthcare services and resource centers. However, because of confidentiality and quality-of-care concerns and a general distrust of the U.S. government, some AI/AN individuals may avoid IHS, limiting their access to needed health care and treatment (CDC, 2015b).

---

years. The annual number of new HIV infections has been declining since the late 1990s, and because of increased access to antiretroviral therapy there are fewer AIDS-related deaths. Although the number of new infections has been decreasing, overall new infection rates are still high and, with the significant reductions in mortality, the number of people living with HIV in the world has increased (Joint United Nations Programme on HIV/AIDS [UNAIDS], 2014b).

At the end of 2013, an estimated 35 million individuals were living with HIV infection, with the global HIV infection rate being 0.8%. Unfortunately, about half of all those infected with the virus do not know their status. Most individuals with HIV live in sub-Saharan Africa (about 24.7 million people, with a prevalence rate of 4.7%), with another 4.8 million living in Asia and the Pacific region (0.2% rate), 1.6 million in Latin America (0.4% rate), 1.1 million in Eastern Europe and Central Asia (0.6% rate), and 250,000 in the Caribbean (1.1% rate). In developed countries (North America and Western and Central

Europe), there were approximately 2.3 million people living with HIV in 2013 (0.2% rate). Worldwide, 2.1 million new infections occurred in 2013, a decrease from the 3.1 million in 2001. Although this decrease is impressive, it still means that more than 6,000 new HIV infections occurred every day in 2013. The number of AIDS-related deaths worldwide has declined 35% since 2005; in 2013, 1.5 million people died from HIV/AIDS-related causes (UNAIDS, 2014b).

In contrast to the incidence in the United States, where most of the cases of HIV are the result of same-sex sexual contact among men, the majority of HIV infections in other regions of the world are the result of heterosexual contact. In areas with high numbers of HIV-positive women, the risk to children being born with or contracting HIV through breastfeeding also becomes an issue. Most children with HIV (91%) live in sub-Saharan Africa. Globally, 3.2 million children live with HIV, with 240,000 new infections occurring among children and 190,000 AIDS-related deaths of children estimated to have occurred in

Gender DIMENSIONS

HIV Among Transgender People

Transgender people are individuals whose gender identity (basic sense of their gender) does not conform to a binary (male or female) classification based on biological sex, external genitalia, or sex assigned at birth. It includes gender-nonconforming people with identities beyond the gender binary who self-identify as male-to-female or transgender women; female-to-male or transgender men; two-spirit; or simply as women or men.

Exact rates of HIV infection among this group in the United States are unknown. Nevertheless, transgender people—especially transgender women—appear to be disproportionately affected by HIV; the CDC reports the percentage of new HIV infections is higher for this group than for either males or females. A review of published studies showed that 27.7% of transgender women tested positive for HIV infection during studies that involved testing, but only 11.8% of transgender women self-reported having HIV. Similar to overall rates and rates in women, most of the new HIV infections occurred in black transgender women (56.3%) compared to white (16.7%) or Latina (16.1%) transgender women. Because of stigma and discrimination, other risk factors also place transgender women at higher risk for HIV. Of those newly diagnosed with HIV, 51% of transgender women had documented substance use, commercial sex work, homelessness, incarceration, and/or sexual abuse in their medical records, compared with 31% of other people who were not transgender. Additionally, individuals may experience attempted suicide, unemployment, lack of familial support, violence, stigma and discrimination, limited

healthcare access, and negative healthcare encounters that can increase their risk for HIV. Discrimination and social stigma can hinder access to education, employment, and housing opportunities. In a study conducted in San Francisco, transgender people were more likely than men who have sex with men (MSM) or heterosexual women to live in transient housing and be less educated. Discrimination and social stigma may help explain why transgender people who experience significant economic difficulties often pursue high-risk activities, including sex work, to meet their basic survival needs (CDC, 2013b).

There are several limitations to efforts directed toward preventing HIV among transgender people. Some current medical systems do not allow individuals to identify as transgender, so these individuals and their experiences may not be well documented. Individuals may also not choose to identify as transgender because of legal or discrimination issues. Additionally, transgender men and their sexual health have been understudied and very little is known about HIV risk in this population. For example, in New York City from 2007 to 2011, 99% of the HIV diagnoses among transgender people were among transgender women (CDC, 2013b).

To adequately address the issue of HIV infection in transgender people, interventions that address multiple co-occurring public health problems—including substance use, poor mental health, violence and victimization, discrimination, and economic hardship—should be developed. Additionally, creating healthcare settings that are sensitive and welcoming to transgender people will increase their likelihood of testing, seeking treatment, and continuing treatment (CDC, 2013b).

2013 (UNAIDS, 2014b). UNAIDS has launched an effort to eliminate new HIV infections in children by 2015. Efforts to reach this goal include increasing access to antiretroviral medication to pregnant and breastfeeding women (UNAIDS, 2014a).

Transmission

HIV is found in large concentrations in two human body fluids: semen and blood. This is related to the large number of white blood cells present in these body fluids. It appears that a concentration of HIV is probably necessary for transmission of the virus from one individual to another. Thus the most common

modes of transmission are those that involve the exchange of semen or blood between individuals. Unprotected penile–vaginal or anal sex with an infected individual is the most common way that infected semen is transmitted.

Approximately half of the estimated AIDS cases in the United States involve men who have sex with men (MSM) (Table 19.2). While sexual risk—specifically, not using a condom during anal sex, and alcohol and drug use that increase this behavior—is the greatest concern, there are other contributing factors. Stigma and homonegativity have a profound impact on the lives of MSM and affect their decision making and risk for HIV (Buot et al., 2014). Racism, poverty, and lack of access to health care are barriers to HIV prevention services. Additional risk factors arise with young gay, bisexual, and other MSM, such as social isolation, lack of relevant sexuality education, and complacency about HIV among young MSM, all of which may affect risk-behavior. Given that young MSM did not experience the severity of the early HIV epidemic, some may falsely believe that HIV is no longer a serious health threat because of treatment advances and decreased mortality (CDC, 2014b).

Of the estimated U.S. adult/adolescent AIDS cases in 2013, approximately 30% appear to be related to heterosexual transmission. In the United States, this transmission category includes individuals who reported heterosexual contact with a person known to have, or to be at high risk for, HIV infection. Heterosexual transmission is of particular concern to women—for them, almost 80% of the 2013 estimated cases were transmitted by heterosexual contact, compared to only 14.1% of male cases (CDC, 2015d). Many women who become infected with HIV through heterosexual contact have partners who are injecting drug users. Women in this category are not necessarily injecting drug users themselves; rather, many become infected through sexual intercourse with partners who are.

The transmission of HIV related to injecting drug use is also of concern. Through December 2013, injecting drug use was associated with HIV transmission in 10.3% of the estimated AIDS diagnoses. Infection in such cases occurs through the sharing of needles contaminated with HIV. Additionally, injecting drug users can transmit the virus to their sexual partners through penile–vaginal or anal sex and, in the case of female injecting drug users, to their infants prenatally, during delivery, or through breastfeeding.

Between 1979 and mid-1985, HIV transmission through blood transfusions was of great concern to health professionals and the public. In the spring of 1985, an HIV antibody test was approved by the FDA for the purpose of screening blood donations. **Antibody** tests do an excellent job of protecting the U.S. blood supply from contamination with HIV. There is, however, still a slight risk that the test will miss HIV antibodies (resulting in a false-negative test result). Additionally, the test may not detect HIV-infected blood because a person who is infected with HIV may not produce a detectable level of antibodies for as long as 3 months after infection. It must be emphasized that this risk is very small. In 1987, the CDC and American Red Cross reported that the risk

Myth vs Fact

Myth: HIV was created in a laboratory by scientists.

Fact: A type of chimpanzee in West Africa has been identified as the source of HIV infection; the chimpanzee version of the immunodeficiency virus (called simian immunodeficiency virus [SIV]) most likely was transmitted to humans and mutated into HIV when humans hunted these chimpanzees for meat and came into contact with their infected blood. Studies show that HIV may have jumped from apes to humans as far back as the late 1800s, then slowly spread across Africa and the world. The virus has existed in the United States since at least the mid- to late 1970s (CDC, 2015a).

Myth: Mosquitoes transmit HIV.

Fact: Scientific experiments have shown that HIV does not multiply in insects. When looking at areas with high rates of HIV infection and high prevalence of mosquitos, epidemiological evidence also supports the hypothesis that transmission by insects does not occur (CDC, 2015e).

Myth: If a person is infected with HIV but the viral load is undetectable, the individual cannot transmit HIV to others.

Fact: While decreased HIV viral loads decrease the likelihood of transmitting the virus to others, it does not eliminate the risk of transmission completely. Individuals should still reduce the risk of transmission through behavioral strategies such as abstaining from sexual activity or using condoms and other latex barriers (CDC, 2015e).

Myth: Serosorting (limiting unprotected sex to partners with the same HIV status) reduces one's risk of becoming infected with HIV.

Fact: In theory, having sex with only HIV-negative people should reduce one's risk; in reality, many

people do not know their HIV status. The CDC does not recommend serosorting as a practice because individuals may have been tested too recently to know about a new infection and individuals may not always be honest about their HIV status. Using condoms or remaining abstinent is a much more effective way to reduce HIV risk (CDC, 2011).

Myth: If two sexual partners are infected with HIV, they do not need to practice safer sex because they already have the infection.

Fact: There is still risk because individuals can get infected with a different type of HIV—a condition called HIV superinfection. The new strain of HIV can replace the originally contracted strain or remain along with the original strain. The effects differ from person to person. In some people, superinfection may cause increased sickness because they are infected with a new strain of the virus resistant to their current HIV medications (CDC, 2015e). Safer sex practices should always be used to reduce risk of HIV transmission—even if both partners are already infected.

Myth: All males should be circumcised to reduce their risk of contracting HIV.

Fact: Male circumcision reduces the risk that a man will get HIV from an infected female partner by 60%; however, studies have not consistently shown that this practice prevents HIV transmission among men who have sex with men. This prevention strategy is being advocated in sub-Saharan Africa and regions where rates of HIV infection among women are high and heterosexual sexual contact is a common form of transmission. Adult men who are considering circumcision should weigh its risks and costs against its potential benefits (CDC, 2013c, 2015e).

---

antibodies A class of proteins secreted by the immune system that bonds with antigens. Antibodies fight off infection-causing organisms.

of contracting HIV through a blood transfusion was 1 in 28,000. Today, more rigorous screening of donors and nucleic acid testing have decreased the risk of contracting HIV through a blood transfusion to 1 in 1.5 million (based on 2007–2008 data) (Zou et al., 2010). There is no risk of becoming infected with HIV by donating blood.

Since 1983, part of the screening process for blood donors was a lifetime ban for men who have ever had sex with another man. This restriction has received much criticism as being discriminatory against gay, bisexual, and other MSM. Based on recommendations from advisory committees to the Department of Health and Human Services and the U.S. Food and Drug Administration (FDA), in 2015 the FDA planned to revise this policy and eliminate the lifetime ban. At the time of this text's publication, the revised policy was unknown, but the advisory committees were recommending a revision that prevents men who have had sex with men in the last 12 months from donating blood (as opposed to a lifetime ban). This change would make U.S. policy more consistent with the policies of many other countries (e.g., the United Kingdom, Finland, Japan, Australia). Some gay activists still consider this type of policy to be discriminatory because it bans anyone who has been sexually active regardless of number of partners, use of condoms, or other factors that affect risk. In September 2015, Argentina adopted a policy that assesses individual risk of MSM instead of imposing a general ban or limitation. Interestingly, some MSM have not been complying with the current ban; Liszewski and colleagues (2014) surveyed attendees of lesbian, gay, bisexual, and transgender festivals in New Orleans and Chicago and found that 42% of MSM had donated blood, with a mean of 4.84 donations per donor, and that 85.9% would be willing to donate if the ban allows them to do so.

The risk of contracting HIV (or other infectious diseases, such as hepatitis B or C) is slightly higher for those individuals receiving an organ donation; however, in 2014, new recommendation guidelines were established to address these concerns (Seem et al., 2013). Screening for HIV, hepatitis B, and hepatitis C is now required; for living donors, this testing should occur within 28 days of the scheduled surgery. In addition, a risk assessment screening of donors should be conducted and if individuals are considered high-risk based on established criteria, nucleic acid testing (NAT) should be performed; NAT is more accurate than antibody screening in reducing the risk of unintentional infection to the organ recipient.

Stages of HIV Infection

Once an individual is infected with HIV, the natural course of the infection progresses in three stages. If untreated, HIV is almost universally fatal, because it eventually overwhelms the immune system. HIV treatment, however, can help people at all stages of the disease by either slowing or preventing progression from one stage to the next. A person can transmit HIV to others during any stage. Figure 19.5 shows rates of HIV infection for U.S. states and dependent areas.

The first stage is **acute HIV infection**. Within 2 to 4 weeks after the initial infection with HIV, an individual may experience flu-like symptoms. This so-called acute retroviral syndrome (ARS) or primary HIV infection represents the body's response to the HIV infection. However, not everyone develops ARS, so some individuals have no indication that they have been infected. Also, many of us get flu-like symptoms frequently enough that few would automatically think, "That is probably acute retroviral syndrome!" Consequently, even if symptoms are present, they are often discounted.

During acute HIV infection, large amounts of HIV are produced in the body and this stage is the most infectious because of it. Eventually, the immune response will begin to bring the amount of virus in

The efforts of the gay community to garner media attention for the HIV and AIDS crisis brought it to the forefront of the U.S. medical agenda during the 1980s. Because of these efforts, HIV and AIDS research and medical funding garnered a far greater percentage of government spending than it would otherwise have, which resulted in a significant reduction of HIV incidence in the mainstream gay community. Unfortunately, gay, bisexual, and other MSM are currently experiencing a resurgence of HIV infections.

acute (primary) HIV infection The initial stage of HIV infection (2 to 4 weeks after exposure) which may or may not include flu-like symptoms.

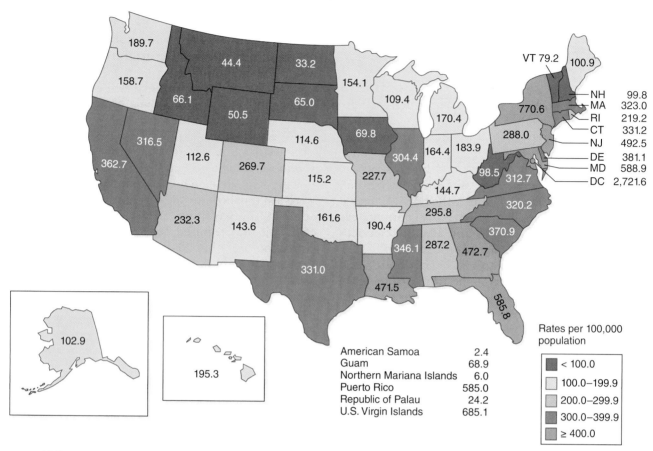

FIGURE 19.5 Rates of adults and adolescents living with diagnosed HIV infection, year-end 2011—United States and six dependent areas.

Note: Data include persons with a diagnosis of HIV infection regardless of stage of disease at diagnosis. All displayed data have been statistically adjusted to account for reporting delays, but not for incomplete reporting.

Source: Reproduced from Centers for Disease Control and Prevention. *Epidemiology of HIV infection through 2012*, Slide 22, 2014. Available: http://www.cdc.gov/hiv/pdf/statistics_surveillance_epi-hiv-infection.pdf.

the body back down to a stable level; CD4 counts will consequently increase but may not return to pre-infection levels (CDC, 2015a).

The second stage of HIV infection is **clinical latency**, which is also called asymptomatic HIV infection or chronic HIV infection. In this stage, HIV is still active, but the virus reproduces at very low levels and infected individuals may not have any symptoms or get sick. People who are on antiretroviral therapy (ART; discussed later in the chapter) may live with clinical latency for several decades. For those not on ART, this period can last up to a decade, although some individuals may progress through this phase faster. Because viral loads are lower in the body (especially

if on ART) during this stage, transmission of HIV is less likely but still possible. Toward the middle and end of this period, the amount of HIV in the body increases and the CD4 cell count begins to drop. As this happens, symptoms of HIV infection may occur as the immune system weakens (CDC, 2015a).

The final stage is AIDS (acquired immune deficiency syndrome). During this stage of infection, the immune system is badly damaged and individuals become vulnerable to infections and opportunistic illnesses. Normal CD4 counts are between 500 and 1,600 cells per cubic millimeter of blood (cells/mm^3). When the number of CD4 cells falls below 200 cells/mm^3 or an individual develops one of the opportunistic illnesses listed in Table 19.1 (regardless of CD4 count), he or she is considered to have progressed to AIDS. Without treatment, people diagnosed with AIDS typically survive about 3 years. Once someone has an opportunistic illness, without treatment, life expectancy decreases to 1 year. People with AIDS need medical treatment to prevent death (CDC, 2015a).

clinical latency Sometimes called asymptomatic HIV infection or chronic HIV infection. HIV is still active during this phase, but the virus reproduces at very low levels. Individuals may not have any symptoms. This phase can last up to a decade (though not for everyone) and several decades for people on antiretroviral therapy.

Although AIDS is classified as a terminal disease, people now live with AIDS for a long time. Newer medication regimens, accompanied by an enthusiastic research agenda, have led many health professionals to consider HIV infection and AIDS to be chronic conditions (like hypertension and diabetes) that can be controlled and perhaps eventually eradicated.

Testing for HIV

Several types of HIV tests are available. Traditional testing (immunoassay) looks for HIV antibodies in either blood, fluid from the cheek, or urine. Antibodies can develop as early as 2 weeks after infection; in some individuals, however, they can take up to 12 weeks to emerge. If antibodies are present, the person is said to be **seropositive**. If no antibodies are present, the person is said to be **seronegative**. However, even though the tests are very accurate, if the results show that HIV antibodies are present, a confirmation test is performed to rule out a "false positive." Follow-up diagnostic testing can take the form of the following: an antibody differentiation test, an HIV-1 nucleic acid test (which looks for the virus directly), or the Western blot or indirect immunofluorescence assay (a more sensitive test for HIV antibodies) (CDC, 2015g).

Some immunoassay tests use oral fluids and urine to test for HIV antibodies. These oral-fluid tests require a person to place a flat inch-long cotton swab attached to a stick between the gum and cheek for 2 minutes. The swab draws fluid from the mucous membrane, which contains HIV antibodies if the person is infected. This test does not use saliva. A follow-up confirmatory Western blot uses the same oral-fluid sample.

Because the level of antibody in oral fluid is lower than it is in blood, blood tests tend to find infection sooner after exposure than do oral-fluid tests. In addition, most blood-based lab tests find infection sooner after exposure than do rapid HIV tests (CDC, 2015g). The sensitivity and accuracy of urine tests for HIV antibodies are less than those of the blood and oral-fluid tests. This immunoassay antibody test also requires a follow-up confirmatory Western blot using the same urine sample.

Rapid tests are also available; these screening procedures produce results in approximately 20 minutes. Rapid tests use blood (often from a fingerstick), or oral fluid to look for the presence of antibodies to HIV. As is true for all screening tests, a reactive rapid HIV test result must be confirmed with a follow-up confirmatory test before a final diagnosis of infection is made. These tests have similar accuracy rates as traditional immunoassay screening tests, although blood-based lab testing may report a positive result sooner.

Some individuals do not want to visit a clinic for an HIV test. Currently, two HIV home collection kits are FDA approved and sold legally in the United States (Home Access HIV-1 Test System and Ora-Quick In-Home HIV Test). Although others may advertise and be sold on the Internet, their accuracy cannot be verified. The Home Access kit allows an individual to take a blood sample and send the sample to a laboratory for testing. The Ora-Quick In-Home HIV Test is a rapid in-home HIV test. This kit tests oral fluid and provides results in 20 to 40 minutes; there is no need to mail anything. The Ora-Quick test is approved for sale to individuals 17 years and older. Studies have shown the test to be highly accurate for people who do not have the virus (only 1 false-positive result will occur for every 5,000 tests in uninfected individuals). However, the accuracy of this testing mechanism with untrained individuals is lower for individuals who are infected with HIV. There will be 1 false-negative result out of every 12 tests performed in HIV-infected individuals. With both the Home Access and Ora-Quick tests, a follow-up confirmatory test is needed for any positive results (CDC, 2015g).

All of the previously discussed tests do not directly test for the presence of HIV. Rather, they test for the presence of antibodies produced in response to HIV infection. Thus it is possible that the infection may not have produced sufficient antibodies to be measured yet, even though the person being tested is, in fact, infected with HIV. Even if it is too early for the antibodies to be present in sufficient numbers to be measured, the person can still transmit the virus.

In addition to the tests that detect HIV antibodies only, tests that can detect both antibodies and antigen (part of the virus itself) are becoming more common. These tests can find recent infections earlier—as soon as 3 weeks after exposure to the virus—than tests that detect only antibodies. Such tests are available only for testing blood, not oral fluid.

RNA tests detect the genetic material of the virus directly. These tests are used in screening the blood supply and for detection of very early infection cases when antibody tests are unable to detect HIV antibodies. Because of their high cost, they are not commonly used in screening for HIV infection, although a clinician may order an RNA test as a follow-up measure (CDC, 2015g).

An individual who receives a positive HIV test result should be given medical and psychological

seropositive The result of a blood test for HIV antibodies that indicates that such antibodies have been found in the blood.

seronegative The result of a blood test for HIV antibodies that indicates no presence of such antibodies.

Total number of new individuals named at each stage of investigation

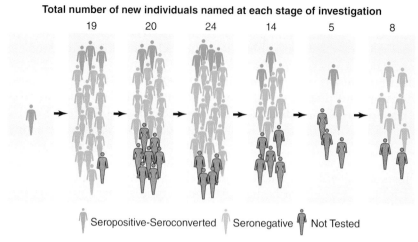

FIGURE **19.6** Partner notification programs can be highly productive, as illustrated by results of a South Carolina investigation that began with one HIV-positive man. Of the 19 sexual contacts he named, all but one were tested, and 3 were seropositive. Those 3 men then named 20 sexual contacts not already identified, leading to the discovery of 2 more HIV-positive men, who in turn named 24 other previously unidentified contacts, and so forth. When the investigation reached its endpoint of no new HIV-positive contacts, it had identified a total of 90 persons at risk, tested 68 of them, and found 12 who either were seropositive or seroconverted 6 months after initial testing.

counseling as well as education intended to prevent HIV transmission to others. Additionally, information about legal obligations surrounding the process of *partner notification*, as well as steps to initiate this process, should be provided. Because treatment for HIV is more successful when initiated early, informing previous partners of their possible infection can help them manage their infection better and prevent them from unknowingly spreading the infection to others should they be infected (Figure 19.6). In addition, some states require partner notification. In some cases, an HIV-infected person may not feel capable of contacting sexual or needle-sharing partners; most

states have a Partner Counseling and Referral Service (PCRS) that can help notify partners without disclosing the name of the infected individual. Four types of partner notification are possible. In *provider referral*, a healthcare provider notifies partner(s). In *self-referral*, individuals notify partners themselves. In *contract referral*, a "contract" is established to notify partner(s) by a particular date. If, by the contract date, the partners have not come in for counseling and testing, the health department will contact them. Finally, in *dual referral*, an individual and the health department notify partner(s) together (U.S. Department of Health & Human Services [DHHS], 2009).

People with HIV must cope not only with the knowledge of their illness but also with society's fear of HIV. Support groups offer emotional support and firsthand advice on coping with the illness.

 Did You Know . . .

HIV can be transmitted from mother to child during pregnancy, labor and delivery, and breastfeeding, and through giving a child pre-chewed food. This perinatal type of transmission is the most common route of HIV infection in children. In 2013, an estimated 107 children acquired HIV through perinatal infection. In recent years, the rate of perinatal transmission has declined dramatically due to the widespread use of ART. When no prevention steps are taken, the risk of transmission from an infected pregnant women to a child is 20%; HIV-infected pregnant women who take antiretroviral medications as recommended, have cesarean sections, and avoid breastfeeding can reduce the risk of transmitting HIV to their babies to less than 1%.

Ethical
DIMENSIONS

Should Recovering Drug Addicts Be Used As Peer Educators for HIV Prevention?

The use of peer educators—individuals like others trained to talk about health issues—is a common strategy in HIV prevention and education efforts. People relate to and are more willing to listen to others who are like them, either in background, culture, or experiences. Successful programs have been used with a variety of communities, including gay, bisexual, and other MSM and African American women. Because of the hidden community and legal aspects of drug use, reaching people who use injectable drugs can be a challenge, however.

In attempts to reach people in this group, peer educators—drug users who are in recovery—have been involved in HIV prevention efforts. However, such efforts raise ethical issues that are not relevant to the other groups. While serving as a peer educator, part of the recovering drug user's work may be to interact with community members and visit places that may have been part of their use history. Prevention programs need to balance beneficence (doing good) with nonmaleficence (doing no harm). In this case, does the dissemination of harm-reduction information and education outweigh the potentially heightened risk for relapse and trauma that a recovering peer educator may experience? Unfortunately, the research studies considering these factors do not provide a consistent answer to this question.

What are your thoughts? Is it ethical to ask people in recovery to place themselves in situations that could trigger challenges to their treatment? Because the risk is not definitive, is the greater good of disseminating life-saving information to others worth the risk to the peer educators? Discuss the issue with a classmate or friend and see if you agree.

Treatment of HIV and AIDS

In 1987, the FDA approved **zidovudine** (also known as azidothymidine [AZT]) as the first drug licensed in the United States for the treatment of patients with AIDS. Zidovudine is an antiviral drug that slows the replication of HIV in human cells. Studies indicate that this agent not only slows the progression of HIV infection when given in early stages, but also prolongs survival and decreases the incidence and severity of opportunistic infections in people living with AIDS. While somewhat effective by itself, zidovudine is no longer the only antiviral medication to combat HIV infection; there are six classes of antiretroviral therapy (ART) used to treat HIV infection (DHHS, 2014b):

1. *Nucleoside/nucleotide reverse transcriptase inhibitors (NRTIs)* (e.g., zidovudine, didanosine, stavudine): These drugs block the action of reverse transcriptase, thereby preventing HIV RNA from reproducing.

2. *Protease inhibitors (PIs)* (e.g., indinavir, nelfinavir, ritonavir, saquinavir): These drugs shut down HIV replication by preventing the viral enzyme protease from cutting other viral proteins into the shorter pieces needed by HIV to make new viral copies for infecting new CD4 cells.

3. *Non-nucleoside reverse transcriptase inhibitors (NNRTIs)* (e.g., delavirdine and nevirapine): These drugs bind to and later alter the reverse transcriptase.

4. *Fusion inhibitors* (e.g.,enfuvirtide): These drugs block HIV from entering the CD4 cell.

5. *Integrase inhibitors* (e.g., dolutegravir, raltegravir): These drugs disable integrase, a protein the HIV uses to insert its viral genetic material into the generic material of an infected cell.

6. *Entry inhibitors* (e.g., maraviroc): These drugs block proteins on the CD4 cells that HIV needs to enter the cells.

In addition to the six classes of antiviral medications, pharmacokinetic enhancers (e.g., cobicistat) are used in HIV treatment to increase the effectiveness of an HIV medication. There are also combination medications that contain two or more anti-HIV drugs from one or more classes of drugs. These medications reduce the number of pills an HIV-infected

zidovudine The first drug (brand name Retrovir; also known as AZT) approved by the FDA for the treatment of AIDS. This antiviral drug slows the replication of the AIDS virus, thereby slowing the course of the syndrome.

individual needs to take (DHHS, 2014b). Because a combination of medications is used to treat HIV, such multidrug therapy is sometimes referred to as "the cocktail," but may also be called antiretrovirals (ARV) or highly active antiretroviral therapy (HAART or ART). Combination therapy makes sense because it attacks the virus at different steps in the life cycle rather than at just one step. This type of treatment significantly strengthens the immune system and improves its ability to fight off infections—outcomes that have resulted in not only a dramatic decrease in opportunistic infections and deaths, but also the ability of HIV-infected individuals to enjoy long, healthy lives (CDC, 2014d).

Early diagnosis is important so individuals can utilize medications that prevent HIV from destroying the immune system. Previously, treatment started when the CD4 count fell to 350 cells/mm^3 or because opportunistic infections began. However, research has shown that it may be easier to maintain higher CD4 counts if HIV treatment is started before the CD4 count drops so low. Currently, strong evidence suggests that it is wise to begin ART if the CD4 count is less than 500 cells/mm^3. Some experts also recommend that HIV-infected individuals with CD4 counts greater than 500 cells/mm^3 start therapy, although the enthusiasm for this treatment may be tempered by the risk of side effects and resulting noncompliance in patients. More research is currently being conducted to better understand the benefits and risks of treating all HIV-infected individuals with ART regardless of CD4 count (DHHS, 2014a).

Although the currently available medications allow many HIV-infected individuals to live longer and have fewer complications, there are limitations to their use. Some individuals do not tolerate certain drugs well, and the body can develop resistance to some medications, so new regimens and medication adjustments are often a component of treatment. In addition, toxicity from the medications can affect other body functions. The CDC (2014c) estimates that only 30% of HIV-infected individuals are currently successfully keeping the virus under control.

From a practical standpoint, many of the drugs are expensive. Average wholesale costs per month range from $350 to $1,200 to more than $3,500 for a fusion inhibitor. The increased costs that individuals must pay out of pocket for these medications (through copayments, coinsurance, and deductibles) are associated with decreased medication adherence and increased drug discontinuation (DHHS, 2014a). For HIV-infected individuals with low incomes, government assistance may be available through Medicaid and Medicare. In addition, AIDS Drugs Assistance Programs (ADAP), which

are federal- and state-funded programs, provide medication to about one-third of all individuals in the United States receiving HIV treatment (Berry, 2011). Unfortunately, many states have waiting lists for these programs, and some individuals do not meet program guidelines. In those cases, many pharmaceutical companies also offer copayment and patient assistance programs to HIV-infected individuals who are not eligible or not enrolled in other programs (Berry, 2011). In spite of these programs, the process of obtaining medications and concerns about payment for medications remain challenging for many HIV-infected individuals in the United States.

Individuals in other countries often must rely on government programs or pharmaceutical assistance programs for medication. Because of the effectiveness of ART, additional efforts have been implemented to increase the availability of these medications worldwide. For example, in sub-Saharan Africa, 86% of those individuals who know they are HIV infected are now receiving ART (UNAIDS, 2014b).

In 2014, several organizations developed HIV prevention strategies specifically for individuals who are already infected with HIV. These strategies focus on linkage and continuation of medical care, the use of ART, increasing adherence to ART, services for partners, and services for pregnant women (CDC et al., 2014). While all of these approaches are important, linkage to medical care deserves special attention. A growing body of evidence indicates that continuing in care during the first year of outpatient HIV medical care is critical. Individuals who continue such care are more likely to start ART than those with early lapses in care, have higher adherence to ART, are more likely to achieve suppression of HIV, and are more likely to practice safer sexual behaviors. Unfortunately, many HIV-infected individuals are not integrated into HIV care (Figure 19.7).

Several strategies have been proposed to increase linkage to care. Clinics and services need to ensure that the infrastructure to support early care (ideally within 3 months of diagnosis) and extended care is in place. Individuals should be informed multiple times—before testing, after preliminary HIV results, and after confirmatory HIV results—about the benefits of starting HIV care and ART early. Healthcare providers and other service workers need to identify facilitators and barriers to linkage and retention; such measures include making referrals to increase access and continuation of care, helping individuals enroll in health insurance or other medical coverage, and collaborating with relevant individuals and organizations to develop the best process of support (CDC et al., 2014).

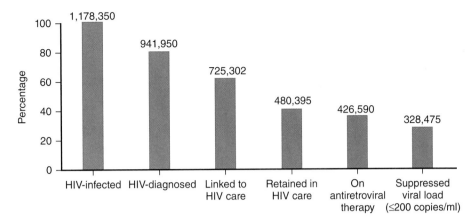

FIGURE **19.7** Number and percentage of HIV-infected persons engaged in selected stages of the continuum of HIV care—United States.

Source: Data from Centers for Disease Control and Prevention. Vital signs: HIV prevention through care and treatment—United States. *Morbidity and Mortality Weekly Report, 60, 47* (2011), 1621.

Prevention of HIV Infection and AIDS

While no cure or vaccine for HIV is currently available, medications and nonmedical strategies are both used for prevention. First, we review progress toward a vaccine.

HIV Vaccine

At this time, a vaccine for HIV is not available. Historically, vaccines have virtually eliminated the spread of infectious diseases such as smallpox, polio, and measles. Because of the success in controlling these other infections, many believe that an HIV vaccine represents the best long-term strategy for ending the HIV pandemic. However, HIV is different from other infectious diseases; the immune system of the human body does not seem capable of effectively preventing the virus from progressing to disease. Some vaccine trials have not shown any promise, whereas others have been able to provide more information useful to vaccine development. The RV144 study conducted in Thailand tested two different vaccines together, ALVAC-HIV and AIDSVAX, in a primarily low- or moderate-risk group. Results showed a short-term protective effect against HIV in about one-third of study participants; however, other analyses were not deemed significant (Rerks-Ngarm et al., 2009). While most researchers consider the study's success to be limited, it does provide hope and some direction for future studies. For example, the vaccine provided in the HVTN100 study launched in 2015 in South Africa is designed to provide greater protection than the RV144 regimen and has been adapted to the HIV subtype that predominates in southern Africa. The HVTN100 study is one of several efforts that hope to capitalize on the success of RV144 (National Institutes of Health, 2015).

Pre-Exposure Prophylaxis

While the vaccine efforts have not been successful, studies have demonstrated that the use of antiviral medication before exposure can reduce the risk of becoming infected with HIV. **Pre-exposure prophylaxis (PrEP)**, consisting of the daily use of a combined pill of emtricitabine and tenofovir (brand name Truvada), has been shown to decrease the risk of HIV infection in high-risk individuals by as much as 92% when the medication is taken consistently and correctly. Effectiveness is much lower if the medication is not taken properly (CDC, 2014d). Daily use of Truvada is associated with side effects such as nausea, vomiting, and dizziness, but these side effects are mild and usually resolve within the first month. For those truly at risk of HIV because of high-risk sexual practices or because of having an HIV-infected partner, the benefit would likely outweigh those risks.

Federal guidelines for the use of PrEP were established in May 2014; these guidelines provide direction for providers in determining who can most benefit from PrEP and how to administer PrEP medications. Individuals may be eligible for PrEP based on their behavior or the HIV status of their partner. Individuals may be defined as being at high risk for

pre-exposure prophylaxis (PrEP) The daily use of a combined pill of antiretroviral therapy (Truvada) that decreases the risk of HIV infection in as many as 92% of individuals with an ongoing high risk of infection.

HIV infection through sexual transmission in one of four ways: (1) in an ongoing relationship with an HIV-infected partner; (2) not in a mutually monogamous relationship; (3) a gay or bisexual man who has had anal sex without a condom or been diagnosed with an STI in the past 6 months; or (4) a heterosexual person who does not regularly use condoms during sex with partners of unknown HIV status who are at substantial risk of HIV infection (e.g., people who inject drugs or have bisexual male partners). Individuals considered to be at high risk for HIV also include those who have injected illicit drugs in the past 6 months and who have shared injection equipment or been in drug treatment for injection drug use in the past 6 months (CDC, 2014d).

PrEP is only for people who are at *ongoing* substantial risk of HIV infection. For people who are concerned about HIV after a single high-risk event—such as unprotected sex, needle-sharing injection drug use, or sexual assault—*post-exposure* prophylaxis is a more appropriate option.

Post-Exposure Prophylaxis

For individuals concerned about HIV exposure after a single high-risk event, **post-exposure prophylaxis (PEP)** is an appropriate prevention strategy. In addition to high-risk behaviors such as unprotected sex and needle-sharing injection drug use, individuals may be exposed to blood or body fluids through an occupational hazard (the risk for healthcare workers is less than 1 in every 100 exposures) or through body fluids during a sexual assault. Typically, two or three medications will be prescribed as part of the PEP regimen. The medications should be taken as soon as possible, but no more than 72 hours after the incident, and must be continued for 28 days. Use of PEP does not guarantee that an individual will not become infected with HIV.

If the potential exposure is work related, worker's compensation should cover the cost of the PEP medications. Individuals who were sexually assaulted and prescribed PEP may be eligible for partial or total reimbursement for medicines and clinical care costs through the Office for Victims of Crime, funded by the U.S. Department of Justice. If an individual is prescribed PEP for other reasons and insurance will not cover its cost, healthcare providers can apply for free antiretroviral medications for the patient through the medication assistance programs run by the drug manufacturers. In many cases, online applications and special phone lines can handle these requests urgently to avoid delays in getting medicine (CDC, 2015f).

Abstinence

In addition to these methods, the best strategy to reduce risk is to refrain from oral, anal, or penile–vaginal sex with an HIV-infected partner and to abstain from sharing needles. This is an important message of HIV and AIDS education efforts—especially for adolescents and young adults who are in a developmental stage at which sexual and drug experimentation is common. Today, such experimentation carries the risk of contracting HIV and AIDS.

Abstaining from sexual activity throughout one's life is impractical and undesirable for most people. For those who are uninfected and sexually active, maintaining a mutually monogamous relationship with an uninfected partner prevents the sexual transmission of HIV. Each partner would also need to abstain from sharing needles during drug or steroid use, another high-risk behavior for HIV transmission.

Understanding of Risk Behaviors

Many people have previously engaged in behaviors that put them at risk of being infected with HIV. People should be considered at risk if they have shared needles or syringes to inject drugs or steroids; are male and have had unprotected anal sex with another male; have had sex with someone they believe may have been infected with HIV; have had another STI; received blood transfusions or blood products between 1978 and 1985; or have had sex with someone who has any of these risk characteristics. In addition, the more sexual partners a person has had, the greater the chances that person will have had contact with an HIV-infected person. The former basketball player Magic Johnson brought this point home to many people when he announced to

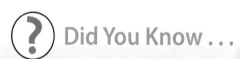

? Did You Know . . .

Worldwide about 2.1 million new infections of HIV occurred in 2013, according to UNAIDS. Of those new infections, 240,000 occurred in children younger than 15 years of age. Furthermore, in 2013, 1.5 million deaths occurred worldwide as a result of AIDS. UNAIDS estimates that an additional 7.6 million deaths have been averted globally since 1995 due to the introduction of antiretroviral therapy (UNAIDS, 2014b).

---

post-exposure prophylaxis (PEP) The use of antiretroviral medicines to reduce the chance of HIV infection after a single potential exposure to HIV.

In November 1991, the basketball star Magic Johnson announced that he had acquired HIV infection through unprotected sexual intercourse with an unknown infected woman. Johnson provides living proof of the effectiveness of the antiretroviral therapy: The level of HIV in his body has been reduced to an undetectable level.

protected, with a 1 in 3 rate among single people (Sanders et al., 2010).

Testing

While knowing one's HIV status has a direct benefit to the person being tested, there are also prevention benefits from testing. In the United States, it is estimated that 1 in 6 individuals who is HIV infected do not know his or her status (CDC, 2015g). The CDC recommends that all patients ages 13–64 be screened for HIV unless the patient declines the test. The objective is for all individuals to be tested at least once in their life. Individuals at high risk for HIV infection should be screened at least once a year, and sexually active gay, bisexual, and other MSM may benefit from testing every 3 or 6 months. The recommendations include an opt-out standard, meaning that once a patient has been told about the test, consent is inferred unless specifically declined. While providers may take this opportunity to counsel patients about prevention and risky behaviors, counseling is no longer required, because it was seen as a barrier to testing for some individuals. Even for those individuals whose results do not show HIV infection, the testing process can provide a valuable "teachable moment."

If there is a positive result, individuals can benefit from more immediate medical intervention to help decrease the viral load in their body, which may in turn decrease the risk of HIV transmission to others. Individuals can also take necessary precautions to prevent transmission by either abstaining from risky behaviors or using condoms. Additionally, the knowledge of a positive result can encourage sexual

the world that he was infected with HIV from unprotected sexual intercourse with a woman he could not identify because of his numerous sexual partners over the years. It is important to remember, however, that unprotected sexual intercourse with just one person is risky if that person is infected with HIV.

Condom and Other Barrier Use

If an individual decides to engage in sexual activity with a person of unknown HIV status or who is infected with HIV, condoms should be used during oral sex on a male, penile–vaginal sex, and anal sex, and latex barriers be should be used during oral sex on a female. Latex condoms have been shown to be a highly effective barrier to HIV (CDC, 2013a). Unfortunately, many people do not use condoms. The most recent nationally representative study of sexual health behaviors in the United States showed that only 1 of 4 acts of vaginal intercourse are condom

HIV infection is determined by a blood test that looks for antibodies produced in response to HIV. Testing may be accompanied by counseling and education to interpret the results and to discuss ways to prevent infection, or to seek treatment if the test is positive.

partners to get tested; if partners' results are positive, the testing may in turn reduce their risk of transmitting the virus to someone else.

Unfortunately, many people do not disclose their HIV status to their partners. Overall rates of disclosure are difficult to determine, and study results vary, especially between countries (Arnold et al., 2008; Obermeyer et al., 2011). A review of U.S. studies showed that 56% to 81% of individuals disclosed their HIV status to sexual partners, but that rate changed significantly for steady partners (74%) compared to casual partners (25%) (Obermeyer et al., 2011). Similar results have been found in HIV-infected youth (Thoth et al., 2014). Given that disclosure can lead to stigmatization and other consequences, it is understandable—though not acceptable—that some HIV-infected individuals might refrain from informing partners or potential partners. However, all individuals deserve the right to make informed decisions about the risk of their sexual activities, and disclosing an HIV infection—or any other type of chronic STI—allows others that opportunity. Interventions that provide HIV-infected individuals with the opportunity to reflect on living with HIV, explore fears of stigma and rejection, and develop communication skills and strategies to disclose (Maiorana et al., 2012), combined with training for providers (including case managers and disease intervention specialists) (Edelman et al., 2014), are needed to help HIV-infected individuals become more comfortable and skilled at disclosing their status.

HIV and Young Adults

Unfortunately, many new HIV infections occur among young adults. In 2013, the estimated rates of infection were second highest among adults 20–24 years of age (35.3 per 100,000); the highest rate was among 25- to 29-year-olds (36.3 per 100,000) (CDC, 2015d). Most of the infections in young adults occur in gay, bisexual, or other MSM and in youth of underserved races and ethnicities. As with overall HIV infection rates, black young adults are disproportionately affected, followed by Hispanic young adults (CDC, 2014a).

A variety of factors place young adults at increased risk of HIV transmission, including low perception of risk, low rates of testing, low rates of condom use, high rates of STIs, older partners, substance use, homelessness, social isolation, and inadequate sexuality education. Given that many young adults do not perceive themselves as being at risk for HIV infection, they are less likely to get tested or use condoms. Approximately 60% of young adults do not know they are HIV infected (CDC, 2014a), and overall rates of testing in this population are low: 12.9%

for high school students (Kann et al., 2014) and 35% for 18- to 24-year-olds (CDC, 2012).

While condom use has increased since the mid-1990s, the rates among young adults certainly do not indicate universal safer sex practices are being followed. Among sexually active high school students, the rate of condom use was 59.1% in a national 2013 survey (Kann et al., 2014). Even fewer college students reported condom or barrier use: Only 50.7% of college students who had engaged in vaginal sex used condoms, with lower rates of condom and barrier use for oral sex (4.6%) and anal sex (27.2%) (American College Health Association [ACHA], 2014). Consistency of condom use among college male students does not appear to differ significantly based on sexual orientation, except for oral sex (Oswalt & Wyatt, 2013). These low rates of condom use are reflected in the higher rates of STIs among young adults. Additionally, the presence of an STI (e.g., syphilis chancre, herpes lesions) increases one's susceptibility to HIV infection when exposed to the virus.

A variety of reasons for not using condoms have been identified, including the following beliefs: that condoms reduce pleasure; that one's partner would not approve of condom use; that condoms are not commonly used in one's social group; that condoms are embarrassing, hard to discuss, and hard to use; and that condoms cause a loss of erection. In addition, some individuals may not have a condom readily available when sex happens. Studies have shown that college students who do not use condoms have high perceptions of invulnerability and low perception of risk associated with their sexual behavior (Thompson et al., 2006). Some students also believe they have the ability to identify a partner's HIV status.

While there is certainly room for improvement in condom use rates, individuals who are using condoms may also need education. Many individuals who are using condoms may not be doing so correctly. Research has revealed a variety of common condom use errors among adolescents and college students, including inaccurate steps, such as putting the condom on after sex has already started or removing the condom before ending sex; not leaving space at the tip; and placing the condom upside down on the penis and flipping it over (e.g., Brown et al., 2008; Crosby et al., 2008; Yarber et al., 2007). Error rates vary; the study reporting the highest rate indicated 93.8% of those surveyed had experienced at least one of the nine errors assessed (Topping et al., 2011).

Other factors can also influence the risk of transmission of HIV among young adults. Substance use is sometimes an issue, as many young adults report the use of alcohol and other drugs before sex; researchers have found that almost 1 in 4 sexually active high

The remarkable AIDS quilt is made up of more than 45,000 panels, each representing a life lost to AIDS. It was created both as a living memorial for those who died and as a brilliant way to help the public visualize the growing toll that AIDS was taking.

school students reported such use before last sexual intercourse (Kann et al., 2014) and that 1 in 5 college students reported unprotected sex within the last year because of alcohol use (ACHA, 2014). Runaways, homeless youth, and youth who have become dependent on drugs are at high risk for HIV infection if they exchange sex for drugs, money, or shelter. For many individuals, there may also be a lack of knowledge about sexual health issues. Young people are not always reached by effective, applicable education, and this may be especially true for gay, lesbian, and bisexual young adults. In addition, these young adults

The Bill and Melinda Gates Foundation has donated billions of dollars to combat HIV infection and AIDS, especially on the African continent.

Global DIMENSIONS

HIV in Africa At the end of 2013, there were 35 million people living with HIV across the globe. Because more people are living longer thanks to antiretroviral therapy, and because new HIV infections continue to occur, this number has been increasing. Since the beginning of the epidemic and continuing today, Africa—specifically, the sub-Saharan region of Africa—has been the most dramatically affected area in the world. Today, more than 70% of all people living with HIV (24.7 million individuals) reside in sub-Saharan Africa; put another way, almost 1 in every 20 adults living with the virus calls sub-Saharan Africa home.

There were 1.5 million new HIV infections in sub-Saharan Africa in 2013, but new infections are on the decline. Among all age groups, there was a 33% drop in the number of new HIV infections in the region between 2005 and 2013; there has been a 19% reduction in this number since 2010.

In terms of these new infections, young women are disproportionately affected, with infections occurring in such individuals at least 5–7 years earlier than in men. Young women aged 15–24 years in sub-Saharan Africa are twice as likely as young men of the same age to be living with HIV. As in the United States, the risk for these girls is not solely related to behavior, but rather is primarily influenced by social factors—for example, gender-based violence, sexual abuse, and lack of access to education and health services all play roles in how well young women are able to protect themselves from HIV.

In tandem with the decline in new infections, the number of AIDS-related deaths fell by 39% between 2005 and 2013 in sub-Saharan Africa. This decline is directly due to the increased number of people on ART; in 2013 alone, an additional 1.7 million people living with HIV received such therapy. In fact, since 1995, ART has prevented 4.8 million deaths in sub-Saharan Africa. In 2013, ART was available to almost 4 in 10 people (37%) living with HIV in the region, with women being more likely to receive treatment (43%) compared to men (33%). Part of this difference may be attributable to the strategic effort to reach women of childbearing age in an attempt to decrease the number of children born with HIV.

However, there are significant differences in HIV outcomes between countries. For example, 19% of AIDS-related deaths in the region in 2013 occurred in Nigeria, where only 2 in every 10 people living with HIV are receiving treatment. In contrast, South Africa—with double the number of people living with HIV—increased treatment coverage from 1 person in 10 in 2010, to 4 people in 10 by 2013; in turn, AIDS-related deaths in the country declined by 48%. South Africa has the highest number of people on HIV treatment—nearly 2.6 million—and has committed to nearly doubling that number in the next few years.

The effect of HIV globally, but especially in Africa, has changed dramatically in the last decade. Theoretically, the rates of HIV infection and death from AIDS should continue to drop as long as there is continued and increased access to antiretroviral medication for infected individuals or as pre-exposure prophylaxis (PrEP) therapy is administered to at-risk populations. Previous rates of HIV had devastating social and economic consequences for many parts of Africa, and the impact on the individuals and families in these nations cannot be underestimated. At the same time, many experts believe that there is now hope of successfully managing the crisis. In fact, a 2014 UNAIDS publication included the heading "The Beginning of the End of the AIDS Epidemic." Perhaps future editions of this text will be able to report on "The End of the AIDS Epidemic."

---

may have some unique risk factors. Many young gay and bisexual men choose older partners, and because older partners are more likely to be infected with HIV, this pattern increases their risk. These young adults may also experience feelings of isolation and may engage in high-risk sexual behavior and/or experience sexual abuse because of these feelings and perceived lack of support. All of these risk factors need to be considered if we are to effectively address the greater risk for HIV among young adults.

While treatment for HIV has turned the infection into a chronic condition rather than a death sentence, there is concern that younger generations appear to lack the knowledge and skills needed to prevent the infection. Additionally, some may take a cavalier attitude toward the infection—considering it similar to other STIs or other manageable health issues. While it is true that the medical gains in relation to HIV and AIDS are impressive, HIV infection is clearly preventable and individuals should strive to remain infection free. Increased and continued testing and education about prevention strategies like condom use and PrEP are needed to further reduce new infections in the United States and around the world.

Gender
DIMENSIONS

Women and HIV   AIDS was originally identified as a disease affecting gay men, and even today gay, bisexual, and other MSM remain the largest group infected with HIV in the United States. However, women account for 20% of the estimated new HIV infections and represent 1 in 4 individuals living with AIDS (CDC, 2015d). Black women are disproportionately affected by this disease, accounting for almost two-thirds of all women living with HIV. Most women (more than 80%) contract HIV through heterosexual contact.

Women are at higher risk for HIV infection for a variety of reasons. Some women may be unaware of their male partner's high-risk behavior (such as injection drug use or having sex with other men) and may not use condoms. For women, there is a biological risk in that transmission of HIV is easier from a male to a female during vaginal sex than from a female to a male. Anal sex without a condom is also a risky behavior for women, and more than 20% of adult women report engaging in anal sex in the last year (Herbenick et al., 2010). Likewise, infection with another STI, such as herpes or syphilis, increases the risk of becoming infected with HIV. Minority communities are also disproportionally affected by some of these STIs, which can in turn increase minority women's risk of HIV infection. Additionally, the larger number of people living with HIV in the black and Hispanic communities and the fact that people tend to have sex with partners from the same race/ethnicity means that women from these communities are more likely to encounter HIV in their sexual partners (CDC, 2015c).

Women who are infected with and at risk for HIV infection face several challenges when trying to access needed services and resources. For example, socioeconomic and structural barriers—such as poverty, cultural inequities, and sexual violence—may detrimentally affect a woman's ability to address her condition. Additionally, many of these women are caring for children, and they may place the needs of their families above their own needs. Among women living with HIV in the United States, 85% have been diagnosed, but only 70% have been linked to medical care, with just 41% in regular care, 36% being prescribed ART, and 26% achieving viral suppression (CDC, 2015c).

Strategies to address HIV infection in women include increased awareness about testing and increased linkage to care for those already infected with the virus. Additional education around mother-to-child transmission is one strategy to encourage testing, as in the CDC campaign emphasizing "One test, two lives." Efforts to address the stigma attached to HIV infection are also critically important.

HIV was once a considered a deadly infection, but today with early and appropriate treatment, it can be a managable chronic condition. Unfortunately, many people in the United States do not know their HIV status. To counteract this lack of information and the risk of infection associated with it, increased testing is needed and, if a person tests positive, antiretroviral therapy should be undertaken. Even among those who are HIV positive, more inidividuals need to be linked to care and treatment to improve their quality of life and life expectancy as well as reduce the risk of infection to others.

Like other STIs, HIV is linked to social determinants of health. Factors related to education, poverty, discrimination, homonegativity, access to health care, healthcare-seeking behavior, and being part of a community with higher prevalence rates of HIV all affect one's risk. While behavior certainly is a risk factor, understanding how these issues influence one's likelihood of contracting HIV is critical if we—as a nation—are to successfully address and control HIV infection in the United States.

Biological Factors

- HIV is contracted primarily through sexual contact and injectable drug use.
- Individuals with another STI have a higher risk of becoming infected with HIV, possibly becasuse the genital lesions of other STIs give the HIV virus ready access to the body.
- Children can become infected with HIV in utero and during breastfeeding.
- While highly effective, antiretroviral therapy can have strong side effects in people who are HIV positive. These side effects need to be managed so that appropriate treatment is continued.

Sociocultural Factors

- Society's unwillingness to discuss sexual issues is a major barrier in responding to the HIV epidemic.
- Stigma and discrimination directed at gay, bisexual, and other MSM contribute to increased rates of HIV.
- Black Americans are disproportionaately affected by HIV relative to people of other ethnicities in the US.
- While abstinence, mutual monogamy with an uninfected partner, and condom use could virtually eliminate risk of HIV infection, these prevention strategies have not been as effective as antiretroviral therapy in actually reducing transmission. By attacking virus replication and reducing viral loads in HIV-infected individuals, the chance of transmitting the virus is significantly lowered.

Psychological Factors

- Individuals infected with HIV may blame themselves for past risk behaviors that led to HIV infection.
- Disclosure to family and friends can be challenging. This is especially true if HIV was contracted through behaviors unknown to the family and friends.
- Psychological stress increases for individuals infected with HIV because they are continally aware of their health and the challenges in handling future sexual relationships (e.g., telling a partner, a partner starting pre-exposure prophylaxis, condom use).
- Additional stress can occur because of the financial burden of HIV care and medication. Concerns about the individual's career or future job prospects can exacerbate this stress.

Summary

- The human immunodeficiency virus (HIV) is transmitted through the transfer of bodily fluids such as semen, vaginal secretions, and blood. HIV infection is contracted primarily through sexual contact such as penile–vaginal sex, oral sex, or anal sex.

- HIV attacks and weakens the immune system of infected individuals.

- Acquired immune deficiency syndrome (AIDS) is the last stage of HIV infection. When it develops, the body is weakened sufficiently to have a severely depleted CD4 count (<200 cells/mm^3) and/or to experience opportunistic infections.

- The death rate from HIV infection has steadily declined, predominantly due to the introduction of antiviral medications that stop the replication of HIV in the body at several different paths. These medications have transformed HIV infection and AIDS into manageable chronic illnesses.

- In the United States, most new HIV infections occur among gay, bisexual, and other MSM. This group also has the greatest number of individuals living with both HIV infection and AIDS. Rates among younger gay, bisexual, and other MSM and black gay, bisexual, and other MSM are higher than among other subgroups within this population.

- Women account for 1 in 4 people living with HIV. More than 80% of women contract HIV from heterosexual contact, with black women being disproportionately affected.

- Several tests are available to diagnose HIV infection. Some screening tests employ blood analysis, whereas others test cheek fluid or urine samples. Two home testing kits have been approved by the FDA for the diagnosis of HIV infection.

- AIDS is treated with one of six classes of antiviral medications: nucleoside reverse transcriptase inhibitors, protease inhibitors, non-nucleoside reverse transcriptase inhibitors, fusion inhibitors, integrase inhibitors, and entry inhibitors. Each class works on a different aspect of HIV infection, such as preventing HIV from reproducing or preventing HIV from invading the cells.

- HIV prevention includes clinical strategies such as pre-exposure prophylaxis (individuals with ongoing high risk of infection taking antiretroviral medication on a daily basis), post-exposure prophylaxis (individuals with a one-time high-risk exposure taking a short course of antiretroviral medication), and increased testing (which allows individuals to know their status, inform partners, modify behavior, and begin treatment, which will decrease viral loads and reduce risk of transmission to others).

- Prevention can also include behavioral strategies such as remaining sexually abstinent, understanding risky behaviors, and using a condom or dental dam.

- Young adults are particularly vulnerable to HIV infection owing to their feelings of invulnerability coupled with lack of condom use during sexual activity.

Discussion Questions

1. Explain the ways HIV is transmitted, the stages of infection, the tests for infection, and how opportunistic illnesses occur as a result of AIDS.

2. Which treatments are available for HIV infection? What limits their worldwide availability?

3. List the safer-sex practices that reduce the risk of HIV transmission.

Application Questions

Reread the chapter-opening story and consider the following questions.

1. On June 25, 1998, the Supreme Court ruled that HIV-infected people are protected by a federal ban on discrimination against the disabled—even if they suffer no symptoms of AIDS. Do you think this ruling affects individuals' willingness to disclose their HIV status? Why or why not?

2. Regardless of the law, if you were an employer making a hiring decision, would the knowledge that the candidate was infected with HIV make a difference? How about if the person were being treated for cancer? Or heart disease? Why should such information make a difference?

3. How would you feel if you knew a fellow classmate or employee were HIV infected?

Critical Thinking Questions

1. Is it fair that the federal government spends a disproportionate share of medical research money on HIV research? Put another way, should federal research money be spent in proportion to the number of people who contract an illness and die of it (such as cancer or heart disease)? Or should the potential threat of a disease becoming more widespread take precedence?

2. You may remember this gender-related issue from another chapter: Men who carry condoms are considered to be "responsible," but women who carry condoms are considered "sluts." Given the need for more condom use to prevent the spread of STIs and HIV, how can this double standard be overcome?

Critical Thinking Cases

Deciding whether to disclose HIV infection is clearly a troubling decision for anyone to make. But do people have an obligation to disclose that information to protect others?

Consider the case of the two-time double–Olympic diving gold medalist Greg Louganis, who was HIV positive during his second Olympics. Louganis did not disclose his HIV status to Olympic officials. During one dive, Louganis hit the diving board with the back of his head and received a wound that bled. A doctor treated him without knowing of the HIV condition—and thus did not take extra precautions. Also, Olympic competitors are required to supply urine samples to test for illegal substances (such as steroids). Because urine would contain HIV, anyone handling Louganis's sample would have also been at risk unless proper precautions were taken.

Should Louganis have been required to disclose his status before the Olympics? What discrimination may result against an athlete who discloses his or her HIV-infected status? Reflecting on the problems Magic Johnson faced when he disclosed his status, do you think there would be similar issues today?

What about typical recreational athletes—people who work out in gyms, play basketball in leagues, fence (saber, epee, or foil), or participate in any recreational activity in which they can be injured accidentally? When do HIV-infected people need to disclose their status?

Exploring Personal Dimensions

Could You Negotiate Safer Sex?

The following items ask you to agree (A) or disagree (D) with the statements presented. Indicate the items about which you are unsure (U) of your response. Compare your responses to those of a friend. Discuss each item about which you said you were unsure of your response. Are there items about which you and a friend disagree? Which changes or adaptations would you or your friend have to make to take on safer practices toward sex with a partner?

I believe that...

_____ 1. I could use a condom or latex barrier effectively.

_____ 2. I could buy condoms or latex barriers without embarrassment.

_____ 3. If my partner did not want to use a condom or latex barrier during sexual activity, I could convince him or her to do otherwise.

_____ 4. Consumption of alcohol or use of other recreational drugs would in no way affect my determination to use a condom or latex barrier or to convince my partner to respect my wishes.

_____ 5. Having to remember to buy, carry, and use condoms or latex barriers would interfere with sexual spontaneity.

_____ 6. If I suggested using a condom or latex barrier, my partner would think that I must have had many previous sexual partners.

_____ 7. I would feel comfortable insisting on using a condom or latex barrier with a new sexual partner.

_____ 8. I would not feel self-conscious about putting a condom on myself (or on my partner).

_____ 9. I would be able to discuss use of condoms or latex barriers with a partner even before we had any physical intimacy such as touching, caressing, or kissing.

_____10. If I suggested using a condom or latex barrier, my partner would think I did not trust him or her.

_____11. Using a condom during oral, penile–vaginal, or anal sex would interfere with sexual pleasure or sexual functioning.

_____12. Using condoms or latex barriers is an activity primarily for people who have many sexual partners.

_____13. Having to use a condom or latex barrier might subsequently prove to be embarrassing to me or my partner if the mechanics of using one resulted in loss of erection.

_____14. I could tactfully remove and dispose of a condom after sexual intercourse.

_____15. I could convince my partner that use of a condom or latex barrier can be a stimulating part of sexual foreplay.

Suggested Readings

Ball, S. C. *Voices in the band: A doctor, her patients, and how the outlook on AIDS care changed from doomed to hopeful*. Ithaca, NY: Cornell University Press, 2015.

Gallant, J. E. *100 questions & answers about HIV and AIDS* (2nd ed.). Burlington, MA: Jones & Bartlett Learning, 2012.

Gifford, A.L, Lorig, K., Laurent, D., & Gonzalez, V. *Living a healthy life with HIV* (4th ed.). Boulder, CO: Bull Publishing, 2015.

Kenworthy, N. J., & Parker, R., eds. *HIV scale-up and the politics of global health*. New York: Routledge, 2015.

Strub, S. *Body counts: A memoir of activism, sex, and survival*. New York: Scribner, 2014.

Web Resources

AIDS.gov
www.aids.gov

This website has three main objectives: (1) to expand the visibility of timely and relevant federal HIV policies, programs, and resources to the American public; (2) to increase the use of new media tools to extend the reach of HIV programs to communities at greatest risk; and (3) to increase knowledge about HIV and access to HIV services for people most at risk for, or living with, HIV. The website includes basic HIV information as well as more complex information regarding strategies for those infected with HIV.

Centers for Disease Control and Prevention: HIV/AIDS
www.cdc.gov/hiv

This website features many different resources, including recommendations, guidelines, fact sheets, FAQs, statistics, and materials for prevention and research partners. It includes sections for everyone as well as specialized sections for healthcare providers, case managers, and infectious disease specialists.

Henry J. Kaiser Family Foundation: HIV/AIDS
www.kff.org/hivaids/

The Kaiser Family Foundation is dedicated to providing trusted, independent information on the major health issues facing the United States and its people. Its website acts as a clearinghouse of news and information for the health policy community and provides extensive information on both the U.S. and global HIV epidemic, federal actions, and U.S. state HIV/AIDS information.

National Institute of Allergy and Infectious Diseases
www.niaid.nih.gov/topics/hivaids

Managed by the federal government, this website presents information pertaining to HIV and AIDS research, including vaccine trials and other prevention strategies. While a basic overview of HIV and AIDS is provided, much of the content focuses on research and research trials.

UNAIDS
www.unaids.org

UNAIDS, the Joint United Nations Programme on HIV/AIDS, works toward achieving universal access to HIV prevention, treatment, care, and support. The website provides country, regional, and global statistics; epidemiological reports; news releases; case studies; and publications on numerous HIV-related topics.

References

AIDS virus gets new name amid feuding. *Medical World News*, 27 (1986), 14–15.

American College Health Association (ACHA). *American College Health Association—National College Health Assessment II: Reference group executive summary, spring 2014*. Hanover, MD: ACHA, 2014. Available: http://www.acha-ncha.org/docs/ACHA-NCHA-II_ReferenceGroup_ExecutiveSummary_Spring2014.pdf.

Arnold, E. M., Riceb, E., Flannery, D. & Rotheram-Borus, M. J. HIV disclosure among adults living with HIV. *AIDS Care, 20, 1* (2008), 80–82.

Berry, J. It's in the cards: Where to get help to pay for your meds. *Positively Aware* (2011, March/April), 67–69. Available: http://issuu.com/positivelyaware/docs/2011 _march_april_clickable.

Brown, L. K., DiClemente, R., Crosby, R., Fernandez, M. I., Pugatch, D., Cohn, S., ... & Project Shield Study Group. Condom use among high-risk adolescents: Anticipation of partner disapproval and less pleasure associated with not using condoms. *Public Health Reports, 123, 5* (2008), 601–607.

Buot, M. L. G., Docena, J. P., Ratemo, B. K., Bittner, M. J., Burlew, J. T., Nuritdinov, A. R., & Robbins, J. R. Beyond race and place: Distal sociological determinants of HIV disparities. *PloS One, 9* (2014), e91711.

Centers for Disease Control and Prevention (CDC). *Serosorting among gay, bisexual and other men who have sex with men*, 2011. Available: http://www.cdc.gov/msmhealth/Serosorting .htm.

Centers for Disease Control and Prevention (CDC). Vital signs: HIV infection, testing, and risk behaviors among youths— United States. *Morbidity and Mortality Weekly Report, 61* (2012), 1–6. Available: http://www.cdc.gov/mmwr/pdf/wk /mm61e1127.pdf.

Centers for Disease Control and Prevention (CDC). *Condoms and STDs: Fact sheet for public health personnel*, 2013a. Available: http://www.cdc.gov/condomeffectiveness/docs /condoms_and_stds.pdf.

Centers for Disease Control and Prevention (CDC), *HIV among transgender people*, 2013b. Available: http://www.cdc.gov /hiv/risk/transgender/index.html

Centers for Disease Control and Prevention (CDC). *Strategy for an AIDS-free generation*, 2013c. Available: http://www.cdc .gov/globalaids/Global-HIV-AIDS-at-CDC/interventions.html.

Centers for Disease Control and Prevention (CDC). *HIV among youth*, 2014a. Available: http://www.cdc.gov/hiv/risk/age /youth/index.html.

Centers for Disease Control and Prevention (CDC). *HIV and young men who have sex with men*, 2014b. Available: http://www.cdc.gov/healthyyouth/sexualbehaviors/pdf /hiv_factsheet_ymsm.pdf.

Centers for Disease Control and Prevention (CDC). *HIV in the United States: At a glance*, 2014c. Available: http://www.cdc .gov/hiv/statistics/basics/ataglance.html.

Centers for Disease Control and Prevention (CDC). *Today's HIV/AIDS epidemic*, 2014d. Available: http://www .cdc.gov/nchhstp/newsroom/docs/HIVFactSheets /TodaysEpidemic-508.pdf.

Centers for Disease Control and Prevention (CDC). *About HIV/AIDS*, 2015a. Available: http://www.cdc.gov/hiv/basics /whatishiv.html.

Centers for Disease Control and Prevention (CDC). *HIV/AIDS among American Indians and Alaska Natives*, 2015b. Available: http://www.cdc.gov/hiv/risk/racialEthnic/aian/.

Centers for Disease Control and Prevention (CDC). *HIV among women*, 2015c. Available: http://www.cdc.gov/hiv/risk /gender/women/facts/index.html.

Centers for Disease Control and Prevention (CDC). Diagnoses of HIV infection in the United States and dependent areas, 2013. *HIV Surveillance Report, 25* (2015d). Available: http:// www.cdc.gov/hiv/pdf/g-l/hiv_surveillance_report_vol_25 .pdf#Page=17.

Centers for Disease Control and Prevention (CDC). *HIV transmission*, 2015e. Available: http://www.cdc.gov/hiv /basics/transmission.html.

Centers for Disease Control and Prevention (CDC). *PEP*, 2015f. Available: http://www.cdc.gov/hiv/basics/pep.html.

Centers for Disease Control and Prevention (CDC). *Testing*, 2015g. Available: http://www.cdc.gov/hiv/basics/testing.html.

Centers for Disease Control and Prevention (CDC), Health Resources and Services Administration, National Institutes of Health, American Academy of HIV Medicine, Association of Nurses in AIDS Care, International Association of Providers of AIDS Care, the National Minority AIDS Council, & Urban Coalition for HIV/AIDS Prevention Services. *Recommendations for HIV prevention with adults and adolescents with HIV in the United States, 2014.* 2014. Available: http://stacks.cdc.gov/view/cdc/26062.

Crosby, R. A., DiClemente, R. J., Yarber, W. L., Snow, G., & Troutman, A. Young African American men having sex with multiple partners are more likely to use condoms incorrectly: A clinic-based study. *Journal of Men's Health, 2* (2008), 340–343.

Edelman, E. J., Cole, C. A., Richardson, W., Boshnack, N., Jenkins, H., & Rosenthal, M. S. Opportunities for improving partner notification for HIV: Results from a community-based participatory research study. *AIDS and Behavior, 18* (2014), 1888–1897.

Food and Drug Administration (FDA). *Blood donor deferral*, 2015. Available: http://www.fda.gov/forpatients/illness/hivaids /safety/ucm117929.htm.

Herbenick, D., Reece, M., Schick, V., Sanders, S. A., Dodge, B., & Fortenberry, J. D. Sexual behavior in the United States: Results from a national probability sample of men and women ages 14–94. *Journal of Sexual Medicine, 7, s5* (2010), 255–265.

Joint United Nations Programme on HIV/AIDS (UNAIDS). *2014 progress report on the global plan*, 2014a. Available: http:// www.unaids.org/sites/default/files/documents/JC2681_2014 -Global-Plan-progress_en.pdf.

Joint United Nations Programme on HIV/AIDS (UNAIDS). *The gap report*, 2014b. Available: http://www.unaids.org/sites /default/files/media_asset/UNAIDS_Gap_report_en.pdf.

Kann, L., Kinchen, S., Shanklin, S. L., Flint, K. H., Hawkins, J., Harris, W. A. et al. Youth risk behavior surveillance— United States, 2013. *Morbidity and Mortality Weekly Report, 63, SS-4* (2014), 1–170. Available: http://www.cdc.gov /mmwr/pdf/ss/ss6304.pdf.

Liszewski, W., Becerril, J., Terndrup, C., West, N., Lavin, B. C., Schieffler, D., & Van Sickels, N. The rates, perceptions, and willingness of men who have sex with men to donate blood. *Transfusion, 54* (2014), 1733–1738.

Maiorana, A., Koester, K. A., Myers, J. J., Lloyd, K. C., Shade, S. B., Dawson-Rose, C., & Morin, S. F. Helping patients talk about HIV: Inclusion of messages on disclosure in prevention with positives interventions in clinical settings. *AIDS Education and Prevention, 24* (2012), 179–192.

National Institutes of Health. *NIH-sponsored HIV vaccine trial launches in South Africa*, 2015. Available: http://www.niaid.nih.gov/news/newsreleases/2015/Pages/HVTN100.aspx.

Obermeyer, C. M., Baijal, P., & Pegurri, E. Facilitating HIV disclosure across diverse settings: A review. *American Journal of Public Health, 101, 6* (2011), 1011–1023.

Oswalt, S. B., & Wyatt, T. J. Sexual health behaviors and sexual orientation in a US national sample of college students. *Archives of Sexual Behavior, 42* (2013), 1561–1572.

Rerks-Ngarm, S., Pitisuttithum, P., Nitayaphan, S., Kaewkungwal, J., Chiu, J., Paris, R., et al. Vaccination with ALVAC and AIDSVAX to prevent HIV-1 infection in Thailand. *New England Journal of Medicine, 361* (2009), 2209–2220.

Sanders, S. A., Reece, M., Herbenick, D., Schick, V., Dodge, B., & Fortenberry, D. Condom use during most recent vaginal intercourse event among a probability sample of adults in the United States. *Journal of Sexual Medicine, 7, s5* (2010), 362–373.

Seem, D. L., Lee, I., Unscheid, C. A., & Kuehnert, M. J. PHS guideline for reducing human immunodeficiency virus, hepatitis B virus, and hepatitis C virus transmission through organ transplantation. *Public Health Reports, 128* (2013), 247–343.

Thompson, S. C., Anderson, K., Freedman, D., & Swan, J. Illusions of safety in a risky world: A study of college students' condom use. *Journal of Applied Social Psychology, 26* (2006), 189–210.

Thoth, C. A., Tucker, C., Leahy, M., & Stewart, S. M. Self-disclosure of serostatus by youth who are HIV-positive: A review. *Journal of Behavioral Medicine, 37* (2014), 276–288.

Topping, A. A., Milhausen, R. R., Graham, C. A., Sanders, S. A., Yarber, W. L., & Crosby, R. A. A comparison of condom use errors and problems for heterosexual anal and vaginal intercourse. *International Journal of STD & AIDS, 22, 4* (2011), 204–208.

U.S. Department of Health and Human Services (DHHS). *Partners*, 2009. Available: https://www.aids.gov/hiv-aids-basics/just-diagnosed-with-hiv-aids/talking-about-your-status/sexual-partners/.

U.S. Department of Health and Human Services (DHHS). *Guidelines for the use of antiretroviral agents in HIV-1-infected adults and adolescents*, 2014a. Available: http://aidsinfo.nih.gov/contentfiles/lvguidelines/adultandadolescentgl.pdf.

U.S. Department of Health and Human Services (DHHS). *HIV overview: FDA-approved HIV medicines*, 2014b. Available: http://aidsinfo.nih.gov/education-materials/fact-sheets/19/58/fda-approved-hiv-medicines.

Yarber, W. L., Graham, C. A., Sanders, S. A., Crosby, R. A., Butler, S. M., & Hartzell, R. M. "Do you know what you're doing?": College students' experiences with male condoms. *American Journal of Health Education, 38* (2007), 322–331.

Zou, S., Dorsey, K. A., Notari, E. P., Foster, G. A., Krysztof, D. E., Musavi, F., et al. Prevalence, incidence, and residual risk of human immunodeficiency virus and hepatitis C virus infections among United States blood donors since the introduction of nucleic acid testing. *Transfusion, 50* (2010), 1495–1504.

CHAPTER 20

Sexual Dysfunction and Therapy

© Gayvoronskaya Yana/Shutterstock

FEATURES

Gender Dimensions
Sexual Issues for Older Men and Women

Communication Dimensions
Discussing Sexual Dysfunction

Multicultural Dimensions
Sexual Dysfunction and Latino Populations

Global Dimensions
Sexual Disorders Around the World

Ethical Dimensions
Should Surrogates Be Used in Sex Therapy?

CHAPTER OBJECTIVES

1 Describe the major male and female sexual dysfunctions. Evaluate what makes the inability to perform sexually a clinical dysfunction.

2 Identify the multidimensional causes of sexual dysfunction, including the physical, psychological, and sociocultural aspects.

3 Compare and contrast the varied approaches to treating sexual dysfunctions. Explain why many different models of therapy exist.

© Gayvoronskaya Yana/Shutterstock

INTRODUCTION

*A*fter he was diagnosed with prostate cancer in 1991, Senator Bob Dole underwent treatment, including surgery. He has since avidly promoted the importance of early detection and encouraged men to speak frankly with their doctors about prostate-related problems.

But it was in May 1998 that Dole made his biggest disclosure: He said on Larry King's talk show that he had been among the men who took part in the trials for the drug Viagra (sildenafil). Viagra is a drug to treat men who have difficulty achieving an erection (erectile dysfunction). In effect, Bob Dole was admitting that he, as do millions of other men, had a sexual dysfunction—specifically, erectile disorder. The next day, Elizabeth Dole, his wife, was asked about the drug during a public appearance. She laughed and said with a beaming smile, "It's a great drug!"

Such public disclosures by celebrities and politicians make taboo topics—such as sexual dysfunctions—the subject of discussion among friends, colleagues, classmates, and even couples. Dole's 1998 public announcement, followed by commercials in March 1999, offered frank and genuine advice: If you have a problem, see a doctor. In the case of erectile disorder, some problems are physical and can be solved with a prescription or a medical procedure. Other disorders, though, have psychological or sociocultural dimensions at their root.

The Viagra story also touches on the socioeconomic and political dimensions of sexuality. In the 1970s, insurers would not have covered treatments for erectile disorder, because the condition was believed to be psychological. Insurers began coverage as research proved there were physical causes as well. Coverage for Viagra is limited generally to 12 pills per month—the recommended dosage.

When the FDA approved Viagra on March 27, 1998, it was not covered under Medicaid. Thus it was unavailable to those in lower economic brackets. But the political ramifications of denying this wonder drug to the poor caused an uproar. Politicians know that older citizens are more likely to vote. Consequently, many states required Medicaid coverage for Viagra. However, under a law signed by President George W. Bush, as of January 2006, Medicaid no longer covers erectile dysfunction medications, and Medicare stopped coverage as of January 2007, though today some supplemental Medicare drug plans offer it as an added benefit.

Data from Why is Mrs. Dole smiling? *Washington Post* (May 9, 1998); Postmarketing safety of sildenafil citrate (Viagra), www.fda.gov/cder/consumerinfo/viagra/viagraupdate721.htm; Stark, K. Will insurers pay? Clamor for Viagra could cinch it, *Philadelphia Inquirer* (April 24, 1998).

Sexual Dysfunction

Are you perfect? What seems a silly question has great importance for sexual functioning. Of course, none of us is perfect. And yet, the occasional inability to function sexually (for example, to achieve and maintain an erection or to secrete adequate vaginal lubrication) leads many of us to conclude that something is drastically wrong with us.

This lack of response may be caused by a number of factors that have no bearing at all on your sexual functioning. For example, the ingestion of alcoholic beverages can interfere with sexual response, as can use of drugs such as hypertension medication, narcotics, and barbiturates. In addition, some people have partners with whom it is difficult to respond sexually. For example, your partner may have poor hygiene; he may know so little about sexual physiology that he attempts penile insertion before sufficient vaginal lubrication; or he may touch the scrotum and handle the testicles in a way that causes pain and discomfort. And yet, if the individuals with these sexual partners do not respond as one would expect under more conducive circumstances, they themselves are sometimes accused of having an "abnormality." It might be more accurate to suggest that those who are sexually responsive to dirty, smelly, clumsy sexual partners are the ones experiencing some abnormality.

The media also help to establish unrealistic sexual expectations that, when not met, may lead people to think of themselves as dysfunctional. For example, when movies portray gorgeous specimens of men and women in romantic settings, who seem to have nothing else on their minds but sex, and who are willing and able to engage in any sexual activity that comes to mind, we and our lovers may not measure up. We might conclude something is wrong with us or our love life, although in reality something is wrong with this portrayal. Suffice it to say here that music videos, movies, plays, advertisements, and the Internet sometimes lead people to decide they are not as sexually adequate as those they see "performing" on satin sheets with unblemished bodies glistening under flattering spotlights.

Beyond the media portrayal of sexual adventures, there are people who experience challenges regarding their sexual activities and who wish their sexual responses could be healthier and more sexually satisfying. They may find it difficult to achieve and/or maintain an erection or to relax enough to allow penile penetration. They may ejaculate too soon, or they may experience disturbing pain during vaginal sex. They may wonder why they do not feel sexually aroused enough or do not experience orgasm. Men and women of all sexual orientations experience these concerns. They may be young or old, African American or white, well-educated or lacking in schooling, and from any socioeconomic group. Sexual dissatisfaction and dysfunction affect people from all walks of life, and this dissatisfaction often affects other aspects of their relationships.

This chapter explores some of these matters. Specifically, it addresses which types of sexual problems people experience, what causes these problems, and how they can be treated. Notice the difficulty in diagnosing particular sexual dysfunctions (even the experts do not always agree about whether a dysfunction exists) and the varied approaches to treating them once they are identified. This, too, is discussed and its implications explored. We begin with a definition of sexual dysfunction.

Sexual dysfunction is a chronic inability to respond sexually in a way that one finds satisfying. This term does not apply to those situations, common to many people, in which they are temporarily uninterested in sexual activity or unable to respond sexually because of exhaustion, excessive use of alcohol, anger, and so on. The key word in our definition is *chronic*—that is, a consistent long-term inability to respond. It applies both to people who have never had satisfactory sexual relations—lifelong dysfunctions—and to people who have had successful sexual relations at some time but are now having chronic difficulty—acquired dysfunction. From a diagnostic perspective, the experience must cause distress for at least 6 months (Sungur & Gündüz, 2014).

The amount of sexual dysfunction prevalent in society is difficult to determine. As noted earlier, experts may disagree on diagnoses and individuals may not seek treatment. In addition, older studies focused on rates within married relationships. More recent reports look at individuals' experiences regardless of relationship status and include international studies. These more recent reports estimate that 40% to 45% of adult women and 20% to 30% of adult men have at least one sexual dysfunction (Lewis et al., 2004; Lewis et al., 2010). For both men and women, the probability of sexual dysfunction occurring increases directly with age; however, distress about sexual issues seems to decrease with age as

People who experience chronic sexual dysfunction often feel shameful and inadequate. Yet, there are successful treatments for most sexual dysfunctions, whether they are caused by physical or psychological factors.

TABLE 20.1

Prevalence of Sexual Problems in U.S. Men and Women (ages 40–80)*

Type of Dysfunction	Men (%)	Women (%)
Pain experienced during sex	3.1	12.7
Sex not pleasurable	11.2	19.7
Unable to experience an orgasm	12.4	20.7
Lack of interest in sex	18.1	33.2
Reaching climax too quickly	26.2	N/A
Unable to maintain an erection	22.5	—
Trouble lubricating	—	21.5

*Percentage includes responses of occasional, periodic, and frequent.

Data from Laumann, E. O., Glasser, D. B., Neves, R. C. S., & Moreira, E., for the GSSAB Investigators' Group. A population-based survey of sexual activity, sexual problems and associated help-seeking behavior patterns in mature adults in the United States of America. *International Journal of Impotence Research, 21* (2009), 171–178. doi: 10.1038/ijir.2009.7.

well (Connora et al., 2011; Lewis et al., 2010). A study examining U.S. adults between 40 and 80 years old indicated that many individuals experienced sexual problems, but fewer than 25% sought help for the issue (Laumann et al., 2009). Table 20.1 details the study's findings for specific disorders.

People who experience chronic sexual dysfunction often feel shameful and inadequate. Yet, there are successful treatments for most sexual dysfunctions, whether they are caused by physical or psychological factors.

The underlying cause of any sexual dysfunction may be either organic (physiological) or psychogenic (psychological). Broadly defined, psychological causes are much more prevalent; however, more studies are demonstrating that sexual dysfunction may be a result of other medical problems (Tan et al., 2012). Some researchers are concerned that there has been a medicalization of sexual health and sex therapy (Bradley & Fine, 2009; Farrell & Cacchioni, 2012; Marshall, 2012; Tiefer, 2010). *Medicalization* is

sexual dysfunction A specific, chronic disorder involving sexual activity.

Gender DIMENSIONS

Sexual Issues for Older Men and Women

Contrary to common belief, older people remain sexually active. Still, as is true with younger men and women, older men engage in sexual activity more often than do older women. In a large-scale study of the sexual behavior and health of older Americans, it was found that 65.5% of men and 45.1% of women older than age 50 participated in a sexual activity (frottage, oral sex, penile–vaginal sex, or anal sex) with a partner at least once during the previous year (Schick et al., 2010). Furthermore, although sexual activity declined as respondents got older, 20% to 30% of respondents older than age 80 still reported engaging in some type of sexual activity with a partner at least once during the previous year.

However, older men and women do report an increase in sexual problems as they age. In another national study (Lindau et al., 2007), the most prevalent sexual problems experienced by older women were low sexual desire (43%), insufficient vaginal lubrication (39%), and inability to achieve an orgasm (34%). The most common sexual problems experienced by older men were erectile dysfunction (37%), lack of interest in sex (28%), premature ejaculation (28%), and performance anxiety (27%).

Lindau, S. T., Schumm, L. P., Lauman, E. O., Levinson, W., Muircheartaigh, C. A., & Waite, L. J. A study of sexuality and health among older adults in the United States. *New England Journal of Medicine, 357, 8* (2007), 762–774. Schick, V., Herbenick, D., Reece, M., Sanders, S. A., Dodge, B., Middlestadt, S. E., & Fortenberry, J. D. Sexual behaviors, condom use, and sexual health of Americans over 50: Implications for sexual health promotion for older adults. *Journal of Sexual Medicine 7, s5* (2010), 315–329.

the process of transforming a personal experience or social situation into one that requires treatment and care by a medical professional. Medicalization may prevent the underlying and causative issues surrounding sexual disorders from being addressed.

In 2000, Leonore Tiefer led a group of advocates to reframe ideas about women's sexual dysfunction. Instead of focusing on the physiological processes (often related to Masters and Johnson's sexual response cycle), Tiefer and associates took a more contextual approach. The group advocated that women's sexual disorders be framed within four categories: sexual problems resulting from (1) sociocultureal, political, and economic factors; (2) partner and relationship factors; (3) psychological factors; and (4) medical factors (Working Group on A New View of Women's Sexual Problems, 2000). We applaud these authors' efforts to reconceptualize female sexual dysfunction and to encourage us as sexual health consumers to critically think about labels, context, and the influence of pharmaceutical companies on our lives. As sexuality educators, we also believe students need to be familiar with the existing ideas and terminology about sexual dysfunction and present that information in this chapter, beginning with sexual dysfunctions experienced by men.

Male Sexual Dysfunctions

Sexual dysfunction in males can be traumatic. In Western culture, gender role expectations dictate that

Although the elderly are often perceived as asexual, that is far from the truth. Almost half of adults 60 years of age and older report engaging in sexual activity at least once a month.

men be experienced and talented in matters of sex. The burden of this expectation is felt most strongly when men have sexual difficulties. In addition to the stress of the sexual dysfunction, they can experience a range of other psychological problems related to self-esteem, feelings of incompetence, and questioning of masculinity.

Along with the impact on psychological health, the relationship can also be affected. A man may not want to initiate or participate in sexual activity when the results may be failure or a demonstration of ineptness. Only a masochist would allow himself to be placed in such a situation continually, and consequently his initiation of sexual activity may become sporadic. His partner may perceive this lack of interest as a reflection on his or her attractiveness, as a result of sexual activity outside of the relationship, or as having some other cause—all of which can affect the relationship as a whole.

However, sexual dysfunction does not have to be exclusively negative. Involvement in sex therapy has been shown to improve ideas about sex and sexual functioning in some aspects. Some studies have shown that even minimal strategies, such as reading materials provided by a sex therapist, can improve sexual functioning (van Lankveld, 2009). Even without therapy, in many cases the sexual dysfunction can be an opportunity for partners to communicate more clearly and openly about their sexual needs and desires. It can also serve as a chance to explore sexual activities that had not been considered previously.

Men experience five main types of sexual dysfunctions: erectile dysfunction, early ejaculation, delayed ejaculation, genito-pelvic pain/penetration disorder, and hypoactive sexual disorder.

Erectile Dysfunction

A man's difficulty in achieving and maintaining an erection used to be called impotence. This term is Latin and means "without power." The word *impotence* is used to connote that a man has lost power—is no longer "manly"—when he cannot achieve or maintain an erection. Furthermore, he has lost power as a lover and has lost his reproductive capacity. Today, the more professional, sensitive, and accurate term for this type of male sexual dysfunction is **erectile dysfunction**. Men who are unable to achieve or maintain erections may be satisfying lovers; they may be very effective at oral sex, manual masturbation, or other activities.

Studies of Western countries estimate that 1 in 5 men will experience erectile dysfunction during their lifetime; however, only a small percentage may experience the issue frequently (Segraves, 2010). As men age, they are more prone to experience erection problems. A review of epidemiological studies shows rates of 1% to 10% for individuals younger than 40 years of age, but for those 60–69 years old the rate increases to 20% to 40%, and for men in their 70s and 80s the rate jumps to 50% to 100%, depending on the study (Lewis et al., 2010). Erectile dysfunction is the most commonly reported concern of men (McCabe & Connaughton, 2014).

Men who have never had an erection sufficient to have sexual activity have **lifelong erectile dysfunction** (also called early-onset erectile dysfunction). Men who have previously been able to maintain an erection long enough to have sexual activity but subsequently have an erection problem have **acquired erectile dysfunction** (late-onset erectile dysfunction). Acquired erectile dysfunction is more prevalent than lifelong erectile dysfunction, which is extremely rare (Gambescia et al., 2009).

Understanding whether the condition is generalized (in that it happens in all circumstances) or situational (in that it only happens in some contexts) is also critical. For example, a male who can achieve and maintain an erection during masturbation may not be able to maintain an erection when attempting penetration. This situational disorder would be considered a dysfunction, assuming that it was persistent and caused distress, even though he can maintain an erection in some contexts.

Making a precise diagnosis of erectile dysfunction is not as easy as one might suppose. Many men—even college-age men—are at times unable to have an erection or lose it before penetration. They may be uninterested in their partner; they may have drunk too much alcohol, which depresses the central nervous system; or they may be using medication that interferes with the erectile reflex. Infrequent erectile difficulties are not cause for alarm. In most cases, the condition needs to be present for 3 to 6 months and occurring 75% of the time to warrant a diagnosis of a dysfunction. Newer definitions also incorporate distress or discomfort about the condition; in the past, sexual disorders were diagnosed on stringent criteria even if the person was not concerned. Today, incorporating the needs and wants of the individual is an important process in diagnosing a disorder, because some men are not distressed by the condition (Segraves, 2010). If a condition is persistent and troubling to you or your partner, then you should seek professional help. If it does not bother either of you, then there is no cause for alarm.

The cause of erectile dysfunction can be psychological, physiological, or some combination of psychological and physiological. Most cases of erectile dysfunction are caused by a combination of psychological and physiological causes (Shamloul & Ghanem, 2013). As men age and experience cardiovascular problems, the likelihood of experiencing

erectile dysfunction The inability of a man to obtain or maintain an erection during sexual activity.

lifelong erectile dysfunction A condition in which an adult male has never had an erection sufficient to engage in sexual activity.

acquired erectile dysfunction A condition in which an adult male has previously had an erection sufficient to engage in sexual activity but no longer has.

It used to be thought that erectile dysfunction was the result of psychological factors. It is now known that most incidents of erectile dysfunction are caused by a combination of physical concerns (such as clogged penile arteries) and psychological issues.

erectile dysfunction increases. Although there are a variety of organic causes, approximately 70% of physical causes relate to blood flow issues (Ghanem & Porst, 2005). Neurologic conditions and hormonal conditions can also affect erectile functioning (Gambescia et al., 2009). Modifiable physical factors that affect cardiovascular functioning have been linked to erectile dysfunction; these include smoking, poor diet, lack of exercise, and obesity. Some medications and recreational drugs can also affect erectile function, including the use of antidepressant medications and medications used to treat cardiovascular disease (Shamloul & Ghanem, 2013).

Since the advent of Viagra and other medications that address erectile dysfunction, there has been increased emphasis on physiological causes. While many men are able to improve their erectile functioning with these medications, researchers caution that psychological factors may be compounding the issue and that treatment with a combination of physiological and psychological methods is often most effective (Althof, 2010; Segraves, 2010).

Early Ejaculation

Early ejaculation, also called premature ejaculation, is a common sexual dysfunction in men. It is estimated that 20% to 30% of men worldwide experience early ejaculation, but some believe this high prevalence rate is a result of imprecise and vague definitions (Althof et al., 2014; Serefoglu & Saitz, 2012).

Years ago, early ejaculation meant the man could not maintain penile insertion without ejaculating within a minimal amount of time (for example, 2 minutes) or could not perform a minimal number of penile thrusts before ejaculating. Masters and Johnson (1970) even proposed a definition that the man's partner had to be satisfied in at least 50% of their coital episodes or it was considered premature. Helen Singer Kaplan (1974) defined premature ejaculation as the man's inability to control his ejaculate voluntarily.

The problems with these definitions were several. The couples in these studies differed in their perception of what was too soon. Some couples were perfectly happy for coitus to last a short period, whereas other couples were dissatisfied with only 2 minutes of insertion or a minimal number of penile thrusts. In addition, Masters and Johnson's definition overlooked the fact that some women do not experience orgasms during coitus and would not achieve orgasm, regardless of the timing of their partner's ejaculation. Kaplan's definition neglected to recognize that men, as a rule, do not possess total voluntary control over ejaculation; this definition would classify most men as sexually dysfunctional.

Newer research considers the desires of the couple in the definition of early ejaculation. Most recently, a group of experts has developed a definition of premature ejaculation as lifelong if the ejaculation has always or nearly always occurred within about 1 minute of vaginal penetration from the first sexual experience, or as acquired if there is a significant reduction in time (typically 3 minutes or less) before ejaculation and the man is unable to delay ejaculation during all or nearly all vaginal penetration experiences. The ejaculate is not classified as early, however, unless it involves negative personal consequences, such as distress, frustration, or avoidance of sexual intimacy (Serefoglu et al., 2014). We define early ejaculation as a condition in which the man ejaculates before he wants to or before his partner wants him to during partnered sexual activity.

Unfortunately, the research on early ejaculation largely focuses on heterosexual men and penile–vaginal sex. Little is known about gay and bisexual men's experiences of early ejaculation or about the experiences of men who engage in other behaviors besides vaginal sex (Althof et al., 2014). In fact, this limitation—a focus on heterosexual men or studies that do not examine the relationship of sexual orientation to male sexual dysfunction—is a limitation of most sexual dysfunction research and a barrier to adequate health care for these men (Štulhofer et al., 2014).

---

early ejaculation Persistent or recurring ejaculation before the person wishes it during partnered sexual activity.

Communication
DIMENSIONS

Discussing Sexual Dysfunction

Two people who love and care for each other can deal with sexual dysfunction together. The key to the resolution of this situation, however, lies in the total relationship, not just the sexual part. Sexual communication is just one form of communication. If the relationship is characterized by ineffective communication in general, assuming that communicating about sex will be different is unrealistic. So, the first step in resolving sexual problems is to develop a relationship of caring, concern, mutual respect, and understanding. For this reason, some sex therapists work with clients to improve their interaction in general and concurrently help them respond to their sexual concerns.

Assuming that the relationship is minimally communicative, the first step is to provide support for each other and the promise of hope: "I still care about you and find you attractive, but something's interfering with my mojo right now." "That's okay, honey; we'll get help and work it out." This form of communication can reduce partners' anxieties that may be interfering with sexual function. Imagine the embarrassment of experiencing a sexual dysfunction and the resulting pressure during

each subsequent sexual encounter. The fear of "failure" and the anticipation of disappointing one's partner can be so frustrating that they can feed on themselves, contributing to, and exacerbating, the sexual problem. Communicating that it is okay, that help can be obtained, that the problem will be faced together, and that there is a commitment to work to make matters better can go a long way in intervening between dysfunctional feelings and resulting dysfunctional sex.

Once counseling starts, the couple needs to continue communicating with each other but now must also begin communicating with the counselor. To be effective, communication with the counselor must be candid. Without candor, the source of the problems may never be uncovered, or at least it will take longer to discover. A commitment is then required to adhere conscientiously to the treatment regimen and remain with it until the problem is resolved.

Certainly, sexual dysfunction puts a strain on both people involved, but caring, supportive lovers can become even closer through facing this problem and overcoming it.

Delayed Ejaculation

For some men, the problem is not ejaculating too soon, but rather being unable to ejaculate at all. This condition is known as **delayed ejaculation**, formerly referred to as retarded ejaculation or ejaculatory incompetence. Delayed ejaculation has a relatively low prevalence—approximately 3% (Perelmen & Rowland, 2006) and is considered one of the least understood sexual male dysfunctions (Michetti et al., 2013). When a man has never ejaculated after sufficient sexual stimulation and is incapable of doing so, he is classified as having lifelong delayed ejaculation. When he has previously been able to ejaculate but can no longer do so, he is classified as having acquired delayed ejaculation. These men may still be able to maintain an erection or stay sexually aroused, or they may be able to ejaculate through masturbation. Sometimes, though rarely, this condition can be specific to only one partner or to specific situations.

Delayed ejaculation is a disorder that may have interesting effects on a relationship. For example, the ability to maintain penile insertion for long periods without ejaculating may be valued by many men and appreciated by their sexual partners. However, the extreme of being unable to ejaculate at all can result

in the partner's questioning her or his own sexual abilities. In this case, the benefit of prolonged insertion quickly dissipates, and frustration and doubt set in. Another effect is that when the man fakes orgasm to prevent his partner from feeling inadequate, not only does he remain sexually unsatisfied, but deceit, rather than trust and openness, can also begin to characterize the relationship as a whole. As with many other sexual dysfunctions, treatment must be directed at the relationship as well as at the specific disorder.

Genito-Pelvic Pain and Penetration Disorders

Painful sexual penetration (formerly called dyspareunia) has not been studied extensively in men. Epidemiological studies show prevalence rates ranging from 1% to 6% (Lewis et al., 2010). During sexual penetration, men may feel pain in the penis, testes, or some other part of the body. Causes of genital pain can be both organic and psychogenic. For example,

> **delayed ejaculation** A condition in which a male is unable to ejaculate or there is marked delay in ejaculation after sufficient sexual stimulation.

Pain during sex can have many different causes, including infection of the sexual organs, uncomfortable positions, allergic reactions to lubricants or spermicidal creams/foams. Any consistent pain should be referred to a clinician.

infections of the penis, foreskin, testes, urethra, or prostate can cause pain. Other causes include a foreskin that is too tight and causes pain when an erection develops; smegma (a cheese-like substance secreted by the glans penis) that has not been washed away from the glans penis and causes an infection or irritates the glans; and Peyronie's disease, in which fibrous tissue and calcium deposits develop in the area around the cavernous bodies of the penis and may cause pain.

Hypoactive Sexual Desire Disorder in Men

Because of cultural expectations, we often assume that men always want sex. In reality, some men may not have a desire for sex Worldwide, 1 in 4 men experiences lack of desire or interest in sexual activity (Lewis et al., 2010), although this rate does drop considerably when asked if it is a persistent condition lasting 6 months or more (Brotto, 2010a). This condition, now called **male hypoactive sexual desire disorder** (HSDD) and previously called inhibited sexual desire, is characterized by a lack of interest in sexual activity or specific sexual activities—for example, vaginal sex, oral–genital sex, or even sexual fantasizing. As with other conditions, it is considered a dysfunction if the condition causes marked distress or interpersonal difficulty. Without this component, it would be extremely difficult to determine a diagnosis. Because each person's interest in sexual activity varies, when is too little interest really "too little"? When

the lack of interest is specific to a sexual partner, is it the partner's fault?

We often compare ourselves—and our relationships—to others. However, when it comes to sexual issues, if one is in a relationship, it is important to consider the context of the relationship. If the degree of interest between two people in a relationship is similar, and the relationship is otherwise healthy, should the couple be concerned? Or should a therapist advise them that they have a problem? Should the therapist attempt to change the couple's degree of interest? What happens when one partner has more interest in a specific activity than the other partner? For example, should an uninterested partner engage in oral sex to satisfy the interest of the partner? Does this situation need to be corrected? These are not easy questions to answer, but they are questions that many individuals struggle with in their relationships.

Male HSDD can have both psychogenic and organic causes. Low testosterone levels have been weakly associated with male HSDD (although the effect seems more prominent in younger men); some medications also affect desire (Weeks et al., 2009). Depression (Brotto, 2010a; Weeks et al., 2009), anxiety, inaccurate beliefs about sex, poor body image, a tendency to fuse sex and affection, and career overload have also been linked with HSDD risk (Weeks et al., 2009).

One additional explanation has been proposed by Bancroft and colleagues (2009). Their concept, known as the dual-control model, postulates that sexual activity is regulated by two competing processes in the brain: the sexual excitation system and the sexual inhibition system. While individuals vary in their predisposition for both sexual excitation and sexual inhibition, most fall in a range that is nonproblematic. However, if those levels are not in normal ranges, arousal disorders or hypersexuality could develop. For example, individuals with a low predisposition for sexual excitation or a high propensity for sexual inhibition could develop an arousal disorder or hyposexuality. Those with a high propensity for excitation or low propensity for inhibition may be more likely to engage in a high frequency of sexual behavior and high-risk sexual behaviors (Bancroft et al., 2009).

Female Sexual Dysfunctions

It was not too long ago that females were first allowed to express their sexual needs and to be viewed as entitled to sexual satisfaction at the same level as men. However, a double standard is still alive and well. Some men consider women suspect if they initiate sexual activity or are vocal in appreciating it. They are still supposed to be coy, letting the man take the lead, for fear of what might be thought of them if they act too assertively. Given this situation, too

male hypoactive sexual desire disorder A disorder characterized by a lack of interest in sexual activity or specific sexual activities.

(?) Did You Know . . .

For years, women's groups have complained about sexist research when it comes to sexually related issues. The issues covered by these complaints range from contraceptive pills to sexual libido. There are sildenafil (Viagra) and tadalafil (Cialis) for men, for example, but no comparable pill to treat women's sexual interest. That situation now appears to be changing.

On August 18, 2015, the Food and Drug Administration (FDA) approved the world's first drug for women designed to treat female sexual interest and arousal disorder. Flibanserin (Addyi) targets neurotransmitters in the brain, whereas Viagra and Cialis increase blood flow to the penis. Another difference between these medications is that Addyi needs to be taken every day, whereas Viagra and Cialis can be taken when sexual intercourse is planned.

However, Addyi is not without controversy. Potential side effects include nausea, dizziness, low blood pressure, fainting, and sleepiness. Given that the benefits of the drug appear to be modest, some experts question whether Addyi should have been approved by the FDA. Opponents of Addyi's approval argue that political concerns (i.e., the FDA's pattern of repeatedly rejecting past drugs to treat female sexual dysfunction) trumped scientific data. In contrast, proponents believe that arousal disorders can be so debilitating to the psychological and social health of women that approval of this drug is warranted, that its side effects can be minimized if it is taken before bedtime, and that its approval will encourage other pharmaceutical manufacturers to pursue research to improve upon this class of medication so that more effective drugs will be available in the future.

---

many women have adopted a passive attitude toward sexual activity and sometimes have developed shame, guilt, or embarrassment about their sexual behavior. For some women, this has progressed into an inability to function in a sexually healthy and satisfying way. Women may experience sexual dysfunctions in the following areas: sexual interest and arousal disorder, female orgasmic disorder, and genito-pelvic pain and penetration disorder.

Female Sexual Interest and Arousal Disorder

While Masters and Johnson's sexual response cycle starts with excitement, the precursors—desire and interest in sex—are critical components. Years ago, to be diagnosed with a desire disorder, women had to lack a physical response, such as a lack of vaginal lubrication or vasocongestion. Today, criteria for the disorder include more subjective components of the sexual experience (Brotto, 2010b). For example, women with **sexual interest/arousal disorder** can experience an absence or reduced frequency of interest in sexual activity or even erotic thoughts or fantasies. They may also find themselves initiating sex less often or being unreceptive to a partner's attempts to initiate. As in male HSDD, these can be very subjective ideas of what is normal or what is normal for you as an individual. Women can also be diagnosed with an arousal disorder if there is a lack of sexual pleasure or genital sensations during sexual activity.

As with other sexual dysfunctions, rates of occurrence are hard to determine. Epidemiological studies show a large range in prevalence rates (17–55%) of women experiencing low levels of desire (Lewis et al., 2010), with most studies typically showing 20% to 30% of women experiencing arousal issues (Brotto et al., 2010). These rates do increase with age: 10% of those younger than 49 years of age experience arousal difficulties, with the rate increasing to 22% for those 50–65 years of age and again doubling to 47% for those 66–74 years of age. Most studies report rates of lubrication difficulties ranging from 8% to 15%, with some reporting higher rates (21–28%) (Lewis et al., 2010).

Possible causes of sexual arousal disorder can be psychogenic or organic. However, sexual arousal disorder is more complicated than it appears initially. Experts have recommended considering the sexual partner and environmental conditions when diagnosing sexual arousal disorder (Brotto et al., 2010; Weeks et al., 2009). For example, sexual dysfunction of a male partner, such as erectile dysfunction or early ejaculation, may have a negative impact on a female partner's sexual desire. Women with low arousal report poorer quality relationships, more dissatisfaction with conflict resolution, and less attraction to and emotional closeness with their partners compared with women who do not have low arousal or desire. Relationships that do not include open communication about sexual needs, wishes, and fears also have a negative impact on the woman's desire to engage in sexual activity. Understanding the interactions of all these factors is critical for successful treatment.

---

sexual interest/arousal disorder A sexual dysfunction that causes a woman to experience little or no erotic pleasure through sexual stimulation.

Some people have strong feelings of anxiety, fear, or disgust when confronted with a sexual opportunity; these symptoms do not indicate a lack of desire but rather a condition previously called *sexual aversion disorder*. In these cases, individuals often experience anxiety-like symptoms and may go so far as to avoid sexual behavior (Brotto, 2010c). Formerly listed as a sexual disorder in diagnostic manuals, sexual aversion disorder was not included in the most recent revision, the DSM-5, because of the lack of evidence supporting the condition as a distinct diagnosis. Many sexual health experts believe this condition overlaps with specific phobias in presentation and treatment methodologies, which means that it should be diagnosed as a phobia, not a sexual disorder (Brotto, 2010c).

Female Orgasmic Disorder

Some women have difficulty experiencing orgasm; women who have a delay or absence of orgasm following normal sexual excitement have a condition called **female orgasmic disorder**. Women who have never had an orgasm are said to have *lifelong orgasmic disorder* or *preorgasmia*. Sometimes preorgasmia is referred to as *anorgasmia*.

However, anorgasmia implies an inability to achieve orgasm, which is not an accurate label for many women. Many women simply have not had an orgasm yet—there is no biological cause preventing them from having one (Trustees of Columbia University, 2012). Those who have experienced an orgasm but are not able to now are said to have acquired orgasmic disorder. Some women have orgasms under certain circumstances but not others—for example, while masturbating but not when stimulated by a partner. This condition is referred to as situational orgasmic disorder. If an orgasm does not occur in any situation, it is considered generalized orgasmic disorder.

As with other sexual dysfunctions, there is a lack of quality data with consistent criteria to estimate prevalence rates (Graham, 2010b). Worldwide, data regarding the incidence of orgasmic disorder in women vary greatly (Lewis et al., 2010), and few of these studies show the age-related increase that is often associated with other sexual dysfunctions. A U.S. study indicated that in women ages 40–80, approximately 20% experience the inability to reach orgasm occasionally, periodically, or frequently (Laumann et al., 2009).

Some studies have found associations between orgasmic responsiveness in women and relationship satisfaction (Mah & Binik, 2001), but the absence of orgasm does not mean that a woman cannot have a satisfactory and enjoyable sexual relationship. In reality, some women do not experience distress about the lack of orgasm (Graham, 2010b), and other research has shown that physical aspects of sex (such as orgasm) are weak predictors of sexual distress compared to relationship and emotional well-being, which are strong predictors (Bancroft et al., 2003). Each woman places a different level of importance on orgasm, and this is likely related to the level of distress experienced (Bancroft, 2009).

Because many women cannot achieve orgasm through vaginal penetration alone (they require clitoral stimulation), they may consider themselves preorgasmic if they have not explored other activities. Being aware of one's own body is critical in understanding stimuli that aid in orgasm. In addition to self-awareness, being in a comfortable and safe relationship that allows honest communication about these issues can facilitate exploration with a partner.

Causes of orgasmic dysfunction seem to be primarily psychological. For women who are preorgasmic, the environment during childhood, such as parental attitudes about sexuality, nudity, and relationships, may affect one's comfort with sexual health issues, body image, communication skills, and other factors. Additionally, stress, levels of fatigue, sexual identity, health, employment situation, and relationship difficulties can affect orgasmic functioning (McCabe, 2009). Much like arousal disorders, if the woman is partnered, considering the relationship quality is critical. Poor intimacy, affection, and communication have been linked with orgasmic disorder, but it is unclear

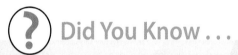 **Did You Know . . .**

Testosterone has been used to increase the sex drives of women. In several well-conducted, randomized trials, testosterone delivered in various ways (e.g., injections, implants, and patches) resulted in an increase in women's sexual desire, sexual responsiveness, and frequency of sexual intercourse (Heiman, 2006). Yet, as with all medications, there are potential side effects of testosterone use for low sexual desire. Among these side effects are unwanted hair growth and the unanswered question regarding the relationship between testosterone administration and the development of breast cancer (Brotto et al., 2010; Davis et al., 2008), insulin resistance, and metabolic syndrome (Brotto et al., 2010). This medication is currently approved for use in women in Europe, but it has not yet been approved by the FDA in the United States.

---

female orgasmic disorder The consistent or frequent inability of a woman to achieve an orgasm.

Cervix

Vagina

Urethra

Vaginal constricting muscle relaxed

Vaginal constricting muscle contracted

Clitoris

Labia

Normal opening

Vaginal opening constricted

Relaxed state

Vaginismic state

FIGURE **20.1** Vaginismus is the involuntary contraction of the muscles in the outer third of the vagina.

whether the relationship problems preceded the sexual dysfunction or whether the sexual dysfunction exacerbated relationship challenges (McCabe, 2009).

Genito-Pelvic Pain and Penetration Disorders

Some women experience pain during sexual intercourse or vaginal penetration. Previously, persistent or recurrent pain associated with sexual intercourse was diagnosed as dyspareunia, but this term is being used less as a diagnosis today. Although all women may experience some pain during some particular sexual episodes (due to position, time of menstrual cycle, lack of adequate lubrication, or other factors), the condition can also be chronic and considered a disorder.

Often the pain manifests as a burning feeling, or cramping and may occur externally (on the vulva), in the vagina, or elsewhere in the pelvis. Because pain can be different symptomatically, many clinicians

and researchers today agree that different syndromes result in dyspareunia. In fact, the pain of dyspareunia can typically be reproduced in nonsexual situations, such as tampon insertion and pelvic exams (Landry & Bergeron, 2009). Two main categories are "superficial" dyspareunia, which includes provoked vestibulodynia (PVD) and vulvovaginal atrophy (VVA), and deep dyspareunia (Binik, 2010). With PVD, women experience pain in the vulva provoked by touch. VVA is a common condition associated with decreased estrogenization of the vaginal tissue. Painful penetration is just one symptom; others include dryness, irritation, soreness, and urinary frequency, urgency, and incontinence. Although VVA can occur at any time in a woman's life cycle, it is more common in the postmenopausal phase (MacBride et al., 2010). Pain during deep thrust vaginal intercourse is called deep dyspareunia.

Another pain-related condition occurs when a woman cannot relax the muscles around the entrance to the vagina enough to allow penetration of an object (e.g., penis, finger, or speculum) and these muscles involuntarily spasm. Women often report that penetration is almost or completely impossible (Meana, 2009). This condition is called **vaginismus** (see Figure 20.1). There is, however, little research supporting vaginal spasms as a criterion for diagnosis, and some experts believe that this symptom may be the severe, phobic end of the dyspareunia continuum (Meana & Binik, 1994; Reissing et al., 2004). One aspect of this condition that appears unique is that the fear of penetration can increase to a phobia (Reissing et al., 2004).

Some women experience pain during intercourse. Possible causes include disorders of the reproductive organs, vaginal infections, or irritation due to the use of some contraceptive products.

vaginismus The involuntary contraction of the muscles surrounding the vaginal entrance so that entry of the penis is prevented.

© JJJ/ShutterStock, Inc.

Although people differ in their interest in sexual activity, when one partner experiences lower sexual desire, the other partner may become frustrated and even angry. Understanding and seeking treatment is necessary at this point.

Studies examining prevalence rates of pain disorders in women show a range of 14% to 27% (Lewis et al., 2010). The large spectrum of symptoms and conditions that can be included in this category may account for the large range. One concern regarding pain disorders is their potential to lead to other sexual disorders. For example, if a woman anticipates pain during vaginal penetration, this anxiety can affect her level of interest and arousal during sexual activity. It is important for any secondary disorders to be considered and treated as well. There is continuing controversy about how to conceptualize and treat these disorders; the uncertainty about best treatment options is complicated by the challenge of dealing with highly distressed patients and the many clinicians who avoid treating these conditions (van Lankveld et al., 2010).

Other Sexual Conditions

Hypersexuality

Hypersexuality is often referred to as sex addiction, and while high levels of sexual fantasies and activities can be a problematic behavior, in the most recent revision of *Diagnostic and Statistical Manual of Mental Disorders* (*DSM-5*), it was not included as a sexual disorder. Among sex therapists and sexuality counselors, there is controversy as to whether sex addiction truly exists as a diagnosis and condition. Some believe that there is enough research to support hypersexuality as a sexual health disorder (Reid & Kafka, 2014), while others believe that normal behaviors—such as sexual behavior—should not be pathologized and that distinguishing between high levels of desire and pathological levels is difficult (Winters et al., 2010). For more on problematic sexual behavior, see the section on sexual addiction in the *Alternative Sexual Behavior* chapter.

Persistent Genital Arousal

Persistent genital arousal disorder (PGAD) is a rare condition in which an individual experiences unwanted, unrelenting, spontaneous genital sensation and arousal. The symptoms do not typically result in orgasm and are considered intrusive and distressful to the individual. This condition is distinct from hypersexuality in that the symptoms occur in the absence of sexual stimuli. Distress and persistency are both critical components of PGAD, as some individuals may experience intermittent symptoms of arousal and find them pleasurable (Facelle et al., 2013). Reported cases of PGAD are higher among women, but men can also experience the condition (Kamatchi & Ashley-Smith, 2013).

Many potential causes of PGAD have been proposed, including psychological origins, medication interactions, and physical—specifically, neurologic and vascular—factors. Recently, PGAD has been associated with other conditions like restless leg syndrome and overactive bladder. For those who experience PGAD symptoms, psychological factors may influence each individual's perception of the symptoms and level of distress. Carvalho and colleagues (2014) found that sexual conservatism influences the severity of symptoms and related distress, such that more sexually conservative individuals experience more distress.

As with the causes of this condition, there is no consensus on best practices for treatment of PGAD. Recommendations include identifying reversible causes and incorporating cognitive therapy such as mindfulness and meditation (Facelle et al., 2013).

Dissatisfaction with Sexual Activity Frequency

Not everyone is as interested in sex as his or her partner. A guest speaker in one of our classes characterized this disharmony as only a matter of the mind. To illustrate his point, he referred to the way he responds to his spouse's occasional "Leave me alone, I've got a headache" when he is "ready and primed to go." Whereas some men would argue or pout, he usually says, "Where does your head ache?" and proceeds to massage her head and temples, cheeks, and neck gently. After a while he moves to her shoulders and asks, "Does this feel good?" One full-body massage later, his spouse's lack of interest has been transformed. Men and women alike can learn to tune into the temporary inhibition, exhaustion, anxiety, or preoccupation that may diminish a partner's sexual interest and learn how that person likes to be treated in such circumstances.

Multicultural
DIMENSIONS

Sexual Dysfunction and Latino Populations

The Hispanic community, as do all subgroups within the United States, has some unique features that need to be considered regarding sexual dysfunction. While the limited research on Hispanic individuals shows similar rates of sexual dysfunction as other groups (Meana et al., 2013), some cultural aspects may preclude Latinos from seeking professional help for sexual dysfunction. One of these is the language barrier. Not speaking English, or not speaking it well, means that if a sexual dysfunction arises, the person's ability to communicate the condition may prevent him or her from seeking help.

There may also be shame, or *verguenza*. Many Hispanic individuals were raised in religious and cultural environments that limited or even forbid conversations about sexuality; this early conditioning may cause experiencing a sexual problem or even discussing sexuality issues to be perceived as shameful (Meana et al., 2013).

Hispanics also view the family as an extended one, not distinguishing between the nuclear family and the extended family. Cousins, aunts, uncles, and other family members are assumed to be part of the family, and advice is traditionally sought from family members as opposed to people outside the family, such as health professionals. However, matters of sexual function are considered inappropriate for a family discussion, and therefore are often ignored.

Hispanics also maintain a sense of fatalism. Expressions such as *que sea lo que Dios quiera* ("it's in God's hands") and *esta enfermedad es una prueba de Dios* ("this illness is a test of God") are examples of this view of health-related problems. Therefore, a sexual dysfunction might be considered a matter for God, not for a sex therapist.

In addition, Latino communities tend to be male dominated, and that condition may interfere with admitting to a sexual dysfunction. In a project to enroll more children in government-sponsored health insurance programs, one of us found that what works for Anglo families does not always work for Hispanic families. In Anglo families, it is the mother who is targeted for improving the health of the family's children. In Hispanic families, we found it necessary to influence the fathers first. This difference arises because of the concept of *machismo* (in which males are projected as strong, virile, powerful, and in control), which manifests itself in male-dominated families. Given the need to maintain this sense of machismo, Hispanic males may be reluctant to admit a "weakness," especially a sexual dysfunction (Meana et al., 2013).

Culturally sensitive approaches are needed in all matters, particularly sexual ones. Sexual dysfunction is no exception.

Regardless of the cause, studies have consistently found that men have a greater desire and stronger motivation for sex than do women (Petersen & Hyde, 2010). However, there is some evidence that sexual desire is influenced and expressed differently between men and women. Women's desire may be influenced more by contextual factors and emotional arousal rather than by genitals. For example, women are more likely than men to report sexual arousal in response to verbal exchanges and nongenital touching (Fisher, 1999).

If there is a difference in sexual interest between partners, this can have a negative impact on other aspects of the relationship. When one person feels he or she is pressuring the other or the other feels pressured, the potential for disagreement is evident. The result may be that both partners feel unloved and guilty. To remedy this problem, the couple must maintain effective communication rather than avoid it. In some cases, the assistance of a sex therapist may be warranted.

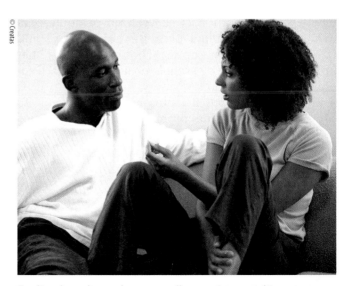

Studies show that males are usually more interested in sexual activity than are women. To resolve these differences, communication is vital for satisfying, long-term sexual relationships to develop.

Sexual Dysfunction and Self-Esteem

Some of us would like to think that sexual functioning is similar to other physical functioning—or that at least it ought to be considered so. If self-worth does not diminish when our digestive functioning goes haywire, why should we think less of ourselves if our sexual functioning is problematic? In reality, sexual functioning is more closely connected to self-esteem than other body processes. Men and women with sexual dysfunctions often feel less confident because they do not function sexually as they want to. Aside from their desire to function sexually for their own satisfaction, some feel they are depriving their partners of satisfaction. Furthermore, they may fear that their partners will seek other sexual partners and/or leave them—fears that further diminish self-esteem. Not surprisingly, the partners of those struggling with a disorder may also lose some self-esteem. They may feel that the dysfunction is due to their own lack of attractiveness, skill, or attention or that the partner no longer cares for them. Evidence shows that heterosexual women are more likely to experience arousal disorders if their partner is also suffering from a sexual dysfunction (McCabe & Goldhammer, 2012).

Therapists and counselors have become increasingly sensitive to the matter of self-esteem for both the person experiencing sexual dysfunction and his or her partner.

■ Causes of Sexual Dysfunction

Sexual dysfunctions can have physical causes, psychological causes, and cultural causes. A combination of factors often influences the condition. Understanding whether the condition is generalized or situational can help an individual or a therapist understand potential underlying causes. Those conditions that are situational have a psychological component. Generalized disorders do not always mean that there is a physical cause, but it increases the likelihood. To prevent and treat sexual problems, these factors need to be understood.

Physical (Organic) Causes

Physical causes can affect many different aspects of sexuality—from desire to the ability to orgasm—in both men and women. Natural physical changes that accompany the aging process are one of the prevalent factors affecting sexual functioning. For example, the physical changes accompanying menopause for women also increase the risk of vaginal atrophy, which could cause an increase in painful penetration. As men age, the risk of coronary heart disease and

blocked blood vessels increases, and this condition can affect penile arteries, causing erectile dysfunction.

Extensive research demonstrates that certain medical conditions and health behaviors represent major risk factors for sexual disorders. For men, diabetes, cardiovascular disorders, hypertension, obesity, smoking, lower urinary tract problems, and prostate disorders all have been positively correlated with males experiencing erectile dysfunction (Shamloul & Ghanem, 2013). For women, chronic illnesses and poor general health status are associated with higher rates of sexual dysfunction. Some conditions, such as diabetes, breast cancer, lower urinary tract problems, multiple sclerosis, and clinical depression, are all consistently connected to increased sexual dysfunction (DeRogatis & Burnett, 2008). A U.S. study has also shown that lack of physical activity is associated with a lack of sexual interest for men and women (Laumann et al., 2009).

Surgery for prostate or bladder cancer has demonstrated an impact on erectile function in men. Similarly, surgical removal of the ovaries affects hormone levels in women, which may cause vaginal atrophy (potentially leading to painful penetration).

Medications can also cause changes in sexual functioning. For example, for both men (Segraves & Balon, 2014) and women, delayed orgasm is the most commonly reported side effect of some antidepressant medications. Approximately 30% to 60% of all persons using selective serotonin reuptake inhibitors (SSRIs) are affected in this way (Graham, 2010a). Medications for a variety of other conditions, such as psychiatric disorders (e.g., bipolar disorder; Nagaraj et al., 2009), hypertension, high cholesterol, heart disease, and allergies, can also affect sexual functioning (Zenilman & Shahmanesh, 2011).

Psychological Causes

Many sexual dysfunctions have no known physiological cause, but rather have a psychological basis. Anxiety is a key factor affecting sexual function. Researchers caution against the broad use of the term *anxiety* and believe that clinicians need to consider differences between general anxiety, sexual anxiety, and performance anxiety as possible factors (McCabe et al., 2010). The level of anxiety combined with the setting also needs to be considered. Moderate anxiety in a safe setting may actually facilitate arousal—for example, the nervousness associated with having a new partner or engaging in a new activity. However, high levels of anxiety combined with less personal control and a history of chronic anxiety may cause dysfunction. Here, imagine feeling anxious plus being critiqued by your partner; in this situation, one is more likely to experience a disorder (Van Minnen & Kampman, 2000).

A previous sexual trauma can lead to a sexual dysfunction if this event is recalled during sex.

Depression also has a link with sexual functioning. This relationship appears reciprocal in that a depressed mood increases the likelihood of sexual dysfunction and sexual dysfunction increases the likelihood of depression. Lower levels of desire caused by antidepressant medication can exacerbate this condition (McCabe et al., 2010).

Many other factors can affect one's sexual functioning. Decreased sexual desire can be caused by traumatic experiences, such as child sexual abuse. Other prior experiences, such as problematic attachments, neglectful or critical parents, restrictive upbringing, physical abuse, and violence, increase the risk that one may experience sexual dysfunction (McCabe et al., 2010).

Many times an individual may experience difficulty functioning sexually, but he or she is able to resolve it relatively quickly and without much difficulty. However, some factors prevent improvement of the condition; these include relationship conflict, performance anxiety, guilt, inadequate sexual information or stimulation, loss of sexual chemistry, fear of intimacy, impaired self-image or self-esteem, loss of sexual confidence, restricted foreplay, poor communication, and lack of privacy.

General stress and stress about the sexual experience can also affect sexual functioning. Stress leads to an increase in the hormone epinephrine in the blood, which in turn can interfere with blood flow to the penis or clitoris. Snegroff (1986) studied stressors associated with nonmarital sexual intercourse and found that males differed in some of these stressors and not in others. For males, the following were of most concern:

1. Can I satisfy her?

2. Is my penis the right size?

3. Will I achieve and/or maintain an erection?

4. Will she want a commitment?

5. Will I perform well?

For females, the following were of most concern:

1. Can I satisfy him?

2. Will he like my body?

3. Will he respect me afterward?

4. Does he love/care for me?

5. Will I have an orgasm?

6. Are my breasts large enough?

While this research was conducted 30 years ago, the issues are still the same today.

It is quite understandable that psychological factors can cause someone difficulty in functioning in an effective manner sexually. Is it any wonder that someone who is self-conscious about his or her body might not function well sexually? Imagine just waiting for a partner to laugh or cringe! Anxiety, guilt, and shame are hardly conducive to healthy sexual functioning.

Cultural Causes

Society also influences sexual functioning. For example, the double standard that judges women as less than moral if they actively seek sexual satisfaction can create shame and guilt, which in turn interfere with normal sexual functioning. Furthermore, if the double standard is interpreted to mean that the male initiates sex and is more expert at it than a female partner, the pressure to behave in this manner can block the male's normal function. However, if females are taught to expect sexual satisfaction in their relationships comparable to that expected by their male partners, they might unintentionally put the onus for their fulfillment on their partners rather than assume that responsibility for themselves. With the onus placed on them, males may succumb to pressure and be unable to function as usual.

The way we perceive sex is also dependent on what our culture has taught us. Someone once said that sex is so "dirty" it should be saved for someone you love. Thinking of sex as dirty can create negative feelings such as embarrassment and guilt, which can result in sexual dysfunction.

Some (Mayo Foundation for Medical Education and Research, 2014) believe that premature ejaculation results from boys' learning by their early teenage years to masturbate. Associated with their masturbatory behavior is guilt that causes them to speed up their orgasm. Having learned to ejaculate rapidly,

Global DIMENSIONS

Sexual Disorders Around the World   The various perspectives and cultural mores of different countries may contribute to the development of sexual disorders, or at least to a diagnosis of a sexual dysfunction. For example, in Uganda and other countries in which homosexuality is considered immoral, gay and lesbian people, thinking every time they engage in sex they are doing something "dirty" and opposed by their society's expectations, might develop a sexual dysfunction. In Islamic countries in which female genital mutilation is customary, women may develop sexual arousal disorders.

In contrast, countries that have more relaxed sexual mores and accept a wider array of sexual behavior as "normal" tend to cultivate a sexually healthier population. For example, Sweden and Denmark have low rates of sexual dysfunction and teenage pregnancy. In Polynesian countries, known for encouraging sexual exploration at young ages, embarrassment and anxiety associated with sex are almost nonexistent.

Where you grew up and where you live now can have a tremendous effect on your sexual health. *What influenced your sexual health? How?*

they have difficulty controlling their ejaculation when they get older.

Religion is also related to sexual function. As one author states: "Rigid adherence to orthodox religious beliefs and practices is a common factor in the backgrounds of men and women with different forms of sexual dysfunction. Strict religious teaching—regardless of the particular religion—often results in negative attitudes toward sexuality. Individuals come to believe that sex is sinful" (Wilson et al., 1996, p. 241). Of course, not all people who hold such religious beliefs develop a sexual problem, and religious beliefs often influence behaviors in a healthy manner.

Another significant cause of sexual dysfunction is related to a lack of information about sexual functioning—for example, not knowing or forgetting that foreplay is necessary to lubricate the vagina before penetration with a penis or a sex toy. Other possible causes are nonsexual problems between sexual partners, ineffective communication (about sex and other matters), and traumatic past sexual experiences (e.g., rape). Thus sexual unresponsiveness might, for instance, be caused by an inexperienced, inept, hasty, or insensitive lover, or by situational factors, such as thoughts of a sick relative or career concerns.

Treating Sexual Dysfunction

In the past few decades, many effective therapeutic approaches to sexual dysfunction have emerged (although love and concern between partners are still important). Because the effectiveness of the various therapeutic approaches is well publicized, not only do more sufferers seek treatment—a positive step—but more people want to become sex therapists. As

might be expected in an emerging field, charlatans and quacks, in addition to well-trained professionals, have set up practice. Therefore, anyone experiencing sexual problems would be well advised to investigate the training and experience of a sex therapist carefully before seeking that person's services. To help people select a professional therapist, the American Association of Sex Educators, Counselors, and Therapists (AASECT) has made public its requirements for certifying individuals as sex counselors or sex therapists. AASECT has also published a code of ethics that provides guidance for sex counselors and sex therapists, as well as for patients. Counselors and therapists whose behavior is inconsistent with this code may be incompetent and/or unethical.

Both single individuals and those in relationships may seek therapy for a sexual dysfunction. A couple that is in a relationship may be first seen together by the therapist or therapists and then be interviewed separately so they will feel free to discuss matters with the therapist that they might not yet feel comfortable discussing with their partner. Once the nature of the problem is identified, instruction and/or counseling can begin. The therapist will address the sexual issue but will often also explore and work on any underlying issues that may be affecting the sexual issue. Depending on the circumstance, the couple may be instructed to abstain from penetrative sex and to learn how to experience pleasure in nongenital touching, with genital fondling and eventually penetrative sex being included. The touching and sexual activity are done in private, away from the therapist's office, without the therapist present or in a room with one-way mirrors. Although rare, sometimes a *surrogate*, or substitute, partner is used to provide instruction, practice, and feedback for an

Ethical DIMENSIONS

Should Surrogates Be Used in Sex Therapy?

In the 1950s, some therapists believed that the use of a substitute sexual partner was a vital and necessary component of sex therapy. This substitute, or surrogate, was an experienced and trained sexual partner who could teach the sexually dysfunctional client effective sexual techniques. The surrogate let the client practice these techniques in a non-threatening situation, because the surrogate was not a person with whom the client had a relationship or whom the client would see after the treatment was complete.

While not commonly incorporated into sex therapy today, some therapists do incorporate sexual surrogates into their therapy model for certain clients. In addition to sexual practices, surrogates may include exercises in basic anatomy, communication, social skills training, sensuality, and sexual touching (Rosenbaum et al., 2014). In addition to the reasons mentioned in the first paragraph, advocates of the use of surrogates believe the therapy to be more effective if the client practices on and receives feedback from a real person. For individuals who do not have a partner, learning techniques related to some sexual dysfunctions—such as premature ejaculation—can be almost impossible by oneself. Likewise, social skills cannot be learned in isolation. For example, one of the authors recently learned of a 50-year-old virgin with physical disabilities who had never been on a date. Part of his experience with the surrogate was to go out to dinner and practice social interactions and chivalry. For individuals using a surrogate, even the ending of the surrogate relationship allows the individual to experience and develop relationship and communication skills relating to feelings and sexuality, by considering such questions as: How does it feel to end this relationship? Are you able to express these feelings to others? How do you reflect on the sexual aspects of this relationship?

Opposition to sexual surrogates is based on a variety of concerns. Opponents note that the knowledge, skills, and attitudes learned with a surrogate may not be readily transferred to another sexual partner. Some people believe that sexual activity between individuals not married to each other is immoral. In addition, because the surrogate is getting paid for engaging in the interaction, the client and the surrogate may be violating prostitution laws. The issue of legality varies by state within the United States, and is often vague. However, surrogacy is legal in some countries; for example, there are counseling clinics in Israel that incorporate surrogacy into the practice (Rosenbaum et al., 2014). In addition to the question of legality, the ethical codes of some professional counseling and therapy organizations do not allow the therapist to facilitate or moderate the relationship between a surrogate and an individual (this triadic approach is recommended); therefore, individuals are not given an opportunity to reflect on how the surrogate relationship is affecting them—either positively or negatively.

Do you think surrogates should be used in sex therapy? Why or why not?

Rosenbaum, T., Aloni, R., & Heruti, R. Surrogate partner therapy: Ethical considerations in sexual medicine. *Journal of Sexual Medicine, 11* (2014), 321–329.

individual with a sexual problem. The use of sexual surrogates is highly controversial, both within the profession and among the public.

Approaches to Sex Therapy

Several models of sex therapy have been proposed. Perhaps a good place to begin a discussion of these models is first to consider a well-regarded stepwise approach to sex therapy.

The PLISSIT Model

Jack Annon (1976) suggested that relatively minor treatment may be effective for some sexual dysfunctions, whereas more intensive treatment may be required for others. Annon's model of sex therapy is known as the **PLISSIT** (*P*ermission, *L*imited *I*nformation, *S*pecific *S*uggestion, and *I*ntensive *T*herapy) model. This model extends from the simplest to the more advanced levels of treatment.

During the Permission stage, the therapist helps people accept their fantasies and desires and, where appropriate, gives them permission to *not* engage in sexual intercourse until they are ready to do so. The therapist helps couples to not compare themselves with other couples or with an idealized sexual relationship.

During the Limited Information stage, the therapist provides factual information that may help the

PLISSIT A model of sex therapy that consists of moving through the stages of giving permission, limited information, specific suggestion, and, if that does not work, intensive therapy.

person become more functional sexually. For example, a person may not realize it is natural to fantasize about sexual activity or perceive sexuality as a natural part of one's life. Information can give clients a more realistic perception, thereby removing an impediment to their sexual functioning. Other kinds of information, such as information about penis size and its limited effect on sexual satisfaction, clitoral sensitivity, or proper hygiene, may be all that is needed to help people overcome their sexual dysfunctions.

Specific Suggestion is the level of therapy at which the therapist actually recommends activities for the clients. For example, self-stimulation, sensate focus, and the squeeze technique may be suggested. Many of these techniques were developed by Masters and Johnson (1970) but have since been modified by other sex therapists. These techniques can help the person reduce sexual anxiety, improve communication between partners, or enhance arousal.

Intensive Therapy may be required when permission, limited information, and specific suggestion are not successful in resolving a sexual problem. Intensive therapy entails a longer-term therapeutic treatment that identifies the deep-seated reasons that interfere with sexual functioning. This therapy has been called *psychosexual therapy* (Kaplan, 1974). Some therapists believe sexual dysfunction is caused by guilt or shame about sex, which leads to sexual anxiety, and the best treatment is intensive therapy to uncover the causes of these feelings.

Myth (vs) Fact

Myth: Sexual dysfunctions occur because someone either has been sexually abused or raped or has masturbated too often.
Fact: It is true that sexual abuse, such as rape and child abuse, can contribute to the development of a sexual dysfunction. Yet, there are many people who experience those traumatic events and never develop a sexual dysfunction. Regarding masturbation, there is no evidence that the frequency of masturbation is in any way related to the subsequent development of a sexual dysfunction.

Myth: Guys who "can't get it up" are not real men.
Fact: Many cases of erectile dysfunction are caused by physiological problems. To classify these men as less than real men is analogous to characterizing any man who has any physical illness as not a real man. The inability to achieve and maintain an erection is in no way related to manliness.

Myth: Women are not naturally interested in sex, so a woman who cannot be sexually aroused is quite normal.
Fact: Males and females have a natural interest in and capacity for sex, although the level of desire and arousal differs between people. When males or females are experiencing less desire or arousal than they would like and this experience distresses them, they should seek professional help.

The Masters and Johnson Model

William Masters and Virginia Johnson advocated a model of sex therapy with several unique components. First, they believed that sexual problems are relationship problems, and therefore that therapy works only with couples. Even seemingly healthy partners can learn how to respond and contribute better to their partner's response through therapy. Second, they believed that if couples are to be treated, the therapy team should be a couple—that is, a male therapist and a female therapist. They believed that such a team can best appreciate the perspectives and best represent the couple in therapy. In addition, Masters and Johnson believed that clients can better identify with a therapist of the same gender, who may understand them better. Third, clients were medically screened for any potential organic causes of their dysfunction and given a complete psychological evaluation. Finally, treatment at the Masters and Johnson Institute was intensive; couples were seen every day for a 2-week period. Masters and Johnson argued that this intensive interaction between the therapists and the clients was necessary initially to reduce anxiety and help the couple concentrate on overcoming the sexual problem.

There are positives and negatives about the approach Masters and Johnson used. Understanding the possible physical causes of sexual dysfunction is critical to successful treatment; today most sex therapists incorporate treatments affecting psychological and medical aspects, if warranted (Althof, 2010). However, less intensive therapies, such as self-help strategies (van Lankveld, 2009) and sex therapy via the Internet (Althof, 2010), are demonstrating success. In addition, the focus on couples and heterosexuals limits the applicability to single people; gay, lesbian, and bisexual individuals; and individuals in consensual nonmonogamous relationships.

Kaplan's Model

Kaplan (1974, 1979, 1983) employed many of the specific techniques of sex therapy recommended by Masters and Johnson. However, Kaplan believed more intensive therapy is required to uncover the reasons for the sexual anxiety that interferes with normal sexual functioning. Kaplan's triphasic model consisted of desire, arousal, and orgasm phases. Desire phase problems are the most difficult to treat because of their association with deep-seated psychological difficulties. Consequently, Kaplan recommended a longer period of therapy to uncover the unconscious rationale for behavior and thought. Kaplan believed that sexual dysfunctions have their roots in multiple causes—some readily accessible and others requiring more intensive therapy to determine them. In addition, Kaplan treated premature ejaculation with the stop–start technique developed by James Semans (1956) rather than the squeeze technique developed by Masters and Johnson. Both the squeeze and the stop–start technique are described later in this chapter.

Other Approaches to Sex Therapy

There are many other ways in which therapists treat sexual dysfunctions. For example, some behaviorists (Leiblum & Pervin, 1980; LoPiccolo, 1977) believe that most sexual problems are learned and, therefore, can be unlearned. Behaviorists use positive and negative reinforcement to encourage healthy behaviors and use gradual approaches to problematic sexual behavior. This latter approach is based on the early work of Joseph Wolpe (1958), who argued that one could not be anxious and relaxed at the same time. Consequently, Wolpe taught his clients deep muscle relaxation (e.g., meditation) and gradually, over time, introduced more and more components of the anxiety-producing behavior. The sensate focus activity described later in this chapter is an example of Wolpe's desensitization technique.

Barbach (1980, 2000, 2001) organized groups of women to treat sexual dysfunction—in particular, orgasmic dysfunction and sexual unresponsiveness. Barbach's methods include exercises for the woman to do for herself. These exercises are also described later in the chapter.

Ellis and Harper (1975, 1979) developed a therapy model called rational emotive therapy. This model is based on the assumption that much of our behavior is a result of our thoughts and interpretations. Sexual problems arise from (irrational) thoughts and interpretations, and these problems can be treated by helping people recognize their irrationality and change these thoughts and interpretations into more rational ones.

Barry McCarthy suggested that in the great majority of cases, the sexual problem stems from a lack of knowledge, communication problems, or psychological difficulties. Consequently, he viewed psychologists, social workers, marriage counselors, and ministers as better suited to working with such patients than physicians. In McCarthy et al.'s (1975) model of sex therapy, a single therapist sees both sexual partners once a week, sometimes together, sometimes apart. This therapist is not a physician. Because a physical examination is a prerequisite to acceptance in the program, McCarthy considered a physician's skills unnecessary during therapy.

Treating Erectile Dysfunction

Erectile dysfunction can have physiological causes, psychological causes, or a combination of physiological and psychological causes. The first step in

Myth (vs) Fact

Myth: Treatment for sexual dysfunctions must entail counseling over the long term to be successful.

Fact: Treatments for sexual dysfunctions vary, depending on the nature of the particular dysfunction and the people involved. In some cases, the cause is a physical one, and medications or exercises can successfully treat it. In other cases, all that may be needed is to educate the couple about effective techniques of sexual arousal. In relatively few cases is long-term counseling necessary.

Myth: Any couple who is not engaging in sexual activities frequently enough, with enough variety, and with orgasm have a sexual dysfunction for which they should seek sexual counseling.

Fact: Most experts believe that for a sexual dysfunction to exist, one or both of the sexual partners must be dissatisfied with the sexual relationship. If both partners are satisfied, regardless of the nature of their sexual relationship, no sexual dysfunction exists.

treatment is to determine the underlying factors. For disorders influenced by physiological factors, the initial treatment plan will likely involve lifestyle modification—specifically, weight reduction for obese men, quitting smoking, and increasing physical activity (Shamloul & Ghanem, 2013). In addition to the lifestyle modifications, the most common treatment is oral medications, specifically phosphodiesterase 5 (PDE5) inhibitors (Gambescia et al., 2009). We commonly know these agents as Viagra (sildenafil), Cialis (tadalafil), and Levitra (vardenafil). Such medications increase the production of cyclic guanosine monophosphate (cGMP) in the muscle cells by blocking the production of PDE5. cGMP is a chemical produced by the body that allows the arteries in the penis to relax and, as a result, increases blood flow. In terms of toxicity, efficacy, and tolerance, all three medications are similar. However, they differ in how long they last; sildenafil and vardenafil are effective for up to 4 hours, whereas tadalafil can last up to 36 hours.

As with all medications, side effects are possible, as are interactions with other medications. Consequently, consultation with a clinician is required before these medications are taken. It is not wise to order Viagra or other medications over the Internet, because potential medication interactions or health conditions may not be reviewed by a qualified health professional and the pills received may contain no medication or a different medication than that ordered. Common side effects of the PDE5 inhibitors include effects on vision, possible temporary hearing loss, and headache. Because of the possible drop in blood pressure, individuals using organic nitrates or nitric oxide should avoid taking PDE5 medications.

Those who have had a recent stroke or myocardial infarction or who have excessively low or high blood pressure or severe liver impairment should also avoid using these medications. One concern with all PDE5 inhibitors is the risk of priapism—that is, a prolonged erection lasting several hours. If the priapism is caused by the blood being unable to leave the penis, the blood in the penis will lose oxygen and become toxic, which can cause damage or destroy tissues. An untreated priapism can result in erectile dysfunction and disfiguration of the penis (Mayo Foundation for Medical Education and Research, 2013).

It is important to note that PDE5 medications will not increase desire, only the erection. Consequently, some therapists are concerned that taking these medications may create unrealistic expectations for a couple about the regularity and duration of sex activity (Rosen et al., 2006). To use a crude analogy, Viagra just cleans the hose of a car—it does not fill the vehicle with gas. Some wonder about women taking Viagra or other medications; several years ago there was even a *Sex in the City* episode about it. In reality, these medications seem to have little effect on women's sexual functioning when used alone because of the complex etiology of women's arousal (Chivers & Rosen, 2010).

In addition to oral drugs, other treatments for erectile dysfunction may include injections, devices, and prostheses. A vasoactive liquid medication or combination of vasodilators can be injected into the corpus cavernosum of the penis, promoting erection. Injections are safe if used properly, but problems with administration, the required extensive education of patients and their partners, and side effects prevent them from being widely used.

Men could also use a vacuum constriction device (VCD), which provides a noninvasive, effective, and safe option for those experiencing erectile dysfunction. The VCD is an acrylic cylinder used with a vacuum pump; the device creates a vacuum that promotes erection. The penis is inserted into the cylinder, and a hand- or battery-operated pump draws air from the cylinder. The reduced air pressure in the cylinder allows increased blood flow to the penis, causing an erection. Blood is trapped in the penis by a tourniquet or other device around the base of the penis. (It is important to remove the tourniquet after sexual activity or there could be damage to the penis.) Many couples find this method inconvenient, which limits its use. As a last option, penile prostheses are available to those men who do not respond

to other medical treatments. This option requires invasive and irreversible surgery that may result in scarring and infection and that frequently does not meet patient or partner expectations.

Although oral medications are successful for more than 65% of men with erectile dysfunction (Shamloul & Ghanem, 2013), it is important to consider psychological factors as well. How does one restart a sexual life after an extended period of abstinence? How does one address partner resistance? What happens when the medication addresses the erectile dysfunction but the partner is now identified as having a sexual concern or dysfunction? Even with medication, how does an individual handle lack of confidence, performance anxiety, depression, relationship issues, or unrealistic expectations? It is estimated that 60% to 70% of those men taking PED5s ultimately stop this treatment (Rosen et al., 2004). However, if strategies address both psychological and physiological issues, success rates are higher (Althof, 2010). Specific counseling strategies and other techniques are described later in this section.

Treating Early Ejaculation

Two behavioral techniques are used to help men control early ejaculation. The first is the **squeeze technique**, developed by Masters and Johnson (Figure 20.2), which entails a gentle squeezing of the penis while the man is experiencing full erection. When the man begins to feel the urge to ejaculate,

FIGURE **20.2** The squeeze technique. The man signals his partner to squeeze when ejaculation is approaching.

---

squeeze technique A method of helping men control early ejaculation whereby the penis is gently squeezed when the man senses ejaculation is imminent.

the partner grasps the penis with the thumb on the underside where the shaft ends and the head begins and two fingers on the opposite side. The partner then squeezes for 3 to 4 seconds, after which the urge to ejaculate will have passed. After 15 to 30 seconds, stimulation is provided to full erection once more and the procedure is repeated as necessary. Eventually the man learns to control his ejaculation without his partner's help.

The second technique for learning ejaculatory control is called the **Semans stop–start method**, named for its developer, James Semans. With this technique, the man lies on his back and concentrates on his feelings and sensations as his partner stimulates his penis manually (Figure 20.3). When he feels ejaculation approaching, he tells his partner to stop stimulating him. The couple repeats the procedure until the man learns ejaculatory control.

Both of these techniques allow the man to recognize mid-level ranges of excitement and to modify his response. Other behavioral strategies include changing the tempo of thrusting, changing the angle or depth of penetration, shifting one's thoughts to other events, talking to oneself ("self-talk"), and focusing on the nongenital aspects of the experience. The use of a condom can also help because the glans penis is not stimulated directly. Alternatively, some men allow a rapid orgasm, or a small orgasm, knowing that the next one will take longer to arrive. If engaging in penetration, ensuring that there is adequate lubrication may help decrease sensitivity of the glans.

Some medications have also been found to control early ejaculation; these include antidepressants, PED5s (either alone or in combination with antidepressants), and tramadol, a pain medication (Althof et al., 2014). Creams designed to decrease sensitivity can be placed on the glans; however, whether the benefit of controlling the ejaculate is worth the price

FIGURE **20.4** Sensate focus allows for nondemanding stimulation.

of reduced sensations (possibly for the partner as well) is a decision that only the man and his partner can make.

Treating Delayed Ejaculation

The therapy for delayed ejaculation includes the technique known as sensate focus (described in the next subsection), which helps the man focus on his sensual feelings and learn to derive pleasure from sexual behavior. Included in this treatment, in a stepwise fashion, is learning to ejaculate by masturbating alone, by masturbating with his sexual partner present, by asking the partner to masturbate him to ejaculation, and by asking the partner to masturbate him to the point just short of ejaculation and then inserting the penis into the partner to ejaculate.

Sensate Focus

Sex therapists treat sexual unresponsiveness in both men and women by teaching the couple a technique termed **sensate focus**. The idea behind this method is to encourage the couple to experience erotic feelings short of penetration so that they will learn to accept sexual pleasuring (both giving and receiving) as part of their lives. The therapist gives the unresponsive partner permission and encouragement to feel nonthreatening sexual feelings, on the assumption that the client has withheld permission from himself or herself (for whatever individual subconscious reason). Eventually the therapy incorporates penetration into the sensate focus program. Figure 20.4 illustrates one of the sensate-focusing positions taught to couples.

FIGURE **20.3** The Semans procedure. The man signals his partner to stop stimulation when he senses that ejaculation is close.

Semans stop-start method A method of controlling early ejaculation (developed by James Semans) in which the man tells his partner to stop stimulating him when he feels ejaculation approaching.

sensate focus A method of alleviating sexual unresponsiveness by procedures designed to encourage erotic feelings and sexual pleasuring.

Barbach's Technique

Barbach's technique, effective in treating both sexual arousal and orgasmic disorders in women, has been widely disseminated to the general public through Lonnie Barbach's book *For Yourself: The Fulfillment of Female Sexuality* (2000). A woman begins the program by setting aside an hour a day for exploring her body visually (with a mirror) and manually (using body lotion or powder), all the time focusing upon feelings and sensations. Next she is led to do a vulva self-examination and vulva self-stimulation with a body lotion or oil. It is important at this stage that orgasm *not* be the goal of the self-stimulation. Rather, the woman is encouraged to become aware of and focus on pleasurable sensations. Eventually the program leads the woman to seek orgasm by using the touching technique she found to be most pleasurable during the self-stimulation stage. The use of a vibrator is recommended for women who still find orgasm elusive after manual stimulation. However, after the woman experiences orgasm with a vibrator, she is encouraged to practice manual stimulation. This transfer is important in helping her to have orgasm with a sexual partner.

Combating Pain Disorders

After a thorough examination and other diagnostic tests to rule out a physical cause, pain disorders are treated by a combination of education and practice. The education component entails instruction about the anatomy and physiology of the human sexual response and reproductive systems. Many pain conditions in women stem from the pelvic floor, with contractions of the muscles of the vagina that prevent penetration; training a woman to control these muscles allows her to relax the muscle when it begins to contract. The best manner in which to carry out this training appears to be teaching the woman to contract and relax the muscles, becoming conscious of the sensations that accompany both contracted and relaxed vaginal muscles. Next slender rods—first a very narrow one and eventually wider ones—are inserted by the woman into the vagina with relaxed muscles. Once this is mastered (about 1 week), the next step is penetration in a partnered sexual activity with the woman controlling the process. Many times a physical therapist who specializes in pelvic

floor dysfunction works with the client to assist with these exercises.

If the pain is a result of insufficient lubrication during penetration, treatment is similar to that used for arousal disorders, such as sensate focus or mindfulness.

Behavior Therapy Model

Joseph Wolpe developed a manner of treating anxiety as the cause of sexual dysfunction. Termed **systematic desensitization**, this model can be applied to people who are anxious about sex. Wolpe reasoned that if people were muscularly relaxed, they could not be anxious at the same time. Consequently, he taught people deep muscle relaxation techniques and then instructed them to think of the anxiety-provoking stimulus. For example, sexually dysfunctional patients might imagine their arms and legs are heavy, warm, and tingly (a relaxation technique called *autogenic training*). Once relaxed, they could imagine the sexual activity about which they feel anxious.

Systematic desensitization also assumes that the gradual introduction of anxiety-provoking stimuli will not produce anxious feelings. Thus this technique involves a fear hierarchy: The initial stimuli are not anxiety provoking, but very gradually more anxiety-provoking stimuli are introduced. For example, the following might be the fear hierarchy of a woman (Ted's partner) who experiences a genital pain disorder:

1. I go out to a movie with Ted.
2. Ted and I return home and are alone.
3. Ted places his arm around me.
4. Ted nuzzles my neck.
5. Ted fondles my breast.
6. Ted takes my clothes off.
7. Ted removes his clothing.
8. Ted stimulates my clitoris and vagina.
9. Ted inserts his finger into my vagina.
10. Ted inserts his penis into my vagina.

The woman is then asked to imagine the first event in the fear hierarchy without feeling anxious—that is, without an increasing heart rate and rapid, shallow breathing. If she can imagine that event for 30 seconds without feeling anxious, she does deep muscle relaxation for 30 seconds. Then she moves to the next event of the hierarchy. The idea is to take very small steps from something that does not make her anxious to the point at which she is involved in

Barbach's technique A method of treating orgasmic dysfunction and sexual unresponsiveness developed by Lonnie Barbach that focuses on awareness of feelings and sensations through self-exploration and stimulation.

systematic desensitization A means of overcoming anxiety by approaching the anxiety-provoking stimulus in small steps.

the activity that was the problem—in the example, allowing penile insertion (Greenberg, 2009).

Behaviorists are concerned with the behavior in question, not the underlying reasons for that behavior. They do not spend a great deal of time analyzing why someone feels or thinks as he or she does. Rather, they begin to manipulate the behavior so it is transformed into the desired behavior. To do this, therapists sometimes employ a technique called *shaping*. Shaping involves rewarding small behaviors along the way to developing the behavior that is the goal of the therapy. For example, if a person becomes anxious on dates, and therefore refuses to accept a date, the therapist might have the person begin by just speaking to a love interest on the telephone. For doing that, he or she would receive a reward (for example, maybe a pass to a movie theater). To receive a reward the next week, however, the patient needs to spend a few minutes in face-to-face contact with that other person—and so on, until the patient goes out on a date without anxiety.

Self-Care Model

Several of the models and techniques of sex therapy can be self-administered. For example, couples can employ the stop–start technique or the squeeze technique, and individuals can try systematic desensitization or shaping by themselves. In this way, they can save some money and whatever inconvenience is associated with attending therapy. A good first step to solving problems associated with sexual functioning, given that any medical cause has been ruled out, is to employ these self-care techniques (van Lankveld, 2009). If they are not successful, the person should consider seeking the help of a trained sexuality counselor or sex therapist. Often the trained eye can observe something that the untrained cannot.

The Next Era of Sex Therapy

You may have noticed that many of the references in the previous treatment sections were older. These methods are effective and used regularly today, but there are new ideas in sex therapy as well. Althof (2010) identified four innovations in sex therapy: combination of medical and psychological treatment, mindfulness, sex therapy via the Internet, and the reconceptualization of genital pain.

While many psychologists and psychiatrists use medications and therapy to treat mental health disorders (think antidepressants and counseling for depression), there is some resistance in the field of sex therapy regarding this approach. Both medical treatment and counseling strategies have their benefits, but by treating these issues from both perspectives the results are more successful for erectile dysfunction

and early ejaculation. Althof (2010) believes that future pharmacologic advancements will address female arousal and other disorders, and practitioners and clients need to be open to combining treatment strategies. Berry and Berry (2013) drew a similar conclusion after conducting a literature review of published intervention strategies over the last three decades; while policies and best practices advocate for a comprehensive approach, continued exploration and model development that incorporates the biological, psychological, and social factors are needed.

Mindfulness is the practice of intentionally being aware of one's thoughts, emotions, and physical sensations without judgment. Brotto and colleagues (Brotto, Basson, & Luria, 2008; Brotto, Heiman, et al., 2008; Brotto et al., 2012) have designed studies that incorporate mindfulness techniques for women who have low desire and arousal disorders. Results have shown that for depressed women and survivors of childhood sexual abuse, the technique of calming the "busy mind" may be especially helpful in increasing desire and interest in sex.

Sex therapy via the Internet is controversial. Benefits of therapy delivery via this mode can include easy accessibility, the removal of constraints related to geographic location and time, and a reduction in embarrassment or humiliation. At the same time, there are concerns related to the subtleties lost in communication without the face-to-face interaction, misinterpretation of written text, and concerns about security and confidentiality of data transmitted via the Internet, as well as professional liability issues. Recent published studies in this area (Hucker & McCabe, 2015; Jones & McCabe, 2011) show promise, and further investigation especially into the use of video chatting is warranted.

The last innovation identified by Althof (2010) is the reconceptualization of genital pain disorders and treatment. Previously, dyspareunia and vaginismus were considered sexual dysfunctions, but recent studies have advocated for practitioners to focus on the pain and not on the function being disturbed (i.e., sex). This reconceptualization incorporates pain management techniques as treatment, which has resulted in moderate success for women.

Other Kinds of Therapy

Other kinds of therapy are also used to treat sexual dysfunction. Some forms of therapy and counseling that are not focused particularly on sexual response can help people with sexual dysfunctions as well, especially when conditions are rooted in a more generalized lack of self-acceptance and self-esteem. Also beneficial in some cases is counseling or therapy directed toward improving communication in the nonsexual aspects of a relationship—for example, marriage counseling, family counseling, or crisis counseling for couples.

If you experience any of the sexual dysfunctions described in this chapter, you may want to ask your instructor or student-health service personnel for a referral to a qualified sex therapist. Paying attention to your sexual responsiveness is part of maintaining total well-being. A dysfunction in the sexual aspect of your life requires the same concern and treatment as any other chronic ailment. We are fortunate to live in a time when effective sex therapy based on sound scientific research is generally available.

Choosing a Sex Therapist

For sex therapy to be effective, the therapist must be qualified. How can you determine this? Someone who claims to be a sex therapist is not necessarily competent in that particular area of expertise. To enhance your chances of choosing a qualified sex therapist, consider the following points:

1. *Does this person have a degree in a recognized profession related to counseling and therapy?* Psychology, marriage and family counseling, pastoral counseling, and social work are examples.

2. *Does this person hold a license or a certification related to counseling and therapy?* Some professions are licensed by the state (psychologists), whereas others are certified by professional organizations (e.g., marriage counselors).

3. *Is this person certified by the American Association of Sex Educators, Counselors, and Therapists (AASECT)?* Certification by this professional organization ensures the person has had training specific to sexuality issues.

4. *Do you know other people who have been helped by this therapist?* Sometimes the best referral is that of someone who has experienced therapy and benefited from it.

To begin choosing a sex therapist, consult local resources. The psychology, counseling, social work, or health education department at your university might be able to help, as might your campus health center. A local health department or sexually transmitted infection clinic may be able to make a referral. Alternatively, you could contact AASECT for a referral in your area.

When first meeting the therapist, or talking with office personnel on the telephone, do not hesitate to inquire about the fee, the therapist's background and qualifications, the licenses and/or certifications the therapist holds, and the usual course of therapy provided for situations such as yours (length of treatment, type of treatment, and so on). Any therapist who objects to you asking these questions should be considered suspect. Reputable therapists should be glad that you are taking such an active interest in obtaining effective treatment—that type of motivation is critical for a successful outcome.

Exploring the Dimensions of Human Sexuality

Case Study

Many sexual disorders are multidimensional. In fact, at different times, there can be different causes. Consider an otherwise healthy male who, after getting too little sleep during the week and ingesting too much alcohol, is unable to achieve and maintain an erection with his partner. The dysfunction here is likely physiological. If he understands that alcohol and lack of sleep are to blame, he will probably be fine. However, if he perceives that he "failed" sexually, he may suffer from performance anxiety during his next sexual encounter.

Partners, too, may blame themselves for sexual dysfunction. When partners call into question their attractiveness or sexual ability, their self-esteem may suffer. Further, they may isolate themselves from sexual situations so as not to "cause" failure again.

Both sexuality education and communication can help couples avoid sexual anxiety. The former would help both partners realize why the initial dysfunction occurred. And communication could help both partner's self-esteem, by letting the other person know that he or she is desired.

Biological Factors

- Some sexual dysfunctions have physiological causes. Age is sometimes a factor, as normal changes in the human body affect sexual desire and arousal.
- Alcohol, drug abuse, and certain medications (e.g., agents used for depression) can interfere with sexual response.

Sociocultural Factors

- The sexual double standard suggests that men be experienced and talented in sexual matters, leading their partners to sexual bliss. Failure to live up to such expectations can lead to psychological problems.
- Mass media create unrealistic sexual expectations that no real person can meet.
- Relationship problems can lead to some disorders.
- Rigid religious convictions that certain sexual activities are immoral may lead to negative attitudes toward sexuality.

Psychological Factors

- Sexual functioning is closely connected to self-esteem. Men and women with sexual dysfunctions may feel less confident and secure because they do not function as well sexually as they wish. Low self-esteem, guilt, or depression can lead to some sexual disorders.
- Gay men, lesbians, and bisexual people seeking treatment for disorders may also confront society's negative attitudes about non-heterosexuals.
- Failure to perform as expected can be devastating psychologically. In turn, such perceived failure could lead to isolation from sexual activities, which would cause further embarrassment. Fear of future sexual inadequacy can be a self-fulfilling prophecy that can result in lowered self-esteem.

Summary

- An individual's sexual desire is not constant; it varies according to situational, emotional, and physical factors. Sexual dysfunction is a *chronic* inability to respond sexually in a way one finds satisfying.

- Lifelong sexual dysfunctions are those in which the person has never been functional in a sexual activity. Acquired sexual dysfunctions are those in which the person was functional at one time but no longer is.

- Male sexual dysfunctions include erectile dysfunction (inability to achieve an erection), early ejaculation (not maintaining penile insertion long enough before ejaculating), delayed ejaculation (inability to ejaculate after sufficient sexual stimulation), male hypoactive sexual desire disorder (low arousal), and genital pain.

- Female sexual dysfunctions include female arousal disorder (not experiencing erotic pleasure from sexual stimulation), orgasmic dysfunction (inability to have an orgasm during sexual activities), and genital pain disorders.

- Both males and females may experience sexual desire dysfunctions, dissatisfaction with sexual frequency, persistent genital arousal disorder (intense unwanted, unrelenting genital arousal that causes distress) and hypersexuality (recurrent intense sexual fantasies, urges, or behaviors that are difficult to control and cause distress).

- Sexual dysfunctions can have physical causes, such as diseases, medications, or blocked blood vessels. They may also be caused by psychological factors, such as low self-esteem, guilt and shame, stress, past sexual abuse, or performance anxiety.

- Among the approaches to treat sexual dysfunctions are the PLISSIT model, teams of cotherapists, the squeeze technique, the stop–start method, sensate focus, surgery, mindfulness, and medication.

Discussion Questions

1. Review the major male and female sexual dysfunctions, including features of diagnosis. What determines what a typical person might consider a sexual problem and what a sex therapist diagnoses as a sexual dysfunction?

2. List the specific physical, psychological, and sociocultural dimensions that can affect sexual performance. Explain how each could have an effect. (Be specific: Religion is a factor, but state the specific religion. Would it affect all members of that religion or only specific people with a high degree of religiosity?)

3. Examine the many types of sex therapy available. Then evaluate which you think would work best for erectile disorder and female arousal disorder. Explain your answer.

Application Questions

Reread the chapter-opening story and answer the following questions.

1. Explain why when a celebrity or a politician discloses a personal problem, it seems easier for the general public to talk about the issue involved. Contrast that with how you might react if a classmate announced in class that he or she had a sexual dysfunction.

2. We know that Elizabeth Dole smiled when asked about Viagra. But if she had been asked about her sex life with Bob before his disclosure, how might she have reacted? Would she have revealed his "dysfunction" (related to prostate-cancer surgery)? If Viagra had not been developed, would either Bob or Elizabeth have realized that there was a dysfunction?

Critical Thinking Questions

1. Masters and Johnson claimed that male and female cotherapists were needed to treat a couple. They reasoned that only a person of the same gender as the client could really understand a sexual problem or dysfunction. Do you agree with Masters and Johnson, or could a couple be successfully treated by one therapist (of either gender)? Explain your answer.

2. The success of the drug Viagra was unprecedented: 36,000 prescriptions in the first week after it became available, 3.6 million prescriptions in the first 4 months. Although it is clear that many of the patients had erectile disorders, there is strong anecdotal information to suggest that some men were experimenting with Viagra to improve their sex life. Consider the physical, psychological, and sociocultural dimensions of such experimentation (e.g., the belief you cannot perform without the pill, the ethics of getting a doctor to write a prescription). Would you take a drug that could possibly improve your sex life, even if it had associated risks?

Critical Thinking Case

Before the 1960s, hardly anyone had heard of sexual dysfunction. However, soon after Masters and Johnson's book *Human Sexual Response* was published in 1966, the prevalence of sexual dysfunctions seemed to skyrocket. Some have argued that there are more sexual problems than in previous years because of the greater emphasis people place on sex today. We can now view sexually explicit material on the Internet, we can purchase erotic print media at the local bookstore or listen to sexually charged music and lyrics, and we can even observe simulated sex during daytime hours on reality TV or on the Internet. This emphasis on sex, the argument continues, has created unrealistic expectations for people, and when they cannot "perform" as they observe others can, they become dysfunctional.

There is another view, however. Perhaps there was as much sexual dysfunction before 1966 as there is today; however, sex was not a topic for conversation, so problems remained undisclosed. The result was that people were unable to achieve sexual satisfaction.

What is your view? Is there more sexual dysfunction now, or has disclosure of sexual problems increased? Is the situation better today, or was it better before 1966? Is there too much pressure for people to "perform" sexually today?

Exploring Personal Dimensions

What Constitutes Sexual Dysfunction?

Perspectives on what constitutes a sexual dysfunction vary. One important consideration is that if you and your partner are satisfied with your sexual relationship, you probably do not have a disorder. If you do not participate in any sexual activity, skip this assessment. With that in mind,

answer the following statements with one of the following responses:

a. Rarely or never

b. Sometimes

c. Often

d. All or most of the time

1. I fantasize about sex.

2. I think about sex.

3. I am able to become aroused.

4. I remain aroused during sexual activities.

5. I enjoy having sex with my partner.

6. I engage in masturbation more than I feel is normal.

7. I worry about my sexual performance.

8. I feel worried about having sexual relations.

Male:

9. I experience pain when I have an erection or ejaculate.

10. I am able to achieve an erection.

Female:

11. I experience pain during vaginal penetration.

12. I have difficulty reaching an orgasm.

This self-assessment is not meant to be scored. Rather, it is intended as a tool to allow you to think critically about sexual performance and dysfunction.

After you have given initial responses to these questions, go back and review them two more times. The first time, consider whether you are satisfied with your initial response. In other words, think about whether you are happy with that particular aspect of your sexuality. The second time, consider whether your partner may be satisfied with your initial response.

For example, a man with a spinal cord injury may not be able to achieve an erection. That situation may still be acceptable to both him and his partner, if they have found other satisfying sexual activities in which to engage.

Suggested Readings

Buehler, S. *What every mental health professional needs to know about sex*. New York: Springer, 2014.

Coady, D., & Fish, N. *Healing painful sex: A woman's guide to confronting, diagnosing, and treating sexual pain*. Berkeley, CA: Seal Press, 2011.

Kleinplatz, P. J., ed. *New directions in sex therapy: Innovations and alternatives* (2nd ed.). New York: Routledge, 2012.

McCarthy, B., & McCarthy, E. *Rekindling desire* (2nd ed.). New York: Routledge, 2014.

Metz, M. E., & McCarthy, B. *Coping with erectile dysfunction: How to regain confidence and enjoy great sex.* Oakland, CA: New Harbinger, 2004.

Moynihan, R., & Mintzes, B. *Sex, lies, and pharmaceuticals: How drug companies plan to profit from female sexual dysfunction.* Vancouver: Greystone Books, 2010.

Web Resources

American Urology Association Foundation: Erectile Dysfunction

www.urologyhealth.org/urology/index.cfm?article=60

The educational arm of the American Urology Association, this website provides detailed information on nonsurgical options for treatment of erectile dysfunction. The site includes visuals to assist in understanding the condition. Links to updated pamphlets are provided.

Medline Plus: Sexual Problems in Men and Sexual Problems in Women

www.nlm.nih.gov/medlineplus/sexualproblemsinmen .html and *www.nlm.nih.gov/medlineplus /sexualproblemsinwomen.html*

Managed by the National Library of Medicine, these websites provide links to an overview of female and male sexual dysfunctions, diagnosis, symptoms, treatment, prevention and screening, coping, management, clinical trials, and others.

Sexual Advice Association

www.sda.uk.net

Operated by a charitable organization in the United States, this website provides information about male and female sexual dysfunctions with links to news and articles and frequently asked questions.

Society for Sex Therapy and Research

www.sstarnet.org

The Society for Sex Therapy and Research (SSTAR) is composed of a broad range of professionals who have clinical or research interests in human sexual concerns. SSTAR's goals are to facilitate communication among clinicians who treat problems of sexual function, sexual identity, and reproductive life, and to provide a forum for exchange of ideas between those interested in research in human sexuality and those whose primary activities are patient care.

References

Althof, S. E. What's new in sex therapy. *Journal of Sexual Medicine, 7* (2010), 5–13.

Althof, S. E., McMahon, C. G., Waldinger, M. D., Serefoglu, E. C., Shindel, A. W., Adaikan, P. G., et al. An update of the International Society of Sexual Medicine's guidelines for the diagnosis and treatment of premature ejaculation (PE). *Journal of Sexual Medicine, 11* (2014), 1392–1422.

Annon, J. S. *The behavioral treatment of sexual problems: Brief therapy.* New York: Harper & Row, 1976.

Bancroft, J. *Human sexuality and its problems* (3rd ed.). Edinburgh: Churchill Livingston/Elsevier, 2009.

Bancroft, J., Graham, C. A., Janssen, E., & Sanders, S. A. The dual-control model: Current status and future directions. *Journal of Sex Research, 46* (2009), 121–142.

Bancroft, J., Loftus, J., & Long, J. S. Distress about sex: A national survey of women in heterosexual relationships. *Archives of Sexual Behavior, 32* (2003), 193–208.

Barbach, L. G. *Women discover orgasm: A therapist's guide to a New Testament approach.* New York: Free Press, 1980.

Barbach, L. G. *For yourself: The fulfillment of female sexuality.* New York: Signet, 2000.

Barbach, L. *For each other: Sharing sexual intimacy.* New York: New American Library, 2001.

Berry, M. D., & Berry, P.D. Contemporary treatment of sexual dysfunction: Reexamining the biopsychosocial model. *Journal of Sexual Medicine, 10* (2013), 2627–2643.

Binik, Y. The *DSM* diagnostic criteria for dyspareunia. *Archives of Sexual Behavior, 39, 2* (2010), 292–303.

Bradley, P. D., & Fine, R. W. The Medicalization of sex therapy: A call to action for therapists. *Journal of Systemic Therapies, 28, 2* (2009), 75–88.

Brotto, L. A. The *DSM* diagnostic criteria for hypoactive sexual desire disorder in men. *Journal of Sexual Medicine, 7* (2010a), 2015–2030.

Brotto, L. A. The *DSM* diagnostic criteria for hypoactive sexual desire disorder in women. *Archives of Sexual Behavior, 39* (2010b), 221–239.

Brotto, L. A. The *DSM* diagnostic criteria for sexual aversion disorder. *Archives of Sexual Behavior, 39, 2* (2010c), 271–277.

Brotto, L., Basson, R., & Luria, M. A mindfulness-based group psychoeducational intervention targeting sexual arousal disorder in women. *Journal of Sexual Medicine, 5* (2008), 1646–1659.

Brotto, L. A., Bitzer, J., Laan, E., Leiblum, S., & Luria, M. Women's sexual desire and arousal disorders. *Journal of Sexual Medicine, 7* (2010), 586–614. doi: 10.1111/j.1743-6109.2009.01630.x.

Brotto, L., Heiman, J., Goff, B., Greer, B., Lentz, G., Swisher, E., et al. A psychoeducational intervention for sexual dysfunction in women with gynecologic cancer. *Archives of Sexual Behavior, 37* (2008), 317–329.

Brotto, L. A., Sealb, B. N., & Rellini, A. Pilot study of a brief cognitive behavioral versus mindfulness-based intervention for women with sexual distress and a history of childhood sexual abuse. *Journal of Sex & Marital Therapy, 38, 1* (2012), 1–27.

Carvalho, J., Verissimo, A. & Nobre, P. J. Psychological factors predicting the distress to female persistent genital arousal symptoms. *Journal of Sex & Marital Therapy, 41* (2015) 11–24.

Chivers, M., & Rosen, R. C. PDE5 inhibitors and female sexual response: Faulty protocols or paradigms? *Journal of Sexual Medicine, 7* (2010), 858–872.

Connora, M. K., Maserejiana, N. N., De Rogatisb, L., Mestonc, C. M., Gerstenbergera, E. P., & Rosena, R. C. Sexual desire, distress, and associated factors in premenopausal women: Preliminary findings from the Hypoactive Sexual Desire Disorder Registry for Women. *Journal of Sex & Marital Therapy, 37, 3* (2011), 176–189.

Davis, S. R., Moreau, M., Kroll, R., Bouchard, C., Panay, N., Gass, M., ... & Studd, J. Testosterone for low libido in postmenopausal women not taking estrogen. *New England Journal of Medicine, 359* (2008), 2005–2017.

DeRogatis, L. R., & Burnett, A. L. The epidemiology of sexual dysfunctions. *Journal of Sexual Medicine, 5* (2008), 289–300.

Ellis, A., & Harper, R. *A guide to rational living.* North Hollywood, CA: Melvin Powers, Wilshire Book Company, 1975.

Ellis, A., & Harper, R. *A new guide to rational living.* Englewood Cliffs, NJ: Prentice-Hall, 1979.

Facelle, T. M., Sadeghi-Nejad, H., & Goldmeier, D. Persistent genital arousal disorder: Characterization, etiology, and management. *Journal of Sexual Medicine, 10* (2013) 439–450.

Farrell, J., & Cacchioni, T. The medicalization of women's sexual pain. *Journal of Sex Research, 49, 4,* (2012), 328–336. doi: 10.1080/00224499.2012.688227.

Fisher, H. *The first sex: The natural talents of women and how they are changing the world.* New York: Ballantine, 1999.

Gambescia, N., Sendak, S. K., & Weeks, G. The treatment of erectile dysfunction. *Journal of Family Psychotherapy, 20* (2009), 221–240.

Ghanem, H. & Porst, H. (2005). Etiology and risk factors of erectile dysfunction. In H. Porst, J. Buvat and The Standards Committee of the International Society for Sexual Medicine (Eds) *Standard Practice in Sexual Medicine,* (pp. 49–58), Malden, MA: Blackwell Publishing, 2005.

Graham, C. A. The *DSM* diagnostic criteria for female orgasmic disorder. *Archives of Sexual Behavior, 39* (2010a), 256–270.

Graham, C. A. The *DSM* diagnostic criteria for female sexual arousal disorder. *Archives of Sexual Behavior, 39* (2010b), 240–255.

Greenberg, J. S. *Comprehensive stress management* (11th ed.). New York: McGraw-Hill Higher Education, 2009.

Heiman, J. R. Treating low sexual desire: New findings for testosterone in women. *New England Journal of Medicine, 359* (2006), 2047–2049.

Hucker, A., & McCabe, M. P. Incorporating mindfulness and chat groups into an online cognitive behavioral therapy for mixed female sexual problems. *Journal of Sex Research, 52* (2015), 627–639.

Jones, L. M., & McCabe, M. P. The effectiveness of an Internet-based psychological treatment program for female sexual dysfunction. *Journal of Sexual Medicine, 8* (2011), 2781–2792.

Kamatchi, R., & Ashley-Smith, A. Persistent genital arousal disorder in a male: A case report and analysis of the cause. *British Journal of Medical Practitioners, 6* (2013), a605.

Kaplan, H. S. *The new sex therapy: Active treatment of sexual dysfunction.* New York: Brunner/Mazel, 1974.

Kaplan, H. S. *Disorders of sexual desire.* New York: Simon & Schuster, 1979.

Kaplan, H. S. *The evaluation of sexual disorders.* New York: Brunner/Mazel, 1983.

Landry, T., & Bergeron, S. How young does vulvo-vaginal pain begin? Prevalence and characteristics of dyspareunia in adolescents. *Journal of Sexual Medicine, 6* (2009), 927–935.

Laumann, E. O., Glasser, D. B., Neves, R. C. S., & Moreira, E., for the GSSAB Investigators' Group. A population-based survey of sexual activity, sexual problems and associated help-seeking behavior patterns in mature adults in the United States of America. *International Journal of Impotence Research, 21* (2009), 171–178.

Leiblum, S. R., & Pervin, L. A. *Principles and practice of sex therapy.* New York: Guilford Press, 1980.

Lewis, R. W., Fugl-Meyer, K. S., Bosch, R., Fugl-Meyer, A. R., Laumann, E. O., Lizza, E., & Martin-Morales, A. Epidemiology/risk factors of sexual dysfunction. *Journal of Sexual Medicine, 1, 1* (2004), 35–39.

Lewis, R. W., Fugl-Meyer, K. S., Corona, G., Hayes, R. D., Laumann, E. O., Moreira, E. D., et al. Definitions/epidemiology/risk factors for sexual dysfunction. *Journal of Sexual Medicine, 7* (2010), 1598–1607.

LoPiccolo, J. Direct treatment of sexual dysfunction in the couple. In *Handbook of sexology*, Money, J., & Masaph, H., eds. Amsterdam: Elsevier/North-Holland, 1977, 1227–1244.

MacBride, M. B., Rhodes, D. J., & Shuster, L. T. Vulvovaginal atrophy. *Mayo Clinic Proceedings, 85* (2010), 87–94.

Mah, K., & Binik, Y. M. The nature of human orgasm: a critical review of major trends. *Clinical Psychology Review, 21* (2001), 823–856.

Marshall, B. L. Medicalization and the refashioning of age-related limits on sexuality. *Journal of Sex Research, 49, 4* (2012), 337–343. doi: 10.1080/00224499.2011.644597.

Masters, W. H., & Johnson, V. E. *Human sexual inadequacy.* Boston: Little, Brown, 1970.

Mayo Foundation for Medical Education and Research. *Priapism*, 2013. Available: http://www.mayoclinic.org/diseases-conditions/priapism/basics/complications/con-20029378.

Mayo Foundation for Medical Education and Research. *Premature ejaculation: Causes*, 2014. Available: http://www.mayoclinic.com/health/premature-ejaculation/DS00578/DSECTION=causes.

McCabe, M. P. Anorgasmia in women, *Journal of Family Psychotherapy, 20* (2009), 177–197.

McCabe, M., Althof, S. E., Assalian, P., Chevret-Measson, M., Leiblum, S. R., Simonelli, C., & Wylie, K. Psychological and interpersonal dimensions of sexual function and dysfunction. *The Journal of Sexual Medicine, 7* (2010), 327–336.

McCabe, M. P., & Connaughton, C. How the prevalence rates of male sexual dysfunction vary using different criteria. *International Journal of Sexual Health, 26* (2014), 229–237.

McCabe, M. P., & Goldhammer, D. L. Demographic and psychological factors related to sexual desire among heterosexual women in a relationship. *Journal of Sex Research, 49* (2012), 78–87.

McCarthy, B. W., Ryan, M., & Johnson, F. A. *Sexual awareness: A practical approach.* San Francisco: Boyd & Fraser, 1975.

Meana, M. Painful intercourse: Dyspareunia and vaginismus *Journal of Family Psychotherapy, 20* (2009), 198–220.

Meana, M., & Binik, Y. M. Painful coitus: A review of female dyspareunia. *Journal of Nervous and Mental Disease, 182* (1994), 264–272.

Meana, M., Oliver, T. L., & Jones, S. C. Assessing sexual dysfunction in Hispanic clients. In L. T. Benuto, ed., *Guide to psychological assessment with Hispanics.* New York: Springer, 2013, 183–199.

Michetti, P. M., Eleuteri, S., Giuliani, M., Rossi, R., & Simonelli, C. Delayed ejaculation and alexithymia: What is the relationship? *F1000 Research, 2* (2013), 81.

Nagaraj, A. K. M., Pai, N. B., & Rao, S. A comparative study of sexual dysfunction involving risperidone, quetiapine, and olanzapine. *Indian Journal of Psychiatry, 51* (2009), 265–271.

Perelman, M. A., & Rowland, D. L. Retarded ejaculation. *World Journal of Urology, 24, 6* (2006), 645–652. doi: 10.1007/s00345-006-0127-6.

Petersen, J., & Hyde, J. S. Gender differences in sexuality. In J. C. Chrisler & D. R. McCreary, eds., *Handbook of gender research in psychology.* (pp. 471–491) New York: Springer, 2010.

Reid, R. C., & Kafka, M. P. Controversies about hypersexual disorder and the *DSM-5. Current Sexual Health Reports, 6* (2014), 259–264. doi: 10.1007/s11930-014-0031-9.

Reissing, E. D., Binik, Y. M., Khalife, S., Cohen, D., & Amsel, R. Vaginal spasm, pain, and behavior: An empirical investigation of the diagnosis of vaginismus. *Archives of Sexual Behavior, 33* (2004), 5–17.

Rosen, R., Janssen, E., Wiegel, M., Bancroft, J., Althof, S., Wincze, J., et al. Psychological and interpersonal correlates in men with erectile dysfunction and their partners. *Journal of Sex & Marital Therapy, 32* (2006), 215–234.

Rosen, R. C., Fisher, W. A., Eardley, I., Niederberger, C., Nadel, A., & Sand, M. The multinational Men's Attitudes to Life Events and Sexuality (MALES) study: I. Prevalence of erectile dysfunction and related health concerns in the general population. *Current Medical Research and Opinion, 20* (2004), 607–617.

Segraves, R. T. Considerations for diagnostic criteria for erectile dysfunction in *DSM V. Journal of Sexual Medicine, 7* (2010), 654–671.

Segraves, R. T., & Balon, R. Antidepressant-induced sexual dysfunction in men. *Pharmacology Biochemistry and Behavior, 121* (2014), 132–137. doi: 10.1016/j.pbb.2013.11.003.

Semans, J. Premature ejaculation: A new approach. *Southern Medical Journal, 49* (1956), 353–358.

Serefoglu, E. C., McMahon, C. G., Waldinger, M. D., Althof, S. E., Shindel, A., Adaikan, G., et al. An evidence-based unified definition of lifelong and acquired premature ejaculation: Report of the second International Society for Sexual Medicine Ad Hoc Committee for the Definition of Premature Ejaculation. *Journal of Sexual Medicine, 11* (2014), 1423–1441.

Serefoglu, E. C., & Saitz, T. R. New insights on premature ejaculation: A review of definition, classification, prevalence and treatment. *Asian Journal of Andrology, 14* (2012), 822–829. doi: 10.1038/aja.2012.108.

Shamloul, R., & Ghanem, H. Erectile dysfunction. *Lancet, 381* (2013), 153–165. doi: 10.1016/S0140-6736(12)60520-0.

Snegroff, S. The stressors of non-marital sexual intercourse. *Health Education, 17* (1986), 21–23.

Štulhofer, A., Šević, S., & Doyle, D. M. Comparing the prevalence and correlates of sexual health disturbances among heterosexual and nonheterosexual men: An overview of studies. *Sexual Medicine Reviews, 2* (2014), 102–111.

Sungur, M. Z., & Gündüz, A. A comparison of *DSM-IV-TR* and *DSM-5* definitions for sexual dysfunctions: Critiques and challenges. *Journal of Sexual Medicine, 11* (2014), 364–373.

Tan, H. M., Tong, S. F., & Ho, C. C. K. Men's health: Sexual dysfunction, physical, and psychological health: Is there a link? *Journal of Sexual Medicine, 9* (2012), 663–671.

Tiefer, L. Beyond the medical model of women's sexual problems: A campaign to resist the promotion of 'female sexual dysfunction.' *Sexual and Relationship Therapy, 25, 2* (2010), 197–205.

Trustees of Columbia University. *What is pre-orgasmic?*, 2012. Available: http://goaskalice.columbia.edu/what-pre-orgasmic.

van Lankveld, J. Self-help therapies for sexual dysfunction. *Journal of Sex Research, 46* (2009), 143–155.

van Lankveld, J. J. D. M., Granot, M., Weijmar Schultz, W. C. M., Binik, Y. M., Wesselmann, U., Pukall, C. F., et al. Women's sexual pain disorders. *Journal of Sexual Medicine, 7* (2010), 615–631.

Van Minnen, A., & Kampman, M. The interaction between anxiety and sexual functioning: A controlled study of sexual functioning in women with anxiety disorders. *Sexual and Relationship Therapy, 15* (2000), 47–57.

Weeks, G. R., Hertlein, K. M., & Gambescia, N. The treatment of hypoactive sexual desire disorder. *Journal of Family Psychotherapy, 20* (2009), 129–149.

Wilson, G. T., Nathan, P. E., O'Leary, K. D., & Clark, L. A. *Abnormal psychology: Integrating perspectives.* Needham, MA: Allyn & Bacon, 1996.

Winters, J., Christoff, K., & Gorzalka, B. B. Dysregulated sexuality and high sexual desire: distinct constructs? *Archives of Sexual Behavior, 39* (2010), 1029–1043.

Wolpe, J. *Psychotherapy by reciprocal inhibition.* Stanford, CA: Stanford University Press, 1958.

Working Group on A New View of Women's Sexual Problems. *A new view of women's sexual problems*, 2000. Available: http://www.newviewcampaign.org/manifesto5.asp.

Zenilman, J. M., & Shahmanesh, M. *Sexually transmitted infections: Diagnosis, management, and treatment.* Burlington, MA: Jones & Bartlett Learning, 2011.

CHAPTER 21

Sexual Consumerism

© Gayvoronskaya Yana/Shutterstock

FEATURES

Communication Dimensions
Feelings About Sexual Themes

Ethical Dimensions
Controlling Cyberspace

Gender Dimensions
Male and Female Use of Pornography

Ethical Dimensions
Should Kids Be Sexualized?

Multicultural Dimensions
"Values" of Prostitution in Other Countries?

Multicultural Dimensions
Organizations for Sex Workers

Global Dimensions
International Differences Related to Prostitution

CHAPTER OBJECTIVES

1 Describe the ways in which sexuality is used in the mass media, including advertising, TV, movies, literature, popular music, and on the Internet.

2 Discuss what constitutes sexually explicit materials, the results of research on their effects, and efforts to control their distribution.

3 Describe the different types of sex workers and the economic factors associated with sex work.

INTRODUCTION

Not long ago, in a human sexuality class, the conversation turned to the relationship between sexuality and money. Some students were surprised when others became very interested in the topic. They seemed to feel that there was nothing to be gained by continuing the conversation because they did not see a relationship between sexuality and money.

The students interested in the topic persisted. One of the communication majors pointed out that in his classes he learned that messages and products related to sexuality are big business. The saying "You've come a long way, baby" definitely applies to this topic for better or worse, he pointed out. He went on to say that we are all bombarded with sexual themes daily; that you cannot turn on TV, pick up a magazine, or see a billboard without being confronted with sexual topics and themes. This use of sexual content, he indicated, is designed to sell even products that have no relation to sexuality.

Some other students warmed up to the discussion. One student, a psychology major, mentioned that commercialism related to sexuality has taken another form as well. Products specifically related to sexuality are available in large numbers and in great variety. Whether you want to put it in, dangle it about, or place it on, there is a store where you can get whatever "it" is.

Several students started arguing about whether the use of sexual themes to influence consumers is good or bad. One health education major argued that the use of sexual themes to sell products unrelated to sexuality is sexploitation, with the potential for sexism. He said this situation could prompt people to view others as sex objects, and it could interfere with personal relationships and sexual satisfaction as well—because when one *compares one's partner against the commercialized ideal seen in the media, one is likely to be disappointed. This could lead to frustration and a mean-spiritedness that might translate into poor communication, sexual and otherwise.*

Another student, a business major, jumped into the fray and added that the pressure to be like people in the ads—sexy, gorgeous, hunky—may cause people to feel inferior and ashamed of their body. Feelings of inferiority and shame, as we learned earlier, can progress to sexual dysfunction.

Still another student pointed out that appearance may not be the only concern. She expressed concern that as the result of observing the sexual prowess of television and movie stars on-screen, we assume that all of us should be able to affect our partners the same way. If they do not swoon at the very thought of a caress from us, if they do not get light-headed when we place an arm around them, if they do not lick their lips when they see us in a state of semiundress, we may believe that we are ineffective lovers. Thus, because of unrealistic depictions of sexual behavior in the movies and TV, ordinary people like us may fear losing our lovers because we cannot sexually satisfy them.

A nursing major argued that some people value sexual commercialization. Whether because idealized views of sexual activity are exciting, because they have potential for improving sexual relationships by indicating new ways to relate, or because they help to desensitize people to an emotionally charged topic (namely, sexuality), these views are considered a positive trend by many people, he said.

The students' discussion was useful in that it covered most of the points that the instructor wanted to raise before starting the chapter on sexuality and commercial activities. Regardless of our points of view, sexual commercialization is probably here to stay. This chapter considers how sexuality is used in a commercial sense and will help you become a better sexual consumer.

▧ Mass Media and the Arts

Advertising

Advertisements in magazines and newspapers that use sexual themes to sell products are abundant. One need only turn at random to any page and more than likely an ad or an article that has some relationship to sex or sexual attractiveness will be evident. In the past, there was a controversy related to ads for condoms. Because of increasing incidence of HIV/AIDS, many people argued that condom ads were needed to help prevent further spread of disease. Many others argued that there should not be condom ads because they feared such ads would encourage more sexual activity—particularly among adolescents and other unmarried people. Little by little, ads for condoms have become more common, and there have not been increases in sexual activity. In fact, in other countries, where condoms have been openly advertised for years, there are lower rates of STIs, lower rates of unwanted pregnancies, and fewer abortions.

After so much controversy about condom ads, it has been interesting to observe the response to ads for Viagra, Cialis, Levitra, and other products with the sole purpose of enhancing sexual pleasure. These ads are found in newspapers, magazines, on the Internet, and on TV. For some reason, there has not been much controversy about these ads. In some cases, well-known celebrities have talked about how well the products work and how they have helped with their relationships. The presence of these ads seems to have made it more acceptable to talk about sexual behavior in general—even for people in older age groups. This is an excellent example of the impact that advertising can have in certain circumstances.

Much of the advertising with sexual themes is fairly obvious if you think about it. But through the years, many advertisers that have used sexual imagery to sell their products intended it to work on the viewer's subconscious—not conscious—awareness. This so-called subliminal advertising might include pictures that look innocent at first, but upon further examination are suggestive of a woman standing somewhere with something shaped like a projectile (such as an airplane or a cigar) aimed at her vagina, or pictures composed to suggest genitals such as a liquor bottle with small round objects on each side suggesting a penis and two testicles. Research has not been conclusive about the effects of subliminal advertising.

Salum (2013) advocated that the Federal Communications Commission should require that advertising relates to the product and does not give a false impression of what will happen if the viewer buys the product. Further, the Advertising Standards Association has indicated that advertisements should not employ sexual appeal in a manner that is exploitative and degrading of any individual or group of people to promote the sale of products or services. In particular, people should not be portrayed in a manner that uses sexual appeal simply to draw attention. According to Salum, each image, situation, and conversation seen in ads is placed precisely and meticulously for a purpose. The descriptor *subliminal* in an advertising context is essentially defined as the unawareness to formulate a conscious or mindful understanding. Effects are meant to show up later, long after the viewing experience has been forgotten.

Subliminal ads can have negative effects on women. The ads can make them feel inferior and

Myth (vs) Fact

Myth: In recent years, there has been an increased and about equal use of male and female body exposure in advertisements.
Fact: There has been an increase in breast and total female body exposure, but female body exposure is about four times more common than male body exposure.

Myth: Women appear more often than men in television beer commercials.
Fact: Men appear twice as often as women in television beer commercials.

Myth: Television is the main source of information about sexuality for teenagers.
Fact: Friends are the main source of information about sexuality for teenagers.

Myth: Fraudulent sexual aids are not among the top sources of health fraud in the United States.
Fact: According to the Food and Drug Administration, fraudulent sexual aids are among the top 10 sources of health fraud in the United States.

subconsciously imply that for women to distinguish themselves as beautiful, they must use this "ideal" product. When we watch an ad, we should evaluate how much it is actually telling us about the product and how much is related to image.

Ads crafted to appeal to basic needs are apparently highly effective, even without the types of manipulation described. For example, some would argue that a beautiful woman washing a car while eating a hamburger is a more recent example of advertising that might be called subliminal advertising, yet appeals to basic needs.

As we shall see in this chapter, we buy many products without fully understanding why. Those selling us these products, though, know that one of the hidden motivations behind our buying habits relates to sexuality. We want to appear sexy, appeal to a potential sexual partner, and feel attractive; knowing this, salespeople use these needs to persuade us to buy products, even though we think we are buying them for reasons totally divorced from sexuality.

Advertisers seem to have made a study of sexual motivation. Since oral–genital activity had become relatively acceptable and widely practiced, it found its way into product advertising. What better way to sell cigarettes to women, for example, than to associate cigarettes with penises? For years cigarettes have been used as phallic symbols. Beginning in the 1930s, cigarette ads featured only men offering cigarettes to women, employing phallic symbolism. Cigarette ads included words such as *longer, firmer, rounder, more satisfying, better tasting,* and *more pleasing* (not to mention *more fully packed*).

Automobile advertisements make obvious use of sexual appeals, along with appeals to such other

Myth (vs) Fact

Myth: There are special exercises and/or creams that are helpful in increasing the size of a female's breasts.

Fact: Breast size and shape are the result of glandular influences and cannot be altered by exercise or by application of anything to the breast.

Myth: Prostitution is illegal in most countries around the world.

Fact: In many countries there are no laws against prostitution. In fact, the United Nations adopted a resolution in favor of decriminalization of prostitution.

Myth: It is illegal to release the names of those accused of using prostitutes or the prostitutes themselves publicly until they have been shown to be guilty in a court of law.

Fact: Although some civil liberties groups object, in some states the identities of prostitutes and their customers are made public as soon as they are arrested—before any court action occurs.

needs as recognition and esteem. When cars were long and well adorned, they were presented as phallic symbols. *Real* men, the ads suggested, wanted long cars. The tips of automobiles were even ornamented.

Victoria's Secret became a multibillion-dollar company by redefining the market for underwear. Here a model shows off the "Angels" line of lingerie at a fashion show. The Victoria's Secret website was inundated with people hoping for a glimpse of more "fashion."

Today, although car companies sell smaller cars as a rule, their ads still associate the product with sexuality, sometimes by posing pretty, well-endowed, scantily clad, and perfectly proportioned females beside cars. At automobile shows, held in coliseums and arenas throughout the United States, companies employ young female models (again scantily clad) to adorn their displays.

Liquor ads are particularly notable for linking sexual imagery to our aspirations for living well. The people depicted as liquor drinkers are attractive, well dressed, sophisticated, flirtatious, and the object of others' unconcealed attention. Readers are supposed to envy the exciting life these attractive people live and, through their choice of liquor purchases, to emulate them.

Whether intended for this purpose or not, advertisements can send sexual messages as well as messages related to gender bias. For example, over several decades there has been a great increase in breast exposure and total female body exposure in ads, even though fashion trends did not account for this. In all types of ads, female body exposure has been about four times more common than male body exposure, in part because women tend to be displayed in underwear and bikinis more often than men.

Reichert et al. (2012) looked at sexual ads appearing in magazines over several decades and found that their numbers are up. "Advertisers use sex because it can be very effective," said these researchers. "Sex sells because it attracts attention. People are hard wired to notice sexually relevant information so ads with sexual content get noticed." Looking at more than 3,200 full-page ads published in *Cosmopolitan*, *Redbook*, *Esquire*, *Playboy*, *Newsweek*, and *Time*, the investigators found sexual imagery in 27% of the ads. Specifically, alcohol, entertainment, and beauty ads were responsible for much of the increase. Out of 18 product categories, those most often using sexual imagery in advertising were health and hygiene (38%), beauty (36%), drugs and medicine (29%), clothing (27%), travel (23%), and entertainment (21%). Products not using sexual themes in their ads included charitable organizations and computer companies. Women were most often used to sell the products presented in sexual ads. Ninety-two percent of beauty ads that contained models used female models. Slightly less than half the ads did not contain models. Of the provocative health and hygiene advertisements that featured models, 31% featured females and 7% featured males.

According to Reichert et al. (2012), things must be more explicit to grab our attention and arouse us than in the past. In the early 1900s, exposed arms and ankles of female models generated the same level of arousal as partially nude models today.

Similar changes in sexually explicit content have also occurred on TV, in movies, in books, on the Internet, and in other forms of media beyond advertising.

Suggett (2015) defined sex in advertising as the use of sexually provocative or erotic imagery (or sounds, suggestions, subliminal messages) that are specifically designed to arouse interest in a particular product, service, or brand. Throughout history, sexuality has been used as a selling tool. As humans, we have a lizard, or reptilian, brain that responds to certain primal urges. Food is one such primal urge; sexuality and reproduction is another. Our preprogrammed disposition to respond to sexual imagery is so strong that it has been exploited for more than 100 years in advertising. The advertising industry, while abusing this biological fact to an increasingly greater extent, would be foolish to ignore the draw of sexual and erotic messaging.

Do sexual themes actually sell? The short answer is "yes." Popular men's magazines have experimented with their covers. Overwhelmingly, when a sexy seminaked woman appears on the cover, the sales of that issue outperform issues carrying the image of a male star, even if that star is someone about whom men want to read. Men respond to sexual images.

If an ad creates a sexual situation, it is likely to get the desired response. Sometimes, however, sexual themes can turn off customers. There is a fine line here, and all too often brands step far over this line. Customers are human, but they are also smart, well-educated people who quickly realize when they are being manipulated. If the product is a shoddy one, the customer may feel cheated or patronized. Once that happens, it will take a much greater effort on the part of the advertiser to regain the consumer's trust.

Clearly, sexual themes are here to stay. As the rules around depictions of sexuality directed at consumers become more relaxed, sexual themes will become an even bigger part of the advertising landscape. Those in advertising would be wise to realize that sexuality,

Many sexual themes are used as part of advertising on TV.

used sparingly and judicially, is a strong selling tool, but if abused, advertisers will ultimately lose out.

Television Advertising and Programming

There have also been some interesting events related to the history of sexual themes on TV (Silver, 2011). For example, back in the 1950s, Ricky and Lucy had separate beds and characters couldn't even use the word "pregnant." Two decades later the title character in the *All in the Family* spin-off *Maude* could decide to have an abortion. In the 1970s the network series *Soap* pushed boundaries with an openly gay main character. Still, in 1989 just the sight of two men in the same bed on *Thirtysomething* caused many sponsors to vanish, along with more than a million ad

 Did You Know . . .

Personal ads in newspapers have been around for many years but are much more prevalent now. They can be found on the Internet, in newspapers, in magazines, and on the radio. A radio station that has a phone-dating service will hook you up with people of a similar demographic and music-taste level. Even legitimate regional magazines, like *Boston*

magazine, carry personal ads. Your choice of whom you want may be partially influenced by where he or she advertises. For example, advertising in *Boston* magazine is much more expensive than advertising in the local newspapers, so such ads may attract a more upscale clientele.

Television is a major source of information about sexuality for people of all ages.

dollars. On the flip side, it was *NYPD Blue's* heterosexual content that aroused the ire of the American Family Association, even before the program hit the air in 1993. The group objected to the show's "steamy sex scenes," and more than 50 ABC affiliates chose not to broadcast the pilot. During its 12-year run the show often flouted authority with its depictions of both male and female bare behinds. In January 2011, a court threw out an FCC fine imposed on ABC for such a shot from an episode that first aired 8 years earlier. Despite ever-changing social mores, nudity on TV can still result in lasting controversies.

Dating shows have become popular in the 21st century. This popularity has shown that people want to observe others in their love and sexual relationships. Not all of the shows are about dating; some deal with personal relationships in general. All of the shows can make love and romance look phony at best, and vicious at worst. However, large numbers of people seem to enjoy these shows. What are the best dating reality shows? See Table 21.1 for the top 25 dating reality shows ever, as voted on by males and females in the United States.

Anyone who has been watching TV for at least a few years knows that the number of sexual scenes on TV has drastically increased, and a high percentage of all shows now include some sexual content. At the same time, only a small percentage of shows include references to sexual risks and responsibilities (such as waiting to have sexual intercourse, using protection, or possible consequences of unprotected sexual activity).

The Parents' Television Council (*TV's newest target: Teen sexual exploitation*, 2013) examined the prevalence of sexually exploitative images in the media and found that these images have become common themes in primetime television. Their major findings included the following:

- Although adult female characters were more likely to have sexualizing dialogue or depictions in their scenes, the likelihood that a scene would include sexual exploitation was higher if the female characters were young adults or younger.

- The likelihood that a scene would include sexual exploitation was highest when the female characters were underage (23.33%).

- Sexually exploitative topics targeting underage girls were more likely to be humorous (42.85%) compared to those targeting adult women (33.02%).

- Topics that targeted underage girls and were presented as jokes included sexual violence (child molestation), sex trafficking, sexual harassment, pornography, and stripping.

- Thirty-seven percent of all sexual exploitation observed during the study period was intended to be humorous.

- The content rose to the level of sexual exploitation in one-third of the shows where females were associated with sexual dialogue and/or depictions.

- Pornography (55%) and stripping (65%) were the two forms of exploitation most likely to be written into the scripts as punch lines.

- Sexually exploitative content was typically presented in the form of dialogue rather than depictions. However, the dialogue was significantly more crude and explicit than the depictions.

Findings from this report revealed that sexual exploitation has become a common topic and a comedic topic on primetime television in shows airing as early as 7 P.M. Central Time. Almost 40% of this content was intended for purposes of humorous entertainment. The researchers pointed out that as society grapples with new levels of tolerance and acceptance of sexual humor, one must ask which elements in the social environment have engendered a collective tolerance for issues and topics that have historically been deemed very serious. Further, if media images communicate that sexual exploitation is neither serious nor harmful, the environment is being

TABLE 21.1

Top 25 Dating and Relationship Reality TV Shows

Male	Female
1. The Dating Game	1. The Bachelorette
2. Rock of Love with Bret Michaels	2. The Bachelor
3. Blind Date	3. The Dating Game
4. Average Joe	4. Blind Date
5. Parental Control	5. It Takes a Church
6. Beauty and the Geek	6. Beauty and the Geek
7. A Shot at Love with Tila Tequila	7. Flavor of Love
8. Next	8. Next
9. Dismissed	9. Date My Mom
10. I Love New York	10. Dating in the Dark
11. Age of Love	11. Room Raiders
12. Singled Out	12. Average Joe
13. The Bachelorette	13. Rock of Love with Bret Michaels
14. Dating in the Dark	14. Parental Control
15. The Bachelor	15. I Love New York
16. Date My Mom	16. Dismissed
17. Flavor of Love	17. Temptation Island
18. Joe Millionaire	18. The Choice
19. Who Wants to Marry My Dad?	19. The Bachelor Pad
20. The Bachelor Pad	20. Take Me Out
21. Temptation Island	21. Who Wants to Marry My Dad?
22. Paradise Hotel	22. Paradise Hotel
23. For Love or Money	23. For the Love of Ray J
24. Take Me Out	24. For Love or Money
25. Ochocinco: The Ultimate Catch	25. Singled Out

Data from The best dating reality shows. *Ranker.com*, 2015. Available: http://www.ranker.com /list/best-dating-reality-shows/tvs-frank?format=GRID&action=tab&type=demographics.

set for sexual exploitation to be viewed as trivial and acceptable.

Many people have protested the television industry's portrayal of sexual themes in everyday life. Although objections to the portrayal of explicit sexual activities and the use of sexual language have been raised for some time, people are objecting to the nature and quality of the sexual relationships enacted—stereotypical roles, sexual violence and hostility, incessant teasing, and more physical than emotional display—and to be concerned about the effects of these views of sexuality on socialization of the young.

A TV rating system was adopted in 1997 (Kalinowski, 2015) that includes age-based symbols like those for movies, such as TV-G (suitable for general audiences, featuring little or no violence, sexual content, or profanity). Shows rated as TV-PG may contain some suggestive dialogue (D), foul language (L), sexual content (S), or violence (V); the "D," "L," "S," and "V" labels are appended to the TV-PG rating accordingly. However, this content is usually negligible. TV-14 programs are not recommended for children younger than age 14; these programs contain more excessive use of the same optional content tags as a TV-PG show. TV-MA broadcasts are intended for audiences older than age 17. In addition, a TV-Y rating means that a program is well suited for children between 2 and 6 years old. These programs are designed specifically for preschoolers, featuring no foul language, violence, or sexual content. TV-Y7 programs are still free of profanity and sexual themes, but may include mild violence best suited for children older than 7 years. Some TV-Y7 programs carry an optional "FV" tag to indicate the presence of fantasy violence.

Television can be an excellent way to educate people about healthy sexual practices. For instance, the Surgeon General of the United States warned that the spread of HIV and AIDS could be slowed only by sexual abstinence or the use of condoms during coitus. Fortunately, in recent years we have seen an increase in condom ads on television.

On cable TV, the fastest-growing segment is adult programming that portrays explicit sexual behavior. As cable TV availability has expanded, even more such programming is available.

Many television programs have been devoted to educating the public about HIV and AIDS, and other programs have focused on such topics as sexual orientation and extramarital sexual activities. Many of these programs follow a talk-show format or are presented as documentaries; however, some sexual topics and issues are dramatized with the intent of entertaining and educating at the same time. For example, one situation comedy depicted a teenager being instructed to use a condom with

Communication DIMENSIONS

Feelings About Sexual Themes

Common communication problems include (1) frame of reference, (2) emotional interference, and (3) physical distractions. Talk with two or three of your classmates about difficulties two people in an intimate relationship might have in these three areas when they are discussing the following topics:

1. Which characters do you think are the sexiest in current television shows? Why?
2. Which ads on TV or in magazines do you find most offensive? Why?
3. What does it take for materials to be considered obscene?
4. Which TV shows and/or movies do you think are most sexually stimulating? Why?
5. If you were a writer for a television series, how would you use sexual themes?

For example, in a discussion about sexy television shows, there could be a difference in which language is considered acceptable or in what might be considered sexy. This could cause emotional interference. Or perhaps one person could not relate to why something is sexually stimulating to another person. Thus one person's frame of reference could cause a problem. Go through each of the five questions with at least two or three other people and see which other possible barriers you can identify. Why do you think these barriers exist? What might be done about them to improve communication?

---

his girlfriend, and another weekly comedy show depicted an unmarried couple living together and the problems they encountered.

Addressing the media in general, a position statement of the Sexuality Information and Education Council of the United States (SIECUS, 2015) indicates that

> *SIECUS believes that the media has a responsibility to present the complexities of human sexuality at all stages of the life cycle in a manner that is medically accurate, sensitive to diversity, and free of exploitation, prejudice, gratuitous sexual violence, and dehumanizing sexual portrayals.*

In 2010, the American Academy of Pediatrics (AAP) revised its policy statement on sexuality, contraception, and the media. Within the statement, the AAP says that new evidence points to the media that adolescents use frequently as important factors in the initiation of sexual intercourse. There is a major disconnect between what mainstream media portray—casual sexual behavior with no consequences—and what children and teenagers need—straightforward information about human sexuality and the need for contraception when having sexual activity. Media content is becoming increasingly sexually explicit, yet information on abstinence, sexual responsibility, and birth control remains rare.

Gilbert (2010), while commenting on the revised AAP policy statement, pointed out that whether the AAP will be successful in its campaign to reduce the sexualization of media available to children remains uncertain. Given the financial interests involved, the answer would likely be "no." Sex sells, it always has, and it sells particularly well to those who do not know any better—the kids.

Barr et al. (2014) reported on the relationship between screen time and sexual behaviors of middle school students. They found that high screen time (3 or more hours per day of TV or recreational computer use) was associated with a number of sexual behaviors, including ever having had sexual intercourse, having sexual intercourse before age 11, and having had three or more partners. The odds of ever having sexual intercourse was 31% higher among those with high TV usage, 43% higher among those with high recreational computer usage, and 54% higher among those with extremely high (6 or more hours) total screen time.

Ybarra et al. (2014) examined sexual media exposure, sexual behavior, and sexual violence victimization during adolescence. Their data came from 1,058 youth 14 to 21 years old who participated in the national online Growing Up with Media study. Forty-seven percent reported that many types of media or almost all or all of at least one type of media they consumed depicted sexual situations. Exposure to sexual media in TV and movies and music was greater than online and in games. All other things being equal, more frequent exposure to sexual media was related to ever having sexual intercourse, coercive sexual victimization, and attempted/completed rape but not risky sexual behavior. The researchers concluded that longer-standing media, such as TV and movies, appear to be associated with greater amounts of sexual media consumption than more recent ones, such as the Internet.

Cox et al. (2015) investigated the things that influence early adolescent attitudes toward sexuality. Among their 1,736 subjects, having a sibling who was a teen parent and greater TV viewing were significantly and positively associated with the probability and extent of favorable attitudes toward sexual activity for females.

Witmer (2015), reporting on a RAND Corporation study, indicated that teens who watch large amounts of TV containing sexual content are twice as likely to begin engaging in sexual intercourse in the following year as their peers who watch little such TV. In addition, the study found that youths who watch large amounts of TV with sexual content are more likely to initiate sexual activities other than intercourse, such as "making out" and oral sexual activity. These adolescents behaved sexually like youths who were 9 to 17 months older but watched only average amounts of TV with sexual content. According to the RAND researchers, the impact of TV viewing was so large that even a moderate shift in the sexual content of adolescent TV watching could have a substantial effect on youths' sexual behavior. TV habits predicted whether adolescents went to "second or third base," as well as whether they had sexual intercourse for the first time. The 12-year-olds who watched a lot of TV with sexual content behaved like the 14- or 15-year-olds who watched the least amount of TV. The researchers indicated that the advancement in sexual behavior they saw among children who watched a lot of sexual TV was striking. They also found that adolescents who watched the most TV with sexual content were twice as likely to initiate sexual intercourse over the next year as adolescents who watched the least amount of TV with sexual content. Adolescents were less likely to initiate sexual intercourse if their parents monitored their activities, if their parents had more education, if they lived with both parents, if their parents did not approve of them having sexual relations, if they were religious, and if they were in good mental health.

Chandra et al. (2008) indicated that teens exposed to high levels of television sexual content are twice as likely to experience a pregnancy in the subsequent 3 years as compared with those with lower levels of exposure. Conversely, Schroeder (2008) pointed out that "We should all raise a skeptical eyebrow whenever any research claims that there's a direct cause–effect relationship between one thing, such as TV viewing, and something as complex as teenage

pregnancy." In other words, maybe the same people who are more likely to become pregnant as teenagers are also the same people who want to watch more sexual content on TV—maybe one doesn't cause the other at all.

It can be difficult to legally determine which sexual content is acceptable on TV and which is not. It is a violation of federal law to air obscene programming at any time or indecent programming or profane language from 6 A.M. to 10 P.M. Congress has given the Federal Communications Commission (FCC) the responsibility for administratively enforcing these laws. The FCC may revoke a station's license, impose a monetary forfeiture, or issue a warning if a station airs obscene, indecent, or profane material. Definitions of important terms can often be tricky. Information about indecent broadcast restrictions, profane broadcast restrictions, determining context, and filing a complaint can be found at http://www.fcc.gov/guides/obscenity-indecency-and-profanity.

Sexuality and the Movies

Any cursory glance at the entertainment section of your local newspaper will show that movies are often marketed to the public by means of sexual themes—and have been for some time. In *The Blue Angel*, a 1930 film starring Marlene Dietrich (1930 was a time when women's bathing suits were much more than three small patches of flimsy cloth precariously held together by string), images of Marlene's bare thighs in a cabaret outfit made men's heads whirl. In *She Done Him Wrong*, when Mae West invited Cary Grant to "come up and see me some time," men's knees knocked. When Clark Gable (Rhett Butler) carried Vivian Leigh (Scarlett O'Hara) up a flight of stairs to her bedroom in *Gone with the Wind*, women swooned; when Marlon Brando appeared in his ripped undershirt in *A Streetcar Named Desire*, they panted. People's imaginations and perceptions, rather than nudity or sexual activity on film, were integral components of cinematic sexuality during the 1930s, 1940s, and 1950s.

By the 1960s and the 1970s, sexual permissiveness and experimentation had permeated the movies, as well as other segments of society. Movies previously shown as stag films (often called blue movies) were elevated to respectable status. With the showing of *I Am Curious (Yellow)*, *Deep Throat*, *Beyond the Valley of the Dolls*, *Vixen*, *The Lickerish Quartet*, and *Behind the Green Door* in movie theaters (in spite of attempts by local communities to ban them), people seemed to be less shocked. Although well-known movie stars had sometimes appeared nude in films in earlier years, a new era began when Marlon Brando

The movie, "Fifty Shades of Grey," had a great deal of impact on the economy. The sex toy industry had increased sales. Mainstream retailers stocked up on blindfolds, whips, handcuffs, and masks. Manufacturers also designed new packaging and products to fit the theme of the film.

appeared in the X-rated *Last Tango in Paris* in the early 1970s. The films of recent years leave little to the imagination and appeal more to the voyeur in us.

To help parents and others make decisions about the appropriateness of a particular movie for themselves or their children, a rating system was developed by the Motion Picture Association of America:

G: Appropriate for the general audience

PG: Appropriate for the general audience; however, parental guidance is advised. There may be brief nudity or some brief moments of sexually explicit language.

PG-13: Parents are advised that some of the material may be inappropriate for younger children.

R: Restricted to people at least 17 years of age or those accompanied by an adult due to sexual content, sexually explicit language, or violence

NC-17: No one under 17 years of age admitted. Extremely sexual in nature, and/ or containing explicit sexual language, or extremely violent (but not necessarily pornographic).

As with television and advertising, some people believe that the sexual explicitness of movies is detrimental to society, and others see this trend as positive. The opponents cite the weak commitments of sexual partners as partly responsible for the soaring adultery and divorce rates by setting poor examples of the meaning of intimate relationships. Those in favor of sexual explicitness in movies see this as just one sign of our increased openness about sexuality and the pleasures inherent in sexual behavior. We must make our own decisions about the appropriateness of this trend.

In an example of regulatory action, the Los Angeles City Council approved a mandate requiring all actors in pornographic films to wear condoms (Medina, 2012). The AIDS Healthcare Foundation had pressed for such legislation for years to help reduce the spread of HIV and to promote the use of condoms. However, the Free Speech Coalition felt that this was an example of government overreaching and intruding into consenting adults' decisions. A unique aspect of the new mandate was its requirement that the police perform spot checks on any movie set once a permit is issued.

Adult film production migrated from California to Nevada after the California law was passed. After voters in Los Angeles County approved the condom requirement in 2012, the number of permits for adult films in Los Angeles dropped dramatically, from 485 in 2012 to 40 in 2013. At the same time, the number of permits for adult films in the Las Vegas area jumped more than 50%, from 226 in 2012 to 343 in 2013. However, in 2015 a similar law was proposed in Nevada. Health officials were particularly concerned when two male performers tested positive for HIV following a video shoot in the state.

Many performers opposed the condom requirement. One male performer noted that condoms can cause friction, irritation, or even infection during scenes that take hours to film before being edited. One female star was opposed to the requirement as well. She said the industry follows strict HIV testing and maintains a database showing pass/fail results. Another reported that she had been in scenes with and without condoms, and called it distracting to have her partner stop to take one off at the end. "We get tested every 14 days," she said. "I trust my performer." Apparently, since 2004 there have been no documented cases of HIV transmission during scenes between professional actors in the database. A representative from the health department said, "We're not against porn. We want it to be safer. We think porn sends the wrong message to young people that the only kind of sex that's hot is unsafe sex" (Ritter, 2015).

The Video Rental Industry

The video rental industry boomed during the 1980s and 1990s. Numerous stores in various communities opened where consumers could buy or rent videocassettes. Toward the end of the 1990s, the industry underwent a significant change with the advent of DVDs. DVDs were sold at lower prices than the videocassettes and could get to the market more quickly. Then, in 1999, Netflix starting renting DVDs through the mail for flat monthly fees to subscribers who could use the Internet to place their orders. This caused the closing of some stores. Today, business people continue looking at the best ways to make video rentals available to people.

Regardless whether it is purchased or rented in a store or obtained from an online source, the availability of sexually explicit material has alarmed some people. They consider these X-rated movies to be pure trash with the potential to instigate sexual violence and to stereotype females as sex objects. They argue that these materials are obscene and pornographic and, as such, should be prohibited. However, others view the openness toward sexual expression of various kinds to be healthy. They argue that a couple's sexual relationship can be enhanced by viewing sexually explicit films, learning about new sexual activities, or being implicitly given permission to act out sexual fantasies. The courts have ruled that people have the right to rent sexually explicit videos and rental shop owners have the right to make such videos available. However, pressure from local groups in some communities has convinced shop owners voluntarily to remove the X-rated videos from their stock. In one view, this expression of community standards is considered healthy and the epitome of the democratic process at work. In another view, it is described as the "uptight" majority's dictating sexual mores to the more sexually comfortable minority. As we learned previously, one's view of sexual morality relates to the valuing of one's ethical principles; this is an example of that process at work.

In 1994 the Entertainment Software Rating Board (ESRB) was formed under heat from Congress to crack down on violent and/or sexual content in video games. It is a self regulating video game industry group. It uses the following rating system:

- EC (Early Childhood—ages 3+) contains no material parents would find inappropriate.

- E (Everyone: ages 6+) contains minimal cartoon, fantasy, or mild violence and/or infrequent use of mild language.

- E10+ (Everyone: ages 10+) contains more cartoon, fantasy, or mild violence, mild profanity, and/or minimally suggestive themes.

- T (Teen: 13+) contains violence, suggestive themes, crude humor, minimal blood, and/or infrequent use of strong language.

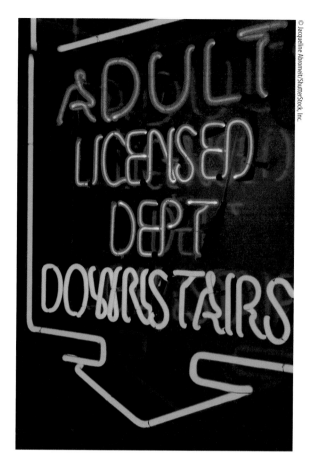

People have various opinions about the legality and availability of sexually explicit materials.

- M (Mature: 17+) contains mature sexual themes, more intense violence, and/or strong language.

- AO (Adults Only: 18+) contains graphic depictions of sex and/or violence.

The mission of ESRB is to empower consumers, especially parents, with guidance that allows them to make informed decisions about the age-appropriateness and suitability of video games and apps while holding the video game industry accountable for responsible marketing practices. Today consumers play games on a variety of platforms and devices, and parental concerns go well beyond content to include interactive elements like user interactions or the sharing of a user's location and personal information. Parents today seem to place equal importance on guidance about interactive elements as they do about the specific content. Consequently, ESRB ratings have three parts: *Rating categories* suggest age appropriateness; *content descriptors* indicate content that may have triggered a particular rating and/or may be of interest or concern; and *interactive elements* relate to users' ability to interact, the sharing of users' locations with other users, or the fact that personal information may be shared with third parties. Packaged or boxed video games available for retail sale or rental in the United States and Canada display the rating category on the front of the package and content descriptors on the back.

It seems that a majority of adult videos are rented by females. They are rented most commonly on weekends and are used by married couples after the kids have gone to bed. Common themes of the sexually explicit videos relate to high levels of sexual desire, diverse sexual activity, many sexual partners being readily available, and pleasure as the main purpose of sexual activity. Video rentals and sales represent multibillions of dollars in sales each year. They are a substantial part of the home-video industry's revenue. Some videos have been produced for use by couples in their homes. Sexologists have made videos that provide explicit graphic instruction to help improve sexual relationships.

Some people wonder about the effects of the video products that are rented or sold. Aubrey et al. (2011) explored the effects of sexually objectifying (treating women as sex objects) music videos on college men's sexual beliefs. Their findings showed that participants who viewed music videos of highly objectified female artists reported more adversarial sexual beliefs, more acceptance of interpersonal violence, and more negative attitudes toward sexual harassment than participants assigned to less sexually objectifying music videos by the same female artists.

Aubrey (2011) pointed out that although sexual objectification is commonplace in media culture, music videos provide the most potent examples of it. She compared sexual objectification across artists' gender and musical genres (R&B/hip-hop, pop, and country). Compared to male artists, female artists were more sexually objectified, held to stricter appearance standards, and were more likely to demonstrate sexually alluring behavior. In addition, sexual objectification was more prominent in R&B/hip-hop and pop videos than in country videos.

Summers and Miller (2014) looked at how the portrayal of sexism in video game magazines has changed in the last 20 years. They examined video game magazines that analyzed the portrayal of female video game characters and determined how this portrayal had changed over time. Their results indicated a growing trend toward a decreased benevolent sexism (favorable attitude toward women, but sexist because women are viewed as weak and in need of protection from men) portrayals and an increase in a hostile sexism (anger and resentment toward women, portraying women as inferior, and their place is "in the kitchen") portrayals over time.

Literature

As with the content of movies, TV programs, and videos, the public has become desensitized to sexually explicit material in books. However, it was not always this way. For example, in 1928 D. H. Lawrence's *Lady Chatterly's Lover* was published. Because of its sexual explicitness, it was banned in the United States until 1959. James Joyce's *Ulysses*, published in 1934, deals with masturbation, prostitution, adultery, and voyeurism. It was not allowed into the United States for years but is now considered to be a masterpiece.

In recent decades thousands of books of varying literary quality that openly treat sexual topics have been published. Sometimes they weave themes related to sexuality into a meaningful story, but other times their authors seem to be gratuitously writing about sexual thoughts and activity as much as possible. Many earlier works appear tame compared to what is now available. What was previously considered risque, if not actually immoral or illegal, has now come to be expected in a bestseller.

Sexually arousing material, of course, has existed for centuries. The ancient *Kamasutra* and *The Perfumed Garden*, Chaucer's *Canterbury Tales* and Boccaccio's *Decameron* (both 14th-century works), Li Yu's *Flesh Prayer Mat*, and the *Memoirs of Casanova* are examples of early erotic literature. However, more and more of our popular literature that is not primarily erotic is at least partly concerned with its characters' sexual activities. For example, romance literature relies on fantasy rather than sexual explicitness; its purpose is to tantalize and to nourish sexual fantasies, rather than to tell a good story. Many mass-market paperbacks are romance novels, read by both women and men.

Magazines have made their mark as well. *Esquire: The Magazine for Men* appeared in 1933. Twenty years later *Playboy* appeared on the newsstands. It offered information about sexuality, an open philosophy toward sexuality, and photographs of nude women along with some stimulating stories. Its approach was followed by many other magazines. In the late 1960s other magazines, such as *Penthouse*, *Oui*, and *Hustler*, published pictures of nude males and females as well as people engaged in assorted sexual activities. Some even had a classified section allowing people to advertise their sexual services or request sexual partners.

As women asked for a more balanced view, magazines such as *Cosmopolitan* and *Playgirl* began printing photos of nude men and stories with appeal for women. Traditionally, women's magazines have focused on two broad topics: what a woman should do to get a man *(Cosmopolitan)* and what a woman should do once she has the man and his children *(Redbook)*. Other magazines have attempted to

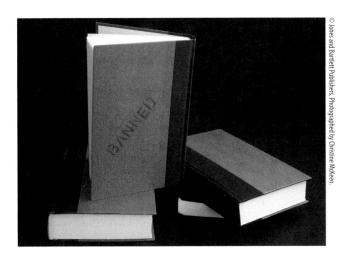

Sexually arousing books and other materials have been available for centuries.

include other aspects of women's lives. For example, *Working Mother* and *Savvy* are aimed at women who work outside the home. *Ms.* magazine, the only women's magazine explicitly dedicated to feminism and the facts about women's sexuality, was founded in 1972. The magazine is published by the Feminist Majority Foundation and has a circulation of 100,000 and a readership of 250,000 women and men. The *Ms.* website indicates that 55% of the female readers identify as feminists, as do 30% of the male readers. A digital version of *Ms.* was launched in 2014 with the introduction of a tablet and mobile device app. Almost 25,000 readers downloaded the app in that first year. The magazine accepts only mission-driven and nonprofit advertising.

Hatton and Trautner (2011) analyzed more than 1,000 images of men and women on *Rolling Stone* covers over a 43-year period. They concluded that representations of both women and men have become more sexualized over time, that women are more frequently sexualized than men, and that the images of women are more intensely sexualized than are those of men. They developed a "scale of sexualization." An image was given points for being sexualized if, for example, the subject's lips were parted or his or her tongue was showing, the subject was only partially clad or naked, or the text describing the subject used explicitly sexual language. The authors said, "We don't necessarily think it's problematic for women to be portrayed as 'sexy,' But we do think it is problematic when nearly all images of women depict them not simply as 'sexy women' but as passive objects for someone else's sexual pleasure."

Adult bookstores specialize in highly sexually arousing books. These stores are adult in the sense that a person must be of legal age to enter. Such establishments also sell sex-illustrated magazines, newspapers, postcards, decks of playing cards, and

videos. Many communities have attempted to outlaw adult bookstores (through the courts and local government statute) or to limit their location to one part of the community. Nevertheless, all major cities have them, as do many smaller cities and towns. Furthermore, many conventional bookstores, recognizing a market for sexually explicit literature, maintain sections devoted to such books and magazines. As with sexuality in the movies, the cost and benefit of adult bookstores versus the risks of censorship is a topic of heated debate.

In addition to sexually explicit fiction, a how-to publishing business has developed to help people reach their sexual potential. Thus we now have countless books about such topics as using sexual techniques, expressing gay and lesbian sexuality, helping ourselves and our partners to be sensuous women or men, improving our overall sexual relationships, and using sexual aids for pleasure.

Popular Music

The mass phenomenon that may affect more young people than any other is popular music. And in this arena, as in most others, blatant sexuality has

Many entertainers use sexual themes to sell themselves and their products.

become a style. Lyrics (words and grunts), performance (movement and costume), and provocative photos on album covers use sexual suggestion and appeal to our sexual fantasies to sell the music and the entertainer.

A major example of sex in music was Elvis ("The Pelvis") Presley, with his gyrating hips. However, both his hips and his songs would be considered tame by today's standards. "Heartbreak Hotel," "Love Me Tender," and "Let Me Be Your Teddy Bear," all recorded in the late 1950s, were sexually appealing mainly because of Presley's soft, sultry voice and innuendo, rather than direct sexual language—a far cry from today's popular music and music videos that contain frequent references to relationships, romance, and sexual behavior. Lyrics about sexuality are mixed with lyrics about love, violence, rejection, and loneliness.

Music videos may be influential sources of sexual information for adolescents because they combine visuals of their favorite musicians with music. Many of the visual elements are sexual. Rap music is particularly explicit about both sexuality and violence.

Groups of citizens have attempted to ban some of this music from local radio stations and have sometimes been successful. Whether sexually explicit music is harmful (in particular, it is argued, to youths in developmental states) is debatable and depends somewhat on our values.

In 1985 the Recording Industry Association of America (RIAA) reached an agreement with the National Parent-Teacher Association and the Parents Music Resource Center. The agreement specified that music releases containing explicit lyrics, including explicit depictions of violence and sex, be identified so parents could make intelligent listening choices for their children. The Parental Advisory Label on music releases informs consumers that recordings with the label may contain strong language or depictions of violence, sex, or substance abuse. Parental discretion is then advised. The label is a nonremovable logo that record companies voluntarily place on products to better inform consumers and retailers while also protecting the rights of artists. The decision about which label to place on a particular sound recording is made by each record company in conjunction with the artist. The industry as a whole and the individual companies take this program seriously. In 1996 the RIAA strengthened the program by revising the logo to apply to both audio and video products. The Parental Advisory standards are reviewed periodically so they are kept up to date. According to the RIAA, the music industry takes seriously its responsibility to help parents determine what is and is not appropriate for their children (*Parental Advisory*, 2015).

Hall et al. (2011) analyzed sexualization in lyrics of popular music over six decades. It is probably no surprise that they found that more recent lyrics were significantly more likely to contain sexualization. Some people are fearful that this may have an impact on adolescent sexual behavior and attitudes.

Technology has made access to music, lyrics, and video easier than ever. Ackerman (2012) summarized findings related to contemporary songs and the sexual content of their lyrics. One researcher analyzed the top songs in a recent year and found that 103 of the 297 songs referenced sexual activity. Out of those, degrading references occurred 65% of the time and non-degrading lyrics occurred 36% of the time. In another study of the top 20 *Billboard* hits during the year, the top 20 songs contained at least 40 references to sex or a sexual act and more than 50 references to a short-term hookup. There was almost no reference to long-term commitments. It was also pointed out that popular music has long been about love, sexual activity, and romance. Even back in 1928, Cole Porter's classic "Let's Do It" begins with "Birds do it, bees do it."

Some studies seem to indicate that adolescents with higher levels of exposure to sexual music lyrics are more likely to have had sexual intercourse. Even 12- to 14-year-olds who had a heavier sexual media diet were found to be twice as likely to have had sexual intercourse. Others point out that it is very difficult to establish a cause-and-effect relationship. According to these sources, perhaps those adolescents who participate in more sexual activity are the ones who are more likely to listen to lyrics with sexual themes, rather than the sexual themes themselves causing more sexual behavior.

Online Material

Advertising, newspapers, books, magazines, television, movies, videos, and music have been around for a long time; a newer entrant on the sexual consumerism scene is online material. An increasing number of people of all ages have access to computers and the Internet, and therefore to countless materials related to sexuality. They can have privacy on computer networks and avoid the embarrassment of getting sexual materials from a public place, and they can download only those images they find most sexually arousing. Discrete storage of sexually explicit images on a computer enables individuals to conceal the images from others. In addition, new computer technologies permit an ever-expanding audience to gain access to the vast amounts of pornography available on the information superhighway.

Pornography has become relatively popular in the workplace. Twenty-five percent of employees who use the Internet visit porn sites during the workday. Hits are higher during office hours than at any other time of day. Some believe that the people who engage in this activity may be looking for an escape and think their bosses are too busy to notice. Another factor is that there is an evolving sense—not universally shared—that porn is no big deal. Many employees have been fired for viewing porn sites while on the job. The threat to companies isn't just the lost hours of work and the risk of sexual-harassment lawsuits, but porn sites expose computers to viruses, adware, and spyware. In one case it was learned that an executive spent many hours a day on adult sites—a fact discovered because his computer was always crashing.

Computer technology has influenced laws as well as behavior. For example, in the 1990s federal legislation banning computer-generated depictions of children engaging in sexual conduct was passed. It outlawed "any visual depiction" that "appears to be of a minor engaging in sexually explicit conduct." This could include scenes from a movie in which an adult portraying a minor is engaged in sexual activity. Although the law was challenged by sex film distributors and the ACLU, a federal judge upheld it in 1997.

For some people, X-rated email can be a problem. Unsolicited email messages that, with a click of a hot-linked universal resource locator (URL), can deliver pornographic websites to your computer screen have become relatively common intrusions online. Some have telltale IDs like "Sue2nite" or "4Hot-Time," but others are more deceptive. For example, in one instance an innocuous-looking message said that clicking on its hot link would provide information on how to fix a computer problem. One click of the hot link revealed a sample of sexually explicit

pictures. This is probably not illegal, but it can be very annoying. The FTC encourages all consumers to forward any unsolicited, unfair, or deceptive spams to its special spam mailbox where investigators keep a database of possibly illegal email solicitations.

On the Internet, people can carry on sensual conversations, play X-rated computer games with each other (for example, they can create the appearance of their characters and engage in a variety of behaviors with characters controlled by other subscribers), obtain recent information on a variety of sexual topics, leave sexual messages for other people on bulletin boards, and obtain and use software designed to help with sexual dysfunction and other problems. Computer bulletin boards and forums exist for just about all sexual interests and fetishes.

In 2005 one of the first studies investigating the characteristics of those who participate in cybersex was reported (Daneback et al., 2005). Cybersex was defined as when two or more people engage in simulated sex talk while online for the purposes of sexual pleasure. It was found that men and women participate in cybersex to a similar extent. Women between 35 and 49 years of age had significantly more experience with cybersex than men of the same age. Men's interest in cybersex seemed to decrease with age, while women's interest stayed almost the same. Women's main reasons for engaging in cybersex were interaction with others and "education" around sexual matters. Gay men were more than four times more likely to have cybersex than were heterosexual men. Cybersex was found not to be primarily a "singles" activity. The amount was about the same for singles as for married people. Married people who participated did not seem to view cybersex as infidelity. Those who engage in cybersex were more likely

Ethical DIMENSIONS

Controlling Cyberspace

Many people believe that attempts to ban sexually explicit materials on the Internet are, in addition to being unconstitutional, unethical. They believe that laws governing obscenity and child pornography already exist and apply to cases involving the Internet. Child pornography is not protected by free speech, so they argue that further control is not needed. In fact, they point out that such control would also deny people of all ages access to needed information about sexuality. Besides, if people want to protect children from certain information, they can do so with Internet-blocking software.

Some people consider it ethical to ban sexually explicit materials in cyberspace. They believe such materials should not be available for viewing by anyone of any age. They also fear that even with Internet-blocking software and well-intended parents, young people will have contact with sexually explicit materials that will be harmful to them. Therefore, it is ethical to ban such materials.

Is it ethical to establish laws to ban sexually explicit materials in cyberspace? Is it ethical to transmit sexually explicit materials in cyberspace? How can the potential need for regulation be balanced with constitutional rights?

Websites like "Persian Kitty's" provide links to free pornographic material and generate a fortune from advertisers for their operators. However, the relative ease of obtaining sexually explicit material that such a site offers raises ethical issues. Should such sites be required to provide age verification? If not, should "Persian Kitty's" be held liable if minors follow the links to sexually explicit material?

to be sexually active offline as well—having had a greater number of sex partners during the past year as compared with those without cybersex experience.

Internet chat rooms related to sexuality are also becoming more common. For example, a person can "sit" with other people or "soak" in a hot tub and discuss sexual fantasies or participate in Internet sexual activities. Flirting and discussion about sexual relationships and desires are everyday occurrences in such chat rooms.

There can be big money involved with Internet and website activities, as Beth Mansfield discovered. In 1995 she was a struggling accountant wondering how she and her husband would ever put their two young children through college. She decided to try her hand at creating a website with adult content. Within 5 months people were clamoring to buy advertising on "Persian Kitty's," a directory of sexually oriented sites she named for her three cats, and soon she grossed more than $900,000 per year.

One of the web's most successful adult-oriented sites was operated by Danni Ashe, a former erotic dancer and nude model. She created and launched her own site in 1995, "Danni's Hard Drive." The site's initial 70,000 hits per day soon grew to more than 5 million per day. Her original staff of one part-time assistant grew to 15 full-time employees in a few years and numbered 45 by 2004, when Ashe sold the website. In 2001, the *Guinness Book of World Records* named her "the most downloaded woman." At that time, Ashe's images had already been downloaded 7 million times. At the time she sold the website, it was making a profit of more than $8 million per year.

Some people feel that the Internet has been a major factor in unleashing women's interest in all things sexual. Women have accounted for more than one-fourth of all visitors to sites with adult content for at least the last 15 years.

In 2011, the board of directors of Internet's key oversight body, the Internet Corporation for Assigned Names and Numbers (ICANN), approved the creation of a red-light district online (.xxx for pornographic websites). This happened after at least a 10-year battle over such a domain. There are various points of view about this development. For example, some pornographers worry that it will ghettoize their content. Although the designation is meant to be voluntary, some fear governmental agencies might try to mandate the domain's use, so that pornographic content is more easily blocked. Some people see this as a positive possibility because it would be easier to block pornographic websites. At the same time, some religious groups are fearful that giving adult websites their own corner of the Internet legitimizes the content.

Traditionally, some people were worried about pornography being transmitted into the home. However, web camera technology potentially inverts this relationship by transmitting activities in the home to outside viewers. One high-profile case occurred when teenagers used their home computers, web cameras, and other web-based commercial establishments such as PayPal to establish and conduct their own home-based, interactive pornography businesses (Soderlund, 2008).

On a related note, "Sex and Tech" (2008) reported that 20% of teens (ages 13–19) and 33% of young adults (ages 20–26) have electronically sent, or posted online, nude or semi-nude pictures or videos of themselves. Sexually suggestive messages were even more common (sent by 39% of teens and 59% of young adults). The term "sexting" has been used to refer to these practices.

Around the country law enforcement officials and educators have struggled with how to deal with minors who sext. When a sexually explicit message includes a participant (subject, photographer, distributor, or recipient) younger than age 18, child pornography laws may apply. In recent years, there have been numerous examples where an elementary or secondary school student has sent nude pictures of himself or herself or of others via cell phone to many others directly or indirectly. Many school districts have banned sexting and have searched for ways to control it. There could be different motivations for sexting, including attention-seeking, sending consensual exchanges, horsing around under the influence of peers or chemical substances, or malicious distribution. Many parents as well as community and school leaders have been struggling to determine the best ways to help protect students from themselves with regard to sexting.

Of course, the Internet also has the potential for abuse with respect to sexuality. Some people have claimed they have been sexually harassed by anonymous participants in computer bulletin boards. Others have been concerned about the transmission of sexual photos of children. There is also concern about uncontrolled access to sexual materials by underage people.

Authorities tell us that at any given time there are thousands of sexual predators online trying to lure unsuspecting young teenagers into interactions. FBI agents often pose as teens to try to snare these predators. The FBI has secured thousands of convictions using this method.

In 2011 the U.S. Attorney General announced the results of an international pornography investigation (Operation Delego) (U.S. Department of Justice, 2011). The operation targeted hundreds of individuals in countries around the world for their participation in "Dreamboard"—a private, membership-only online bulletin board that was created and operated to promote pedophilia and the sexual abuse of very young children. Dreamboard's members traded graphic images and videos of adults molesting young children—often violently—and created a massive private library of images of child sexual abuse. Members were required to upload pornography portraying children 12 years old or younger. As a result of Operation Delego, 72 defendants were charged. It was the largest prosecution in history of people who participated in an online child exploitation enterprise operated for the sole purpose of promoting child sexual abuse and disseminating child pornography.

Many people use the Internet to meet others through online ads. Padgett (2007) surveyed 740 women who had met in person with a man who answered their online personal ads. She found that women used email prior to a face-to-face meeting to negotiate such issues as safety, boundaries, sexual preferences, history of STIs, and condom use. Thirty percent of respondents engaged in sexual activity on their first encounter. Seventy-seven percent did not use condoms for their first sexual encounter. The large amount of email communication prior to meeting seemed to accelerate the intimacy for people involved and may have affected women's decisions to engage in risky sexual behaviors.

Simon and Daneback (2013) conducted a thematic literature review to determine what is known about adolescents' experiences with sexuality education. They identified four major themes in the literature: (1) Adolescents report engaging with sexuality information online; (2) adolescents are interested in a number of topics, including sexually transmitted infections and pregnancy; (3) the quality of adolescent-targeted sexuality information online may be lacking, but adolescents can evaluate these sources; and (4) Internet-based interventions can increase adolescents' sexual health knowledge.

Revenge porn is sexually explicit media that is publicly shared online without the consent of the pictured individual. The vast majority of the victims are females, and many of the pictures have been taken by the pictured persons themselves (selfies). More than three-fourths of the states in the United States either have laws against revenge porn or are considering passing such laws. The most recent status of these states can be found at http://www.cagoldberglaw.com/states-with-revenge-porn-laws/. In 2015, Twitter banned revenge porn. The social media giant had previously come under fire for it lax controls against cyberbullying, but new policies targeting revenge porn added to Twitter's efforts to crack down on cyberbullying.

The Internet has been used in many ways related to sexuality—some positive and some negative. Mustanski et al. (2015) examined the feasibility of recruiting youth in same-sex relationships into an online sexual health intervention. A sample (202) of 16- to 20-year-old LGBT youth completed a pretest, intervention, and post-test assessments. The results, which covered the topics of sexual orientation identity and self-acceptance, sexual heath knowledge, relationship variables, and safer sex, demonstrated that an online comprehensive sexual health program could be very effective for LBGT youth.

Technology has even allowed people to find out what music others like to use during their sexual activity (Condliffe, 2015). The music streaming service, Spotify, sifted through 2.5 million user-made playlists mentioning sex in their title—to see what music gets streamed during sexual activity. Spotify then assembled the most popular songs into a playlist that others can use. It also did the same exercise for the word "love."

Previously, we discussed sexual addiction. We also listed some symptoms of cybersex addiction, which could relate to this discussion as well. You may want to refer to them again to see if they apply to you or anyone you know.

Another example of positive use of the Internet related to sexuality occurred when the New York City Health Department launched a Facebook page to promote condom use. In just one afternoon, 1,500 Facebook messages, called e-condoms, were sent through the website. One more example occurred when the U.S. Department of Justice unveiled new public-service announcements to educate people about potential dangers that children face online and, for the first time, warned potential online predators that exploiting a child online is a serious federal offense.

Sex toys are just one part of the commercialization of sexuality. It is estimated that the U.S. sex industry generates $9 billion in annual sales. With so much money at stake, do you think it would be difficult to control and regulate such an industry?

Sexual Aids

Another aspect of the commercialization of sexuality is selling the promise (and sometimes the reality) of more satisfying sexual activity through the use of sexual devices and other aids. There is a big business in the manufacture and sale of sexual aids and enhancers. Some, such as penile implants and vibrators, are used in treating sexual dysfunctions. Videos on techniques for achieving orgasm and enhancing the sexual experience are often used by sex therapists as an adjunct to their treatment programs.

Previously we discussed some of the uses of vibrators. They come in a variety of colors and shapes and can be electrically or battery operated. They can be used by males or females for solitary masturbation or as a part of heterosexual or LGBTQ encounters. Many are sold in ordinary retail outlets for massage purposes.

One vibratorlike device, called the Eroscillator, even has its own website. It points out that the Eroscillator is *not* a vibrator. "It provides a totally unique, gentle 'oscillating' motion which moves naturally and softly from side to side rather than up and down like a vibrator." If you believe the ad, the Eroscillator has three different levels of intensity, is completely safe, is specifically designed to meet your needs, and has no risk of irritation.

Magazines and newspapers are full of ads claiming that women may add extra inches to their breasts with only a few minutes of specific exercise daily or by using creams, massage, or worthless gadgets—all for a price. Just as the Eroscillator does, a breast cream called Enhancia has its own web page. One woman claims she noticed a difference in about 2 weeks: an increase of almost 1 inch around her bust.

In fact, breast size and shape are the result of glandular influences that cannot be altered by applying anything to the breast. It is also impossible to increase breast size through exercise. The effect of exercise is to enlarge muscle tissue. Because there is no muscle tissue in the breast, exercise cannot enhance the breast. Only injections or implants can enlarge the breast. These procedures are controversial and expensive, and they can have dangerous long-term effects.

Underclothing that particularly emphasizes the genitals is manufactured to satisfy a range of tastes. It is sold by mail-order businesses, by email, and by expensive boutiques. Other sexual products are more exotic. A few examples of these products will demonstrate their nature:

1. Some manufacturers have gone beyond the standard type of vibrator that therapists recommend to enhance sexual pleasure. For example, one manufacturer advertises a 7-inch vibrator with various attachments: natural veined penis, French tickler, fuzzy tongue, and others.

2. A variety of aphrodisiacs and lotions are available: Motion Lotion, Joy Jelly, Korean Ginseng capsules, Man Power capsules, Spanish Fly Sugar powder, or Wild Passion Ginseng capsules. They are unlikely to be effective.

3. A man dissatisfied with the size of his penis may be persuaded to buy a "penis enlarger vacuum," and a female dissatisfied with the size of her breasts can buy a "breast enlarger."

4. Penis extenders are used by those who want to give their partner the sensation of penetration by a larger penis. They are worn at the tip of the penis and are held in place by a condom or straps. Penis erectors vary in design, but many are like splints designed to support a nonerect penis. Another variety is a "cock ring," which fits around the base of the penis after erection and maintains the erection while it is in place. Also available is an artificial penis attached to a motor that moves the penis in a thrusting manner.

5. Artificial vaginas are available for males for masturbatory purposes; artificial penises (dildos) can be used by either males or females for insertion into the vagina or anus.

6. Another product advertises by asking men whether they have ever experienced fellatio while driving a car. If they have and enjoyed the sensation, or would like such an experience, they are invited to buy the Auto Suck Vagina. The product resembles an automobile vacuum and thus, the ad reassuringly advises, keeps its user out of trouble with the highway police should he be stopped "at the moment of climax."

Herbenick et al. (2009) studied the lifetime and recent popularity of women's vibrator use during masturbation and sexual activity with partners. More than half of the 2,000 respondents reported vibrator use. Vibrator users were significantly more likely to have had a gynecologic exam during the past year and had more positive function. Nearly three-fourths of the vibrator users reported no genital symptoms with vibrator use.

Reece et al. (2009) explored the lifetime and recent prevalence rates for vibrator use by men in the United States. Forty-five percent of the men had integrated vibrators into sexual activities during their lives. Those who had used vibrators were more likely to report participation in sexual health–promoting behaviors, such as testicular self-exam. Men who had used vibrators recently also received higher scores on erectile function, intercourse satisfaction, orgasmic function, and sexual desire.

Rosenberger et al. (2012) found a high prevalence of sex toy use among gay and bisexual men, including a diverse range of products being used and incorporation of sex toys in a variety of sexual behaviors. Although not directly measured, the data implied the possibility that gay and bisexual communities have responded to ongoing public health messages encouraging men to speak openly with sexual partners and take responsibility for their sexual health.

Sexual aids used to be sold almost exclusively out of "porno-sleaze" shops in such places as New York's Times Square, but they have become such big business that they are now sold in women's sex-toy boutiques. Many of these boutiques run a very profitable catalogue business. An example of this type of organization is the Xandria Collection. Through its catalogue one can purchase dildos, vibrators that fit over the penis for self-stimulation, prosthetic penis aids, penis extensions, clitoral stimulators, penis rings, and Ben-Wa balls (small balls to insert into the vagina that move around, thereby stimulating the woman), not to mention the various lotions and potions and underwear with holes in just the right places. In addition, the Xandria Collection sells educational books such as *Complete Guide to Sexual Positions*, *Ride 'Em Cowgirl*, *Tickle His Pickle*, *Tickle Your Fancy Book*, and *Toy Gasms Book*.

Another means of selling sexual aids has as its model the famous Tupperware parties. Here is how it works: Someone volunteers the use of her house for the party and invites a group of friends, and a saleswoman shows a variety of sexual aids, ranging from soft leather to French ticklers (penis sleeves with ribs to stimulate the vagina). Thousands of women are supplementing incomes and sometimes even becoming wealthy by selling sex products at home demonstrations. Passion Parties is one of the largest such companies. Good Vibrations is an example of a company that advertises numerous sexual toys. Its representatives will come to private homes to host parties and sell sex products. As an example of the company's advertising on the Good Vibrations website it indicates you can "make it a birthday party or bridal shower they'll never forget." Fisher et al. (2010) used online questionnaires to interview 1,197 women who facilitate in-home sex-toy parties. They found that the parties seem to provide an effective avenue through which to increase adult sexual literacy.

In-home sex toy parties can be sexuality education opportunities to promote sexual functioning by opening discourses around pleasure and desire. The parties allow women to purchase products such as lubricant and vibrators. Facilitators may also provide sex therapists with a new means of reaching women. The women who attend these parties are often not able to be contacted using traditional outreach methods, as they may feel shy voicing sexual concerns (Schick et al., 2013).

As you can see, the use of sex to sell products, combined with the manufacture and sale of sexual aids, is significant. You can hardly open a magazine or newspaper, read a book, watch television, attend the theater, or listen to popular music without encountering sexual themes; sexual explicitness (and implicitness) is part of our everyday existence.

We need to be aware of its presence so that we can better control its effect on our behavior and attitudes. By way of example, knowing that the scantily clad model has no relation to our need to own a new car, we might be better able to ignore the sexual appeal of the ads and purchase a car that is suited to our needs and financial constraints.

Being aware of the uses of sexuality in the marketplace can make you a better consumer, a more enlightened citizen, and a healthier person sexually.

Sexually Explicit Materials

Terminology is critical, but somewhat confusing, in relation to sexually explicit materials. You may hear different people use the same terms to describe different things, so it is important to establish definitions. **Pornography** is visual and written material that is used for purposes of sexual arousal. It has been said that pornography, as is beauty, is in the eye of the beholder. Opinions about what it is, its possible uses, and its legal status are extremely varied.

Definitions

The legal definition of *obscenity*, established by the Supreme Court in 1973, is that for something to be obscene it must meet all three of the following conditions:

1. The average person, applying contemporary community standards, would find that the work, taken as a whole, appeals to **prurient** interest.

2. The work depicts or describes, in a patently offensive way, sexual conduct specifically defined by the applicable state (or federal) law.

3. The work, taken as a whole, lacks serious literary, artistic, political, or scientific value.

Therefore, although sexually explicit materials are legal in the United States, obscenity is not. Taking the three Supreme Court criteria just listed together, a reasonable definition of **obscenity** is a personal or societal judgment that something is offensive. Therefore, one person may consider obscene something that another does not.

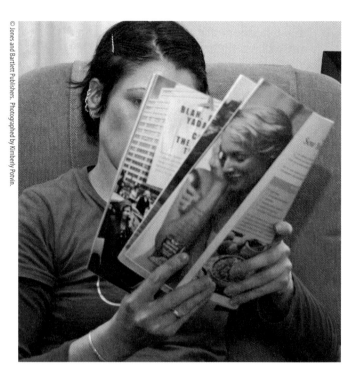

Sexually explicit materials are easily available to people of all ages.

Another important term is **erotica**, which usually describes sexually oriented material that can be evaluated positively, in contrast to obscenity, which is offensive. Erotica consists of "depictions of sexuality which display mutuality, respect, affection, and a balance of power". Some people will differentiate between pornography and erotica by indicating that pornography provides a degrading or demeaning portrayal of human beings. In contrast, erotica is not degrading or demeaning anyone. Therefore, a person may find pornography to be unacceptable and erotica to be acceptable based upon this differentiation.

Effects of Sexually Explicit Materials

Traditionally many people have been opposed to sexually explicit materials. Perhaps this is because they feared that the materials had many undesirable effects, such as causing people to participate in sexual activity they might not otherwise have engaged in, increasing the number of sexual offenses, and corrupting the minds of children. It is difficult to do research in an area where there are so many personal and social variables, but a brief look at research findings about the effects of sexually explicit materials may be helpful.

The report of the Commission on Obscenity and Pornography (1970), sponsored by the federal government, and a review of this report by two researchers at Johns Hopkins University (Money & Athanasiou, 1973) give us some information about the effects of pornography. Although this research

pornography Visual and written materials used for the purpose of sexual arousal.

prurient Characterized by lustful thoughts or wishes.

obscenity Personal or societal judgment that something is offensive.

erotica Sexually oriented material that may be artistically produced or motivated.

summary is almost 50 years old, it still represents a valid summary of the effects of sexually explicit materials. According to these sources, the following appear to be true:

1. There is little, if any, difference in males' and females' sexual responses to sexually explicit materials.

2. People are stimulated only by portrayals of sexual ideas or acts that turn them on. In other words, sexually explicit materials do not seem to plant in people's minds ideas or desires that they do not already have.

3. Exposure to sexually explicit materials does not seem to alter a person's sexual behavior patterns in the long run.

4. Continued exposure to sexually explicit materials tends to lead to indifference and boredom. Stimuli in sexually explicit materials are effective for 2 to 4 hours. After this time a person becomes either more selective or indifferent to the stimuli.

5. Filling out questionnaires on responses to sexually explicit material may be more stimulating than the material itself. (Perhaps this is best explained by human beings' great capacity to fantasize.)

6. Convicted sex offenders have been exposed to fewer sexually explicit and sexuality education materials during their life than nonoffenders. This fact contradicts the common belief that exposure to sexually explicit materials causes people to commit sexual offenses.

The Society for the Scientific Study of Sexuality (What scientists know about pornography, 2007) provides the following summary regarding effects of exposure to sexually explicit material:

- In general, when exposed to nonviolent erotica, men and women show small, short-term increases in the sexual behaviors they already are used to engaging in, but generally they do not add anything new to their sexual repertoire.

- Both men and women are sexually aroused by erotic material, but women report more negative emotional reactions than men, and women seem to be less likely to access sexually explicit materials.

- Findings on the effects of exposure to violent pornography are more mixed. Some researchers have found that exposure to sexually violent materials increases the

Gender DIMENSIONS

Male and Female Use of Pornography

According to Covenant Eyes (2015), 9 out of 10 boys and 6 out of 10 girls are exposed to pornography before the age of 18. The first exposure to pornography among males is at age 12 years, on average. Fifty-one percent of male and 32% of female students first viewed porn at age 12 or younger. Approximately 64% to 68% of young adult men and 18% of women view porn at least once every week. Another 17% of men and another 30% of women view porn 1 or 2 times per month. Two-thirds of college-age men and half of college-age women say viewing porn is an acceptable way to express one's sexuality.

Barber (2013) pointed out that 30% of Internet pornography users are women. Clearly, women are not less sexual than men. Other research has shown that women's bodies are capable of experiencing a great deal of sexual pleasure. Contrary to gender stereotypes, many women are interested in pornography, and it is probably no accident that young women are drawn to cyberporn that can be enjoyed in private.

In a study carried out by Knibbs (2014), 21.3% of women and 1.8 % of men were reported to prefer same-sex porn to heterosexual porn. Seventy percent of men and 14% of women watched activities on porn they would not attempt in real life. Two-thirds of men reached orgasm faster while watching porn than they did from real-life sexual activity. Sixty-three percent of women were not bothered by their male partner's porn-watching habits, as long as this activity did not interfere with the relationship.

Pornography statistics: Annual report 2015. *Covenanteyes.com*, 2015. Available: http://www.covenanteyes.com/pornstats/.: Barber, N. Women flock to pornography. *PsychologyToday.com*, 2013. Available: http://www.covenanteyes.com/pornstats/. Knibbs, K. This survey shows how men and women view porn differently. *Time.com*, 2014. Available: http://time.com/author/kate-knibbs/.

acceptance of rape myths (beliefs that ascribe responsibility to women who are the victims) and increases men's self-reported likelihood of raping a woman. Other studies have found just the opposite. Still others have found no association between use of sexually explicit media and negative attitudes toward women.

Rich (2008) summarized research related to the effects of relatively violent pornography on adolescents. Male adolescents were more likely to believe women enjoy forced sexual activity after seeing an excerpt in which a woman was shown as aroused by nonconsenting intercourse. Males who watched films that portrayed violence against females as justifiable and with positive consequences showed increased belief in rape myths and acceptance of violence against women as compared with males who saw films with no sexual violence. Females had the opposite reaction to the same films. Both male and female viewers reported they were more sexually aroused by nonaggressive rather than aggressive sexually explicit materials.

Kingston et al. (2009) looked at pornography's influence on sexually aggressive behavior. They found that pornography use can be a risk factor for sexually aggressive outcomes, principally for men who rate high on other risk factors and who use pornography frequently.

Albright (2008) surveyed more than 15,000 men and women related to pornography. Seventy-five percent of men and 41% of women had intentionally viewed pornography. Women reported more negative consequences, including lowered body image, their partner being critical of their body, increased pressure to perform acts seen in pornographic films, and less actual sexual behavior. Men reported being more critical of their partners' body and less interested in actual sexual behavior.

Sun et al. (2014) examined the role that pornography plays in real-world sexual encounters between a man and a woman. They found that the more pornography a man watches, the more likely he is to use it during sexual activity, request particular pornographic sex acts of his partner, deliberately conjure images of pornography during sexual activity to maintain arousal, and have concerns over his own sexual performance and body image. Higher pornography use was negatively associated with enjoying sexually intimate behaviors with a partner.

Braithwaite et al. (2015) found that more frequent viewing of pornography is associated with a higher incidence of "hooking up" and a higher number of unique hookup partners. They also found that more frequent viewing of pornography is associated with having more previous sexual partners of all types, more one-occasion partners ("one-night stands"), and plans to have a higher number of sexual partners in the future.

It is important to point out that, as with other topics in this book, a relationship between two things does not show causation. In other words, in this case we do not know if viewing pornography changes behaviors in any way, or if it just that those people who view more pornography are the same people who would engage in those behaviors anyway.

For years some people have suggested that sexually explicit materials might be stimulating to men, but not to women. Today we know that such materials can be stimulating to both sexes, but that there are individual differences in responses. We also know that in most cases exposure to pornography does not influence long-term behaviors or change interests in most sexual behaviors one way or the other.

Watson and Smith (2012) reviewed literature summarizing both negative and neutral-to-positive findings about the effects of sexually explicit materials. They found that despite widespread beliefs that such material causes or contributes to violence, sexual deviance, degradation of women, destruction of relationships, public health concerns, and moral decay, there is little evidence to support such broad claims. When considering the neutral-to-positive impacts of sexually explicit materials, they pointed out that proponents of sexually explicit materials have long held that greater access to information about sexuality/sexual health may diminish anxieties and that encouragement of sexual expression may enhance individual enjoyment and relational connection. Their literature review seems to support these points. Although it is always important to properly prepare and use educational materials, the literature reviewed by Watson and Smith supported the use of sexually explicit material to provide information about sexuality and male and female bodies, to help individuals understand differences in arousal and fantasy, to open lines of communication, and to share thoughts and ideas about sexual topics.

Child Pornography

So far we have considered sexually explicit materials about adults for adults. There is increasing concern about the use of children in pornographic materials and, more recently, about continued eroticization of young children in the print media, on the Internet, and on television.

The use of minors in sexually explicit media—**child pornography**—is now prohibited. In the past,

child pornography Use of minors in sexually explicit media.

People who might support the availability of sexually explicit materials for adults usually do not condone child pornography.

many magazine publishers and film producers used their own children in sexually explicit materials they developed. Others advertised in magazines catering to readers of pornography. Still, in spite of the law, magazines and films that depict children in sexually erotic conditions are produced and sold. Given the current societal concern for child abuse (sexual and otherwise) and for missing children, law enforcement agencies have organized to crack down on the kiddie porn industry.

In 1984, the National Center for Missing and Exploited Children was established by the federal government. In 1997, an Exploited Child Unit was established within this agency to deal with child pornography and other crimes. In 1998, the CyberTipline was launched to have a means of reporting incidents of child sexual exploitation including the possession, manufacture, or distribution of child pornography; online enticement; child prostitution; child sex tourism; extrafamilial child sexual molestation; unsolicited obscene material sent to a child; and misleading domain names, words, or digital images. The Cyber-Tipline (*www.cybertipline.com*) is staffed 24 hours a day, 7 days a week. More than 33 million reports of suspected child sexual exploitation were made to the CyberTipline between 1998 and 2015. In 2002, a Child Victim Identification Program was established with a dual mission. The program provides two types of assistance:

- It helps federal and state law enforcement agencies and prosecutors with child pornography investigations.

- It assists law enforcement in identifying child victims so these personnel can locate and rescue the children from exploitative situations.

In 2006, the Sex Offender Registration and Notification Act was passed. It was passed for two reasons: (1) to establish a national database that tracks the location and movements of people convicted of a criminal offense against a victim who is a minor, have been convicted of a sexually violent offense, or are sexually violent predators, and (2) to register and verify the addresses of sex offenders who reside in states without a "minimally sufficient" sex offender registry program. (Today all 50 states have minimally

Ethical DIMENSIONS

Should Kids Be Sexualized?

There has been a great deal of discussion related to whether to control the routines of high school bands, cheerleaders, and dancers. A Texas legislator sponsored a bill to ban "sexually suggestive" cheerleading in the public schools. A school superintendent in Alabama told bands to clean up their acts. These actions prompted a variety of responses.

On the one hand, one Alabama parent said, "As long as they're not taking any clothes off, I don't see anything wrong with it." A PTA president said, "If we're going to limit our children doing their routines, then take the Dallas Cowgirls off TV."

On the other hand, one band director said, "It is a family show, and high school girls shouldn't be doing college-girl dance routines." A school superintendent said, "It would be much more appealing to have fine sounds produced by the bands than vulgar routines."

Is it ethical for high school bands, cheerleaders, and dancers to be allowed to do suggestive routines? Is it right to have legislation, such as that in Texas, designed to ban "sexually suggestive" cheerleading? Who should decide what is right or wrong related to the possibility of sexualizing students in public schools?

Technological advances have made controlling access to sexually explicit materials very difficult. Debates continue about whether or not it should be controlled at all.

sufficient programs.) Guidelines for this act can be found at http://ojp.gov/smart/pdfs/final_sornaguidelines.pdf.

Under federal legislation, child pornography is defined as any visual depiction where a minor is used to engage in sexually explicit conduct, or a technological image is used that is indistinguishable from that of a minor, or it appears that a minor is engaging in sexually explicit conduct. It is a federal crime to knowingly produce, distribute, receive, or possess with intent to distribute, a visual depiction of any kind, including a drawing, cartoon, sculpture, or painting that meets these criteria. A minor is defined as a person younger than the age of 18.

In 2014, Japan finally passed a bill to ban the possession of child pornography (Hellmann, 2014). Under the new law, people found with explicit photos or video of children can be imprisoned for up to 1 year and fined up to $10,000. Prior to this time, Japan had been known as an international hub for the production and trafficking of child pornography. It was the last Organization for Economic Cooperation and Development nation to make possession of such materials a punishable offense.

Child pornography exists in multiple formats and is transmitted on various platforms on the Internet.

The Control of Sexually Explicit Materials

Should sexually explicit materials be censored and controlled? There are varying opinions. In an attempt to keep sexually explicit materials on the Internet away from the 16 million users younger than 17 years old in the United States, Congress passed the Child Online Protection Act, which forced websites to require a credit card number or some other

adult ID. The law made it a crime to knowingly communicate to a minor "for commercial purposes" any online material that is "harmful to minors." Penalties included fines up to $50,000 per day for each violation and up to 6 months in prison. (Head, 2012). This law has been controversial. Some people believe that it is in society's best interest to protect children from sexually explicit materials. Free speech advocates, in contrast, challenge the law on constitutional grounds, arguing it would affect everybody on the web.

In 2009, the long legal drive to shield children from sexually explicit material on the web ended. The Supreme Court struck down the law on free-speech grounds. Judges said parents can protect their children in their own way by installing software filters on their computers.

The Child Pornography and Protection Act was passed in 1996 (High court to hear arguments on child porn amendment, 2001). Since then supporters have claimed that the act was an essential tool to prevent pedophiles from preying on children. Those who disagree have argued that it is so vaguely worded that there is no way to know what is over the line and what is not. The U.S. Supreme Court struck down the law in 2002 for being overly broad.

A major related event occurred in June 2003 when the U.S. Supreme Court upheld a federal law requiring public library personnel to install pornography filters on all computers providing Internet access as

Myth vs Fact

Myth: There is no difference between obscenity and pornography.

Fact: Yes, there is. Obscenity is not protected by the Constitution. It follows the Supreme Court definition, but pornography is material designed to arouse and has no legal or consistent definition.

Myth: Sexually explicit material causes violence against women.

Fact: No reputable research in the United States, Europe, or Asia finds a causal link between pornography and violence.

Myth: Men watch pornography and imitate it or force women to do what they see.

Fact: Violence and intimidation existed for thousands of years before commercial pornography. People do not mimic what they

read or view in knee-jerk fashion. Men do not learn coercion from sexual pictures.

Myth: Pornography degrades women.

Fact: Sexism, not sexual behavior, degrades women. Opponents of sexual speech do not understand that it is in everyone's interest to allow a variety of pleasurable materials that enhance well-being and sexual fulfillment.

Myth: Pornography is only for men.

Fact: Half the adult videos in the United States are bought or rented by women alone or women in couples. AIDS and other STIs have made it a public health necessity to encourage sexual fantasy material that offers women and men safe alternatives to unhealthy sexual contact.

a condition of continuing to receive federal subsidies and grants (Greenhouse, 2003). The law, enacted in 2001, had been blocked by a lower court and never taken effect. Under the law, filters are required for all library users, not just children. The law authorizes, but does not require, librarians to unblock Internet sites at the request of adult users. Many opinions exist about the wisdom of this law and how it relates to First Amendment rights to free speech.

Certain segments of the public are very concerned about the increased availability of sexually explicit materials and have organized to combat this trend. They point out that many X-rated movies, CDs, and DVDs are purchased and rented. They talk about the popularity of cable television channels, such as the Playboy Channel, that specialize in sexual broadcasts; they also emphasize the success of such sexually explicit magazines as *Penthouse* and *Playboy*.

The interesting aspect of the organized opposition to sexually explicit materials is that it has united diverse groups. National conservative groups as well as some national feminist groups have joined a loose network of local groups to fight the "Porn War." Among the conservative organizations are the American Family Association, the Citizens for Decency Through Law, the National Center on Sexual Exploitation, and the Citizens for Legislation Against Decadence. Among the feminist groups are Feminists Against Pornography and Women Against Violence Against Women.

The objections of these groups to sexually explicit materials are several. Some consider an explicit description or image of sexual acts immoral and irreligious. Others object to women being portrayed as sex objects and believe this view of women will be generalized to "real life." Still others perceive that women in sexually explicit materials are treated violently and fear that this type of portrayal might cause more violence toward women. For example, one group demanded that sexually explicit materials be prohibited from depicting rape, whipping, or bondage. They believed that such depictions lead men to feel superior to women and extend that idea of superiority to nonsexual relationships (such as those in the workplace). Others concentrate predominantly on music and advertising, asserting that commercial degradation of women fosters sexism.

Many groups of women are most vocal in their opinions. However, though not organized, men also suffer from sexploitation. When men are shown performing violent acts on women, they are being taught to be powerful and dominant over the other sex. They are learning that sexual relationships require a measure of forcefulness that in actuality interferes with sexual arousal rather than enhances it. When men learn to treat women as sexual objects, their relationships suffer. Depictions of men and women sharing equally in sexual and loving relationships would teach both sexes that sexual fulfillment is a mutual responsibility; the results would be a decrease of pressure on men to know what to do and how to do it and fewer sexually frustrated women.

The ACLU says that it is no accident that freedom of speech is the first freedom mentioned in the First Amendment. It is not limited to "pure speech"—books, newspapers, leaflets, and rallies. It also protects "symbolic speech"—nonverbal expression whose purpose it is to communicate ideas. It exists precisely to protect the most offensive and controversial speech from government suppression. The best means to counter obnoxious speech is speech. Persuasion, not coercion, is the solution. The ACLU also indicates that the innovation and citizen empowerment inspired by online communications will be lost if civil liberties do not also apply in cyberspace. Furthermore, there are three reasons freedom of expression is essential to a free society: (1) The right to express one's thoughts and to communicate freely with others is the foundation of self-fulfillment. (2) It is vital to the attainment and advancement of knowledge and the search for the truth. (3) It is necessary to our system of self-government and gives the American people a "checking function" against government excess and corruption.

Feminists for Free Expression (FFE) is a leading voice opposing state and national legislation that threatens free speech. This organization

Myth (vs) Fact

Myth: Women in pornography are exploited or victimized.
Fact: Women are exploited and harassed in all fields, including pornography. Exploitation will stop when it is vigorously prosecuted everywhere it occurs. Some women in pornography say their work gives them independence and a sense of accomplishment; banning it would worsen their lives.

Myth: As an aid to masturbation, pornography is action that is not protected by the First Amendment.
Fact: Pornography may lead to masturbation much as a novel or film may lead to tears or laughter. Feminists for Free Expression does not believe policing masturbation is the proper business of government or well-meaning committees.

Myth: Banning sexual material will protect or help women.
Fact: Historically, censorship has hurt women. It has prevented them from getting information about sexuality and reproduction. The best protection for women's ideas is the constitutional protection of free speech. The answer to bad pornography is good pornography, not no pornography.

defends the right of free expression in court cases, supports the rights of activists whose works have been suppressed or censored, and provides expert speakers. On the topic of sexually explicit materials, FFE published *Feminism and Free Speech: Pornography* to aid in the understanding of pornography, its uses and benefits, and its relation to violence. An overview of its scientific and cross-cultural research is provided in the Myth vs Fact box about pornography on the previous page. Relatedly, there is more erotica being developed that is not sexist but feminist and gender friendly. It is designed to portray equitable relationships.

The increased easy access to sexually explicit materials has raised an interesting issue: What should we be allowed to watch in public? (Richtel, 2012). For example, is it okay to play explicit materials in the back seat of a car or on buses that could be viewed by others in the vehicle or on the road? Should airlines police what people watch on planes? How about in an Internet cafe or a restaurant? This can be a thorny issue because not everyone agrees on what might be considered offensive. Also, people don't agree on what is acceptable to view in private as opposed to in public settings.

In October 2002 the Museum of Sex opened in New York City. The purpose of the museum is to preserve and present the history, evolution, and cultural significance of human sexuality. Not everyone approves of it. William Donohue, president of the Catholic League for Religions and Civil Rights, denounced the museum for celebrating "smut as sex." He accused the museum of championing or associating with racists, pornographers, and individuals who "exhibit pathological characteristics." On the other side, June Reinisch, a historian adviser to the museum and director emeritus of the Kinsey Institute, characterized it as a serious endeavor, in the sense that it wants to inform and educate as well as to entertain. "Sexuality is a very important part of individual life and to culture," she said. "To not understand it is to be handicapped in your understanding of human relations and culture" (James, 2002). Over a recent 7 year period the Museum of Sex generated 16 exhibitions and 5 virtual installations, each in keeping with its mission of advocating open discourse surrounding sexuality as well as presenting to the public current scholarship unhindered by self-censorship. The museum is committed to addressing a wide range of topics while highlighting material and artifacts from different continents, cultures, time periods, and media.

Finally, the position of the Sexuality Information and Education Council of the United States on sexually explicit materials is as follows:

SIECUS believes that sexually explicit visual, printed, or online materials can be valuable educational or personal aids when sensitively used in a manner appropriate to the viewer's age and developmental level. Such materials can help reduce ignorance and confusion and contribute to a positive concept of sexuality while supporting the sexual rights of all. However, the use of violence, exploitation, or degradation, or the portrayal of children in sexually explicit materials is reprehensible.

SIECUS believes that adults should have the right to access sexually explicit materials for personal use. Legislative and judicial efforts to prevent the production or distribution of sexually explicit materials endanger constitutionally guaranteed freedoms of speech and press, and could be employed to restrict the appropriate professional use of such materials by sexuality educators, therapists, and researchers.

Sex Workers

An important consideration in the study of sexual commercial enterprises is the topic of sex work, or prostitution. The term **prostitution** refers to any situation in which one person pays another for sexual gratification. Sex workers may be males as well as females, but primarily sex workers have been and are females. Women do sex work mainly to make money, but other factors can also motivate them. For example, the lack of education of most sex workers limits their job opportunities. In addition, some women think sex work will be exciting and glamorous, whereas others are motivated to become sex workers because they do not like the discipline and boredom of regular jobs. Some women who are drug addicts turn to sex work to support their habit. The background of many sex workers has included emotional deprivation and sexual abuse—even within the family. Some sex workers therefore feel that by providing sexual pleasure they can gain intimacy and attention.

Is prostitution a victimless crime? Lowen (2015a) pointed out that the opposing attitudes of many men and women regarding prostitution reveal one of the widest gender gaps in male–female relationships. Many men see nothing wrong with it because it is legal in some other countries and in Nevada. However, what a prostitute endures on any given workday ranges from rape and physical violence to life-threatening abuse at the hands of her pimp or her customers (johns). The act of selling one's body as a commodity and the associated mental health

---

prostitution Participating in sexual activity for pay or profit.

Because of their visibility, streetwalkers are the most frequently arrested sex workers.

risks are significant factors that can stand alone in disproving the "victimless crime" idea.

What explanations are given for adult involvement in sex work? McCarthy et al. (2014) indicated that two approaches are often taken to address this issue. One approach highlights a variety of negative experiences in childhood and adolescence, including physical and sexual abuse, family instability, poverty, associations with "pimps" and other exploiters, homelessness, and drug use. An alternative approach recognizes that some of the above factors may be involved, but underscores the contribution of more immediate circumstances, such as current economic needs and employment opportunities. In their research, McCarthy et al. found that both immediate circumstances and negative experiences from early life were independently associated with adult sex work, as were limited education and employment experience, adult drug use, and marital status.

Dank et al. (2014) sought to determine the scale of the underground sex economy in eight major U.S. cities. Their findings were eye-opening:

- The underground sex economy was estimated to involve revenues between $39.9 million and $290 million per year.

- The pimps and traffickers interviewed by the researchers took home between $5,000 and $32,000 per week.

- Most pimps believed that media portrayals exaggerated violence. Although they

indicated that the physical violence involved in prostitution is less than what people generally believe, they did cite frequent use of psychological coercion to maintain control over their employees.

- Pimps used a variety of tactics to recruit and maintain employees. Some credited their entry into pimping to a natural capacity for manipulation.

- Some pimps and sex workers had family members or friends who exposed them to the sex trade at a young age, normalizing their decision to participate in it.

- The Internet is changing the limitations of the trade. Prostitution is decreasing on the street, but thriving online. Pimps and sex workers advertise on social media to attract customers and new employees.

- The underground sex economy is perceived as low risk. While they had some fears of prosecution, pimps, traffickers, and child pornography offenders believed that their crimes were low risk.

- Policy and practice changes can help combat trafficking and prostitution. Among them are efforts geared toward imposing more fines for ad host websites, consistently enforcing the laws against offenders to diminish the low-risk perception, and increasing awareness among school officials and the general public about the realities of sex trafficking to deter victimization and entry into this environment.

Types of Sex Workers

It is difficult to estimate the number of persons who currently work or have ever worked as sex workers because there are various definitions of prostitution and because sex work is usually illegal. There are many types of sex workers; the major types are call girls, house prostitutes, streetwalkers, massage parlor prostitutes, and bar girls and strippers.

Call Girls
Call girls are at the top of the profession. They do not solicit; rather, their "dates" are arranged by personal referral or by another person. They have regular clients who pay high fees and also pay their bills.

call girls Highly paid female sex workers who work by appointment only.

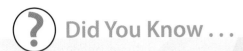

Did You Know . . .

Did you know that there is a historical connection between Santa Claus and sex workers? In the third century, a rich and good-hearted Turkish man named Nicholas saved poor girls from prostitution by throwing bags of gold coins through their windows or down a chimney. Over the next 700 years, with a little help from Dutch settlers in America and a poet named

Clement Clarke Moore, Saint Nicholas was transposed into a merry old gent with a white beard and red suit who spends most of Christmas giving toys to good little girls and boys.

Darvas, M. "Real" Santa Claus fought sex trafficking, 2012. Available: http://mattdarvas.com/2012/12/17/real-santa-claus-fought-sex-trafficking/.

House Prostitutes

House (brothel) prostitutes work in more structured conditions in brothels (houses in which prostitutes work) and serve more men at cheaper rates than call girls would charge. Brothels are legal in some counties of Nevada but are illegal in all other areas of the United States.

Streetwalkers

Streetwalkers are more independent than house prostitutes but lack the contacts or ability to become call girls. They stand or stroll on streets and approach passing males. Because of their visibility, streetwalkers are the most frequently arrested sex workers.

The ratio of on-street prostitution to off-street prostitution in cities varies with local law, police, and custom. For example, in larger cities experts seem to think that street prostitution is about 10–20% of the prostitution, but in smaller cities (with more limited indoor opportunities), street prostitution might be as much as 50% of the total.

Many women who engage in street sex work experience pregnancies and become mothers. They report that being pregnant or parenting while regularly working the street caused them to feel ashamed of themselves and their work and anxious for their own and their children's safety. Pregnancies and parenting responsibilities also alter their working productivity and practices.

Massage Parlor Sex Workers

Some **massage parlors** offer only massages, but at others a client can find many "extras." The environment offers an indoor place to work that is safer than the streets, and massage parlor workers may be motivated to earn extra money by providing sexual favors. Fellatio is popular among both customers and masseuses. Many men claim they cannot get their regular partners to participate in fellatio. The masseuses appreciate it because it is efficient. They are trying to earn as much money as they can, and with this technique they can service a large number of men in a short period.

Bar Girls and Strippers

Bar girls and strippers are supposed to act available so men will buy them drinks, thereby profiting the house. This helps the establishment make more on the sale of liquor. Sometimes paid sexual activity is also offered.

Examples of this type of activity can be found in many countries. For example, an increasing number of Cambodian "beer girls," who sell international beers, wines, and liquors at outdoor eateries and in bars, are also selling sexual activity. If the women refuse a client's offer of sexual activity for money, they may lose a beer sale. Because they depend heavily on commissions, they feel they have to do something to convince the client to buy.

Japan's sex trade, estimated at $13 billion per year, is one of the nation's fastest-growing industries. Record unemployment has forced many women to work at brothels euphemistically known as fashion, health, soapland, pink salons, or telephone clubs.

Stripping can be a springboard either to something better or to an abyss of drugs, alcohol, abuse, and prostitution. Sometimes stripping is just a living—the rent. Many dancers say they love what they do, if not for the money then for the attention, or for the power they wield over men who are "stupid enough to pay to see you naked." Most dancers seem to aspire to something else—being an actress, a model, a good mother, or a successful career person.

There has been greater female attendance at strip clubs in recent years. Some dancers have incorporated female patrons into a sexualized space traditionally designed for men. They have tailored their lap dances for a female patron. In this way, the strip

---

house (brothel) prostitutes Sex workers who work in brothels.

streetwalkers Sex workers who work on the streets.

massage parlors Places where sex workers can be hired to perform sexual acts under the guise of giving a massage.

bar girls Sex workers who are supposed to act available so customers will buy them drinks.

club becomes a potential space for engaging in same-sex eroticism that includes elements of play.

Male Sex Workers

Whereas the majority of sex workers are women, some men also sell sexual services to women or to other men. **Gigolos** provide escort and sexual services for women, and **hustlers** are male sex workers who perform gay acts for pay. Male sex workers may be classified as female sex workers are, but the differences are often not obvious.

Percentages of male and female sex workers vary from city to city. Estimates in some larger cities suggest that 20% to 30% of sex workers are male.

In Bangkok, Thailand, a nonprofit group called Swing provides services—including education about condom use—to male sex workers (*Bangkok Post* profiles group providing services for male commercial sex workers, 2005). It is the first organization to focus on Thailand's approximately 4,000 male sex workers. Swing offers English classes, Internet access, and places to nap and shower. The group plans to offer exercise equipment and medical assistance. Although Thai society has become "more tolerant" of female sex workers, it is "less accepting" of male sex workers. People look down on them because they think they are lazy and terrible people. Male sex workers also have experienced stigma in doctors' offices and sometimes avoid being treated for STIs if a doctor or nurse makes them feel uncomfortable. Swing establishes relationships with doctors to make "appropriate referrals" for its clients, and the group plans to have its own in-house physician.

Few studies have examined male clients who pay for sexual activity with males. Grov et al. (2014) found that almost 88% of clients are white/Caucasian, 90% are HIV negative, 71% are employed full-time, 59% are single, and their mean age is 54. Three-fourths of clients were gay, 18% bisexual, and 4% heterosexual. The median rate paid was $250 per hour, with a modal appointment time of 1 to 2 hours. Oral sexual activity was common (89% gave, 69% received), 30% reported anal insertive sexual activity, and 34% reported anal receptive sexual activity. Few (12%) reported unprotected anal sexual activity. Satisfaction with encounters was high.

Pimps

The people who set up sex workers with clients are called **pimps**. Sex workers give the money they earn to their pimps in exchange for affection, concern, and love. Pimps recruit newcomers into sex work, they manage the sex workers' business and provide them counsel, bail them out of jail when necessary, and regulate the streetwalking prostitution enterprise (without a pimp, streetwalking sex workers might be in danger in certain neighborhoods).

Although most sex workers are women, it is thought that as many as 20% to 30% of sex workers are men.

Little is known about the magnitude of prostitution or changes in its incidence. Because prostitution is an illegal (except in rural Nevada) and socially stigmatized profession in the United States, the amount of reliable information is very limited.

Lowen (2015b) indicated that of the estimated 1 million individuals who have worked as prostitutes in the United States, the overwhelming majority are women. Statistics are grim for sex workers. Prostitutes have a significantly greater risk of experiencing violence, rape, physical abuse, and death than other women in the general population. Two characteristics are especially notable among prostitutes: A high percentage have been sexually abused as children, and a high percentage will be physically abused or raped after entering the sex trade.

gigolo A man who is paid to provide escort and sexual services, usually for wealthy, middle-aged women.

hustler A male sex worker who performs homosexual acts for pay.

pimps Individuals who set up female sex workers with clients.

Lowen (2015c) also indicated that for women who are prostitutes, rape is every bit as traumatic as it is for women who are not sex workers. It may even be more painful, as the act may unearth buried memories of previous assault and abuse. Eighty-two percent of respondents reported having been physically assaulted since entering prostitution. Of those, 55% had been assaulted by customers. Eighty-eight percent had been physically threatened while in prostitution, and 83% had been physically threatened with a weapon. Sixty-eight percent reported having been raped since entering prostitution. Forty-eight percent had been raped more than five times. In addition, 57% reported a history of childhood sexual abuse by an average of 3 perpetrators.

Phone Sex Workers
Why do people (mostly women) work as phone sex workers? Some of them believe they have an important social role. Some think they might keep potentially violent men from enacting real-life crimes. Some believe they can help educate others about their sexuality. Some like the casual environment and being able to work from home before settling down in a more serious career. The main motivation is the money—phone sex workers report that they made more than most felt they could earn elsewhere. However, the income came at a price because they could not be honest with people about what they did to make money.

Jameson (2014) looked at the reality of being a phone sex operator. The fact that a job in the sex industry can pay far better than a minimum-wage job is a major motivator for many women. Many college students are finding this practice is a convenient way to help pay for high college costs, and the number of mothers pursuing phone sex jobs recently increased by 400%.

But what is the reality of being a phone sex operator? One college senior said that, like any job, it has its ups and downs. It can take a great deal of effort when you are tired or in a bad mood and have to say dirty things to some random person, but it can also be fun and interesting. The same student reported that working at this job was without doubt the easiest money she ever made.

One good thing about the job, according to phone sex workers, is that they really do leave it all behind at the end of the day. No one has to know what the worker does to make money. Indeed, many workers would hate it if people recognized them on the street and thought they knew the type of person they were because of their professional role.

Another phone sex worker noted that there is a huge difference between working as a phone sex operator and being a porn star, so it is silly to lump them together. Nevertheless, this type of work is not for everyone. Most phone sex operators last only 3 months or so. If they do not have the right attitude, these workers can find it very challenging to maintain a healthy outlook on sexuality. If individuals are feeling vulnerable for whatever reason, they may struggle with low self-esteem. The perception that "I am just a vessel for a stranger's sexual gratification" can have a negative effect unless the worker has sufficient internal strength.

Most phone sex workers do it for the money, but some enjoy the male attention. They deal with the job in different ways, and most do other things while they chat with their customers—such as painting their nails, email friends, or even knit.

Public Health Perspective
The issue of commercial sex work causes a lot of debate among public health professionals. Historically, public health professionals focused on sex workers as disease vectors—those who could spread STIs to the wider population. Interventions, therefore, focused not on the health of the sex workers but rather on their role in shaping the health of society. More recently, the World Health Organization indicated that interventions can have a positive impact on both the spread of disease and the lives of those involved in sex work. Paying more attention to the health of sex workers involves adopting a nonjudgmental attitude, respecting sex workers' human rights, involving sex workers in program development, and recognizing that sex workers are part of the solution. This kind of model can be controversial because it seeks to improve conditions and health without necessarily eliminating potentially harmful behavior or behavior that some people would feel is wrong or immoral.

Sexual Slavery

Human rights groups estimate that between 12.3 million and 27 million people are enslaved in forced or bonded labor, child labor, sexual servitude, and involuntary servitude at any given time. Human trafficking is estimated to generate $9.5 billion in annual revenue. Although there are many different kinds of trafficking, women and girls make up the majority of human victims (66% and 13%, respectively). Sex trafficking appears to be growing in scope and magnitude. It is estimated that only about 5% of trafficking cases are ever reported. Those most vulnerable to trafficking include impoverished and drug-addicted women and runaway girls. Children as young as 1 and 2 years old have been found in brothels. Organized crime is largely responsible for the proliferation of human trafficking. Women and

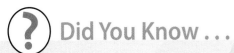

Did You Know . . .

Obtaining the services of a sex worker has changed with the advent of the Internet. For example, one can search under "prostitutes" and "[name of city]" and get a listing of the best spots to find a sex worker. Local police monitor such sites as well. Also, one can link up with an "escort" service via the Internet, ordering these services online.

girls are lured with promises of love, marriage, educational opportunities, and a better life. Sex trafficking of women and girls has astronomical costs, both to the women and girls who are its primary victims, and to society as a whole (The new face of slavery, 2010).

The trafficking Victims Protection Act of 2000 and its reauthorizations in 2003, 2005, 2008, and 2013 define a human trafficking victim as a person induced to perform labor or a commercial sex act through force, fraud, or coercion. There are an estimated 27 million slaves worldwide—more people are enslaved now than at any other time in history. Together human trafficking and slavery are among the most lucrative criminal enterprises. The Victims Protection Act was put in place to combat international trafficking in persons, to combat trafficking in persons in the United States, and to provide funding to assist with these efforts. Among other things, the 2013 reauthorization prevents U.S. foreign aid from going to countries that use child soldiers, strengthens the tools needed to combat human trafficking both in the United States and abroad, improves the means by which trafficking can be prevented, protects victims, and enhances prosecutions.

Chong (2014) made some interesting observations related to ethnicity and race issues in human trafficking. She noted several interrelated themes: Racist and sexual stereotypes of women are exploited in the sex industry, traditional patriarchal culture has a strong influence on setting up stereotyped female passivity and submissiveness, and racialized and ethnicized peoples are prone to experience violence in numerous ways, including sexual exploitation.

According to Warren (2015), most of us really do not want to know the truth about human sex trafficking. We do not want to know that 2 million children are victims of the sex trade each year, that the average girl being forced into prostitution in the United States is 13 years old, and that more than 80% of confirmed sex trafficking in the United States involves American-born citizens. We cannot

fathom that an estimated 20.9 million people are enslaved in the world, many of whom are forced to engage in sexual activity for the profit of someone else. The truth is that human sex trafficking is the fastest-growing criminal industry in the world, accounting for an estimated $150 billion in revenues each year.

Warren (2015) has pointed out that, in the interest of humanity, there are three simple things we can do to help fight sex trafficking in our communities:

- Education and awareness are important. We must admit that sex trafficking is happening, be willing to acknowledge the data, and listen to the many emotionally charged stories of survivors. We have to be affected by the reality.

- We must talk about sex trafficking—honestly and openly. The more we can start a dialogue about the realities of sex trafficking, the more likely we can do something about it as a global community.

- As the truth is acknowledged, we have to *do* something. In addition to talking about this issue, we need to be involved in prevention efforts in our communities. Whether we take a moment to sign a petition that supports legislation to help end trafficking, attend an awareness event, or talk to friends about this difficult topic, collective efforts can make a difference.

The U.S. Department of State has an Office to Monitor and Combat Trafficking in Persons. Annually, it publishes a *Trafficking in Persons Report*. Organizations that work on the issue of sex slavery include the International Justice Mission (*www.ijm.org*) and Free the Slaves (*http://freetheslaves.net*).

Opinions About Sex Work

The subject of sex workers produces strong emotional reactions. Some people believe sex workers should have the right to do their work. Others believe that this practice maintains a world where women are subordinate and sex workers reinforce broad patterns of discrimination. From an economic perspective, it has been argued that sex work helps many women escape poverty and hunger. They get paid much more than they could earn by doing anything else, so they can better help their families. Also, legalizing sex work would make it easier for sex workers to organize into unions as other workers have, which could help improve their working conditions, raise the status of their profession, and promote respect for their human rights.

**"Values" of
Prostitution in
Other Countries?**

In Russia, tens of thousands of female college students work as prostitutes or carry on exclusive relationships with so-called sponsors to pay for college. The Russian Internet is replete with websites that offer free search engines that match potential clients with students. Most sites provide the woman's age, body measurements, types of sex she practices, corresponding costs, and even reviews by former clients. One girl used to work as an elementary teacher earning the equivalent of $60 per month. Now she works as a prostitute and earns the equivalent of $200 to $300 for a night of sexual activities. Of course, the women have expenses such as paying for a madam (agent) and use of an apartment or other appropriate facility. When asked how her parents feel about her work, one student said, "We tell them we work as waitresses. They don't ask any questions."

In some situations, prostitutes are very concerned about their rights. For example, in Paris hundreds of prostitutes wearing white masks with tears painted on them rallied in front of the French Senate to protest a high-profile government crackdown on their livelihood.

Of course many people would argue against sex work on moral grounds. Perhaps they feel that sexual activity should be restricted to marital relations or that it is immoral for sex workers to participate in sexual activity with many different people.

In contrast to those who organize against sex work, the North American Task Force on Prostitution (NTFP) was founded in 1979 to act as an umbrella organization for prostitutes and prostitutes' rights organizations. It is a network of sex workers and their supporters that advocates for the rights of sex workers to organize on their own behalf, work safely and without legal repression, travel without legal restrictions, have families and raise children, and enjoy the same rights, responsibilities, and privileges as other people. The goals of the NTFP are to (1) repeal the existing prostitution laws; (2) ensure the right of prostitutes and other sex workers to bargain with their employers, when they work for third parties, to improve their working conditions; (3) inform the public about a wide range of issues related to prostitution and other forms of sex work; (4) promote the development of support services for sex workers, including HIV, AIDS, and STIs and violence-prevention projects, as well as health and social support services for sex workers (including supportive programs to deal with STIs, violence, and substance abuse), legal assistance projects, and job retraining and other programs to assist prostitutes who wish to change their occupation; and (5) end the public stigma associated with sex work.

There are other examples of giving a louder voice to a business that has thrived in silence. The Sex Workers Outreach Project—USA (SWOP; http://www.swopusa.org/) is a national social justice network dedicated to the fundamental rights of sex workers and their communities, focusing on ending violence and stigma through education and advocacy. At its most basic, SWOP is an antiviolence campaign. As a multistate network of sex workers and advocates, SWOP addresses at local and national levels the violence that sex workers experience because of their criminal status. It works to educate policy makers and the public on the institutional harms committed against sex workers, and advocates for alternatives. Among its other activities, SWOP operates a 24/7 helpline where current and former sex workers can access direct support, provides sponsorship and funding to local sex worker initiatives, organizes media and advocacy outreach, and assists with interorganizational research and projects.

In one large city, a center has been established where prostitutes sometimes meet to plan political moves related to their status. In another, a magazine for people in the sex industry has been published. On the Internet, prostitutes are able to find one another, form online communities, and connect with groups in other communities. The ultimate goal for many in the movement is decriminalization of prostitution. They say there are safe ways to work—that sex work is only a risk when it is illegal. They also argue that prostitution is a viable source of income for many people, and that sexual activity between adults for money should be treated as any other form of legal labor. However, some former prostitutes oppose this movement because they see prostitution as inherently exploitative and degrading.

Controlling Sex Work

Some officials have tried various ways to manage sex work. For example, San Francisco took a laissez-faire

Multicultural
DIMENSIONS

Organizations for Sex Workers

Call Off Your Tired Ethics (COYOTE) is an organization for sex workers that was founded in 1973. It works for the rights of all sex workers of all genders and persuasions. COYOTE supports programs to assist sex workers if they choose to change their occupation, works to prevent the scapegoating of sex workers for AIDS and other STIs, and educates sex workers, their clients, and the general public about safer sex.

Prostitutes of New York (PONY) is a support and advocacy group for all people in the sex industry. PONY advocates the decriminalization of prostitution and calls for an end to illegal police activity in the enforcement of existing laws. It provides legal and health referrals to sex workers and encourages members to recommend doctors, therapists, and other professionals who provide high-quality service to sex workers. PONY encourages all people who sell sex or profit from sex to learn about the

diversity of their industry, to promote professional standards in their sector, and to learn more about the history of the world's oldest profession (and its allied industries).

There are similar groups in other countries. One example is the Prostitutes Collective of Victoria (PCV) (Australia), which is a community-based organization developed to include and represent sex-industry workers' concerns about the issue of prostitution as a part of a worldwide prostitutes' rights movement. It works for basic human rights and occupational health and safety rights for all prostitution workers.

The Network of Sex Work Projects (NSWP) was formed in 1991. It consists of sex workers and organizations that provide services to sex workers in more than 40 countries. The NSWP focuses on issues similar to those of interest to the other groups and aims to facilitate opportunities for the voices of sex workers to be heard in relevant international forums.

approach. As a result, sex work is highly visible in tourist sections in the form of massage parlors, escort services, bar sex workers, hotel sex workers, and call girls (or boys). The major benefit of this approach has been to restrict sex work to nonresidential parts of the city. The control model—whereby certain neighborhoods strictly enforce laws against sex work—has been employed in North Dallas; the results have been reductions in crime and in visibility of sex workers. The regulation model—whereby sex work is legalized and subject to certain regulations—has been tried in rural Nevada, where it has resulted in a minimal amount of crime and where, for the most part, sex work is limited to controlled brothels. Finally, there is the zoning model—whereby sex work is tolerated but legal only in certain parts of the city. With this model, sex workers are supposedly visible only in a certain part of the city, and crime associated with sex work is limited to that area. None of these approaches has been totally successful, and each has advantages and disadvantages.

Another method of trying to control sex work has been making public the identities of sex workers and their customers. For example, in 1997 "John TV" started in Kansas City. Every Wednesday morning viewers of the local government cable TV channel saw the names, photographs, dates of birth, and addresses of people—mostly men—who were arrested for visiting sex workers. Above each picture was this

disclaimer: "This person is innocent until found guilty by a court." The ACLU objected to this practice because it targeted people before they were convicted of a crime and used a government-controlled medium to deliver its message of humiliation.

"John TV" has been used in other places as well. In Oklahoma, its goals include to expose and identify those who have preyed upon women lost to drug addiction and street prostitution, use those caught and published as an example to dissuade others, and to forward the ideology of decriminalization of 100% private, consensual and nonorganized prostitution so that the community's limited resources can be focused on street, forced, and organized prostitution and trafficking. More detail is available about John TV at http://johntv.com.

Another method of controlling sex workers involves organizations that provide help and support for sex workers who desire to change their life and stop being sex workers. One such organization is the Council for Prostitution Alternatives in Portland, Oregon. Its goal is to help women who want to leave the sex industry find alternatives to lives in prostitution. A number of services are provided, including education, health care, referrals to services when needed, legal assistance, mentoring, and hospitality. More information can be found at www.prostitution-alternatives.org. Children of the Night is a similar organization located in San Francisco.

International Differences Related to Prostitution

From a selection of 100 countries inclusive of major religions, geographical regions, and policies towards prostitution, prostitution is legal in 49 of the countries, of limited legality in 12 of the countries, and illegal in 39 of the countries. Countries where prostitution is legal include Argentina, Austria, Belgium, Brazil, Chile, Denmark, Ecuador, Finland, Greece, Germany, Hungary, Ireland, Israel, Italy, Mexico, the Netherlands, New Zealand, Poland, Portugal, Switzerland, Turkey, and the United Kingdom. Countries where prostitution is illegal include Afghanistan, the Bahamas, China, Cuba, Egypt, Haiti, Iran, Jamaica, Kenya, North and South Korea, Liberia, the Philippines, Romania, South Africa, Thailand, Uganda, and the United Arab Emirates. Countries with limited legality include Australia, Bulgaria, Canada, Iceland, India, Japan, Norway, Spain, Sweden, and the United States.

The percentage of men who have paid for sexual activity at least once varies quite a bit among countries. For example, in the United States estimates are between 15% and 20%. At the higher end are Cambodia (59–80%), Thailand (75%), Italy (17–45%), Spain (27–39%), and Japan (37%). At the lower end are Australia (16%), Sweden (8–14%), Finland (10–13%), Norway (13%), and the United Kingdom (7–9%).

Data from Prostitution. ProCon.org, 2015. Available: http://prostitution.procon.org/view.resource.php?resourceID=000772 and http://prostitution.procon.org/view.resource.php?resourceID=004119.

The federal government has tried another way to control sex work. Since 2003 all foreign nongovernmental organizations seeking U.S. global HIV/AIDS funds have been required to pledge their opposition to prostitution and sex trafficking to be eligible to partner with the U.S. government in combating HIV/AIDS in the developing world. In 2005 the rule was extended to American organizations as well.

Some people feel that many agencies are severely restricted by the policy. For example, some projects advocate the empowerment of sex workers to help them develop better lives. Other projects assist trafficked persons and sex workers in various ways. Some help sex workers to obtain high school diplomas so they can get other employment. As one project administrator said: "How can we ask prostitutes to take a position against themselves?" As a result of the governmental policy, those in a number of worthwhile projects decided to turn down the money. This meant they could not help as many people.

Arguments about the pros and cons of controlling sex work and its safety will probably continue for many years to come. Schmidt (2011) summarized the research and the beliefs of other researchers. He pointed out that some research indicates that Nevada's legal model is a better solution than criminalization. Women working in Nevada brothels do so under the protection of other brothel employees in rooms equipped with intercoms and panic buttons. It seems that women in Nevada brothels are far safer than those engaged in street prostitution or, for that matter, many women in the ordinary dating scene. Some researchers found no evidence "that selling sex is harmful to women." Other researchers, however, feel that women in Nevada's legal brothels are vulnerable to violence, STIs, and a host of other ailments; that some women were placed in the brothels by their pimps as punishment for not earning more money elsewhere; that some women appear to have been trafficked into Nevada's brothels; and that many working in them appear to be brainwashed.

The Law and Prostitution

Should prostitution be legal? This question has been argued for many years. Some people believe there are potential benefits of legalizing prostitution, such as increased human rights protection and health precautions. They argue that prostitution always has been and always will be. Legalization would increase condom use and, in turn, lead to a reduction of HIV and AIDS and other STIs. They feel prostitutes have the right to choose the way they earn their income; therefore, how can society stand in the way of someone's earning a good living?

Opponents of prostitution argue that most prostitutes are forced into sexual slavery. They suggest that legalization would give rise to a black market that would be frightening and abusive. For some opponents to prostitution, the issue is a moral one because prostitution gives rise to dehumanizing, unsafe, illegal activities. It is morally reprehensible, they say, for prostitutes to be treated as too many are treated. They conclude that the abuses and potential threat for ongoing abuse far outweigh any potential benefits of legalization. And the argument continues.

It has been pointed out that a large number of those who would be governed by legislation on commercial sexual activity don't identify with such legislation or consider it useful to their lives. Even in those places in the world where sex workers can legally register and operate within the law, many do not bother to do so because they fail to see any benefit. Few sex workers join trade unions or interest groups where they exist.

Is prostitution safer when it is legal? This question was debated by eight experts in 2012 (Is prostitution safer when it's legal?, 2012). The main points raised included:

1. Labor laws, not criminal laws, are the answer. Prostitutes should be allowed to protect themselves, organize, and advocate.

2. Legality leads to more trafficking. The presence of an adult sex industry increases the rates of child sexual exploitation and trafficking. The argument that legalizing prostitution makes it safer hasn't been borne out in countries implementing legalization.

3. Prostitution should not be illegal, but the buying of sexual activity should be criminalized. (The customers should be prosecuted, but not the prostitutes.)

4. The legalization of prostitution would likely make things a little better for those women who have few options to begin with. If options are not good, the focus should be on education, skills training, and job creation.

5. In legal brothels, employees report that they feel safe, are free to come and go, and are bound only by their contract. The police, employers, and coworkers are there to protect them. Legality brings protection and better care.

6. The way to address oppression is to end it—not legalize, regulate, or make it more tolerable. Prostitution teaches people that other people can be rendered into sexual commodities that can be bought or sold for sexual use and abuse.

7. Legal brothels can be coercive. Some have been like prisons or detention camps.

Child Prostitution

A particularly disturbing feature of sex work is the presence of minors selling sexual activity. Child prostitution has become more common in recent years. Children may be forced by adults to perform sexual acts, but sometimes they may wrongly appear to be selling sexual activity by their own choice.

Cultures exist around the world in which children, as belongings, are property to be bought and sold. In some developing countries, boys outnumber girls on the streets because girls are often put into brothels. These children are prostituted or sold to prevent their families from starving. The customers who purchase the children or their services are adults who are commonly pedophiles or sadists.

In some instances there can be links between child prostitution and child pornography. For example, costumed children might act out a customer's fantasy in special surroundings while filming is done. The acting might be done as part of a story, such as an abduction of a virgin or a "schoolgirl tease," or the action might simply be rape and torture. There is money to be made from both the prostitution activities and the selling of videos.

© Kuzma/ShutterStock, Inc.

To survive on the streets, adolescents who have run away from home often sell drugs or their bodies.

In the United States a large number of adolescent sex workers are runaways who are looking for companionship, friendship, love, and approval, as well as a way of supporting themselves financially. Unfortunately, many of them are ideal targets for gangs, drug pushers, and pimps. To survive on the streets, runaways often sell drugs or their bodies, and a large number turn to other types of crime to support themselves.

Some U.S. children engage in commercial sexual activity while living at home and generally find customers among their peers. Those children at highest risk for commercial sexual exploitation are those who run away or are thrown out by their relatives. Fewer than 25% are members of impoverished families. A significant number of their customers are married men, many with children of their own. Other children at higher risk to become victims of commercial sexual activity include female gang members who get involved to raise money for the gang; foreign children; and teenagers living along the Canadian or Mexican borders who cross into those countries specifically to solicit sexual activity.

The fact that runaways make up a significant percentage of adolescent sex workers creates a particularly difficult problem for law enforcement personnel. When they arrest a child sex worker, it does little good to send the child back to a poor home environment. In fact, there have been reports of children setting up their own prostitution rings, while living at home, to earn spending money.

In response to childhood sex work, law enforcement personnel have attempted to crack down on pimps of adolescent sex workers and at the same time better coordinate with other law enforcement agencies to recognize and help runaways when possible. Service programs for runaways have incorporated a medical component to treat the physical and mental health needs of runaways who have turned to sex work (and of other runaways, too). Runaway shelters provide services to help reduce the need for runaways to turn to sex work. Such services include medical services, crisis intervention services, individual and group counseling, vocational training and job placement, legal services, independent living skills training, and support and friendship. The hope is that the many shelters and service centers around the United States will help convince young people that they need not turn to pimps and sex work to meet their needs.

A survey of 56 county social service providers showed that the exploitation of children for money, whether it is pornography or prostitution, is an often unseen but very real problem (Invisibility, 2011). For example, 87% of the respondents said children who are sexually exploited are working for a pimp or are being pimped by a parent, many of the pimps are members of the child's family, an equal number of blacks and whites were involved, and a little over half of the young people were homeless. The vast majority of those surveyed said there were no programs in place designed to specifically help the young people.

Research about all forms of sex work has changed more in recent years than at any time in the past. We now know more about the extent of sex work and its changing nature worldwide, but particularly in the West. We also have a better grasp of the reasons some people enter the sex industry. With the growth of sex-worker organizations, there is greater access to research subjects. The existence of a pool of volunteers willing to contribute to both their own research projects and those of others has the potential of adding greatly to our knowledge about this area of human sexual behavior.

Exploring the Dimensions of Human Sexuality

Marketing of sexual products and use of sexual imagery to market nonsexual products are multibillion-dollar businesses. The alluring imagery may draw attention to the product but does not necessarily result in a sale unless the product is sexually related, such as a product to enhance one's appearance.

As marketers attempt to target certain groups (typically younger populations) with sexual imagery, they need to be aware that other people may find their ads offensive.

Marketing of sexually explicit materials to consumers in conditions of privacy (i.e., at home) has driven the markets for DVDs and the Internet.

But marketers also face legal challenges to distributing sexually explicit material. Because "community standards" are used to judge whether material is obscene, a website operator in one state can be charged with obscenity under the community standards of a person in another state who downloads the materials.

Marketing of any sexually explicit material involving children is prosecuted harshly. Even just downloading such material is a violation of the law.

Biological Factors

- Prostitutes in general have a much higher rate of HIV infection. Many New York City streetwalkers are infected with HIV.
- No externally used products can enlarge the penis or breasts.

Sociocultural Factors

- Fraudulent sexual aids are among the top 10 sources of health fraud in the United States.
- Prostitution is outlawed in every U.S. state except Nevada (and even there it is legal in only a few counties).
- Many countries allow prostitution. South Korea issues identification cards to prostitutes that serve as hotel passes. South Korea and Thailand consider prostitution of young girls to be a tourist attraction.
- Some countries, such as Iran and China, have attempted to ban distribution of sexually explicit materials. Laws govern distribution and possession of sexually explicit photos of children.
- Media often fail to depict safer sexual practices in books, articles, TV shows, movies, and on the Internet.
- Sexually explicit materials helped create and expand the market for home videos, movies, DVDs, and the Internet.

Psychological Factors

- Media images may negatively impact body image and self-esteem.
- Many ads use sexual imagery to attract attention and stimulate senses.

Summary

- Countless advertisements in magazines, in newspapers, and on TV and the Internet use sexual themes to sell products. Advertisers have made a careful study of sexual motivation.

- The sexual content of TV programs has increased immensely in the past few decades. TV can be an excellent way to educate people about healthy sexual practices, but it is rarely used that way.

- The sexuality content of movies has also increased greatly in the past few decades. Some people believe the sexual explicitness is detrimental to society, whereas others see this trend as positive.

- The availability of sexual material in DVDs, video games, and on the Internet continues to increase. Businesses related to these products have grown by leaps and bounds.

- The mass phenomenon that may affect more young people than any other is popular music. Blatant sexual themes in music are very common today.

- Sexual content available on the Internet has raised many interesting issues. Among them is whether and how to apply censorship, whether and how to control access to the Internet for children, and how to deal with sexual predators on the Internet.

- Sexually explicit materials have been around for centuries and have often spawned controversy. Some people believe it is necessary to strictly control such materials, but others feel they are not harmful if used by adults. Most agree that child pornography should be prohibited.

- There are many types of sex workers, including call girls, house prostitutes, streetwalkers, massage parlor sex workers, bar girls, gigolos, hustlers, and pimps. In addition, in more recent years new types have emerged—phone and Internet sex workers, sex shop operators, and owners of stores that sell toys and devices related to sexuality.

- Sexual slavery has become a huge international problem. Millions of people around the world are trapped in virtual prisons on farms, in sweatshops, or in brothels.

Discussion Questions

1. Analyze the value of sexuality in selling products. Discuss sexually oriented ads, including the ways sex helps sell products (bikini-clad women in calendars, sexually explicit rap music, "dirty" classic literature, and so on).

2. Create a legal standard for distributing sexually explicit materials. Include in the standard what constitutes art, child pornography, literature, and the like.

3. Compare and contrast the varied types of sex workers. Then describe efforts to control sex work.

Application Questions

Reread the chapter-opening story and answer the following questions.

1. Of the students who had opinions about sexual consumerism, with whom do you agree? Explain your answer, citing contemporary examples.

2. In what ways do actor portrayals of sexuality—or models with "perfect" bodies—make us feel inferior? Could those same images be said to promote erotic feelings and thus have value?

3. Does the use of naked flesh make ads sexier? Or have ads from the past, albeit with less flesh, been just as sexually oriented?

Critical Thinking Questions

1. When planning an ad campaign, a marketer needs to think about all audiences who will view the ad. Consider the anecdotal story that has appeared in various advertising publications about the former first lady Nancy Reagan and her daughter, Patty Davis: During the early 1990s, the two women were waiting in a hotel lobby when the conversation turned to sexual consumerism. Mrs. Reagan, showing her daughter a perfume ad in a magazine, said that she did not like having to look at a nearly naked man in the ad. Her daughter replied, "Well, I sure do!" They both laughed.

   Clearly, the marketer was targeting the demographics of Reagan's daughter. But should a marketer have to be concerned about offending people in other demographics—older and more conservative people as well as minors? Describe the steps a marketer should have to take before placing ads.

2. Although it is billed as the "world's oldest profession," prostitution is not legal in the United States except in a few counties in Nevada. Should prostitution be legalized? Consider the social, legal (including tax ramifications), health, moral, and other dimensions of sexuality of both clients and prostitutes in your answer.

3. Former stars of sexually explicit films, such as Linda Lovelace and Traci Lords, described the world of porn films as one of physical abuse (actual and threatened) and drugs. If an actress participated in explicit sexual activity under such coercion, does that constitute rape? Should distribution of such movies be illegal?

4. Distribution of photos of naked minors is illegal. But prominent "art" photographers often take photos of naked minors, and such photos are distributed in photo anthologies through major bookstore chains. How is it possible to differentiate between art and child pornography?

5. China, Iran, and other countries limit Internet access for their citizens. Two major concerns are antigovernment rhetoric and sexually explicit material. Given the ease with which minors can access sexually explicit material, should the U.S. government restrict the Internet access of U.S. citizens? Should the Internet be regulated?

Critical Thinking Cases

In parts of Japan, December 24 is the "hottest" night of the year. Societal pressure is strong for every unmarried person to have a date on Christmas Eve and for that date to include an overnight stay. In this respect December 24 is not dissimilar to prom night here in America. Just about every major hotel in Tokyo is sold out for that night months in advance. The Japanese describe Christmas Eve as a night to make love and refer to it as "H-Day" (for "hormone," the Japanese euphemism for sex).

This evening is quite expensive for young Japanese, as the cost typically exceeds $1,000. Men are expected to buy their date a present ($215), take her to Tokyo Disneyland ($100), provide dinner at a fancy restaurant ($385), take a room at a nice hotel (between $350 and $650), have breakfast the next morning ($35), and rent a limousine ($150)— all of this in a country less than 1% Christian and where December 25 is a normal working day.

1. Discuss H-Day in terms of the dimensions of sexuality. Include safer-sex practices, the psychological implications of engaging in sexual activity with someone because of societal pressure, religion, culture, and other factors.

2. Which cultural factors would prevent H-Day from being accepted in the United States? (Assume that the date would be changed from December 24.)

Exploring Personal Dimensions

Are You a Good Sexual Consumer?
Answer the following statements with one of the following responses. When you are finished, total your points and find out how good a sexual consumer you are.

1. Rarely or never

2. Sometimes

3. Often

4. All or most of the time

_____ 1. I make sure the date on any product (such as condoms or oral contraceptives) has not expired.

_____ 2. I am not influenced by sexually alluring images to purchase products.

_____ 3. I am aware of whether any sexually explicit material I view involves minors.

_____ 4. I make sure that any sexually explicit material I view is kept away from minors.

_____ 5. I understand that sharing sexual aids (or toys) with others is a high-risk activity, capable of transmitting STIs and AIDS.

_____ 6. I am aware that sexual contact with sex workers or former sex workers is a high-risk activity because of the potential for STI and/or HIV transmission.

_____ 7. I believe that aphrodisiacs offer no sexual help physiologically, and I consider their side effects before using them.

_____ 8. I evaluate "research" claims made by marketers before buying a product.

_____ 9. I consider the source of sexual health information before purchasing any product.

_____10. I have sought recommendations from friends for whom to consult in case of sexually related healthcare needs.

_____11. I have regular exams by a physician.

_____12. I understand that certain prescription drugs (such as antibiotics) can affect the effectiveness of oral contraceptives.

_____13. I read labels of health products and follow directions.

_____14. I do a monthly breast or testicular self-exam.

_____15. When friends state a sexual myth as though it were a fact, I use knowledge from this course to correct them tactfully.

Scoring

0–15   Your sexual consumer skills are weak.

16–30   Your sexual consumer skills are below what they should be.

31–45   Your sexual consumer skills are good but can stand improvement.

Suggested Readings

Brief history: Sex on TV. _Time, 177, 5_ (February 7, 2011), 19.

Finklea, K., Fernandes-Alcantara, A. L., & Siskin, A. _Sex trafficking of children in the United States: Overview and issues for Congress._ Congressional Research Service, 2015. Available: http://fas.org/sgp/crs/misc/R41878.pdf.

Jantz, G. L. Is porn the most prevalent drug? _PsychologyToday.com,_ 2015. Available: https://www.psychologytoday.com/blog/hope-relationships/201501/is-porn-the-most-prevalent-drug.

McCarthy, B., Benoit, C., & Jansson, M. Sex work: A comparative study. _Archives of Sexual Behavior, 43, 7_ (2014), 1379–1390.

Minichiello, V., Scott, J., & Callander, D. (2013). New pleasures and old dangers: Reinventing male sex work. _Journal of Sex Research, 50, 3–4_ (2013), 263–275.

Oliveira, C., Laja, P., Carvalho, J., Gomes, A. Q., Vilarinho, S., Janssen, E., & Nobre, P. J. (2014). Predictors of men's sexual response to erotic film stimuli: The role of affect and self-reported thoughts. _Journal of Sexual Medicine, 11, 11_ (2014), 2701–2708.

Roberts, R., Jones, A., & Sanders, T. Students and sex work in the UK: Providers and purchasers. _Sex Education: Sexuality, society and Learning, 13, 3_ (2013), 349–363.

Sorbring, E., Hallberg, J., Bohlin, M., & Skoog, T. (2015). Parental attitudes and young people's online sexual activities. _Sex Education: Sexuality, Society and Learning, 15, 2_ (2015), 129–143.

Web Resources

The Dove Foundation
www.dove.org

The Dove Foundation supports efforts to move Hollywood in a more family-friendly direction. It provides film reviews for consideration by consumers.

The Free Speech Museum
www.spectacle.org/musm.html

The Free Speech Museum is intended to serve as a permanent Internet resource on the freedom of speech. It is very concerned that many current efforts are designed to cut down or eliminate free speech.

Good Vibrations
www.goodvibes.com

Good Vibrations considers itself the place to go for sex toys, sex education, erotic and informative books, adult DVDs, and more.

National Coalition for the Protection of Children and Families
www.colsoncenter.org/connections/ministry-partners/12382-national-coalition-for-the-protection-of-children-a-families

The Coalition's mission is to move the people of God to embrace, live out, preserve, and advance the biblical truth of sexuality. It wants to educate the Christian community on sexual ethics according to a biblical worldview, encourage and challenge Christians to live sexually pure lives, engage Christians in public policy relative to sexual ethics, and embrace those harmed by pornography and help restore them to sexual wholeness.

Prostitution Research and Education
http://prostitutionresearch.com/#

The goal of Prostitution Research and Education is to abolish the institution of prostitution while at the same time advocating for alternatives to trafficking and prostitution—including emotional and physical health care for women in prostitution. Its strategy is to focus on providing knowledge and advocacy for good policy and the promotion of public awareness about the commercial sexual exploitation of women through prostitution, pornography, and trafficking.

Veronica's Voice

www.veronicasvoice.org/#!

The mission of Veronica's Voice is to empower women to exit from, to prevent entry into, and to end all demand for prostitution/sex trafficking in the United States through survivor-informed leadership.

References

Ackerman, T. Popular song lyrics contain sex, alcohol and no regrets. *Deseret News*, 2012. Available: http://www.deseretnews.com/article/865553547/Popular-song-lyrics-contain-sex-alcohol-and-no-regrets.html?pg=all.

Albright, J. M. Sex in America online: An exploration of sex, marital status, and sexual identity in Internet sex seeking and its impacts. *Journal of Sex Research, 45,* 2 (April–June 2008), 175–186.

American Academy of Pediatrics (AAP). *Policy statement: Sexuality, contraception, and the media,* 2010. Available: http://pediatrics.aappublications.org/search?fulltext=sexuality%2C+contraception%2C+and+the+Media&submit=yes&x=39&y=9.

Aubrey, J. S. Sexual objectification in music videos: A content analysis comparing gender and genre. *Mass Communication and Society, 14,* 4 (2011), 475–501.

Aubrey, J. S., Hopper, K. M., & Mbure, W. G. Check that body! The effects of sexually objectifying music videos on college men's sexual beliefs. *Journal of Broadcasting & Electronic Media, 55,* 3 (2011), 360–379.

Bangkok Post profiles group providing services for male commercial sex workers. *Kaiser Daily HIV/AIDS Report* (January 5, 2005). Available: http://www.kaisernetwork.org.

Barr, E. M., Moore, M. J., Johnson, T., Merten, J., & Stewart, W. P. The relationship between screen time and sexual behaviors among middle school students. *Health Educator, 46,* 1 (2014), 6–13.

Braithwaite, S. R., Coulson, G., Keddington, K., & Fincham, F. D. The influence of pornography on sexual scripts and hooking up among emerging adults in college. *Archives of Sexual Behavior, 44,* 1 (2015), 111–123.

Chandra, A., Martino, S. C., Collins, R. L., Elliott, M. N., Berry, S. H., Kanouse, D. E., & Miu, A. Does watching sex on television predict teen pregnancy? Findings from a national longitudinal survey of youth. *Pediatrics, 122,* 5 (November 2008), 1047–1054.

Chong, N. G. Human trafficking and sex industry: Does ethnicity and race matter? *Journal of Intercultural Studies, 35,* 2 (2014), 196–213.

Commission on Obscenity and Pornography. *The report of the Commission on Obscenity and Pornography.* New York: Bantam, 1970.

Condliffe, J. These are the songs you have sex to, according to Spotify. *Gizmodo.com*, 2015. Available: http://gizmodo.com/these-are-the-songs-you-have-sex-to-according-to-spoti-1685616372.

Cox, R. B.; Schreffer, K. M.; Merten, M. J.; Schwerdtfeger, G. K.; and Dowdy, J. L. (2015). Parenting, peers, and perceived norms: What predicts attitudes toward sex among early adolescents? *Journal of Early Adolescence 35,* 1 (Jan 2015), 30–53.

Dank, M., Khan, B., Downey. P. M., Lotonias, C., Mayer, D., Owens, C., Pacifici, L., & Yu, L. (2014).

Fact sheet: Trafficking Victims Protection Reauthorization Act. Alliance to End Slavery & Trafficking, 2015. Available: http://www.endslaveryandtrafficking.org/legislative_updates/fact-sheet-trafficking-victims-protection-reauthorization-act.

Fisher, C., Herbenick, D., Reece, M., Dodge, B., & Fischtein, D. Exploring sexuality education opportunities at in-home sex-toy parties in the United States. *Sex Education, 10,* 2 (May 2010), 131–144.

Gilbert, S. Sex in the media: A new study finds troubling links to teens. *DailyFinance.com*, 2010. Available: http://www.dailyfinance.com/2010/09/04/sex-in-the-media-a-new-study-finds-troubling-links-to-teens/.

Greenhouse, L. Justices back law to make libraries use Internet filters. *The New York Times* (June 24, 2003). Available: http://www.nytimes.com.

Grov, C., Wolff, M., Smith, M. D., Koken, J., & Parsons, J. T. Male clients of male escorts: Satisfaction, sexual behavior, and demographic characteristics. *Journal of Sex Research, 51,* 7 (2014), 827–837.

Hall, P. C., West, J. H., & Hill, S. Sexualization in lyrics of popular music from 1959 to 2009: Implications for sexuality education. *Sexuality & Culture.* DOI: 10.1007/s12119-011-9103-4.

Hatton, E., & Trautner, M. N. Equal opportunity objectification? The sexualization of men and women on the cover of *Rolling Stone. Sexuality and Culture, 15,* 3 (September 2011), 256–278.

Head, T. The Child Online Protection Act (COPA) of 1998. About.com Civil Liberties, 2012. Available: http://civilliberty.about.com/od/freespeech/p/copa1998.htm.

Hellman, M. Japan finally bans child pornography. *Time.com*, 2014. Available: http://time.com/2892728/japan-finally-bans-child-pornography/.

Herbenick, D., Reece, M., Sanders, S., Dodge, B., Ghassemi, A., & Fortenberry, D. Prevalence and characteristics of vibrator use by women in the United States: Results from a nationally representative study. *Journal of Sexual Medicine, 6,* 7 (2009), 1857–1866.

High court to hear arguments on child porn amendment. *The Birmingham News* (October 28, 2001), 20A.

Invisibility. Youth and Family Services Network, 2011. Available: http://media.al.com/spotnews/other/Invisibility.final.revised%281%29.pdf.

Is prostitution safer when it's legal? *The New York Times* (April 19, 2012). Available: http://www.nytimes.com/roomfordebate/2012/04/19/is-legalized-prostitution-safer.

James, M. S. Museum of Sex to debut in New York (2002). Available: http://www.ABCnews.com.

Jameson, E. What's it really like to be a phone sex operator? *Huffington Post*, 2014. Available: http://www.huffingtonpost.com/ella-jameson/phone-sex-operator_b_5275952.html.

Kalinowski, R. Definition of TV ratings. *ehow.com*, 2015. Available: http://www.ehow.com/facts_5208683_definition-tv-ratings.html.

Kingston, D. A., Malamuth, N. M., Federoff, P., & Marshall, W. L. The importance of individual differences in pornography use: Theoretical perspectives and implications for treating sexual offenders. *Journal of Sex Research, 46, 2 & 3* (March 2009), 216–232.

Lowen, L. Is prostitution a victimless crime? Answer exposes gender gap. *Womensissues.about.com*, 2015a. http://womensissues.about.com/od/prostitution/a/VictimlessCrime.htm.

Lowen, L. Prostitution and sex workers: Prostitutes in the sex trade. *Womensissues.about.com*, 2015b. Available: http://womensissues.about.com/od/violenceagainstwomen/p/ProstitSexTrade.htm.

Lowen, L. Prostitution statistics and rape: Physical abuse of prostitutes common. *Womensissues.about.com*, 2015c. Available: http://womensissues.about.com/od/rapesexualassault/a/Wuornos.htm.

McCarthy, B., Benoit, C. & Jansson, M. Sex work: A comparative study. *Archives of Sexual Behavior, 43, 7* (2014), 1379–1390.

Medina, J. Los Angeles mandates use of condoms for sex films. *The New York Times* (January 17, 2012). Available: http://www.nytimes.com/2012/01/18/us/los-angeles-makes-condoms-mandatory-for-adult-film-actors.html.

Money, J. Pornography in the home. In *Contemporary Sexual Behavior*, Zubin, J., & Money, J., eds. Baltimore: Johns Hopkins Press, 1973.

Money, J., & Athanasiou, R. Pornography: Review and bibliographic annotations. *American Journal of Obstetrics and Gynecology, 115* (January 1973), 130–146.

Mustanski, B., Greene, G. J., Ryan, D., & Whitton, S. W. Feasibility, acceptability, and initial efficacy of an online sexual health promotion program for LGBT youth: The Queer Sex Ed intervention. *Journal of Sex Research, 52, 2* (2015), 220–230.

The new face of slavery. *Soroptimist International*, November, 2010. Available: http://www.soroptimist.org/whitepapers/WhitePaperDocs/WPNewFaceSlavery.pdf.

Padgett, P. M. Personal safety and sexual safety for women using online personal ads. *Sexuality Research & Social Policy, 4, 2* (June 2007), 27–37.

Parental Advisory. Recording Industry Association of America, 2015. Available: http://riaa.com/toolsforparents.php?content_selector=parental_advisory#background.

Reece, M., Herbenick, D., Sanders, S. A., Dodge, B., Ghassemi, A., & Fortenberry, J. D. Prevalence and characteristics of vibrator use by men in the United States. *Journal of Sexual Medicine, 6, 7* (2009), 1867–1874.

Reichert, T., Childers, C. C., & Reid, L. N. How sex in advertising varies by product category: An analysis of three decades of visual sexual imagery in magazine advertising. *Journal of Current Issues & Research in Advertising, 33, 1* (2012).

Richtel, M. He's watching that, in public? Pornography takes next seat. *The New York Times* (July 21, 2012). Available: http://www.nytimes.com/2012/07/21/us/tablets-and-phones-lead-to-more-pornography-in-public.html?pagewanted=all.

Ritter, K. Nevada considering strict condom regulation for porn films. *Yahoo.com*, 2015. Available: https://www.yahoo.com/movies/s/nevada-considering-strict-condom-regulation-porn-films-092700837.html.

Rosenberger, J., Schick, V., Herbenick, D., Novak, D., & Reece, M. Sex toy use by gay and bisexual men in the United States. *Archives of Sexual Behavior, 41, 2* (2012), 449–458.

Salum, E. *Sexual subliminal advertising*, 2013. Available: https://prezi.com/q5sssqysl4gl/sexual-subliminal-advertisements/.

Schick, V., Herbenick, D., Jozowski, K. N., Jawed-Wessel, S. & Reece, M. The sexual consumer: Characteristics, expectations, and experiences of women attending in-home sex toy parties. *Journal of Sex & Marital Therapy, 39, 2* (2013), 160–175.

Schmidt, P. Scholars of legal brothels offer a new take on the "oldest profession." *Chronicle of Higher Education 58, 5* (September 23, 2011), A14–A15.

Schroeder, E. Blaming TV for teen pregnancy is a convenient excuse. *New York Daily News* (November 28, 2008). Available: http://www.nydailynews.com/opinion/blaming-tv-teen-pregnancy-a-convenient-excuse-article-1.339238.

Sex and Tech. Washington, DC: National Campaign to Prevent Teen and Unplanned Pregnancy, 2008. Available: http://www.thenationalcampaign.org/sextech/PDF/SexTech_Summary.pdf.

Silver, A. Brief history—sex on TV. *Time, 177, 5* (February 7, 2011), 19.

Simon, L., & Daneback, K. Adolescents' use of the Internet for sexuality education: A thematic and critical review of the literature. *International Journal of Sexual Health, 25, 4* (2013), 305–319.

Sloss, C., & Harper, G. When street sex workers are mothers. *Archives of Sexual Behavior, 33, 4* (August 2004), 329–341.

Soderlund, G. Journalist or panderer? Framing underage webcam sites. *Sexuality Research & Social Policy, 5, 4* (December 2008), 62–72.

Suggett, P. Sex in advertising. *About.com*, 2015. Available: http://advertising.about.com/od/advertisingprojects/a/Sex-In-Advertising.htm.

Summers, A., & Miller, M. K. From damsels to distress to sexy superheroes. *Feminist Media Studies, 14, 6* (2014), 1028–1040.

Sun, C., Bridges, A., & Johnason, J. Pornography and the male sexual script: An analysis of consumption and sexual relations. *Archives of Sexual Behavior.* (2014). doi: 10.1005/s10508-014-0391-2.

TV's newest target: Teen sexual exploitation. Parents' Television Council, 2015. Available: http://w2.parentstv.org/main/MediaFiles/PDF/Studies/sexploitation_report_20130709.pdf.

U.S. Department of Justice. Attorney Holder announces results of international child pornography investigation at Operation Delego press conference, August 3, 2011. Available: http://www.justice.gov/iso/opa/ag/speeches/2011/ag-speech-110803.html.

"Unusual" FDA order requiring corrections to Yaz ad campaign. National Partnership for Women & Families, *Daily Women's Health Policy Report* (February 11, 2009).

Warren, C. S. The naked truth about human sex trafficking. *PsychologyToday.com*, 2015. Available: https://www.psychologytoday.com/blog/naked-truth/201501/the-naked-truth-about-human-sex-trafficking.

Watson, M. A., & Smith, R. Positive porn: Educational, medical, and clinical uses. *American Journal of Sexuality Education, 7, 2* (2012), 122–145.

What scientists know about pornography. Allentown, PA: Society for the Scientific Study of Sexuality, 2007.

Witmer, D. Teens who watch a lot of TV with sexual content have sex sooner. *About Parenting*, 2015. Available: http://parentingteens.about.com/od/teensexuality/a/teen_sex8.htm.

Ybarra, M. L., Strasburger, V. C., & Mitchell, K. J. Sexual media exposure, sexual behavior, and sexual violence victimization in adolescence. *Clinical Pediatrics, 53, 13* (2014), 1239–1247.

Sexual Ethics, Morality, and the Law

© Gayvoronskaya Yana/Shutterstock

FEATURES

 Ethical Dimensions
Extramarital Sex

 Gender Dimensions
The "Umbrelly"
(A Little Humor)

 Global Dimensions
Marital Age Around
the World

 Communication Dimensions
The Morality of
Requesting a Variety
of Sexual Behaviors

CHAPTER OBJECTIVES

1 Define *ethics, morals, ethical principles, ethical dilemmas, values,* and the five ethical principles that serve as a basis for deciding whether a decision is moral.

2 State the ethical considerations of such sexually related topics as sexually transmitted infections, sexual activity between unmarried partners, sexting, sodomy, contraception, abortion, amniocentesis, fetal tissue implantation, prostitution, in vitro fertilization, genetic engineering, and sexual responsibility to a partner.

3 Identify the rationale for laws pertaining to homosexuality, obscenity and pornography, rape, statutory rape, marriage, polygamy, adultery, and divorce.

INTRODUCTION

Wendy Weaver was a well-respected high school philosophy teacher and girls' volleyball coach in the Nebo, Utah, school district (Associated Press, 1998). Concerned about her student athletes, in the summer of 1997 she telephoned each one to ask about her summer camp schedule. That is when it happened. A student asked, "Are you gay?" Weaver answered that she was, eliciting a response from the student that she would not play on Weaver's volleyball team in the fall. When school district officials heard what Wendy Weaver disclosed to the student, they immediately fired her from her coaching responsibilities and instructed her not to speak of her sexual orientation to either students or school staff, in or outside school.

The Nebo school district officials believed they were right to protect young people in their school from what they perceived to be disclosure of immoral behavior. They believed that homosexuality was wrong and that it was sinful.

Wendy Weaver, however, believed that she had a moral right to express her sexuality in any way she sought, as long as she did not impose it on her students. After all, she argued, heterosexual teachers are not forbidden to disclose their sexual orientation. Therefore, she asserted that it was wrong—immoral—to forbid her to do so.

Eventually a judge determined the legal issues involved in this case. In November 1997, U.S. District Court Judge Bruce Jenkins ruled that Wendy Weaver's rights of free speech, equal protection under the law, and due process were violated. He ordered that the gag order be lifted and that Wendy Weaver be reinstated as coach of the girls' volleyball team. In his ruling Judge Jenkins stated, "Although the Constitution cannot control prejudices, neither this court nor any other court should, directly or indirectly, legitimize them."

This case includes issues of morality, ethics, and law. The school officials believed that they were acting morally by protecting young people from a teacher they thought might inappropriately affect their sexual orientation. Wendy believed she was acting morally when she answered the team member honestly and when she asserted her constitutional rights. And the judge believed he was acting morally when he applied a law designed to prevent prejudice from depriving a person of her rights in a democratic society. Certainly everyone could not be right; nor could everyone be wrong. Certainly, everyone was not purposefully acting immorally. We shall see in this chapter how complex issues of morality really are and how a systematic approach can manage some of this complexity when these issues relate to matters of sexuality. Furthermore, we shall see how the law is used to codify societal consensus about morality and how it is applied to express societal mores.

Many ethical dilemmas relate to sexuality. For example, whether women should use intrauterine devices (IUDs) as a means of contraception that may prevent fertilized ova from successfully implanting on the uterus's endometrial lining involves the moral question of when life begins. Whether fetal tissue or stem cells—that is, from aborted fetuses—should be made available as a treatment for such conditions as Parkinson's disease concerns the moral issue of the sanctity of the human body.

These and other questions of sexual morality are pervasive. They affect every one of us, if not directly and daily, then certainly as members of a society wrestling with their resolutions. They are also emotionally charged. This point should not go unnoticed. When issues evoke emotional reactions—as sexual issues tend to do—these emotions too often interfere with a rational investigation. Consequently, people argue their own viewpoints while ignoring other perspectives, and that method of argument is not conducive to learning.

This chapter explores the morality and ethics of particular sexually related behaviors or decisions in a unified, systematic manner. In addition, it highlights the importance of considering the ethics and morality of all sexual matters.

Talking about sexual morality is not easy. Whose morality should we focus on? Which morals, if any, should we advocate? How can we prevent offending people whose morals differ from ours? It would be arrogant for us to insist that everyone adopt a single set of sexual morals, and it would be particularly impertinent to suggest that our own morals be the ones adopted.

The story of Wendy Weaver illustrates the multidimensional facets of ethics, morality, and the law.

Therefore, in this chapter, rather than advocating a particular set of morals or ethical principles, we describe the process of moral reasoning. We sketch our society's moral stance on STIs, contraception, in vitro fertilization, rape, prostitution, and so on, and describe the background and enforcement of some laws. Along the way we acknowledge some of the religious, philosophical, cultural, family-related, and experiential reasons for the differences in sexual morality among individuals and among societies.

■ Ethics: The Basis for Making Decisions

To begin investigating sexual morality, we need to distinguish between the terms *ethics* and *moral*. **Ethics** refers to a *system* by which we determine whether some action is moral or immoral. An action is **moral** if it is judged to be *good* or *right*; it is **immoral** if it is judged to be *bad* or *wrong*. To guide the decision of whether an action is moral or immoral, the system of ethics employs **ethical principles**. These ethical principles provide answers to abstract questions—they are general guidelines, not meant for individual cases. With regard to abortion, for example, ethicists would be more concerned with the general question of when life begins or with a woman's right to control her own reproductive capacity than with whether abortion is appropriate in a particular case. Decisions about what is moral are determined by many different experiences and influences. Religious beliefs and values, social mores, humanistic views, education, culture, and friends and family are but a few of these influences.

When a set of ethical principles is available and accepted by a society, the people of that society know how they are expected to behave. Professional societies attempt to develop guiding principles—or *codes of ethics*—to govern their members' behaviors. The code of ethics developed by the American Association of Sex Educators, Counselors, and Therapists, for example, sets guidelines for its members.

Ethical Principles

Table 22.1 introduces five examples of ethical principles that can be used to make moral decisions. As will be discussed, though, these kinds of principles may be in opposition to one another in any given situation.

Nonmaleficence

Is it moral to convince someone else to engage in sexual intercourse in spite of his or her reluctance? One ethical

TABLE 22.1	
Selected Ethical Principles	
1. Nonmaleficence	Whatever else, do no harm. This includes preventing harm, not inflicting harm, and removing harm when it is present.
2. Beneficence	Not only should one not do harm, but one is also obligated to do good.
3. Autonomy/liberty	People should be free to decide their own course of action as long as they do not harm others.
4. Justice/fairness	Each person should be treated fairly.
5. Social utility	The greatest good for the greatest number should be considered. What is best for society may outweigh what is best for the individual.

principle that speaks to this issue is maleficence—the act of committing harm or evil. The principle of *nonmaleficence* is that whatever is moral—right or good—can be determined by asking whether it does any harm. If it does harm, it is not moral. Does coercing someone to engage in sex do physical, psychological, or spiritual harm? If so, that behavior is immoral.

Beneficence

For some ethicists, doing no harm is not enough. For an action to be moral, it has to do good. That is

---

ethics A system that uses ethical principles to make decisions about morality.

moral What is judged to be right according to a system of ethics.

immoral What is judged to be wrong according to a system of ethics.

ethical principles Guides by which we can judge an action or decision as moral or immoral.

Ethical DIMENSIONS

Extramarital Sex   Actually making a decision regarding sexual morality may help you comprehend the rather abstract material to come. Consider, for example, *extramarital sex*—that is, sex between a married person and someone other than his or her spouse. In all cultures, consensual sexual intercourse is acceptable within marriage. However, when it comes to sexual intercourse outside of marriage, some cultures take a cavalier attitude, whereas others have made it illegal. In fact, in some countries, *any form of sexual activity* outside of marriage is illegal. Among these countries are Saudi Arabia, Pakistan, Iran, Kuwait, Maldives, Morocco, Oman, Mauritania, United Arab Emirates, Sudan, and Yemen.

Even when it is not illegal, extramarital sex without the approval of the partner is often considered *unethical*. Yet the issue of consent is not the determining ethical consideration in all cultures. Some cultures consider extramarital sex ethical if the spouse consents, whereas others view sexual intercourse outside of marriage as unethical, with or without consent.

Albert Ellis, a prominent psychologist, argued that there is even a *healthy adulterer*. Although Ellis's argument was presented a number of years ago, it is as applicable today as it was then. Ellis wrote (1977, 374–375):

1. The healthy adulterer is nondemanding and noncompulsive. He prefers but he does not need extramarital affairs. He believes that he can live better

with than without them, and therefore he tries to have them from time to time. But he is also able to have a happy general and marital life if no such affairs are practicable.

2. The undisturbed adulterer usually manages to carry on his extramarital affairs without unduly disturbing his marriage and family relationships or his general existence. He is sufficiently discreet about his adultery.

3. He fully accepts his own extramarital desires and acts and never condemns himself or punishes himself because of them, even though he may sometimes decide that they are unwise and may make attempts to bring them to a halt.

4. He faces his specific problems with his wife and family as well as his general life difficulties and does not use his adulterous relationships as a means of avoiding any of his serious problems.

5. He is sexually adequate with his spouse as well as with others and therefore has extramarital affairs out of sex interest rather than for sex therapy.

Although the adulterer who lives up to these criteria may have other emotional disturbances and may be having extramarital affairs for various neurotic reasons, Ellis argues that there is also a good chance that this is not true.

Do you believe there is such a thing as a healthy adulterer?

what is meant by the ethical principle of *beneficence*. School officials who banned Wendy Weaver from coaching volleyball thought they were doing good for the students in that school. Therefore, they thought they were acting morally. Those who opposed the ban believed they were doing good by upholding the right of people to acknowledge their sexuality in an appropriate and honest manner, regardless of their particular sexual orientation. Therefore, they thought they were acting morally. We will soon discuss how these contradictions can be resolved.

Autonomy/Liberty

The ethical principle of *autonomy* or *liberty* requires people be free to decide an issue for themselves before that decision can qualify as moral. That does not mean that every decision made freely is a moral one, only that any decision made under coercion is

immoral. Was the decision to bar Wendy Weaver made freely by school officials, or was it coerced by a small group of vocal parents? Was Weaver allowed to decide freely whether she would discuss her sexual orientation, as could heterosexuals teaching in that school, or was she being coerced by school officials? The way you answer these questions will help you determine which actions you think were moral in this case.

Justice/Fairness

Some ethicists believe that for an action to be moral, it must treat people fairly. They term this ethical principle *justice* or *fairness*. That does not mean that people must be treated equally. For example, our culture has determined that homosexuals and heterosexuals may be treated differently by different segments of society. That is, in private clubs or homes, or in certain churches or synagogues, gays may be excluded. However, our society has determined that excluding gays from public facilities is not just or fair—it is immoral—and has codified that decision by making a law defining that behavior illegal/unconstitutional.

Social Utility

Sometimes there is a clash between individual rights and the rights of a large group of people. In these instances, some ethicists use the ethical principle of *social utility* to determine the morality of various actions being contemplated. Social utility defines the moral decision as the one that is best for society (or the large group) rather than what is best for the individual (or the small group). School officials in Nebo, Utah, determined that removing Wendy Weaver from coaching was the greater good for the greater number of people (the students). Whether they were aware of it or not, they were using social utility to justify their decision. Of course, others might argue that the greater number of people in this instance ought to have been the gay community throughout the United States whose rights have been violated for far too long.

Ethical Dilemmas

We often experience situations in which one ethical principle clashes with another. We call these clashes **ethical dilemmas**. For example, consider your response to the question of adultery in the Ethical Dimensions box. Suppose you held the following ethical principles: Marriage should be a sexually monogamous relationship and people have a right to a satisfying, fulfilling sexual life. Obviously if you were in a marriage in which you were sexually unfulfilled for some reason, these two ethical principles would conflict. In such a situation which principle would be operative? Which one would take precedence over the other? Sometimes religion or culture provides answers to ethical dilemmas. For instance, in Islamic countries adultery is opposed by tradition and the law; such a society has resolved our ethical dilemma—at least officially—by placing the higher value on fidelity within marriage. Where there are no such prohibitions, individuals must rank their own values to make a choice.

The existence of such dilemmas has led to the development of situation ethics, in contrast to rule ethics. **Rule ethics** are exhaustive principles intended to guide people in their moral decision making in all situations. These principles are explicit, specific, and all-encompassing. People who hold to the letter of the law and proponents of religious dogmas are rule ethicists. **Situation ethics**, in contrast, are based

on the premise that all situations are unique, and therefore no one set of rules is applicable in all cases. Consequently a situation ethicist faced with a moral decision carefully reviews, analyzes, and evaluates each specific situation to determine which principles are applicable; a rule ethicist applies a given principle, regardless of the specific circumstances. As an example, a rule ethicist believes abortion is wrong in all cases. A situation ethicist may also believe abortion is wrong but may also believe it is moral in the case of a 12-year-old rape victim who becomes pregnant.

Trying to decide which viewpoint—rule ethics or situation ethics—is correct is itself an ethical dilemma. When we narrow our focus to sexual behavior, we can see that the rule/situation dichotomy has relevance. Are there general rules to guide sexual behavior, or does each situation require its own set of rules? Which rules, if any, will guide your behavior? Given your intuitive responses to the questions we raise in this chapter, see whether you consider yourself a rule or situation ethicist.

■ Moral Decision Making and Sexual Behavior

What influences the decisions we make about sexuality? Such factors as our knowledge or lack of knowledge; our sense of who we are; our ideals regarding fidelity and responsibility; our desire to express affection, passion, and delight; the emotional excitement we experience while facing the decision; and external cultural influences such as the double standard are all involved. The questions one asks in making moral decisions about sexuality or any other area of life are, What is *right*? What is *good*? What is *wrong*? What is *bad*? If it is right or good, it is moral! If it is wrong or bad, it is immoral! Thus morals relate to concrete decisions in particular situations.

To determine whether an action or decision is moral or immoral, we use our system of ethics. This system of ethics involves our ethical principles, which are guides by which we can judge an action or decision as moral or immoral. If the decision is inconsistent with our ethical principles, it is immoral; if it is consistent with them, it is moral.

ethical dilemma When two or more ethical principles work in opposing fashion in a particular situation, resulting in bewilderment regarding what is moral and what is immoral.

rule ethics Guiding principles used in all situations to arrive at moral decisions, which are considered applicable to all situations.

situation ethics A belief that no one set of rules can apply to all situations and each specific situation must be analyzed to determine which ethical principles are applicable.

Deciding whether a rule should be applied to a particular ethical issue, or whether the situation is unique and requires a unique decision, is a dilemma faced by ethicists.

Ethical principles specific to sexual matters include the following:

1. Sexual behavior should not be forced on anyone.

2. Sexual behavior between consenting adults is acceptable.

3. Fidelity (faithfulness) in marriage is a must.

4. Marriage partners and loved ones must be responsive to each other's needs.

Unfortunately, most situations are not so cut and dried. Applying ethical principles is often a complex matter because they provide only guidance, not ready-made answers. If our principles are in conflict, we must examine our personal values to rank conflicting ethical principles in order of importance. By personal *values* we mean the worth or importance we assign to our ethical principles. If we personally value our commitment to a monogamous relationship more than we value sexual fulfillment, for example, then we resolve a conflict between the two by choosing not to have extramarital relationships. If we value sexual fulfillment more highly, then we resolve the same conflict differently.

To summarize, then, we decide the morality of an action or decision after identifying and ranking ethical principles in order of our personal values. Most people learn that the many moral decisions they make about sexual behavior are ultimately based on their personal values.

Our intention is to help you explore your own values and ethical principles so you may apply them in specific situations, and thereby act morally.

Commonly Accepted Ethical Principles

This discussion is not intended to convey the notion that *anything goes*. Although we value and recognize the need for diversity, as a society we have reached agreement on a set of ethical principles. For example, we have societal consensus that caring, respect, honesty, responsibility, and trust ought to guide our decisions regarding morality. In fact, a whole educational movement that seeks to convey these principles to school-aged children and youth has sprouted. That movement is called *character education*. Its objectives are consistent with the societal consensus regarding ethical principles described: respect for the rights of all people regardless of their race, religion, gender, age, and sexual orientation; understanding, sympathy, concern, and compassion for others; and personal integrity and honesty. These are principles to which all citizens should adhere, and to emphasize their importance, society has passed laws specifying sanctions for acting contrary to them. For example, we have laws against discrimination by gender, race, ethnicity, and sexual orientation. And we have laws punishing those who sexually abuse others. If someone lies to a sexual partner about his or her HIV status and infects that partner, we have laws to punish that behavior. If someone takes advantage of someone else by engaging in coitus with that person while he or she is incapable of deciding freely to participate (for example, if intoxicated

Although people may value ethical principles differently, there is agreement on a set of common principles such as caring, respect, and honesty.

or mentally impaired), we have laws punishing that behavior. And if someone fires someone else from a job solely because of that person's sexual orientation, we have laws to punish that behavior (as the school officials who fired Wendy Weaver found out).

In matters of sexuality and sexual morality, it is important to keep these consensually agreed-on ethical principles in the forefront. Certainly we, as the writers of this chapter, value diversity and recognize the influence of different experiences and values as they play out in various ethical dilemmas. Still, these consensually accepted ethical principles are ones to which we are committed. The problem arises when behaving consistently with one or more of these principles means violating one or more of the others. This is what we earlier described as an ethical dilemma. Ethical dilemmas apply to human sexuality, as we shall now see.

Government Control and Regulation

As will be evident in the rest of this chapter, each sexual ethical issue can be controlled or regulated by government. The broader issue, then, is how much control should we expect the government to exert through regulation, and how much should individuals be allowed to decide these issues for themselves. Laws are a reflection of moral judgments. For example, we judge stealing from another to be immoral so we pass laws penalizing those who steal. Because many sexual ethical issues are controversial, passing regulations or laws to control sexual behavior can be problematic. Whose morals should be the basis for law? How will the minority view of morality be protected? These are important, but not easily answered, questions. The government has an obligation to pass laws to regulate behaviors believed to be harmful—that is, to protect the health of its citizens. Where should the line between individual freedoms and governmental protections be drawn?

To resolve many of these sexual ethical issues raised by government regulations, as manifested in laws, these laws are juxtaposed against constitutional protections. The U.S. Constitution is the arbiter of issues that divide the populace. It offers guidance to lawmakers and others to help them protect the public without infringing on their rights. As you will soon see, it is not unusual for the government to pass laws pertaining to sexual behavior (for example, sodomy) or other sexually related issues (such as abortion), only to have these laws challenged, and sometimes overturned, by the U.S. Supreme Court.

Sexually Transmitted Infections

To treat sexually transmitted infections (STIs) effectively on a large scale, health care workers often ask their patients to identify their sexual contacts. The purpose is to inform these contacts that they have been exposed to a disease and encourage them to seek treatment. Generally the carrier is inclined, at least fleetingly, to protect the anonymity of his or her sexual contacts (and perhaps his or her own identity and reputation). One of the ethical principles commonly underlying such a reaction is probably, *One should not discuss other people's private sexual behavior.* However, a competing ethical principle might be, *People should not intentionally harm the health of others.* Most individuals would probably value the second principle over the first and would therefore identify their sexual contacts. Observers who also value health over confidentiality would judge this decision to be moral. If the infected person is married and has contracted the disease through nonconsensual extramarital activity, the principle of not harming others becomes harder to apply. In this situation the patient would have to decide whether the health of the marriage partner was more valuable than potential damage to the marital relationship and the family and whether the couple had an agreement regarding fidelity that had been breached.

An important ethical issue raised by the HIV and AIDS epidemic is whether to require pregnant women to be tested for HIV. With modern medications and medical regimens, approximately 75% to 80% of HIV and AIDS can be prevented in babies born to infected mothers. Consequently, using the ethical principle of beneficence, some medical experts argue that all pregnant women should be required to be tested for HIV, thereby identifying mothers who ought to be treated before their babies' births and newborns who ought to be treated as soon after birth as possible. However, others argue that requiring all pregnant women to be tested would actually harm newborns (maleficence). They believe that if pregnant women are required to be tested they will refrain from identifying themselves as pregnant, thereby depriving their babies of the prenatal care that can prevent all kinds of health problems, not just HIV and AIDS. This would, in turn, increase the infant mortality rate, which is already too high, especially in low-socioeconomic-status populations. Therefore, opponents of mandatory pregnancy testing for HIV believe testing ought to be voluntary (autonomy/liberty) with educational campaigns to communicate the advantages of being tested.

There are other ethical issues related to HIV and AIDS. For example, should research funds be used for treating AIDS patients or for finding a cure or for developing a vaccine? What is the appropriate balance in this funding? Are funds best used for education about HIV and AIDS to prevent the greatest possible number of cases?

These questions are more than issues for academic consideration: Decisions are being made on a regular basis by research institutes, the government, and insurance companies. Are these decisions being made ethically? Are they moral decisions? Your answers to these questions depend on the way you value your ethical principles. Although no one answer will meet with everyone's approval, society adopts a consensus view of morality as a matter of necessity. That is, *something* must be decided, even if the decision is to ignore the situation. Further, because we are citizens in a society that allows for our input, we are contributing to this ethical exercise by our votes, letters, and attitudes (as determined by opinion polls).

Sexual Activity Between Unmarried Partners

Whether to participate in sexual activity without being married is another common moral decision. Those who decide that such behavior is immoral might value the following ethical principle: *Marriage is a unique relationship blessed by God and allowing for a total expression of love.* Those who consider sexual intercourse to be moral in any circumstance, unless one participant is harmed in some way, might value another principle more, such as *You should experience life fully.* However, decisions regarding premarital or nonmarital sexual behavior are usually more complicated than a choice between two principles. Situation ethicists pondering the morality of premarital sex in a given situation might ask the following questions:

1. How old are the people involved? Seventeen? Forty-five?

2. What do the people feel for each other?

3. Is their intention to marry or enter into a union? Soon?

4. What are their religious beliefs?

5. In which society (country, culture) do they live?

In your own situation, which special considerations are or were relevant to your decisions about the morality of your sexual behavior?

Sexting

Sexting is sending sexually explicit messages—text messages, photos, or videos—by cell phone or instant messaging (Matte, 2015). In the first study to quantify

© Digital Vision/Thinkstock

One ethical dilemma is whether sexual intercourse between unmarried partners is moral. Should the age of the partners matter? Should the quality of the relationship matter? What other factors do you think need to be considered when deciding on the morality of coitus between unmarried partners?

the extent of sexting by teenagers (13 to 19 years of age) and young adults (20 to 26 years of age), a significant number were found to have engaged in sending sexually explicit messages and/or photos (National Campaign to Prevent Teen and Unplanned Pregnancy, 2008). Twenty percent of teens have sent or posted nude or semi-nude pictures or videos of themselves (22% of girls and 18% of boys). Even more young adults are sending nude or semi-nude pictures or videos of themselves: 33% overall, including 36% of women and 31% of men. Sexually explicit messaging is even more prevalent: 39% of teens (37% of girls and 40% of boys) and 59% of young adults (56% of women and 62% of men) have sent such messages. Another study (Drouin & Landgraff, 2012) found that 67% of college students had sent sexually explicit text messages and 54% had sent sexually explicit photos and videos.

Many problems can arise as a result of sexting. What you post online never truly disappears. Potential employers, parents, friends, or enemies may be able to find your past posts, even after you delete them. In addition, you never know who has already copied an explicated photo and posted it elsewhere. Another issue relates to the legality of sexting. Alarmingly, 20% of youth who engaged in sexting without any demonstrable harm to others were arrested (Peskin et al., 2013).

Aside from the legal ramifications, several ethical issues are associated with sexting. Forty percent of teens and young adults report they have had sexually explicit communications that were meant to be private shown to them, and 20% admitted they had shared such messages with someone other than the

---

Sexting Sending sexually explicit messages—text messages, photos, or videos—by cell phone or instant messaging.

person to whom they were originally sent. Is sharing such a text, photo, or video with someone else without the sender's permission moral? In one sense, the ethical principle of autonomy applies: I am free to do as I choose. On the other hand, the concept of nonmaleficence applies: Do no harm to others.

Another ethical concern is how truthful to be when sexting. A study of college students (Drouin et al., 2014) found that 48% had lied to their committed partner during sexting about what they were wearing, doing, or both. Women reported lying more than men (45% of women compared to 24% of men). Is it moral to lie to someone with whom you have a committed relationship? Does it matter that 67% of respondents stated they lied to serve their partners in an effort to make their partners happy? How about the 33% who lied to serve themselves (for example, they were bored)? Which of these two groups is more moral, or does the reason why they lied even matter?

Sodomy

It is impossible to define the term **sodomy** because states lump together those sexual activities they consider immoral and codify their views by passing laws that make these sexual behaviors illegal. Usually sodomy laws refer to such sexual activities as anal intercourse, oral–genital sexual behavior, homosexual activities, and any sexual behavior with animals. In earlier years, some states defined *sodomy* as any sexual activity of anyone other than a married couple. In fact, as late as 1990, a bill was proposed by a Washington state legislator that would allow the state to prosecute anyone younger than 18 years old who was "necking" or "petting." The proposed penalty was a maximal sentence of 90 days in jail and a $5,000 fine.

Most sodomy laws were applied primarily against homosexuals. The penalties varied from state to state, ranging from a $200 fine to 20 years of imprisonment. Violators of sodomy laws have been imprisoned, lost their jobs and homes, lost custody of their children, and even been beaten and killed. One test of the constitutionality of sodomy laws occurred in 1986. In the *Bowers v. Hardwick* case, an Atlanta man was arrested after police officers entered his home at the request of his roommate regarding another matter and found him in bed with another man. When this case finally reached the U.S. Supreme Court, the Court upheld Georgia's sodomy law in spite of recognizing that the Constitution creates "zones of privacy." Dissenting from this decision was Justice Harry A. Blackmun, who wrote that the Court mistakenly refused to recognize "the fundamental interest all individuals have in controlling the nature of their intimate associations with

others." However, on June 26, 2003, in a landmark ruling on sexuality and privacy, the U.S. Supreme Court overturned *Bowers v. Hardwick*. In *Lawrence v. Texas*, the Court found that *Bowers* "was not correct when it was decided, is not correct today, and is hereby overruled." Further, the *Lawrence* decision states, "When homosexual conduct is made criminal by the law of the State, that declaration in and of itself is an invitation to subject homosexual persons to discrimination both in the public and private spheres… Its continuance as precedent demeans the lives of homosexual persons."

Contraception

People who oppose so-called artificial methods of contraception for religious reasons are usually guided by the ethic, *All life is sacred*. They argue that prevention of a conception that would occur without interference is interference with God's creation of life. Proponents of modern birth control, in contrast, are often guided by the ethic, *Every child deserves to be wanted and loved*. They argue that when unwanted children are born, the quality of life diminishes for the parents and the society, and the children themselves often have difficult lives as well.

In 1914 Margaret Sanger began publishing her newspaper, *The Woman Rebel*, in which she argued that women should be free to choose whether to bear children. Sanger had witnessed the death of a young woman who tried to perform an abortion on herself and cited this incident as her motivation for working for a woman's right to control her fertility.

For some people, certain types of fertility-control methods are acceptable and others are not. For example, methods that prevent a fertilized egg from implanting on the endometrial lining of the uterus might be unacceptable to people who believe life begins at conception. For others, any action taken before birth is acceptable because they believe that birth is when human life begins.

Then there is the issue pertaining to who should be responsible for contraception. Some people wonder why most methods of contraception are designed to be used by women. Accompanying these methods of contraception are potential side effects that can have significant health implications. Why aren't men subjected to the same risks, some wonder (see Gender Dimensions). Is it moral to subject women to health risks disproportionate to the risk expected of men so as to prevent conception?

sodomy A term that specifically refers to anal intercourse, but is often used to refer to almost any sexual behavior that might not be considered normal.

Gender DIMENSIONS

The "Umbrelly" (A Little Humor)

Critics of research on contraceptive technology argue that research is immoral—that is, sexist. It focuses on female techniques, largely ignoring male methods of contraception. Others argue it is the characteristics and complexities of the male reproductive system that make the development of effective male contraception difficult. In an attempt to have males develop a greater appreciation for how the critics view the morality of contraceptive research, the following facetious description of a new male contraceptive was written:

> The newest development in male contraception was unveiled recently at the American Women's Surgical Symposium held at the Ann Arbor Medical Center. Dr. Sophia Merkin, of the Merkin Clinic, announced the preliminary findings of a study conducted on 763 unsuspecting male grad students at a large Midwest university. In her report Dr. Merkin stated that the new contraceptive—the IPD—was a breakthrough in male contraception. It will be marketed under the trade name "Umbrelly."
>
> The IPD (intrapenal device) resembles a tiny folded umbrella that is inserted through the head of the penis and pushed into the scrotum with a plunger-like instrument. Occasionally there is perforation of the scrotum but this is disregarded, since it is known that the male has few nerve endings in this area of his body. The underside of the umbrella contains a spermicidal jelly, hence "Umbrelly."
>
> Experiments on a thousand white whales from the Continental Shelf (whose sexual apparatus is said to be closest to man's) proved the Umbrelly to be 100% effective in preventing production of sperm and eminently satisfactory to the female whale, since it doesn't interfere with her rutting pleasure.
>
> Dr. Merkin declared the Umbrelly to be statistically safe for the human male. She reported that of the 763 grad students tested with the device, only two died of scrotal infection, only 20 experienced swelling of the tissues, three developed cancer of the testicles, and 13 were too depressed to have an erection. She stated that common complaints ranged from cramping and bleeding to acute abdominal pain. She emphasized that these symptoms were merely indications that the man's body had not yet adjusted to the device. Hopefully the symptoms would disappear within a year.
>
> One complication caused by the IPD and briefly mentioned by Dr. Merkin was the incidence of massive scrotal infection necessitating the surgical removal of the testicles. "But this is a rare case," said Merkin, "too rare to be statistically important." She and the other distinguished members of the Women's College of Surgeons agreed that the benefits far outweighed the risk to any individual man.

Source: Unknown.

Lastly, different cultural groups view the morality of contraception differently. Some countries' health insurance plans will not reimburse its subscribers for contraceptive devices or pills. In other countries, contraceptive services are part of reimbursable expenses. Countries with large Hispanic populations, such as in Latin America, with a strong belief in Catholicism, may not be as accepting of contraception as non-Catholics. Once again, morality is influenced by many variables and, therefore, what one person determines to be moral, another may determine to be immoral.

Emergency Contraception

A more recent contraceptive development pertains to *emergency contraception*. This is the use of oral contraceptives after unprotected sexual intercourse has occurred and there is a fear of pregnancy. For example, emergency contraception can be used in the case of rape or condom failure to prevent conception. The oral contraceptives must be taken within 72 hours of intercourse.

One of the issues debated was whether to allow women access to emergency contraception without a physician's prescription. An expert Food and Drug Administration (FDA) panel recommended the FDA approve emergency contraception to be disbursed by pharmacists. The FDA asked the panel to gather more information and did not follow through on its recommendation. Some accused the FDA of bowing to political pressure from social conservatives (Kaufman, 2005). They argued that making emergency contraception available through pharmacists would make emergency contraception more effective. Their reasoning was that since it has to be used within 72 hours of coitus, why jeopardize that time frame by requiring a physician be contacted and a prescription be written. Further, they argued, studies have shown emergency contraception to be safe and effective.

Others, though, considered emergency contraception to be an abortion pill. That is, it prevents a fertilized egg from developing into a fetus and, eventually, a baby. They were opposed to any action that interfered with a pregnancy. They also believed that with emergency contraception available as a back-up, people (in particular, youth) might engage in riskier sexual behavior. Studies, however, have found this fear to be unfounded (Kaufman, 2005). Whether and how emergency contraception should be available elicits more debate. As a responsible citizen, you should keep abreast of this debate and let your elected representatives know your views.

Abortion

Is induced, or voluntary, abortion simply a method of fertility control and as such the right of every woman, or is it taking of life that has a right to exist? Can it be both? If so, how can the dilemma be resolved? Some people seek to solve the problem by looking for evidence—or a definition—of when life begins. Does it begin at conception or does it begin when a fetus is capable of living outside the mother (at birth, or shortly before)? Others seek to solve it by asking who controls a woman's reproductive capacity. One must decide whether preserving the life and quality of life of the living is more or less important than maintaining the existence or viability of the unborn. This ethical dilemma is one of the most divisive issues in modern society. Laws are no sooner made than they are challenged. Some of these laws seek to limit abortions or encourage women to reconsider before deciding to abort. For example, some states require a waiting period before abortions can be done. Other states are seeking to require women to view sonograms of the fetus, obtain parental consent if a minor, or prohibit government funds from supporting organizations (such as Planned Parenthood) that support a woman's right to abort. What is your view of the morality of these legal strategies? The morality of abortion is a subject of ongoing debate in many arenas of modern life—from the purely personal to the political.

Amniocentesis

Amniocentesis involves withdrawing, via a needle inserted into the uterus through the abdominal wall, a small amount of amniotic fluid surrounding the fetus. The procedure is recommended for women whose risk of producing babies with birth defects is greater than average (for example, women older than 35 years or women who have previously given birth to babies with birth defects). The moral question arises because if the test shows that the fetus will be deformed, mentally retarded, or seriously ill, the parents can choose to have an abortion rather than let the pregnancy run its course. Is it moral to take the risk (for example, of miscarriage) of having the test at all? Other issues are raised as well. For example, the sex of the fetus can be determined through amniocentesis. Is abortion moral when parents who have, say, four sons discover that their unborn child is a boy? Should the genes of an unborn baby be manipulated to conform with the parents'—or society's—idea of a superior human being? How much genetic manipulation is consistent with our ethical principles and values? As science becomes more sophisticated in this area, new ethical dilemmas arise.

Fetal Tissue Implantation

Parkinson's disease patients suffer tremors, muscular rigidity, and loss of balance as a result of a lack of the brain neurotransmitter dopamine. Research has discovered that fetal brain tissue, if implanted within the brain of Parkinson's patients, can produce enough dopamine to relieve many of the symptoms. However, the potential for abuse of this knowledge has prompted many groups and individuals to oppose the use of fetal tissue for implantation, or even for research purposes. One of the concerns is that a woman will become pregnant with the intention to abort the fetus and use its brain tissue for a family

In 1990, Mary and Abe Ayala were told that the only chance to save their 17-year-old daughter Anissa from dying of leukemia was for her to have bone marrow transplantation. With no matching donors, the Ayalas decided to have another child (Marissa Eve) to use his or her bone marrow. Did the Ayalas act in a moral way? Did their physicians? What would you have done faced with such a dilemma?

Global DIMENSIONS

Marital Age Around the World

It is not surprising that different countries with different cultures have different views of ethical issues. One of these issues is age at marriage. In the United States, it is believed to be immoral for a 13-year-old girl to marry, especially an older man. We even maintain legislation defining this as a violation of law. However, in other countries, the morality of early marriage, even to an older man, is not called into question. Worldwide, more than 700 million women alive today were married as children. More than 1 in 3—or some 250 million women—were married before the age of 15. Girls living in the poorest 20% of households are more likely to get married at an early age than those living in the wealthiest 20%. For example, in Peru, 45% of women were married by age 18 among the poorest 20% of the population, compared to 5% among the richest 20%. Women with primary education were significantly less likely to be married as children than those who received no education. In Zimbabwe, 48% of women who had attended primary school had been married by the age of 18, compared to 87% of those who had not attended school.

Parents choose to marry off their daughters early for a number of reasons. Poor families may regard a young girl as an economic burden and her marriage as a necessary survival strategy for her family. They may think that child marriage offers protection for their daughter from the dangers of sexual assault or, more generally, offers the care of a male guardian. Child marriage may also be seen as a strategy to avoid girls becoming pregnant outside of marriage. Gender discrimination can also underpin child marriage. Girls may be married young to ensure obedience and subservience within their husband's household and to maximize their childbearing.

UNICEF argues that child marriage can have serious harmful consequences for children, including *denial of education* (once married, girls tend not to go to school), *health problems* (including premature pregnancies, higher rates of maternal and infant mortality, and STIs, including HIV/AIDS), and *abuse* (a practice common in child marriages; children who refuse to marry or who choose a marriage partner against the wishes of their parents are often punished or even killed by their families in so-called honor killings).

Data from UNICEF. *Child marriage.* New York: UNICEF, 2014. Available at: http://www.unicef.org/protection/57929_58008.html. UNICEF. Child protection from violence, exploitation and abuse: Child marriage. 2009. Available: http://www.unicef.org/protection /index_earlymarriage.html. UNICEF. *The state of the world's children 2009: Maternal and newborn health.* New York: UNICEF, 2009. Available: http://www.unicef.org/sowc09/docs/SOWC09Figure-2.4-EN.pdf.

member suffering from Parkinson's disease. Others argue that using human tissue in this manner defiles the sanctity of the human body.

Stem cell research has the potential to result in cures for debilitating diseases, but it is fraught with moral potholes. What do you think the policy ought to be regarding stem cell research and the appropriate source of stem cells?

Yet there are those who strongly support the use of fetal tissue to relieve Parkinson's and other diseases. They point to the socially acceptable practice of donating and transplanting organs such as hearts, livers, kidneys, lungs, and corneas.

In 1988, the federal government banned the use of federal funds for research involving aborted fetal tissue implantation. Believing this policy deprives certain patients from receiving adequate care, the American College of Obstetrics and Gynecology and the American Fertility Society in February 1991 established a private advisory body to guide scientists conducting fetal tissue and fertility research. This board, the National Advisory Board on Ethics in Reproduction, sets uniform standards, reviews proposed projects, advises researchers, and serves as a clearinghouse of information.

By 1993, the federal government's ban on research with fetal tissue implantation was lifted. Since then the National Institutes of Health (NIH) has awarded millions of dollars in grants for research involving

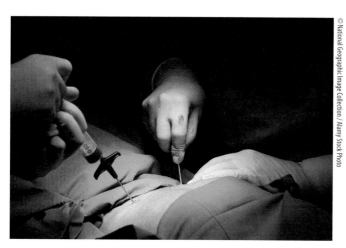

Doreen Flynn is the mother of three young girls with an incurable blood disorder called Fanconi anemia. They will all need bone marrow transplants to survive. Their mother fears there will not be a match for her girls when the time comes or, even worse, that if a match is found, he or she will not follow through and donate. She has reason to worry: Some experts say that nearly half of donors do not follow through with donation. The National Organ Transplant Act in 1984 made it illegal to buy and sell organs and organ parts. In an effort to save her daughters' lives, Doreen Flynn has become the lead plaintiff in a case that she hopes will change medical history and make it legal to pay bone marrow donors.

the study, analysis, and use of human fetal tissue. Today research continues on the potential of fetal tissue in treatment of not only Parkinson's disease but also Alzheimer's disease, Huntington's disease, diabetes, multiple sclerosis, epilepsy, blindness, leukemia, hemophilia, sickle cell anemia, spinal-cord injuries, deficiencies of the immune system, birth defects, and pain (Kenney, Reinholtz, & Angellini, 1997). Supporting this research are the Alzheimer's Association, the Epilepsy Foundation of America, the Cystic Fibrosis Foundation, the Parkinson's Disease Foundation, and the Society for Pediatric Research.

Part of the remaining ethical issues regarding the use of human fetal tissue pertains to the finding that tissue from miscarriages and ectopic pregnancies appears rarely to be suitable for transplantation. However, tissue from induced abortions is effective when transplanted. Researchers argue that legal barriers to harvesting tissue from induced abortions stand in the way of building up the supply of usable fetal tissue.

Stem Cell Research

Stem cells are cells that can be found in embryos, fetuses, and adults. In adults, stem cells are specialized and can evolve into more cells of their own kind. In embryos, however, stem cells have the capacity to evolve into many different types of tissues and

organs, depending on a complex of biological instructions. However, scientists think that tissues derived from embryonic and adult stem cells may differ in the likelihood of being rejected after transplantation. It is not yet known whether tissues derived from embryonic stem cells will cause transplant rejection, because the first-phase clinical trials involving embryonic stem cells have only recently been approved by the U.S. Food and Drug Administration (FDA). However, adult stem cells, and tissues derived from them, are currently thought to be less likely to initiate rejection after transplantation. This is because a patient's own cells could be expanded in culture, coaxed into assuming a specific cell type (differentiation), and then reintroduced into the patient. The use of adult stem cells and tissues derived from the patient's own adult stem cells would mean that the cells are less likely to be rejected by the immune system. This represents a significant advantage, because immune rejection can be circumvented only by continuous administration of immunosuppressive drugs, and the drugs themselves may cause deleterious side effects (National Institutes of Health Resource for Stem Cell Research, 2011).

Embryonic stem cells are taken from embryos at the blastocyst stage of development (4 or 5 days after conception) when they are, in essence, a "blank page." Scientists are working on ways of instructing stem cells to develop into specific tissue—for example, into insulin-producing pancreatic cells for implantation in diabetics.

The moral debate about stem cells involves a number of complex issues. For example, is it moral to use stem cells from aborted fetuses? Will this practice encourage more abortions? Is it moral to use stem cells from embryos created specifically for their stem cells? Is this the destruction of one human life to benefit another human life? Should scientific research, and consequently money that is devoted to scientific research, be concentrated on developing techniques for using adult stem cells rather than on embryonic stem cells? What should be the government's role in regulating and/or supporting stem cell research? Given the potential for stem cells to contribute to cures and/or treatments for Parkinson's disease, Alzheimer's disease, diabetes, heart disease, and arthritis, among others, should scientific research be entailed by governmental restrictions? Is that moral?

In 2001, President George W. Bush approved a regulation that would provide government funding for limited stem cell research. Bush, a conservative politician, tried to walk the fine line between what he believed to be morally justified and the potential for the enhancement of a large number of American lives—another moral consideration. He decided that,

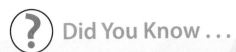

Did You Know . . .

Fetal brain tissue is not the only type of fetal cell that has potential for medical use. Early in development, the fetus's blood cells are produced by stem cells in the liver. Eventually these blood cells move into the fetus's bones and become bone marrow. Therefore, injecting fetal liver cells intravenously into patients is, in effect, giving them immune system transplantation.

Fetal liver transplants hold promise for such conditions as certain leukemias, sickle cell anemia, aplastic anemia, AIDS, and severe combined immunodeficiency disease.

Diabetics have also been given fetal insulin-producing pancreas cells, and fetal brain tissue's potential to aid in the treatment of Alzheimer's disease is very real.

on the one hand, stem cell research had a great deal of potential to cure diseases that affect large numbers of Americans. On the other hand, he believed that developing "human life" (embryos) to harvest their stem cells was immoral. Consequently, Bush decided that the government would provide funding for scientific research that used only adult stem cells or embryonic stem cells that had already been harvested. Bush estimated that there were about 60 of those groups of embryonic stem cells around the world. Staunch conservatives viewed this decision as immoral because it did not make a statement about the sanctity of life and allowed "immorally produced" embryonic stem cells to be used for research purposes. Scientists considered this decision immoral because it limited research to a small number of embryonic stem cells that were thought to be too homogenous to produce wide-scale cures (for example, many of these existing colonies of embryonic stem cells were obtained from white populations). Furthermore, scientists argued, adult stem cells do not have the capacity to develop into a range of tissue as do embryonic stem cells but are, instead, tissue specific. That limits their potential for a scientific breakthrough.

When Americans were surveyed, a majority supported stem cell research (Stem cell research, 2005). When asked if they favored or opposed stem cell research using embryonic stem cells, 58% were either strongly or somewhat in favor, 29% were either strongly or somewhat opposed, and 13% had no opinion. Of those opposed to the use of embryonic stem cells for research, 57% were opposed on religious grounds. Furthermore, 78% stated they thought the United States should be the global leader in medical and scientific research, in general. However, this is not the case when it comes to stem cell research. Whereas the federal government has restricted funding, several other countries have proceeded vigorously in stem cell research. They believe that, aside from developing techniques to cure many of the diseases plaguing humankind today, embryonic stem

cell research is both moral and has tremendous economic potential for these countries' economies.

In 2009, bringing a different perspective to this issue, President Barack Obama lifted the restriction on federal funding of human embryonic stem cell research.

If you were the person deciding the role government ought to play in stem cell research, what would you decide? Which moral justifications would you offer to support that decision?

Prostitution

Prostitution is the selling of sexual gratification. Examples of prostitution were recorded even in ancient times, so contemporary society can take neither credit nor blame for inventing this trade—only for the way in which it treats it.

People who consider prostitution immoral often argue that it degrades sexual intercourse, which is sanctified within marriage as an expression of love, into a mere animalistic act. Centuries ago Christianity adopted the Persian view, that the demands of the spirit and flesh were in conflict with each other, rather than the Greek view, which saw no conflict and allowed for prostitution (so long as the prostitutes were male). Nevertheless making some allowances for the flesh, Christianity developed incentives for marriage and deemed sexual intercourse within marriage appropriate and outside it sinful. Our culture has largely adhered to this view of who is a legitimate and morally acceptable sexual partner. To make a judgment about prostitution, a person must decide whether the desire for sexual services and sexual outlets is more important than the principle that coitus outside marriage is immoral.

In Vitro Fertilization

In 1980 the first "test-tube" baby clinic in the United States was approved by the state of Virginia. Located at the Norfolk General Hospital in Norfolk, Virginia, this clinic offers its services to couples who wish to conceive but are infertile as a result of blocked, missing, or damaged fallopian tubes of women. (It does not treat male infertility.) The clinic, officially named the In Vitro Clinic (for **in vitro fertilization**), had a waiting list of from 1 to 2 years just 1 week after gaining state approval.

Some people believe using in vitro fertilization to produce babies is immoral. For example, in March 1987 the Catholic Congregation for the Doctrine of the Faith issued "Instruction on Respect for Human Life in Its Origin and on the Dignity of Procreation," a document that defined generation of human life outside the body as "morally illicit." In addition to in vitro fertilization, other biomedical breakthroughs were condemned as immoral. Among these were genetic engineering, surrogate motherhood, cloning, and manipulations to produce human beings according to sex or other predetermined qualities. According to the document, the only approved method of human procreation is "the act of conjugal love."

Other ethical issues pertain to in vitro fertilization. For example, what will be its effect on the population of the world? Will it produce too many people for the available resources? What would that mean for the quality of life of the world's population? What should be done if the fetus develops defectively once it has been implanted in the uterus? When choosing to have a baby by artificial means, should parents be allowed to select the baby's sex, eye color, intelligence, and so on? These issues need societal attention; we as citizens need to inform our representatives of our judgments regarding what is moral and immoral relative to in vitro fertilization.

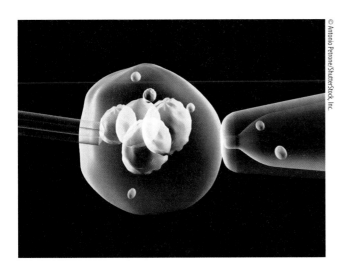

© Antonio Petrone/ShutterStock, Inc.

What is the appropriate and/or moral use of reproductive technologies such as in vitro fertilization? Should reproduction remain a natural phenomenon, or should medical advancements and techniques be used to enhance conception?

Genetic Engineering

In vitro fertilization evokes images of genetic manipulation to some people. Of course, that is not its intent. However, as science progresses and reproductive technology develops new ways to manage and enhance reproduction, fears of Huxley's *Brave New World* emerge. There are hundreds of biotechnology companies devoted to identifying genes and their functions with the hope of obtaining patents for these genes and the ways in which they can be put to use. It is envisioned that these genes will lead to designer medicines, engineered foods, and eventually custom-made kids (Achenbach, 1998), and the companies that own these patents will make a lot of money. Even the U.S. government staked out a claim to this research by funding the largest scientific project, the Human Genome Project. The $3 billion Human Genome Project, in collaboration with the private firm Celera Genomics, decoded the entire human genetic code in 2003.

All this research raises the possibility that a new generation will be genetically manipulated so that parents will be able to select the color of their babies' eyes, height, athletic and intellectual abilities, and artistic talents. Some experts are concerned about this possibility. Jeremy Rifkin, the eminent futurist, argues that in a few generations babies will be "engineered." The biologist Lee Silver believes that the human race will be divided into two distinct species, the "Naturals" and the "GenRich" (Achenbach, 1998).

There are other experts who disagree. They argue that although a sheep (Dolly) has been cloned, researchers are a long way from being able to clone humans, and even if it were possible, scientists are too ethical to do it. However, there are groups of scientists who are attempting to clone a human as of the time of this writing. Experts who do not see a "Brave New World" on the horizon expect that as we approach new and more sophisticated reproductive technological advancements, ethicists, clergy, philosophers, politicians, and others will intervene to develop gene-technology protocols that are acceptable to our societal values and mores.

Whether we will have "designer babies" is still an open question. As citizens in a democratic society we need to keep abreast of the latest developments in this area, because the very nature of the human race may be at issue. The uses of this new technology may be as much a function of the will of the people as it is the interests of the scientists, and, if so, every person has a responsibility to become involved in some way.

> **in vitro fertilization** The creation of a pregnancy in a laboratory by uniting the sperm and egg outside the womb; sometimes termed the "test-tube" baby technique.

The issue of bioethics is recognized throughout the world. The United Nations (UN) Commission on Human Rights adopted the first international guidelines on bioethics and the human genome. The "Universal Declaration on the Human Genome and Human Rights," cosponsored by 86 countries, sets standards for people researching and using genetic information and techniques. Although it specifically recognizes the rights to freedom of research and freedom of thought, it states that "practices which are contrary to human dignity, such as reproductive cloning of human beings, shall not be permitted." The United States is one of the countries that support the UN declaration.

Sexual Responsibility to a Partner

The last sexual ethical dilemma we discuss is, What degree of responsibility do we have, sexually, with respect to others? Should our sexual behavior achieve our own ends, regardless of the desires of our sexual partners? Conversely, are we under an obligation to subjugate our own sexual needs to the needs of our sexual partners? Given that two individuals are involved, just what is moral sexual behavior?

The issue of sexual responsibility, as are all the issues discussed so far, is complex. Certainly we are all responsible for ourselves and our own behavior, but when we take care of ourselves by involving someone else, the issue becomes clouded. As an example, imagine that a typical couple, Paul and Paula, who love each other and are engaged to be married. Paula wants to share coitus with Paul, but Paul considers sexual intercourse outside marriage immoral. Should Paula attempt to convince Paul that they should have intercourse? Would it be reasonable for her to threaten to date someone else if he refuses? Should Paul go against his beliefs and give in to Paula? What is their responsibility to themselves? To each other? To their future? To their relationship? These questions are not easy to answer. However, when sexual behavior involves someone else, there is always potential for manipulation or coercion. The moral nature of such behavior should be explored.

Even when a decision is the individual's alone, ethical dilemmas may arise. For example, should sexually active people use some means of contraception, even if their partners do not care? If not, are they behaving responsibly? What if one's religion opposes the use of contraception but one is sexually

active and unwilling to risk pregnancy? As with all the issues we have explored, the means of resolving these questions is to rank the conflicting ethical principles according to our personal values.

Laws Regulating Sexual Behavior

Laws formalize moral decisions for a society. Our laws regarding sexual behavior developed from a general acceptance of specific ethical principles, values, and judgments about behaviors such as those we have explored. They have their roots in experience, in religious dogma, and in economics and politics.

Consensus—or general agreement—about which sexual actions should be considered permissible has not always been easily achieved. Indeed, communities have sometimes had to devise ingenious compromises to keep peace among their various moral factions. Consider, for example, the "Combat Zone" in Boston, Massachusetts. To meet the needs of people who frequented bars featuring topless dancers, attended X-rated movies, and so forth, but also to protect citizens opposed to such activities from exposure to them, the municipal government restricted the bars and theaters in question to a specific part of the city, nicknamed the "Combat Zone." The Combat Zone has subsequently been abolished. For similar reasons, some European countries have established red-light districts, in an attempt to limit prostitution to a single section of town.

However, even when consensus is achieved and codified into city, state, or federal law, it is by no means stable. State laws prohibiting prostitution, which were widely acceptable when they were enacted, are periodically under attack and may well someday be modified or rejected. Supreme Court rulings on abortion and on pornography have not settled those issues. Changes occur—albeit slowly—when there is a conflict between existing law and new morality. An illegal activity might begin to be seen as moral; a legal act, as immoral.

We will see in this discussion that sexual laws develop through a societal consensus of the valuing of ethical principles. The process of devising such laws involves identifying ethical principles, valuing them to define moral behavior, and then encoding laws to enforce that behavior (or prohibit it if defined as immoral). Because our values may change over time, however, we periodically reassess and change our laws governing sexual behavior.

Obscenity and Pornography

Some issues continue to be debated even in the face of definitive opinions from the Supreme Court. An example involves the definitions of **obscenity** and **pornography**. The Comstock Act of 1873, the first

obscenity Something offensive to modesty or decency; often sexually related.

pornography Sexually arousing music, art, literature, or films; a determination that may vary from individual to individual and from community to community.

Myth (vs) Fact

Myth: Morality is morality. What is right is right, and what is wrong is wrong.

Fact: Most people agree that what is moral in one society may not be moral in another. Furthermore, what is considered moral in one situation may not be considered moral in another situation.

Myth: There is no systematic way in which to resolve ethical and moral issues. It is mostly a matter of intuition and subjective judgment.

Fact: Ethics is a system that uses ethical principles to determine the morality of a situation or decision. Ethical principles are valued according to many factors, including experience, religious teachings, cultural background, education, and family values.

Myth: In our diverse society, there are no commonly accepted ethical principles. Different groups have different values and different views of morality.

Fact: Although it is true that in a country with many different cultural groups living together there are many different views of morality, there are some ethical principles that we can all agree on. These include caring, respect for others, honesty, responsibility, and trustworthiness.

Myth: There are some situations about which there is no disagreement regarding morality. For example, there is no disagreement about HIV and AIDS, because AIDS is such a serious and deadly disease.

Fact: HIV and AIDS provide a good example of how complex moral decisions can be. For example, there is disagreement regarding whether condom advertisements should be allowed on television and whether needle-distribution programs for intravenous drug users should be developed.

major law concerning obscenity in the United States, prohibited the mailing of obscene or lewd material. The interpretation of what was obscene or lewd was left to the Postal Service. In 1957 the Supreme Court attempted to clarify the issue by ruling that sexuality-related material and obscene material were not one and the same. Rather, sexual material was ruled obscene (and therefore outside the protection of the First Amendment) only when sexual behavior was presented in a lewd and lascivious manner. But how was it to be determined whether some particular material was lewd or lascivious? The Supreme Court stated that the standard to be applied was whether the average person would judge it as such.

Further rulings between 1957 and 1968 (55 separate legal opinions in 13 obscenity cases) attempted to define obscenity more explicitly. As a result, the phrase "utterly without redeeming social value" was added to the definition. In 1973 the Court rejected its own "utterly without redeeming social value" criterion and defined the standards of obscenity that are currently in effect:

1. Whether the average person applying contemporary community standards would find that the work, taken as a whole, appeals to the prurient (lustful) interests

2. Whether the work depicts or describes, in a patently offensive way, sexual conduct specified by state law

3. Whether the work, taken as a whole, lacks serious literary, artistic, political, or scientific value.

Despite the history of legal activity, a consensus in the society as to the definition of obscenity has yet to be reached. With the advent of the Internet and the access it provides to sexually explicit material, the problem is exacerbated.

Rape

Although there is considerable debate about the psychological, sociological, and cultural causes of rape, the chief legal issue involves achieving consensus on a set of standards for enforcing the laws against rape. The legal definition of forcible rape is sexual intercourse against one's will, but because anyone might accuse another of rape, society has had to define acceptable evidence. Until recently a prosecutor had to prove that semen was present—on the woman's body or clothing—to gain a conviction of rape. However, many female victims do not have a medical exam after rape; others bathe or shower before being examined; and in many cases of true rape, the rapist fails to ejaculate. Because many rapists have been pronounced innocent because of a lack of such evidence, the presence of semen is no longer considered the sole evidence of forcible rape; bruises, the presence of a weapon, and even threats of force may now be accepted.

Defense attorneys have often focused on the victims, attempting to show that they were promiscuous and thus responsible for provoking sexual attacks. New laws reflect society's growing concern with protecting victims from unfair questioning, as well as with ensuring conviction when rape has actually occurred. These laws now prohibit questions regarding the victim's sexual experience during a rape trial. Thus the focus of the trial is on determining the guilt or innocence of the accused, not on the moral character of the victim.

Statutory Rape

Statutory rape is placed in a different legal category from forcible rape, and a situation ethicist might also put it in a different moral category. Statutory rape is sexual intercourse with a person below the legal age of consent, which varies from state to state. The statute is designed to protect children considered too immature to make sexual decisions for themselves. Even if boys or girls willingly participate in sexual intercourse,

Communication
DIMENSIONS

The Morality of Requesting a Variety of Sexual Behaviors

In some sexual relationships, one partner desires more variety in sexual activities than the other. For example, one partner may prefer anal sexual intercourse, and the other may object. Or one partner may be extremely excited by oral–genital sex, and the other may be turned off by it. One person may think of certain sexual activities as immoral, another as exciting. Too often, these conflicts result in anger and resentment, thereby interfering with other aspects of the relationship, not merely the sexual part. Consequently, partners should discuss differing sexual desires and resolve these issues. Fortunately, there are ways to do just that.

To begin, each person's thoughts and feelings should be expressed. A comment like "That's sick!" short-circuits any meaningful communication. The initial part of the conversation should be devoted to understanding the viewpoint of the other person, and that requires listening. There is time to express an opposing point of view, but not until one person has had the chance to be understood. Once one person has expressed his or her viewpoint, the other should. Refrain from arguing or disagreeing at this point. Merely listen.

Once both points of view have been aired, points of agreement should be identified. For example, both partners might agree that sex is a normal and desirable part of their relationship; that variety of sexual behaviors enhances the sexual relationship and thereby positively influences other aspects of their life together; that each cares about the other's feelings and sexual satisfaction; and that they want to make each other happy.

The part of communication regarding conflicts of ethics and morality that is most difficult is finding a compromise with which both persons are satisfied. Identifying areas of agreement provides a starting point in this process. Perhaps one partner is willing to try a particular sexual activity because he or she has identified a concern for making the other person happy. Perhaps the other is willing to forgo a particular sexual activity because it will make the other unhappy. The goal is to maintain the relationship as a stimulating one, not to engage in specific behaviors. The original focus on the behaviors is what is "wanted," whereas the real issue is the "need" for excitement and stimulation. That need can be met in ways that satisfy both partners with a little ingenuity and creativity.

Remember, though, no one should be forced, coerced, or manipulated to behave in any way that he or she considers immoral. That will result only in guilt, shame, or embarrassment and will not be healthy for the person or the relationship. If your partner is trying to manipulate you, the relationship is probably not worth saving.

---

their consent is ignored for legal purposes. And even if they appear to be of age or lie about their age, the laws still apply, with few exceptions. In some states the exception is that a child proved to be sexually promiscuous or a prostitute may be considered an adult.

Adultery

Adultery, or extramarital intercourse, is quite prevalent in the United States. Kinsey reported back in 1948 that more than one-third of the men in his study reported extramarital coitus; in 1953 he reported that half of the men and 26% of the women he studied had extramarital sexual intercourse by age 40 years. Many suspect that the incidence of extramarital coitus has increased since Kinsey's studies. However, Hicks and Leitenberg (2001) report that men are engaging in fewer instances of extramarital sexual intercourse. They report the incidence for men at 28%, similar to women (29%). Other researchers

Myth (vs) Fact

Myth: As long as two adults agree, any sexual activity in which they engage is legal, as long as it is done in private.

Fact: Not long ago, most states had sodomy laws that made certain sexual activities illegal even though they were consensual and performed by adults. These laws have since been declared unconstitutional.

have found the prevalence of adultery to be even lower, between 20% and 25% (Smith, 2006; Atkins, Baucom, & Jacobson, 2001). More recently, it has been reported that 22% of men and 14% of women have been adulterous at least once (Statistic Brain Research Institute, 2014). Even so, our concept of morality vis-à-vis marriage still leads us to sustain the laws against it. Adultery is frequently a legal ground for divorce. When adultery is the basis of divorce and custody of children is challenged in court, the adulterous partner often loses custody.

Polygamy

Two popular television programs have brought the practice of polygamy to the forefront. *Sister Wives*, a reality show broadcast on the TLC network, documented the life of a polygamist family living in Lehi, Utah. The family consisted of a husband living with his four wives and their 16 children. *Big Love*, another television show broadcast on HBO, was about a fictional fundamentalist Mormon family in Utah that also practiced polygamy.

Polygamy is when one man is married to more than one woman at the same time. The women know each other and are aware they are sharing one husband. Polygamy has been practiced in the United States over a long period of time, although currently it is illegal. Many Native American tribes practiced polygamy, as did some Scottish, Irish, and Welsh settlers. Some polygamous marriages also occurred in the southern United States shortly after the Civil War. Today, the most prominent polygamous group is the Fundamentalist Church of Jesus Christ of Latter-Day Saints (FLDS), a sect of the Mormon Church. FLDS members practice polygamy in arranged marriages that often, though not always, involve young girls with older men. FLDS members can be found primarily in Hildale, Utah, and Colorado City, Arizona. Other FLDS communities exist in Canada, Texas, and other areas of western North America.

In 2001, Tom Green, a fundamentalist Mormon, was convicted and sentenced to 5 years in prison for polygamy. He had five wives and 30 children, despite the fact that the Mormon Church and the state of Utah are formally against the practice of polygamy. One of Green's wives was only 13 years old when he first had intercourse with her, Green argued he was being singled out among an estimated 30,000 polygamists in the United States. Another publicized case occurred in 2008. Texas officials took 436 children into temporary legal custody after a 16-year-old girl called authorities claiming that she had been beaten and forced to become a wife of an adult man. The raid occurred at the YFZ Ranch, which is owned by the FLDS. The children ranged in age from infants to teenagers, including teenage mothers and pregnant teens.

Should men be able to decide how many wives they wish to have at one time? For that matter, should women also be able to decide to have more than one husband at the same time (autonomy/liberty)? Or is there a societal interest in preserving the current legal standard of one husband being married to only one wife at the same time (social

Although it is illegal for a typical person to photograph and publish nude photos of minors, many "artists" seem to have few problems getting away with it. Many bookstores sell photo albums that contain full nudity of clearly underage boys and girls, without prosecution. Is it possible to distinguish ethically or legally between nude photos of minors that are taken for the purpose of arousal from those that are taken as "art"?

utility)? Does polygamy do harm to those involved; husbands, wives, and children (nonmaleficence)? Do you believe the law should be changed, or vigorously enforced?

Divorce

Laws involving divorce have been reformed over the years. Originally marriage and divorce laws in the United States were based on Judeo-Christian ethical principles involving the sanctity of the family and of parenthood. These laws reinforced the idea that the family was an economic necessity, both for the individual and for the society. Consequently divorce was granted by law only if misbehavior was proved in court. In other words, one of the marriage partners had to be at fault by being adulterous, mentally

polygamy When one man is married to more than one woman.

Polygamist Tom Green with his "family."

Some people argue that no-fault divorce laws have led to more divorces (a bad thing); others say they have led to happier people (a good thing). Another way of looking at the prevalence of divorce—regardless of fault—is to argue that we should make marriage laws stricter, rather than making divorce laws looser. People would then have to work harder to get married, and those without a strong commitment to each other would be unlikely to follow through.

Alimony is money that a judge orders the partner who earns more to pay on the granting of a divorce to the partner who earns less or no money. As are other matters related to divorce, alimony is being reevaluated. Previously alimony was handled as punishment for divorce, and the husband was forced to make payments to his wife. Today judges are more likely to assess the particular circumstances in a case and award alimony to either the man or the woman, on the basis of their respective resources and contributions to the marriage.

or physically cruel, and so on. When the number of divorces increased, and it became a common belief that people wishing to be free of each other should not be forced to remain married, many states adopted **no-fault divorce**. No-fault divorce statutes allow courts to dissolve marriages when no fault is cited and both partners agree to end the marriage.

no-fault divorce The granting of divorce without either partner's proving the other was the cause of the marriage's failure.

alimony Money a divorced person is ordered by the courts to pay regularly to his or her ex-spouse.

Exploring the Dimensions of Human Sexuality

At the center of many ethical and moral dilemmas are cultural underpinnings—especially religious and political beliefs.

However, sometimes those cultural underpinnings clash. Consider the woman who unexpectedly finds herself pregnant. Raised as a member of the Roman Catholic religion—with its antiabortion doctrine—the woman has also been raised as a feminist, with a pro-choice doctrine. Further, consider the rights of her partner, who may have a different set of sociocultural doctrines to rely on for making moral decisions.

On a more personal level, it is important to make moral decisions regarding sexual relationships before becoming sexually involved. During a state of sexual arousal and response, it is often hard to put moral feelings ahead of intense physiological feelings.

States may pass specific laws dealing with sexuality; however, such laws must not conflict with federal laws and may be challenged for their constitutionality.

Biological Factors

- Alcohol and drugs can blur decision-making ability.

Sociocultural Factors

- Religions often establish codes of ethics, which state for members beliefs on matters including abortion, premarital sexual activity, extramarital sexual activity, same-gender sexual relations, and nonintercourse sexual activities.
- Political beliefs often suggest ethical standards. Although there are exceptions, in Democrats and feminists generally take a pro-choice stance (not always), and Republicans and fundamentalist Christians take an antiabortion stance. Laws in the United States ban discrimination based on race, religion, gender, age, and sexual orientation for public organizations, but private organizations can still discriminate. In many Islamic countries, adultery is illegal—even punishable by death. Gender selection through female infanticide or amniocentesis coupled with abortion is tolerated in some countries.

Psychological Factors

- During the state of sexual arousal and response, it is often hard to make moral judgments that conflict with intense physiological feelings.

Summary

- Ethics is a system on which we base our moral decisions. Ethical principles provide guidelines for abstract questions, not solutions to individual cases.

- When ethical principles clash, we have an ethical dilemma. Ethical dilemmas are resolved by placing a value on the competing ethical principles, with the principle carrying the highest value being the one that guides the decision.

- Rule ethics uses ethical principles to guide decisions in all situations. Situation ethics is based on the premise that all situations are unique and, therefore, there are no ethical principles that can be used the same way to guide all moral decision.

- If a decision or action is moral, it is *good* or *right*. If a decision is immoral, it is *bad* or *wrong*.

- Laws represent the encoding of generally accepted societal views of morality. Laws regarding sexual behavior develop from a general consensus of specific ethical principles, values, and judgments about behavior. When laws are not representative of societal views of morality, they are not followed and often need to be changed.

- Sexual morality is a consideration in such sexually related areas as sexually transmitted infections, sexual activity among unmarried persons, emergency contraception, abortion, amniocentesis, fetal tissue implantation, stem cell research, prostitution, in vitro fertilization, genetic engineering, sexting, and sexual responsibility to a partner.

- Among laws pertaining to sexual behavior are those regarding obscenity and pornography, rape, statutory rape, marriage, polygamy, adultery, and divorce.

Discussion Questions

1. Differentiate between ethics and morals. Apply the ethical principles of nonmaleficence, beneficence, autonomy/liberty, justice/fairness, and social utility to issues in human sexuality.

2. Discuss commonly accepted ethical principles and ways they can be applied in situations involving sexual behavior.

3. Which types of sexual behavior are regulated by laws? What is the basis of those laws?

Application Questions

Reread the chapter-opening story and answer the following questions.

1. Consider the ethical principles of nonmaleficence, beneficence, autonomy/liberty, justice/fairness, and social utility as they relate to the opening story. Which of the ethical principles did Wendy Weaver and the Nebo school district follow? Then explain how the case might have been affected if Weaver and the school district had followed other principles.

2. Was it ethical for Weaver to disclose her sexual orientation to a minor student? Should Weaver have considered the student's possible religious (70% of Utah residents are Mormon) objections to homosexuality before answering?

Critical Thinking Questions

1. Is practicing safer sex an ethical issue or a legal issue? For example, is it unethical not to have STI and HIV tests before starting a new relationship? Can this become a legal issue?

2. An unmarried woman who has been in a steady sexual relationship for 5 months discovers she is pregnant. Is it ethical, moral, or legal for the male to decide whether the female should have the child and keep it, give the child up for adoption, or have an abortion? What if the couple breaks up before she finds out she is pregnant? What rights, if any, does the man have in relation to the baby he helped create?

3. The ethics and morality of creating (or re-creating) life sometimes reflect technological innovations of the times. As the age of electricity dawned in the 1800s, Mary Shelley's *Frankenstein* (1818) provoked ethical and moral concerns about the use of electricity. Today, the use of electricity in the defibrillator to save a heart attack patient is accepted as ethical, moral, and legal. In fact, it would be considered unethical, immoral, and illegal not to use a defibrillator when a life could be saved. During our current age of genetic research (beginning with the 1950s discovery of DNA), Michael Crichton's *Jurassic Park* provoked similar concerns about the misuse of genetic engineering. However, even as you read this question, new technological applications are being devised that can and will save lives. Do you think people in 200 years will look back at *Jurassic Park* and wonder why we feared genetic research?

The ability to select the gender of a child has for years been the source of ethical debate. In some countries, cultures approve of female infanticide or amniocentesis coupled with abortion. However, the cultural morals of the United States do not favor such methods.

Would the current U.S. culture accept a scientifically based method of gender selection? The Genetics and IVF Institute (Fairfax, Virginia) announced in September 1998 that it had found a way to separate male and female sperm cells. Using specialized technology, its personnel are able to sort out 85% of X-bearing sperm (females) and 65% of Y-bearing sperm (males). Using artificial insemination, the Institute can give parents potential for gender selection, in proportion to the sperm-sorting abilities.

The technique has been used for some time on animals, which are easier to sort by gender. Testing with humans began in 1998. Human applications include preventing the birth of children with rare genetic sex-linked diseases (such as X-linked hydrocephalus) or "balancing" families with an opposite-sex sibling. The Institute is not planning to market the sorting procedure to first-time parents who simply have a dream of a specific-gender child.

Do you think that sperm-sorting technology is ethically acceptable in the case of raising farm animals? How about in the name of protecting endangered species from extinction?

As far as human applications are concerned, do you find it ethical to use sperm sorting to prevent the birth of a child who has a genetic sex-linked disease? How about to have an additional child to provide needed bone marrow for transplantion to a current child? Finally, is it ethical to use sperm sorting to have a third or fourth child of the opposite gender?

Determining Your Ethical Compass
Several ethical dilemmas are presented in this activity to help you determine which ethical principles you use to guide your behavior and your view of morality. Choose the one option for each dilemma that best represents your views, even though you might agree with more than one.

1. Juan and Maria decide to live together and share a sexual relationship. They are thinking that they may marry in the future, but not anytime soon.

   a. Juan and Maria should not move in together because we know that when men and women live together, they are not equals. Women tend to take on more of the household chores than men.

   b. Juan and Maria should be free to decide what is best for them.

   c. Juan and Maria should not live together because Maria will suffer if she does not eventually marry Juan. She will be perceived as immoral by her family and her community.

   d. No good will come of Juan and Maria's living together. In fact, it might harm society by encouraging sexual relations between people who are not married to each other.

2. Evan and Rhonda place their 2-year-old son in child care so they can both work outside the home.

   a. This is unfair because Evan and Rhonda are placing their interests above the welfare of their son.

   b. Each couple should be able to decide what is best for their family unit.

   c. Without the direct and extensive contact with one of his parents, Evan and Rhonda's son will not grow and develop to his potential.

   d. Society will suffer if this becomes a common practice because of the emotional cost and health effects that the community will eventually have to absorb.

3. Although Kevin and Latisha have a sexual relationship, Kevin has not disclosed to Latisha that he has herpes. Kevin argues that their relationship is not "serious" and, therefore, he should not have to divulge his STI to Latisha. Furthermore, Kevin states, he refrains from having intercourse with Latisha when he has noticeable sores.

   a. Because Kevin knows about his STI and Latisha does not, Kevin is treating Latisha unfairly. He has more information than she, and that is not right.

   b. Kevin has a right to decide to whom information about his health is released, as well as the nature of that information.

   c. Lacking knowledge of Kevin's herpes, Latisha is likely to engage in behavior that can cause her harm.

   d. If Kevin continues to withhold information about his health and infects other sexual partners, society will suffer, health premiums will be raised for the rest of us, and hospital and medical staff resources may have to be redirected from other health issues.

4. Frankie and Lynn had been married for 10 years when Frankie began a sexual relationship with his coworker Flo.

a. It is not fair that Frankie engages in sex outside his marriage whereas Lynn refrains because of her vows of fidelity. If Frankie engages in extramarital sex, why should Lynn not have affairs as well?

b. Frankie may have many reasons for deciding to have a sexual relationship with Flo. He is an adult and should be free to decide whether the risk outweighs the benefits he derives from the relationship with Flo.

c. If Lynn ever found out she would be devastated, and their marriage might end. If they have children, even more harm would be done.

d. Society cannot allow extramarital affairs to be unpunished; otherwise, we would have chaos, unstable families, and dysfunctional children growing into dysfunctional adults.

5. Rose and Amber are lovers who are often seen by their neighbors holding hands as they enter their apartment building. Several of the more conservative tenants have complained about being "confronted by two lesbians flaunting their relationship to everyone else."

a. It is not fair that heterosexual tenants can hold hands but gay couples are expected to refrain from doing so.

b. Rose and Amber should be able to do whatever they choose. It is a free world. The other residents are free to look away.

c. Raising this issue with Rose and Amber might make them self-conscious and lead to their questioning whether they are welcome in that apartment building. Furthermore, the strain of this confrontation might lead to stress that could harm their health.

d. It is harmful to young children, who are impressionable and in the process of developing their own sexual orientation, to see outwardly gay couples' being accepted by society. For the good of the total society, gay couples should be more discreet.

If you found yourself selecting choice (a) more often than the other choices, you are predominantly guided by the ethical principle of *justice*, believing people ought to be treated fairly. If you selected choice (b) over the others, you are guided by *autonomy*, believing people ought to be free to make their own choices without interference from others. However, if you selected choice (c) most often, you are guided by the ethical principle of nonmaleficence, believing no harm ought to be done, and, when it is, the decision is immoral. And, if you found yourself most often selecting choice (d), you are guided by *social utility*, believing a decision needs to be considered in terms of the benefit or harm to society.

Suggested Readings

Ali, K. *Sexual ethics in Islam*. London, UK: Oneworld Publications, 2011.

Buss, M. J., & Stipe, N. M. *Good sex: A Christian and a pagan discuss sexual ethics*. Eugene, OR: Wipf and Stock, 2014.

Ellison, M. M. *Making love just*. Kitchener, ON: Fortress Press, 2012.

Freedman, E. B. *Redefining rape*. Cambridge, MA: Harvard University Press, 2013.

MacKinnon, B., & Fiala, A. *Ethics: Theory and contemporary issues*. Independence, KY: Cengage Learning, 2014.

May, W., Boyle, J., & Lawler, R. *Catholic sexual ethics: A summary, explanation, & defense* (3rd ed.). Huntington, IN: Our Sunday Visitor, 2011.

Panza, C., & Potthast, A. *Ethics For Dummies*. Indianapolis, IN: For Dummies, 2010.

Greenberg, J. *The code of ethics for the health education profession: A case study book*. Boston: Jones and Bartlett, 2001.

Piderit, J. *Sexual morality: A natural law approach to intimate relationships*. Cary, NC: Oxford University Press, 2011.

Salzman, T. A., & Lawler, M. G. *Sexual ethics: A theological introduction*. Washington, DC: Georgetown University Press, 2012.

Teutsch, D. A. *Family and sexual ethics (guide to Jewish practice)*. Wyncote, PA: Reconstructionist Rabbinical College Press, 2010.

Twomey, V. *Moral theology after Humanae Vitae: Fundamental issues in moral theory and sexual ethics*. Dublin, Ireland: Four Courts, 2010.

West, I. *Transforming citizenships: Transgender articulations of the law (sexual cultures)*. New York: NYU Press, 2013.

Web Resources

The Feminist Sexual Ethics Project
www.brandeis.edu/projects/fse

Explores sexual ethics within Judaism, Christianity, and Islam, and presents how the toleration of slavery in the early teachings of these religions affects the lives of women today. Among the links are those dealing with Jewish sexual ethics, Christian sexual ethics, and Muslim sexual ethics.

United Nations High Commissioner for Human Rights (UNHCHR)

www.ohchr.org/EN/Pages/WelcomePage.aspx

The Office of the High Commissioner for Human Rights (OHCHR) is a department of the United Nations Secretariat. It is mandated to promote and protect the enjoyment and full realization, by all people, of all rights established in the Charter of the United Nations and in international human rights laws and treaties. The mandate includes preventing human rights violations, securing respect for all human rights, promoting international cooperation to protect human rights, coordinating related activities throughout the United Nations, and strengthening and streamlining the United Nations system in the field of human rights. Among these rights are those that pertain to sexual issues—for example, female clitoral mutilation.

Sexual Ethics in Psychology

www.rotten.com/library/sex/sexual-ethics-in-psychology

Presents case studies to discuss the American Psychological Association's code of ethics that governs the interaction between therapists and patients. The sexual interaction between clinician and patient is emphasized.

Human Rights Campaign

www.hrc.org

The Human Rights Campaign is America's largest civil rights organization working to achieve gay, lesbian, bisexual, and transgender (GLBT) equality. HRC seeks to improve the lives of GLBT Americans by advocating for equal rights and benefits in the workplace, ensuring families are treated equally under the law, and increasing public support among all Americans through innovative advocacy, education, and outreach programs. The website includes links to legislation, laws, work life, religion and faith, employment opportunities, and other subjects.

Sexual Ethics in Islam and in the Western World

www.al-islam.org/sexualethics/

Offers chapters from a book describing sexual ethics as it relates to Islam. Chapters explore traditional sexual ethics, sexual ethics as conceived by modern thinkers; proposed new sexual freedom; a critical examination of the theoretical basis of the proposed new sexual freedom; the basic need for humane conditioning of natural instincts and desires; and love, sexual discipline, and chastity.

References

Achenbach, J. Splice of life. *The Washington Post Magazine* (November 29, 1998), 12–19, 27–30.

Associated Press. Lesbian can resume coaching, judge rules. *Washington Post* (November 27, 1998), A12.

Atkins, D. C., Baucom, D. H., & Jacobson, N. S. Understanding infidelity: Correlates in a national random sample. *Journal of Family Psychology, 15* (2001), 735–749.

Catholic Church. *Encyclical of Pope Paul VI, humanae vitae, on the regulation of birth, and Pope Paul VI's credo of the people of God.* Glen Rock, NJ: Paulist Press, 1968.

Drouin, M., & Landgraff, C. Texting, sexting, and attachment in college students' romantic relationships. *Computers in Human Behavior, 28* (2012), 444–449.

Drouin, M., Tobin, E., & Wygant, K. "Love the way you lie": Sexting deception in romantic relationships. *Computers in Human Behavior, 35* (2014), 542–547.

Ellis, A. Healthy and disturbed reasons for having extramarital relations, in *Encounter with family realities*, Powers, E. A. & Lees, M.-W., eds. St. Paul, MN: West, 1977, 374–375.

Hicks, T., & Leitenberg, H. Sexual fantasies about one's partner versus someone else: Gender differences in incidence and frequency. *Journal of Sex Research, 38* (2001), 43–50.

Kaufman, M. Morning-after pill study contradicts claim by foes: Easy access did not lead to riskier behavior. *Washington Post* (January 5, 2005), p. A09.

Kenney, J. W., Reinholtz, C., & Angellini, P. J. Ethnic differences in childhood and adolescent sexual abuse and teenage pregnancy. *Journal of Adolescent Health 21, 1* (1997), 3–10.

Matte, C. What is sexting and why is it a problem? *About Parenting*, 2015. Available: http://familyinternet.about.com/od/computingsafetyprivacy/a/sexting_what.htm.

National Campaign to Prevent Teen and Unplanned Pregnancy. *Sex and tech: Results from a survey of teens and young adults.* Washington, DC: National Campaign to Prevent Teen and Unplanned Pregnancy, 2008.

National Institutes of Health Resource for Stem Cell Research. Stem cell information: Stem cell basics. 2011. Available: http://stemcells.nih.gov/info/basics5asp.

Peskin, M. F., Markham, C. M., Addy, R. C., Shegog, R., Theil, M., & Tortolero, S. R. Prevalence and patterns of sexting among ethnic minority urban high school students. *Cyberpsychology, Behavior, and Social Networking, 16* (2013), 454–459.

Smith, T. W. American sexual behavior: Trends, socio-demographic differences, and risk behavior. GSS Topical Report no. 25. Chicago, IL: National Opinion Research Center, University of Chicago; 2006.

Statistic Brain Research Institute. *Infidelity statistics*, 2014. Available: http://www.statisticbrain.com/infidelity-statistics/.

Stem cell research: What Americans think. *Parade* (July 10, 2005), p. 5.

Epilogue: Taking Responsibility for Your Sexual Health

THE SEXUAL FUTURE

It was a morning of unmatched brilliance; the sun shone brightly, the robins were singing, and the spring air was morning fresh. It was a typical morning in the year 2099 for Todd and his housemates Keri, Karen, and Jerry.

Excuse me. I am being impolite. I forgot that you were from another time. I should have introduced you to our way of life before mentioning my friends. Of course we have made lots of technological advances, as you will soon see. But given what was going on in your day, you could probably see that coming, even if you could not foresee the form. Beyond that, however, we have changed our attitudes and values, our ways of doing work, and our social, sexual, and family relationships. For example, in 2099 we are altogether more respectful of individual differences than you were in your time. Questions of morality do not dominate our way of life as they did yours, and much ignorance has been dispelled. Is it a good or bad time, you ask? Let me describe our ways to you and you can answer for yourself.

Keri, Karen, Jerry, and Todd range in age from 21 to 41 years, but they are not rushing off to work today. In fact they never rush off to work, because they all work at home. Most people do. It is the computer and all the other technological and communication advances, you see. Of course, as you did in the early part of this century, we all have computers, smartphones, and tablets at home, and we use them for work and play, as well as for banking, shopping, and communicating with one another over long and short distances. We play games on them and can program our devices to play music for us. The difference between our time and yours, however, is that we have perfected computers such that no one needs to travel anywhere. Just about everyone works from home, shops from home, and we even date and experience virtual sex from home. Our physicians use them to diagnose illnesses and prescribe medication. (Wait until you hear about the medication we have!) Anyway, why do you think the morning air is so fresh? No cars to pollute it! In fact, there is very little transportation as you knew it. We have little need to go anywhere. Our computers meet most of our needs. Life really is easy.

Family life, as you can imagine, is also quite different from home life as you knew it. Long ago we realized that marriage was archaic—it just did not make sense in a rapidly changing society to expect two people to live together forever. People change as the society changes, but not all marriage partners change at the same pace. Once we understood this, we changed our laws to allow for a number of different marriage styles. The styles are not really new, but the legal and social ease of choosing and changing *is*. For example, we have repeating monogamous marriages (RMMs), wherein one maintains only one partner at a time but, when the marriage becomes stale, one can dissolve the marriage easily and marry another partner. Some people marry 10 or more times in this manner. Polygamy (one person married to several people at the same time) is also common, as are multiple marriage partners (MMPs). MMPs allow several males to share several female marriage partners, and vice versa.

In spite of all our attempts to adapt marriage to our society, however, most people never marry. Rather they establish informal arrangements of convenience. Some live together, some raise children together (their own or those of others), and some just share particular events together. I, for example, have an informal arrangement with Betty for sexual play, with Tina for computer game play, and with Tasha for sharing of thoughts and important feelings.

By the way, we laugh when we hear stories of your struggle with sexual equality. In 2099 we cannot imagine that males would be treated differently from females. I guess our attitude evolves partly because the need for physical strength continued to decrease, just as it was in your day, and that eliminated the male's biological advantage. You see, robots do all our strenuous work, and competitive sports (other than computer games) have long since been outlawed. They were thought to contribute to warlike attitudes that, with the existence of weapons that could destroy the world, were deemed intolerable. But really that only partly explains our sexual equality. We realize that people who are discriminated against eventually revolt. It is only a matter of time—treat a group unfairly and it eventually rebels, disturbing the peace. Furthermore, our scientists have discovered treatments that allow everyone, male and female, to feel however they wish and to acquire almost any trait they want or need. Because people can change themselves nearly at will, how could we believe any one or any group to be inferior?

Scientists have made other important advances, too. Most diseases are curable now—your dreaded cancer and heart diseases among them. But perhaps the single most significant advance has been the discovery of K25W. Added to our water supply by our leaders (all of whom are scientists rather than politicians), K25W is a chemical that prepares the mind to receive and accept subliminal messages.

What are subliminal messages, you ask? Just a little trick of the media trade. The subliminal messages are verbal messages delivered so quickly and at such a low volume that those who receive them are not even aware that messages have been conveyed. Subliminal messages can be visual, too, images relayed so quickly along with other broadcast material that viewers remain unaware of them. Your society experimented with a crude form of subliminal messages when, for instance, voices were hidden beneath the pleasant music that department store customers heard while shopping reminding customers to be polite and not to shoplift. But you did not have K25W in your water! We use subliminal messages to plant many ideas, one of which is sexual equality, in the minds of our citizens.

The one problem we are still wrestling with is how to solve the discontent of our elderly. Having eradicated many of the diseases that plagued you, plus eliminating traffic accidents, we have lengthened the life span of most people, and so the size of our elderly population has grown enormously. By the way, we do not think of 70-year-olds as elderly; people live now to the ages of 120, 130, even 140 years. Mind you, our old people are quite happy (remember K25W) and able to care for themselves (remember our medications). Still, they tell stories of their past, and young people wonder whether our society is really better than the one the old folks recall. There is much ambivalence in those recollections. The old ones speak of illness, on the one hand, and the joy of life, on the other hand; of cruelty and war, on the one hand, and the Peace Corps, on the other hand; of nursing homes, on the one hand, and growing old with families to care for you, on the other hand. No small wonder the younger ones are confused. But our scientists are working on this issue even as we speak. Before long it will be clear to all that our new society is developing in the right direction. After all, do we not live longer? Have we not eliminated sexual bias? Can we not take a pill and acquire just about any trait we want?

Well, that gives you a quick overview of some major areas of our life. Now let me tell you about my friends to show you examples of how some personal relationships work.

Todd is an Edibilist. His job relates to developing new strains of foods and nutrients. Because many of our citizens live to be 130 years old, world population has skyrocketed, and all the life-sustaining resources (food, energy, oxygen) are at a premium. Todd is married to Jerry (homosexual marriage is not uncommon among us, because people do not marry primarily to have babies). His recreational needs are met by Keri and his intellectual needs by Karen. Jerry is also Karen's sexual mate. As a matter of fact, they had a scare recently. No, not an unwanted pregnancy. That is no longer a problem. We have an enormous range of effective contraceptives (male contraceptives that prevent sperm development or immobilize sperm and female contraceptives are taken only once a year).

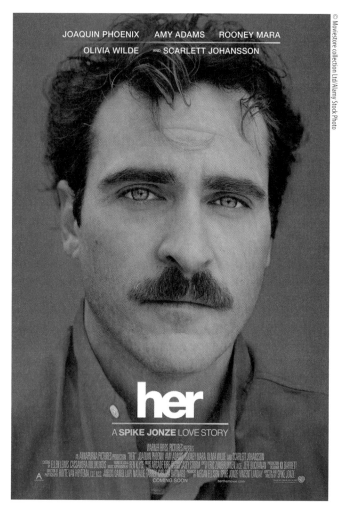

In the Academy Award–nominated film *Her*, starring Joaquin Phoenix and Scarlett Johansson, a man develops a love relationship with an advanced computerized operating system he purchased to run his life. He finds it easier to relate to this "unreal" woman than to the other "real" women he encounters in his life. What are the missing dimensions of sexuality in this scenario? Which elements of this plot are farfetched and which elements can be anticipated as futuristic possibilities?

Furthermore, someone who misuses reproductive privileges—by becoming pregnant without written approval from the Population and Parenthood Screening Bureau—is liable to be sterilized by court order. As you can imagine, population control is a major concern, and reproductive control is therefore a governmental issue. At least we have no need for abortions!

No, Jerry and Karen's problem pertained not to pregnancy but to sexual dysfunction. We have eliminated the kinds of sexual dysfunction you were familiar with. Pills are available that eliminate inhibitions to sexual response. They can also lubricate vaginas, make penises erect, and even increase sexual desire. Jerry and Karen's problem arose when she popped a "desire" pill and Jerry did not want

to take his. As yet it is not a matter of policy to add these chemicals to the water supply, as we do with K25W, to make people's sexual desires compatible. The controversy is ongoing as to whether controlling sexual desire should be left to individual discretion. At present the *dysfunction of the sexual union*, the term for our form of sexual dysfunction, is subject to the whims of the sexual partners. Opponents of adding desire chemicals to the water supply suggest that if one person drank a glass of water, felt a rush of desire, and could not find his or her partner, hysteria, frustration, violence, or a change of partner could ensue. Well, Jerry finally took his "desire" pill and the dysfunction was eliminated. It is my guess that if this incompatibility recurs, they will be looking for new mates.

Speaking of new mates, Keri is presently looking for one. Her old mate is raising her child and Keri would like a new mate with a drastically different endowment than the last. Keri's child was a dream come true, but only after some medical intervention. The Population and Parenthood Screening Bureau tested Keri both physiologically and psychologically to determine her qualifications for parenthood and approved her application. She chose John as the father because of his blond hair, blue eyes, impressive height, and high intelligence. Several months after conception, the amniotic fluid tests revealed that the fetus was male and had brown eyes and a cleft palate—not at all like John. You can imagine how quickly Keri ordered a genetic manipulation (GM)! When her daughter was born with blue eyes and devoid of any defects, Keri was elated and decided to keep her.

Keri's friend Josie is an interesting case. In fact, her situation would make a good riddle for you: How can someone be both the biological mother and the biological father of the same child? Well, Josie was not always Josie; she was once Joseph! Joseph was born a male and as a young adult deposited sperm in one of our neighborhood sperm banks. Joseph then decided that his maleness was unsuited to his disposition (unfortunately, his mother had not ordered a GM but had let nature take its course), and he had a sex-change operation. Joseph's male genitals were surgically removed and replaced with two ovaries, two fallopian tubes, a uterus, and a vagina. Once recuperated, Joseph, now Josie, used the deposited sperm to fertilize the ovum during her ovulation period. Hence when the baby was born, its mother and father were one and the same.

But enough of unusual stories. Josie's situation is unique. Keri's case is more common. Perhaps she can soon choose another accurately genetically analyzed mate to make the kind of child she wants. If not, the GM people should be able to help, although, because

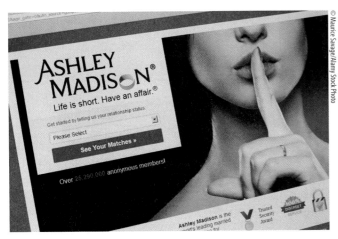

Ashley Madison is an online dating and social networking service marketed to people who are already in a relationship but want to meet other people for sex. Ashley Madison's slogan is "Life is short. Have an affair." A similar website, IllicitEncounter.com, is an online dating service in the United Kingdom for married people and has a reported 900,000 subscribers. What does the popularity of these websites say about future sexual and marital relationships? Is the availability of these websites a positive sign for our future or a symbol of impending catastrophe?

they are in such demand, we encourage our citizens to do their genetic planning as much beforehand as possible (even though, as Keri's case indicates, this may result in something short of perfection).

By the way, the birthing process has changed much since your time. In 2099 women neither experience pain nor use unnatural chemicals during the delivery of babies. Instead we use endorphins. These substances were discovered more than a century ago but were not put to much use right away. Maybe you remember that endorphins are chemicals naturally produced by the human body that decrease pain and are related to relaxation. Since their discovery in the human brain, we have learned how to produce them synthetically. We administer these synthetic endorphins during childbirth (which, by the way, occurs in people's homes rather than in birthing factories—hospitals, I think you called them). Thus the birth of a baby involves nothing but joy—more joy than we have been able to develop with our medications.

For women too busy to carry the unborn for the 6 months required (we sped up the gestation process for convenience), surrogate mothers are available to do the job. A surrogate receives the fertilized ovum in her uterus and goes through the birth process as usual. The baby is then presented to the original parents and the surrogate is paid according to the birth weight and health of the baby (consequently surrogates do not smoke cigarettes, drink alcohol, or use drugs, and they monitor their nutrition carefully). Other options are available for parents of lesser

financial means—animal uteruses serve as surrogate fetal development sites, as does the womb simulator (a machine in which a fetal development is maintained). These options allow the original mother to continue her usual routine unimpeded by pregnancy. However, the price she pays for this convenience is losing the joy of birthing. Moreover, a certain detachment often characterizes the mother–child relationship in such cases.

As you could probably guess, infertility does not exist today. We have so many ways of fertilizing ova and so many ways of organizing embryo and fetal development that our only problem is in restricting birth to a number that does not draw too heavily upon our society's resources.

Before you leave us, take with you the knowledge that sexual infections need not exist—it does not for us. As you can gather, I am sure, we are quite active sexually. And yet we managed to eliminate sexually transmitted infections by the year 2047. We finally found the link among all the causative agents of STIs, including AIDS. We termed this link the *Syphgon factor*, after syphilis and gonorrhea, although a more appropriate name might be *basic biological matter–thwarting factor*. Soon after the link was found, a vaccine was developed to immunize people against STIs. Originally injected into the bloodstream, this chemical is now in pill form and is designed to dissolve under the tongue. Regarding cancer—breast, uterine, vaginal, testicular, and others—we have been able to teach people, using no medication, to control the flow of T lymphocytes to the cancerous area, thereby eliminating the cancer. Of course, to allow the technique to work, early detection is imperative; the required monthly screening (consisting only of passing through a sensitive doorway similar to that used by your generation to screen airline passengers) serves this purpose. Cancer has virtually been eliminated.

What? You want to know how we arrive at ethical and moral decisions? I am afraid you can only get into trouble asking these questions. Do you not remember the trouble they caused in your time? We leave ethical issues to our leaders. You ask why our leaders are scientists and not ethicists, philosophers, clergy, psychologists, or sociologists? Well, would you have nonscientists leading this highly technical society? We have to trust our leaders to do what is best for us.

To be honest, though, the questions you ask trouble me, too. For us, however, the opportunity to make some other choices has passed. Our society is what it is. It is, you might say, a snowball rolling downhill picking up more and more snow. But take a look at your time. Are not the seeds of our society already planted? Perhaps you still have the chance to nurture the humanizing aspects of your society and to prevent its dehumanizing aspects from developing and taking over your future.

Commentary

Interestingly, the scenario you just read was written in the mid-1980s to promote discussion about the future and dimensions of sexuality (Greenberg & Bruess, 1986). As we reread this in preparation for its inclusion in this book, it struck us just how on target our predictions were. It made us think that we should be advising people on which stocks to invest in. Let us take a closer look at the future we projected two decades ago, at the characteristics of that future that already have come to pass and those that have not.

Social Dimensions

We described the year 2099 as one in which fewer people left their home and family to travel to work. Rather, they worked from home with the help of new technologies. We do not have to wait for 2099 for that to occur; it is already happening today. With the advent of the computer, smartphones, tablets, and telecommunications capabilities, more people are "telecommuting" than ever before. As in the scenario, more and more people are shopping, banking, and communicating from home. If you want a book, you need only go to the website of Amazon.com or Barnes and Noble. If you want to switch money from one bank account to another, you can hit a few keys on your home computer or a few numbers on your smartphone and the transfer is completed. And, if you want to communicate with someone, you can do so by email, instant messaging, or iPhones and Androids. The result should be more time for the family and for people about whom we care. However, this does not seem to be a social benefit we have as yet derived from technological advances. Too many people spend too much time at their computers or on their smartphones, checking out Internet sites, receiving and sending email messages, or playing computer games.

Physical Dimensions

We also guessed right about the ability of physicians to use computers to treat patients better. Today, physicians can call on experts from afar, using computers and telecommunications to read X rays, computed tomography (CT) scans, and magnetic resonance imaging (MRI) results and make a diagnosis that a local physician may be incapable of making.

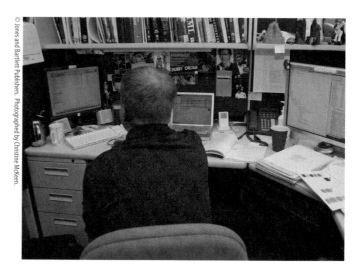

Many people telecommute, working from their homes with new technology. With decreased human contact, will our society change? For the better or for the worse?

Robots are even conducting surgeries managed from afar. This technology has tremendous potential for the diagnosis and treatment of sexually transmitted infections and other sexual illnesses.

In 2099, sexual dysfunction is not one of those matters about which citizens are concerned; they have a "desire pill." In a way, this is not much different from today's Viagra and Cialis and other drugs that treat sexual dysfunctions. In addition, microsurgical techniques are available to alleviate some sexual dysfunctional problems.

However, in 2099 the reason the "desire pill" is not added to the water supply is that a person who took a drink and experienced sexual desire might form a "sexual union" with a stranger who happened to be nearby and available. Today, we have a different variable serving as a barrier to "haphazard" sexual unions: HIV and AIDS. The fear of contracting HIV has led to a decrease in casual sex and an increase in condom use when sexual activity does take place. Still, research to develop an HIV and AIDS vaccine, if successful, might once again lead to a more cavalier attitude toward sex and a reemergence of the sexually free attitude of the 1960s. And yet, many Americans and others around the world are not waiting for a vaccine. Too many refuse to adopt responsible sexual behavior and engage in safer-sex practices.

Marital Dimensions

In the year 2099, there is a new form of marriage—repeating monogamous marriage (RMM). Today, with the divorce and remarriage rates as they are, we have a de facto RMM system. We have even

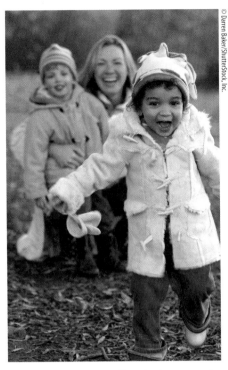

Blended families, as well as the large number of international adoptions, are having a dramatic effect on the families in the 21st century.

Some countries value male babies for their ability to support the family. This has resulted in infanticide in the form of female babies being aborted. How do you imagine females feel in such societies?

developed a name for the convoluted family structure possible when remarriage occurs (possibly several times for the same parent): *blended families*. As of 2009, gay and lesbian marriages have been legalized in most states and in 2015 the Supreme Court ruled that gay marriage is constitutional. However, we have not institutionalized polygamy as was described in the scenario. We still believe in the fidelity of one marital partner to the other, although some might argue that the prevalence of extramarital sex provides evidence of a trend in the opposite direction. And today, as in the scenario, it is common for people to live together and not be married to each other. Young couples move in together to determine whether a long-term relationship is feasible for them. In many states, gay couples live together as unmarried, in the eyes of the law at least, because legislators in many states have proscribed gay marriage. And elders cohabit because our society reinforces that arrangement through our tax codes and social welfare programs. Many Americans choose to remain unmarried, and those who do marry do so at a later age.

Gender Dimensions

We have discussed gender dimensions of sexuality throughout this book, and in 2099 attention is paid to this issue as well: Gender equality is a reality. In present-day society we have made great strides toward gender equality. It is no longer unusual for a female to be a physician or a lawyer. It is no longer unusual for a male to assume such household chores as cooking, cleaning, and child rearing. And yet, women are still paid less than men even when they do the same job; also, although men do more household chores when they and their spouses work full-time outside the home, women still assume a disproportionate share. And female genital mutilation is still practiced in many parts of the world. We have yet to discover a way to remedy the disparity in the way we treat our females and males in a manner that is best for women, men, children, and the rest of society, as they did in 2099 with the magical K25W. Still, we are headed in the right direction; the trend is toward greater gender equality and fairness. We hope that we will not have to wait until 2099 to see their full development.

Pregnancy and Childbearing Dimensions

In 2099, there are no unintended pregnancies. That is certainly not where we are today. More than half of all pregnancies in the United States are unintended, and our teenage pregnancy rate is one of the highest among developed countries. As in 2099, we have a wide range of effective contraceptives. The difference is that too few Americans use them or use them irregularly or incorrectly. That leads to a greater number of unwanted births, abortions, and adoptions than would otherwise be the case.

Perhaps our descendants in 2099 have the right idea with the Population and Parenthood Screening

Bureau. Today, we have too many children who are abused and neglected. We have too many children who are taken from their birth parents and placed in foster care with the intent of having them adopted, although many never do get a stable family and remain in the foster care system until they become of emancipated age. Perhaps we need to pay as much attention to enhancing parenting skills as our descendants do in 2099.

One area in which we do not have to wait for 2099 is that of genetic manipulation. With medical scientific advances, it is possible to perform surgery on fetuses in the womb to remedy structural abnormalities. Soon we will be able to apply different genes to influence eye color, intelligence, or other traits. Researchers have already isolated stem cells from embryonic tissue that can eventually be used to grow human replacement parts for transplantation. People wonder, if Dolly the sheep has been cloned, will humans eventually be cloned? The ethical implications of rapidly developing scientific advances have outstripped our society's ability to develop laws that will assure that technology will be used to enhance our culture rather than diminish it.

Want a boy baby? No need to engage in abortion or infanticide, as in some countries. Just use sperm-separation techniques to improve the odds. No, this is not part of the 2099 scenario. This is occurring today. Want a child who is likely to be an athlete or a musician? Just be selective at the sperm bank, careful to choose sperm from a male who has the characteristics you want for your child. No, this is not part of the 2099 scenario. This is occurring today. The future is here!

Tonow

As the 21st-century narrator of our story implies, being aware of present trends and considering what personal and social agreements about sexuality may be like in the future can be fun, but it can also be a responsibility.

As our society evolves, we must not lose sight of our heritage and what we have learned from it. To that knowledge we must add new information—information filtered through ethical and moral awareness and values. As citizens of today and of the future, we can ill afford to shirk our responsibility to help shape our sexual society.

The physician Bernie Siegel worked with cancer patients—"cancer survivors," he called them. Knowing they probably had little time left to live, he helped them live "well" during the time left to them. This is a lesson that all of us could profit from. Siegel was fond of speaking of today, tomorrow, and "tonow." Using Siegel's terminology, many sexual futuristic issues are actually occurring tonow.

A woman is judged guilty of a criminal act and is considered to be a poor mother, so a judge prevents her from having other children. He offers her a choice of going to jail or having a contraceptive implant (Norplant) surgically placed on her arm. Tonow.

A society experiments on itself. Its children grow up with the majority of their mothers working full-time outside the home. In many cases, a male figure is absent from the home because of desertion, death, or divorce. What will the effects be? Tonow.

A country changes dramatically. What were once "minorities," when grouped together, become the majority. In many areas of the United States, Hispanic, Asian American, and African American populations have increased in numbers and in percentage of population. What will be the effects on sexuality? On attitudes toward sexual issues? On views of censorship, morality, abortion, and family life? Many believe the country will profit from this diversity. Will it? Tonow.

During the sexual revolution of the 1960s, individuals fought for free sexual expression. Today people wrestle with potentially serious consequences of their sexual choices—including sexually transmitted infections, HIV/AIDS, and unplanned and unwanted pregnancies. Will sexual behavior change as a result? How many instances of these consequences will it take for that to happen? Will relationships ever be the same? Tonow.

It is our hope that this book helps to prepare you for your sexual tonow and your sexual tomorrow. Most likely your instructor hopes your sexuality course will have the same effect. No one can predict the future, but we can anticipate trends and prepare for them. How will you prepare? When will you start?

Discussion Questions

1. Vaccines were one of the greatest wonders of the 20th century and eradicated several major diseases. However, a small percentage of people contract the disease through the vaccine and are left disabled or dead. Would you be willing to take such a risk to be vaccinated for STIs or HIV? Would you subject your infant children to such vaccines to protect their future? Explain why or why not.

2. Over the time you have taken this course, you have undoubtedly heard news stories about current research that could affect your future sexuality. Relate some of the more interesting research projects, and discuss whether they are feasible, given the biological, psychological, and sociocultural dimensions of sexuality.

Application Questions

Reread the chapter-opening scenario and answer the following questions.

1. Would you prefer to live in your current world or in the world of 2099 described in the scenario? Explain your answer.

2. Allowing government control over subliminal messages (and lacing the drinking water with K25W) would give the government complete control of the population. How could government be regulated so that only positive messages (for example, gender equality) would be conveyed? What if the government decided to convey messages like "Don't vote for the opposing political party"—or worse?

Critical Thinking Questions

1. As our society continues to accept the ideal of diversity, we seem less and less likely to unify as a nation on any issue—especially sex! Consider the use of stem cells in the United States. Which sociocultural groups are likely to be in favor of their use? Which groups would be against it? Under which circumstances do you think the federal government should approve the use of embryonic stem cells?

2. Aldous Huxley, in *Brave New World*, portrayed a government that kept control of its people by granting them unrestrained sexual pleasures. George Orwell, in *1984*, took the opposite position: The government keeps control by discouraging sexual contact among spouses and forbidding it among nonmarried people. Compare and contrast these methods given what you know about the many dimensions of human sexuality.

Critical Thinking Cases

What Is "Quality of Life"?

The year 2099 seems to have some attractive features. Diseases are curable. Computers do a lot of the work, and the remainder can often be done at home. Cars do not pollute air. People live longer and establish numerous relationships—each designed to meet a specific need.

And yet some of the citizens in the year 2099 seem disenchanted. Their marriages often do not last very long. They cannot have children whenever they want. They cannot engage in competitive sports. Their mind is manipulated as a result of K25W in their water supply.

Given these and the other conditions we have described, would you want to live in the year 2099? Why or why not?

What in life is important to you aside from *how long you live?*

What is present and what is absent in 2099 that you need to be happy sexually?

Exploring Personal Dimensions

The form below might be used in our fictional story set in 2099. In our story, those individuals wishing to conceive may have to answer questions very much like those in the form. Their answers determine whether they are given permission to have a child, as well as specifying the gender and appearance of the child. As you read through this form, consider whether it is ethical to ask such questions of potential parents. What would be the effects on the sociocultural dimensions of sexuality of applying such rules to parenting?

POPULATION AND PARENTHOOD SCREENING BUREAU

Parenthood Application

Name: _____

Mate's Name: _____

Address: _____

Computer Access Number: _____

Answer all of the following questions:

1. How long have you been mating? _____

2. List all illnesses/diseases experienced within the last year by the female mate: _____
   _____
   _____

3. List all illnesses/diseases experienced within the last year by the male mate: _____
   _____
   _____

4. On the breakup of your relationship, what do you plan for your child?
   _____
   _____
   _____
   _____

5. What time is best for you to be interviewed by our psychological team?
   _____
   _____
   _____
   _____

6. List those traits you want ensured in your child:
   a. Sex: _____

   b. Eye color: _____

   c. Hair color: _____

   d. Intelligence quotient: _____

   e. Height: _____

   f. Special abilities (for example, athletic, mathematical, artistic):
      _____
      _____

7. Which method of birth control do you employ?
   _____

8. Do you have any other children? _____

9. Which method of birthing do you plan?
   _____

10. How will your child be cared for during the workday? _____
    _____
    _____

11. List any parenting training you and your mate have received: _____
    _____
    _____

12. Will you agree to amniotic fluid screening during the pregnancy?
    _____
    _____

Special Note: Be aware that approval will not be granted to individuals who already have a child, who are untrained for parenthood, who do not agree to amniotic fluid screening, who have not planned for the daily care of their child-to-be, or who have not prepared for the breakup of their relationship.

Glossary

69 Two partners' simultaneous stimulation of each other's genitalia orally. The numerals 6 and 9 visually describe the body positions.

abortifacient A medical method that causes an embryo or fetus to die.

abstinence Avoidance of any type of sexual intercourse.

acquaintance rape Rape by a friend, acquaintance, or date; also known as *date rape*.

acquired erectile dysfunction A condition in which an adult male has previously had an erection sufficient to engage in sexual activity but no longer has.

acquired immune deficiency syndrome (AIDS) A syndrome caused by the human immunodeficiency virus (HIV), characterized by a depressed immune system and the presence of one or more opportunistic diseases.

active listening Paraphrasing what someone has said to demonstrate interest and understanding.

acute (primary) HIV infection The initial stage of HIV infection (2 to 4 weeks after exposure), which may or may not include flu-like symptoms.

adipose Pertaining to fat tissue in the body.

afterbirth Delivery of the placenta.

aggressiveness Standing up for one's basic rights, but at the expense of someone else's basic rights.

alimony Money a divorced person is ordered by the courts to pay regularly to his or her ex-spouse.

amenorrhea The absence of menstruation in a woman who should be menstruating.

amniocentesis Withdrawal by syringe of amniotic fluid to determine the presence of fetal abnormalities.

amniotic fluid The fluid inside the amniotic sac in which the fetus floats; it acts as a shock absorber, maintains the fetus at a constant temperature, and serves as a nutrient.

amniotic sac A fluid-filled membrane that surrounds the developing infant in the uterus.

ampulla The enlarged portion of the vas deferens where sperm are provided nutrients from the seminal vesicles; also, the part of the fallopian tube of women containing the cilia.

anal intercourse Insertion of the penis into the anus.

analgesics Substances that decrease pain locally, such as topical creams.

analingus Licking of the anus.

androgens Male sex hormones.

androgynous Exhibiting a combination of masculine and feminine traits as defined by the society.

anesthetics Substances that elicit unconsciousness and thereby relieve pain.

annular Type of hymen that surrounds the vaginal opening.

anorexia nervosa A condition in which an individual severely limits caloric intake.

antiandrogen drugs Chemicals that reduce the sex drive by lowering the testosterone level in the bloodstream.

antibodies A class of proteins secreted by the immune system that bonds with antigens. Antibodies fight off disease-causing organisms.

areola The darkened part of the breast immediately surrounding the nipple.

asexual One who does not experience sexual attraction. Some asexuals may experience attraction but feel no need to act out that attraction sexually.

asphyxiophilia Desire for a state of oxygen deficiency to enhance sexual excitement.

assertiveness Standing up for one's basic rights without violating anyone else's rights.

assisted reproductive technologies (ART) Procedures in which the clinician handles both the sperm and the egg.

aversion therapy Pairing an undesirable sexual behavior with a painful response.

bar girls Sex workers who are supposed to act available so customers will buy them drinks.

Barbach's technique A method of treating orgasmic dysfunction and sexual unresponsiveness developed by Lonnie Barbach that focuses on awareness of feelings and sensations through self-exploration and stimulation.

Bartholin's glands Small glands located within the labia minora that secrete a few drops of fluid during sexual arousal.

basal body temperature A woman's body temperature immediately upon waking.

basal body thermometer A special thermometer used to measure changes in basal body temperature.

behavior therapy Applying learning principles to help people change behavior.

bestiality Sexual contact with animals—also called *zoophilia*.

binge-eating disorder (BED) Eating disorder characterized by recurrent binge eating but not by inappropriate weight-control measures.

biopsy (open biopsy) Usually referred to as an open biopsy, a minor surgical procedure during which tissue of a tumor is removed and examined for presence of cancer.

birthing room A homelike birth setting now available in some hospitals.

blended orgasm An orgasm in a female in which there are contractions of the muscles in the outer third of the vagina as well as breath holding; a combination of the vulval and uterine orgasms.

bloody show Expelling of the mucus plug (often streaked with blood) that has closed off the cervix during pregnancy.

body composition The percentage of fat versus lean tissue.

body image The mental image we have of our own physical appearance

body mass index (BMI) Weight in kilograms divided by the square of the height in meters.

bondage perversion Getting sexual pleasure from being bound, tied up, or otherwise restricted.

bonding A process of developing a close physical and psychological relationship with one's caregiver; a sense of close emotional attachment.

Braxton-Hicks contractions Weak and slow uterine contractions that occur during the last few months of pregnancy.

breast abscess Infection of the breast characterized by redness, swelling, and a painful or tender mass.

breast budding First stage of breast development in females, whereby breast tissue elevates as a small mound.

breast cancer The second most common type of cancer in women.

breast self-examination (BSE) A periodic self-care procedure that involves feeling the breast for any abnormalities. The test is performed once every menstrual cycle or every month after menopause.

breech delivery A delivery in which the infant is born with another body part first, rather than head first. This form of delivery can be hazardous for both mother and infant.

bulbocavernosus muscle A muscle that encircles and supports the vagina.

bulimia nervosa A condition in which the individual periodically binges and purges, with an obsessive fear of becoming fat.

bypassing When misunderstandings result from missed meanings.

calendar method Charting of the length of a woman's periods for several months to determine the days she is most likely to be fertile.

call girls Highly paid female sex workers who work by appointment only.

candidiasis A common form of vaginitis, sometimes called a yeast infection, which is caused by the fungus *Candida albicans*.

carcinoma A type of cancer emanating from epithelial cells.

case study In-depth study of individual(s) or small groups.

causation A relationship in which one event causes another event to occur.

cerebral cortex The part of the brain called the gray matter that controls higher-order functioning such as language and judgment.

cervical cap Shallow rubber cap, smaller than a diaphragm, that covers the cervix to prevent sperm from entering the uterus.

cervical secretions Normal fluids from the cervix that change consistency during the month.

cervix The mouth of the uterus, through which the vagina extends.

cesarean section (C-section) Surgical intervention to deliver the fetus, placenta, and membranes through an incision in the walls of the abdomen and uterus.

chancre A painless lesion that is symptomatic of the primary stage of syphilis and appears at the site of contact.

change-of-life baby A baby born to a menopausal woman who, in spite of not menstruating regularly, ovulated.

chemotherapy Use of chemicals (medication) to treat disease; may be oral, intravenous, intramuscular, or topical.

child pornography Use of minors in sexually explicit media.

child sexual abuse Any sexual abuse involving fondling, erotic kissing, oral sexual activity, or genital penetration between an adult and a child, including pedophilia and incest.

chlamydia A term that encompasses several major diseases caused by *Chlamydia trachomatis*, including genitourinary tract infection, a type of conjunctivitis in newborns, a type of pneumonia in infants, lymphogranuloma venereum, and trachoma.

Chlamydia trachomatis An intracellular parasite that causes chlamydial infections.

chloasma A yellow to brown patch of skin pigmentation that may appear on the faces of pregnant white women; sometimes referred to as the "mask of pregnancy."

chorionic villi sampling (CVS) A technique for prenatal detection of genetic defects that involves removal of some of the villi growing on the outer surface of the chorion and examining their chromosomes.

cilia Hairlike structures that guide objects, such as ova, moving past them.

circumcision Surgical removal of the foreskin covering the glans penis.

clinical breast exam A breast examination conducted by a physician to detect any abnormalities.

clinical latency Sometimes called asymptomatic HIV infection or chronic HIV infection. HIV is still active during this phase, but the virus reproduces at very low levels. Individuals may not have any symptoms. This phase can last up to a decade (though not for everyone) and several decades for people on antiretroviral therapy.

clitoral hood The skin covering the clitoris.

clitoridectomy Surgical removal of the clitoris.

clitoris The structure located at the upper part of the labia minora that is homologous to the penis and is very sensitive to stimulation.

cognitive development Explains the ability to think concretely or abstractly.

cohabitation Situation in which people who live together and share a sexual relationship are not married.

coitus interruptus The Latin term for *withdrawal*, which means "interrupted intercourse."

colostrum The yellow fluid secreted by the breasts just before and after childbirth until milk production begins.

colposcopy An examination of the vagina and cervix using an instrument—a colposcope—to detect abnormal tissue growth.

combined pill or combined oral contraceptive (COC) Oral contraceptive containing estrogen and progestin.

come out Accept and make LGBTQ orientation public.

common-law marriage The recognition by some states that heterosexual couples who have lived together for a specified period and have represented themselves as married are in fact legally married.

conception The union of the sperm and ovum; also called *fertilization*.

conceptual identity Who am I in my world?

conceptus The fertilized ovum; the product of conception.

condom A sheath that covers the penis.

conformity with peers Desire to be like everyone else.

consensual In this context, a married person's engaging in extramarital sexual activity with the knowledge and permission of the spouse.

contraception Means of preventing pregnancy.

contraction The shortening or tension of uterine muscles during labor.

control group In an experiment, the group not subjected to a particular event or condition.

coprophilia Sexual pleasure associated with feces.

coronal ridge (corona) The raised ridge where the glans penis ends and the penile shaft begins.

corpora cavernosa A cavernous structure located within the clitoris or the penis that fills with blood during sexual excitement, causing erection.

corpus The upper two-thirds of the uterus.

corpus luteum A yellowish structure that develops in the Graafian follicle at the discharge of an ovum and that produces progesterone and estrogen.

corpus spongiosum A spongy body in the penis that contains a network of blood vessels and nerves.

correlation A relationship between two events; a statistical measure that shows how variables are naturally related to each other.

cosmetic surgery Surgery done for the sole purpose of improving the appearance.

Cowper's glands Two pea-sized glands adjacent to the urethra that secrete a lubricating fluid before ejaculation.

cribriform Type of hymen that creates a sievelike covering for the vaginal opening.

critical thinking Thinking that avoids blind acceptance of conclusions or arguments and closely examines all assumptions.

crowning The presentation of the baby's head at the vaginal opening.

cunnilingus Stimulation of the female genitalia by the mouth, lips, and/or tongue of the sexual partner.

cystic mastitis Known also as fibrocystic disease, a condition characterized by fluid-filled lesions (cysts) that are tender and believed to be related to estrogen activity.

date-rape drugs Sedative hypnotic drugs used to incapacitate victims who are then sexually molested or raped.

decoding Translating the message from its symbol form into meaning.

delayed ejaculation A condition in which a male is unable to ejaculate or there is marked delay in ejaculation after sucient sexual stimulation.

delivery The stage of childbirth characterized by the expulsion of the infant and the placenta.

Depo-Provera (DMPA) An injectable progestin-only contraceptive.

dermoid cyst A type of benign ovarian cyst commonly found in young women.

desire phase The first stage of the sexual response cycle, as described in Helen Singer Kaplan's model, which consists of psychologically becoming interested in sex before any physical changes occur.

diaphragm Shallow rubber cap that covers the cervix and prevents sperm from entering the uterus.

digital rectal examination (DRE) A rectal examination whereby a physician inserts a finger into the rectum of a male patient to check for any abnormalities of the prostate.

dilation In childbirth, the gradual opening of the cervix during labor.

dilation and evacuation (D&E) Surgical procedure that involves dilating the cervix, scraping the walls of the uterus, and removing the endometrial lining with suction.

dildos Artificial penises.

disorders of sexual development Anomalies of the sex chromosomes, the gonads, the reproductive ducts, and the genitalia.

douche Cleansing of the vagina by inserting a nozzle that secretes a recommended cleansing substance, a controversial procedure.

duration How long something occurs or has occurred.

dysmenorrhea Painful menstruation.

early adolescence First stage of adolescence, defined by pubertal changes—usually ages 9–13 years for females and ages 11–15 years for males.

early ejaculation Persistent or recurring ejaculation before the person wishes it during partnered sexual activity.

eclampsia Pregnancy-induced hypertension accompanied by swelling of the face, neck, and upper extremities, plus convulsions or coma, which may be fatal.

ectopic pregnancy The attachment and development of the zygote in a location other than in the uterus.

ejaculation The ejection of semen from the penis during orgasm.

Electra complex Freud's theory that 3- to 5-year-old girls want to take their father away from their mother.

electronic fetal monitoring A technique used during labor whereby a physician places an electrode on the woman's abdomen to monitor the fetal heart rate for signs of fetal distress.

embryo The developing fetus during the 2 months after conception.

embryonic stage The stage of prenatal development that includes the first 8 weeks of pregnancy.

emergency contraception (EC) The use of oral contraceptives or insertion of an IUD after unprotected sex has occurred at midcycle.

encoding Converting an idea into words or gestures to convey meaning.

endocrine glands Glands that secrete their products into the bloodstream.

endometriosis The growth of the endometrium uterine lining at a location other than in the uterus.

endometrium The innermost layer of the uterus, to which the fertilized egg attaches and by which it is nourished as it develops before birth, which is partly discharged (if pregnancy does not occur) with the menstrual flow.

epididymis The location where sperm are stored in the testes and where nutrients are provided to help the sperm develop.

episiotomy Incision between the vulva and anus to enlarge the vaginal opening at the time of birth.

erectile dysfunction The inability of a man to obtain or maintain an erection during sexual activity.

erection The extension of the penis and its engorgement with blood when the male is sexually stimulated.

erotica Sexually oriented material that may be artistically produced or motivated.

essentialism Belief that once the cultural and historical aspects are taken away, the essence of sexuality is biological.

estrogen A hormone produced by the ovaries whose level in the blood helps control the menstrual cycle.

ethical dilemma When two or more ethical principles work in opposing fashion in a particular situation, resulting in bewilderment regarding what is moral and what is immoral.

ethical principles Guides by which we can judge an action or decision as moral or immoral.

ethics A system that uses ethical principles to make decisions about morality.

ethnicity The degree of identification an individual feels with a particular ethnic group.

excitement phase The second stage of Kaplan's model of sexual response, which consists of physiological arousal and changes and, possibly, orgasm.

exhibitionism Achievement of sexual gratification by exhibiting the genitals to observers.

expected date of confinement (EDC) Due date for normal pregnancy that is usually estimated by Nägele's rule.

experiment Observation of behavior (or effects) under controlled conditions.

experimental group In an experiment, the group subjected to a particular event or condition.

external urethral sphincter The valve that closes during the emission stage, resulting in a buildup of semen, and that opens during the ejaculation stage, allowing semen to be expelled.

fallopian tubes (oviduct) The routes through which eggs leave the ovaries on their way to the uterus, in which fertilization normally occurs.

feedback When the receiver responds verbally or nonverbally.

fellatio Oral contact with a male's penis.

female condom A polyurethane or synthetic rubber sheath with flexible inner and outer rings worn inside the vagina.

female orgasmic disorder The consistent or frequent inability of a woman to achieve an orgasm.

femininity Those qualities characteristic of and suitable for girls and women according to the rules and expectations of a society.

fertility-awareness methods (FAMs) See *natural family planning*.

fertility-awareness-combined methods Calculation of a woman's fertile times and use of a barrier or withdrawal on fertile days.

fetal alcohol spectrum disorders (FASD) The full spectrum of birth defects that are caused by prenatal alcohol exposure.

fetal alcohol syndrome (FAS) Impaired psychological and physical characteristics common in infants born to alcoholic women.

fetal stage Period from the ninth week of pregnancy to birth.

fetishism Paraphilia in which there is a disorder with pathological assignment of sexual fixation, fantasies, or behaviors toward an inanimate object.

fetus The developing child from the ninth week after conception until birth.

fibroadenoma A benign (noncancerous) tumor that is firm, round, and somewhat movable.

fimbriae The fingerlike ends of the fallopian tubes that catch the ova when they are discharged from the ovaries.

flaccid The relaxed, unerect state of the penis.

flooding Experiencing something so frequently that you no longer are aroused by it. This is a technique used to become more comfortable with sexual terminology.

focus group A form of research where a group of 6 to 10 people are asked about a topic and then discuss related issues.

follicle-stimulating hormone (FSH) A hormone, secreted by the anterior portion of the pituitary gland, that "instructs" the ovaries to prepare an egg to be released from a follicle.

follicular phase The part of the menstrual cycle during which menstruation occurs and the pituitary increases the production of FSH so the follicles mature: a combination of the menstrual and proliferative phases.

foreplay Physical contact preceding sexual intercourse.

foreskin (prepuce) The covering of the glans penis, which is removed during circumcision.

frequency How often something occurs or has occurred.

frottage Obtaining of sexual pleasure from rubbing or pressing against another person.

functional identity What adult roles will I play in the world?

functional cyst An ovarian cyst that occurs on the follicle or corpus luteum, usually caused by the failure of the follicle to rupture and release an egg.

fundus The upper end of the uterus closest to the opening of the fallopian tubes.

gay Male or female homosexual. (Gay used alone probably refers to a male, though it is acceptable to refer to a gay female.)

gender constancy The concept that people's sex does not change—even if they change their dress or behavior.

gender dysphoria Feeling trapped in the body of the "wrong" sex.

gender identity The awareness and acceptance of one's gender.

gender role Complex groups of ways males and females are expected to behave in a given culture.

gender-role stereotyping Expectation that individuals will behave in certain ways because they are male or female.

gender schema A grouping of mental representations about male and female physical qualities, behaviors, and personality traits.

gender stereotypes Beliefs about how each gender should behave, which may be overgeneralized or rigidly held.

gender typing The process whereby children develop behavior that is appropriate to their sex.

generalization The ability to conclude that the same results would be obtained outside the study.

genital herpes An STI characterized by tiny fluid-filled blisters that appear on the genitals and in the genital tract.

gigolo A man who is paid to provide escort and sexual services, usually for wealthy, middle-aged women.

glans penis The head of the penis.

gonadotropins Sexual hormones secreted by the pituitary that stimulate the gonads to produce their hormones.

gonads The male testes and the female ovaries, which produce gonadotropin hormones responsible for the development of secondary sexual characteristics.

gonorrhea An STI that commonly starts with inflammation of the mucous membrane lining of the openings of the body (e.g., mouth, vagina).

Graafian follicle A part of the ovary from which a mature egg ruptures, allowing the corpus luteum to develop in the location where the egg was released.

Grafenberg spot (G spot) An area located along the anterior wall of the vagina, several inches into the vaginal canal, that when stimulated in some women may result in sexual excitement and/or orgasm.

gynecologist A physician specializing in women's reproductive health.

gynecomastia Glandular tissue development in the breasts of males.

herpes simplex virus (HSV) The virus that causes oral and genital herpes infections.

heterosexist An attitude that reinforces heterosexuality as the privileged and powerful norm.

homologous Organs that differ but that developed from the same tissue—for example, the glans penis and clitoris.

homophobia An irrational fear of homosexuality.

hormone A chemical substance secreted by a ductless gland, which is carried to an organ or tissue where it has a specific effect.

hormone therapy Form of treatment for cancer that uses hormones to combat cancer cell growth.

hot flashes Intermittent sensations of heat reported by menopausal women, possibly caused by decreased estrogen production.

house (brothel) prostitutes Sex workers who work in brothels.

human chorionic gonadotropin (HCG) A hormone secreted by the placenta whose presence in a woman's urine is the most common medical method of determining pregnancy.

human immunodeficiency virus (HIV) A retrovirus that causes AIDS.

human papillomavirus (HPV) A persistent STI caused by any of a group of viruses associated with the development of cervical cancer and/or genital warts.

human sexuality A part of your total personality. It involves the interrelationship of biological, psychological, and sociocultural dimensions.

hustler A male sex worker who performs homosexual acts for pay.

hymen A thin connective tissue covering the opening of the vagina.

hyperthyroidism Excessive functional activity of the thyroid gland.

hyperventilation Deep and rapid breathing that occurs during sexual excitation.

hypogonadism Decreased activity of the gonads that may result in retardation of growth and sexual development.

hypothalamus A structure in the brain that controls the pituitary gland and is directly connected by nerve pathways to various organs of the body.

hypothesis Tentative proposal or an educated guess about the results of a research study.

hypothyroidism A deficiency of thyroid activity.

"I" statement Statement that begins with an "I" to express personal feelings.

imaginary audience Belief in early adolescence that other people are looking at you as if you are onstage.

immoral What is judged to be wrong according to a system of ethics.

in vitro fertilization The creation of a pregnancy in a laboratory by uniting the sperm and egg outside the womb; sometimes termed the "test-tube" baby technique.

incest Sexual behavior between relatives who are too closely related to be married.

induced abortion Purposeful termination of a pregnancy.

infants Babies from birth to 1 year old.

infertility The inability to reproduce.

informed consent Document required to participate in a research study after the purposes, risks, and benefits of the study have been explained.

internal urethral sphincter The valve that prevents urine from entering the urethra and sperm from entering the bladder during ejaculation.

interstitial cells The cells (sometimes called Leydig's cells) between the seminiferous tubules, where testosterone is produced.

interstitial-cell-stimulating hormone (ICSH) A hormone, secreted by the anterior portion of the pituitary gland in males, that stimulates the production of sperm.

interview Oral research method designed to gather information.

intrauterine device (IUD) Synthetic device that is inserted into the uterus to prevent the sperm from fertilizing the ovum.

intrauterine insemination (IUI) Introduction of semen into the uterus by noncoital means.

introitus The vaginal entrance.

invasive cervical cancer Cancer that has invaded a wide area of cervical tissue.

Kamasutra Ancient sex manual from India.

Kegel exercises Exercises to help women develop greater control of muscles supporting the genitalia.

klismaphilia Sexual arousal produced by the use of enemas.

labia majora Two large folds of skin whose main function is to protect the external genitalia and the opening of the vestibule (defined later).

labia minora Two folds of skin lying inside the labia majora, which contain numerous blood vessels and nerve receptors.

labor The process of expelling a child by uterine contractions, dilation of the cervix, and bearing-down pressure.

lactation Production of breast milk.

lactobacilli Bacteria in the vagina that aid in keeping it healthy; also called *Doderlein bacilli*.

lactogen A hormone that stimulates the production of milk, the principal one being prolactin.

Lamaze method An approach to childbirth in which exercise and breath control are central to reducing anxiety and discomfort.

laparoscopy Female sterilization procedure that involves inserting a narrow viewing instrument—a laparoscope—through an incision in the abdomen and then performing ligation or applying clips or rings to block the fallopian tubes.

late adolescence Period of transition to adulthood, beginning usually at age 16 years for females and age 17 years for males.

late luteal phase dysphoric disorder (LLPDD) A type of premenstrual syndrome in which mental and emotional symptoms occur the week before menstruation. This is the name given to that condition by the American Psychiatric Association.

late (tertiary) syphilis The final stage of syphilis, which is characterized by systemic complications including damage to the nervous and circulatory systems, and possibly death. This stage is rare because of widespread use of antibiotics to treat syphilis.

latency period Outdated Freudian theory that children aged 6–12 years old have no sexual feelings or interest.

latent genital herpes The stage of genital herpes characterized by inactivity of the herpes virus, during which an infected individual is asymptomatic and transmission of the virus is rare.

latent syphilis A stage of syphilis that may last for years. Early latent syphilis typically lasts 1 to 4 years and individuals can still be infectious. Late latent syphilis also lasts multiple years, but individuals are not infectious to others except for transmission in utero to the fetus.

latex A synthetic rubber.

lesbian Female homosexual.

letdown The tingling sensation in the breasts when milk is forced out about 30 to 60 seconds after the infant begins to suckle.

libido Sexual desire or drive.

lifelong erectile dysfunction A condition in which an adult male has never had an erection sufficient to engage in sexual intercourse.

ligation The tying of the fallopian tubes to prevent the sperm–egg union.

limbic system The part of the brain referred to as the "seat of emotions," which produces emotions in response to physical and psychological signals.

liposuction A technique for removing adipose tissue with a suction-pump device.

locus of control Refers to an individual's perception of the main causes of events in life. More simply, is life's destiny controlled by the self (*internal locus*) or by external forces such as fate or other people (*external locus*)?

lumpectomy Removal of a lesion, benign or malignant.

luteal phase The same phase of the menstrual cycle as the secretory phase, which includes ovulation and the production of LH from the corpus luteum.

luteinizing hormone (LH) A hormone, secreted by the anterior portion of the pituitary gland, that stimulates ovulation.

male climacteric Sometimes termed "male menopause," which occurs at about the same age that women experience menopause, when men experience slightly decreased testosterone production and begin to question the directions in which their lives are headed.

male hypoactive sexual desire disorder A disorder characterized by a lack of interest in sexual activity or specic sexual activities.

mammary glands Milk-secreting glands located in the female breast.

mammography An X ray of the breasts to detect any abnormality before it is visible or palpable.

manual vacuum aspiration (MVA) A variation of vacuum aspiration that uses nonelectric suction instruments and can be used from the time of detection of pregnancy through 12 weeks.

masculinity Those qualities characteristic of and suitable for boys and men according to the rules and expectations of a society.

massage parlors Places where sex workers can be hired to perform sexual acts under the guise of giving a massage.

mastectomy Removal of the breast and/or other tissue. Simple: Removal of only the breast (sometimes with removal of lymph nodes under the arm). Modified radical: Removal of the breast, lymph nodes, lining of the chest muscle, and sometimes part of the chest wall. Radical: removal of the breast, lymph nodes, and chest muscle.

masturbation Self-stimulation of the genitals.

meatus The opening of the urethra in the head of the penis, where both seminal fluid and urine are passed.

medical abortion A procedure that uses drugs to induce abortion.

menarche The time when a female begins her first menstrual cycle, usually at 8 to 16 years of age.

menopausal hormone therapy (MHT) Replacement of hormones that a woman's ovaries stop making at the time of menopause, easing some of the symptoms of menopause.

menopause The time when a woman's menstrual cycle ceases, usually between 40 and 55 years of age.

menstrual phase The part of the menstrual cycle during which the endometrial lining is sloughed off as the menstrual flow.

menstruation The cyclical emission of the blood-enriched endometrium when pregnancy does not occur.

metastasis Spread of cancer from a primary site to other parts of the body.

methotrexate A drug that blocks the hormone progesterone, which is needed to maintain a pregnancy.

middle adolescence The typical "teenage years," usually ages 13–16 years for females and ages 14–17 years for males.

midlife crisis A time of life, usually between 40 and 50 years of age, during which men question the path their lives have taken and make plans for changing their goals.

midwifery The practice by nonphysicians of assisting in the process of pregnancy and childbirth. Lay midwives are not trained healthcare professionals; nurse midwives are registered nurses who have received advanced training and often certification in the techniques of the birthing process.

mifepristone A drug that blocks the hormone progesterone, which is needed to maintain a pregnancy.

minilaparotomy Female sterilization procedure that involves a small incision in the abdomen through which the fallopian tubes are pulled so they can be blocked.

minipill (POP) A progestin-only birth control pill.

misoprostol A prostaglandin that causes uterine contractions.

mons pubis (mons veneris, mount of Venus) The rounded, soft area above the vaginal opening that becomes covered with hair at puberty.

moral What is judged to be right according to a system of ethics.

morning sickness The condition of nausea and vomiting that is common in early pregnancy; thought to be caused by hormonal changes.

motility The ability to move spontaneously, which is required for fertilization.

multiple orgasms Orgasms that occur without the need for a refractory, or recovery, period.

muscle dysmorphia A disorder whereby a bodybuilder in top shape considers himself or herself to be puny.

myometrium The middle layer of the uterus, consisting of smooth muscle that aids in the pushing of the newborn through the cervix.

myotonia Muscle tension occurring during sexual arousal.

natural childbirth Drug-free childbirth; sometimes called *prepared childbirth*.

natural family planning (NFP) Calculation of a woman's fertile times and abstention from penile–vaginal sex on fertile days.

necrophilia Sexual relations with a dead person.

needle biopsy Insertion of a needle into a lump in a breast to see whether fluid (which indicates a cyst rather than a tumor) can be removed.

Neisseria gonorrhoeae The bacterium that causes gonorrhea; also known as *gonococcus*. Street names include "clap" and "drip."

neonatal intensive care A medical specialty that focuses on the care of premature infants.

no-fault divorce The granting of divorce without either partner's proving the other was the cause of the marriage's failure.

nonassertiveness Giving up one's basic rights so others may achieve theirs.

nonconsensual In this context, a married person's engaging in sexual intercourse without the consent of the spouse.

nongonococcal urethritis (NGU) Inflammation of the urethra caused by *Chlamydia trachomatis, Ureaplasma urealyticum, Mycoplasma hominis, Trichomonas vaginalis,* herpes simplex virus, and unknown organisms.

nonoxynol 9 (N-9) The major spermicidal ingredient in U.S.-made products.

nuclear family A father and mother and their children.

nymphomania An excessive, insatiable sexual drive in women.

objectivity Being sure the results are the same no matter who asks the questions or records the answers.

obscenity Personal or societal judgment that something is offensive. Something offensive to modesty or decency; often sexually related.

observation Watching subjects in a particular setting.

obstetrical analgesia A nondrug pain reliever used in delivery (e.g., hypnosis).

obstetrician A physician who specializes in the care of pregnant women and the process of childbirth. Because these physicians are also gynecologists, they are often referred to as obstetrician–gynecologists or OB–GYNs.

Oedipus complex Libidinal feelings of a child toward the parent of the opposite gender and hostile or jealous feelings toward the parent of the same gender.

open marriage A marriage in which partners allow each other to have intimate and emotional relationships with others.

opportunistic infections A major manifestation of AIDS, diseases that occur in the presence of a suppressed immune system.

oral contraceptive (OC) A daily pill taken to prevent pregnancy.

orgasm The peak release of sexual tension, accompanied by sensory pleasure and involuntary rhythmic muscular contractions; ejaculation in the male.

orgasmic platform The narrowing of the outer third of the vagina during orgasm caused by contractions of the muscles in that area.

orgasmic reconditioning Increasing sexual arousal to socially appropriate stimuli.

os The opening to the uterus.

osteoporosis A condition of weakened bones resulting from decalcification (loss of calcium) of bone that increases in the absence of estrogen and is of particular concern in postmenopausal women.

ovarian cancer Cancer of the ovaries that causes more cancer deaths than any other cancer of the female reproductive system.

ovary A structure of the female genitalia that houses ova before their maturation and discharge and that produces estrogen and progesterone.

ovist Adherent to the 17th-century belief that the preformed baby was contained within the female body and that the male's sperm simply activated its development.

ovulation The part of the menstrual cycle when the ovum is discharged from the ovary.

ovulation methods Observation of signs of ovulation to calculate fertile days.

oxytocin A pituitary hormone that stimulates the breasts to eject milk so that breastfeeding may occur after childbirth.

pansexual One whose sexual orientation includes all kinds of sexual expression and sexual relationships that can exist in humans.

Pap smear A test of the tissue of the cervix for cervical cancer (named after its founder, Dr. Papanicolaou).

paracervical block An anesthetic used during childbirth that blocks pain sensations in the pelvic area, in which injections are given at positions around the cervix.

paraphilia Literally meaning "love (*philia*) beyond the usual (*para*)," this term refers to various sexual behaviors previously referred to as deviant.

partialism Paraphilia in which sexual arousal is associated with a particular body part.

parturition The process of giving birth.

pediculosis lice Also known as crabs, of three common types: *Pediculus corporis*, a body louse; *Pediculus capitis*, a head louse; and *Pediculus pubis*, a pubic louse.

pedophilia Sexual behavior in which a child is the sexual object.

peer marriage Relationship in which partners have equal status.

pelvic inflammatory disease (PID) Infection of the reproductive organs, particularly the uterus, fallopian tubes, and pelvic cavity.

penetrative behaviors Any behavior whereby penetration occurs—for example, penile–vaginal sex, oral sex, or anal sex.

penile strain gauge A wire or cuff placed around the penis to measure physiological changes over time.

penis Structure of the male external genitalia consisting of the root, shaft, and glans; also contains the urethra, through which urine is excreted.

perfect use The ability of a method of contraception to prevent pregnancy as measured by consistent and correct use.

perimenopause (climacteric) The period just before menopause when the production of estrogen and progesterone is decreasing, usually a 5- to 10-year period.

perimetrium The outermost layer of the uterus, sometimes termed the *serosa*, a very elastic layer that allows the uterus to accommodate a growing embryo and fetus.

pheromones Substances that when secreted have a specific scent found to be sexually arousing.

phimosis Condition resulting when penile erection causes pain because the foreskin is too tight.

pimps Individuals who set up female sex workers with clients.

pituitary The "master gland," an endocrine gland located at the base of the brain that stimulates the other endocrine glands to produce their hormones.

placenta An organ of interchange between mother and fetus; oxygen, nutrients, and waste are exchanged through its cells.

plethysmograph A laboratory measuring device that charts physiological changes over time.

PLISSIT A model of sexual therapy that consists of moving through the stages of giving permission, limited information, specific suggestion, and, if that does not work, intensive therapy.

polygamy When one man is married to more than one woman.

polyurethane A type of plastic.

population The group being studied in a research project.

pornography Visual and written materials used for the purpose of sexual arousal.

post-exposure prophylaxis (PEP) The use of antiretroviral medicines to reduce the chance of HIV infection after a single potential exposure to HIV.

precocious puberty Pubertal development before the age of 7 years.

preeclampsia Pregnancy-induced hypertension; symptoms include swelling of the face, neck, and upper extremities; and excess levels of protein in the urine.

pre-exposure prophylaxis (PrEP) The daily use of a combined pill of antiretroviral therapy (Truvada) that decreases the risk of HIV infection in as many as 92% in individuals with an ongoing high risk of infection.

premature or preterm birth Infants born that have not reached 37 completed weeks of gestation.

premenstrual syndrome (PMS) Marked mood fluctuation during the week before menstruation, accompanied by physical symptoms.

prenatal care Care given to an expectant mother before the birth of her child that typically consists of monitoring fetal development, screening for high-risk pregnancy, and providing education for pregnancy and childbirth.

primary amenorrhea A condition in which a woman of age 18 years or older has never menstruated.

primary dysmenorrhea Painful menstruation, the cause of which is unknown.

primary genital herpes The first stage of a genital herpes infection; it begins with infection by the herpes virus and the formation of antibodies. Common symptoms include painful lesions in or around the genital area, a sluggish feeling, fever, and possibly swollen lymph nodes.

primary syphilis The first stage of syphilis most generally manifested by the appearance of a painless lesion called a *chancre*.

procreation Sexual intercourse for the purpose of reproduction.

prodrome Itching, tingling, or burning sensations that occur where a herpes lesion will appear.

progesterone A hormone secreted by the corpus luteum signaling the endometrium to develop in preparation for a zygote.

prolactin A pituitary hormone that stimulates the production of milk from the mammary glands.

proliferative phase The first part of the menstrual cycle, during which FSH production is increased and the follicles are maturing.

prostaglandins Hormonelike substances produced by body tissue that may cause dysmenorrhea.

prostate gland A structure of the male internal genitalia that secretes a fluid into the semen before ejaculation to aid sperm motility and prolong sperm life.

prostatitis Infection of the prostate gland.

prostitution Participating in sexual activity for pay or profit.

prurient Characterized by lustful thoughts or wishes.

psychosexual development The blending of sexual aspects of one's development with other psychological factors.

pubic lice A parasite, commonly referred to as crabs; a louse that grips the pubic hair and feeds on tiny blood vessels of the skin.

pubococcygeal muscle A muscle that encircles the vagina and supports it.

questionnaire Written instrument designed to gather information.

quickening Movements of the fetus felt by the mother; usually occurs about the fourth month of pregnancy.

radiation therapy A form of treatment for cancer that uses carefully directed radiation to destroy cancer cells.

random sample A sample that represents the larger population and that is chosen without bias, so that every member of the larger population had an equal chance to be selected.

rape Forcible sexual intercourse with a person who does not give consent.

rape trauma syndrome A two-phase reaction to rape. An acute phase involves intense emotional responses for several weeks. The long-term phase may last several years and involves reorganization and establishment of control.

recurrent genital herpes The stage of a genital herpes infection that is characterized by a reactivation of the virus and the appearance of blisters on the skin. Not all people with herpes have recurrences.

refractory (recovery) period The time needed by males for recovery between orgasms.

releasing factors Chemicals released from the hypothalamus that affect the function of various body parts.

resolution phase A stage of the sexual response cycle consisting of a return to the prearoused state.

reticular activating system (RAS) A network of nerves that connect the cortex and the subcortex—the connection between mind and body.

retroviruses A group of viruses consisting of ribonucleic acid (RNA) surrounded by a protein coat that can convert their RNA into deoxyribonucleic acid (DNA) once they have invaded a living cell, allowing them to take over the cell and reproduce themselves.

Rh factor The presence of Rh agglutinogens (antigens) in the blood, which indicates that a person is Rh positive, whereas its absence designates the person as Rh negative.

rhinoplasty Surgery done to change the shape of the nose.

rule ethics Guiding principles used in all situations to arrive at moral decisions, which are considered applicable to all situations.

saddle (epidural) block An anesthetic used during childbirth that blocks pain sensations in the buttocks, perineum, and inner thigh.

same-sex marriage A marriage between two people who perceive themselves to be of the same sex.

sample A segment of the larger population.

satyriasis An excessive, insatiable sexual drive in men—also called *Don Juanism*.

scabies Skin irritation caused by a tiny mite that is transferred from one person to another by close contact, sexual or otherwise.

scientific method Research conducted in an atmosphere free from bias.

scrotum (scrotal sac) A sac of skin that contains the testes and spermatic cords.

secondary amenorrhea A condition in which a woman has ceased menstruating after menarche.

secondary dysmenorrhea Painful menstruation caused by some identifiable condition such as endometriosis.

secondary sexual characteristics Changes occurring during adolescence—such as growth of pubic hair, breast development, and testes and penile development.

secondary syphilis The second stage of syphilis, often characterized by a rash.

secretory phase The second part of the menstrual cycle, during which ovulation occurs and the production of LH stimulates the development of the corpus luteum.

self-esteem Sense of personal worth.

self-report data The respondents' descriptions of something.

Semans stop–start method A method of controlling premature ejaculation (developed by James Semans) in which the man tells his partner to stop stimulating him when he feels ejaculation approaching.

semen The male ejaculate, which contains sperm and other secretions.

semenarche First ejaculation of semen for boys.

seminal vesicles Two sacs of the male internal genitalia that secrete nutrients to nourish sperm.

seminiferous tubules The structures located within the testes that actually produce the sperm.

sensate focus A method of alleviating sexual unresponsiveness by procedures designed to encourage erotic feelings and sexual pleasuring.

septate Type of hymen that bridges the vaginal opening.

seronegative The result of a blood test for antibodies to HIV that indicates no presence of such antibodies.

seropositive The result of a blood test for antibodies to HIV that indicates that such antibodies have been found in the blood.

sex flush A darkening of the skin of the neck, face, forehead, or chest during sexual stimulation.

sexism The prejudgment that because of sex a person will possess negative traits.

sexology The study of sexuality.

sexting Sending sexually explicit messages—text messages, photos, or videos—by cell phone or instant messaging.

sexual abuse The psychological exploitation or iniction of unwanted sexual contact on one person.

sexual cognition Attitudes, expectations, beliefs, and values framing one's sexual experiences.

sexual dysfunction A specific, chronic disorder involving sexual performance.

sexual fantasies Thoughts, images, and daydreams of a sexual nature.

sexual harassment Unwelcome verbal, physical, or sexual conduct that has the effect of creating an intimidating, hostile, or offensive environment.

sexual identity Inner sense of oneself as a sexual being, including one's identification in terms of gender and sexual orientation.

sexual interest/arousal disorder A sexual dysfunction that causes a woman to experience little or no erotic pleasure through sexual stimulation.

sexual masochism Sexual gratification that results from experiencing pain.

sexual orientation One's erotic, romantic, and affectional attraction to the same gender, to the opposite gender, or to both.

sexual preference Term formerly used to describe sexual orientation that is now outdated, because sexual orientation is no longer commonly considered to be a conscious individual preference or choice, but to be formed by a complicated network of factors.

sexual response cycle The sequence of physiological and psychological reactions as a result of sexual arousal.

sexual sadism Sexual gratification that results from inflicting pain on another person.

sexual self-concept Who am I as a sexual being?

sexually healthy relationship Consensual, non-exploitative, honest, mutually pleasurable, safe and protected from unwanted pregnancy, STIs, and other harm (National Guidelines Task Force, 2004).

sexually related diseases (SRDs) Diseases of the reproductive system that can occur in either sexually active or sexually inactive individuals.

sexually transmitted infections (STIs) Infections that are primarily contracted through sexual contact.

single-parent family For whatever reason, only one parent who is living with a child or children.

situation ethics A belief that no one set of rules can apply to all situations and each specific situation must be analyzed to determine which ethical principles are applicable.

situational homosexuality Homosexual behavior limited to circumstances in which members of the same sex are deprived of contact with the other sex.

Skene's glands Glands located along the walls of the vagina that are thought to be analogous to the male prostate gland, and the site from which some women eject a fluid during orgasm.

smegma A cheeselike substance secreted by the glans penis that must be removed from below the foreskin of uncircumcised males to prevent irritation and/or infection.

social cognition Ability to see a situation from another person's point of view.

social constructionism The belief that sexual identities are acquired from and influenced and modified by an ever-changing social environment.

social training Improving a person's social skills.

socialization The process of guiding people into socially acceptable behavior by providing information, rewards, and punishments.

sodomy A term that specifically refers to anal intercourse, but is often used to refer to almost any sexual behavior someone might not consider normal.

sonogram A diagnostic picture revealing the fetal outline. In ultrasonography, sound waves are bounced off the fetus. With a scanner, the image is then projected onto a computer screen, revealing whether certain defects are present.

speculum A metal (or plastic) instrument that is inserted into the vagina to hold the walls apart, allowing for medical examination.

spermatic cord The cord from which the testicle is suspended that contains the vas deferens, blood vessels, nerves, and muscle fibers.

spermatocytes Cells that develop through several stages to form sperm.

spermatogenesis The manufacturing of sperm in the seminiferous tubules.

spermatorrhea (wet dreams, or nocturnal emissions) Emission of semen during sleep.

spermatozoa (sperm) The mature male sperm cell.

spermicide Chemical detergent compound that immobilizes or kills sperm on contact; as a barrier, prevents sperm from entering the uterus through the cervical os.

spirochete A spiral-shaped bacterium, one of which—*Treponema pallidum*—causes syphilis.

spontaneous abortion (miscarriage) The natural termination of a pregnancy.

squeeze technique A method of helping men control premature ejaculation whereby the penis is gently squeezed when the man senses ejaculation is imminent.

statistical significance The likelihood that a study's results are due to the relationship uncovered between the study's variable as opposed to chance.

statutory rape Intercourse with a person younger than the legal age of consent.

Stein–Leventhal syndrome Reproductive malfunction in women; a syndrome of endocrine origin that involves ovarian cysts, amenorrhea, and infertility.

stepfamily A family with children that is formed as a result of remarriage.

stereotyping The expectation that individuals will exhibit certain characteristics or behaviors.

sterilization A procedure that makes a person biologically incapable of reproducing.

steroids Synthetic versions of the male hormone testosterone that promote tissue growth.

stranger rape Rape of a person by an unknown person.

streetwalkers Sex workers who work on the streets.

survey Research in which people complete questionnaires or are personally interviewed.

swinging Swapping of mates for sexual activities.

symptothermal method A combination of natural family planning methods, in which both temperature and signs of ovulation are observed and charted.

syphilis An STI caused by the spirochete *Treponema pallidum*.

systematic desensitization A means of overcoming anxiety by approaching the anxiety-provoking stimulus in small steps.

tachycardia An increase in heart rate that occurs during sexual activity.

Tanner scale Scale developed by Dr. John Tanner for measuring pubertal development in boys and girls.

teratology The study of causative factors of birth defects.

testes Male gonads contained within the scrotal sacs that produce sperm cells and the male sex hormone testosterone. Singular form: testicle.

testicular cancer Cancer of the testicles; the most common form of cancer in men aged 29 to 35 years.

testosterone The male sex hormone produced in the testes that is responsible for the development of male secondary sexual characteristics.

thriving Normal physical and psychological pattern of weight gain, neuromuscular development, and other developmental attributes of infants.

toxemias of pregnancy Hypertensive conditions, subdivided into preeclampsia and eclampsia.

toxic shock syndrome (TSS) A syndrome caused by *Staphylococcus aureus* bacteria in which symptoms include high fever, nausea, vomiting, diarrhea, and a drop in blood pressure; a potentially fatal syndrome that has been linked with the use of superabsorbent tampons.

transgender A general term used when one's identity does not match one's physical/genetic sex. It includes such diverse categories as transsexualism and transvestism.

transsexual A person whose gender identity does not match her or his biological sex; also a person who wishes to have, or has had, his or her sex surgically altered to conform to his or her gender identity.

transudation The process of vaginal lubrication resulting from engorgement of blood that creates pressure that forces moisture to seep from the spaces between the cells.

transvestite A person who achieves sexual satisfaction from wearing clothes usually worn by the other gender.

tribadism Rubbing genitals against someone's body or genital area.

trichomoniasis (trich) A type of vaginitis that can be an STI or an SRD. Symptoms include a foul-smelling, foamy white or yellow-green discharge that irritates the vagina and vulva. Urethritis may also be present.

troilism Having sexual relations with another person while a third person watches.

true labor Characterized by regularly spaced contractions of the uterus, thinning and dilation of the cervix, and a descending of the presenting part of the fetus into the vagina.

tummy tuck (abdominoplasty) Extensive surgical procedure that removes excess skin and fat from the abdomen.

typical use The ability of a method of contraception to prevent pregnancy as actually used at home by people not being monitored.

umbilical cord The lifeline between mother and fetus, which contains two arteries and one vein. Food, oxygen, and chemicals are transported to the child through the arteries, and waste is returned to the mother through the vein.

urethra The tube through which the bladder empties urine outside the body and through which the male ejaculate exits.

urine The body-waste product stored in the bladder and eliminated through the urethra.

urophilia Sexual pleasure associated with urine.

uterine orgasm An orgasm in a female that can occur only in the presence of penile penetration and that involves a woman's holding her breath just before orgasm and then exhaling when the climax occurs.

uterus A pear-shaped hollow structure of the female genitalia in which the embryo and fetus develop before birth.

vacuum aspiration Surgical procedure that uses a suction tube to evacuate the contents of the uterus, which can be used through the first weeks of the second trimester.

vagina A hollow, tunnel-like structure of the female internal genitalia whose reproductive functions are to receive the penis and its ejaculate, serve as a route of exit for the newborn, and provide an exit for menstrual flow.

vaginal plethysmography Insertion of a probe into the vagina to measure changes in blood volume.

vaginismus The involuntary contraction of the muscles surrounding the vaginal entrance so that entry of the penis is prevented.

validity, validation Demonstration that tests measure what they are designed to measure.

values Those beliefs to which we attach the most worth.

variable A measurable event that varies or is subject to change.

vas deferens The duct, through which sperm stored in the epididymis is passed, that is cut or blocked during vasectomy.

vasa efferentia The duct through which sperm produced in the seminiferous tubules travel to the epididymis.

vasectomy Cutting or cauterizing of the vas deferens to prevent sperm from being ejaculated; a means of sterilization.

vasocongestion Increased blood flow to an area of the body; occurs in the pelvic area during sexual arousal.

vasovasectomy Reversal of a vasectomy, so that sperm can be ejaculated.

vestibule The area containing the vaginal and urethral openings.

viral shedding HSV is excreted from the body even though an infected individual experiences no signs or symptoms.

volunteer bias Characteristics of volunteers that are likely to influence research results.

voyeurism (scopophilia) Obtaining of pleasure from watching people who are undressing or engaging in sexual behavior.

vulva The female external genitalia.

vulval orgasm An orgasm in a female that includes the contractions of the orgasmic platform, which is not sexually satisfying and, as a result, allows another orgasm to occur almost immediately.

withdrawal Removing the penis from the vagina before ejaculation.

zidovudine The first drug (brand name Retrovir; also known as AZT) approved by the FDA for the treatment of AIDS. This antiviral drug slows the replication of the AIDS virus, thus slowing the course of the syndrome.

zoophilia Sexual contact with animals—also called *bestiality*.

zygote A fertilized egg.

Index